Differential Diagnosis of Fracture

Yingze Zhang
Editor

Differential Diagnosis of Fracture

PMPH PEOPLE'S MEDICAL PUBLISHING HOUSE

Springer

Editor
Yingze Zhang
Department of Orthopaedics
The Third Hospital of Hebei Medical University
Shijiazhuang
China

ISBN 978-981-13-8338-0 ISBN 978-981-13-8339-7 (eBook)
https://doi.org/10.1007/978-981-13-8339-7

The print edition is not for sale in the Mainland of China. Customers from the Mainland of China please order the print book from: People's Medical Publishing House Co. Ltd.

This Springer imprint is published by the registered company Springer Nature Singapore Pte Ltd.
The registered company address is: 152 Beach Road, #21-01/04 Gateway East, Singapore 189721, Singapore

Preface

Fracture is the most common injury in the orthopedic clinical practice, and most of them are not difficult to be diagnosed. Since Wilhelm Roentgen discovered the X-ray more than 100 years ago, the diagnosis of fractures has completely departed from the era of "touch and track." Therefrom, most fractures can be recognized by radiography. However, the limitations of radiograph in diagnosing fractures, as well as the complexity of fractures, have been gradually revealed by the development of medical imaging techniques, especially the extensive application of the computerized tomography and the magnetic resonance imaging. Precise evaluation of complicated fractures according to radiographs alone is quite challenging even for experienced orthopedic surgeons and radiologists and often requires other diagnosing tools. For instance, the differential diagnosis of pathological fractures, which may be secondary to benign, or malignant, or metastatic bone tumors, should be backed up with the result of pathological examination; patient's medical history is very important for differentiating between insufficiency fractures and fatigue fractures; the involvement of the epiphysis and the age and location of ossification centers, as well as their interactions, should be considered comprehensively in pediatric fracture cases; and, there are variations in number, size, and location of sesamoids, so attention should be paid to distinguish bi- or tripartite patella from patella fractures. Clinical practitioners should deal with these cases carefully, utilizing their comprehensive clinical knowledge and competence of differential diagnosis.

It is the basic professional literacy for orthopedic surgeons to diagnose and differential diagnose fractures. Combining various imaging techniques cannot only prevent misdiagnosis and missed diagnosis by identifying injuries which may not be fully revealed on radiographs but also provide reliable basis for surgical planning. For complicated fractures, especially the pelvic, spinal, wrist, and intra-articular fractures, CT and/or MRI scanning with three-dimensional reconstruction, fat suppression, or diffusion-weighted imaging are often applied, in order to choose appropriate treatment methods.

The purpose of writing this book is to remind vast orthopedic surgeons that the way of we think need to be updated and the evaluation of fractures, especially the comminuted fractures in specific areas, should be based on integrated imaging examinations. This is essential to obtain effective treatment and optimal outcomes in patients with fractures. In this book, plenty of fracture cases that were diagnosed in our institute with CT and/or MRI rather than X-ray alone were summarized and illustrated by the combination of imaging pictures and diagrams, so as to briefly demonstrate the importance of comprehensive analysis and evaluation of fractures using multiple diagnostic tools. I sincerely hope that the readers of this book can benefit from our successful experiences and failures. In particular, I hope that orthopedic surgeons will always take the responsibility of taking good care of our patients, with the effort of adopting new thoughts, concepts, and methods to make correct and thorough diagnosis and treatment plan.

The editorial board of this book was consisted of orthopedists and radiologists who bear heavy clinical work everyday. Writing manuscripts was an add-on task taking up a lot of their spare time, and every chapter was composed with their great efforts and contributions. Hereon,

I would like to express my sincere appreciation to all the editors for their hard work! *Differential Diagnosis of Fracture* is finally published. The proposed opinions and suggestions may be biased on the basis of our limited experiences and perceptions. We sincerely welcome and greatly appreciate any comments from experts, peers, and vast readers!

Shijiazhuang, China
July 25, 2019

Yingze Zhang

Contents

Part IV Fracture of Axial Skeleton

Part V Cartilage and Epiphysis Injury

About the Editor

Yingze Zhang academician of Chinese Academy of Engineering and doctoral supervisor, is currently the vice chairman of Chinese Medical Doctor Association (CMDA), the chairman of Chinese Orthopaedic Association (COA), the chairman of Chinese Association of Orthopaedic Surgeons (CAOS), and visiting professor at the University of Colorado and other three universities. He was awarded three second prizes of National Science and Technology Progress and Invention Award as the first completer, six first provincial prizes, and Science and Technology Progress Award of the Ho Leung Ho Lee Foundation in 2015. He has obtained more than 70 invention patents and 3 US invention patens as the first inventor and/or patentee, among which 10 items have been issued registration certificates and converted into products and 3 items have been also registered in the US Food and Drug Administration (FDA). He published more than 500 papers as first/corresponding author (170 SCI papers), edited and translated 34 monographs, and founded the *Chinese Journal of Geriatric Orthopedics and Rehabilitation* serving as the chief editor. He is also the chief editor of *The Journal of Bone and Joint Surgery*, Chinese version.

Contributors

Wei Chen Department of Orthopaedics, The Third Hospital of Hebei Medical University, Shijiazhuang, Hebei, China

Jianling Cui CT/MRI Center, The Third Hospital of Hebei Medical University, Shijiazhuang, Hebei, China

Zhiyong Hou Department of Orthopaedics, The Third Hospital of Hebei Medical University, Shijiazhuang, Hebei, China

Xiaodong Lian Department of Orthopaedics, The Third Hospital of Hebei Medical University, Shijiazhuang, Hebei, China

Yake Liu Department of Orthopaedics, The Third Hospital of Hebei Medical University, Shijiazhuang, Hebei, China

Zhigang Peng CT/MRI Center, The Third Hospital of Hebei Medical University, Shijiazhuang, Hebei, China

Jiashen Shao Department of Orthopaedics, The Third Hospital of Hebei Medical University, Shijiazhuang, Hebei, China

Tao Sun Department of Orthopaedics, The Third Hospital of Hebei Medical University, Shijiazhuang, Hebei, China

Yingcai Sun CT/MRI Center, The Third Hospital of Hebei Medical University, Shijiazhuang, Hebei, China

Bo Wang Department of Orthopaedics, The Third Hospital of Hebei Medical University, Shijiazhuang, Hebei, China

Juan Wang Department of Orthopaedics, The Third Hospital of Hebei Medical University, Shijiazhuang, Hebei, China

Wenjuan Wu Department of Radiology, The Third Hospital of Hebei Medical University, Shijiazhuang, Hebei, China

Xin Xing Department of Orthopaedics, The Third Hospital of Hebei Medical University, Shijiazhuang, Hebei, China

Bing Zhang Department of Orthopaedics, The Third Hospital of Hebei Medical University, Shijiazhuang, Hebei, China

Li Zhang CT/MRI Center, The Third Hospital of Hebei Medical University, Shijiazhuang, Hebei, China

Qi Zhang Department of Orthopaedics, The Third Hospital of Hebei Medical University, Shijiazhuang, Hebei, China

Yingze Zhang Department of Orthopaedics, The Third Hospital of Hebei Medical University, Shijiazhuang, Hebei, China

Zekun Zhang CT/MRI Center, The Third Hospital of Hebei Medical University, Shijiazhuang, Hebei, China

Zhanle Zheng Department of Orthopaedics, The Third Hospital of Hebei Medical University, Shijiazhuang, Hebei, China

Part I

General Introduction

1 General Introduction

Yingze Zhang

1.1 Definition of Bone Fracture

Bone fractures are defined as complete or partial break of the bone structure. Fractures can be divided into traumatic, stress, and pathological fractures based on the mode of injury and underlying pathological features of the bone.

Traumatic fractures (Fig. 1.1) are classified into direct and indirect injuries according to the pattern of injury. A direct injury fracture is a bone fracture at stressed area caused by a direct force blow, for instance, a fracture sustained at the site of external force, hit by a heavy object or person. This type of injury often causes comminuted fracture, accompanied by soft tissue injury, bruises, blisters, and abrasion. An indirect fracture is one that occurs at a distant location away from the force due to longitudinal conduction, leverage, or torsional action. For example, as jumping off from a moving bicycle, the feet are suddenly stopped and fixed on the ground while the body still keeps inertial forwards, which can result in a spiral fracture of distal 1/3 of tibia with posterior malleolus fracture due to torsional transmission of force.

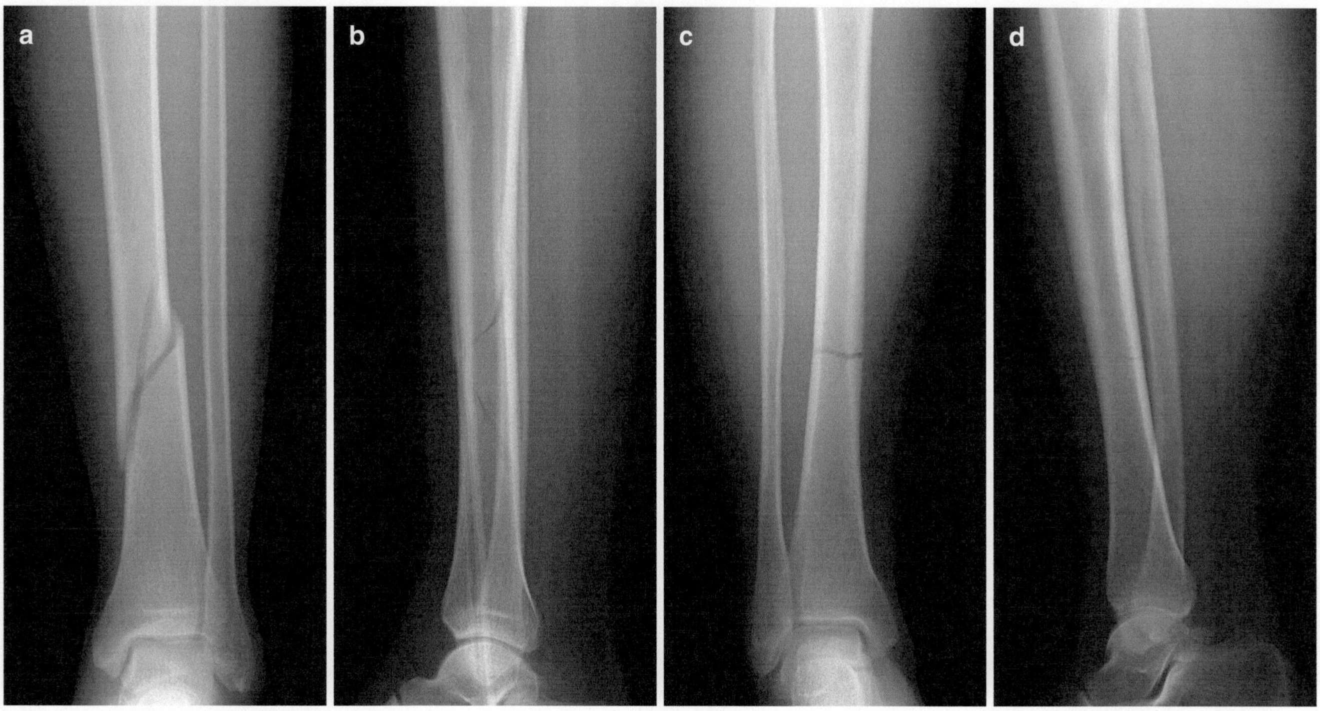

Fig. 1.1 Traumatic fracture of the tibia X films (**a**, **b**) show the spiral fractures of distal 1/3 of tibia, and (**c**, **d**) show the transverse fractures of distal 1/3 of tibia

Y. Zhang (✉)
Department of Orthopaedics, The Third Hospital of Hebei Medical University, Shijiazhuang, Hebei, China

Y. Zhang (ed.), *Differential Diagnosis of Fracture*, https://doi.org/10.1007/978-981-13-8339-7_1

Stress fractures include fatigue fractures and insufficiency fractures. Fatigue fractures (Fig. 1.2) are attritional cracks in bones, caused by a long-term repeated stress acting directly or indirectly to a certain part of the limb. For example, long distance walking is prone to cause fractures of the second and third metatarsals in the foot, and fractures of the distal 1/3 of the tibia shaft. Insufficiency fractures arise when there is a stress on a bone with reduced bone strength due to various causes. The difference between fatigue fracture and insufficiency fracture is that the former is caused by increased stress force on bones with normal structure whereas the latter is caused by a normal stress applying on abnormal bone tissue with reduced bone mineral density or lower elastic resistance. Insufficiency fracture occurs in a number of diseases including rheumatoid arthritis and osteoporosis.

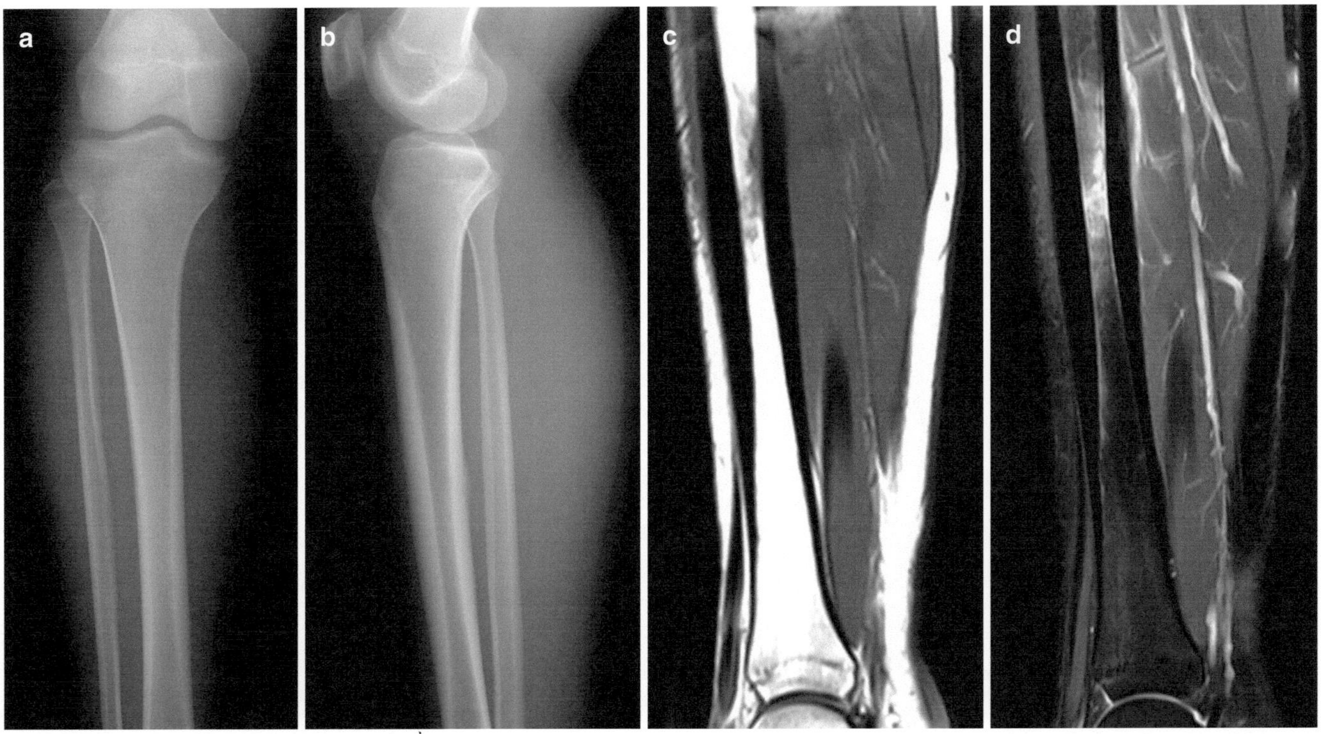

Fig. 1.2 Fatigue fracture of the tibia (**a**, **b**) X films show the periosteal thickening of the posterior to the middle tibia, and (**c**, **d**) MR T1W1 and T2W1 images showed periosteal thickening of the posterior to the middle tibia, long T1 and long T2 signals in the bone cortex, and edema in the surrounding bone marrow

Pathological fractures (Fig. 1.3) occur in bones with underlying lytic lesions. The most common cause of this is bone erosion and destruction caused by primary or metastatic bone tumors, which leads to a weakened bone structure with lower strength. In this situation, bone is prone to get fractured when exposed to a slight external force, sometimes due to its own gravity. Other factors that may lead to reduced bone strength include osteoporosis caused by various diseases, including endocrine disorders of the parathyroid hormone and gonadotropin, as well as dysplasia of bone and cartilage. According to the definition of pathological fracture, the insufficiency fracture could also be classified as generalized pathological fracture (Fig. 1.3).

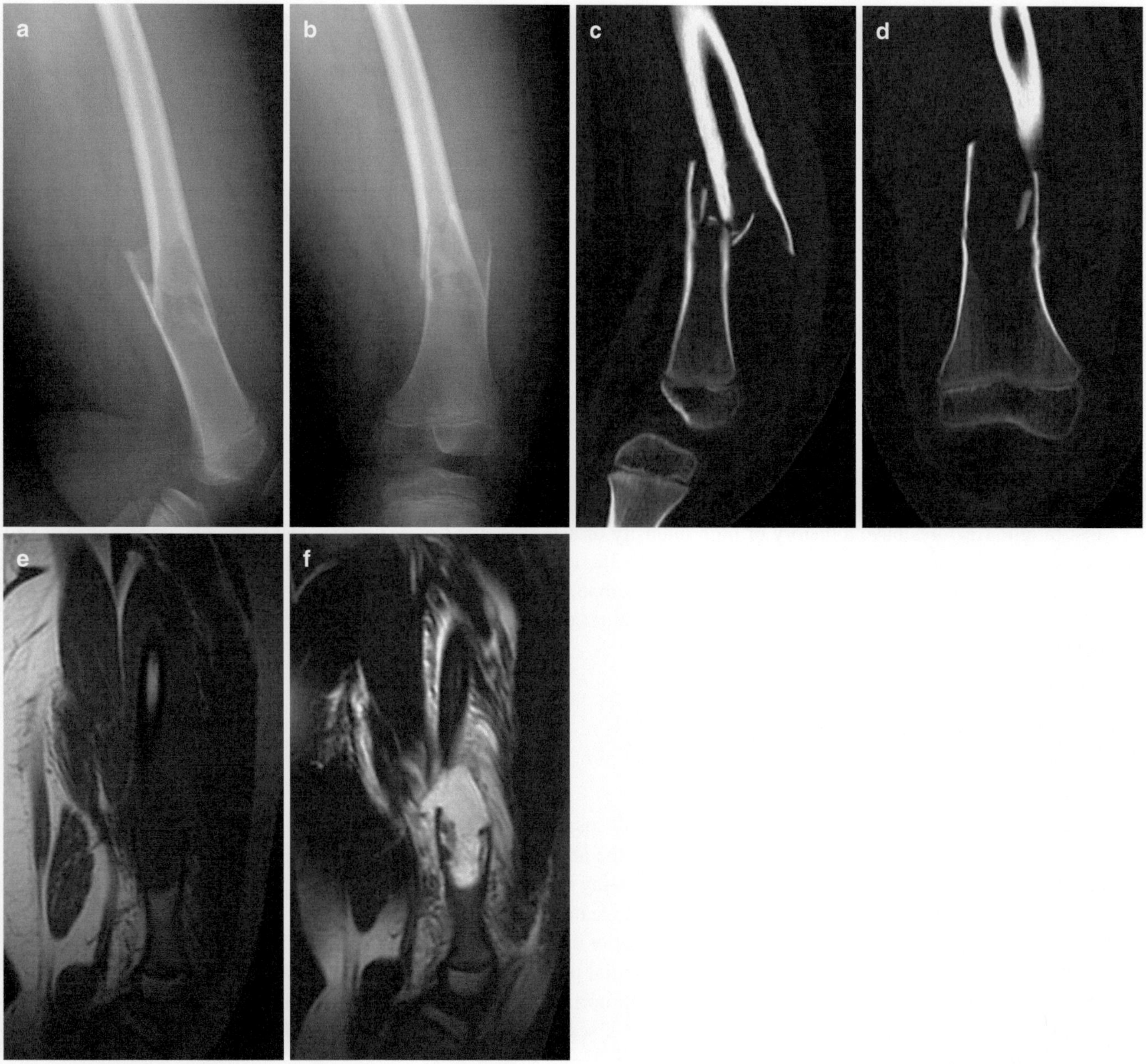

Fig. 1.3 Pathological fracture of the tibia (**a**, **c**) X-ray showed pathological fractures of the distal femur; (**b**, **d**) CT reconstruction showed pathological fracture of femur and collapse of fracture slice; (**e**, **f**) MRI showed long T1 and long T2 signal of femur damage, pathological fractures and the swelling of surrounding soft tissue

1.2 Diagnosis of Bone Fracture

The diagnosis of fracture is mainly based on clinical history, symptoms, and image examination.

1.2.1 Clinical Examination

Traumatic fractures display an obvious history of trauma. The locations of pain and stress mode are clues when assessing the fracture sites. Characteristic of physical signs of fracture include:

(1) Deformity and displacement of the fracture end, which can change the shape of the affected limb, mainly manifesting as shortening, angulation, and extension;
(2) Abnormal activity: the part of the body which cannot move under normal circumstances; thus fractures induce abnormal activity.
(3) Bony crepitus or two fracture ends rub against each other after a fracture, resulting in bony crepitus or bone grinding sensation.

Fractures can be diagnosed if one of the above three signs is found; however, the possibility of fracture cannot be ruled out given none of these signs is present, such as in the case of impacted fracture and fissured fracture. Severe trauma can be accompanied by systemic manifestations, such as.

(1) Shock: In the case of multiple fractures, pelvic fractures, femoral fractures, spinal fractures, and severe compound fractures. Patients often suffer from shock due to extensive soft tissue injury, massive bleeding, severe pain, or visceral injury.
(2) Fever: There is a large amount of internal bleeding in the site of fracture when the hematoma is absorbed, the body temperature will rise slightly, which is usually not higher than 38 °C. The possibility of infection should be considered when the temperature is elevated in the case of open fracture.

Most fatigue fractures have a history of high intensity of exercise in the recent times. The pain appears to be increased during the day, relieved after a night's rest and has a specific location during a specific activity.

In pathological fracture, the bone with the fracture is abnormal. For instance, the external force leading to the fracture is very light, yet the pain in the site exists before the fracture; therefore, the possibility of a pathological fracture should be suspected.

1.2.2 Selection of Imaging Evaluations

(1) X-ray evaluation

X-ray evaluation should be routinely performed in all suspected fractures, such as incomplete fractures and fractures in deep region, which helps detect the fractures given the above are difficult to detect in clinical examinations. Even if it has been shown to be an obvious clinical fracture, X-ray investigation is often useful in helping to understand the type and displacement of the fracture, and has significant meaning in guiding clinical therapy (Fig. 1.4).

When taking X-ray projections, both anteroposterior and lateral radiographs should be taken—adjacent joints must be included. Radiographs of oblique position, tangential position, or healthy contralateral parts should also be taken for comparison and evaluation. This is particularly appropriate in the emergency rooms. The complementary projection should be selected as far as possible, when whereby CT scanning is unavailable, which help to make up for the shortcomings of conventional position.

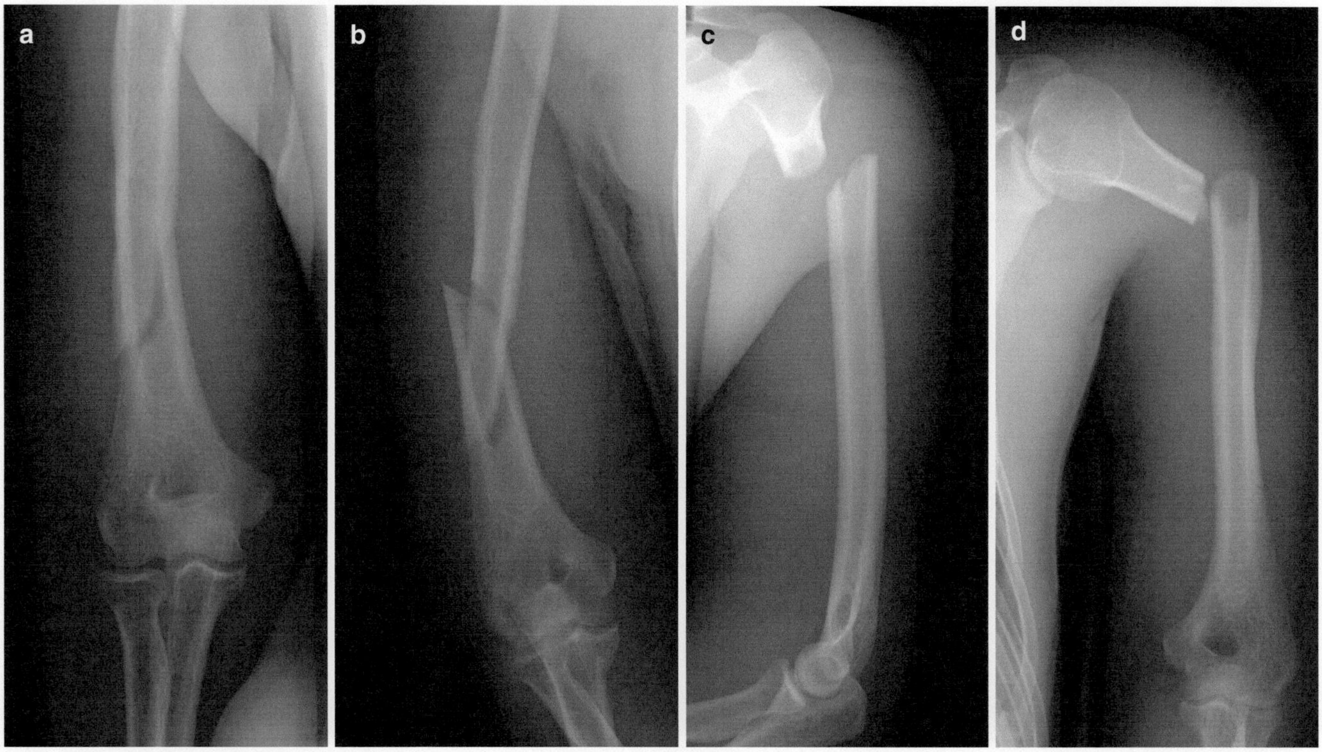

Fig. 1.4 X-ray plain film showing humerus shaft fracture. X-ray plain film (**a** and **b**) showing spiral fracture of the distal humerus, slight malposition, angulation. X-ray plain film (**c** and **d**) showing oblique fracture of the proximal humerus, malposition, angulation

(2) CT scanning

The diagnosis of a fracture is usually considered simple and direct-viewing; however, in some situations misdiagnosis and missed diagnosis of fracture can occur due to the complication and overlap of anatomical structures, in conspicuous displaced fracture, and small fracture fragments. The rates of misdiagnosis and missed diagnosis of fractures by routine X-ray plain film differ according to different sites: It has been reported that the rate of misdiagnosis and missed diagnosis of spinal fracture diagnosed with X-ray plain film can be as high as 30–60%. Therefore, to reduce or avoid misdiagnosis, CT scanning should be performed routinely on patients with fractures of the spine and pelvis, or fractures in other complex anatomical sites and complex fracture types. Fractures located in the metaphysis of the extremities and articular surface should also undergo CT scanning (Fig. 1.5) routinely. Multi-planar reconstruction in multi-slice spiral CT has efficacy in cases of complex anatomy. 3D CT reconstruction can be more visualized and convenient for the fracture classification, which is beneficial to guide the selection of treatment.

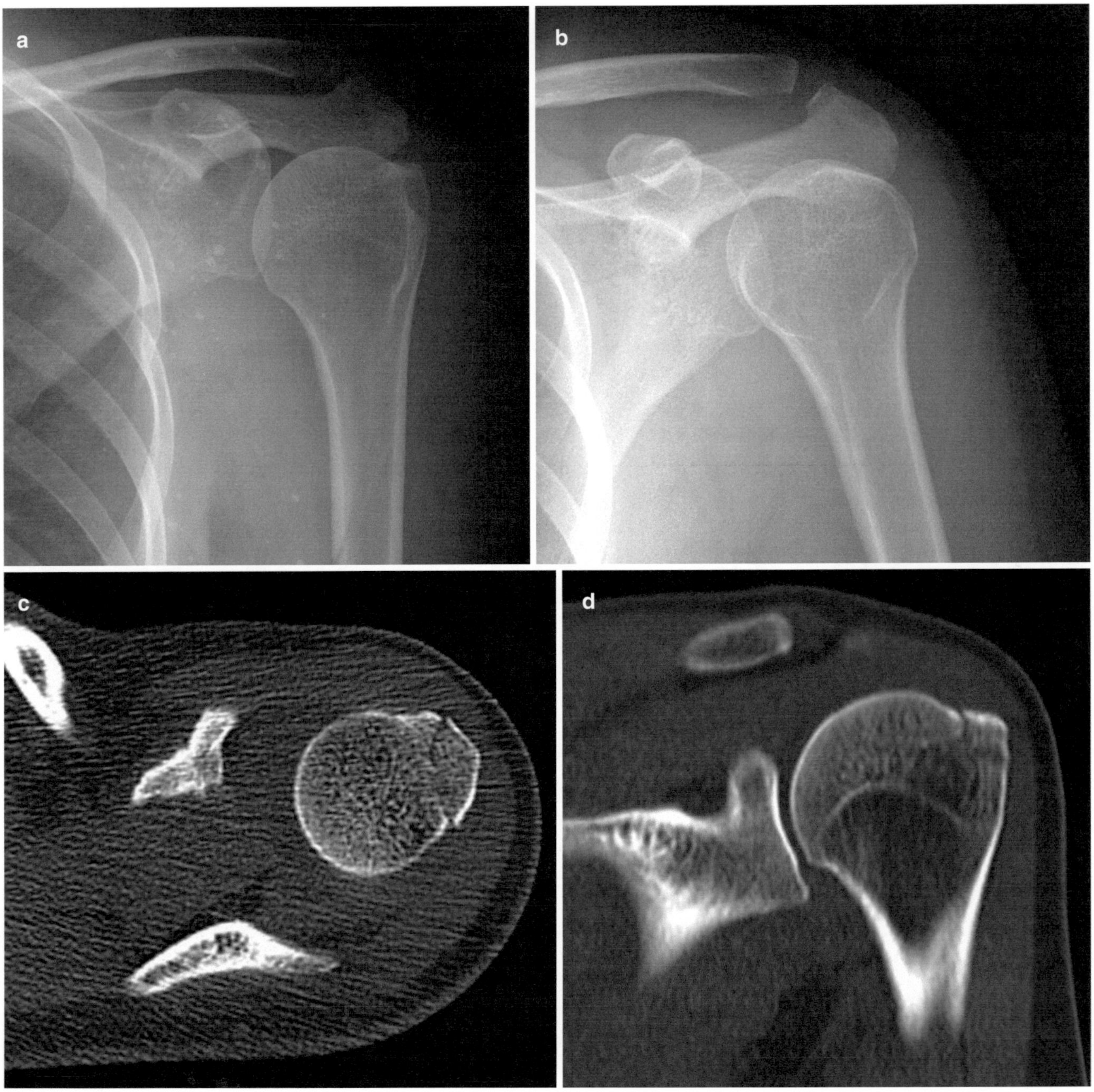

Fig. 1.5 CT scan showing greater tuberosity fracture of the humerus. X-ray plain film (**a** and **b**) showing irregular shape of greater tuberosity of left humerus and no clear signs of fracture. Cross-sectional and coronal image of CT (**c** and **d**) showing greater tuberosity fracture of humerus and no displacement of bone fragment

(3) MRI scanning
Though MRI is not as good as the CT evaluation in regards to showing the fracture lines, but it has advantages in spine trauma, by illustrating combined injuries in spinal cord, intervertebral discs, ligaments, and other soft tissue. It can show the level and range of the injured spinal cord segment, and distinguish whether it is a simple contusion swelling or combined with spinal hemorrhage, which is important for the prognosis and treatment. MRI scanning should also be the first choice for joint ligament and articular cartilage injury (Fig. 1.6).

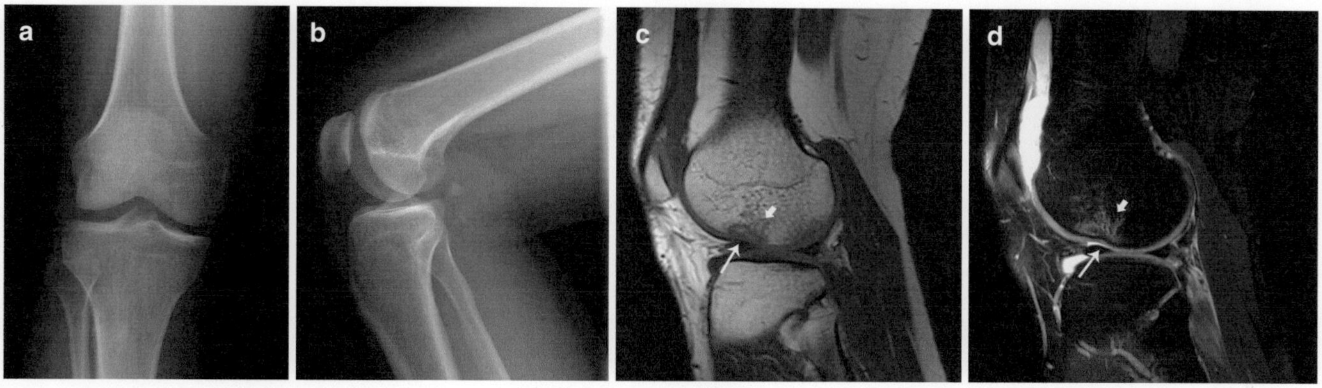

Fig. 1.6 MRI scan showing depressed fracture of articular cartilage on the femoral condyle. X-ray plain film (**a** and **b**) showing that no obvious abnormal bone mass was observed. MRI sagittal T1WI (**c**) and fat inhibition T2WI (**d**) showed fracture depression of cartilage and bone cortex of external condyle of femur (fine white arrow) and surrounding bone marrow edema (coarse white arrow)

Part II

Upper Limb Fracture

Shoulder Fracture

2

Li Zhang and Yingze Zhang

2.1 Proximal Humerus Fractures

The proximal humerus include the humeral head, the greater tuberosity, the lesser tuberosity, and the surgical neck. The surgical neck is the narrowing below the tuberosities and is frequently the site of fracture of the proximal humerus. The greater tuberosity, situated lateral to the head, has three areas of muscle insertions: the supraspinatus superiorly, the infraspinatus in the middle, and the teres minor inferiorly. Situated in front of the head is the lesser tuberosity, into which the tendon of the subscapularis attached [1]. A proximal humerus fracture accounts for 4.04% of total fractures, and for 39.70% of adult humeral fractures.

The proximal humerus is in a lateral position, and there are fewer overlapping tissues around it. Therefore, conventional X-ray of the proximal humerus fracture can help formulate an accurate diagnosis. CT is mainly used for both minor avulsion fractures at the insertion of the ligament, and details of the fracture of a joint surface. MR scan is essential for diagnosing tendon and soft tissue injury around the shoulder joint, rotator cuff injury, and an injury of the labrum of the scapula.

The AO/OTA classification of proximal humeral fractures is divided into three groups: extra-articular unifocal fractures, extra-articular bifocal fractures, and intra-articular fractures. Extra-articular unifocal fractures are sub-grouped into greater tuberosity fractures, surgical neck-impaction fractures, and surgical neck displacement fractures. The greater tuberosity fractures account for 12.99% of humeral fractures, while surgical neck fractures account for 15.88% of humeral fractures, and surgical neck displacement fractures account for 3.79% of humeral fractures. Extra-articular bifocal fractures are sub-grouped into surgical neck-impacted fractures, surgical neck non-impaction fractures, and extra-articular fractures with glenohumeral joint dislocation. Surgical neck-impaction fractures account for 3.11% of humeral fractures. The surgical neck non-impaction fractures account for 1.63% of the humeral fractures, and the extra-articular fractures with glenohumeral joint dislocation account for 0.49% of the humeral fractures. Intra-articular fractures are divided into fractures with slight displacement, fractures with marked displacement, and intra-articular fractures with dislocation. The fractures with slight displacement account for 1.05% of humeral fractures. The fractures with marked displacement account for 0.31% of humeral fractures. The intra-articular fractures with dislocation account for 0.46% of the humeral fractures.

A brief introduction to the differential diagnosis of proximal humeral fractures is presented as follows.

2.1.1 Identification of Injury Mechanism

The proximal humerus fracture has a certain relationship with osteoporosis, so the age of patients is an important factor, thus, doctors need to pay more attention to identification. Elderly patients often suffer from indirect injuries, by which it is either mild or moderate. The commonest mechanism of injury is a fall from standing: a fall on the outstretched arm, thrust of the

L. Zhang
CT/MRI Center, The Third Hospital of Hebei Medical University, Shijiazhuang, Hebei, China

Y. Zhang (✉)
Department of Orthopaedics, The Third Hospital of Hebei Medical University, Shijiazhuang, Hebei, China

Y. Zhang (ed.), *Differential Diagnosis of Fracture*, https://doi.org/10.1007/978-981-13-8339-7_2

hand or elbow, indirect force upward applied at the point of cancellous bone and cortical bone near the proximal humerus, which could result in a fracture. On the other hand, young patients have high bone strength and hardness. Proximal humerus fractures are mostly caused by direct or severe injuries. The direction of force is mostly from the lateral or anterior lateral side. It is difficult for mild injuries to cause a fracture. There are many associated injuries during fractures, such as the injuries of chest and head.

Pathological fracture identification: The injury is often trivial. Cases, such as a patient occurred unexpected fracture when moving a flower vase, should be highly suspected pathological fracture.

2.1.2 Identification of Symptoms and Clinical Signs

The most obvious symptoms of the proximal humerus fractures are pain, swelling, and limited mobility. These symptoms are not specific, which cannot be exclusively used for diagnosis.

Due to the shoulder joint muscle tissue being thicker, the deformity is not prominent when the fracture is simple; therefore, greater attention should be paid when identifying the fracture.

Careful identification of clinical signs becomes critical when fracture dislocation is present at the same time: (1) When an anterior shoulder dislocation is present, the normal contour of the deltoid is lost and acromion is prominent posteriorly and laterally—square shoulder deformity, palpable fullness below the coracoid process. (2) When a posterior dislocation of the humeral head is present, the shoulder will show fullness posteriorly whereas flatness anteriorly.

When examining the patients, attention should be paid to the texture of the skin on the lateral side of the shoulder. If there is a sensory disturbance, axillary nerve injury should be highly suspected; however, if the skin on the lateral side of the shoulder feels normal, axillary nerve injury cannot be ruled out. Early deltoid muscle contraction is difficult to perform due to the patient experiencing pain, so after the pain is relieved, the ability for the deltoid muscle to contract should be examined again to avoid missing diagnosis of an axillary nerve injury.

2.1.3 Imaging Differential Diagnosis

Conventional X-ray scans can provide a basic diagnosis for a proximal humerus fracture. However, with the wide application of CT, some researchers questioned the accuracy of conventional X-ray diagnosis. The following points should be noted: (1) Significant signs of a fracture can't be seen in a conventional X-ray scan, forasmuch as clinical symptoms and signs are distinct, CT or MR scans should be ordered; (2) Conventional X-ray scans can show simple transverse, oblique, and spiral fractures, but after a CT scan, multiple fragments of fractures were found. (3) Conventional X-ray scan is used to clearly diagnose an extra-articular fracture, but following a CT scan, it was found to be a complete intra-articular or partial intra-articular fracture; (4) Conventional X-ray confirmed a partial intra-articular fracture, however, after a CT scan was conducted, it was presented an intra-articular comminuted fracture; (5) Conventional X-ray scan of a fracture found a disarrangement of the bone structure. CT or MR scans should be ordered to exclude pathological fractures. Therefore, we should closely combine the clinical history with the diagnosis of fractures in adjacent joints, and carefully analyze the signs following an X-ray, if suspected, further CT or MR scans are necessary.

1. Differential diagnosis between greater tuberosity fracture and non-fracture
   1.1 X-ray (Fig. 2.1a, b)

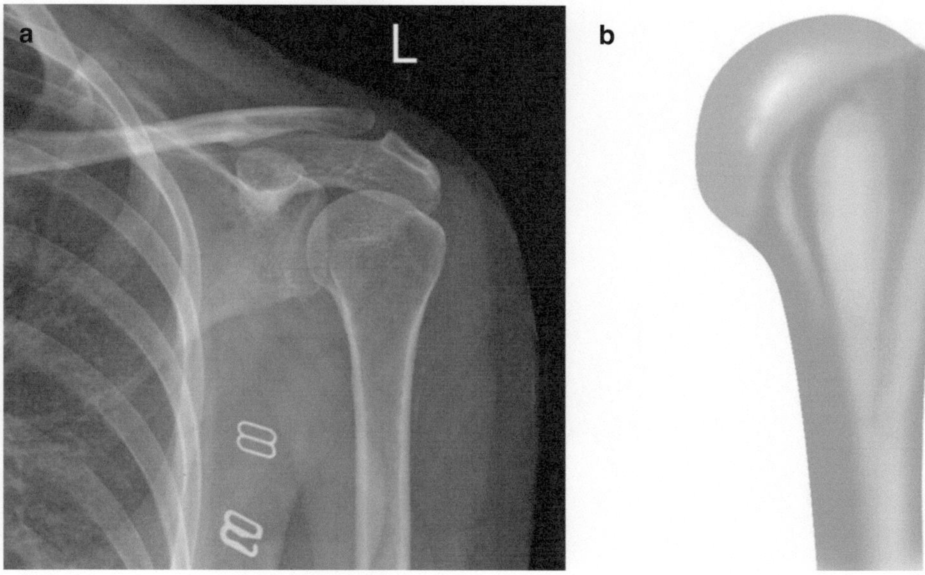

Fig 2.1 X-ray film (**a**) shows that the position of the bones of the left shoulder joint is normal, the cortical bone is continuous, no clear fracture signs are seen, but the patient has significant pain. Therefore, a further CT scan was performed (**b**)

   1.2 CT scan (Fig. 2.1c–e)

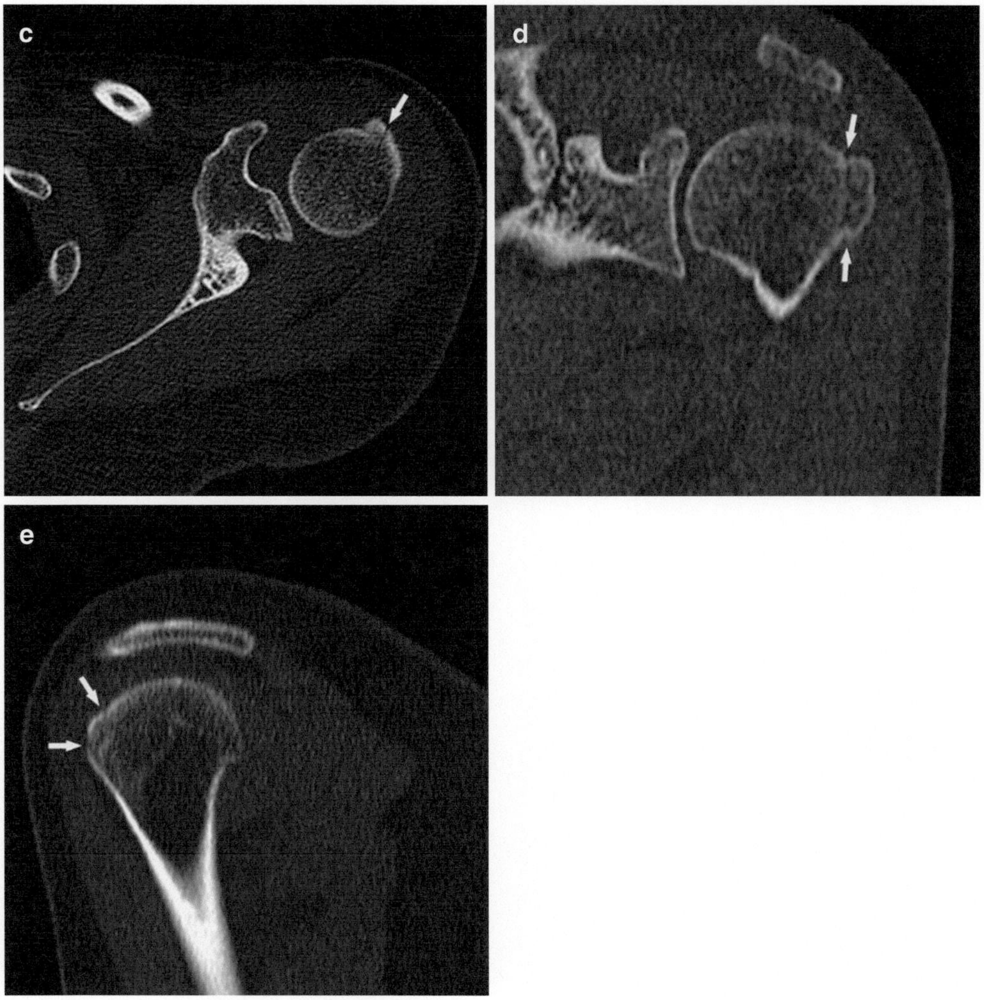

Fig. 2.1 CT cross section (**c**), coronal reconstruction (**d**), and sagittal reconstruction (**e**) showed the linear fracture (arrow) of the greater tuberosity, without displacement

1.3 MR scan (Fig. 2.1f, g)

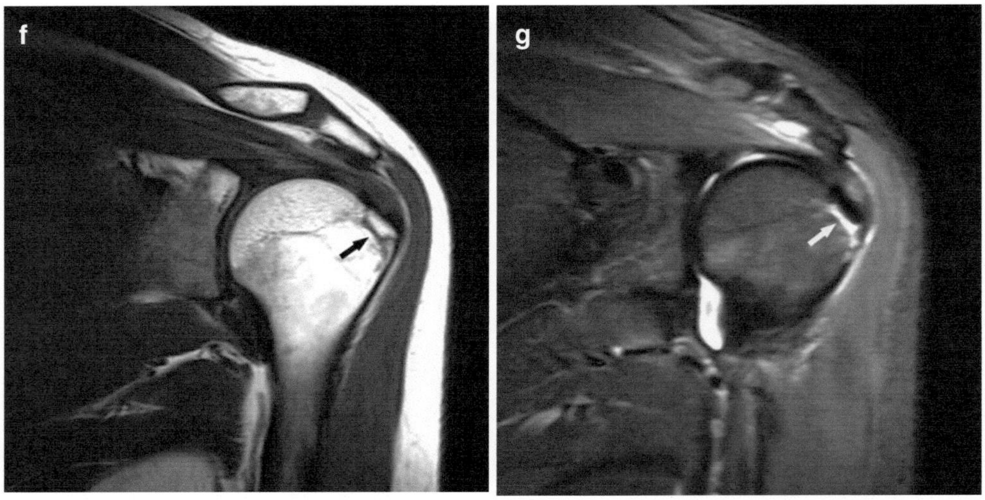

Fig. 2.1 Further results of MR coronal T1WI (**f**) and T2WI (**g**) showed that the continuity of the greater tuberosity was interrupted, and the long linear T1 and T2 signal (arrow) and multiple fragments shadows were observed, together with the surrounding edema of bone marrow

2. Differential diagnosis of greater tuberosity comminuted fracture from suspected fracture
   2.1. X-ray (Fig. 2.2a, b)

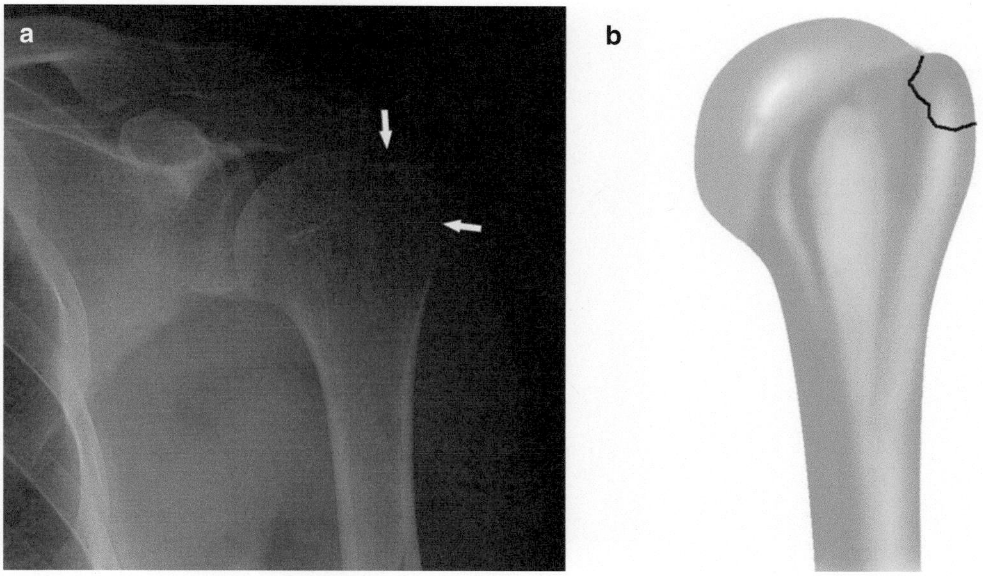

Fig. 2.2 X-ray plain film (**a**) shows the disorder of bone structure of the left greater tuberosity, irregularity (arrow), greater tuberosity suspicious fracture, and schematic diagram (**b**)

   2.2. CT scan (Fig. 2.2c–e)

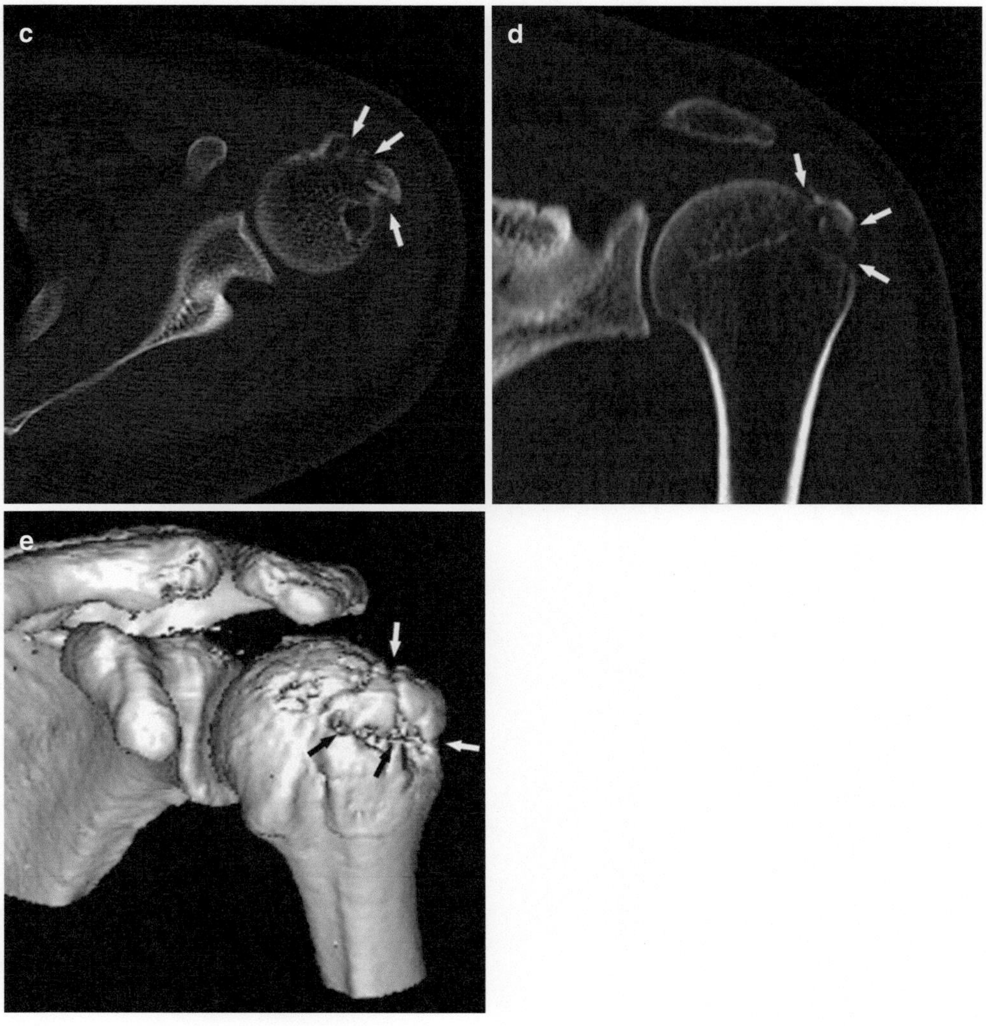

Fig. 2.2 CT cross section (**c**), coronal reconstruction (**d**), and three-dimensional reconstruction (**e**) show that the greater tuberosity of the left humerus is shattered (arrow), with local displacement

3. Differential diagnosis of the greater tuberosity comminuted fracture and simple fracture
   3.1. X-ray (Fig. 2.3a, b)

Fig. 2.3 X-ray plain film (**a**) shows the longitudinal fracture (arrow) of the greater tuberosity of the right humerus, with slightly displaced, which is a simple fracture. Schematic diagram (**b**)

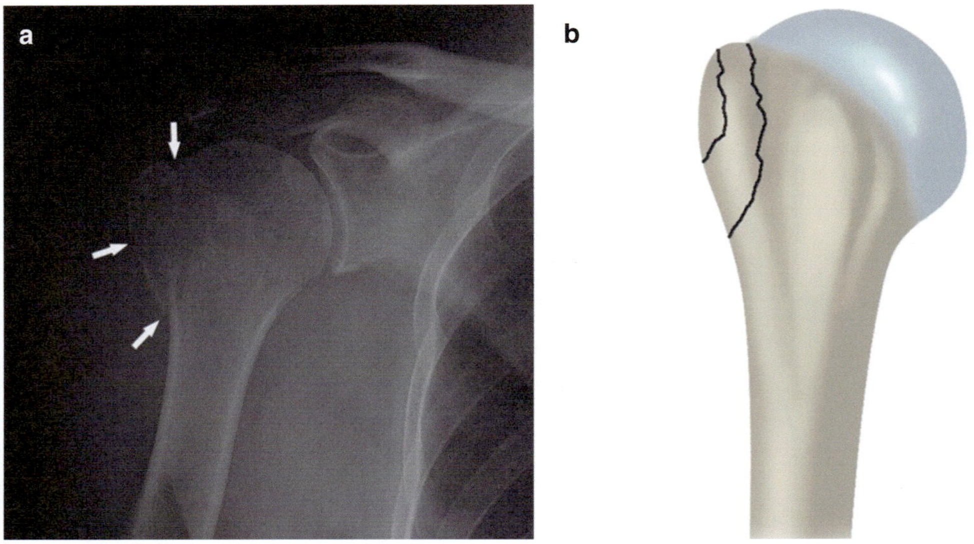

   3.2. CT scan (Fig. 2.3c–e)

Fig. 2.3 CT cross section (**c**), coronal surface (**d**), and three-dimensional reconstruction (**e**) showed that the fracture of greater tuberosity (arrow) with multiple bone fragments and displacement

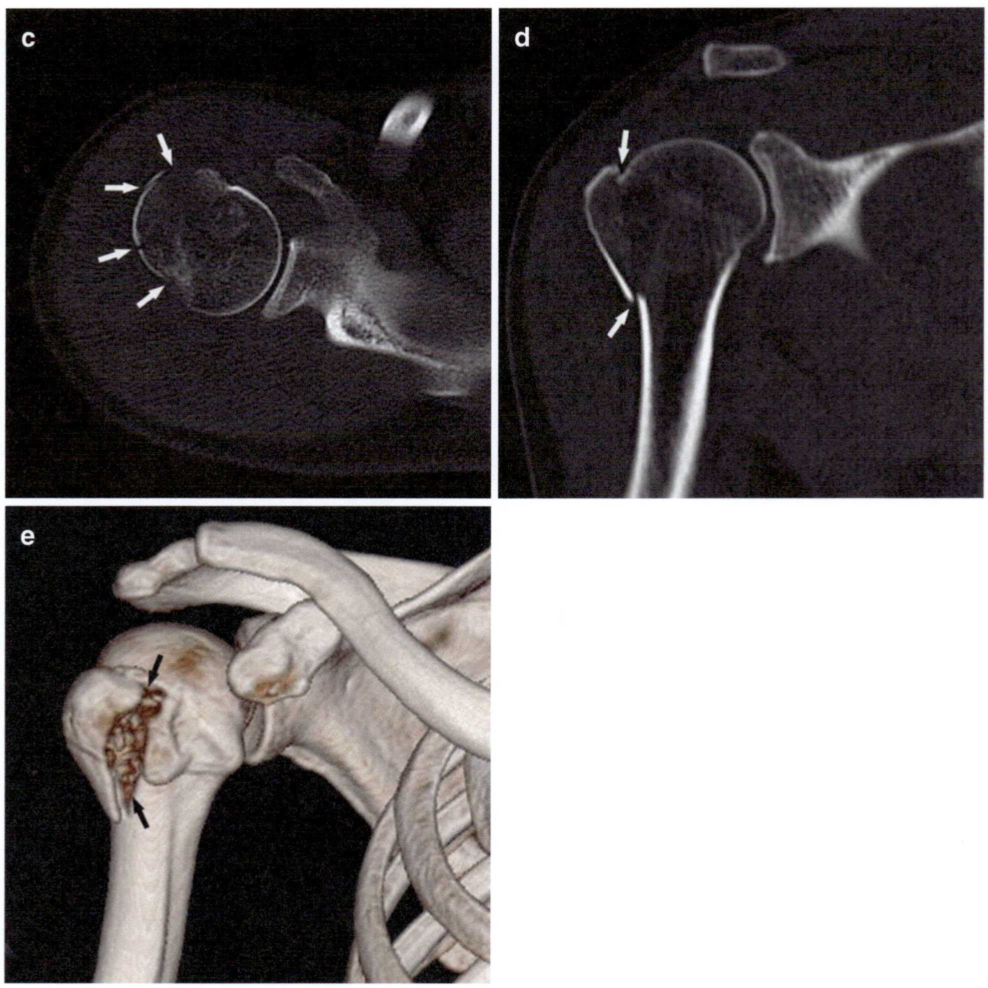

4. Identification of the simple greater tuberosity fractures and suspected fractures
   4.1. X-ray (Fig. 2.4a–d)

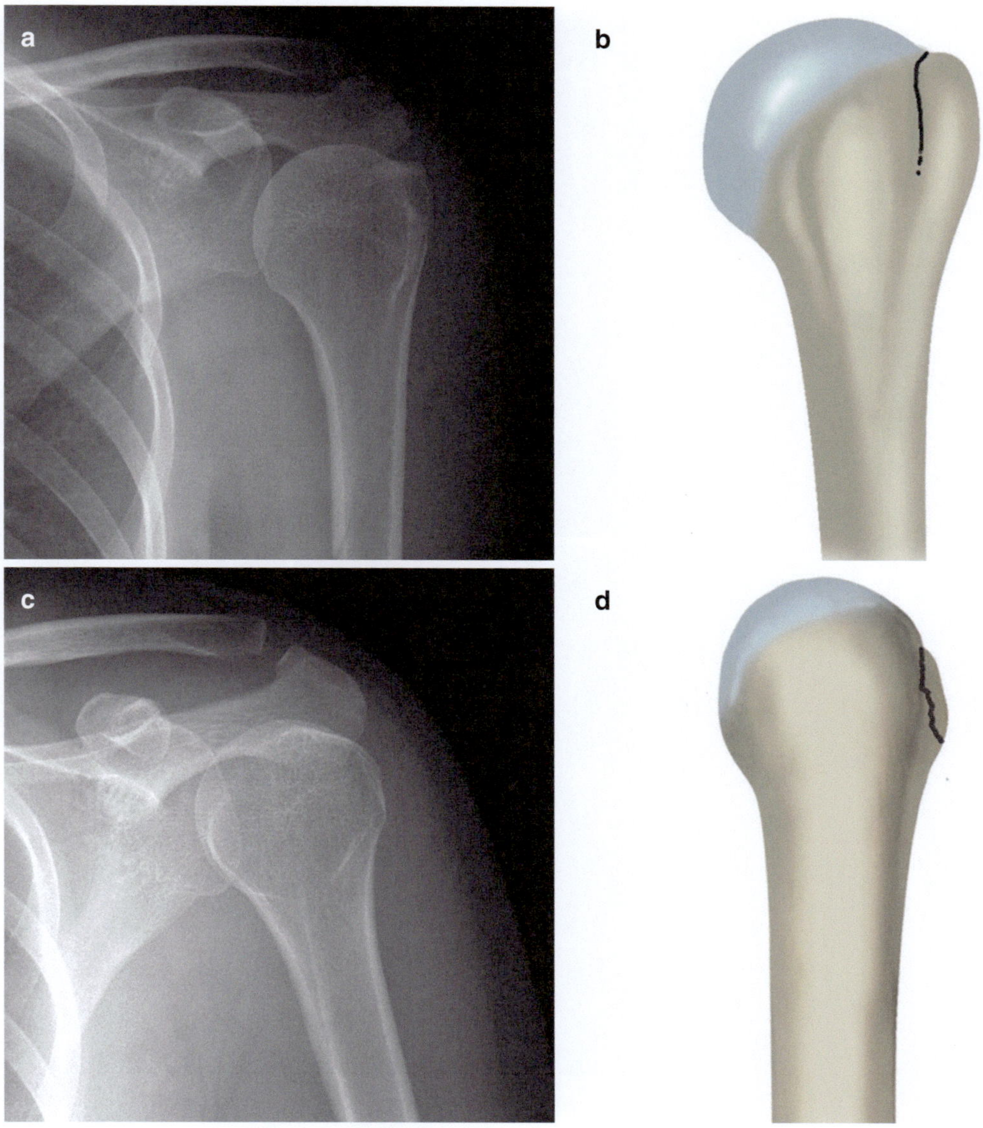

Fig. 2.4 X-ray plain film (**a**, **c**) shows the position of all the bones of the left shoulder joint. The bone structure of the greater tuberosity is slightly disordered, and the fracture is suspected (**b**, **d**)

   4.2. CT scan (Fig. 2.4e, f)

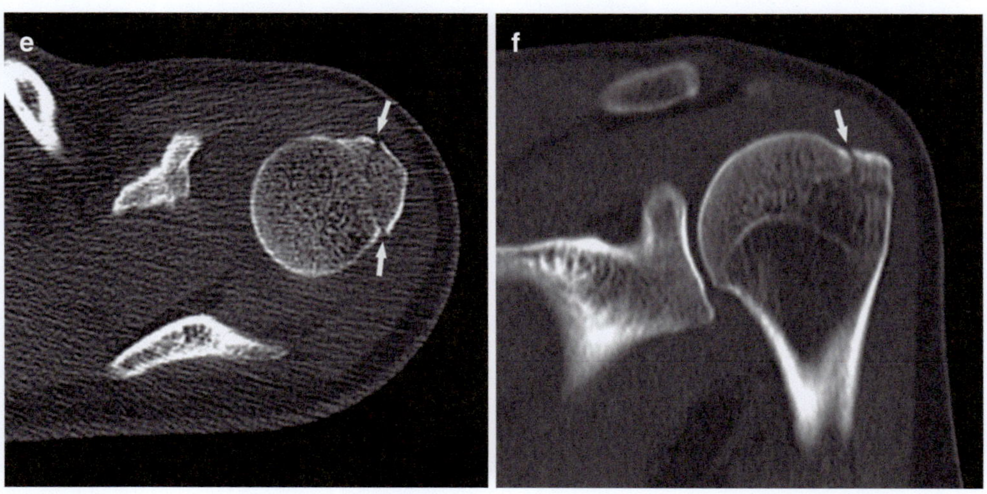

Fig. 2.4 CT cross section (**e**) and coronal reconstruction (**f**) showed that the fracture of the greater tuberosity (arrow), with no displacement, was a simple fracture

5. Differential diagnosis between proximal humerus impaction fracture and linear fracture
   5.1. X-ray (Fig. 2.5a–d)

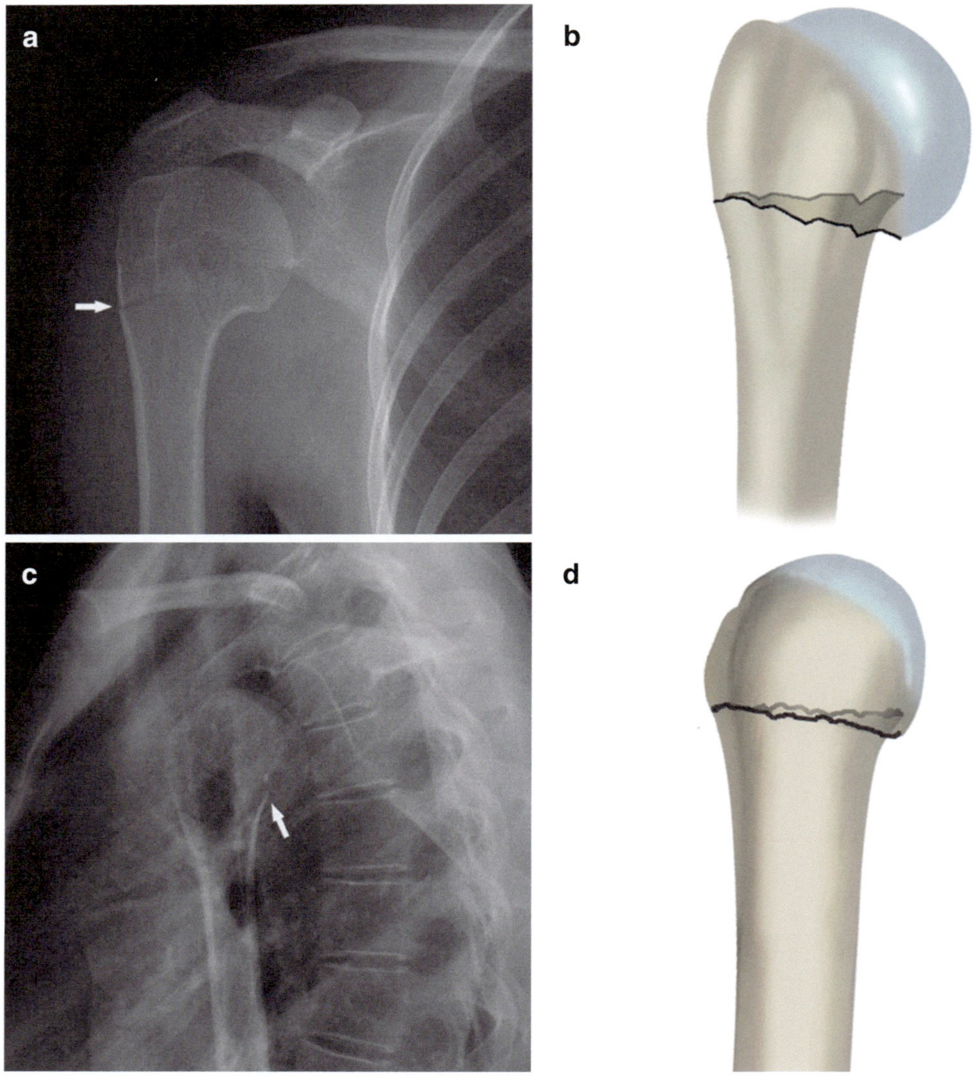

Fig. 2.5 The anteroposterior position of shoulder joint (**a**, **c**) X-ray film showed the linear fracture of right surgical neck of humeral (arrow), with no obvious displacement, continuity of medial humeral margin is normal, and schematic diagram (**b**, **d**)

   5.2. CT scan (Fig. 2.5e, f)

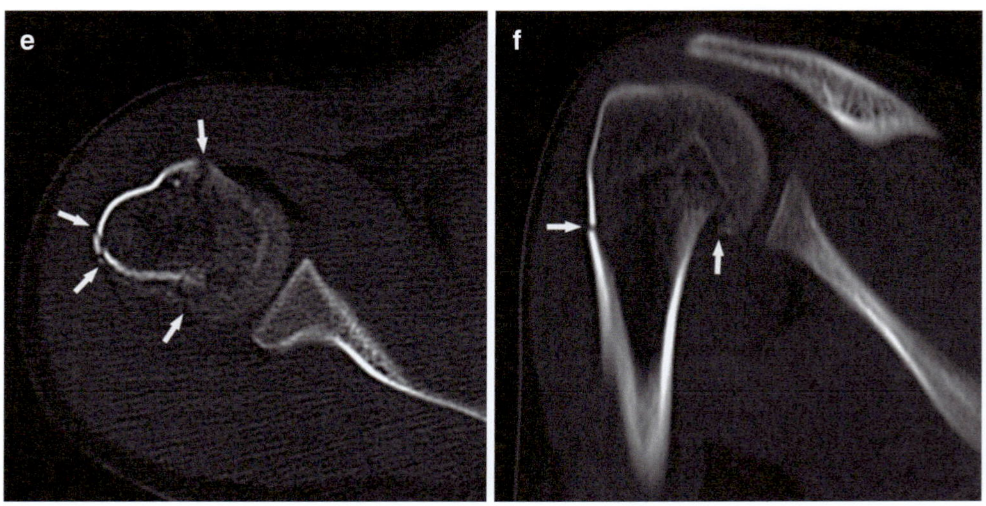

Fig. 2.5 CT cross section (**e**) and coronal reconstruction (**f**) showed that the fracture of the humeral surgical neck (arrow) was embedded into the humeral head, and the medial humerus edge was distinctly broken

6. Differential diagnosis of proximal humerus impaction fracture and comminuted fracture
   6.1. X-ray (Fig. 2.6a, b)

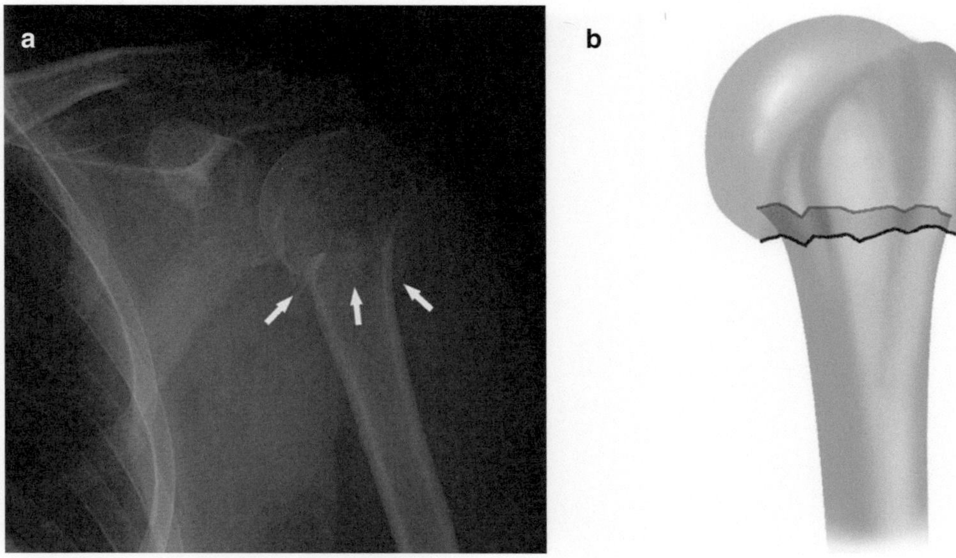

Fig. 2.6 The X-ray of the shoulder joint (**a**) shows the fracture of the left humeral surgical neck (arrow), with multiple bone fragments, and the schematic diagram (**b**)

   6.2. CT scan (Fig. 2.6c)

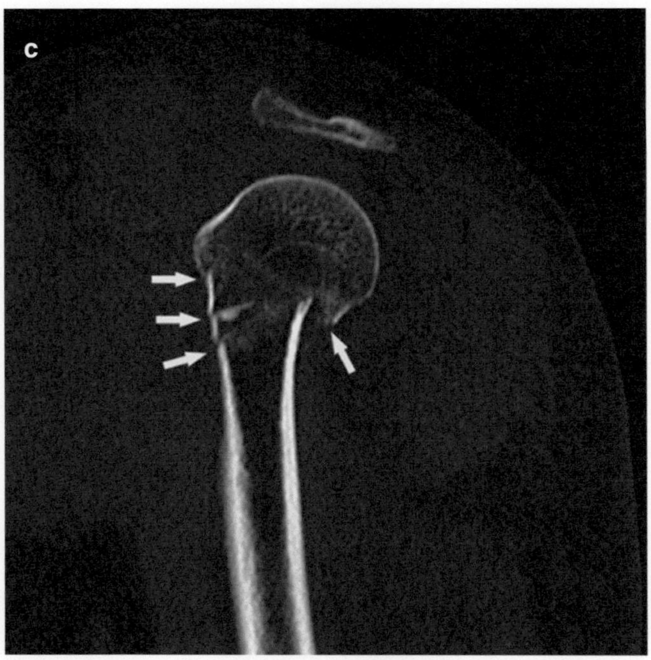

Fig. 2.6 CT sagittal reconstruction (**c**) shows the fracture of the surgical neck (arrow) and the impaction fracture in humeral metaphysis

7. Differentiation of proximal humeral non-displaced fracture and displaced fracture
   7.1. X-ray (Fig. 2.7a, b)

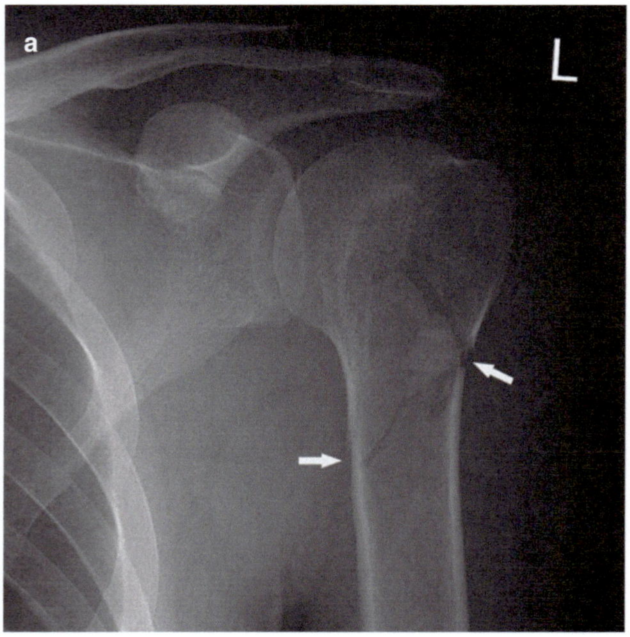

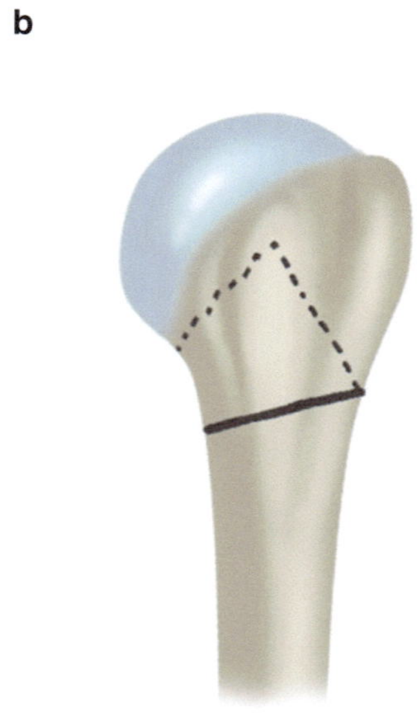

Fig. 2.7 The anteroposterior position of shoulder joint (**a**) X-ray flat film shows the left humeral surgical neck fracture (arrow), no displacement, and schematic diagram (**b**)

   7.2. CT scan (Fig. 2.7c)

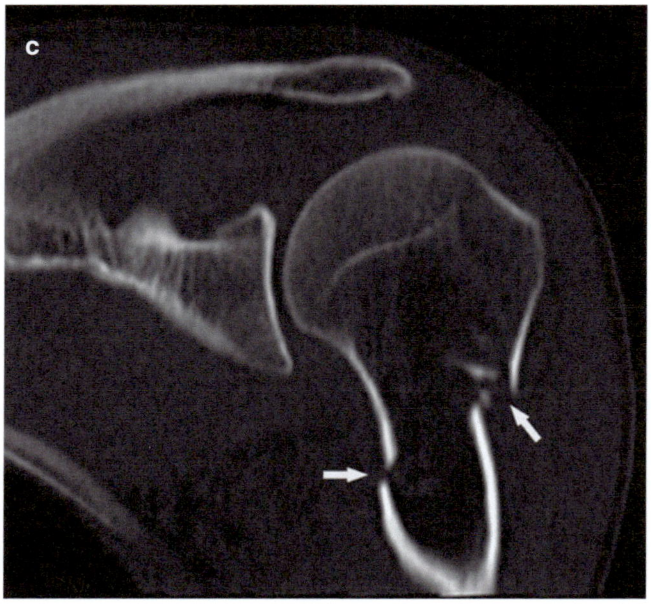

Fig. 2.7 CT coronal reconstruction (**c**) shows the fracture of surgical neck in the humerus, with marked displacement (arrow)

8. Differential diagnosis of proximal humeral comminuted fracture and fracture with displacement
   8.1. X-ray (Fig. 2.8a–d)

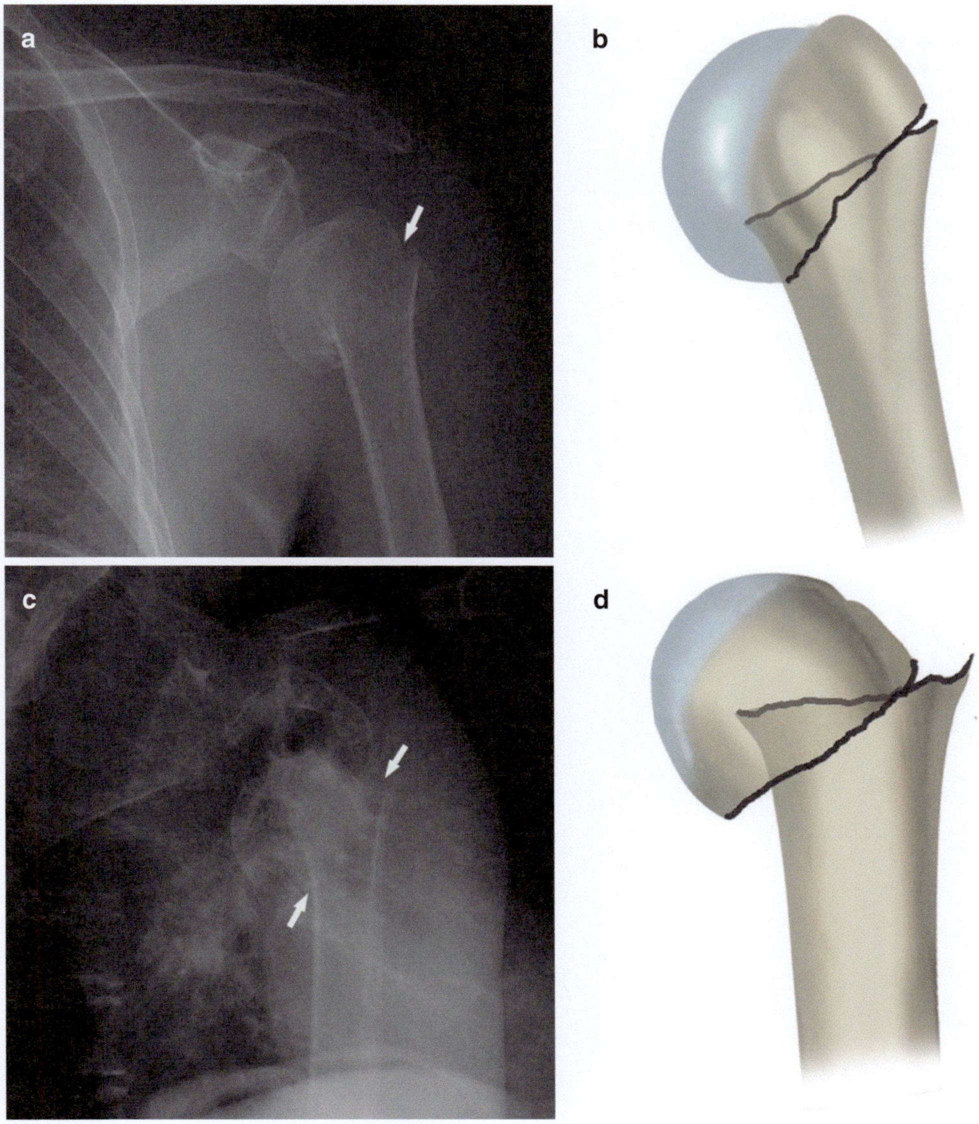

Fig. 2.8 The anteroposterior position of shoulder joint (**a**, **c**) X-ray film showed the fracture of surgical neck (arrow) in the left humerus, with marked displacement, and the schematic diagram (**b**, **d**)

   8.2. CT scan (Fig. 2.8e, f)

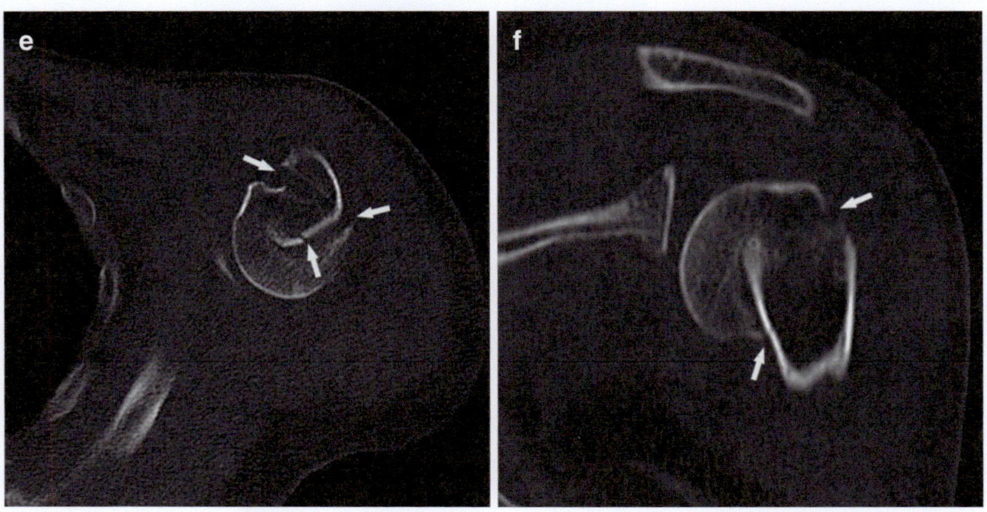

Fig. 2.8 CT cross section (**e**) and coronal plane (**f**) reconstruction showed that the surgical neck of the humerus was fractured, with marked displacement and impaction (arrow)

9. Differential diagnosis of proximal humerus comminuted fracture and simple fracture
   9.1. X-ray (Fig. 2.9a–d)

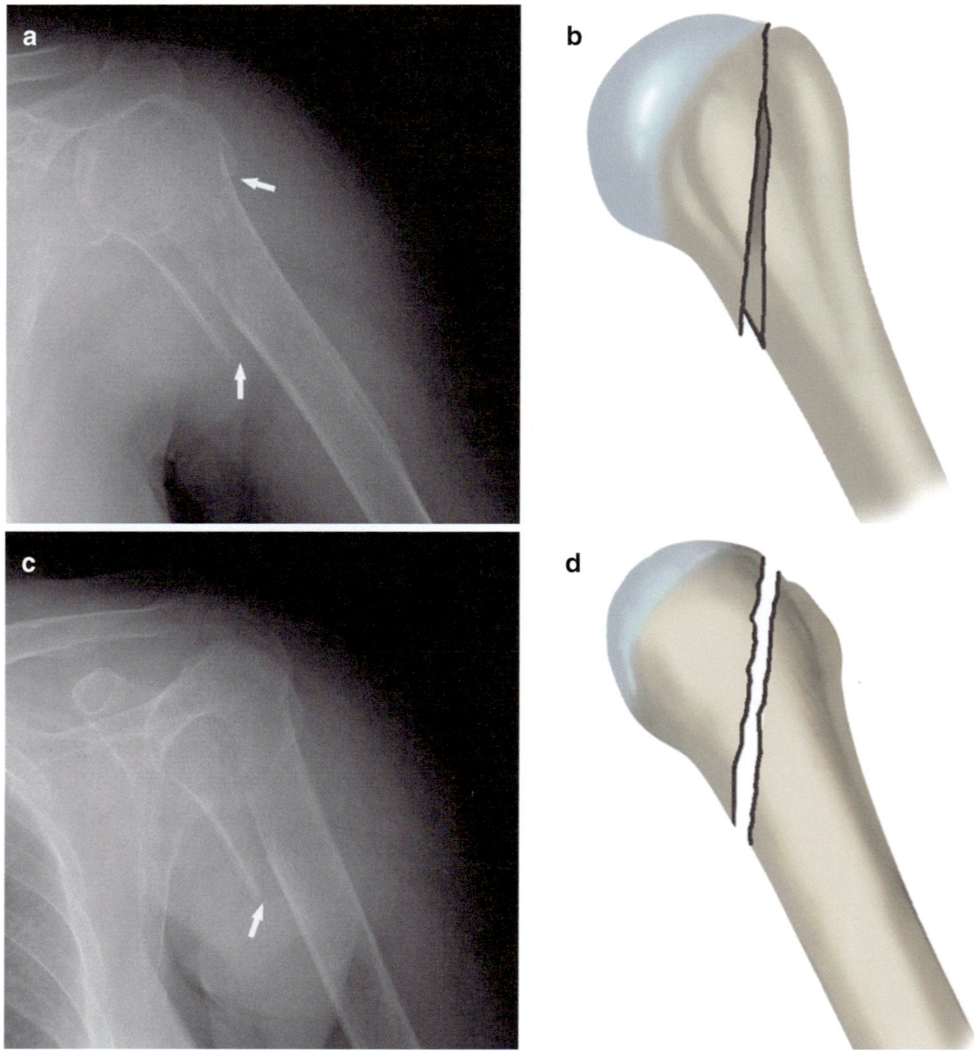

Fig. 2.9 The anteroposterior position of the shoulder joint (**a**, **c**) shows the left humeral surgical neck fracture (arrow), and the fracture end is obviously displaced (**b**, **d**)

   9.2. CT scan (Fig. 2.9e, f)

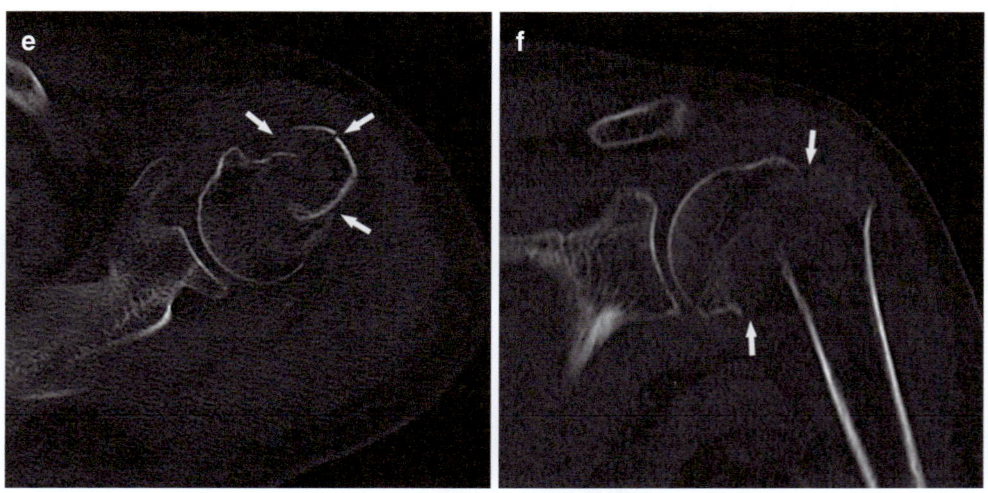

Fig. 2.9 CT cross section (**e**) and coronal plane (**f**) reconstruction showed: fracture of the surgical neck of the humerus (arrow), with multiple bone fragments, marked displacement

10. Differential diagnosis between proximal humerus comminuted impaction fracture and simple impaction fracture
    10.1. X-ray (Fig. 2.10a–d)

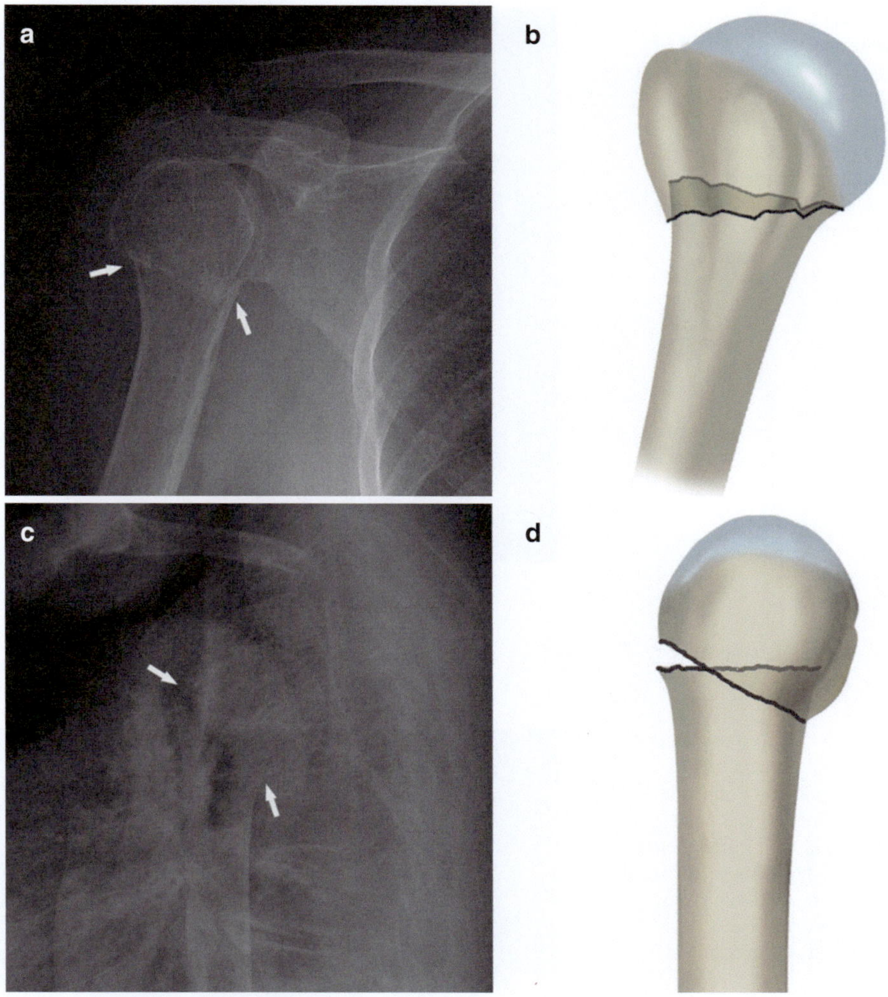

Fig. 2.10 The anteroposterior position of shoulder joint (**a**, **c**) X-ray film shows the right humeral surgical neck fracture (arrow), the fracture end is displaced, slightly impacted, schematic diagram (**b**, **d**)

    10.2. CT scan (Fig. 2.10e, f)

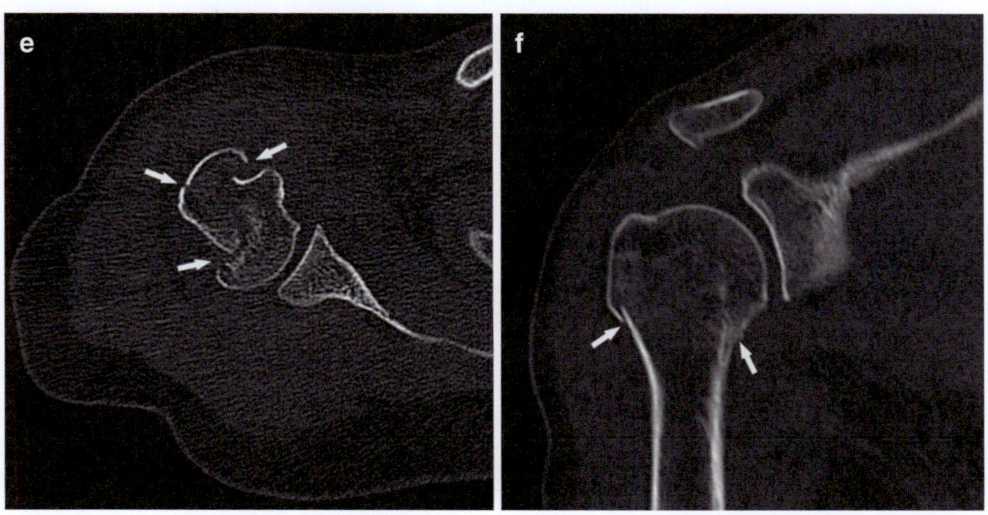

Fig. 2.10 CT cross-sectional (**e**) and coronal (**f**) reconstruction showed: fractures of the surgical neck (arrows) with multiple bone fragments, with rotating, displaced, and embedded

11. Differential diagnosis between proximal humerus comminuted displaced fracture and simple displaced fracture
    11.1. X-ray (Fig. 2.11a, b)

Fig. 2.11 The anteroposterior position of shoulder joint (**a**) X-ray film shows the fracture of the surgical neck (arrow) in the right humerus, and the fracture ends are displaced and overlapped schematic diagram (**b**)

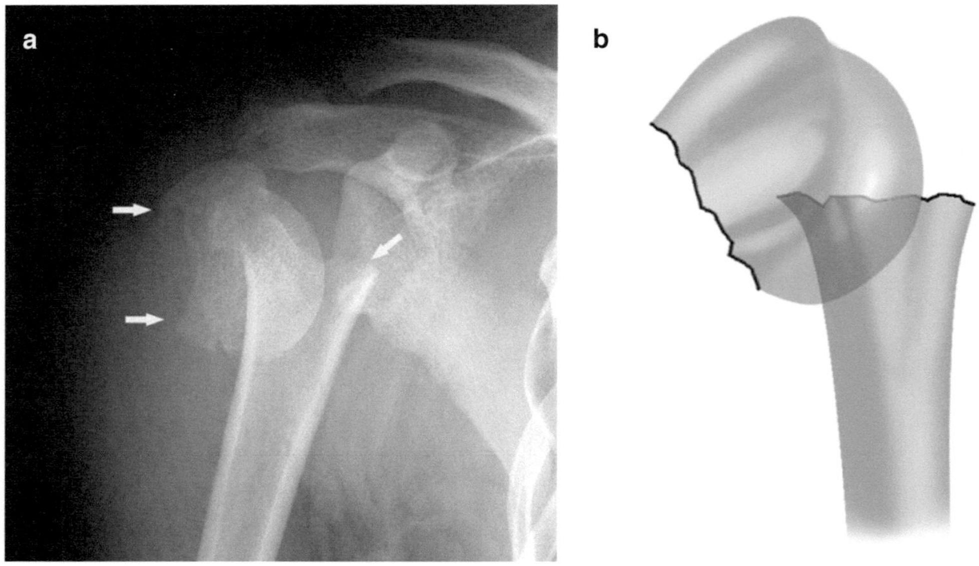

    11.2. CT scan (Fig. 2.11c–e)

Fig. 2.11 CT cross sections (**c**, **d**) and coronal surface reconstruction (**e**) showed: fracture of surgical neck (arrow) in the right humerus, multiple bone fragments were easy seen, and the broken ends were obviously displaced and overlapped

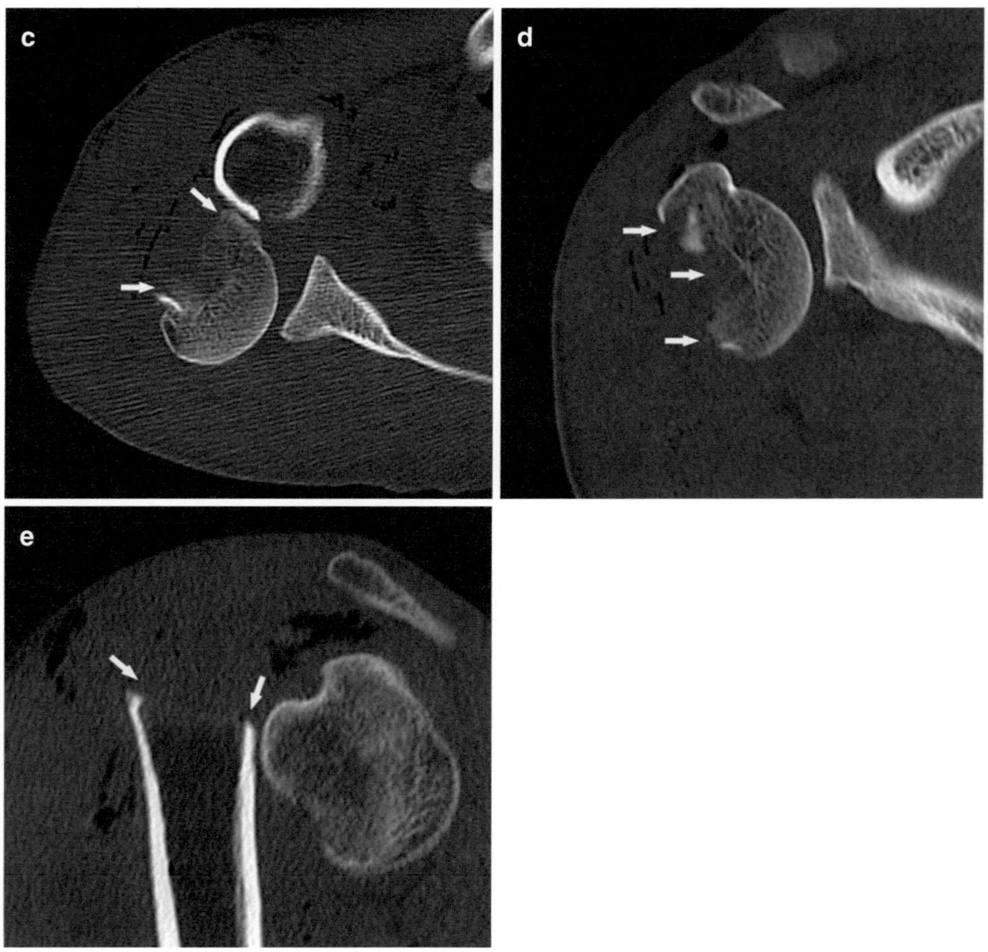

12. Differential diagnosis of proximal humeral comminuted fracture with the greater tuberosity and comminuted fracture
    12.1. X-ray (Fig. 2.12a–d)

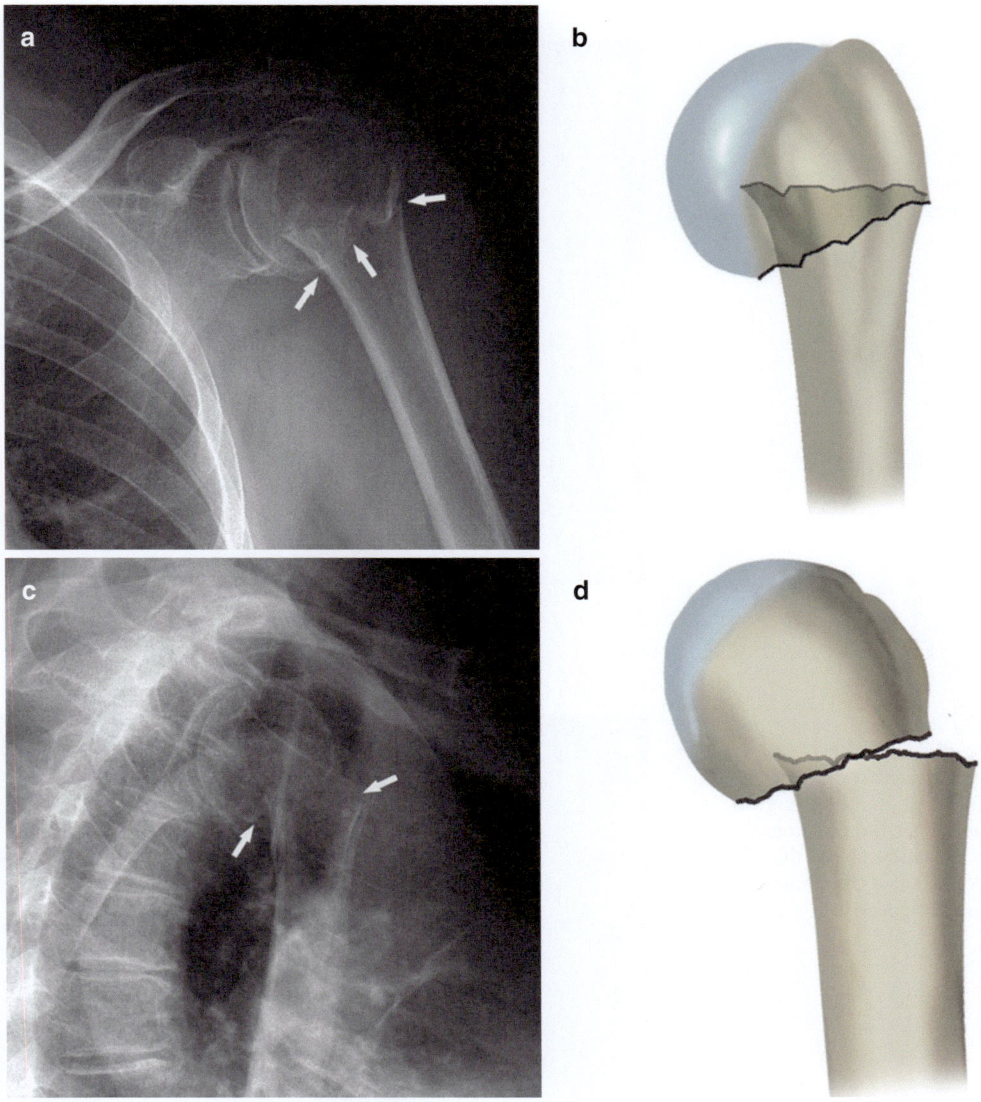

Fig. 2.12 The anteroposterior position of shoulder joint (**a**, **c**) X-ray film shows the fracture of surgical neck bone (arrow) in the left humerus, and the impaction of fracture end schematic diagram (**b**, **d**)

    12.2. CT scan (Fig. 2.12e, f)

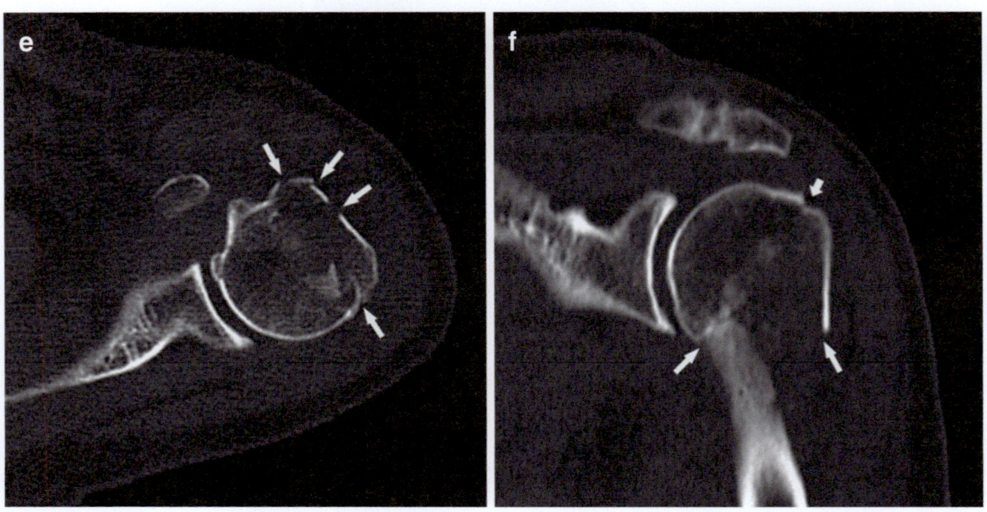

Fig. 2.12 CT cross section (**e**) and coronal plane (**f**) reconstruction showed: humeral surgical neck fracture (arrow), with the impaction of fracture end, and the greater tuberosity fracture

13. Differential diagnosis of proximal humerus fracture with greater tuberosity fracture and metaphyseal comminuted fracture
    13.1. X-ray (Fig. 2.13a, b)

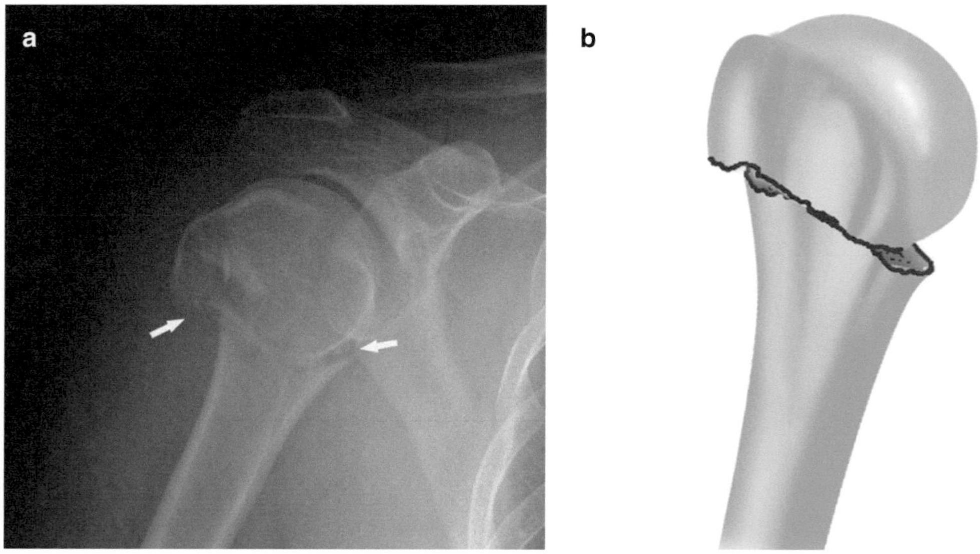

Fig. 2.13 The anteroposterior position of shoulder joint (**a**) X-ray shows the fracture of humeral surgical neck (arrow) in the right side, and the impaction of fracture ends schematic diagram (**b**)

    13.2. CT scan (Fig. 2.13c–e)

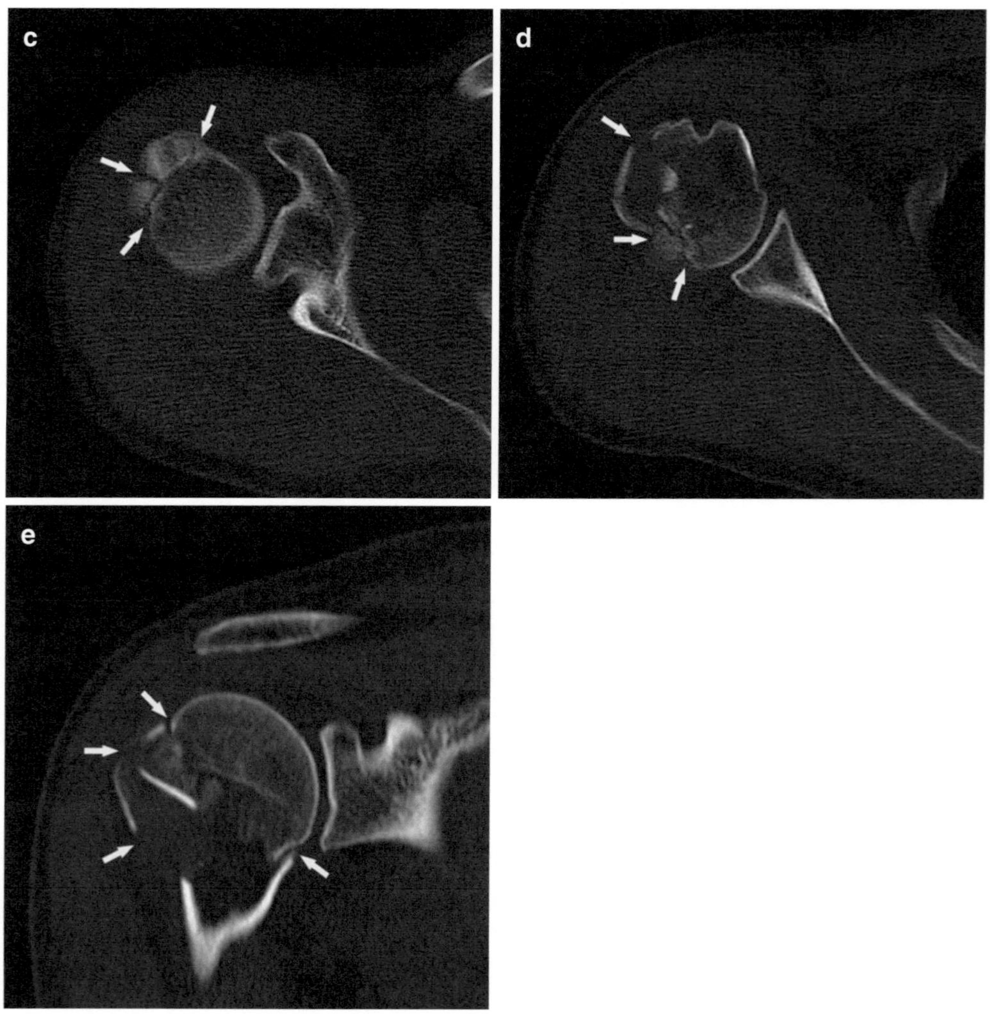

Fig. 2.13 CT cross-sectional (**c**, **d**) and coronal (**e**) reconstruction showed: fracture of humeral surgical neck bone (arrow), impaction of fracture end, and the comminuted fracture of greater tuberosity

14. Differential diagnosis of humeral surgical neck fracture with lesser tuberosity fracture and simple surgical neck-impaction fracture
    14.1. X-ray (Fig. 2.14a, b)

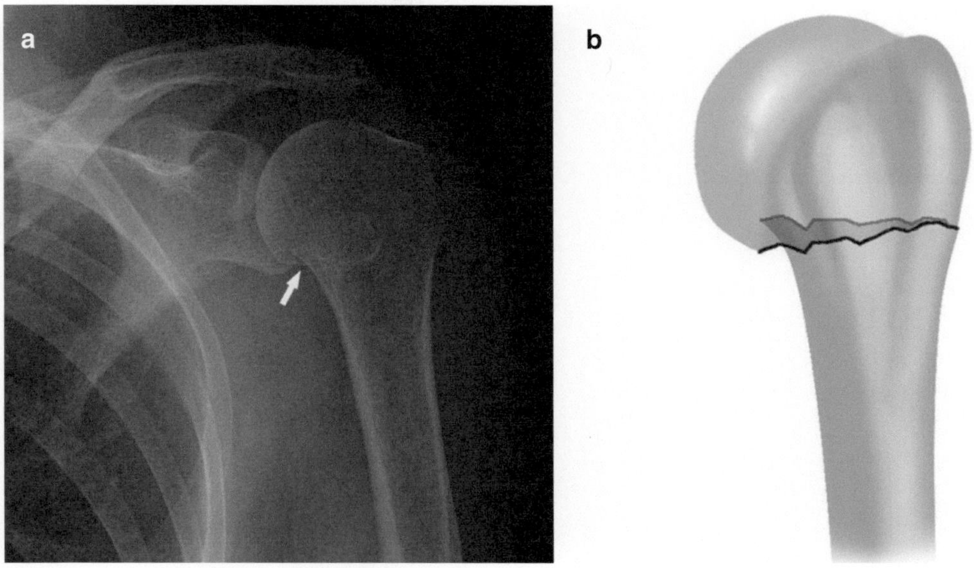

Fig. 2.14 The anteroposterior position of the humerus (**a**) X-ray shows the fracture of the left humeral surgical neck (arrow), the fracture end is impacted, without lesser tuberosity fracture schematic diagram (**b**)

    14.2. CT scan (Fig. 2.14c–e)

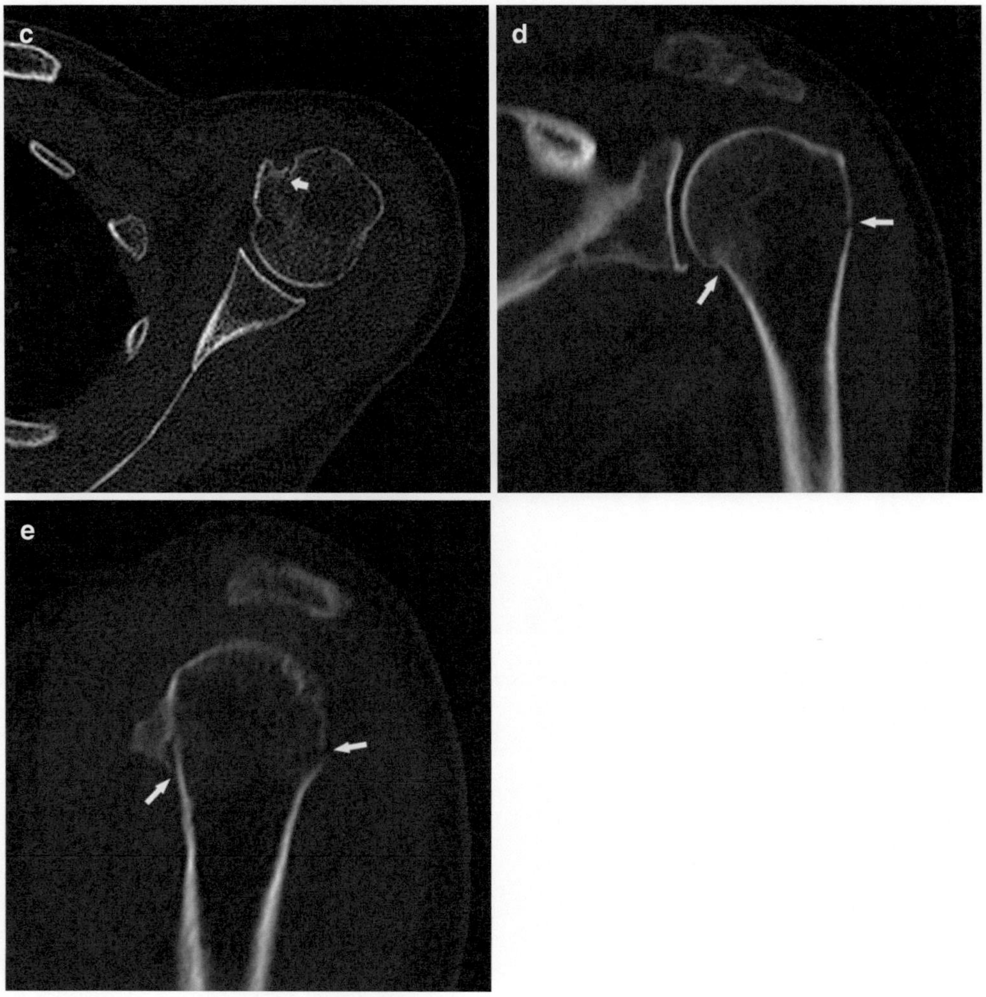

Fig. 2.14 CT cross section (**c**), coronal plane (**d**), and sagittal plane (**e**) reconstruction showed that surgical neck fracture (arrow) and lesser tuberosity fracture (arrow). It should be vigilant for missing diagnosis of such fracture

15. Differential diagnosis of humeral surgical neck fracture with lesser tuberosity fracture and simple surgical neck-impaction fracture
    15.1. X-ray (Fig. 2.15a, b)

Fig. 2.15 The anteroposterior position of shoulder joint (**a**) X-ray shows the fracture of surgical neck (arrow) in the left side, and the fracture end is displaced and impacted (**b**)

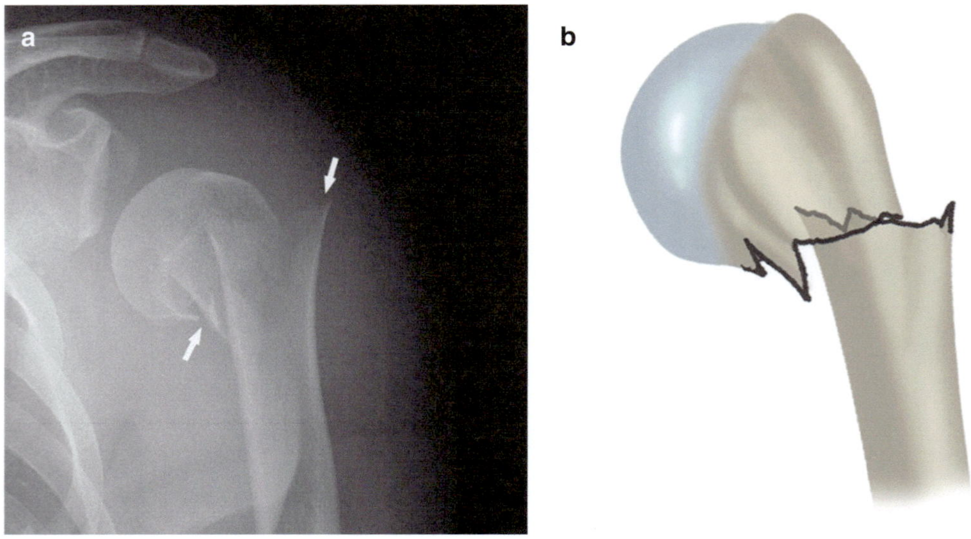

    15.2. CT scan (Fig. 2.15c)

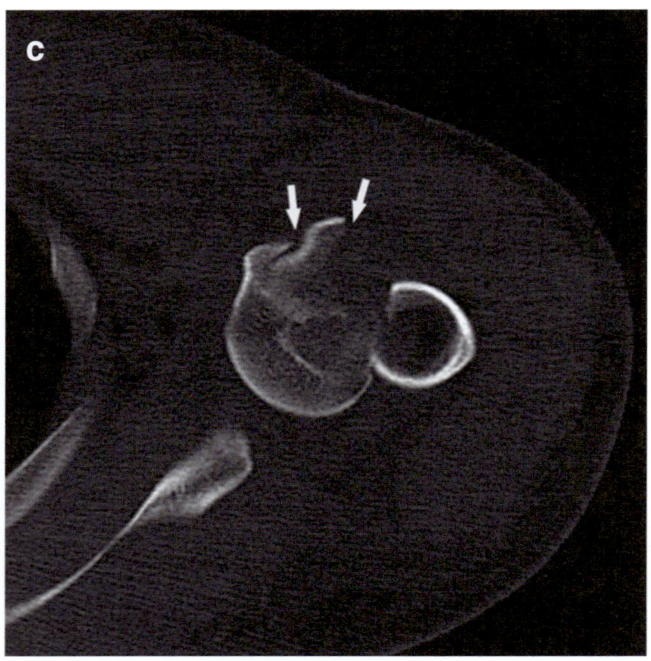

Fig. 2.15 CT cross-sectional (**c**) shows: fracture of humeral surgical neck (arrow), displacement of fracture end, impacted slightly, fracture of lesser tuberosity

16. Differential diagnosis of humeral surgical neck fracture with lesser tuberosity fracture and simple surgical neck displaced fracture
    16.1. X-ray (Fig. 2.16a–d)

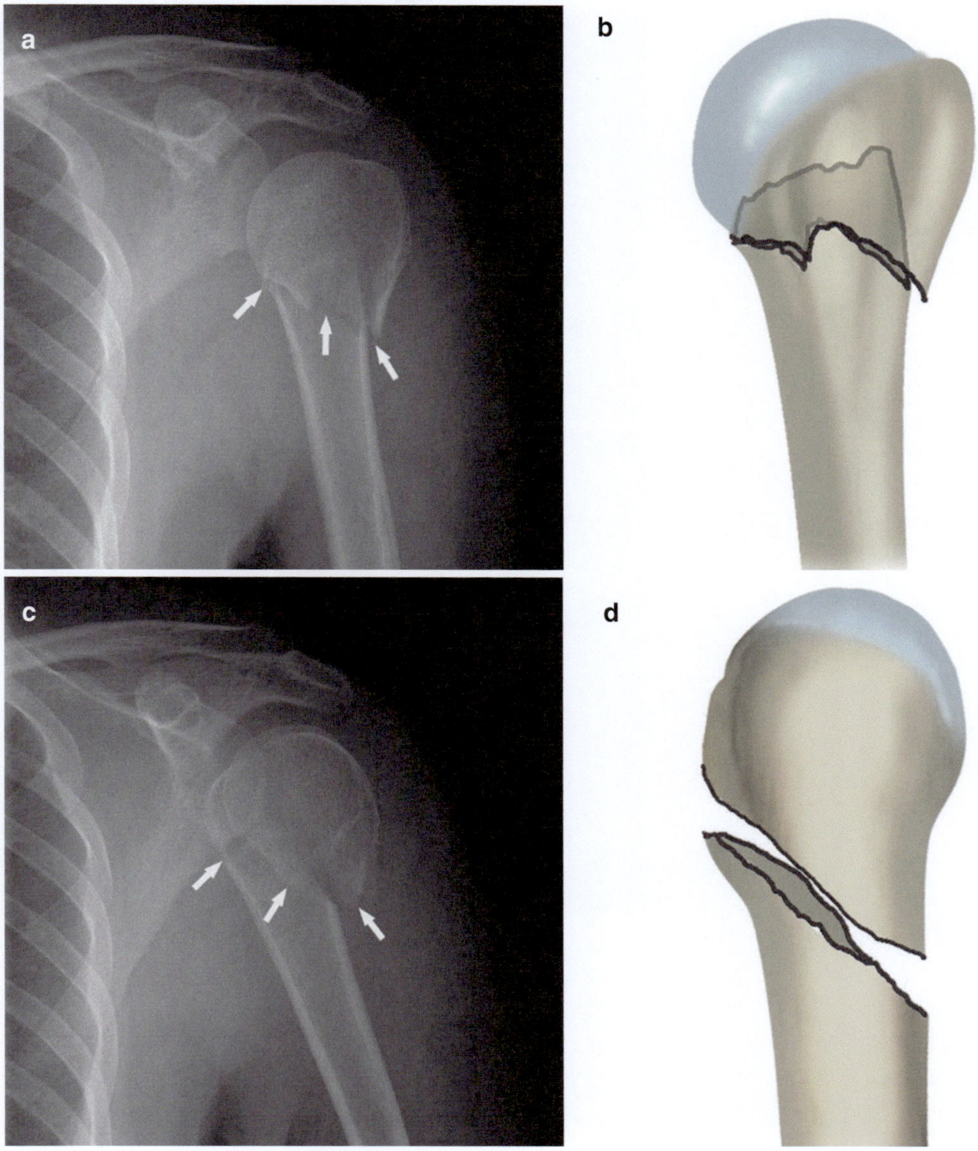

Fig. 2.16 The anteroposterior position of shoulder joint (**a**, **c**) X-ray shows the displaced surgical neck fracture (arrow) of left side schematic diagram (**b**, **d**)

16.2. CT scan (Fig. 2.16e–h)

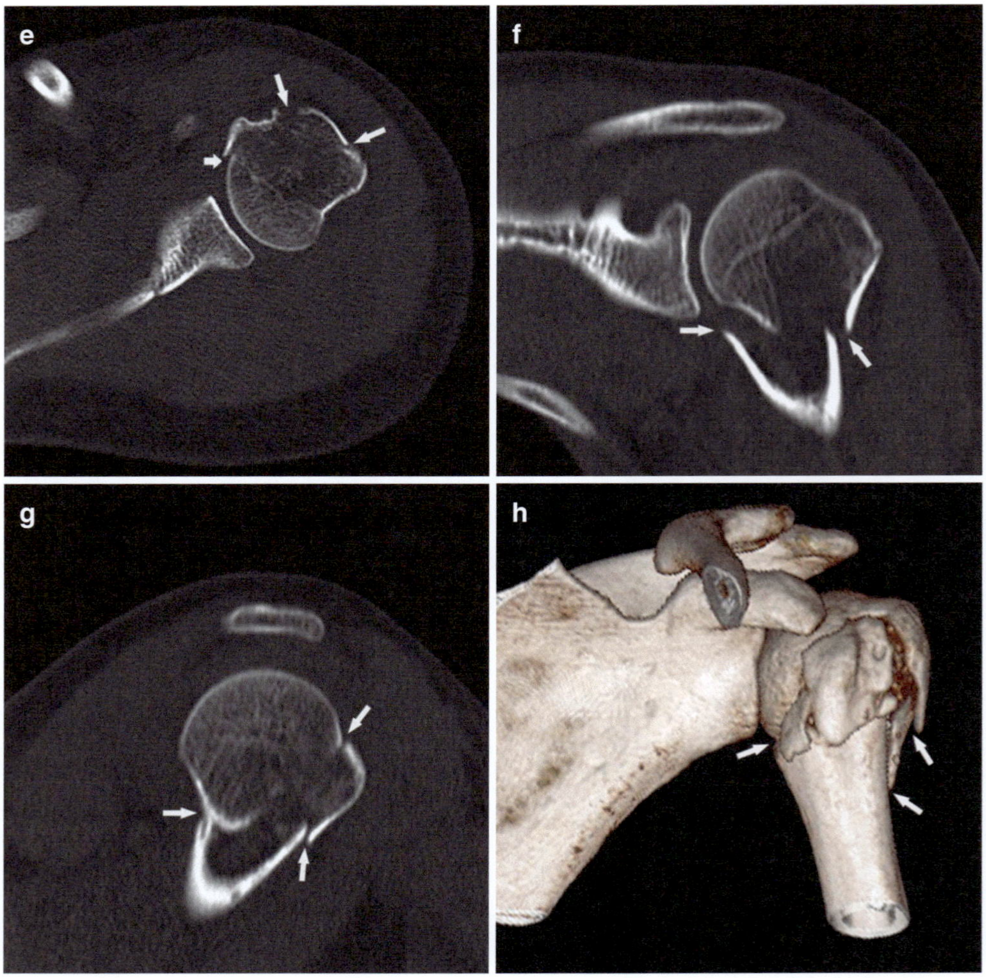

Fig. 2.16 CT cross sections (**e**), coronal plane (**f**), sagittal plane (**g**), and 3D reconstruction (**h**) show: fracture of humeral surgical neck (arrow), with lesser tuberosity fracture (arrow). The anteroposterior position of the X-ray often fails to accurately show the lesser tuberosity fracture

17. Spatial localization of proximal humeral comminuted fracture with humeral head dislocation by CT
    17.1. X-ray (Fig. 2.17a, b)

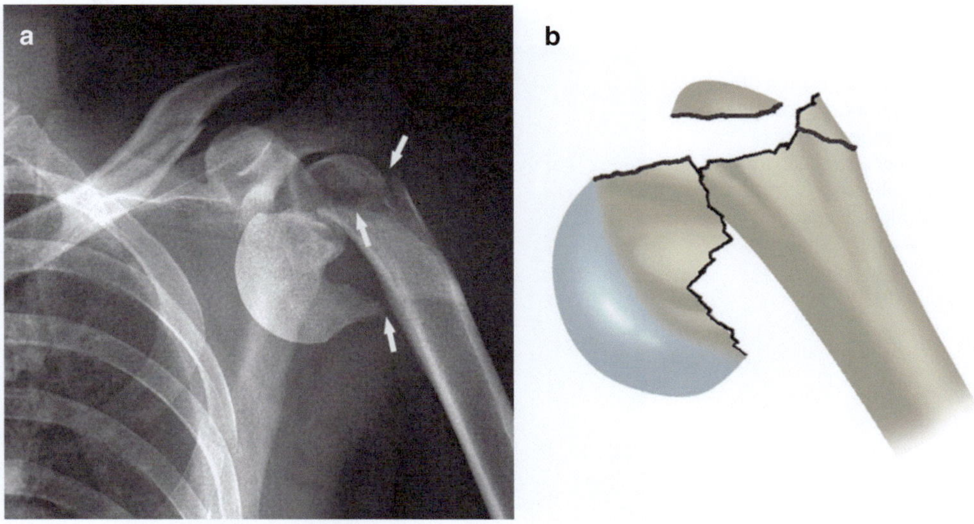

Fig. 2.17 The anteroposterior position of shoulder joint (**a**) X-ray shows the dislocation of the head of the left humerus, the fracture of the surgical neck and greater tuberosity (arrow), the displacement of the fracture end, the fracture of the middle clavicle with no displacement schematic diagram (**b**)

17.2. CT scan (Fig. 2.17c–e)

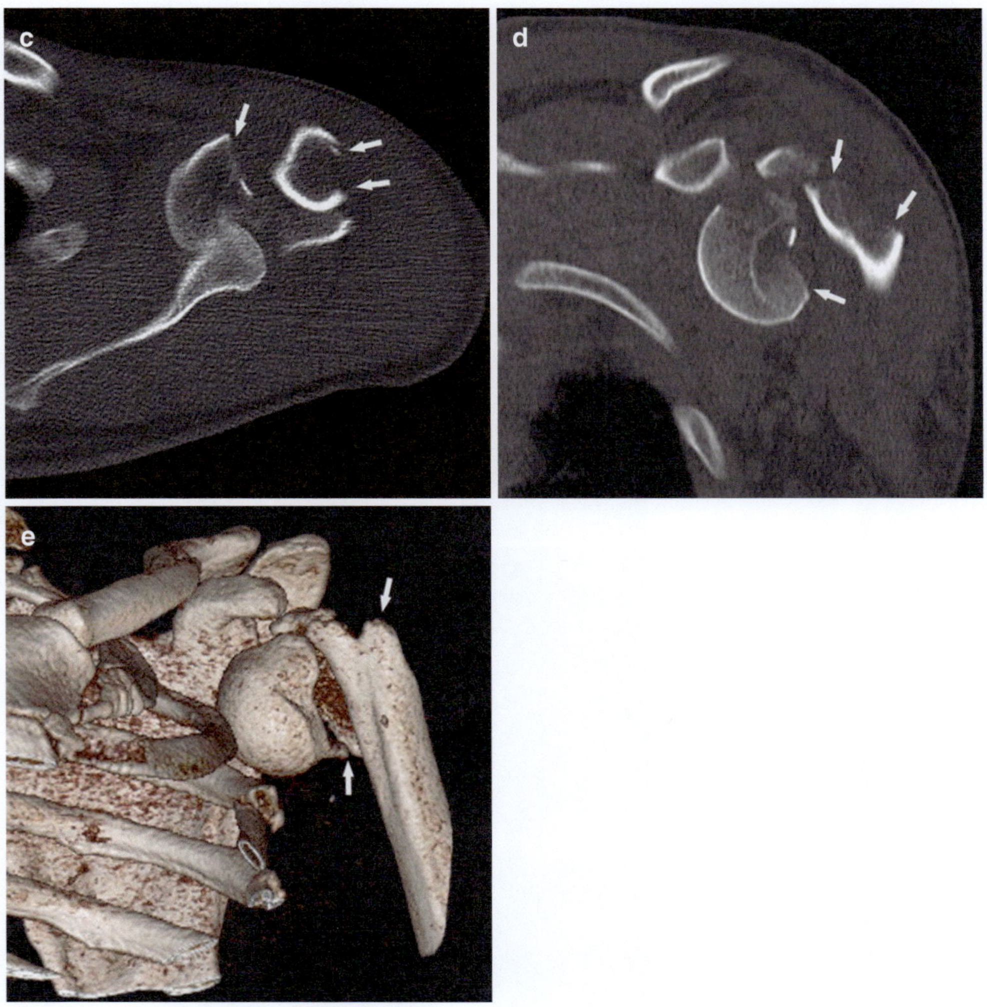

Fig. 2.17 CT cross-sectional (**c**), coronal CT (**d**) and 3D reconstruction (**e**) showed the dislocation of humeral head, with the fracture of surgical neck (arrow) and greater tuberosity fracture

18. Differential diagnosis between surgical neck fracture with greater tuberosity comminuted fracture and surgical neck simple fracture with greater tuberosity fracture
    18.1. X-ray (Fig. 2.18a, b)

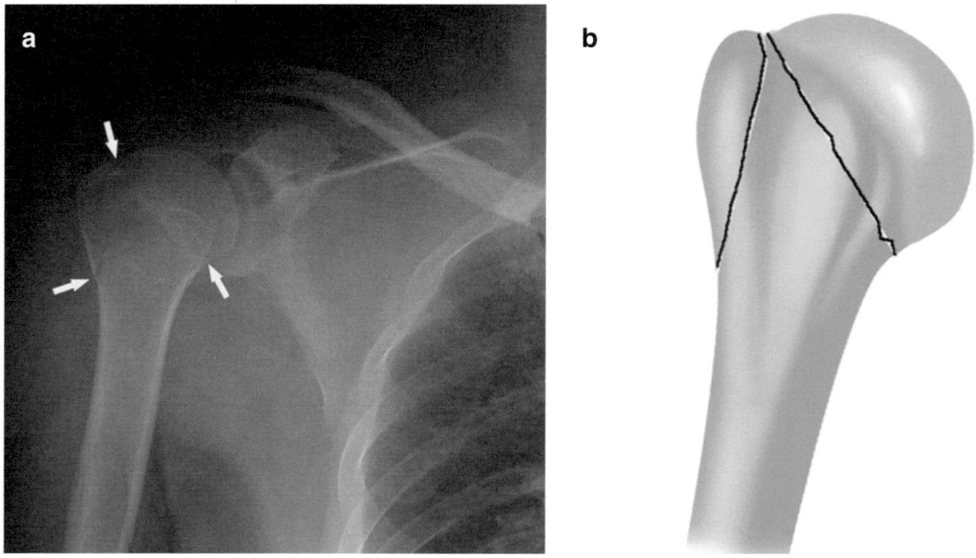

Fig. 2.18 The anteroposterior position of shoulder joint (**a**) X-ray plain film shows the fracture of right humeral surgical neck (arrow), without displacement. Greater tuberosity simple linear fracture schematic diagram (**b**)

    18.2. CT scan (Fig. 2.18c–e)

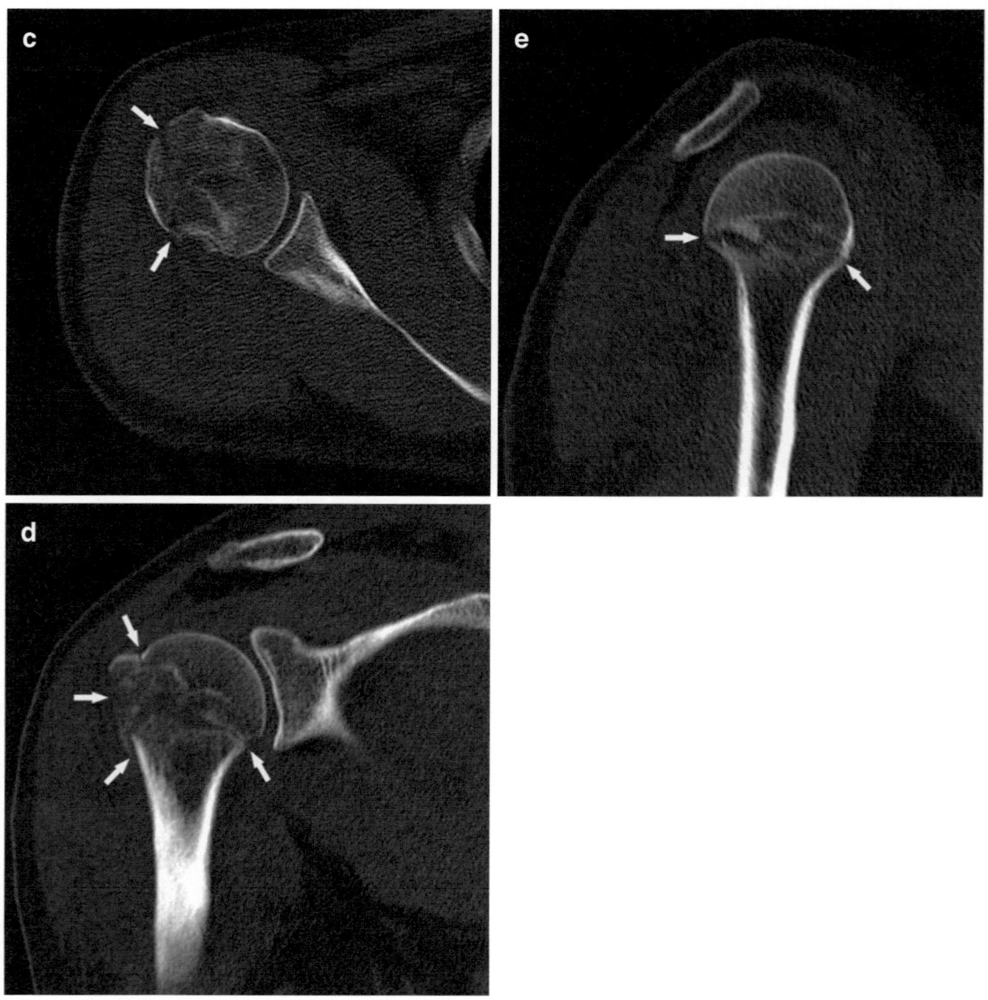

Fig. 2.18 CT cross section (**c**), coronal plane (**d**), and sagittal plane reconstruction (**e**) show: humeral anatomical neck fracture (arrow), without displacement (arrow), greater tuberosity comminuted fracture

19. Differential diagnosis of surgical neck fractures with greater and lesser tuberosities fracture and simple surgical neck fractures
    19.1. X-ray (Fig. 2.19a, b)

Fig. 2.19 The anteroposterior position of shoulder joint (**a**) X-ray shows the surgical neck fracture (arrow), no displacement is seen (**b**)

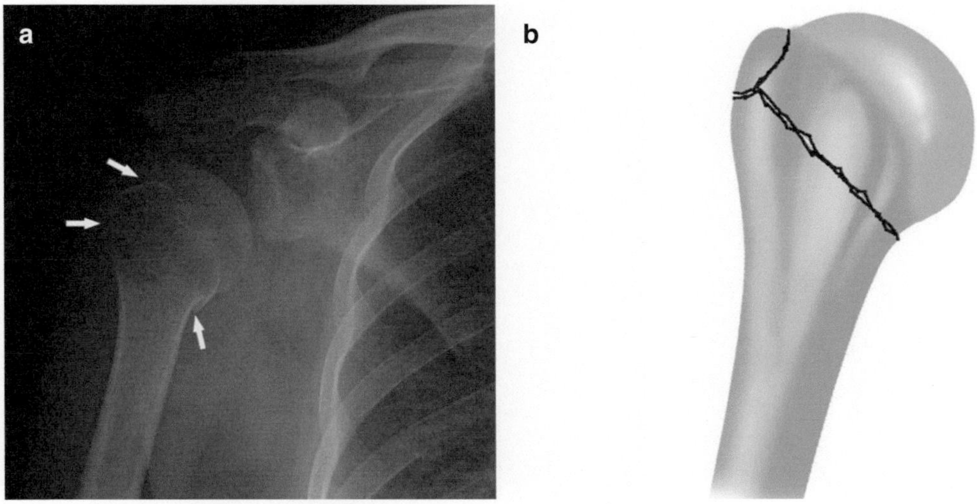

    19.2. CT scan (Fig. 2.19c–e)

Fig. 2.19 CT cross section (**c**), coronal plane (**d**) and sagittal plane, (**e**) reconstruction shows: fracture of humeral surgical neck (arrow), combined with fracture of tuberosities (arrow)

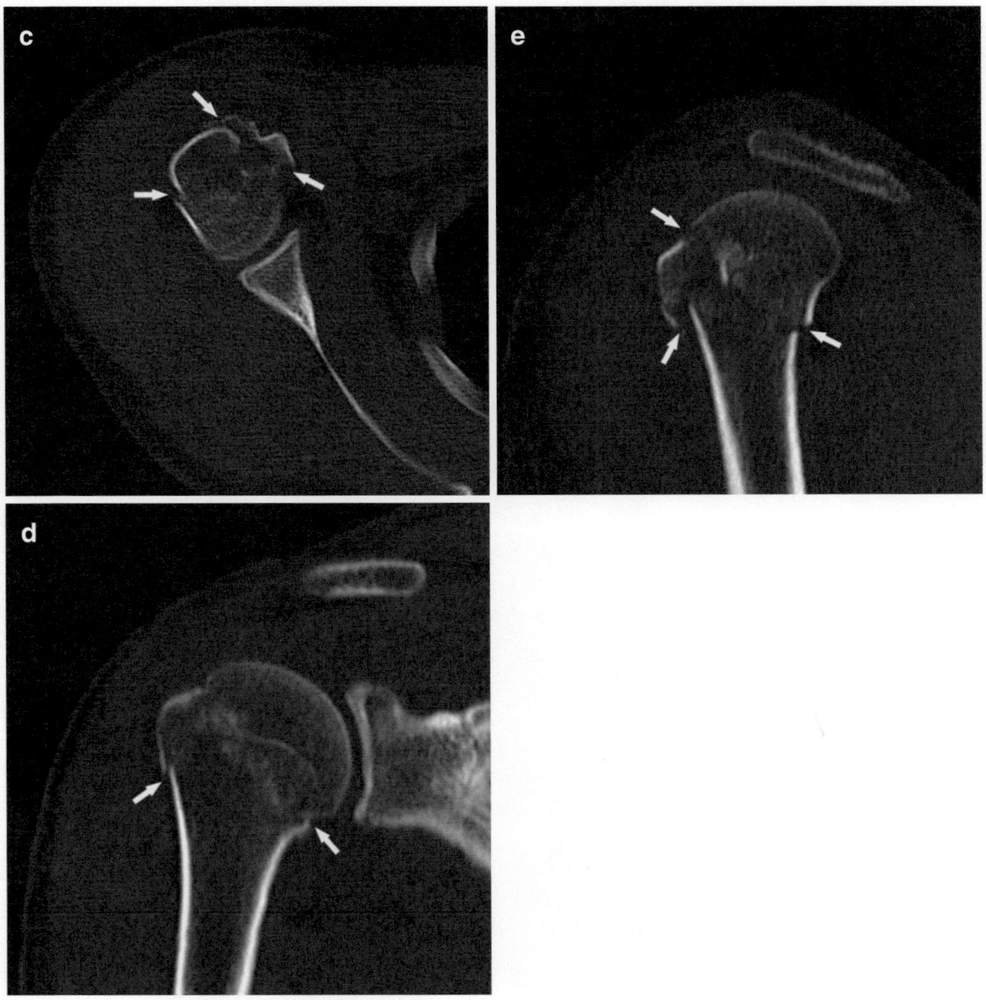

20. Differential diagnosis of surgical neck fracture with greater tuberosity fracture and surgical neck simple fracture
    20.1. X-ray (Fig. 2.20a, b)

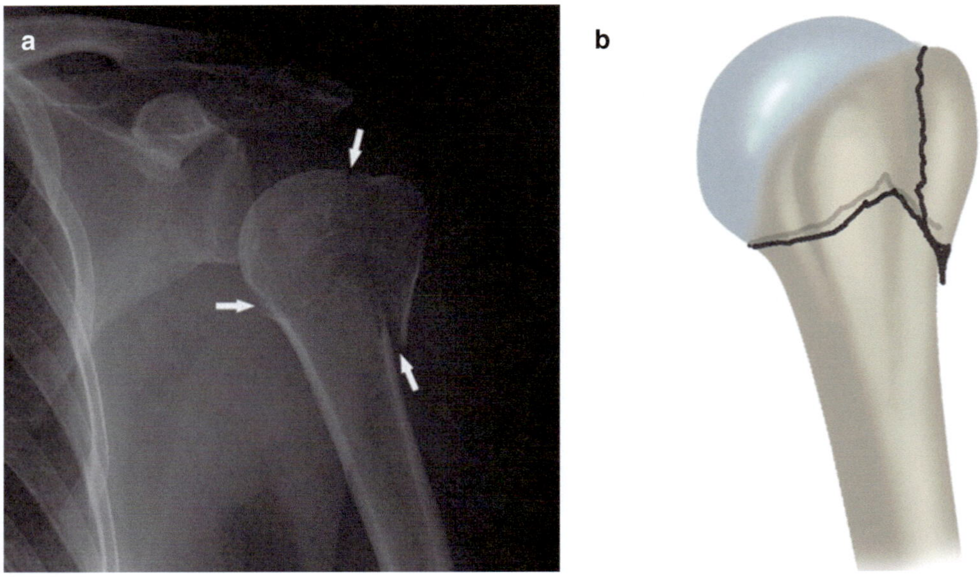

Fig. 2.20 The anteroposterior position of shoulder joint (**a**) X-ray shows fracture of the left humeral surgical neck (arrow), with slightly displaced (**b**)

    20.2. CT scan (Fig. 2.20c–e)

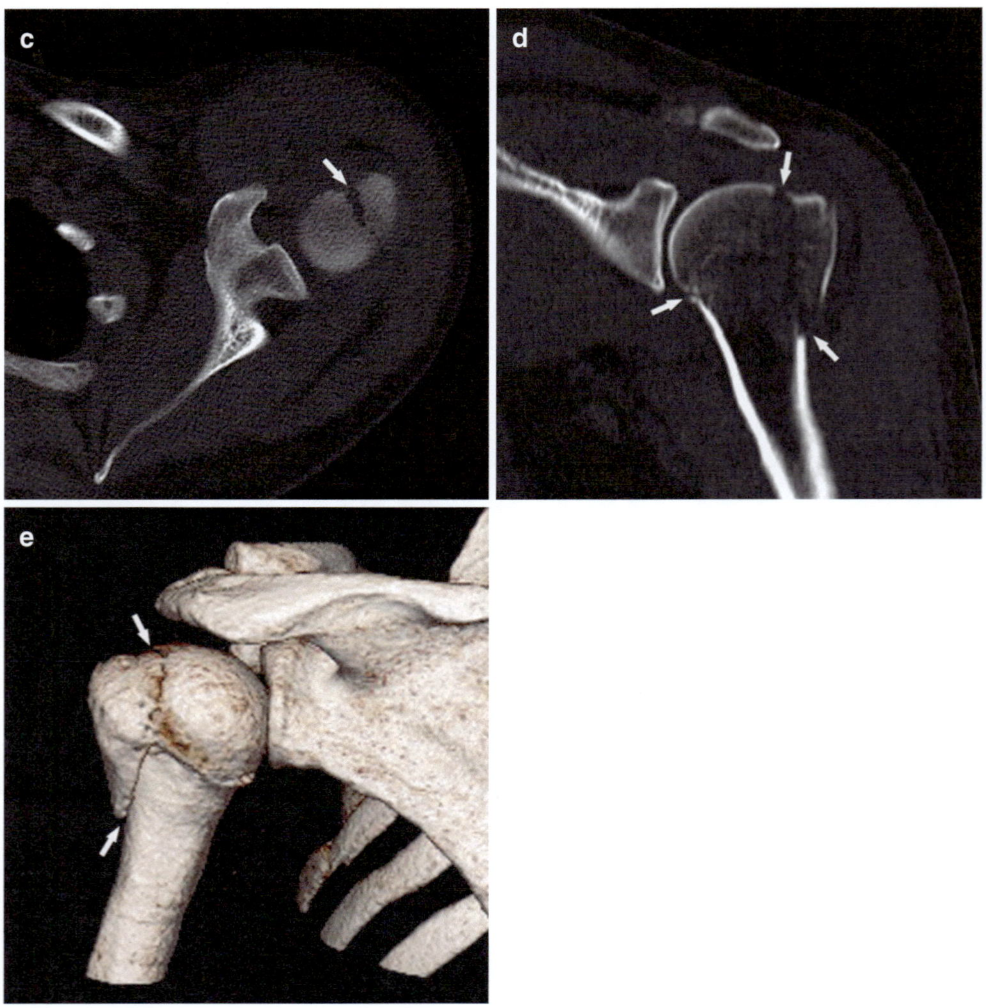

Fig. 2.20 CT cross section (**c**), coronal plane (**d**), and three-dimensional reconstruction (**e**) show: humeral anatomical neck fracture with greater tuberosity fracture (arrow), with slightly impacted

21. Differential diagnosis of humeral anatomical neck comminuted fracture and impacted fracture
    21.1. X-ray (Fig. 2.21a–d)

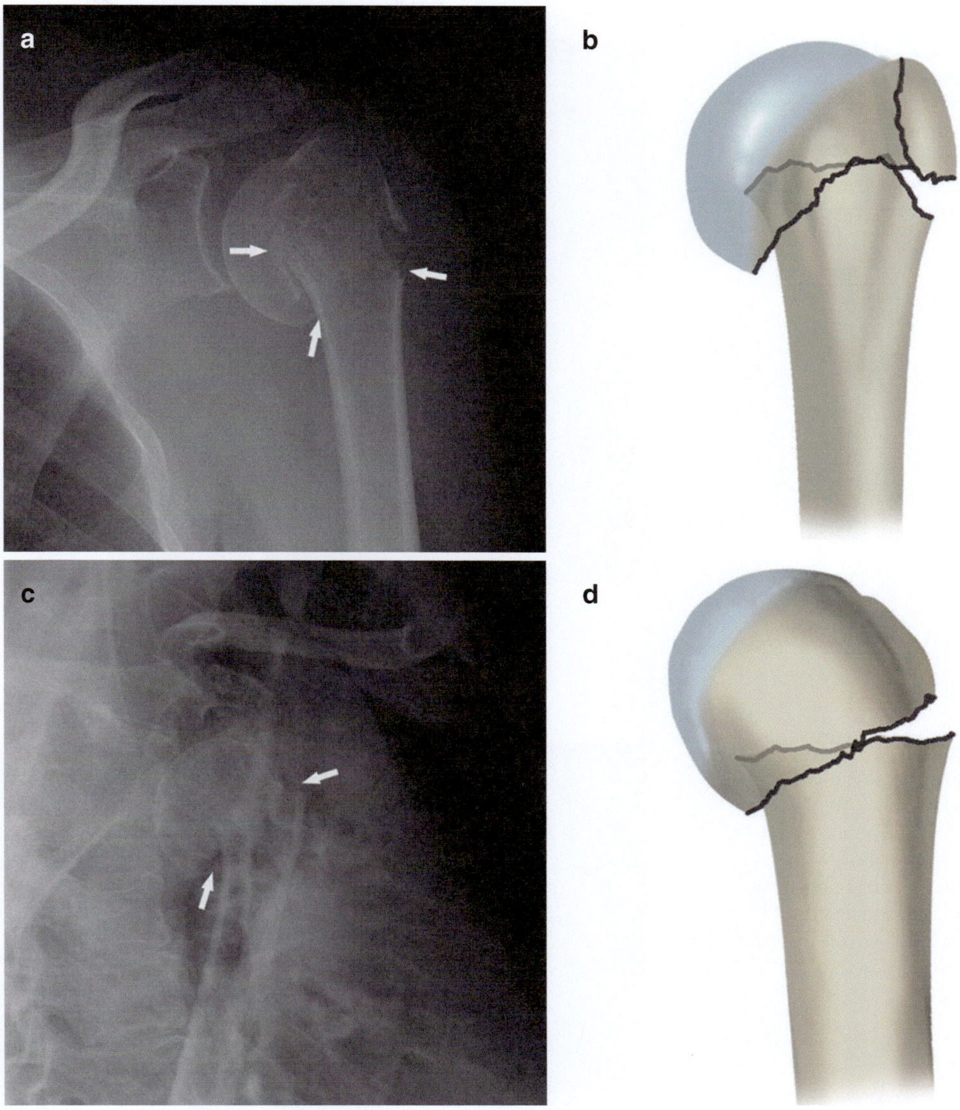

Fig. 2.21 The anteroposterior position of shoulder joint (**a**, **c**) X-ray shows the left humeral anatomical neck-impacted fracture and the greater tuberosity fracture (arrow) schematic diagram (**b**, **d**)

    21.2. CT scan (Fig. 2.21e, f)

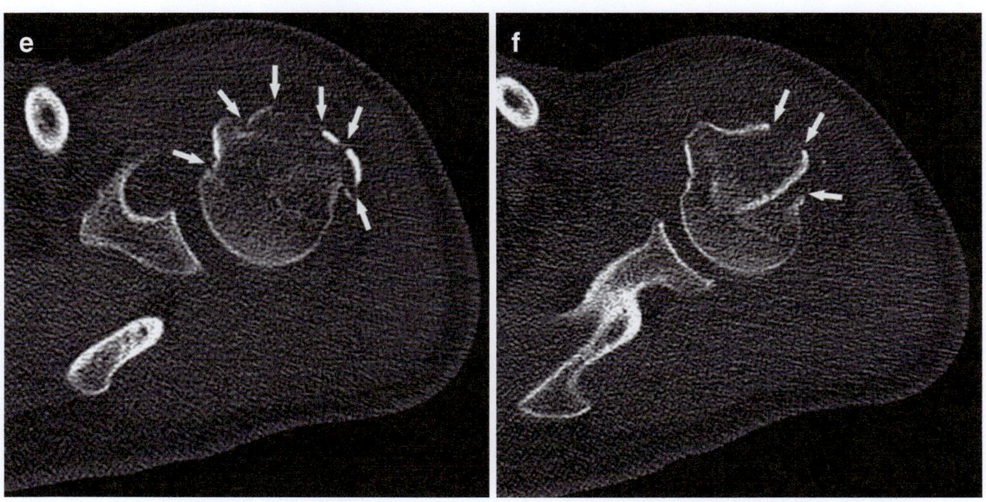

Fig. 2.21 CT cross section (**e**, **f**) shows: humeral anatomical neck comminuted fracture (arrow), with lesser and greater tuberosity fracture (arrow)

22. Differential diagnosis of surgical neck comminuted fractures with humeral head dislocation and surgical neck displaced fractures
    22.1. X-ray (Fig. 2.22a, b)

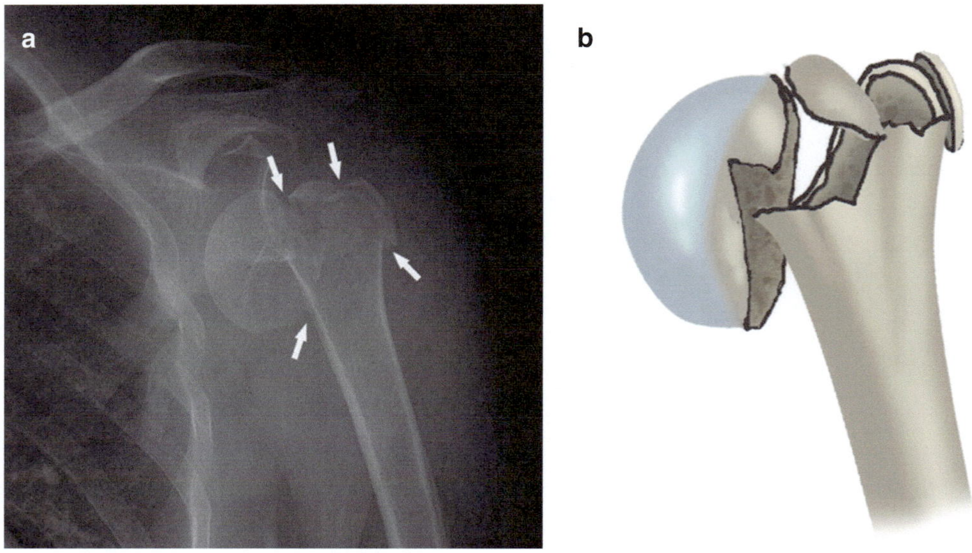

Fig. 2.22 The anteroposterior position of shoulder joint (**a**) X-ray film shows the anatomical neck fracture of the left humerus and greater tuberosity fracture (arrow) schematic diagram (**b**)

    22.2. CT scan (Fig. 2.22c–e)

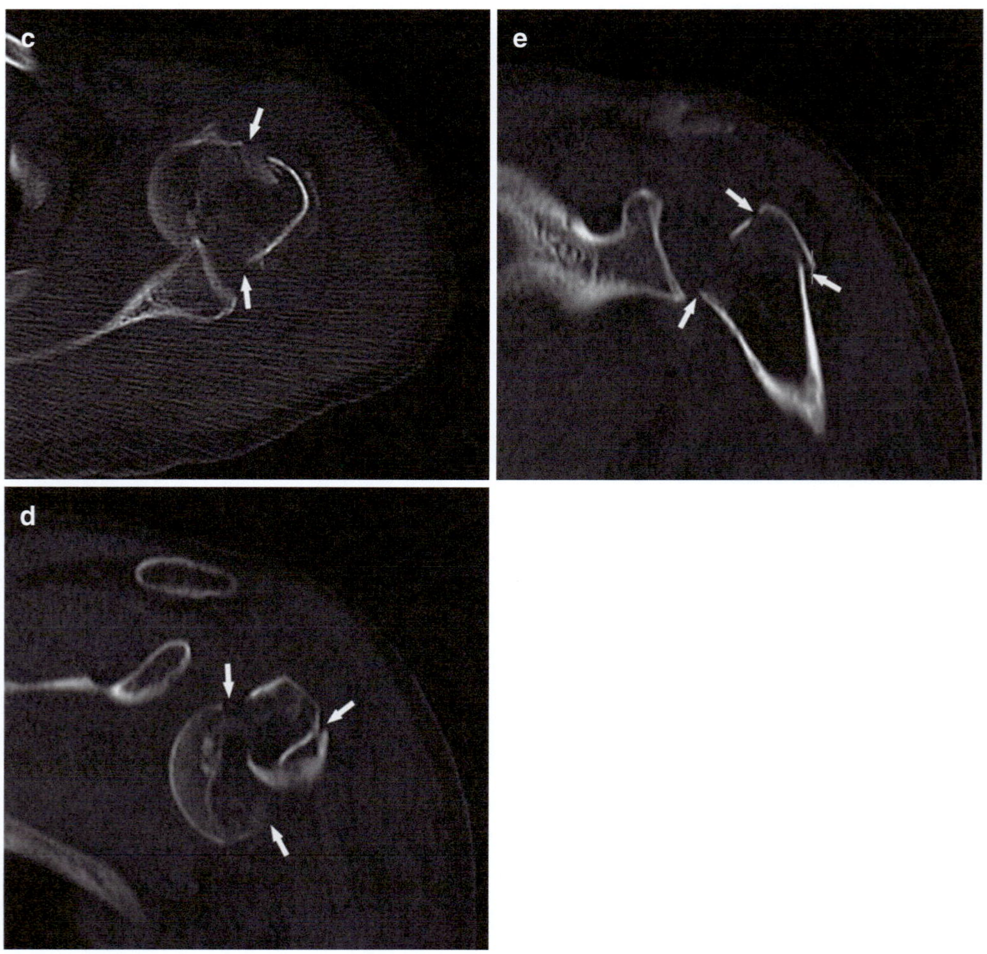

Fig. 2.22 CT cross section (**c**) and coronal plane reconstruction (**d**, **e**) show: humeral anatomical neck fracture (arrow), with dislocation and impaction, humeral head anterior dislocation (arrow), greater tuberosity fracture

2.2 Scapular Fracture

Scapular fractures account for approximately 0.91% of total fractures. The scapula is an irregular bone. There are three protrusions on the lateral side: Acromion, coracoid process, and scapula glenoid cavity. These overlap each other. X-ray scan often leads to misdiagnosis and missed diagnosis. Therefore, CT scan is remarkably necessary. MR scanning is essential for the diagnosis of tendon and soft tissue injury around the shoulder, especially rotator cuff injury and scapula labrum injury. The AO/OTA classification of scapular fractures is divided into extra-articular fractures, partial intra-articular fractures, and complete intra-articular fractures. The extra-articular fractures are also divided into acromial fractures, coracoids fractures, and scapular body fractures. Acromial fractures account for 9.52% of scapular fractures. The coracoids fracture accounts for 3.40% of the scapular fractures, and the scapular body fracture accounts for 43.54% of the scapular fractures. Some intra-articular fractures were divided into anterior cruciate fracture, posterior cruciate fracture, and subtalar fracture. The anterior margin fracture of glenoid cavity accounts for 4.59% of the scapular fracture. The posterior margin fracture accounts for 3.06% of the scapular fracture. The inferior margin fracture accounts for 3.74% of the scapular fracture. Complete intra-articular fractures were divided into scapular neck fracture, intra-articular fracture combined with scapular neck fracture, intra-articular fracture combined with scapular body fracture. Scapular neck fracture accounts for 25.34% of the scapular fracture, intra-articular fracture combined with scapular neck fracture accounts for 4.08% of the scapular fracture, intra-articular fracture combined with scapular fracture accounts for 2.72% of the scapular fracture.

2.2.1 Identification of Injury Mechanism

The scapula is covered by thick muscles that provide support and protection for the scapula. Indirect and direct violent blow on the scapula can cause scapular fractures. When patients fall, the force passes through the glenohumeral joint to the scapula, which causes a fracture. Direct violence is mostly caused by traffic injuries or high-altitude fall injuries. Violence directly applied on the scapula causes fractures. It often involves chest, head, and vascular or nerve injuries. These injuries tend to be more severe, and often result from missed diagnosis of scapula fractures because of the focus on the treatment for combined injuries.

Identification of pathological fractures: The scapula can cause bone destruction due to tumors and other reasons, and pathological fractures will occur. Special attention should be paid to the diagnosis and treatment for this situation.

2.2.2 Identification of Symptoms and Signs

Scapular fractures are characterized by pain, swelling, limited mobility. These symptoms are not specific and often do not help with diagnosis.

Because of the deep position of the scapula, malformations are often difficult to be noted, so this sign does not helped with diagnosis.

2.2.3 Imaging Differential Diagnosis

The scapula is an irregular bone. There are three protrusions on the lateral side, which overlap each other. X-ray scan often leads to misdiagnosis and missed diagnosis; therefore, CT scans become necessary. MR scan is essential for the diagnosis of tendon and soft tissue injury around the shoulder, especially for rotator cuff injury and scapula labrum injury. The following attention should be paid to identify: (1) the conventional X-ray did not see clear signs of fracture, but the patient has significant clinical symptoms and signs, CT or MR scan should be used; (2) The routine X-ray diagnosis of a fracture, but local bone structure disarrangement should be closely combined with clinical history. If it is caused by trivial trauma, the pathological fracture should be excluded by CT or MR scan.

1. Differential diagnosis of acromion fracture and no fracture
    1.1. X-ray (Fig. 2.23a, b)

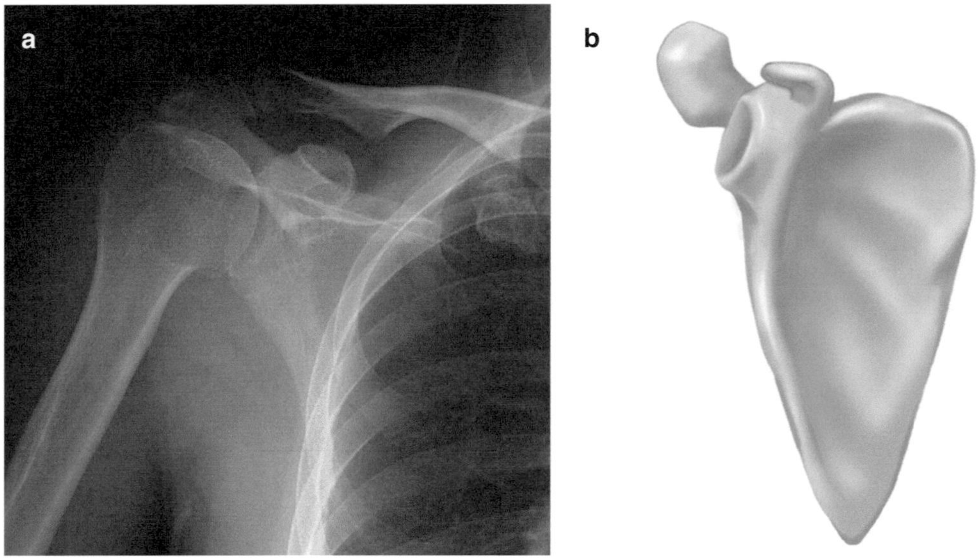

Fig. 2.23 X-ray plain film (**a**) showed no clear fracture sign on the right scapula, and slightly disarranged bone trabecula schematic diagram (**b**)

    1.2. CT scan (Fig. 2.23c–e)

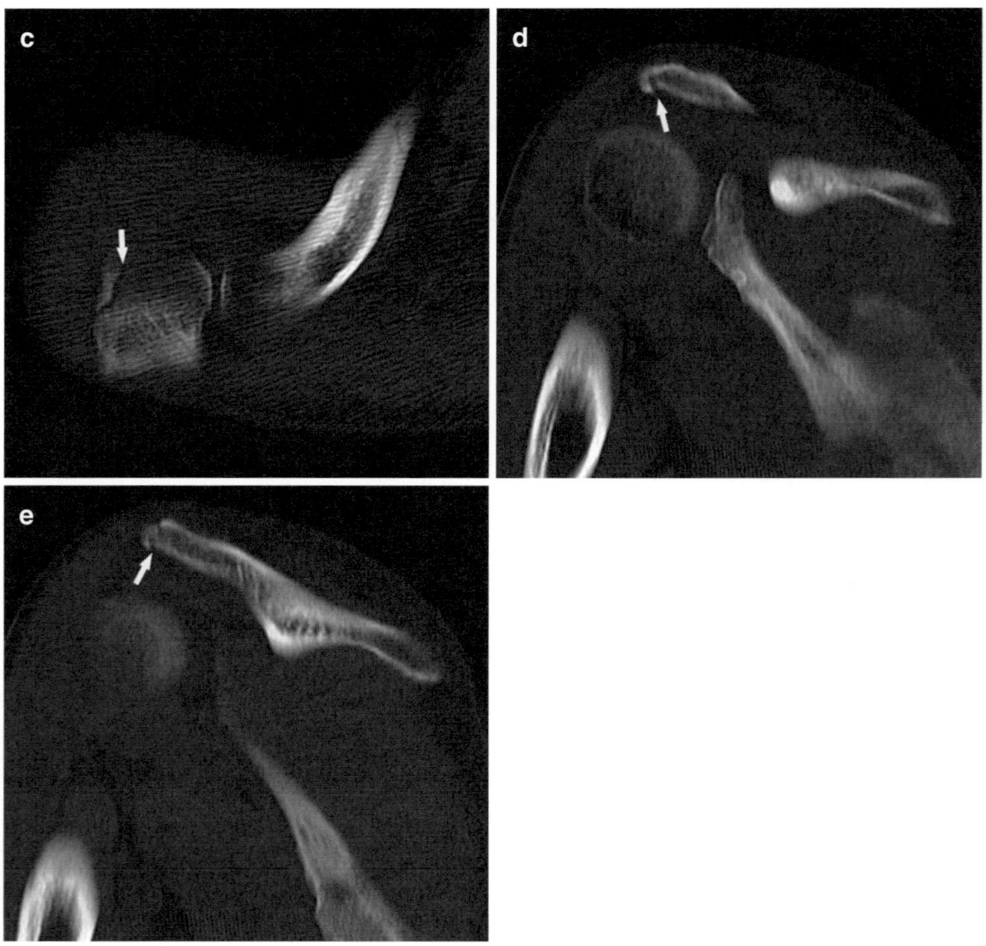

Fig. 2.23 CT cross section and reconstruction (**c**–**e**) showed that the irregularity of acromion with small fragment shadow (arrow) and slightly displaced

2. Differentiation of acromial basement fractures and mesoscapula fractures
   2.1. X-ray (Fig. 2.24a–d)

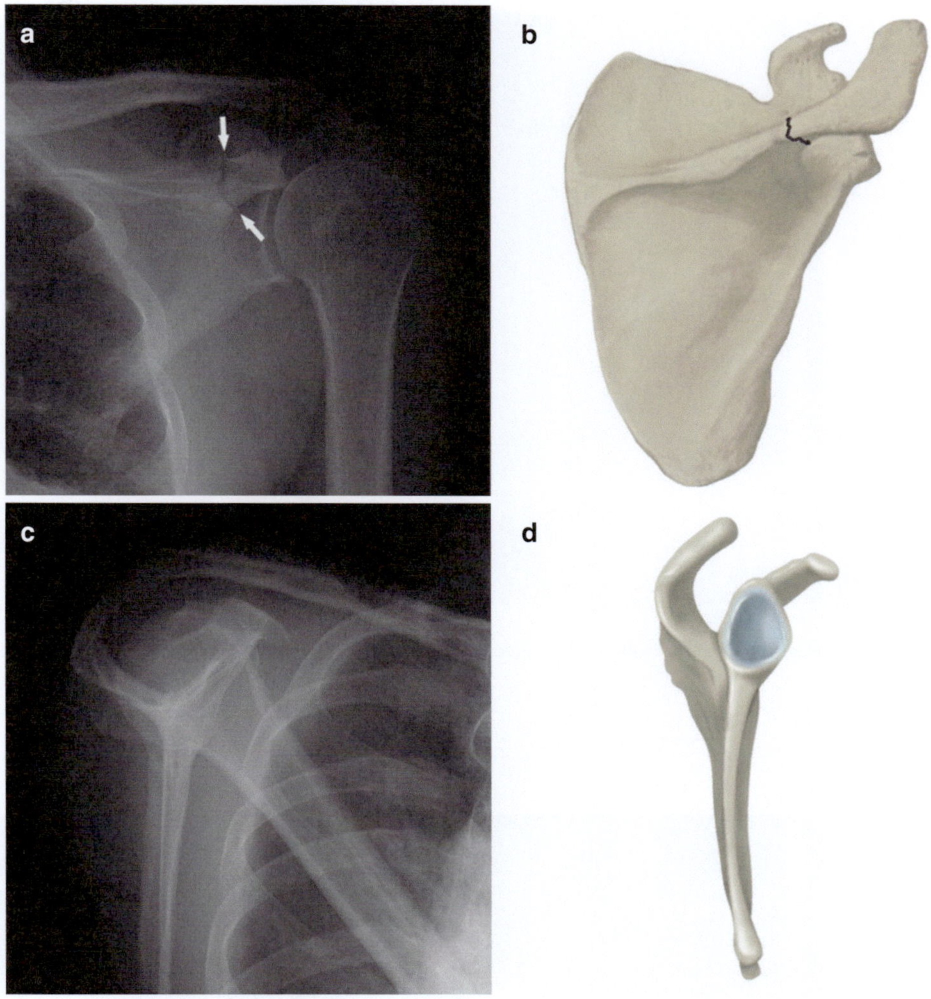

Fig. 2.24 The anteroposterior position of shoulder joint and "Y" position plane (**a**, **c**) show linear low-density shadow (arrow) at the overlap between left mesoscapula and acromion basement, without displacement schematic diagram (**b**, **d**)

   2.2. CT scan (Fig. 2.24e, f)

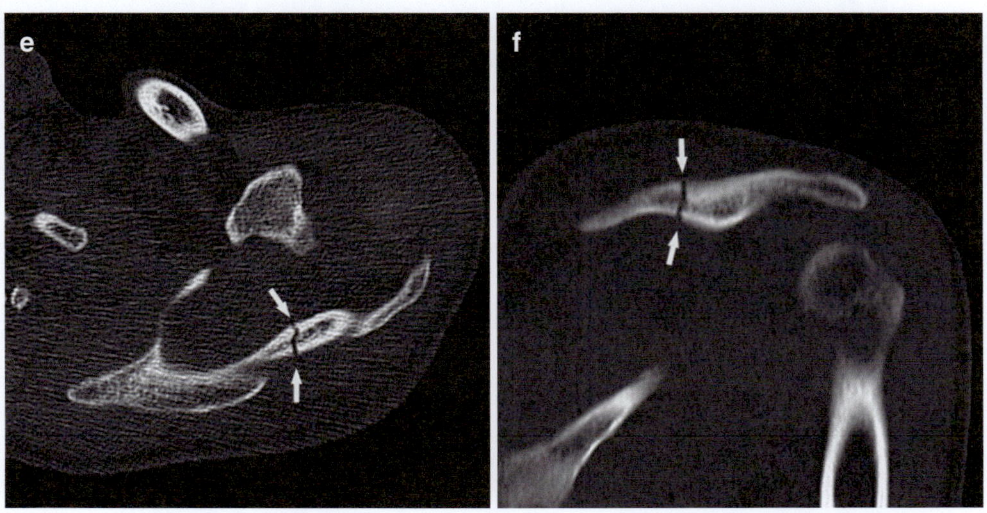

Fig. 2.24 CT cross section and reconstruction (**e**, **f**) showed: fracture of basement of acromion (arrow), no displacement

3. Differentiation of basement of acromion fracture and no fracture
   3.1. X-ray (Fig. 2.25a, b)

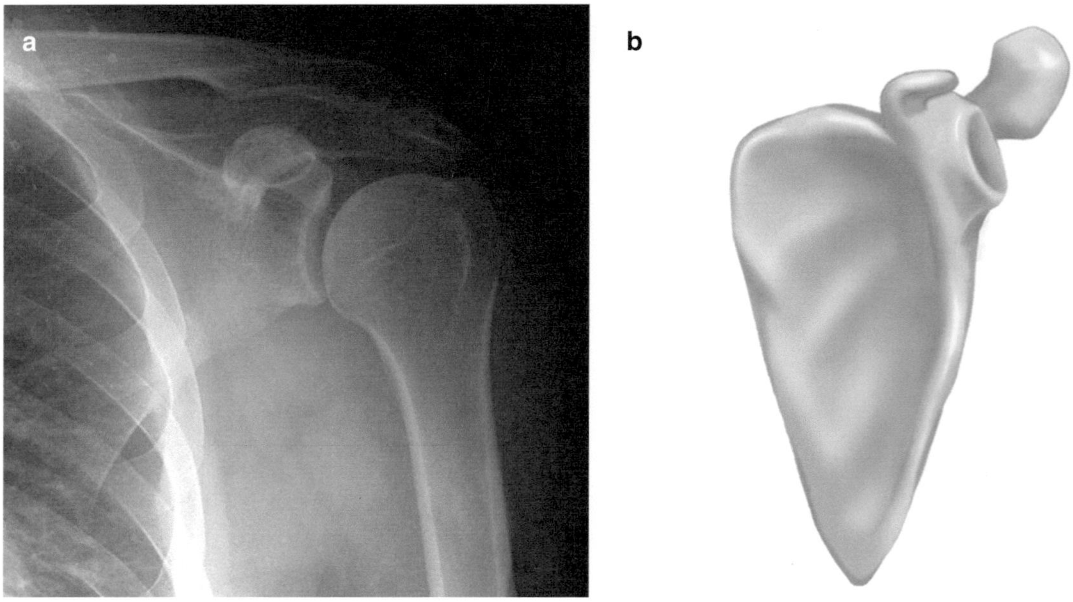

Fig. 2.25 The anteroposterior position of shoulder joint (**a**) shows no definite fractures in the bones of the left shoulder joint schematic diagram (**b**)

   3.2. CT scan (Fig. 2.25c, d)

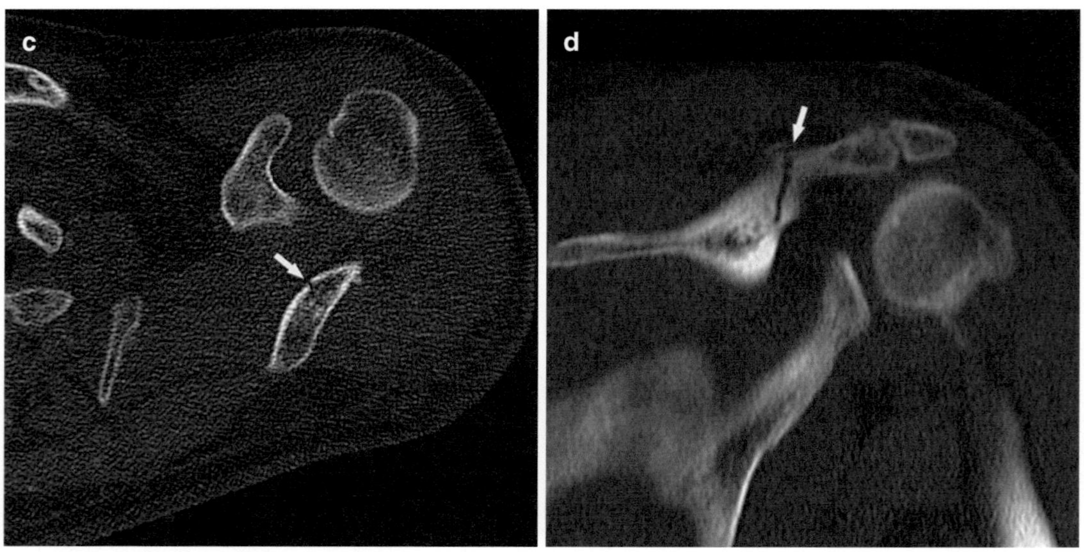

Fig. 2.25 CT cross section and reconstruction (**c**, **d**) showed: fracture of acromion (arrow), without displacement

4. Differentiation of acromion displaced fracture and non-displaced fracture
   4.1. X-ray (Fig. 2.26a, b)

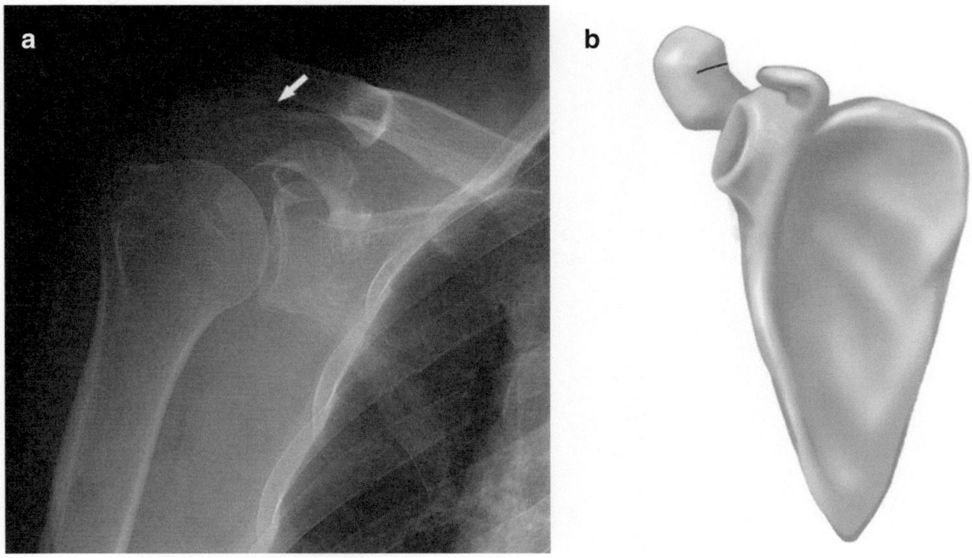

Fig. 2.26 The anteroposterior position of shoulder joint (**a**) shows linear low-density shadow (arrow) at the acromion without displacement schematic diagram (**b**)

   4.2. CT scan (Fig. 2.26c–e)

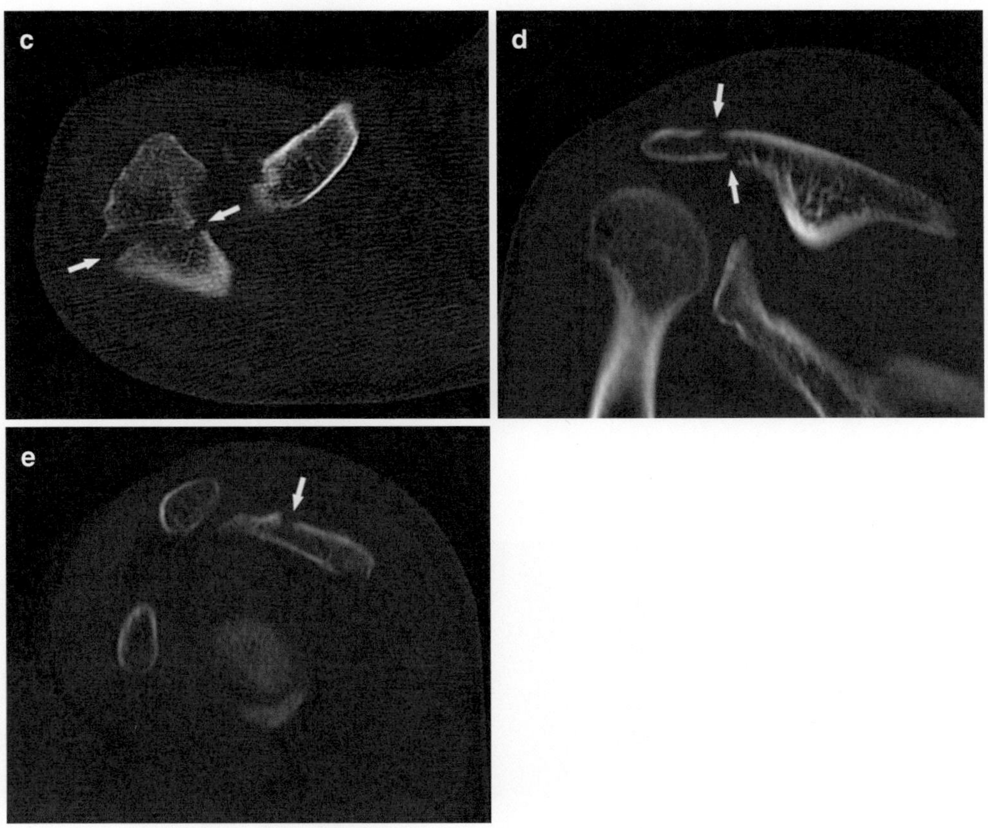

Fig. 2.26 CT cross section and reconstruction (**c–e**) showed: fracture (arrow) of acromion, with slight displacement

5. Differentiation of scapular coracoid process fractures and non-fracture
   5.1. X-ray (Fig. 2.27a–d)

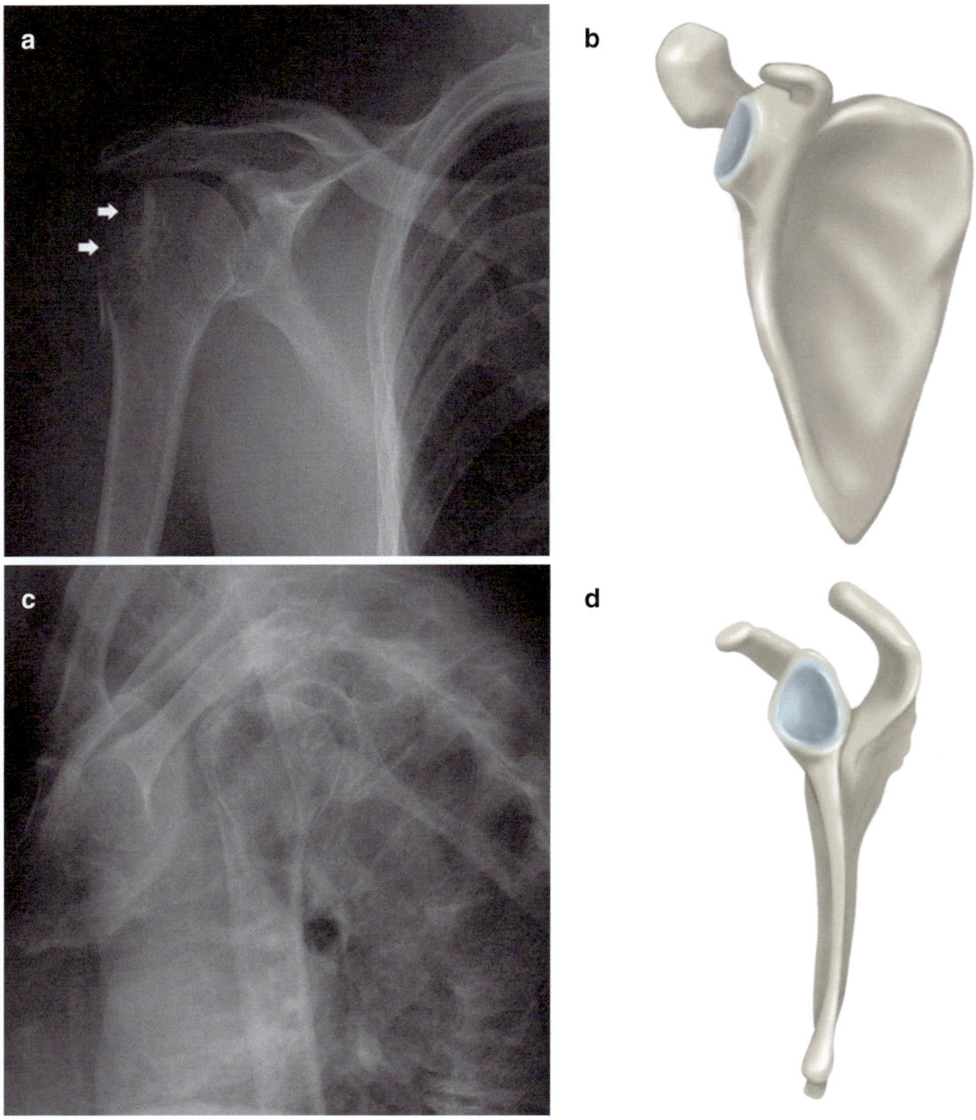

Fig. 2.27 The anteroposterior position of shoulder joint (**a**, **c**) showed greater tuberosity of right humerus (short arrow). No obvious fracture sign was seen in the coracoid process of right scapula schematic diagram (**b**, **d**)

   5.2. CT scan (Fig. 2.27e, f)

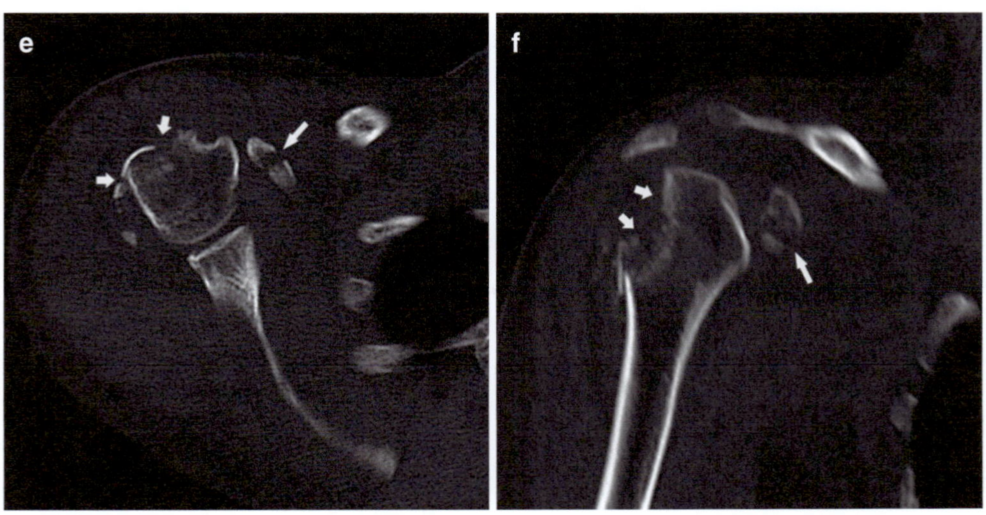

Fig. 2.27 CT cross section and reconstruction (**e**, **f**) showed: greater tuberosity fracture of humerus, scapula coracoid process fracture with slightly displaced

6. Differentiation of displaced scapula coracoid process fractures and suspected fractures
    6.1. X-ray (Fig. 2.28a, b)

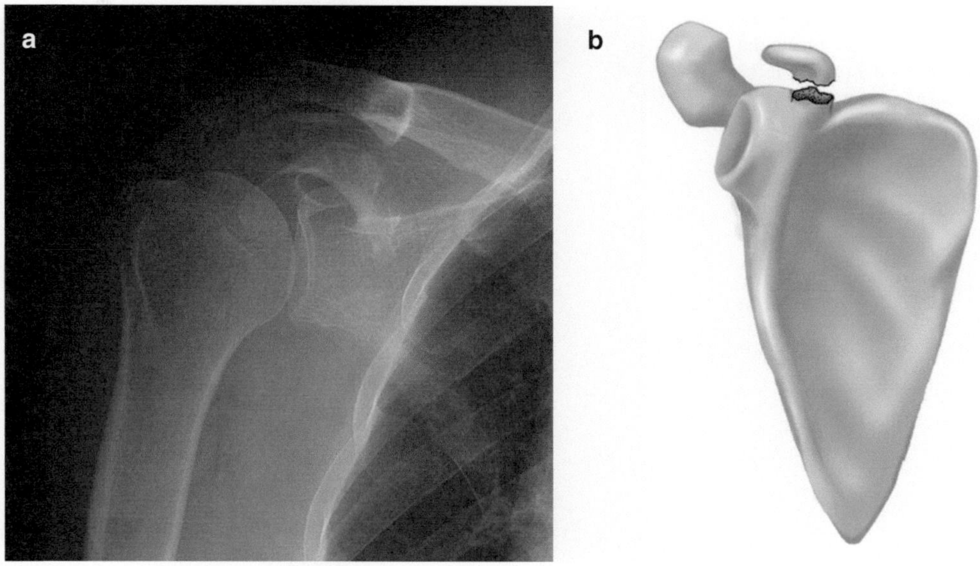

Fig. 2.28 X-ray plain film (**a**) shows the irregular contour of the coracoid process of the right shoulder, and low-density linear shadow can be seen at the basement of scapula schematic diagram (**b**)

    6.2. CT scan (Fig. 2.28c–e)

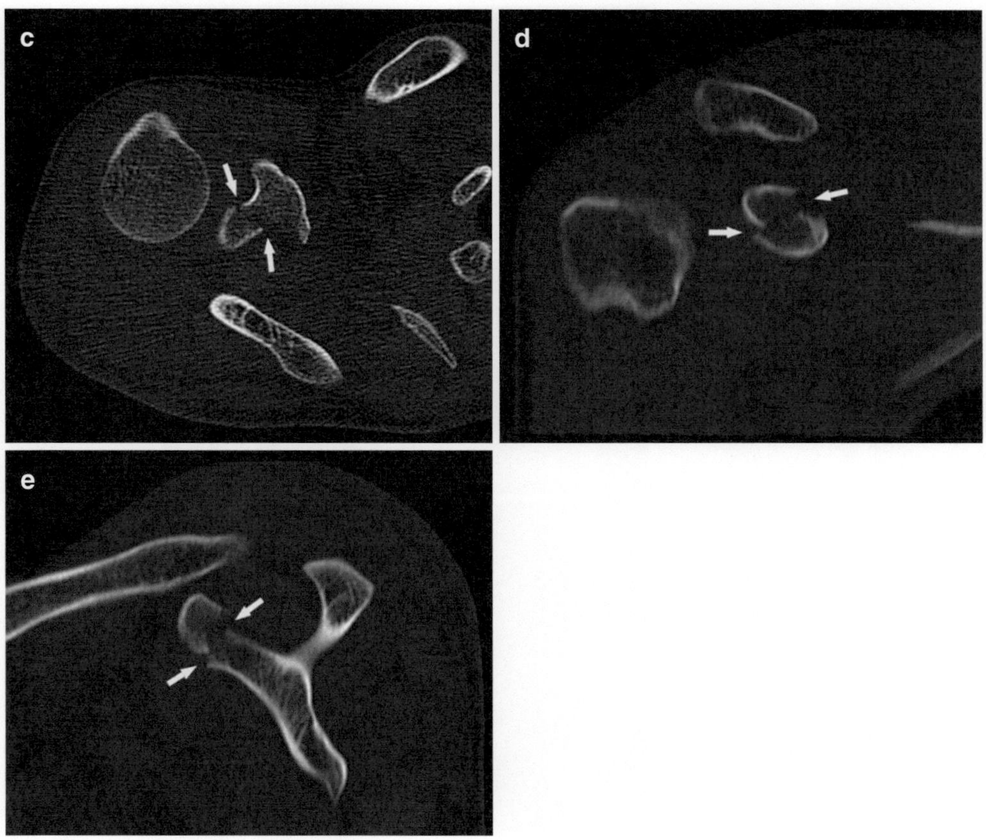

Fig. 2.28 CT cross section and reconstruction (**c**–**e**) showed fracture of coracoid of scapula (arrow) with slight displacement

7. Identification of basal fracture of scapula coracoid and suspected fracture
   7.1. X-ray (Fig. 2.29a, b)

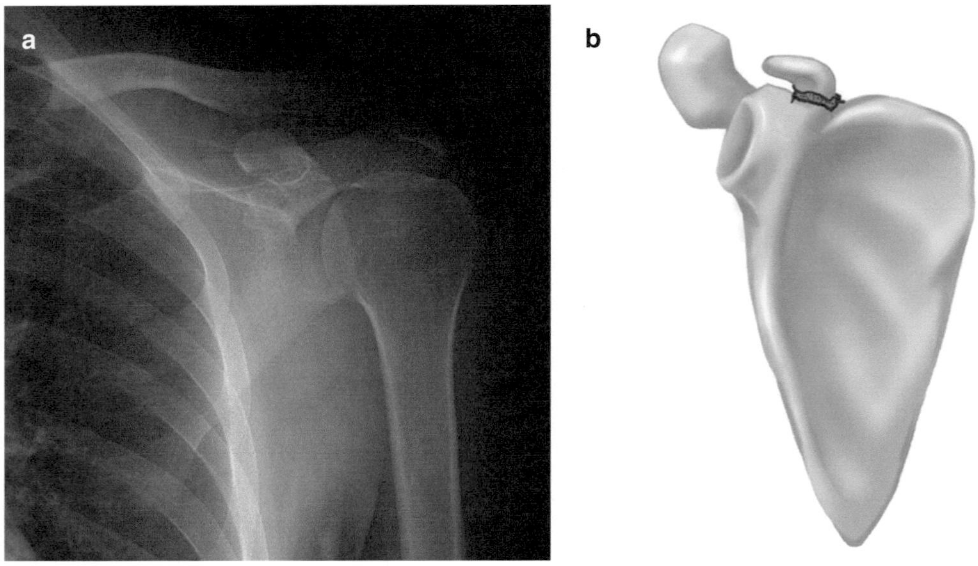

Fig. 2.29 X image, X-ray film, (**a**) shows an irregular contour at the base of left coracoid process, interrupted bone cortex continuity, a strip of fragment sit over the superior border. Schematic diagram (**b**)

   7.2. CT scan (Fig. 2.29c–e)

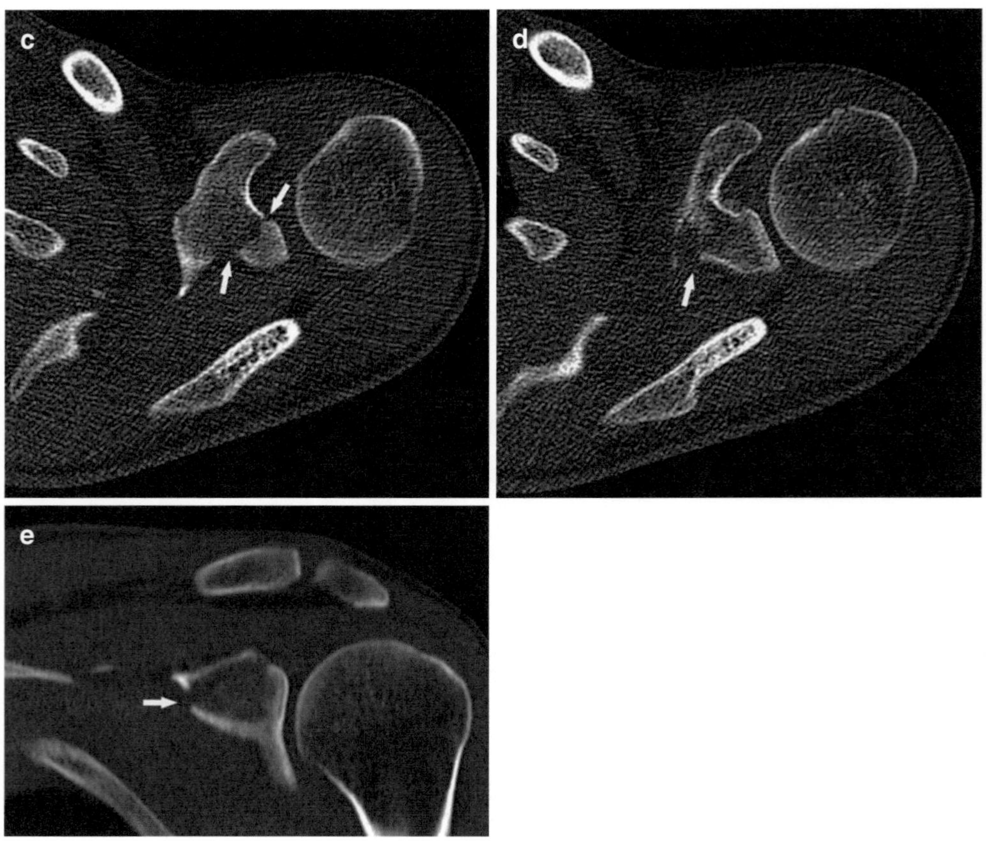

Fig. 2.29 CT cross section and reconstruction (**c**–**e**) showed: basal fracture (arrow) of the coracoid of scapula, no obvious displacement, the fracture was involved in the upper margin of scapula, no fracture sign was found in the glenoid cavity

8. Differentiation of scapular fractures from non-fractures
    8.1. X-ray (Fig. 2.30a–d)

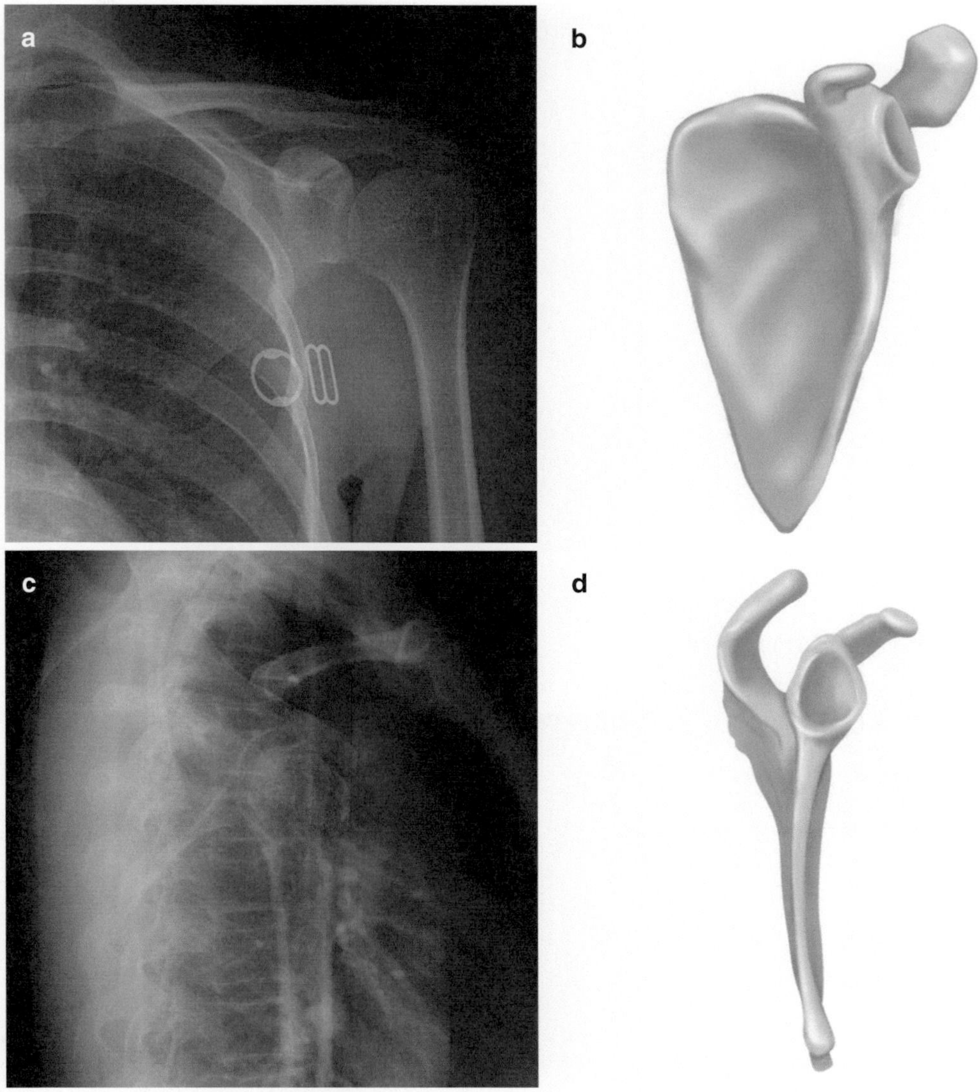

Fig. 2.30 The anteroposterior position of shoulder joint (**a**, **c**) showed no obvious fracture sign on the left scapular. Schematic diagram (**b**, **d**)

    8.2. CT scan (Fig. 2.30e, f)

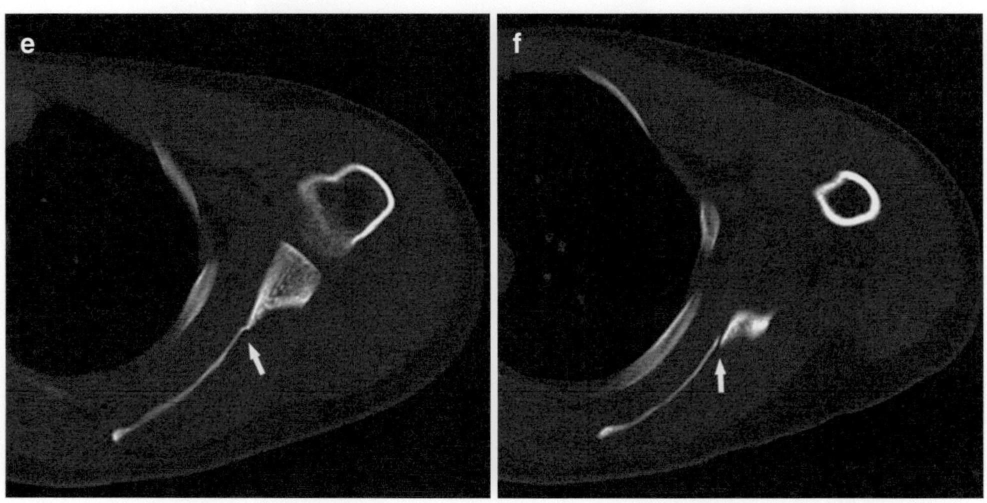

Fig. 2.30 CT cross section (**e**, **f**) shows: fracture of scapula (arrow), with slight displacement

9. Differentiation of inferior angle of the scapula fractures from non-fractures
   9.1. X-ray (Fig. 2.31a, b)

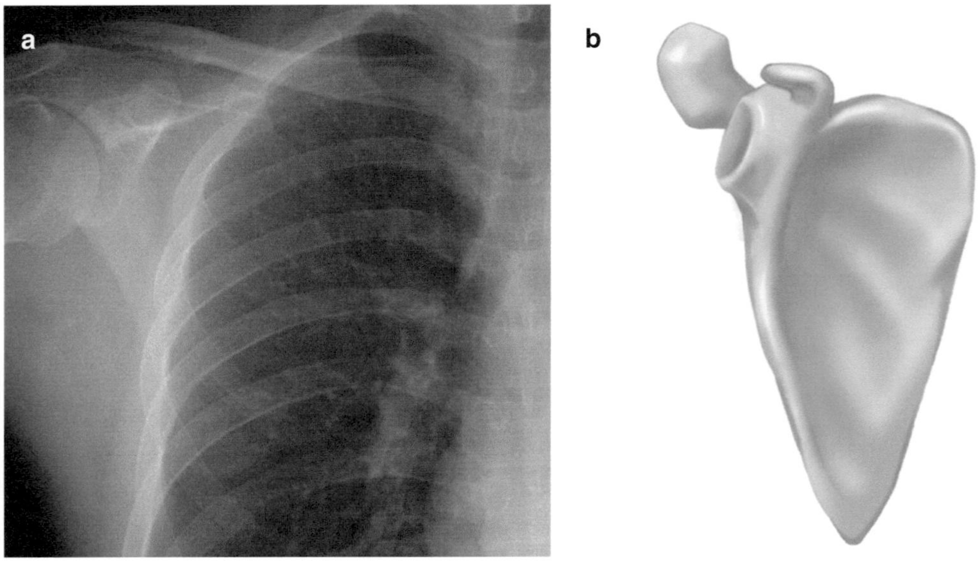

Fig. 2.31 The anteroposterior position of shoulder joint (**a**) shows no obvious fracture sign on the right scapula (**b**)

   9.2. CT scan (Fig. 2.31c–e)

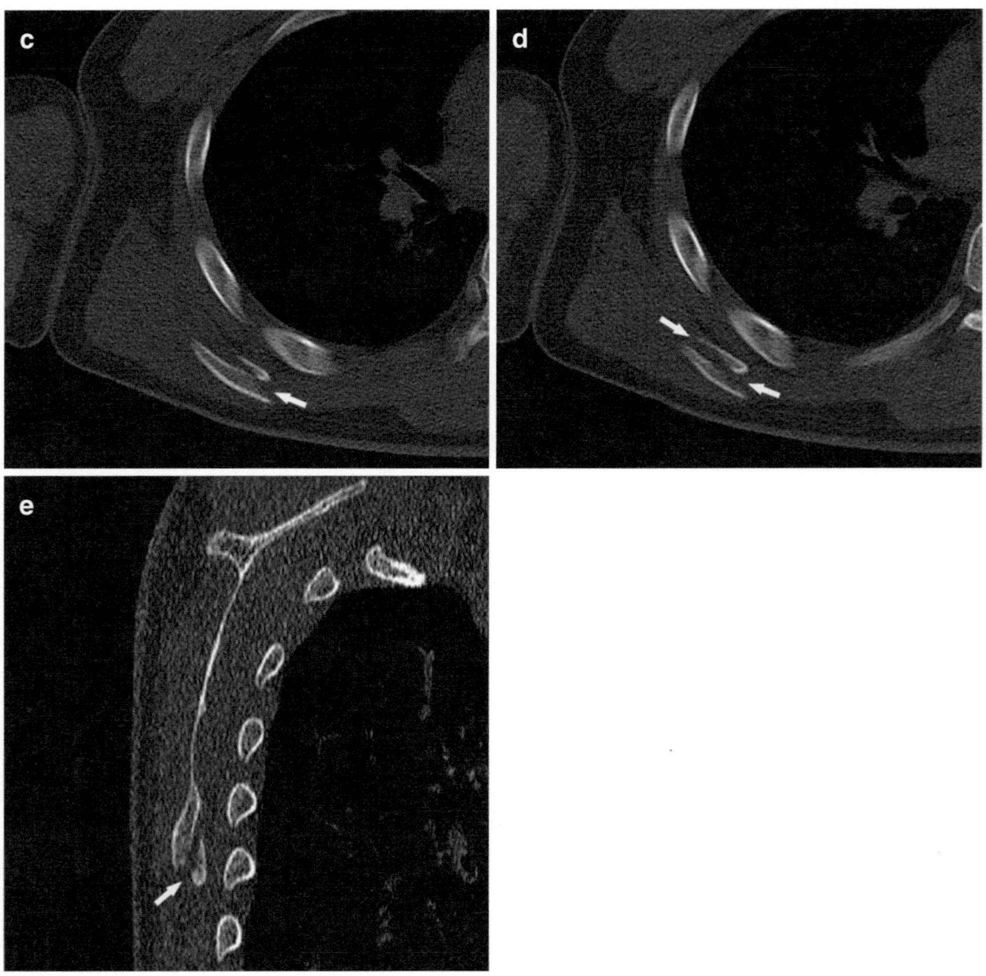

Fig. 2.31 CT cross section and reconstruction (**c**–**e**) showed the oblique fracture (arrow) of the inferior angle of scapula, with displacement

10. Differentiation of comminuted scapular fractures from simple fractures
    10.1. X-ray (Fig. 2.32a, b)

Fig. 2.32 The anteroposterior position of shoulder joint (**a**) shows fracture (arrow) of the right scapula body (**b**)

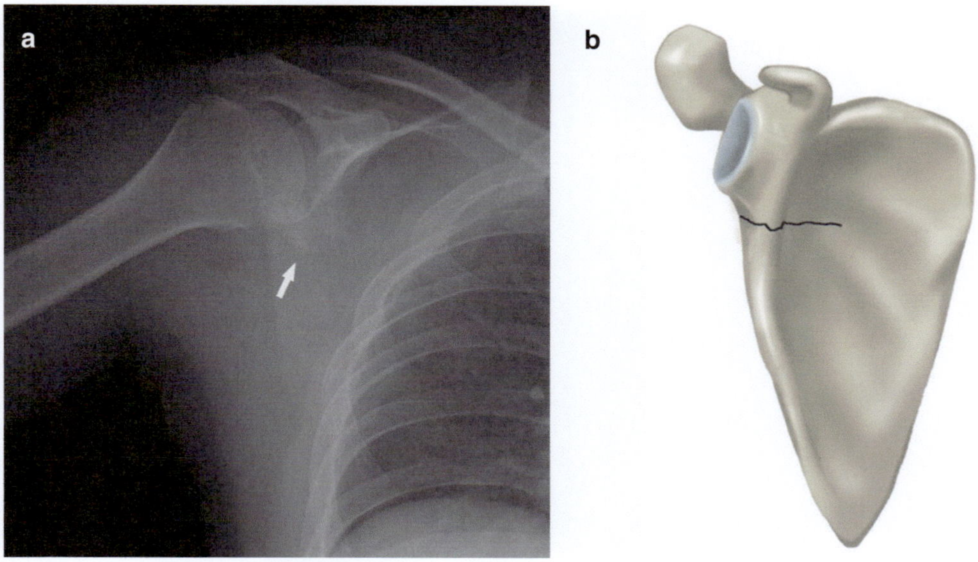

    10.2. CT scan (Fig. 2.32c–e)

Fig. 2.32 CT cross section and reconstruction (**c–e**) showed: fracture (arrow) in the body of scapula, multiple fragments were visible, and the fracture was displaced

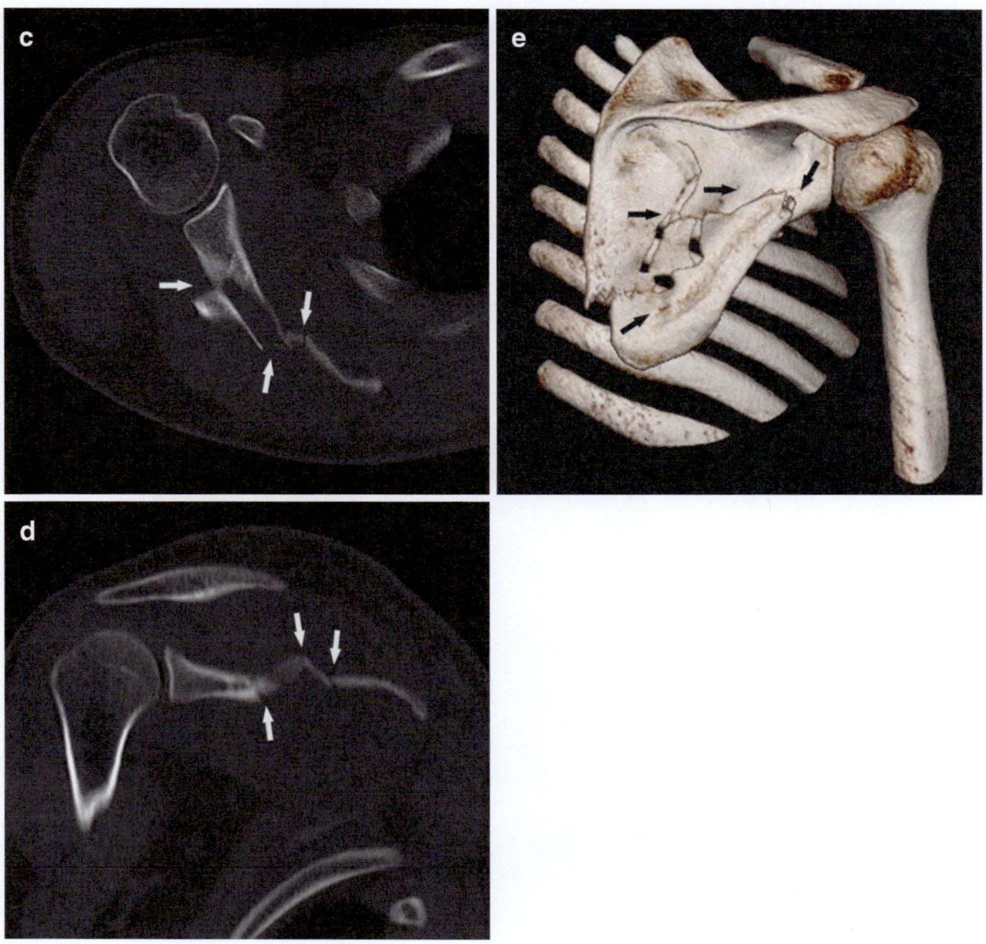

11. Differentiation of scapular glenoid cavity fractures from suspected fractures
    11.1. X-ray (Fig. 2.33a, b)

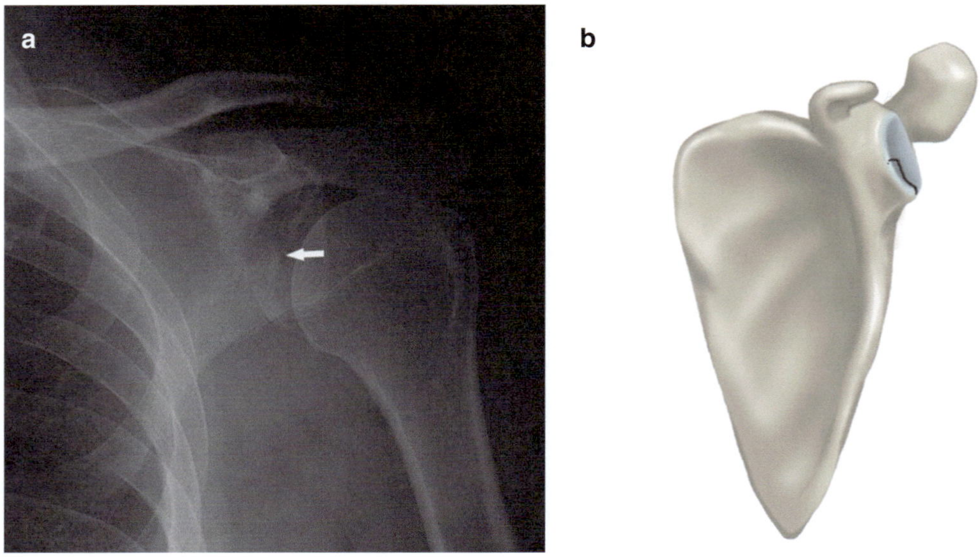

Fig. 2.33 The anteroposterior position of shoulder joint (**a**) shows fracture (arrow) of the scapular glenoid schematic diagram (**b**)

    11.2. CT scan (Fig. 2.33c–e)

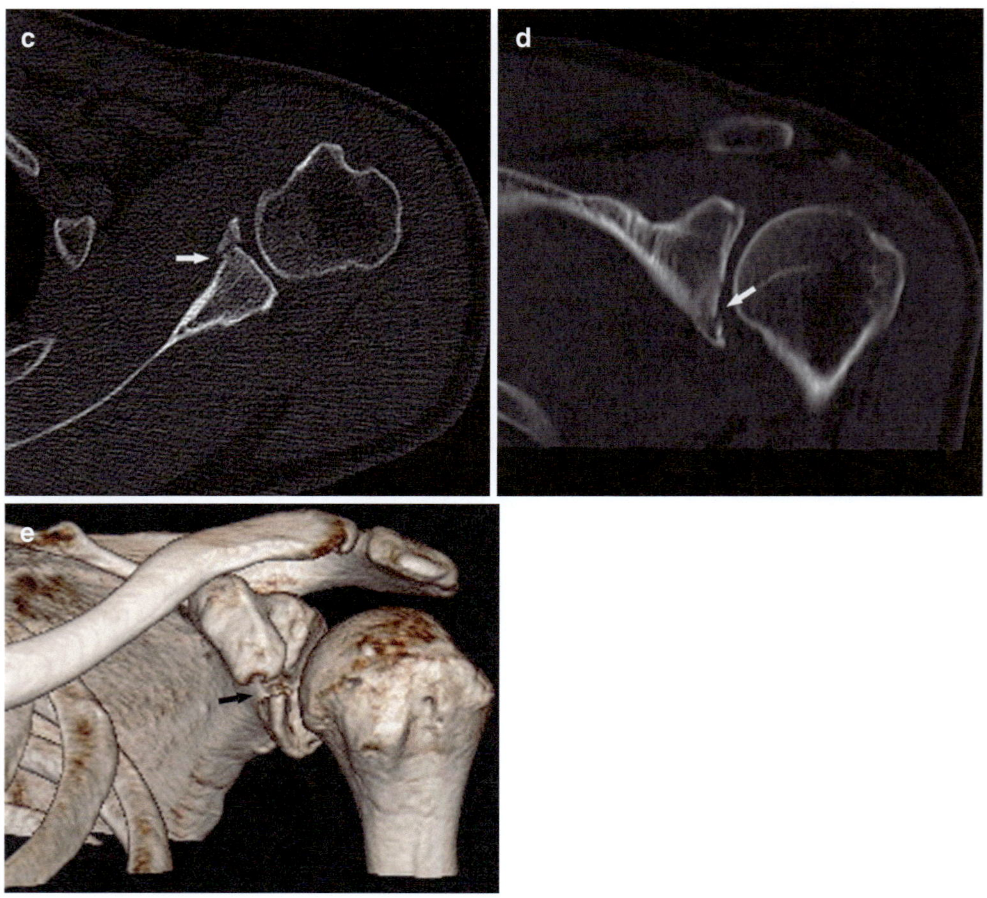

Fig. 2.33 CT cross section and reconstruction (**c**–**e**) showed: fracture (arrow) at the anterior margin of the glenoid of scapula and irregular articular surface

12. Differentiation of displaced scapula glenoid cavity fractures from suspected fractures
    12.1. X-ray (Fig. 2.34a, b)

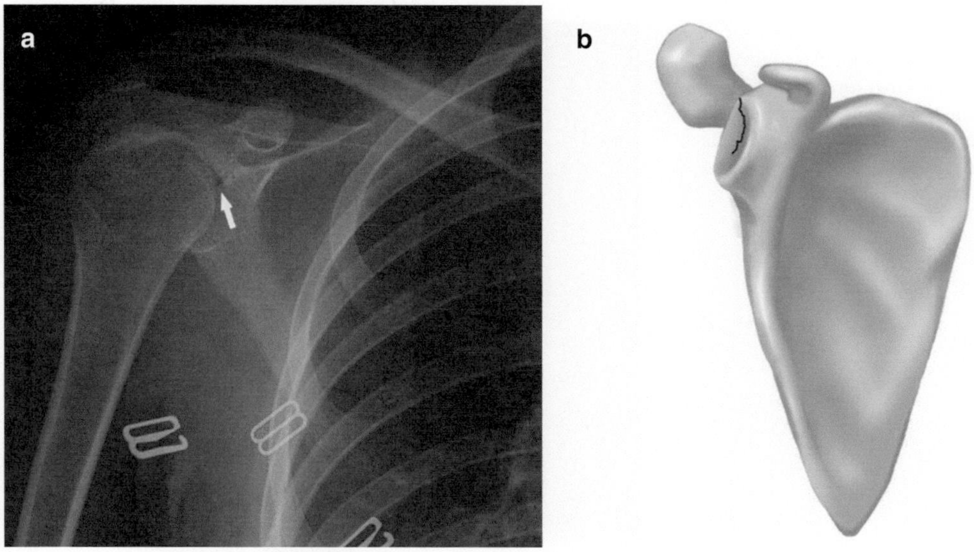

Fig. 2.34 The anteroposterior position of shoulder joint (**a**) shows irregularity (arrow) of the glenoid margin of scapula schematic diagram (**b**)

    12.2. CT scan (Fig. 2.34c)

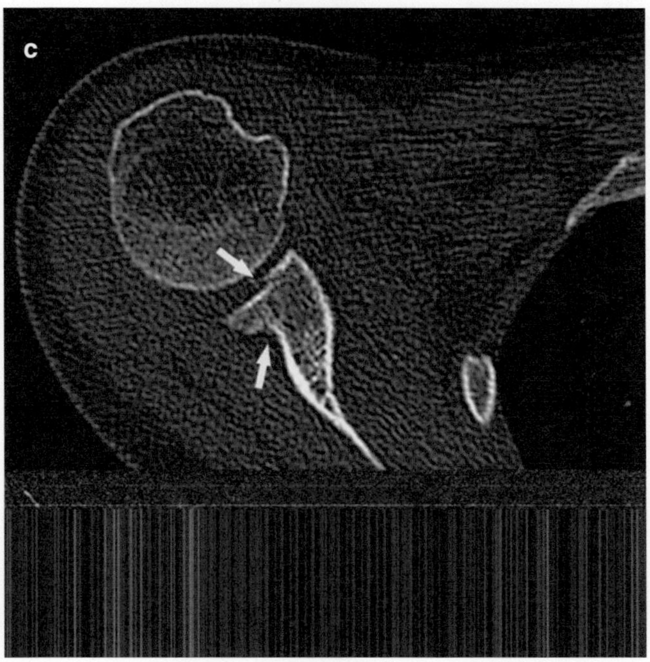

Fig. 2.34 CT cross section (**c**) shows: fracture (arrow) at the posterior margin of the scapula glenoid, disrupted inner surface continuity of the glenoid cavity with slightly displaced

13. Differentiation of glenoid and body displacement of scapula and suspected fracture
    13.1. X-ray (Fig. 2.35a–d)

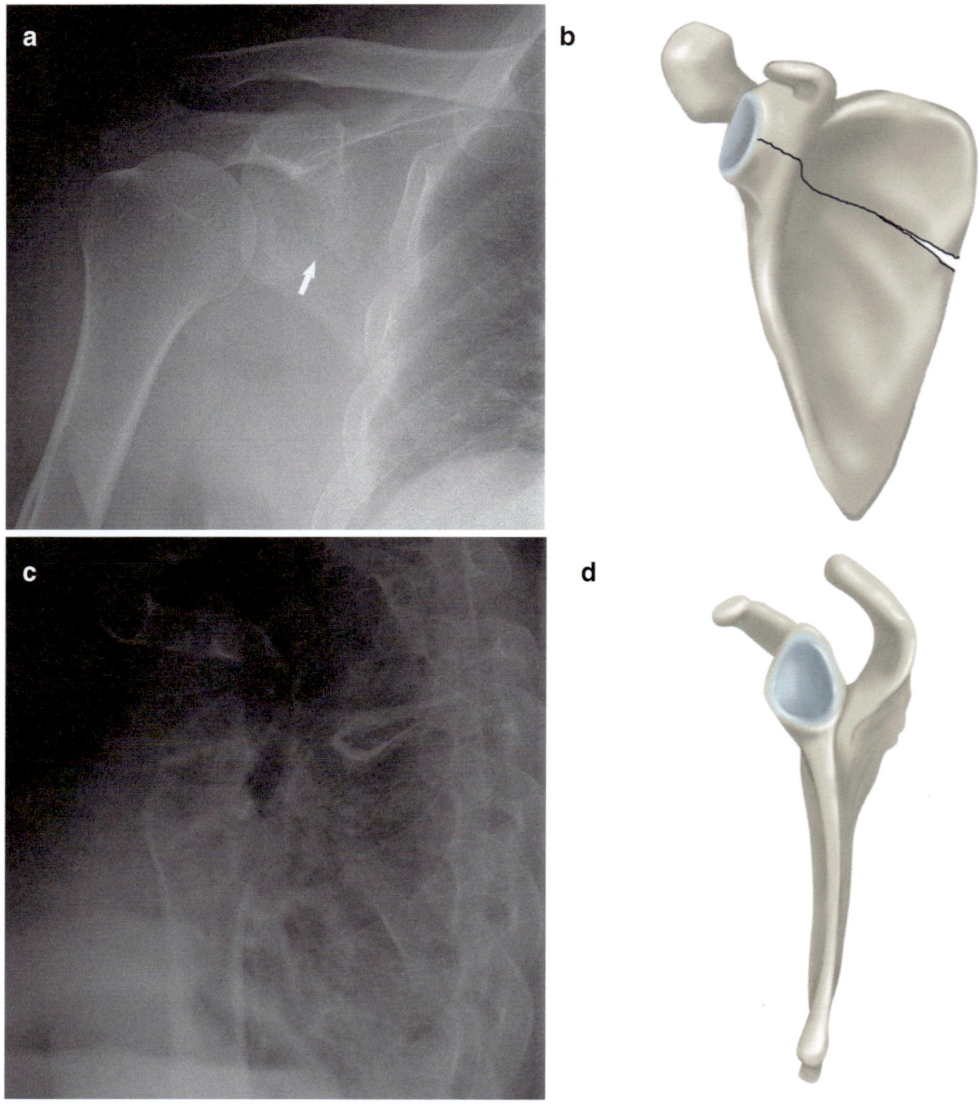

Fig. 2.35 The anteroposterior position of shoulder joint (**a**, **c**) shows low-density shadow (arrow) on the glenoid and body of scapula schematic diagram (**b**, **d**)

13.2. CT scan (Fig. 2.35e–h)

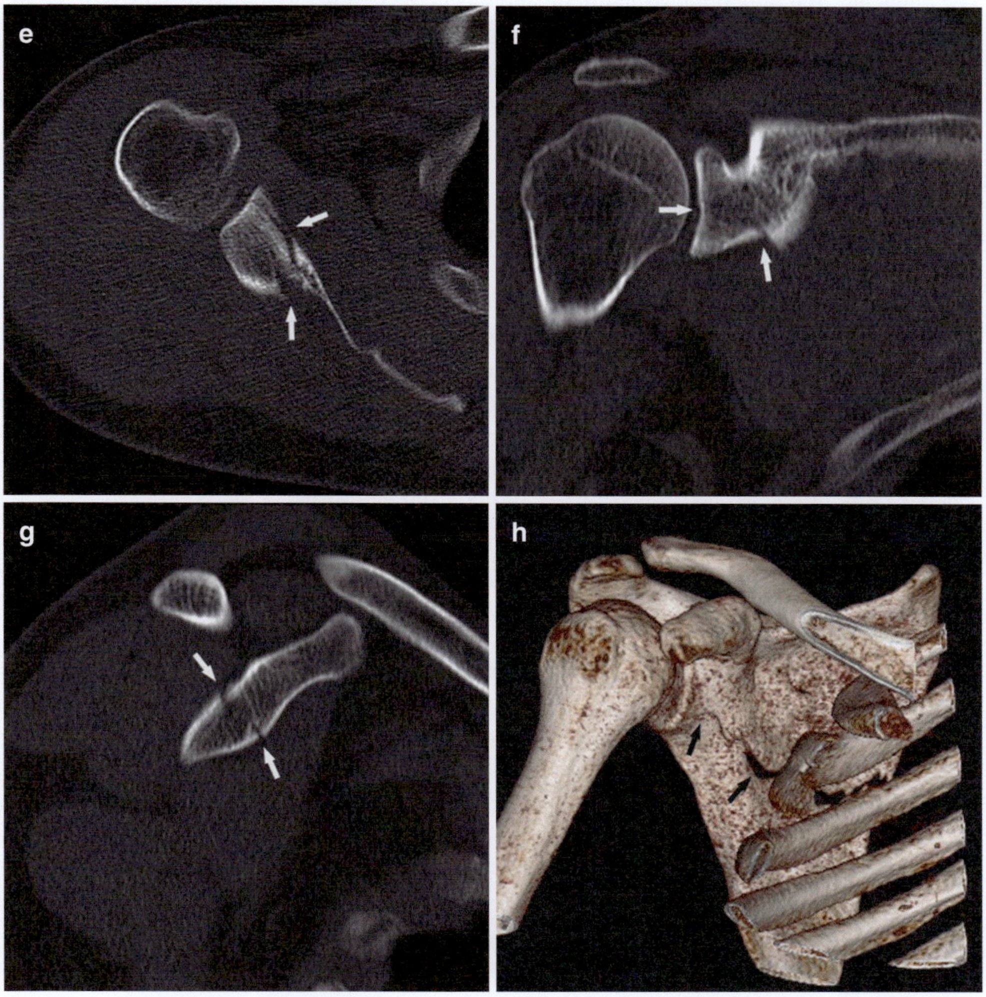

Fig. 2.35 CT cross section and reconstruction (**e**–**h**) showed: fracture of scapula glenoid (arrow), fracture line involved the articular surface and scapula body, slight displacement

2.3 Clavicle Fracture

The clavicle is the only bony structure that connects the scapula to the body, which plays an important role in the stability of the upper limb. Clavicular fractures account for about 2.20% of total fractures. Classification of clavicle fractures is numerous, but the Allman classification is most commonly used, namely: type I, fractures of the 1/3 middle clavicle; type II distal 1/3 clavicle fractures, type III proximal 1/3 clavicle fractures. Type IV, accounts for 61.96% of the clavicle fractures; type V, accounts for 34.87% of the clavicle fractures; type VI, accounts for 3.17% of clavicle fractures.

2.3.1 Identification of Injury Mechanism

The clavicle is thin and curved, and the 1/3 of the distal clavicle changes from tubular to flat. The external force of the upper limb or shoulder produces shearing force. Therefore, most of the clavicular fracture occurs at the distal 1/3. The injury mechanism of the patient has a certain differential diagnosis. The most common injury mechanism of the middle third clavicle fracture is that the elbow is in the extension position during the fall, the external force is transmitted upward along the upper limb, causing the fracture at the clavicle; the distal clavicle fracture tends to be injured on the lateral side of the shoulder, and the shoulder and scapula are fractured by the downward violence. The fracture of the inner end of the clavicle is caused by indirect external force acting on the distal part of the clavicle.

Pathological fracture differentiation: the clavicle may cause bone damage due to infection or tumor, and the fracture is highly suspected to be pathological fracture when the injury violence is very mild, such as when lifting heavy weights.

2.3.2 Identification of Symptoms and Signs

The most obvious symptoms after clavicular fracture are pain, swelling, and limited mobility, these symptoms lack of specificity, and difficulty in definitive diagnosis.

Because the clavicle is located under the skin, the soft tissue is thin, and the severe fracture is seen as an apparent diagnosis. It can be used as a diagnosis basis, but the fracture or mild displacement fracture is not distinct and should be identified.

When examining the patients, you should pay attention to whether there is an abnormal activity or bone grinding, which can be used to confirm the diagnosis.

2.3.3 Imaging Differential Diagnosis

Conventional X-ray can basically diagnose clavicular fractures, but with the wide application of CT in clinical practice, the accuracy of conventional X-ray diagnosis is questioned. Clinical and imaging physicians should pay attention to the following points: (1) No obvious fracture signs are seen on conventional X-ray. However, the clinical symptoms and signs are prominent, CT or MR scan should be performed; (2) If Type I clavicular fracture has a fracture line running through the coronal plane, diagnosis is easily missed when the fracture is not displaced. At this time, the clavicle tangential view can be added to clearly show the fracture; Type II clavicle fractures should pay attention to the no-displaced fracture occurred between the trapezoid ligament and the conoid ligament, as well as the intra-articular fracture involving the distal joint surface of the clavicle. It should be identified that the difference between intra-articular fracture and acromioclavicular joint separation. (3) Conventional X-ray indicated fracture, whereas local bone structure disarranged, this should be closely related with clinical history, especially caused by trivial injury. Further CT or MR scan should be done to rule out pathological fractures. It is necessary to pay great attention to the type III proximal clavicle fracture, which has a low morbidity rate. Radiographically the proximal clavicle overlaps with thoracic ribs and thoracic vertebrae, so it has a high rate of missed diagnosis if only investigated by plain X-ray film, and more importantly, the morbidity rate of pathological fractures occurs more higher in proximal fractures.

In the same case, three different scanning methods, including plain film, CT, and MRI, showed that the fracture performance was not completely consistent, which would affect the accurate judgment of fracture classification. Therefore, the three imaging methods should complement each other. The following cases noted that the plain film, CT, and MRI show differences in different fractures.

1. Differentiation of clavicle fractures from non-fracture
   1.1. X-ray (Fig. 2.36a–d)

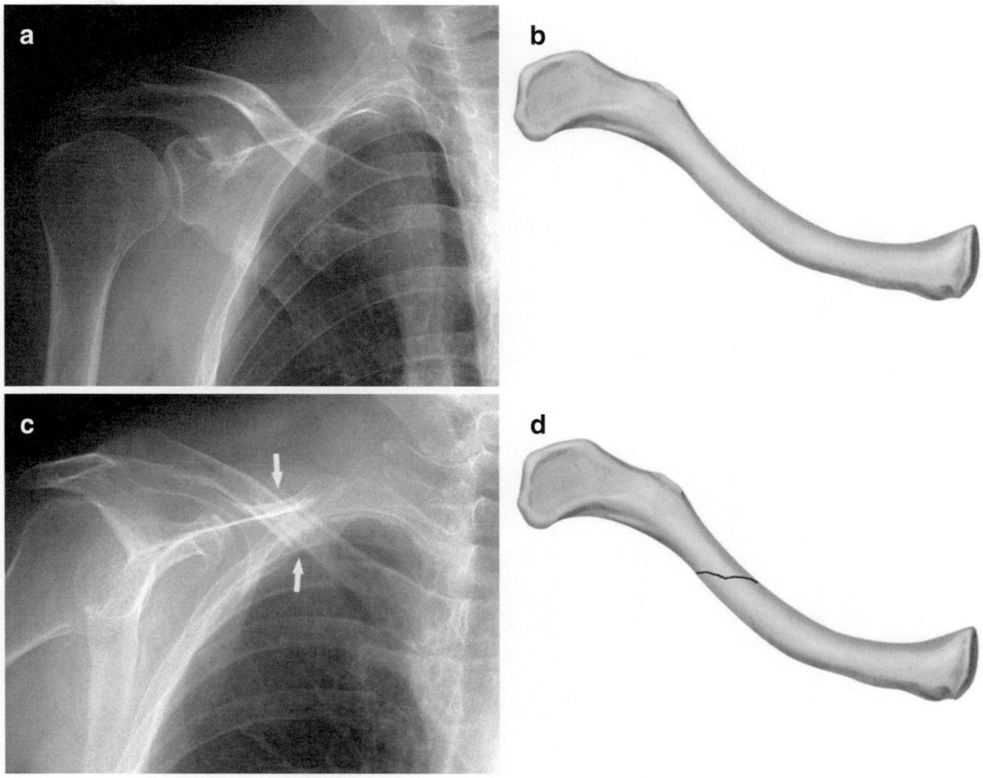

Fig. 2.36 No clear sign of clavicle fracture was found in the anteroposterior plane of right shoulder (**a**). After a week (**c**), X-ray showed: fracture of the middle part of the clavicle on the right side (arrow), with displacement (**b**, **d**)

   1.2. CT scan (Fig. 2.36e, f)

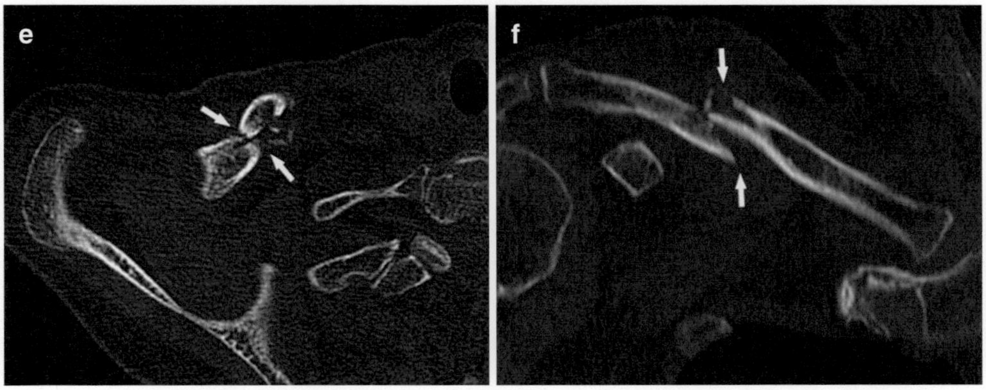

Fig. 2.36 CT cross section and reconstruction (**e**, **f**) showed fracture (arrow) in the middle part of the right clavicle, with obvious displacement and surrounding callus formation

2. Differentiation of distal clavicular fractures from suspected fractures
   2.1. X-ray (Fig. 2.37a, b)

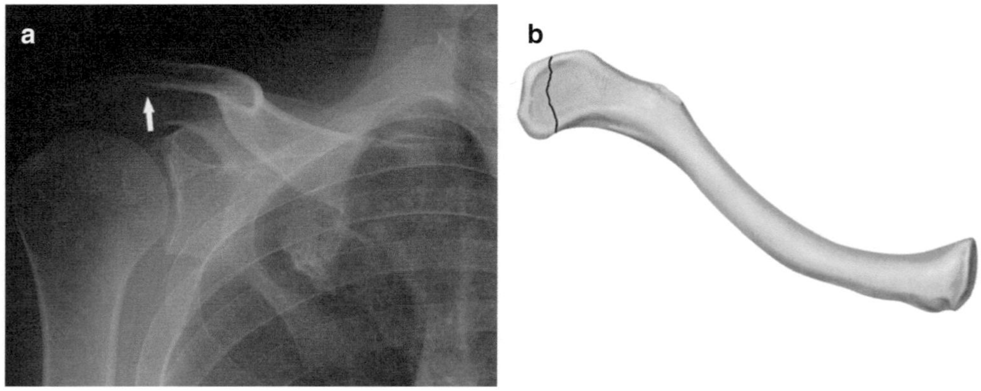

Fig. 2.37 X-ray plain film (**a**) shows slightly disarranged bone trabecula (arrow) at the distal of the right clavicle, without obvious displacement (**b**)

   2.2. CT scan (Fig. 2.37c–e)

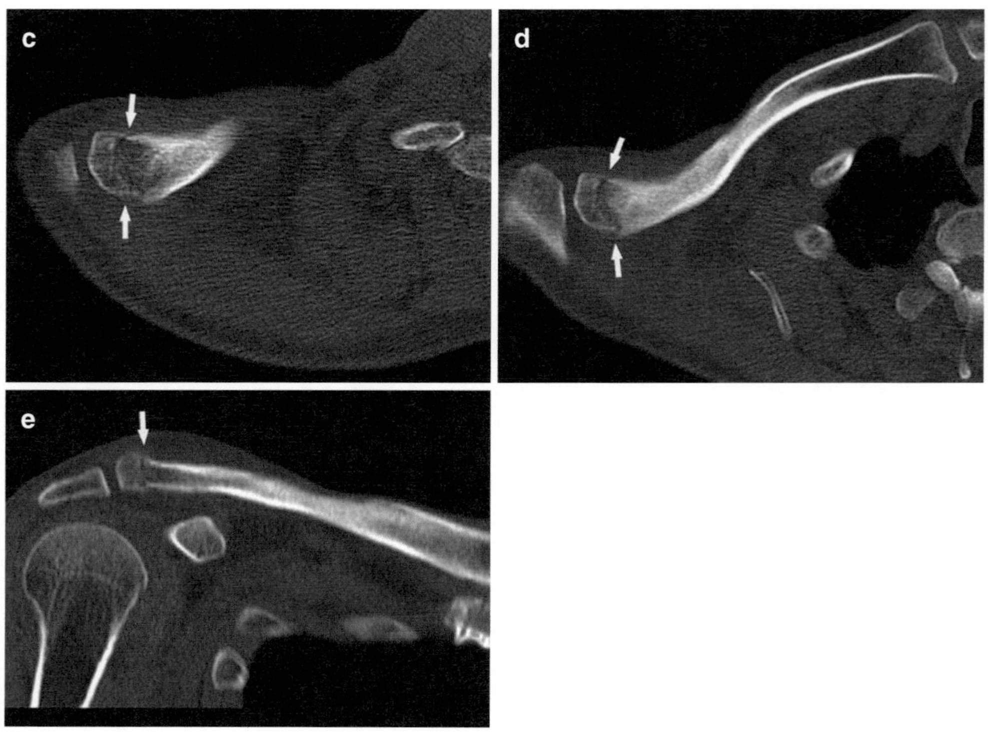

Fig. 2.37 CT cross section and reconstruction (**c**–**e**) showed: fracture (arrow) in distal clavicle, without displacement

3. Identification of clearly displaced clavicle fractures and un-displaced fractures
   3.1. X-ray (Fig. 2.38a, b)

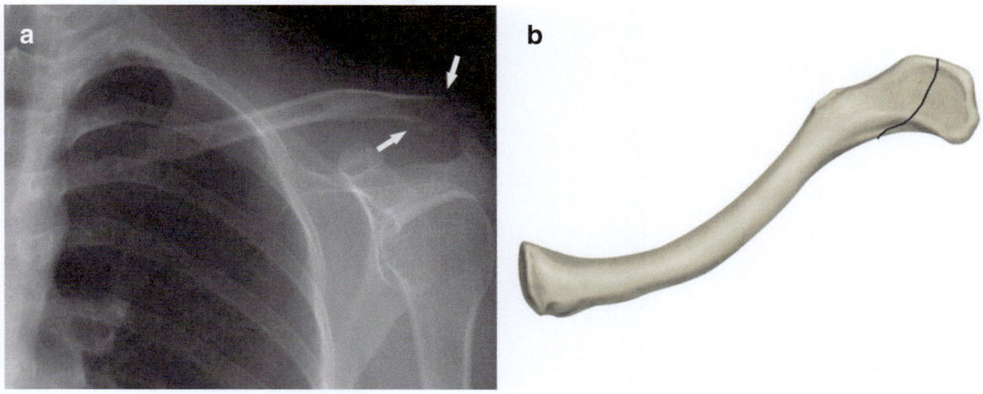

Fig. 2.38 X-ray plain film (**a**) shows fracture (arrow) at the left distal clavicle without displacement (**b**)

   3.2. CT scan (Fig. 2.38c–e)

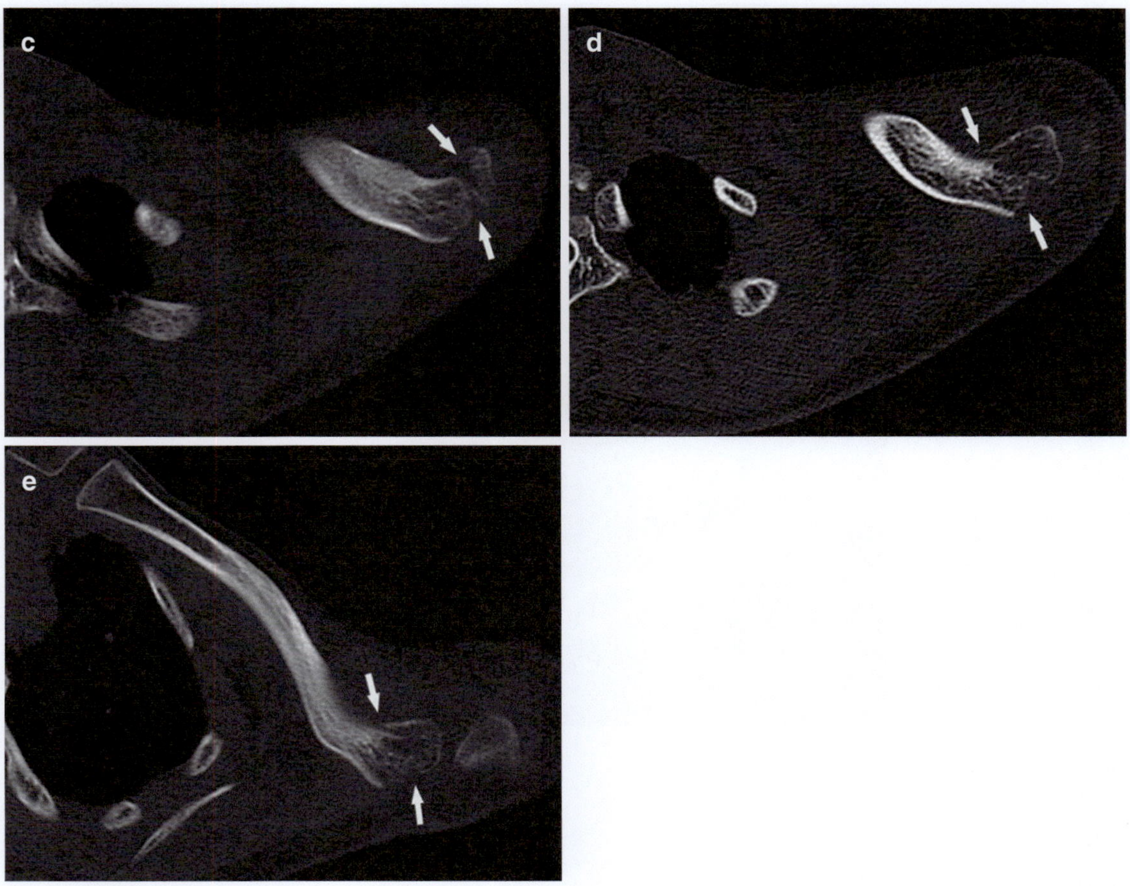

Fig. 2.38 CT cross section and reconstruction (**c**–**e**) showed the distal fracture of the clavicle, with displacement

4. Differentiation of proximal clavicle comminuted fractures from simple fractures
   4.1. X-ray (Fig. 2.39a, b)

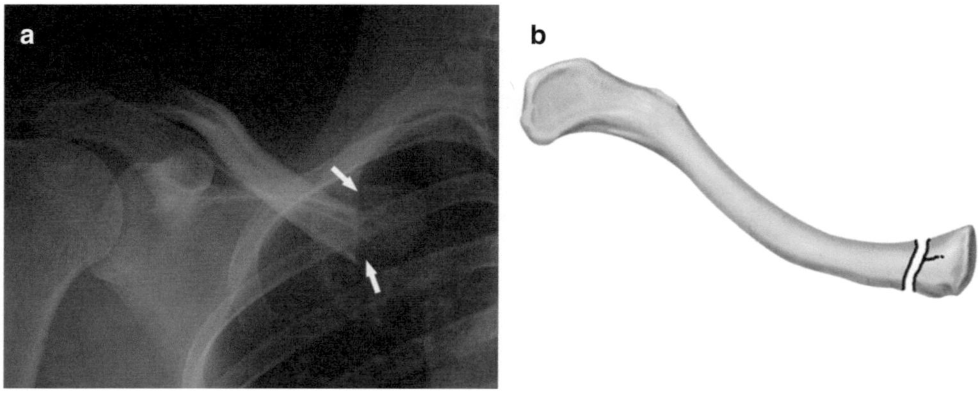

Fig. 2.39 X-ray plain film (**a**) shows the fracture (arrow) at the proximal of the right clavicle, with obvious upward displacement (**b**)

   4.2. CT scan (Fig. 2.39c–e)

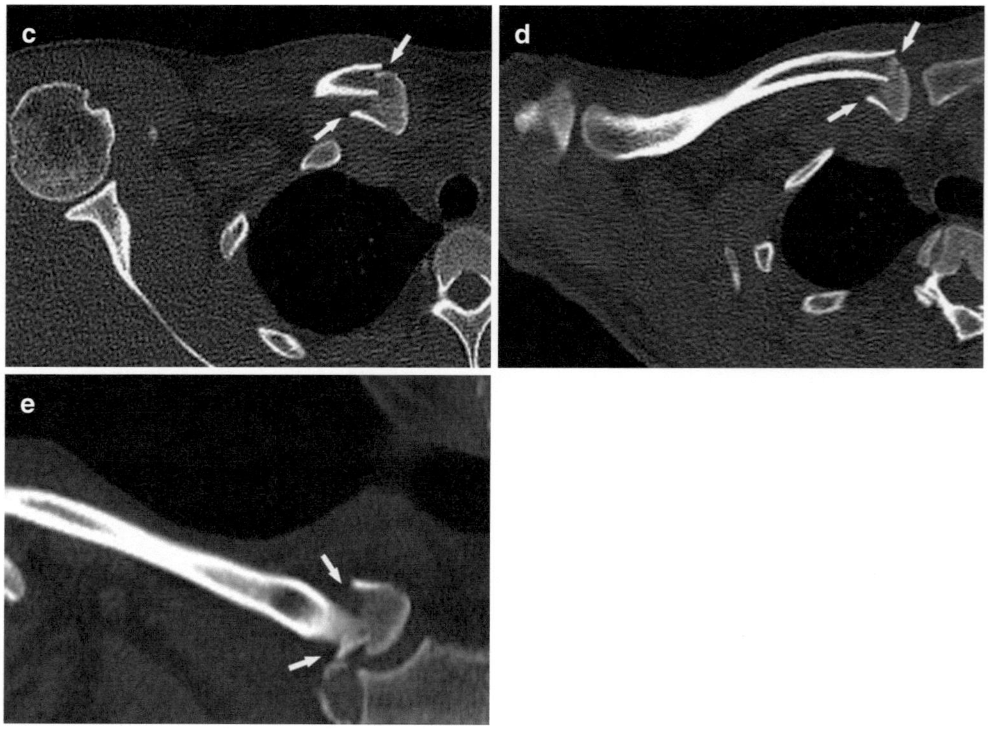

Fig. 2.39 CT cross section and reconstruction (c–e) showed: fracture of proximal clavicle, with multiple fragments (arrows) and obvious displacement

5. Differential diagnosis of proximal clavicular comminuted fractures and no fractures
   5.1. X-ray (Fig. 2.40a, b)

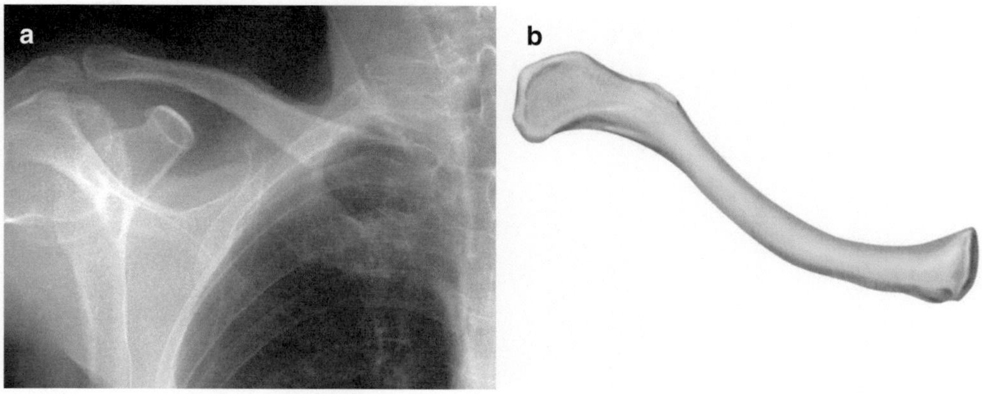

Fig. 2.40 X-ray plain film (**a**) shows no clear fracture sign at the proximal end of the right clavicle (**b**)

   5.2. CT scan (Fig. 2.40c, d)

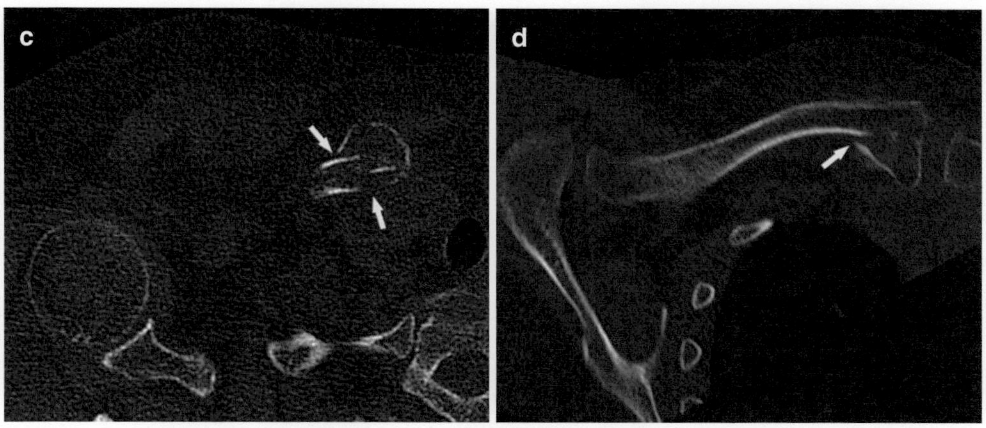

Fig. 2.40 CT cross section and reconstruction (**c**, **d**) showed: fracture (arrow) at the proximal clavicle, with impacted and displaced

6. Differential diagnosis of proximal clavicle comminuted fractures and no fractures
   6.1. X-ray (Fig. 2.41a, b)

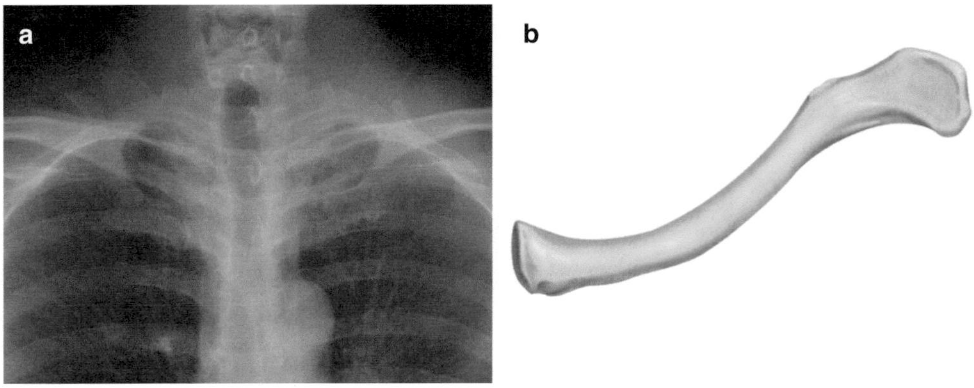

Fig. 2.41 X-ray plain film (**a**) showed no clear fracture sign at the proximal of the left clavicle (**b**)

   6.2. CT scan (Fig. 2.41c–e)

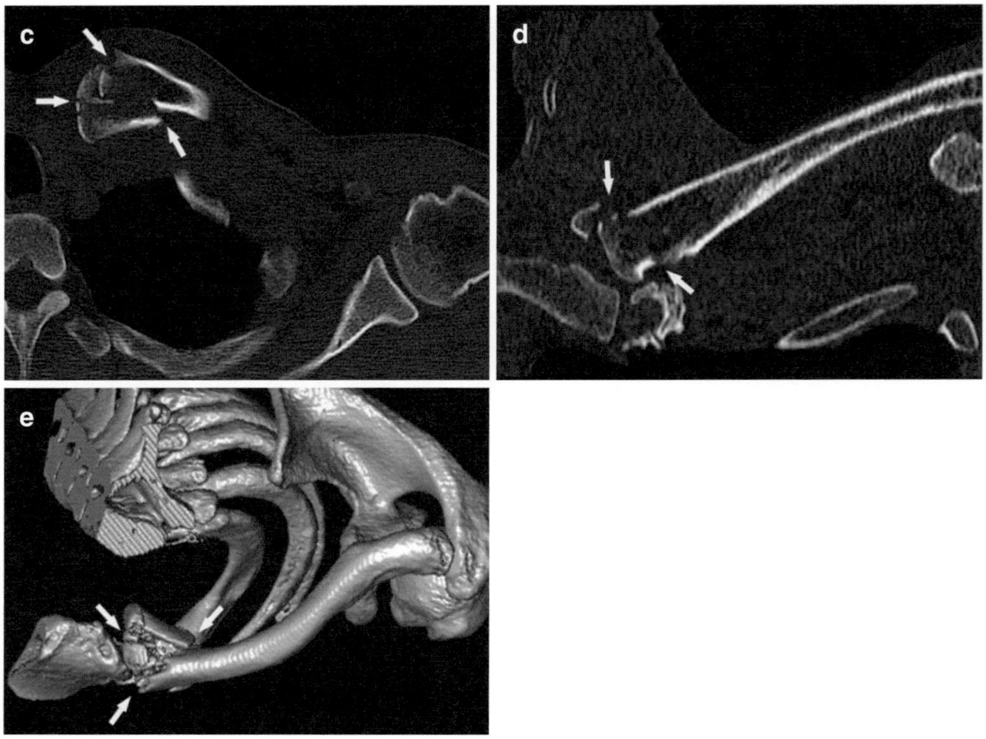

Fig. 2.41 CT cross section and reconstruction (**c**–**e**) showed: fracture (arrow) at the proximal clavicular bone, with multiple fragments and the fracture was involved in the articular surface

2.4 Summary

1. The scapula; an irregular bone, belongs to the pectoral girdle. The difference in body thickness between the glenoid and the scapula body is distinct, and the projections of the ribs, clavicle, and other tissues of the thorax overlap, which makes the X-ray show the details of the entire bone structure very difficult. Therefore, CT + multi-planar reconstruction and three-dimensional reconstruction have great advantages in the display of fracture, and should be examined as a clinical routine.
2. Humeral tuberosities are attached to the rotator cuff, and avulsion fractures often occur. Glenohumeral dislocation is often accompanied by the fracture of the humeral head, or the edge of scapula. The evaluation of proximal humeral comminuted fracture requires the addition of CT and three-dimensional reconstruction.
3. MRI is used to evaluate tendon and soft tissue injuries around the shoulder, especially rotator cuff injuries, labrum injuries, and humeral head cartilage injuries.

Reference

1. Zhang Y, et al. Clinical epidemiology of orthopaedic trauma. New York: Thieme; 2016.

3 Elbow Fracture

Jianling Cui and Yingze Zhang

3.1 Distal Humerus Fracture

Distal humerus fractures account for 23.21% of adult humerus fractures. The AO/OTA classification of distal humerus fractures are divided into the following: extra-articular fracture, partial intra-articular fracture, and complete intra-articular fracture. Furthermore, extra-articular fractures are divided into avulsion fracture of the condyles, simple fracture of the metaphysis, and comminuted fracture of the metaphysis. The avulsion fracture of the condyles accounts for 4.96% of the adult humerus fracture, the simple fracture of the metaphysis accounts for 7.63% of the adult humerus fracture, and the metaphyseal fracture of the metaphysis accounts for 1.08% of the adult humerus fracture. Moreover, partial intra-articular fractures are sub-divided into lateral condyle sagittal fractures, medial condyle sagittal fractures, and coronal fractures. Lateral condyle sagittal fractures account for 3.57% of adult humerus fractures. Medial condyle sagittal fractures account for 2.00% of adult humerus fractures, coronal fracture accounts for 0.28% of adult humerus fractures. Complete intra-articular fractures are divided into simple intra-articular fractures with simple metaphyseal fractures; simple intra-articular fractures with comminuted metaphyseal fractures, and intra-articular comminuted fractures. The simple intra-articular fractures and simple fracture of the metaphysis account for 1.32% of the adult humerus fracture. The simple intra-articular and comminuted metaphyseal fractures account for 1.85% of the adult humerus fractures, and the intra-articular comminuted fracture accounts for 0.52% of the adult humerus fracture.

3.1.1 Injury Mechanism Identification

The supracondylar fracture of the humerus is usually caused by indirect violence. According to the mechanism of injury, it can be divided into two types: straight type and flexion type. A common cause of a straight supracondylar fracture is force exerted onto the palm when used as support during a fall, whilst the elbow is hyperextended with the forearm anteriorly rotated. The distal end of the fracture is located posterior to the proximal end of the fracture.

The flexion type fracture: the elbow joint is in a flexion position when the injury occurs. The violence comes from the rearmost end, thus, the distal part of the fracture is located in front of the proximal fracture.

Most fractures of the humeral condyle are caused by avulsion force of the collateral ligament; however, some can be caused by direct violent blow.

3.1.2 Symptom and Sign Identification

The symptoms typically manifest as pain, swelling, limited mobility, yet these symptoms lack specificity, which cannot be solely used to formulate an accurate diagnosis. If the fracture is obviously displaced, a sensation of bone grinding can be

J. Cui
CT/MRI Center, The Third Hospital of Hebei Medical University, Shijiazhuang, Hebei, China

Y. Zhang (✉)
Department of Orthopaedics, The Third Hospital of Hebei Medical University, Shijiazhuang, Hebei, China

Y. Zhang (ed.), *Differential Diagnosis of Fracture*, https://doi.org/10.1007/978-981-13-8339-7_3

examined. Therefore diagnosis is confirmed. Distal humeral fractures are often combined with neurovascular injury, thus special attention should be paid when examining the body to prevent a missed diagnosis.

3.1.3 Image Differential Diagnosis

Using a conventional X-ray helps confirm an accurate diagnosis of a distal humuerus fracture in an adult. However, a distal humerus injury of the children is difficult to diagnosis, in some cases; comparison of the fracture with a normal joint of the contralateral side is needed for diagnosis. CT is mainly used for identifying a small tear of the ligament attachment, and the fragments relationships as well as for observing joint articular surface details. A CT scan for diagnosing a distal humerus fractures in children is helpful, but the radiation of CT scan is considerably large. MR scanning is essential for the diagnosis of tendon and soft tissue injury around the distal humerus, especially in children with epiphysis injury and elbow ligament injury. The humerus lateral condylar fracture should be differentiated from the humeral capitulum fracture, given the humeral capitulum fracture only affects the articular surface and its supporting bone, whilst the lateral condylar fracture includes the articular surface and the non-articular surface, which often involves the radial part of the humerus trochlea.

1. Distal humeral epicondylar fracture and epiphysis fracture
    1.1. X-ray film (Fig. 3.1a–d)

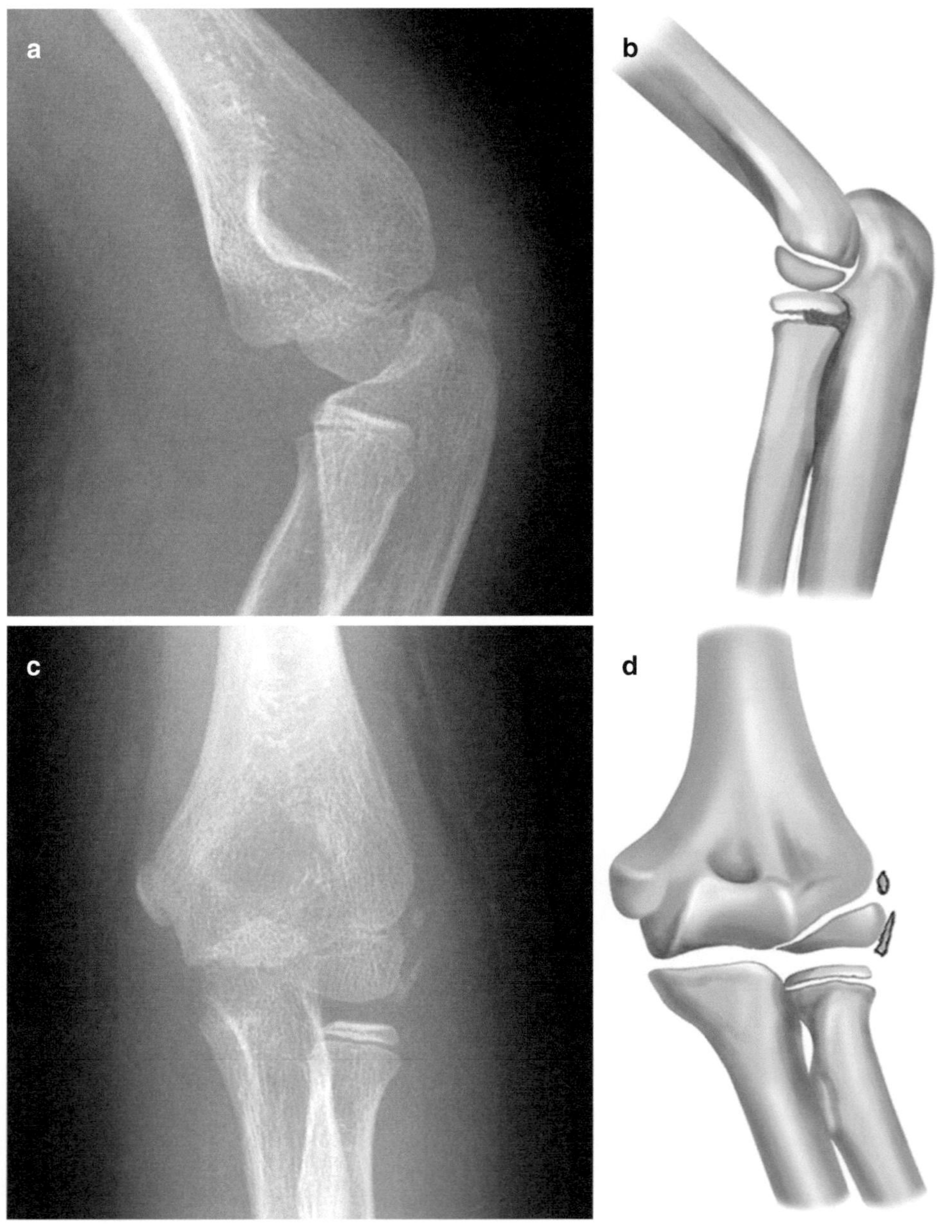

Fig. 3.1 Identification of the fracture of the lateral condylar and the fracture of the epiphysis. (**a**, **c**) Lateral X-ray films show no clear fracture signs. The X-ray films show that the outer edge of the lateral condylar of the humerus could be viewed as a curved fragment. The position of the bone was lower than that of the normal lateral epicondyle, and the surrounding soft tissue was swollen. (**b**, **d**) Schematic

1.2. CT scan (Fig. 3.1e, f)

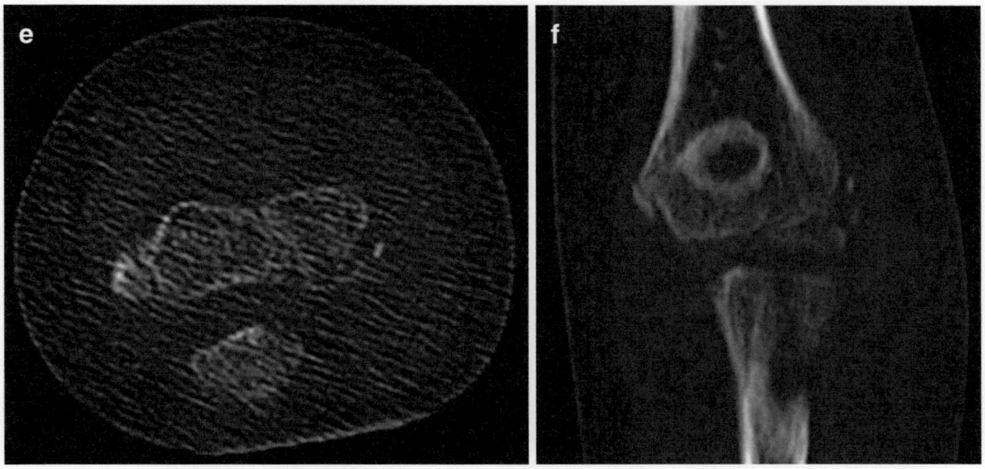

Fig. 3.1 (**e**, **f**) CT cross-section and coronal reconstruction showed osteophyte fragmentation of the lateral humerus condylar, showing multiple small bone shadows, surrounding soft tissue swelling

2. Identification of humerus lateral epicondyle epiphyseal separation and fracture
   2.1. X-ray film (Fig. 3.2a–d)

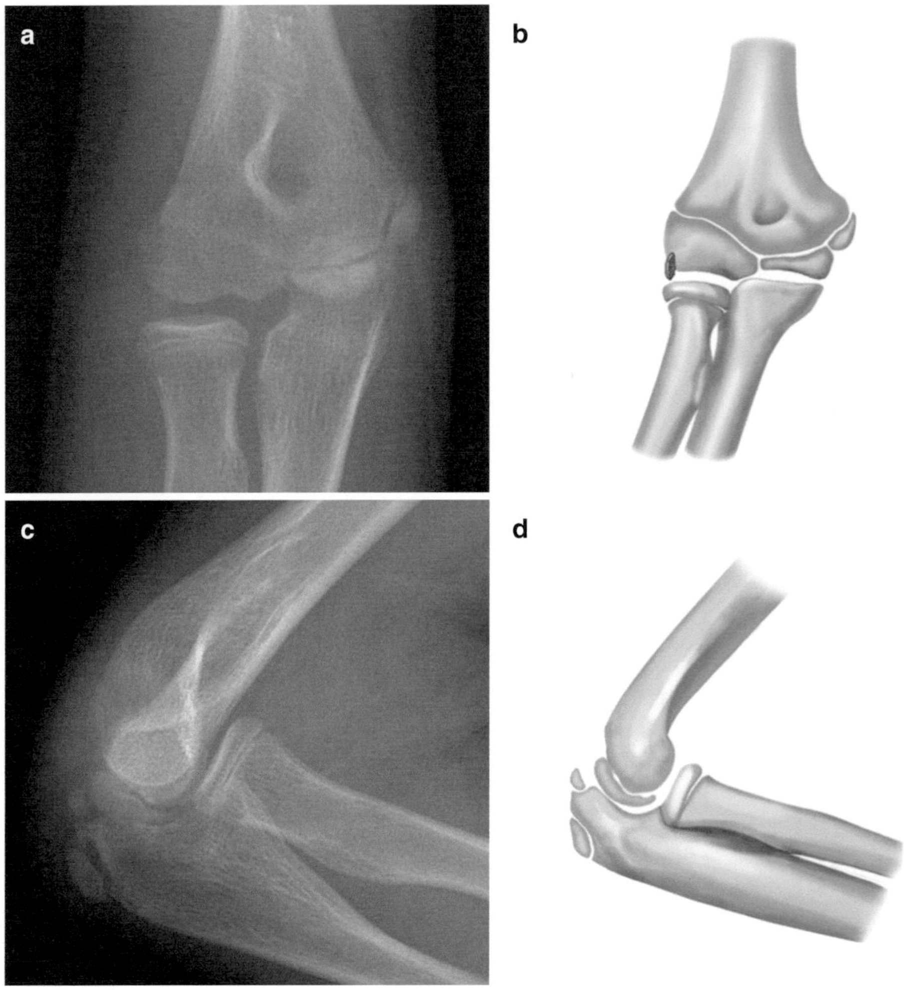

Fig. 3.2 Identification of the humerus lateral epicondyle epiphyseal separation with fracture. (**a**, **c**) Anteroposterior position X-ray showed irregular shape of the lateral epicondyle of humerus, and the joint surface of the lateral condylar humerus was like the fracture piece. There was no obvious fracture in the lateral X-ray film; (**b**, **d**) Schematic

   2.2. CT scan (Fig. 3.2e, f)

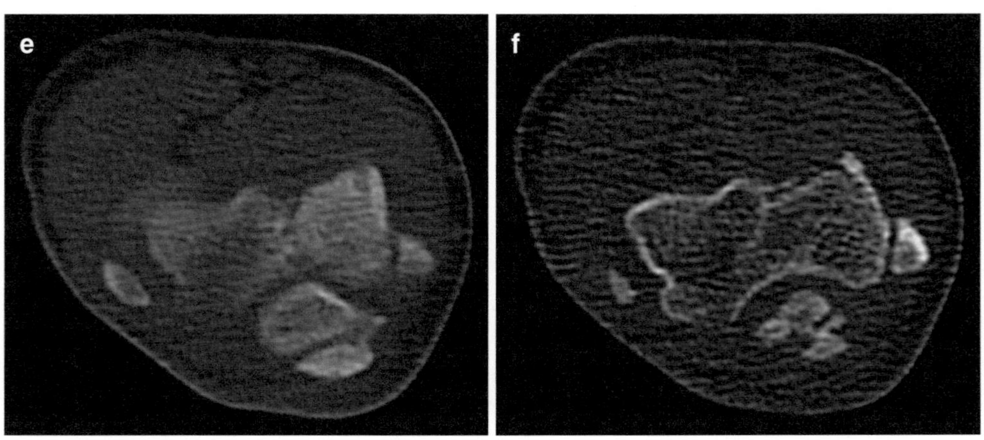

Fig. 3.2 (**e**, **f**) CT cross-section shows the lateral epicondyle of the humerus shifts to the lateral side, and the epiphyseal line is widened

3. Identification of partial fractures of the humerus medial epicondyle and epiphysis
   3.1. X-ray film (Fig. 3.3a–d)

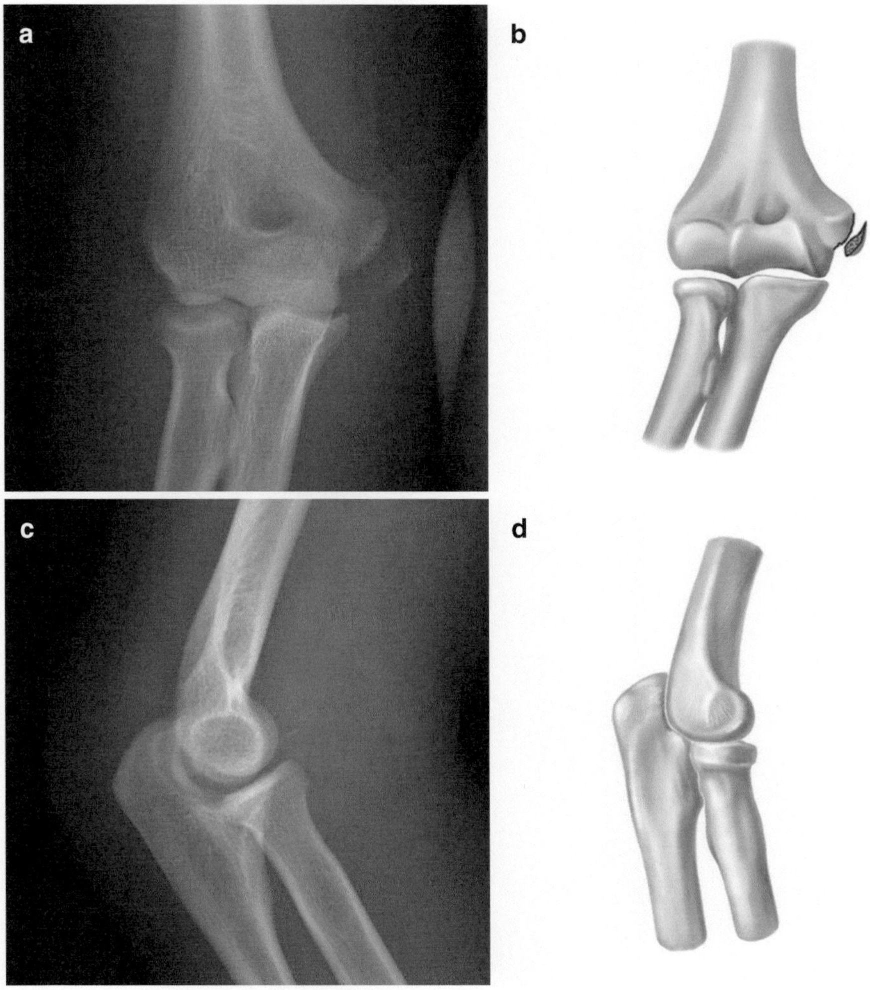

Fig. 3.3 Identification of partial fractures of the humerus medial epicondyle and epiphysis. (**a**, **c**) Anterior–posterior X-ray film shows the shape of the humeral medial epicondyle is intact, the bone block shadow can be seen inside and below, the edge is sharp, and there is no fracture sign in the lateral X-ray film; (**b**, **d**) Schematic

   3.2. CT scan (Fig. 3.3e, f)

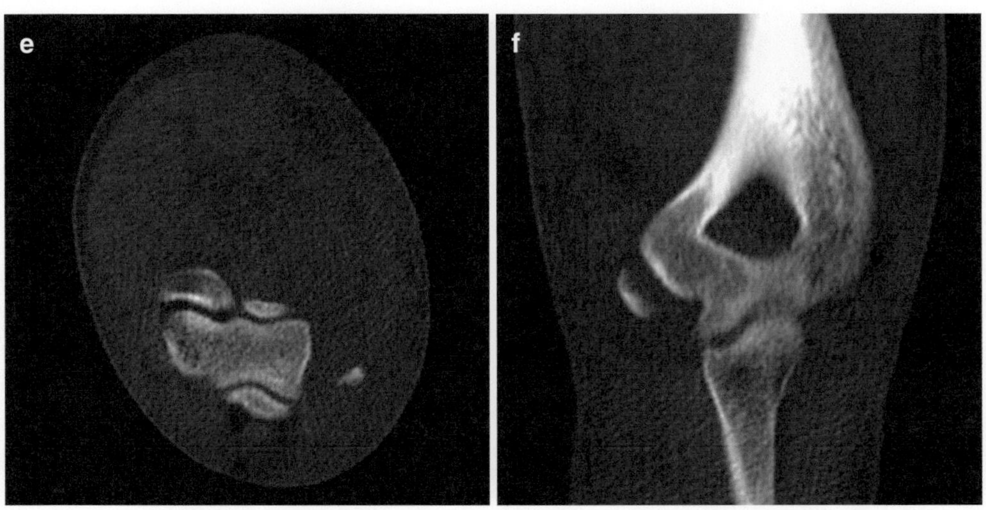

Fig. 3.3 (**e**, **f**) CT cross-section, coronal reconstruction shows fracture of the humeral medial epicondyle. The fracture block is displaced inward and downward

4. II degree separation and fracture identification of the humeral medial epicondyle
   4.1. X-ray film (Fig. 3.4a–d)

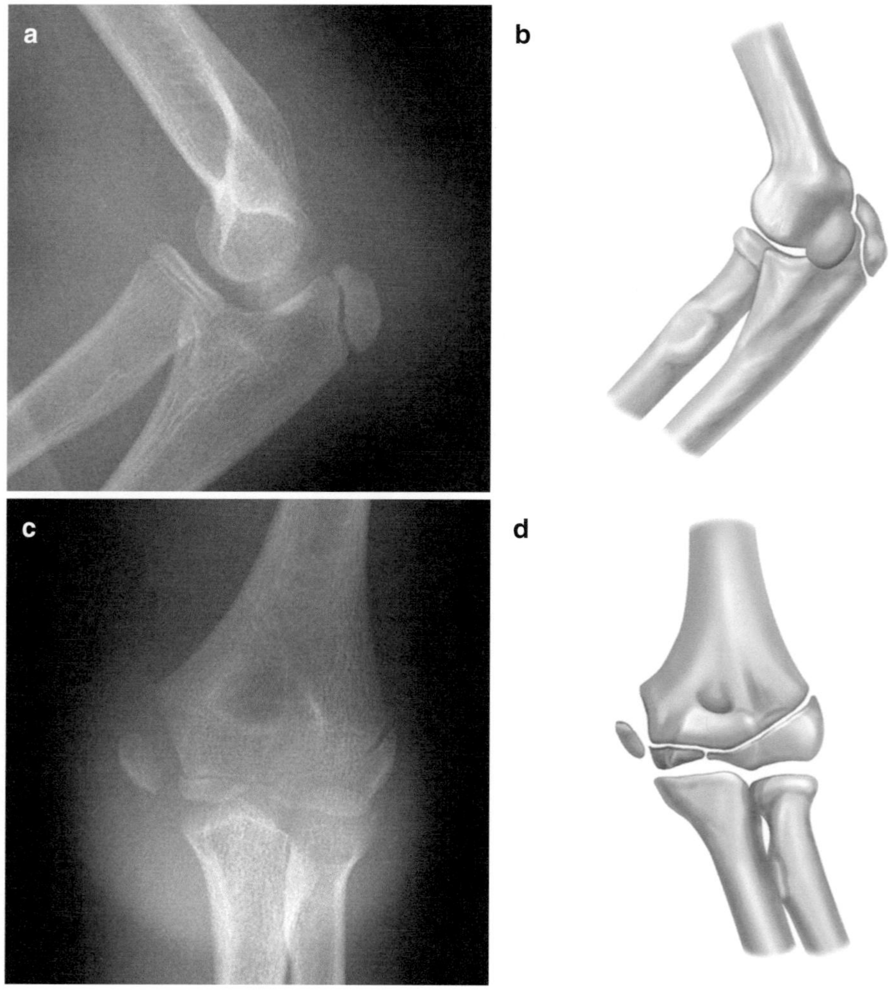

Fig. 3.4 II degree separation and fracture identification of the humeral medial epicondyle. (**a**, **c**) X line shows that the humeral medial epicondyle is displaced inward and downward, the epiphysis line is widened, and the surrounding soft tissue is swollen; (**b**, **d**) Schematic

4.2. CT scan (Fig. 3.4e–h)

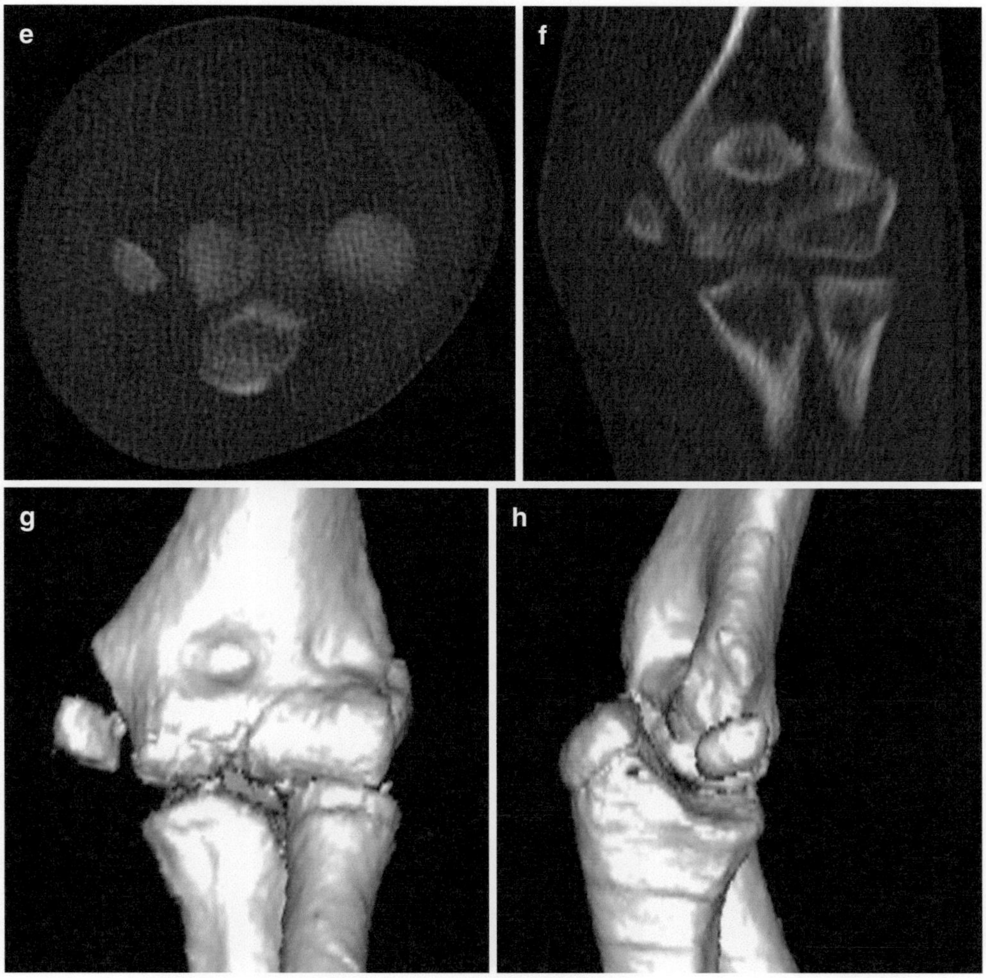

Fig. 3.4 (**e**–**h**) CT cross-section, coronal reconstruction, and three-dimensional reconstruction show that the humerus was displaced forward, inward, and downward, and the epiphysis line was widened

4.3. MR scan (Fig. 3.4i, j)

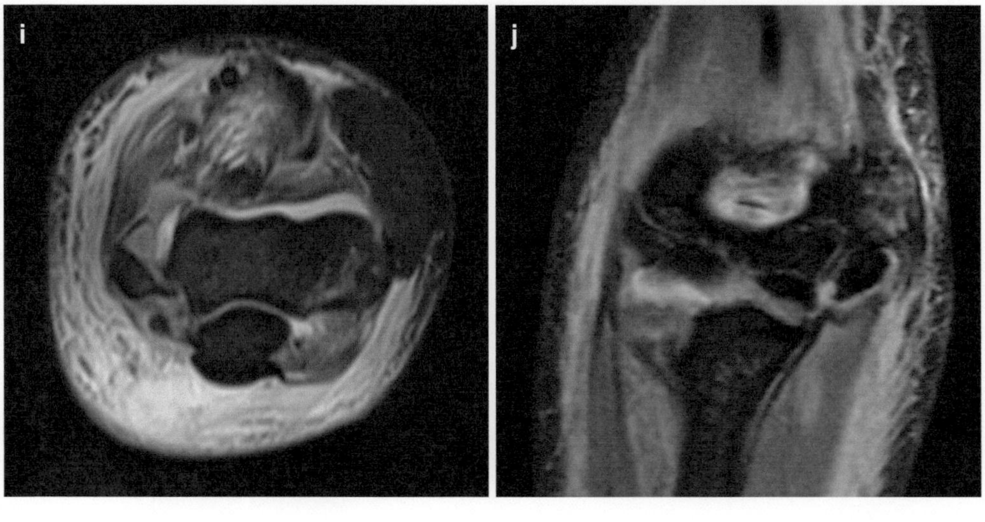

Fig. 3.4 (**i**, **j**) MR cross-section T2WI and coronal T2WI show that the humeral medial epicondyle was displaced forward, inward, and downward, and shows the surrounding soft tissue edema

5. Identification of the third degree separation of the medial epicondyle and the intra-articular loose body in the humerus
    5.1. X-ray film (Fig. 3.5a–d)

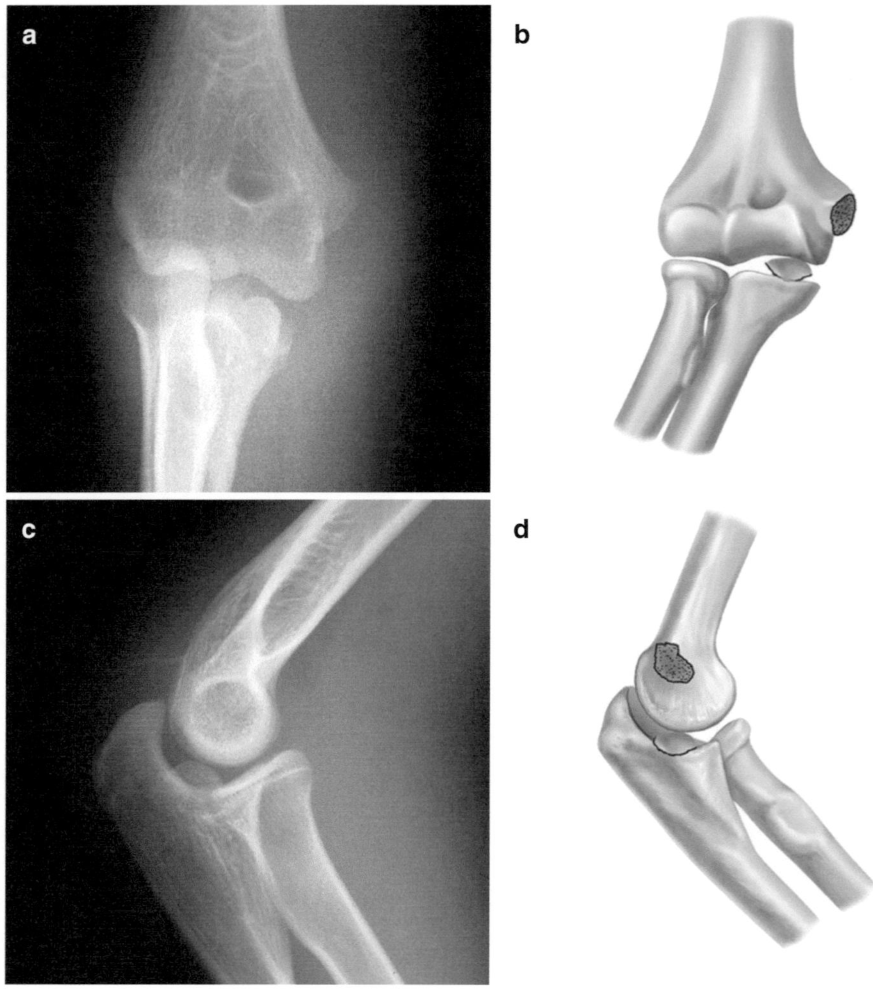

Fig. 3.5 Identification of the third degree separation of the medial epicondyle and the intra-articular loose body in the humerus. (**a**) CX line shows the defect of the medial epicondyle of the humerus; the half-moon shape of the bone in the humeroulnar joint should not be misdiagnosed as the loose body in the joint, the elbow joint components' relative position is abnormal; (**b**, **d**) Schematic

5.2. CT scan (Fig. 3.5e–j)

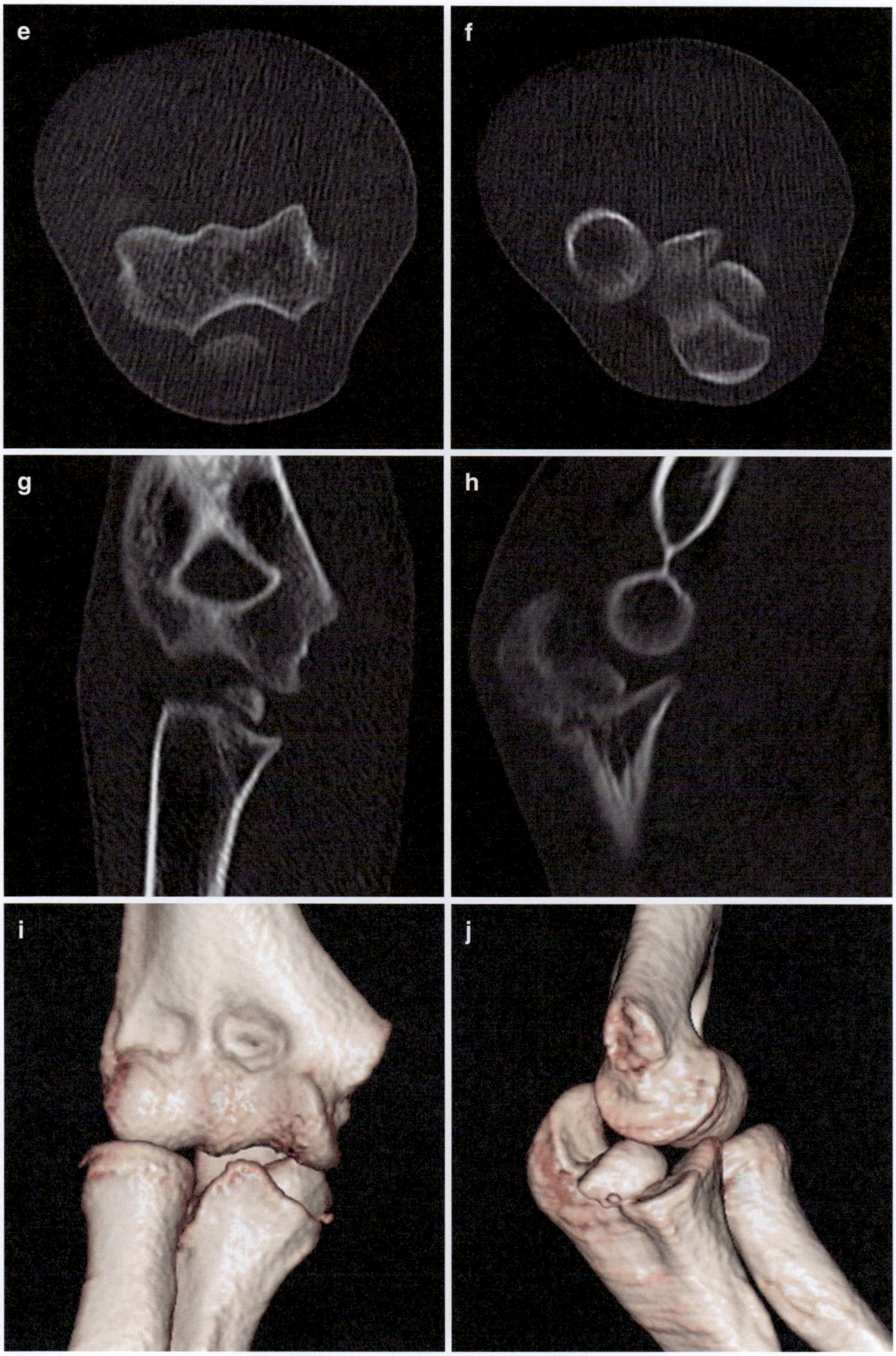

Fig. 3.5 (e–j) CT cross-section, coronal reconstruction, sagittal reconstruction, and three-dimensional reconstruction of the medial epicondyle of the humerus, the fracture end is obviously displaced, inserted in the humeroulnar joint space, elbow subluxation

6. Identification of the impaction fracture of the humerus supracondylar ridge with the linear fracture
   6.1. X-ray film (Fig. 3.6a–d)

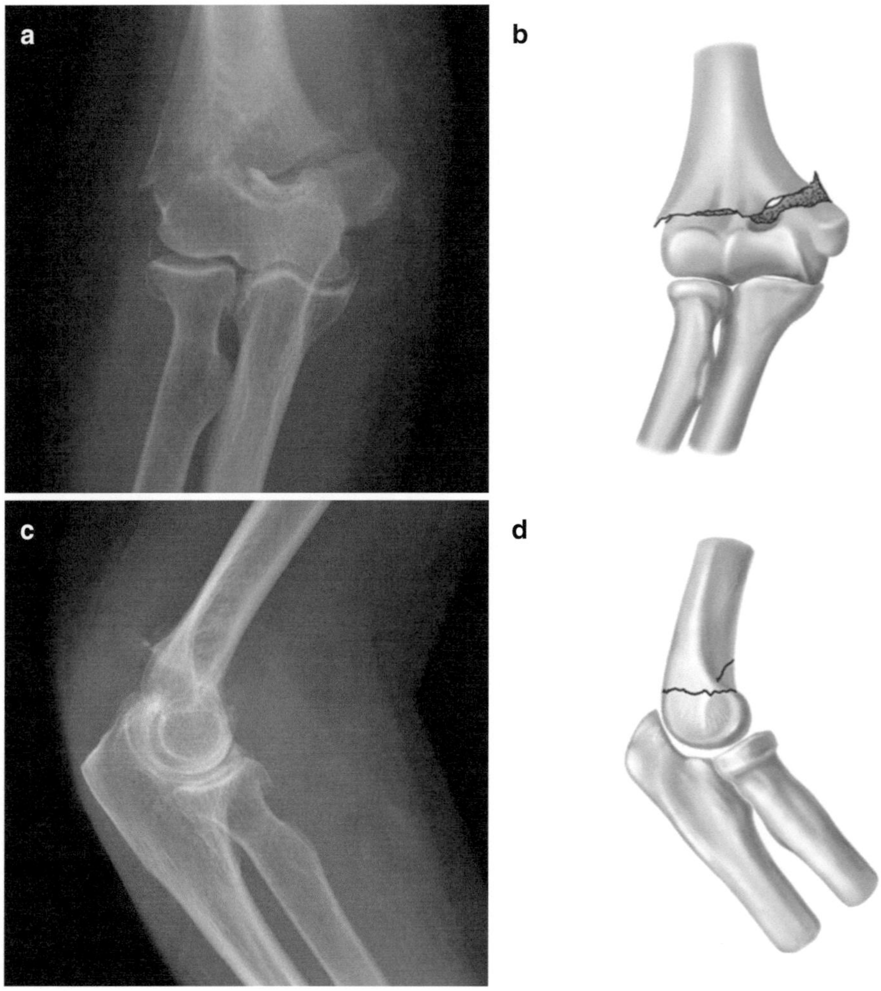

Fig. 3.6 Identification of the impaction fracture of the humerus supracondylar ridge with the linear fracture. (**a**, **c**) X line shows the transverse linear fracture on the humerus supracondylar ridge, the displacement of the broken end is not obvious; (**b**, **d**) Schematic

   6.2. CT scan (Fig. 3.6e, f)

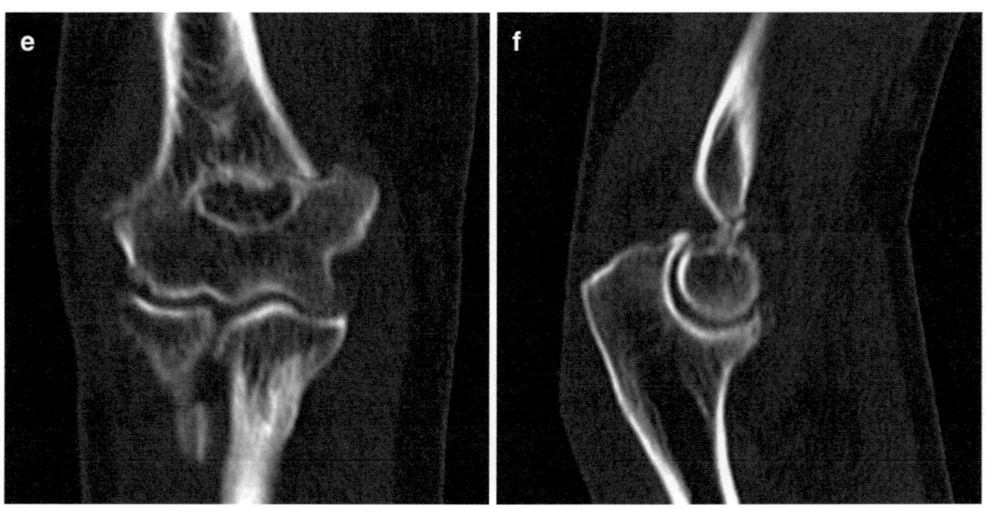

Fig. 3.6 (**e**, **f**) CT coronal reconstruction and sagittal reconstruction of the humerus supracondylar ridge, the transverse linear fracture. The proximal fracture part inserted into the distal part

7. Identification of supracondylar fracture of the humerus with the suspicious fracture
   7.1. X-ray film (Fig. 3.7a–d)

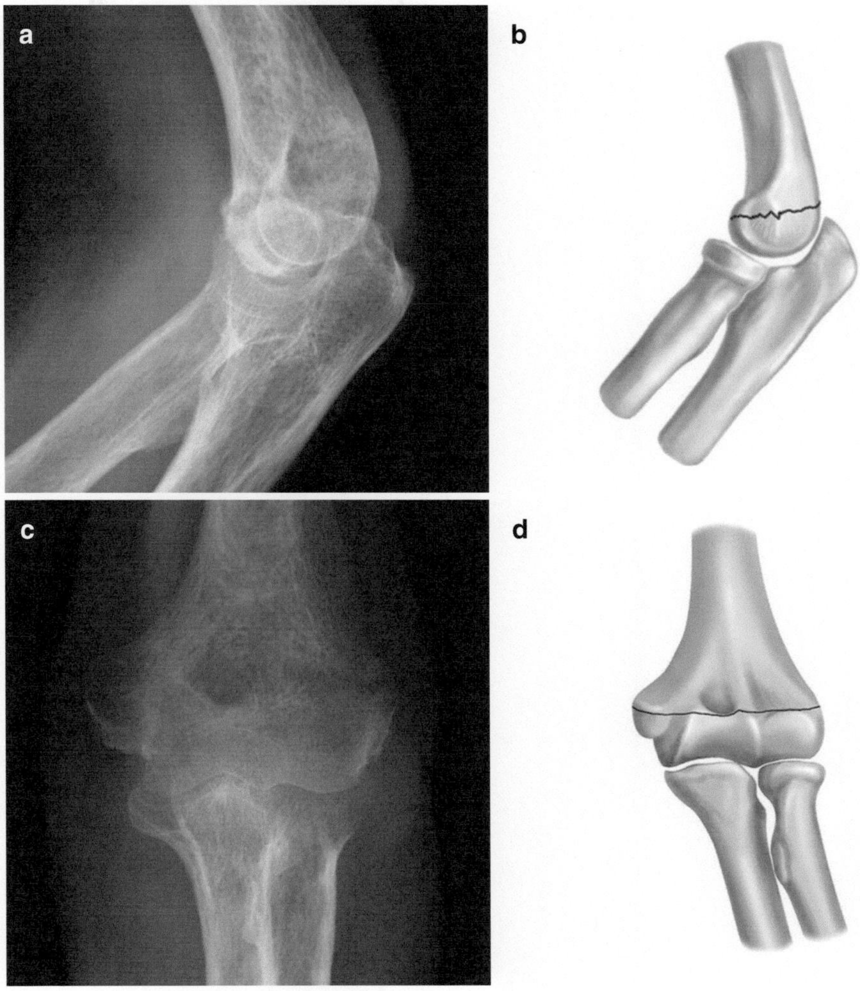

Fig. 3.7 Identification of supracondylar fracture of the humerus with the suspicious fracture. (**a**, **c**) X-ray shows obvious osteoporosis of the elbow joint bones, trabecular bone trabecular structure disarranged, suspicious fracture; (**b**, **d**) Schematic

   7.2. CT scan (Fig. 3.7e, f)

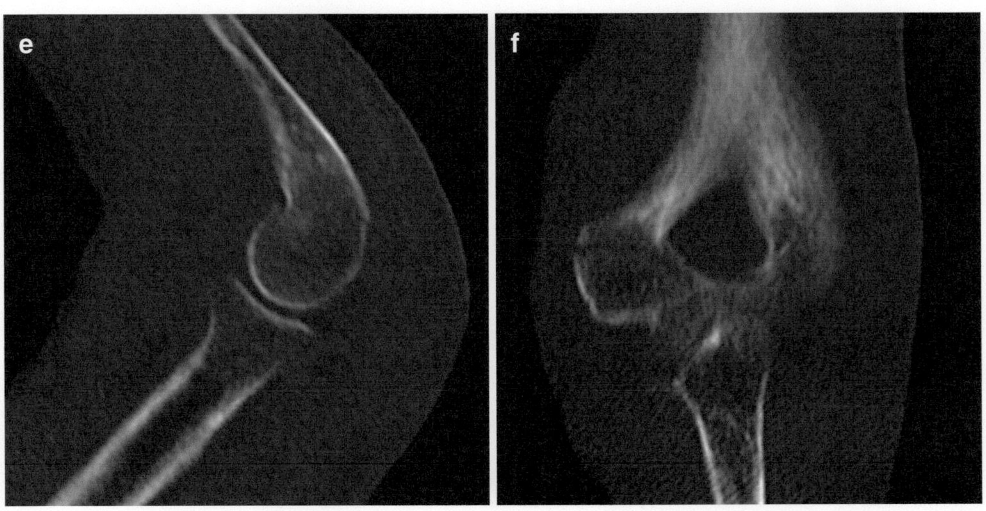

Fig. 3.7 (**e**, **f**) CT sagittal reconstruction and coronal reconstruction showed elbow joint osteoporosis is obvious, fracture of the humerus supracondylar ridge, the fracture end is slightly inserted, and the fracture line is not involved in the articular surface

8. Comparison X-ray films with CT of comminuted fracture of the humerus supracondylar
   8.1. X-ray film (Fig. 3.8a–d)

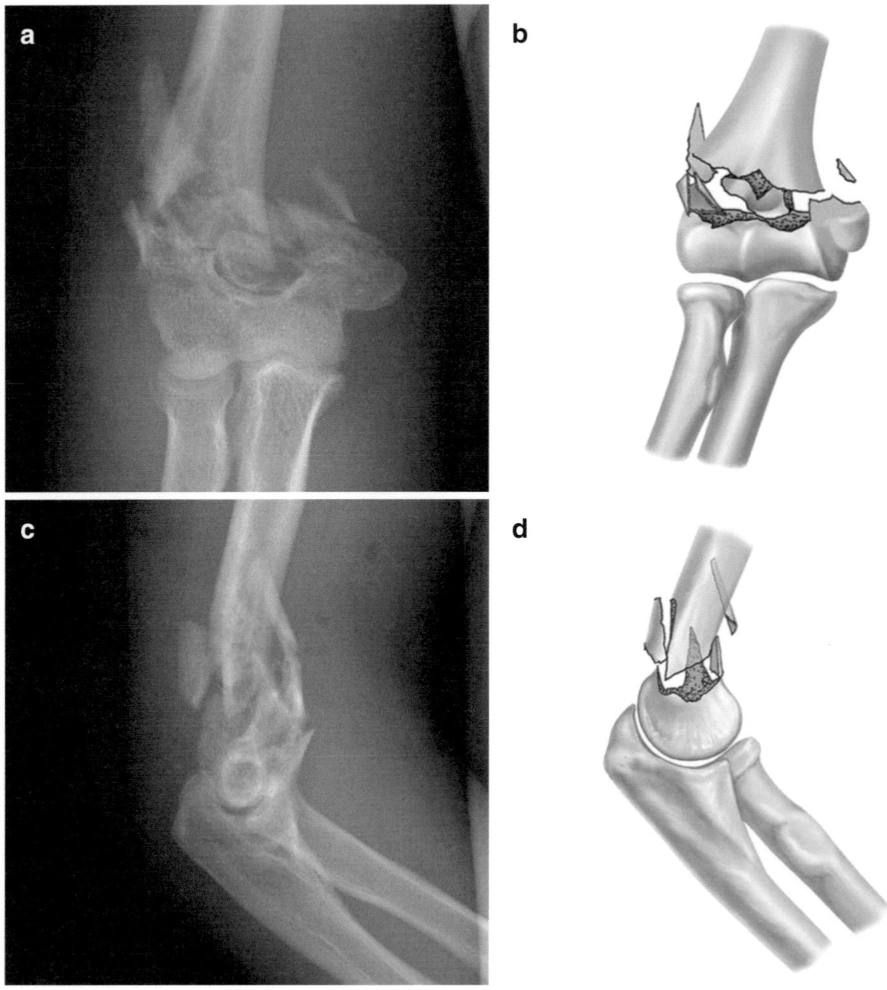

Fig. 3.8 Comparison of X-ray films with CT of comminuted fracture of the humerus supracondylar. (**a**, **c**) X-ray shows bone fracture of the humerus supracondylar ridge, dislocation of the broken end, angular deformity; (**b**, **d**) Schematic

   8.2. CT scan (Fig. 3.8e, f)

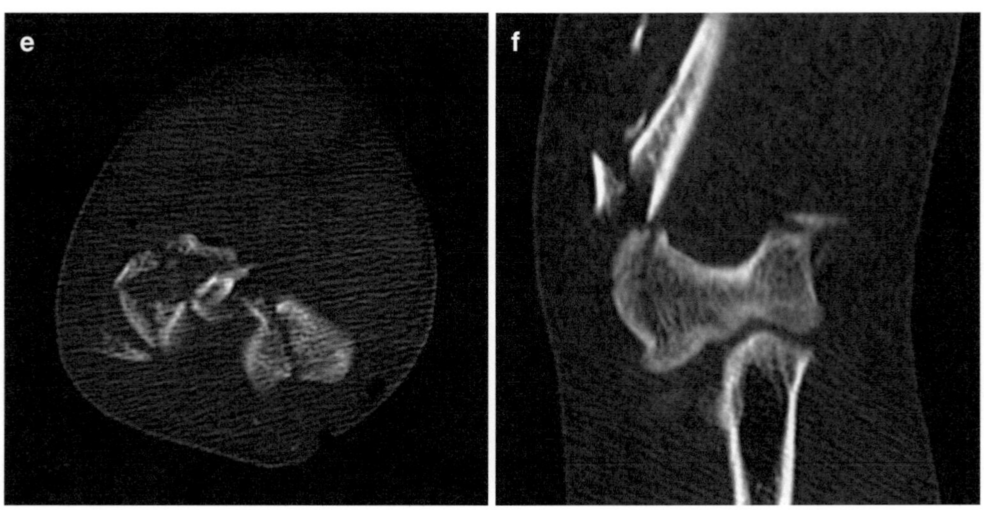

Fig. 3.8 (**e**, **f**) CT cross-section and coronal reconstruction showed fracture of the humerus supracondylar, dislocation, angled, fracture does not involve the articular surface, soft tissue swelling, visible gas density shadow

9. Identification of the lateral condylar sagittal fracture with the lateral epicondyle fracture
   9.1. X-ray film (Fig. 3.9a–d)

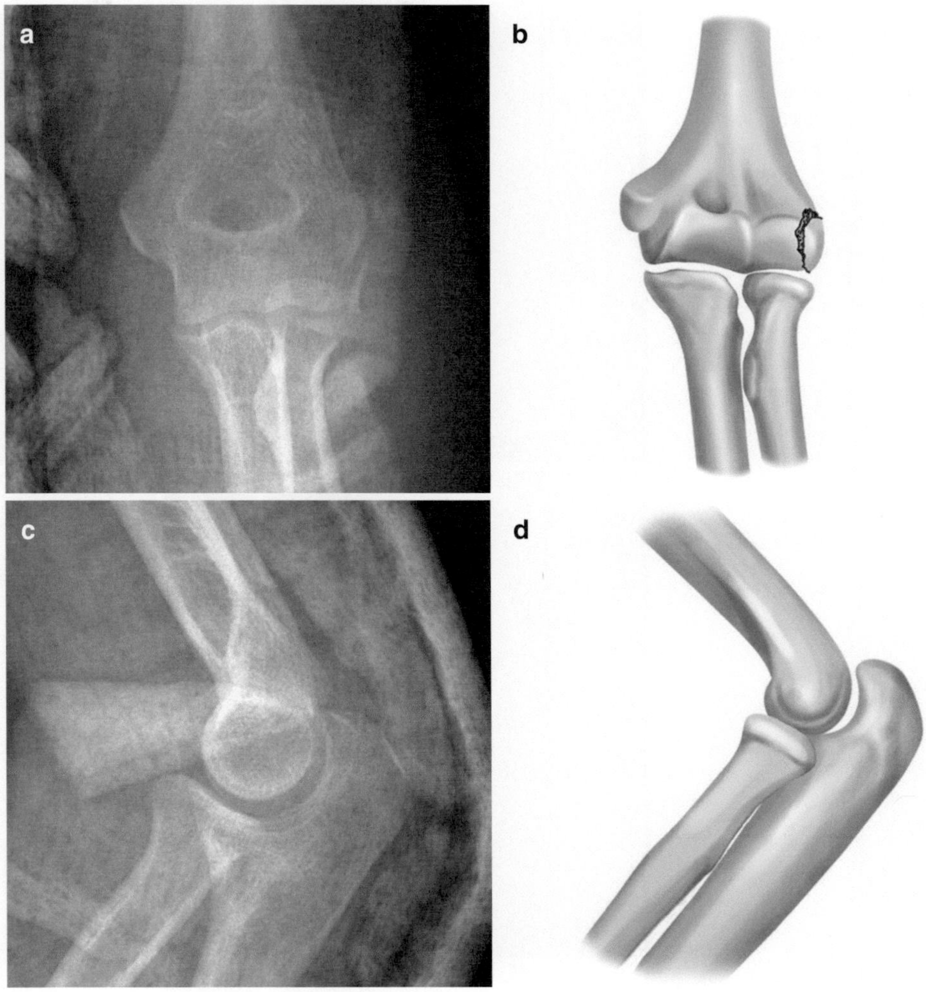

Fig. 3.9 Identification of the lateral condylar sagittal fracture with the lateral epicondyle fracture. (**a**, **c**) X-ray shows longitudinal fragment's shadow on the outer edge of the humerus lateral condyle, the fracture line involves the articular surface, the lateral epicondylar is normal; (**b**, **d**) Schematic

9.2. CT scan (Fig. 3.9e–h)

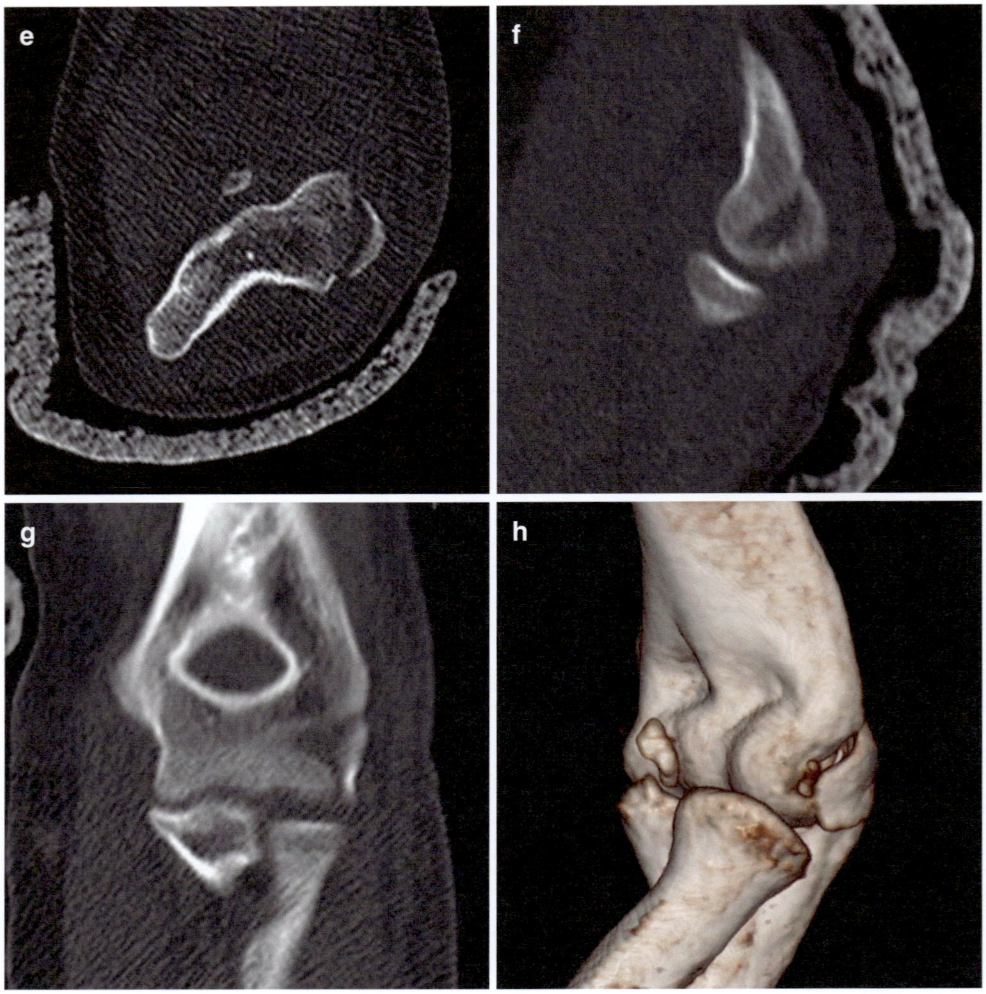

Fig. 3.9 (**e–h**) CT cross-section, sagittal reconstruction, coronal reconstruction, and three-dimensional reconstruction showed a sagittal fracture of the lateral condylar of the humerus. The bone piece was curved, the fracture line involved the lateral condyle joint surface of the humerus, and the ulnar coronoid process was irregular

10. Identification of the comminuted lateral humerus condyle fracture with simple linear fracture
    10.1. X-ray film (Fig. 3.10a–d)

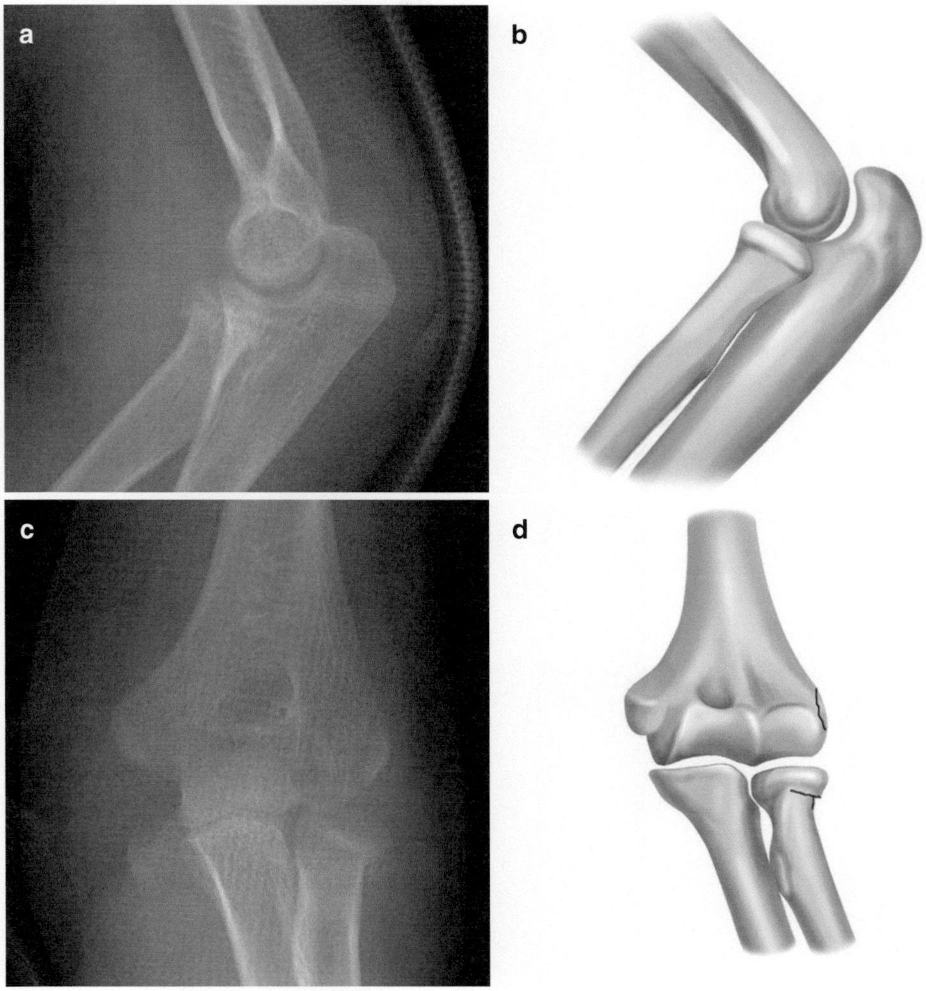

Fig. 3.10 Identification of the comminuted lateral humeral condyle fracture with simple linear fracture. (**a**, **c**) X-ray shows that the outer edge of the humerus lateral condyle is like a longitudinal translucent shadow, the head of radius is inclined to the outside, the outer edge of the radial neck is broken, slightly inserted; (**b**, **d**) Schematic

    10.2. CT scan (Fig. 3.10e, f)

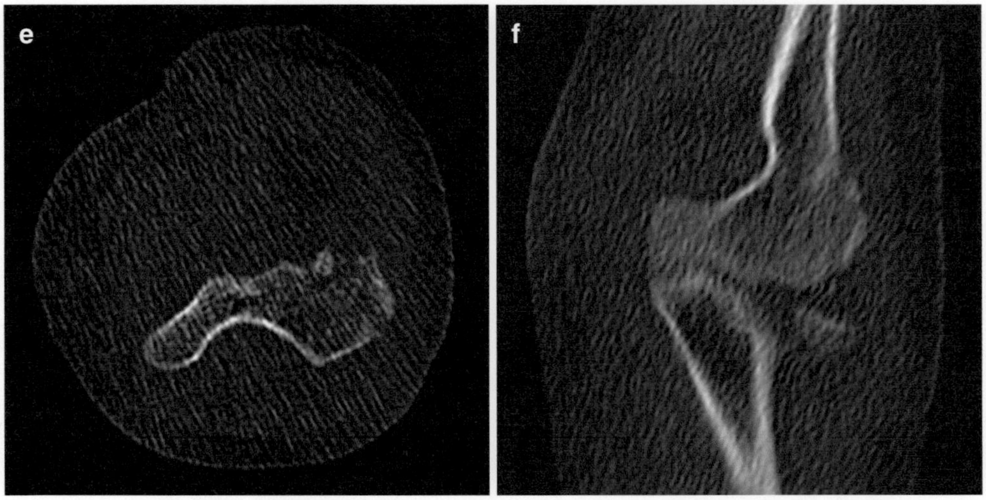

Fig. 3.10 (**e**, **f**) CT cross-section and coronal reconstruction showed that the outer edge of the lateral condyle humerus was fractured, and multiple bone fragments were seen. The fracture line involved the articular surface

11. Identification of sagittal comminuted fractures and linear fractures of the lateral condyle
    11.1. X-ray film (Fig. 3.11a–d)

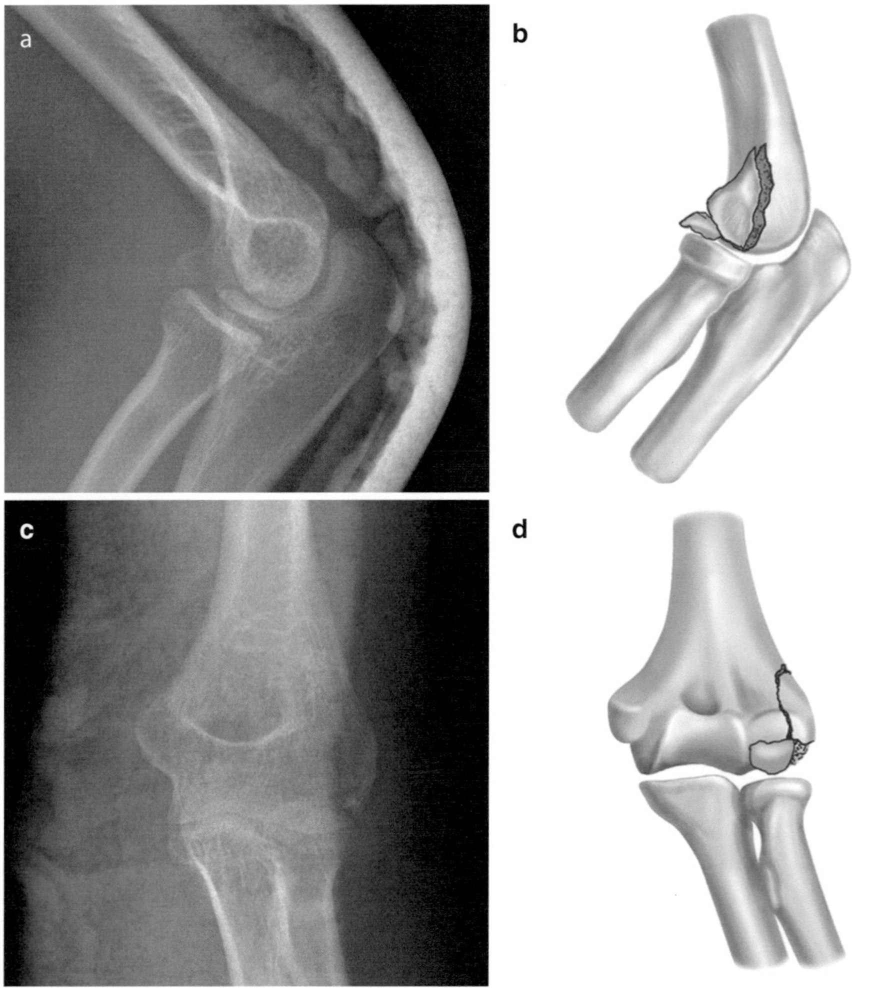

Fig. 3.11 Identification of sagittal comminuted fractures and linear fractures of the lateral condyle. (**a**, **c**) X-ray shows irregular outer edge of the humerus lateral condyle, bone formation in front of the humerus condyle; (**b**, **d**) Schematic

11.2. CT scan (Fig. 3.11e–h)

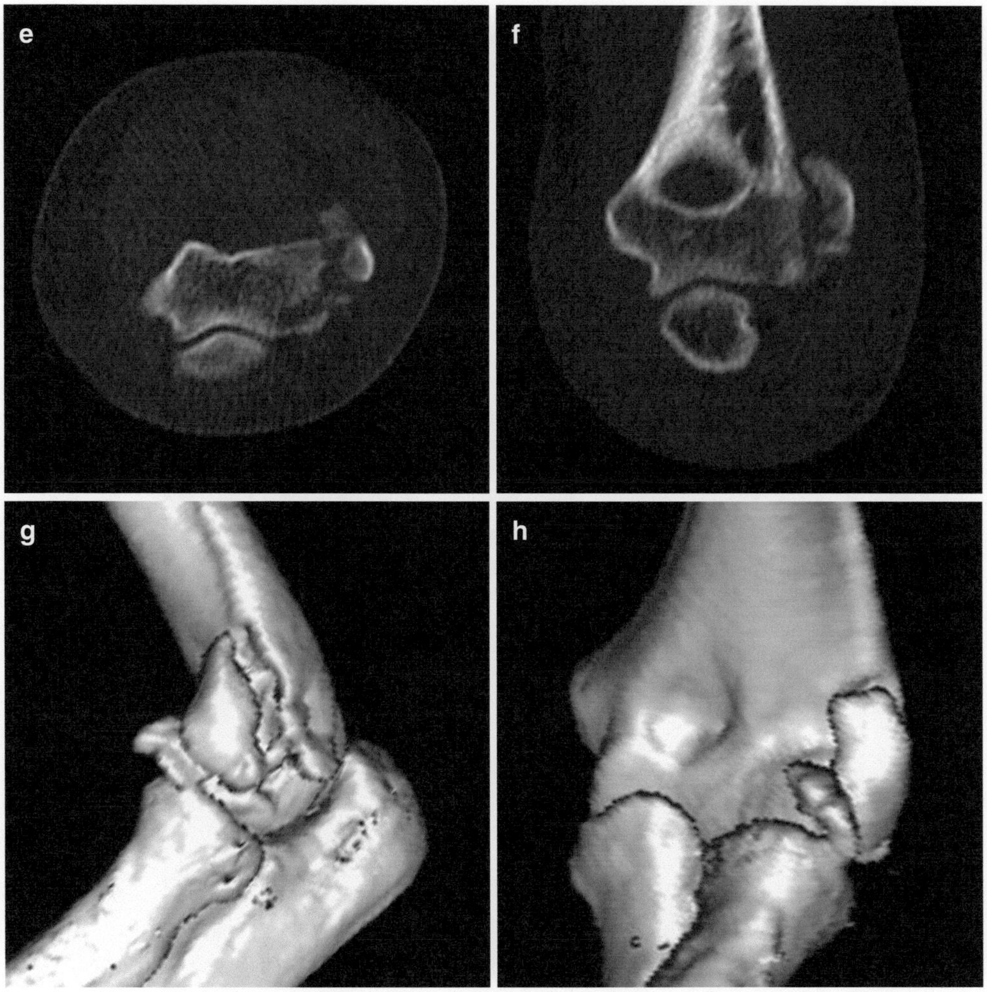

Fig. 3.11 (**e**–**h**) CT cross-section, coronal reconstruction, and three-dimensional reconstruction showing the fragmentation of humeral lateral condyle, visible multiple bone shadows, fracture lines involving the articular surface

12. Identification of sagittal comminuted fractures and linear fractures of the lateral condyle
    12.1. X-ray film (Fig. 3.12a–d)

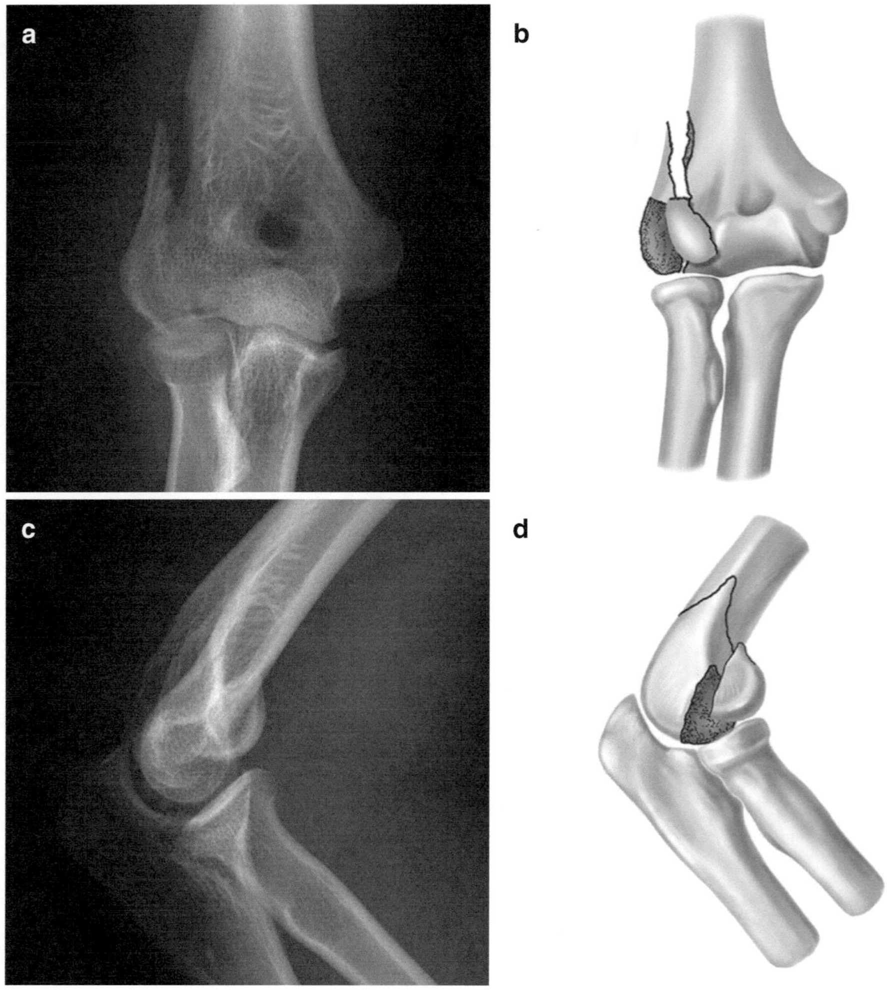

Fig. 3.12 Identification of sagittal comminuted fractures and linear fractures of the lateral condyle. (**a**, **c**) X-ray shows longitudinal fracture of the lateral humerus condyle, fracture line involving the articular surface, there is a dislocation; (**b**, **d**) Schematic

    12.2. CT scan (Fig. 3.12e, f)

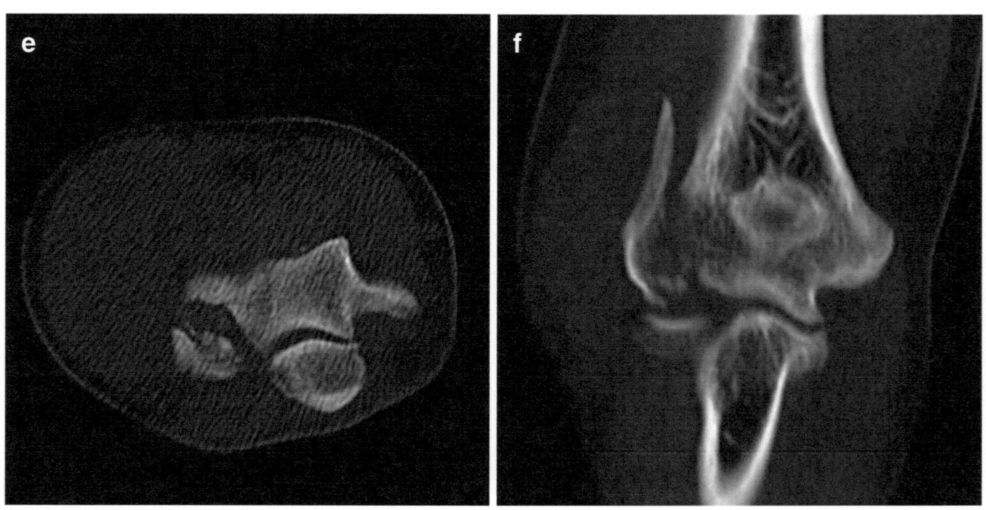

Fig. 3.12 (**e**, **f**) CT cross-section, coronal reconstruction showed humeral lateral condyle longitudinal fracture, humerus lateral condyle articular surface fracture, articular surface collapse

13. Identification of the coronal humerus lateral condyle comminuted fracture with the linear fracture
    13.1. X-ray film (Fig. 3.13a–d)

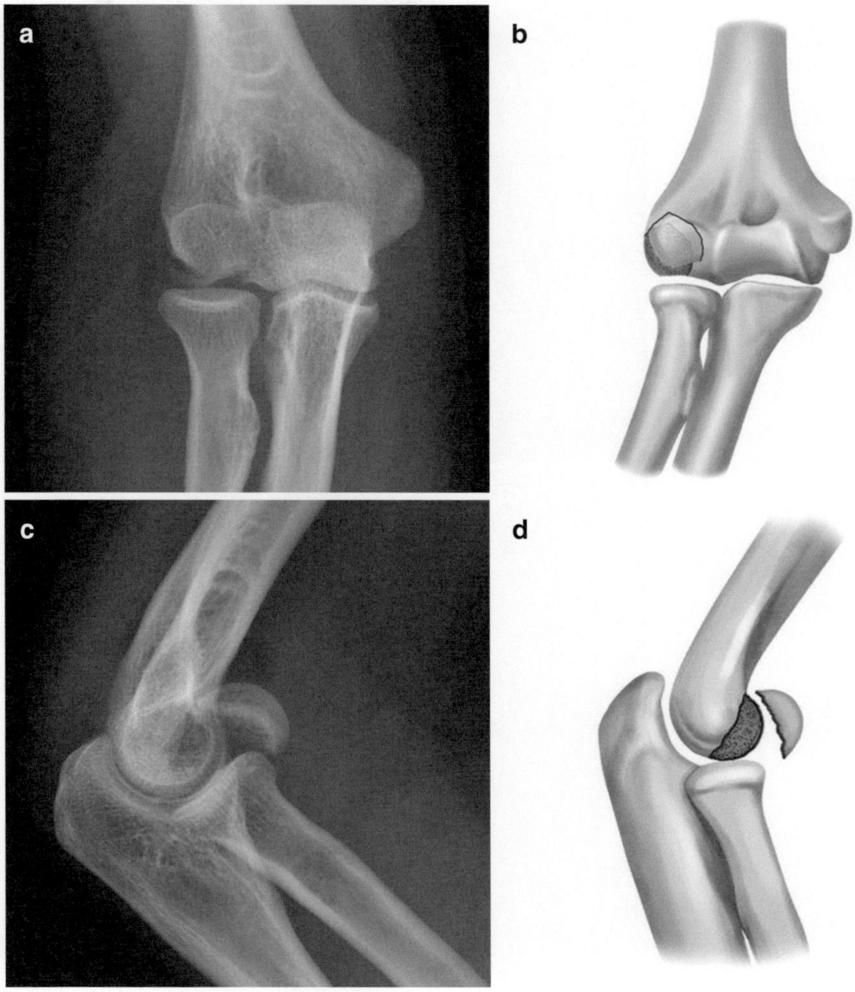

Fig. 3.13 Identification of the humerus lateral condyle comminuted fracture with the linear fracture. (**a**, **c**) X-ray shows an elliptical overlapping shadow at the humeral capitulum, the articular surface is discontinuous, and the lateral humeral capitulum coronal fracture block is semi-circular, rotating upward and forward; (**b**, **d**) Schematic

13.2. CT scan (Fig. 3.13e–h)

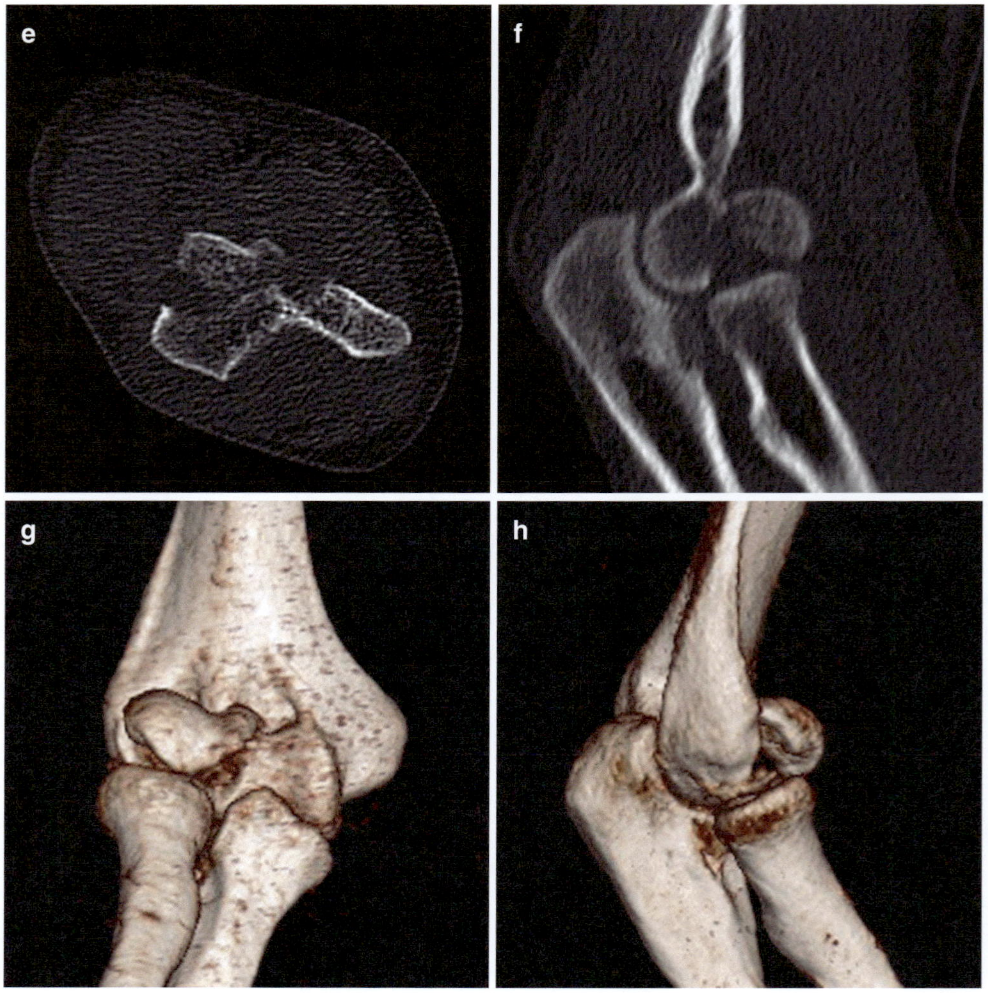

Fig. 3.13 (**e**–**h**) CT cross-section, sagittal reconstruction, and three-dimensional reconstruction showed 1/2 coronal split across the humeral capitulum. The anterior bone was rotated forward and upward. The fracture line was widened and small bones were visible. The fracture line involved the lateral edge of the humerus trochlea

14. Identification of the distal humeral coronal comminuted fracture with the linear fracture
    14.1. X-ray film (Fig. 3.14a–d)

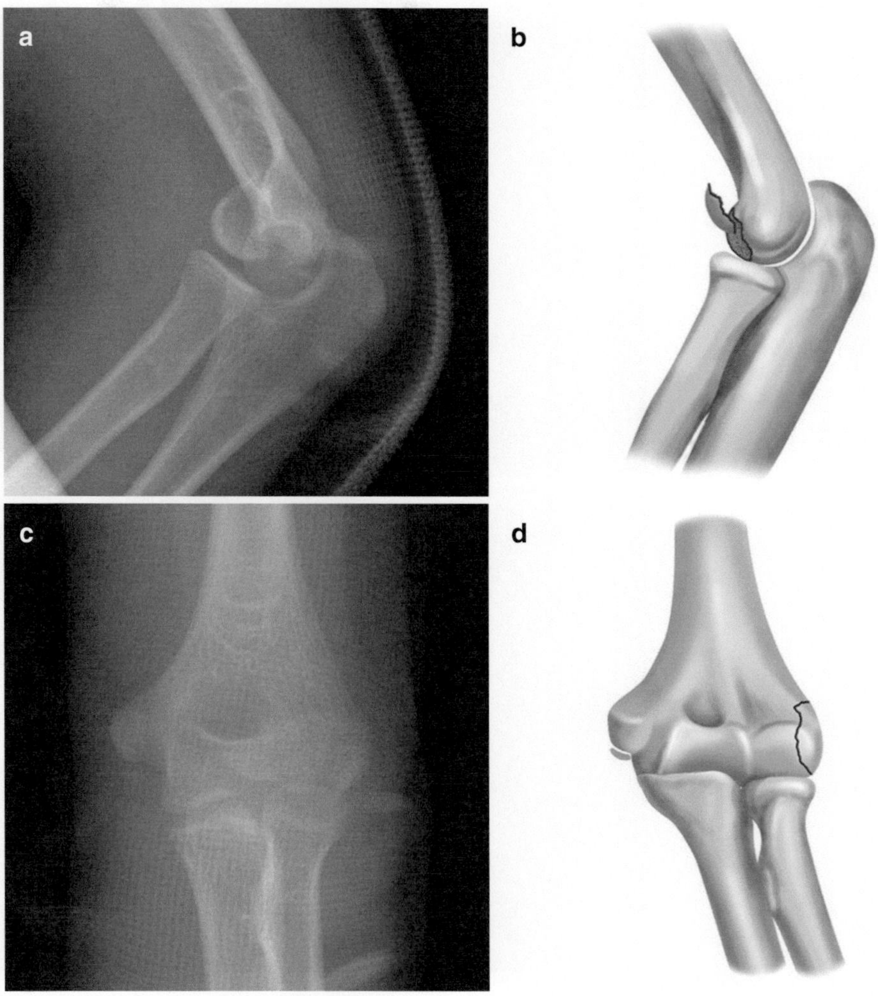

Fig. 3.14 Identification of the distal humeral coronal comminuted fracture with the linear fracture. (**a**, **c**) Anterior–posterior X-ray shows that the irregular bone segments can be seen on the overlap of humerus lateral condyle, the bone fragments can be seen under the medial epicondyle of the humerus. In the lateral view, humerus lateral coronal fracture, the fracture fragment is displaced upward; (**b**, **d**) Schematic

14.2. CT scan (Fig. 3.14e–h)

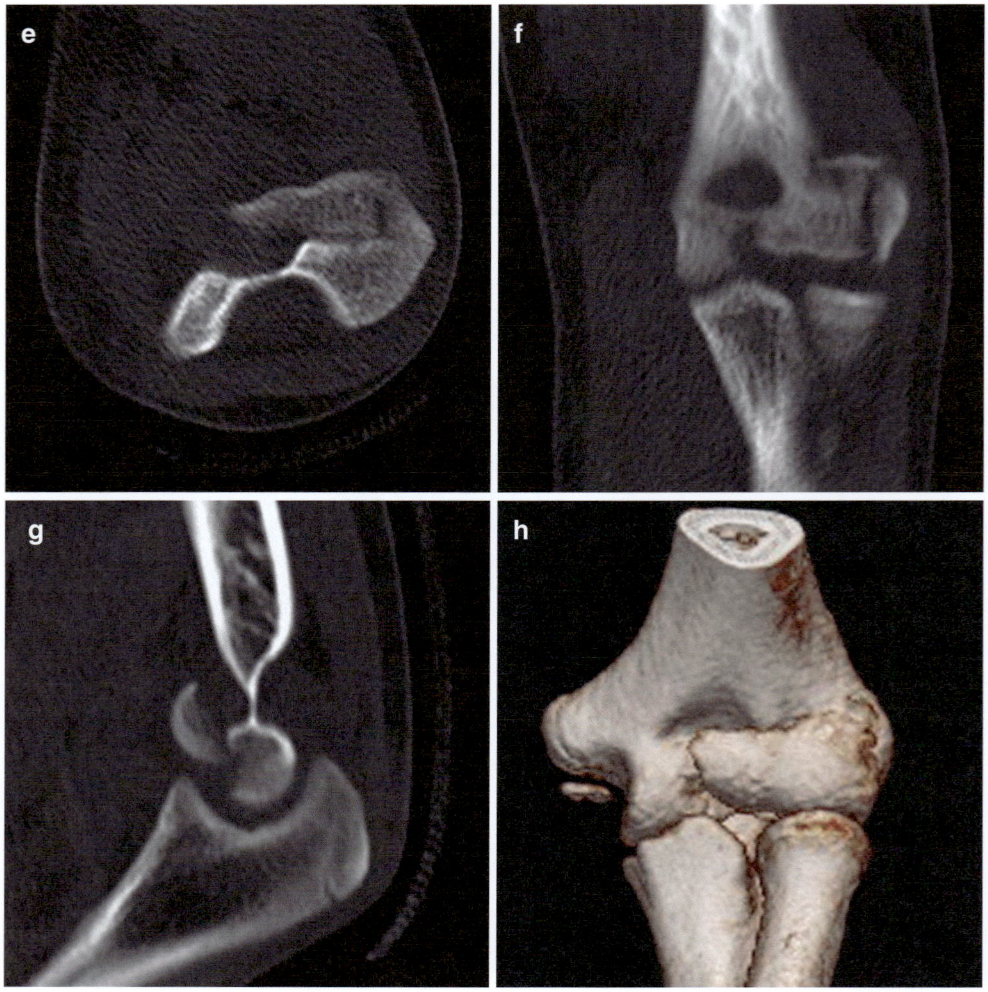

Fig. 3.14 (**e**–**h**) CT cross-section, coronal reconstruction, sagittal reconstruction, and three-dimensional reconstruction showed that comminuted fracture at the anterior distal humerus coronal, visible multiple fragments, fracture line involving the humerus trochlea, upward displaced fragment, another fragment can be seen under the humerus medial epicondyle

15. Identification of the distal humerus intra-articular comminuted fracture with the partial intra-articular fracture
    15.1. X-ray film (Fig. 3.15a–d)

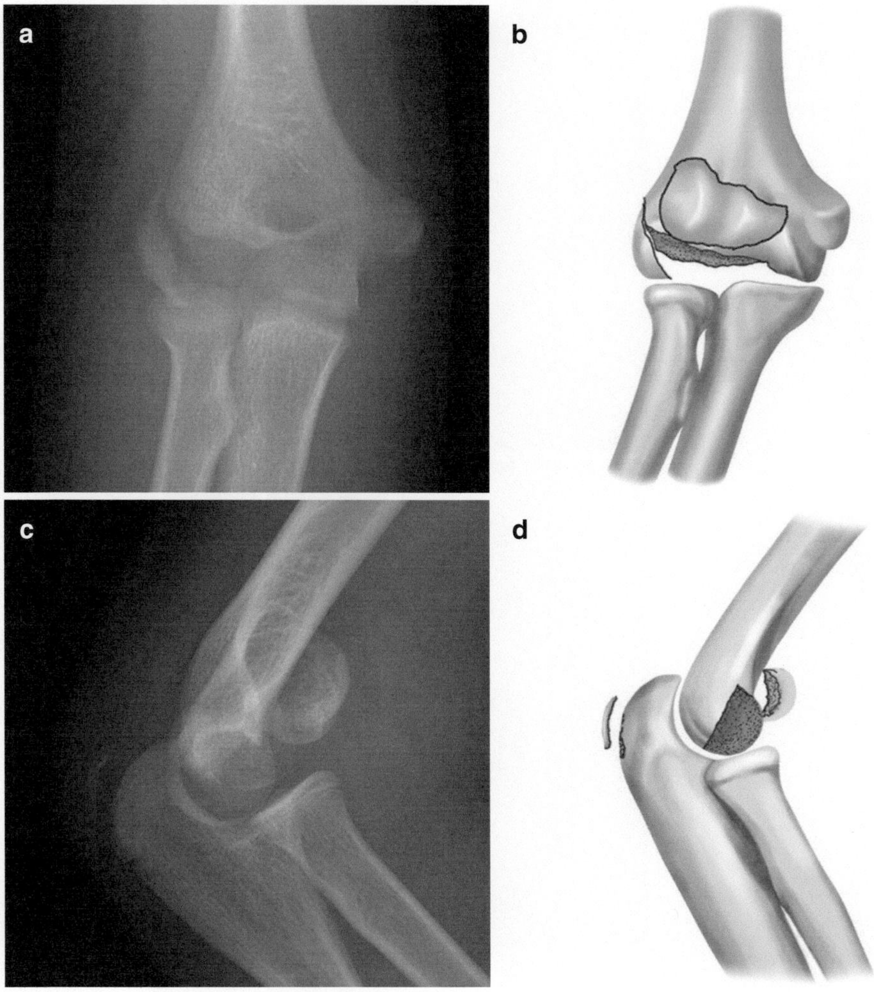

Fig. 3.15 Identification of the distal humerus intra-articular comminuted fracture with the partial intra-articular fracture. (**a**, **c**) X-ray shows fracture of the humerus lateral condyle, the fragment is displaced upward, fragment displaced anteriorly, bone fragments are visible at the olecranon; (**b**, **d**) Schematic

15.2. CT scan (Fig. 3.15e–h)

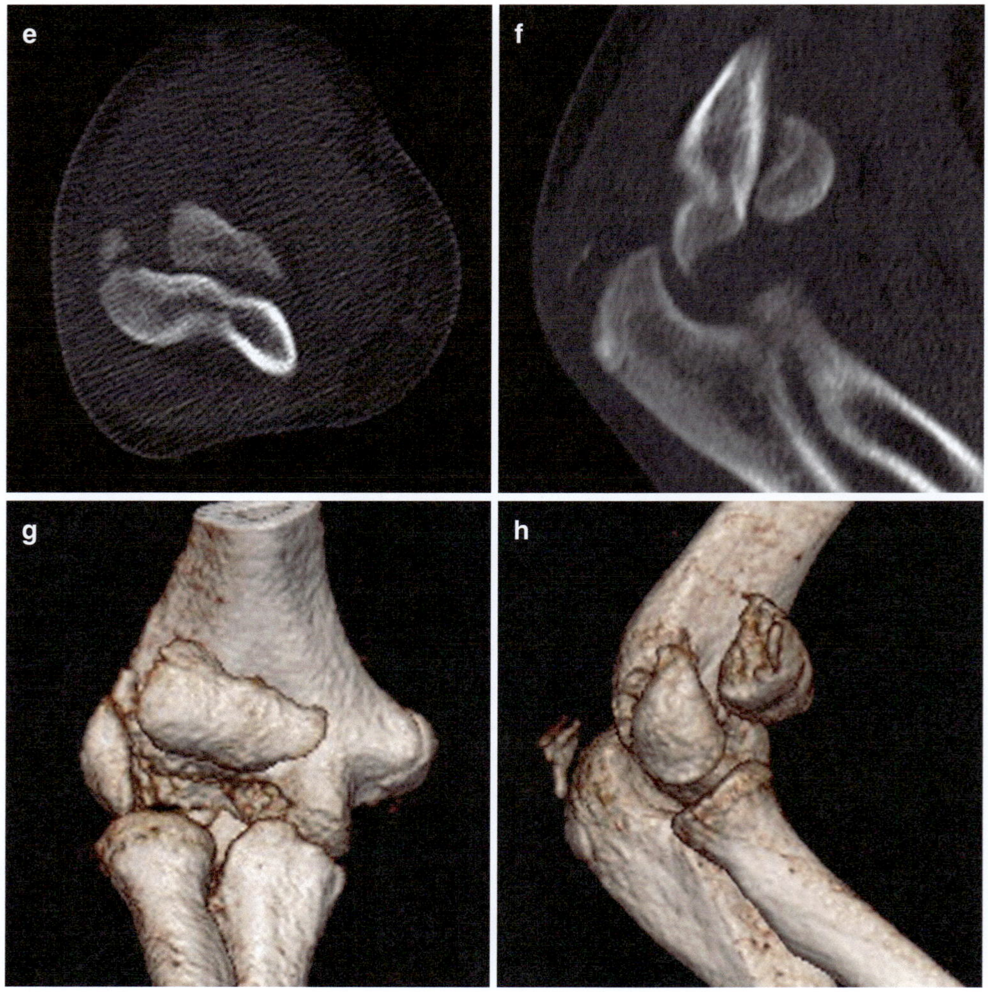

Fig. 3.15 (**e**–**h**) CT cross-section, sagittal reconstruction, and three-dimensional reconstruction showed fracture of the humerus lateral condyle and multiple fractures involved in the articular surface. Coronal and sagittal fractures were noted. The coronal fracture block was displaced upwards, involving the humerus trochlea. Another clear displaced fragment was seen at the olecranon

16. Identification of the humerus distal partial intra-articular fracture with the extra-articular fractures
    16.1. X-ray film (Fig. 3.16a–d)

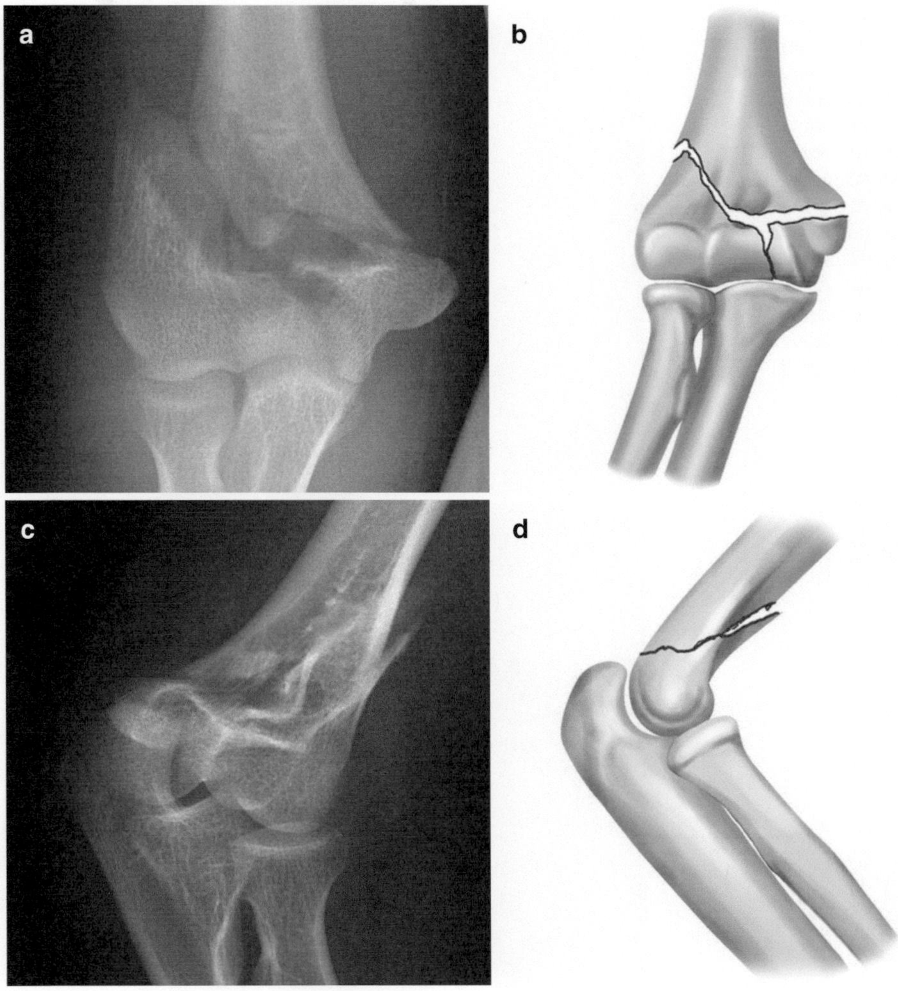

Fig. 3.16 Identification of the humerus distal partial intra-articular fracture with the extra-articular fractures. (**a**, **c**) X-ray shows the oblique fracture of the humeral condyle, dislocation, low-density radiolucent was seen at the distal humerus; (**b**, **d**) Schematic

    16.2. CT scan (Fig. 3.16e, f)

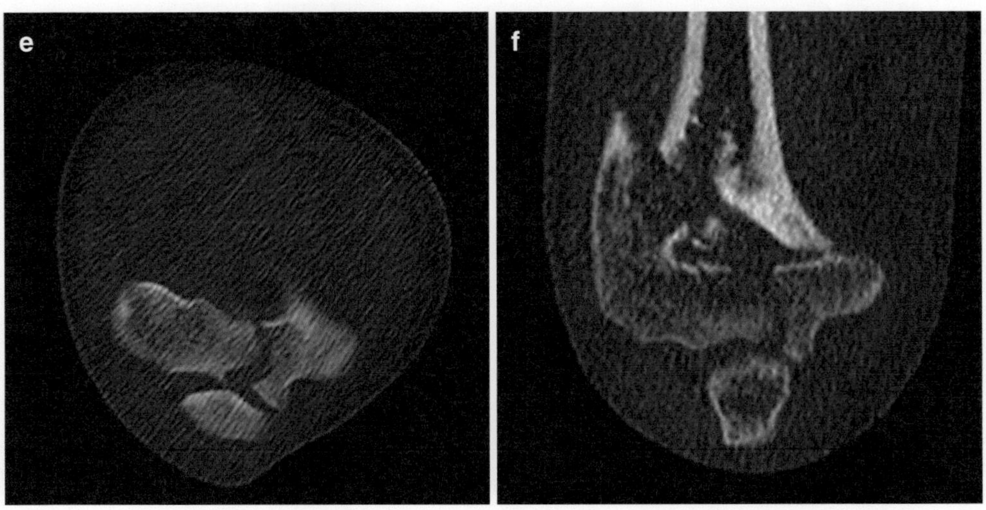

Fig. 3.16 (**e**, **f**) CT cross-section, coronal reconstruction to show the fracture at humerus supracondylar ridge, the broken end is inserted into the dislocation, the small bone shadow is visible locally, the humeral intercondylar fracture, the fracture line involves the joint surface of the trochlear, and the joint surface is slightly dislocated

17. Identification of the distal humerus partial intra-articular fracture and intra-articular comminuted fracture
    17.1. X-ray film (Fig. 3.17a–d)

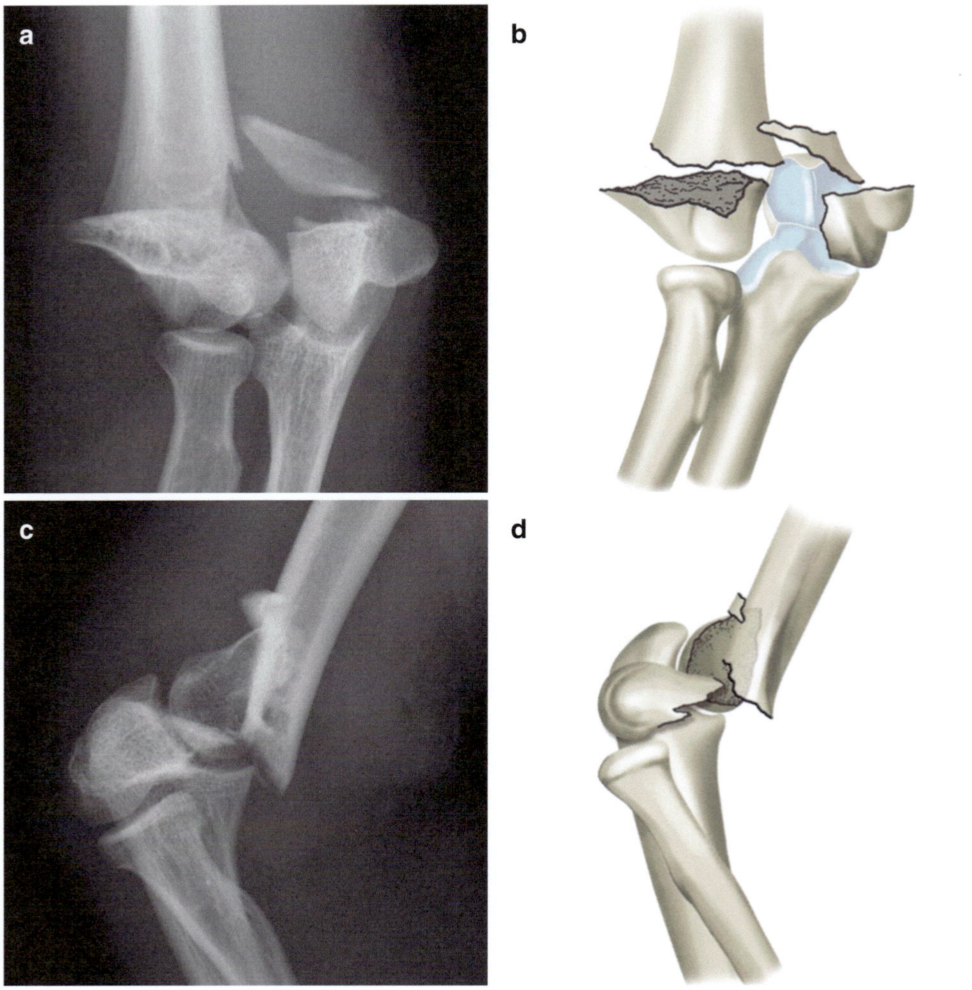

Fig. 3.17 Identification of the distal humerus partial intra-articular fracture and intra-articular comminuted fracture. (**a**, **c**) X-ray shows fracture of the humerus condyle, showing multiple bone fragments, dislocation of the broken end, angular deformity, fracture of the articular surface of the distal humerus, disarranged structure, dislocation of the articular surface; (**b**, **d**) Schematic

    17.2. CT scan (Fig. 3.17e, f)

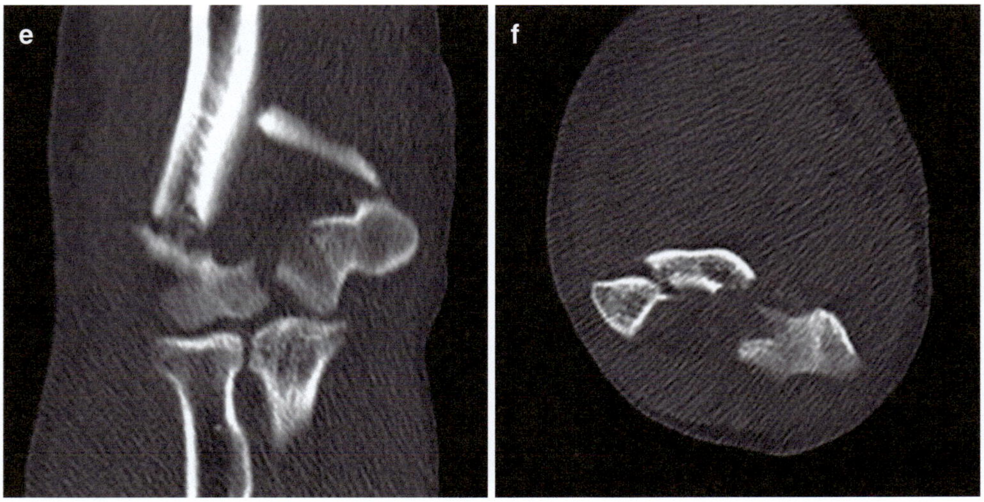

Fig. 3.17 (**e**, **f**) CT coronal reconstruction, cross-section showing dislocation of the fracture of the humerus condyle, with angulation, simple longitudinal fracture line across the inter-condyle humerus, and marked joint dislocation

18. Identification of the distal humerus partial intra-articular fracture with the intra-articular comminuted fracture
    18.1. X-ray film (Fig. 3.18a–d)

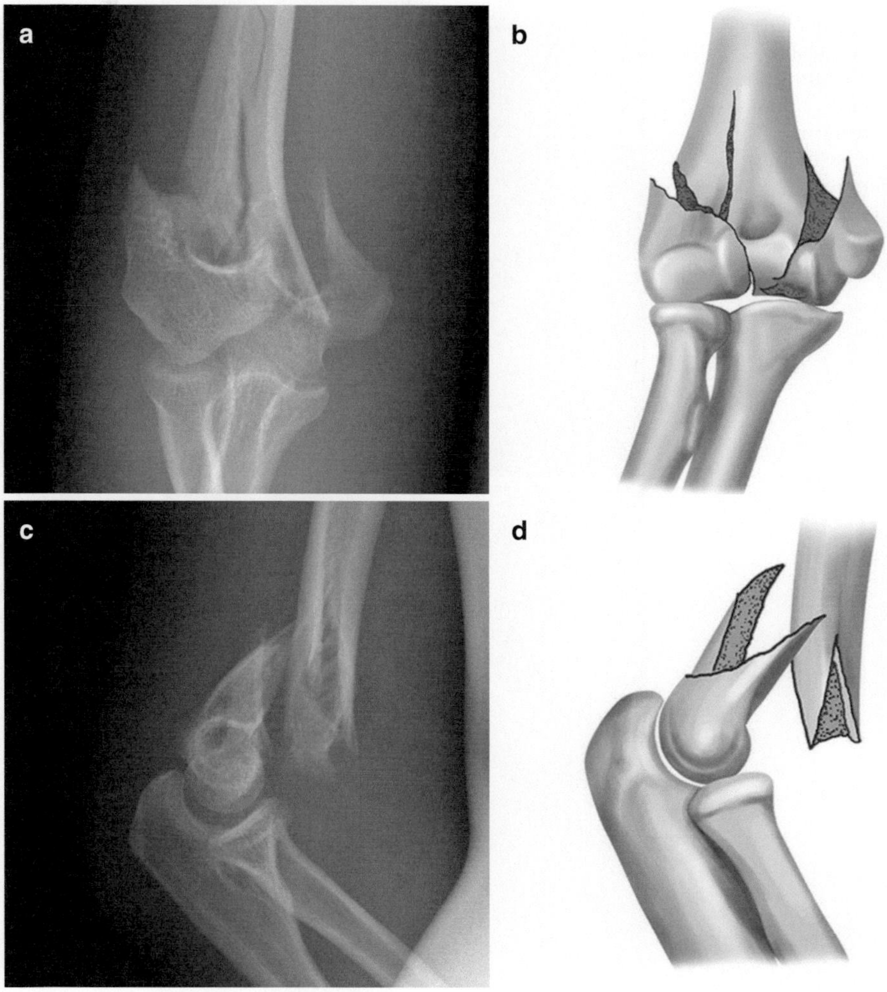

Fig. 3.18 Identification of the distal humerus partial intra-articular fracture with the intra-articular comminuted fracture. (**a**, **c**) X-ray shows fracture of the humerus condyle, showing multiple bone fragments, dislocation of the broken end, angular deformity, fracture line involving the distal articular surface of the humerus, local structural disarrangement, joint surface dislocation; (**b**, **d**) Schematic

18.2. CT scan (Fig. 3.18e–h)

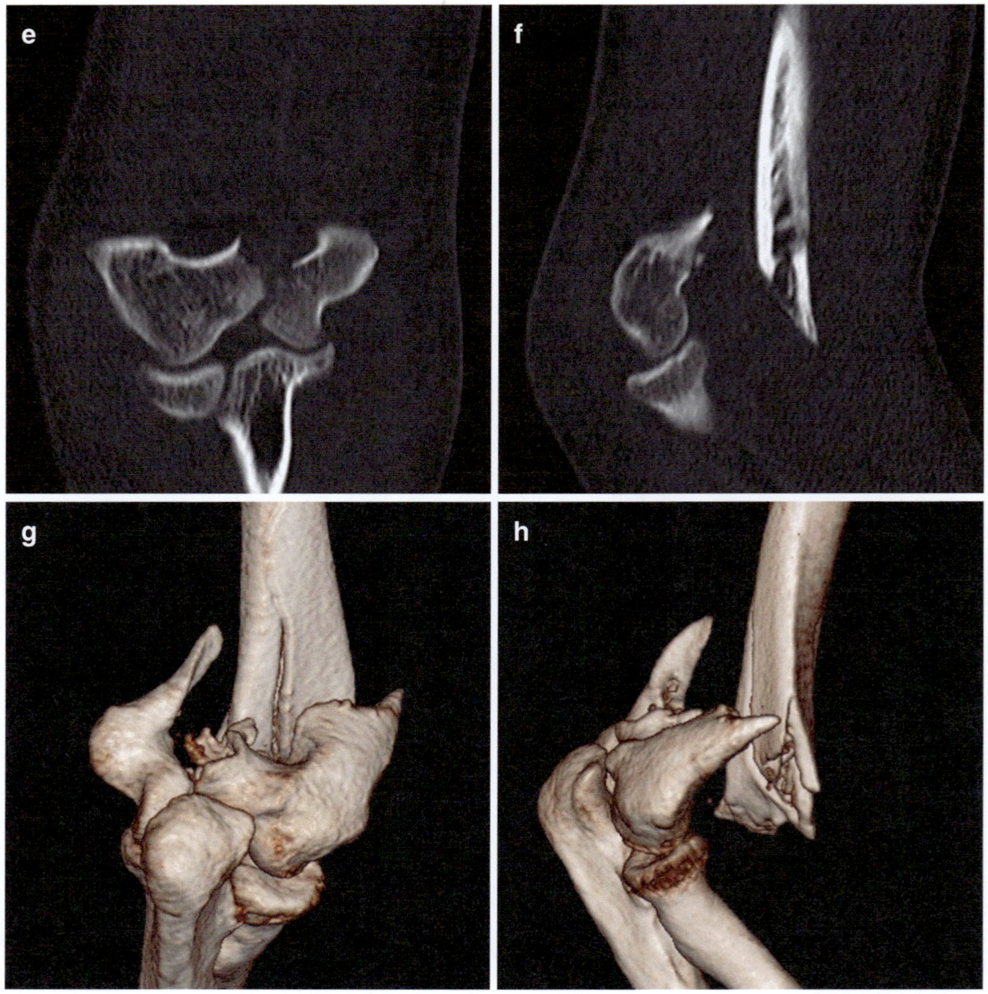

Fig. 3.18 (**e–h**) CT coronal reconstruction, sagittal reconstruction, and three-dimensional reconstruction showed humeral supracondylar fracture, dislocation of the broken end, angular deformity, longitudinal fracture of the humerus trochlea, and dislocation of the articular surface

19. Identification of the distal humerus intra-articular fracture with the intra-articular comminuted fracture
    19.1. X-ray film (Fig. 3.19a–d)

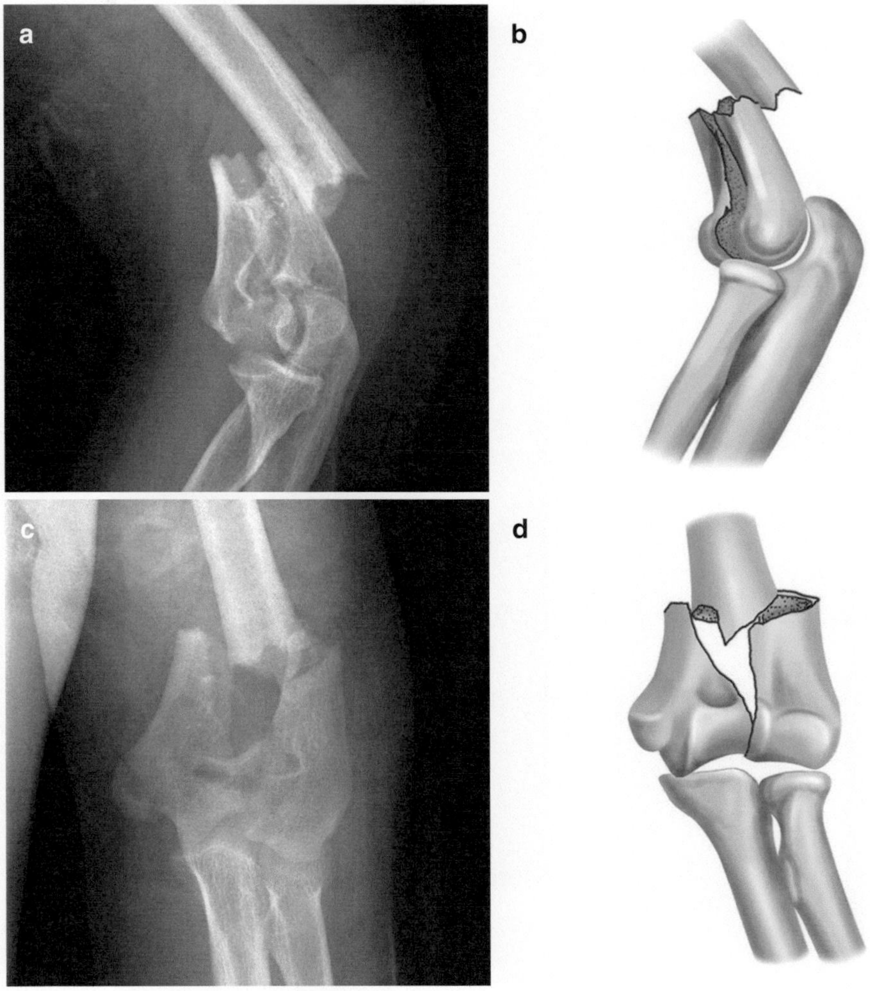

Fig. 3.19 Identification of the distal humerus intra-articular fracture with the intra-articular comminuted fracture. (**a**, **c**) X-ray shows T-shaped fracture of the distal humerus, the fracture end is distinct dislocated, the articular surface is irregular, dislocation; (**b**, **d**) Schematic

    19.2. CT scan (Fig. 3.19e, f)

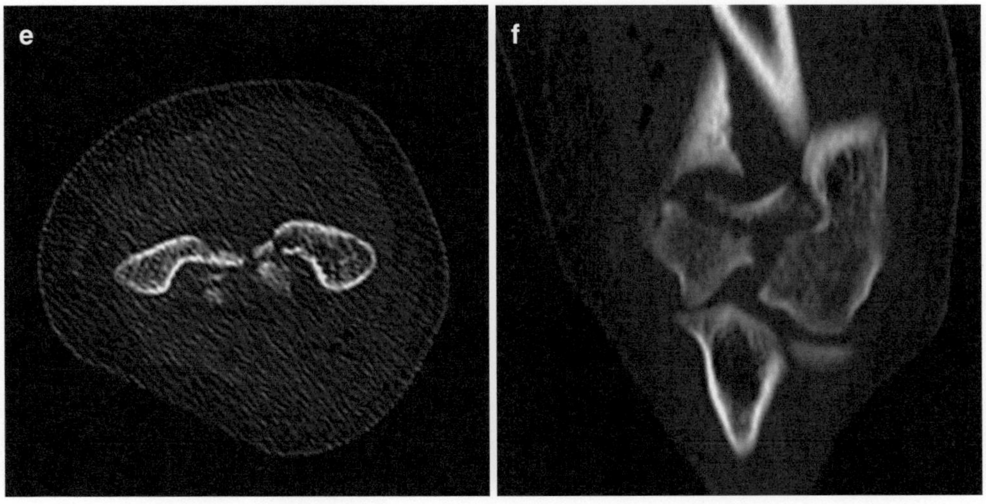

Fig. 3.19 (**e**, **f**) CT cross-section, coronal reconstruction shows the fracture of the humeral condyle, dislocation of the fracture end, longitudinal fracture line was across the humerus intra-condyle, simple fracture of the humerus trochlea, dislocation of the articular surface

20. Identification of the distal humerus intra-articular comminuted fracture with the intra-articular simple fracture
    20.1. X-ray film (Fig. 3.20a–d)

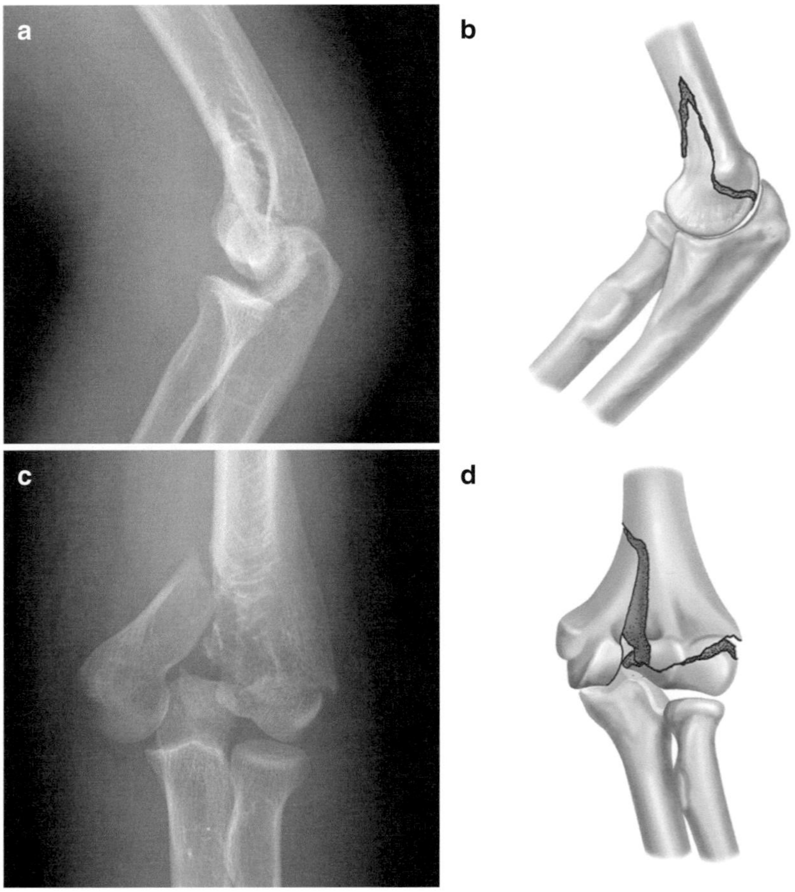

Fig. 3.20 Identification of the distal humerus intra-articular comminuted fracture with the intra-articular simple fracture. (**a**, **c**) X-ray shows fracture at the distal end of the humerus, joint surface dislocation, separated, multiple small fragments; (**b**, **d**) Schematic

20.2. CT scan (Fig. 3.20e–h)

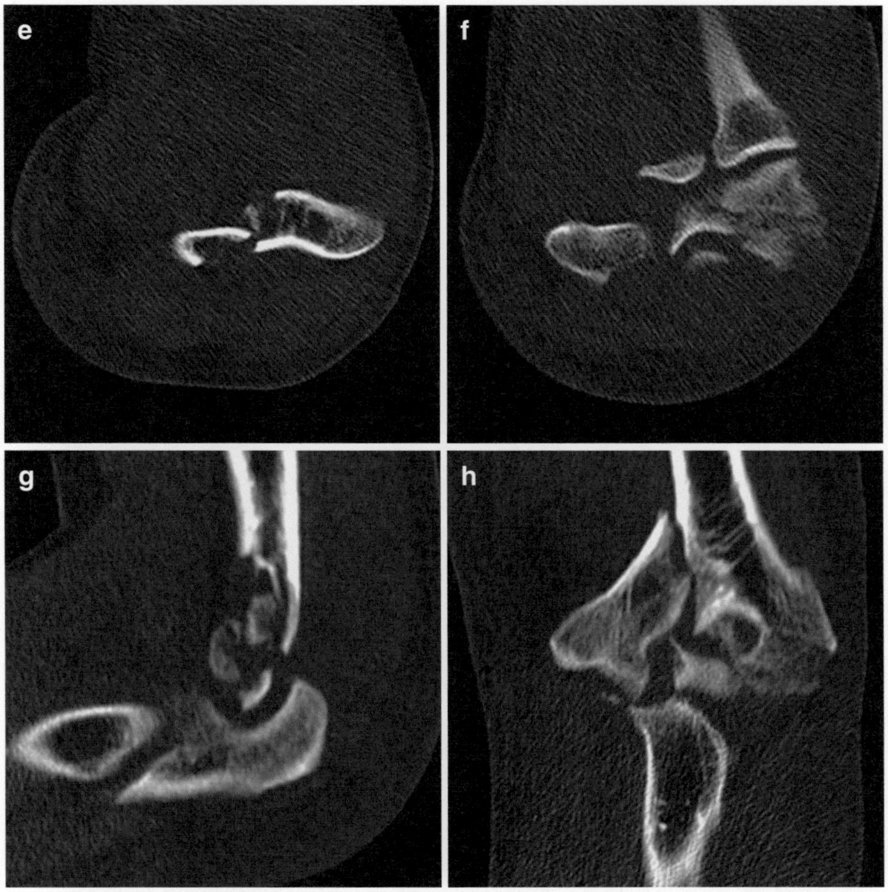

Fig. 3.20 (**e**–**h**) CT cross-section, sagittal reconstruction, and coronal reconstruction showed humeral epiphysis fracture, dislocation at the end of the fracture, fracture of the articular surface of the distal humerus, dislocation

21. Identification of the distal humerus intra-articular comminuted fracture with the intra-articular simple fracture
    21.1. X ray (Fig. 3.21a–d)

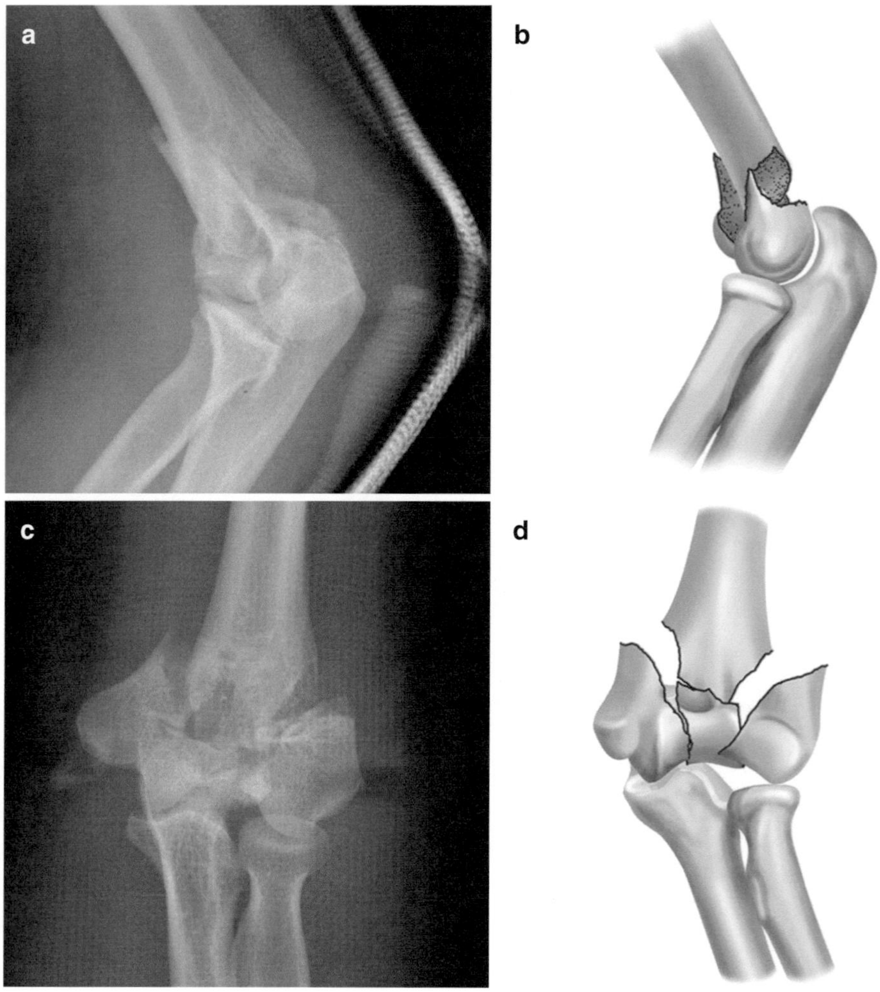

Fig. 3.21 Identification of the distal humerus intra-articular comminuted fracture with the intra-articular simple fracture. (**a**, **c**) X-ray shows the fracture of the distal humerus, the end of the fractures was inserted with each other, the joint surface dislocation, visible multiple segments; (**b**, **d**) Schematic

21.2. CT scan (Fig. 3.21e–h)

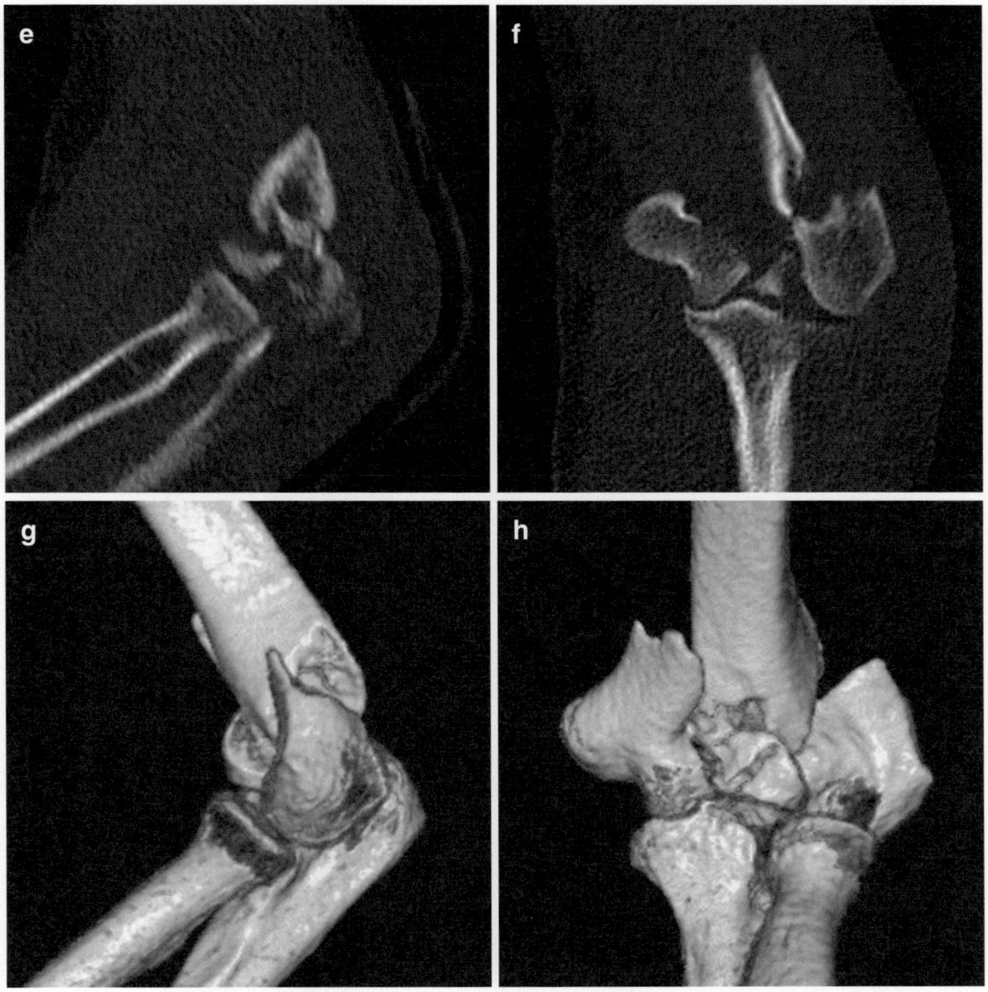

Fig. 3.21 (e–h) CT sagittal reconstruction, coronal reconstruction, and three-dimensional reconstruction showed fractures of the humerus supracondylar ridge, and the end of the fractures was impacted. The bone of the distal humerus joint surface was comminuted and dislocated

22. Identification of the distal humerus intra-articular comminuted fracture with the intra-articular simple fracture
    22.1. X ray (Fig. 3.22a–d)

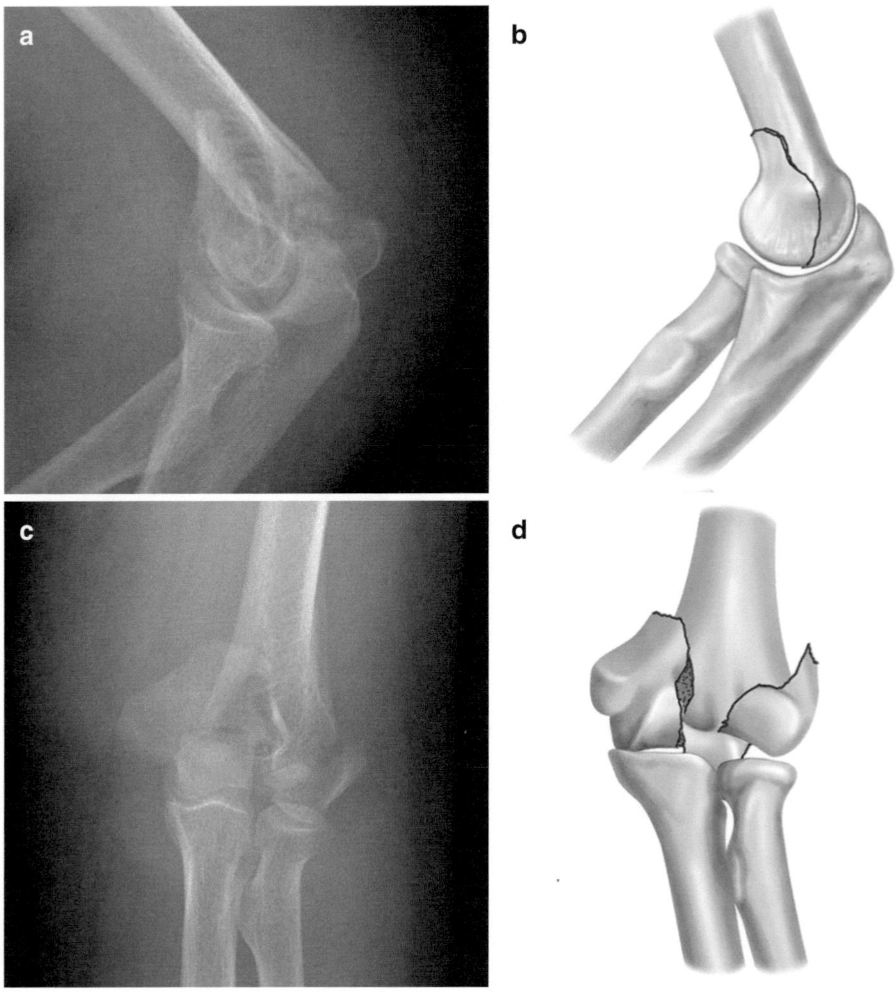

Fig. 3.22 Identification of the distal humerus intra-articular comminuted fracture with the intra-articular simple fracture. (**a**, **c**) X-ray shows the fracture of the distal humerus, the impaction of the broken end, the fracture of the articular surface, the dislocation of the broken end; (**b**, **d**) Schematic

22.2. CT scan (Fig. 3.22e–h)

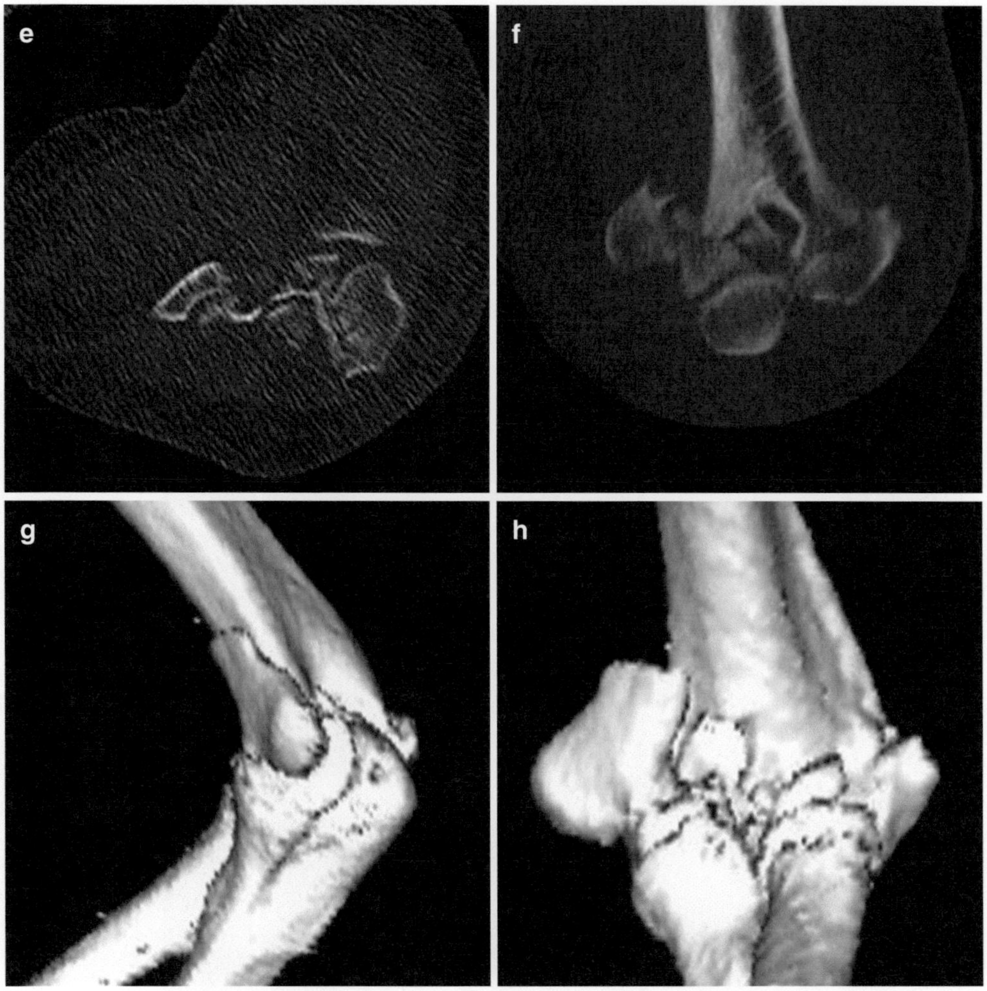

Fig. 3.22 (**e**–**h**) CT cross-section, coronal reconstruction, and three-dimensional reconstruction show the humerus epicondyle fracture, impaction at the end of the fracture, comminuted fracture at the distal joint surface of the humerus, obvious dislocation

23. Identification of the distal humerus intra-articular comminuted fracture with the intra-articular simple fracture
    23.1. X ray (Fig. 3.23a–d)

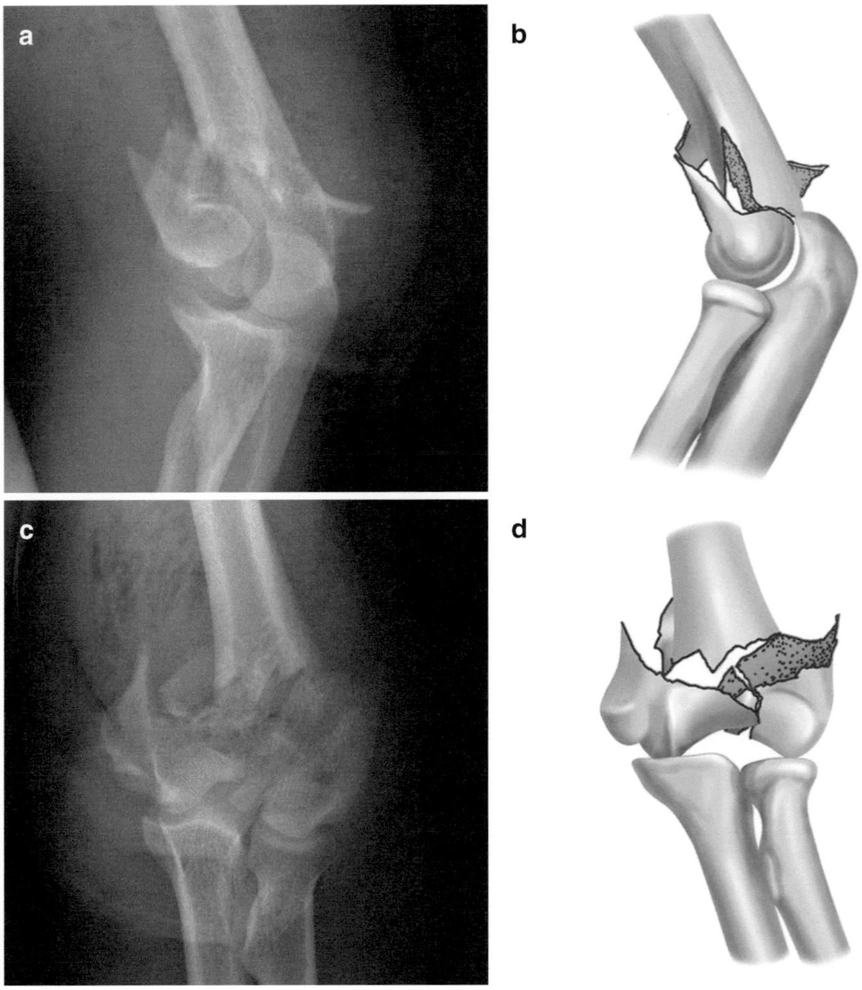

Fig. 3.23 Identification of the distal humerus intra-articular comminuted fracture with the intra-articular simple fracture. (**a**, **c**) X-ray shows comminuted fracture of the distal humerus, multiple bone masses on the distal articular surface and epicondyle of the humerus, joint surface fracture dislocation; (**b**, **d**) Schematic

23.2. CT scan (Fig. 3.23e, f)

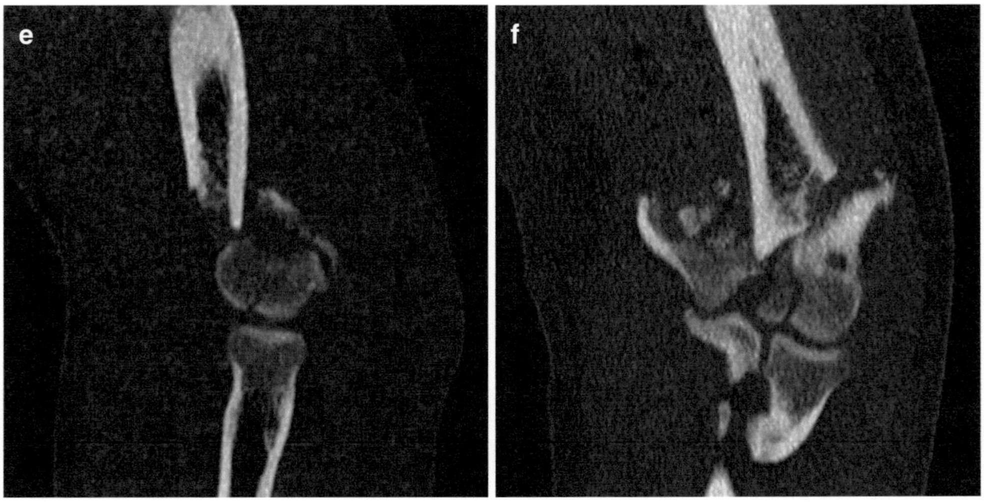

Fig. 3.23 (**e**, **f**) CT sagittal reconstruction and coronal reconstruction show the fracture of the humerus epicondyle, the impaction of the broken end, the fracture of the articular surface of the distal humerus, and dislocation

24. Identification of the distal humerus intra-articular comminuted fracture with the intra-articular simple fracture
    24.1. X ray (Fig. 3.24a–d)

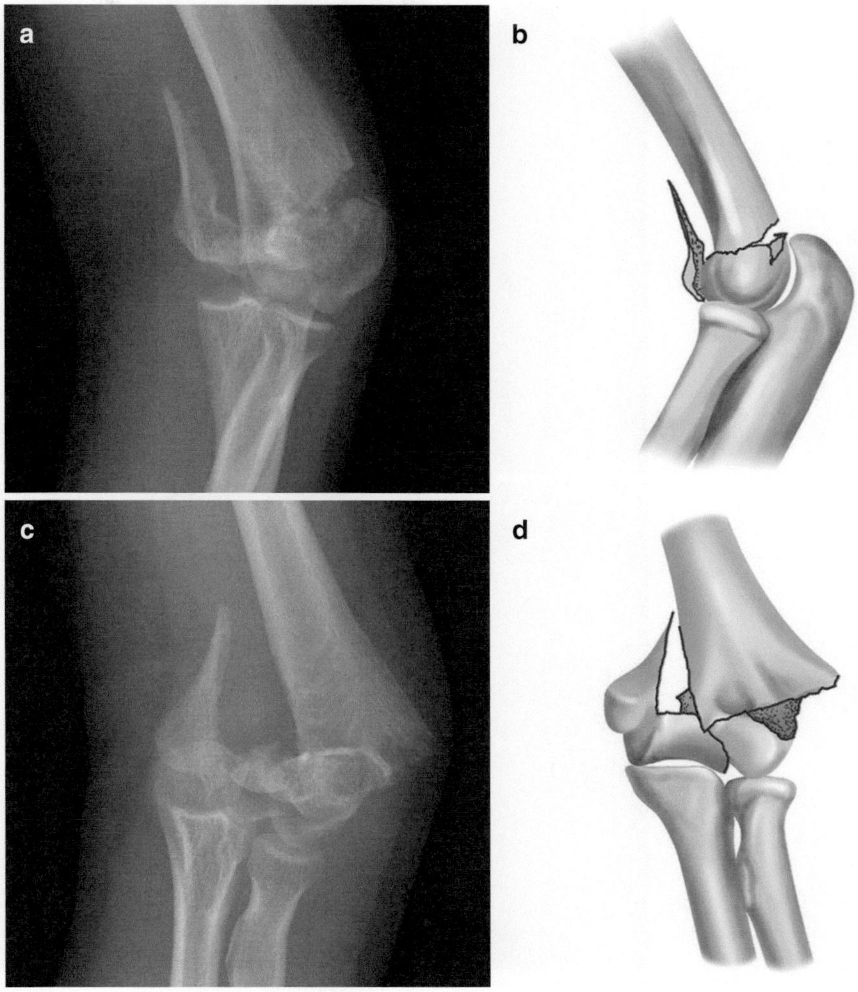

Fig. 3.24 Identification of the distal humerus intra-articular comminuted fracture with the intra-articular simple fracture. (**a**, **c**) X-ray shows comminuted fracture of the distal humerus, multiple bone masses on the distal articular surface, and the humerus epicondyle, joint surface dislocation; (**b**, **d**) Schematic

24.2. CT scan (Fig. 3.24e–h)

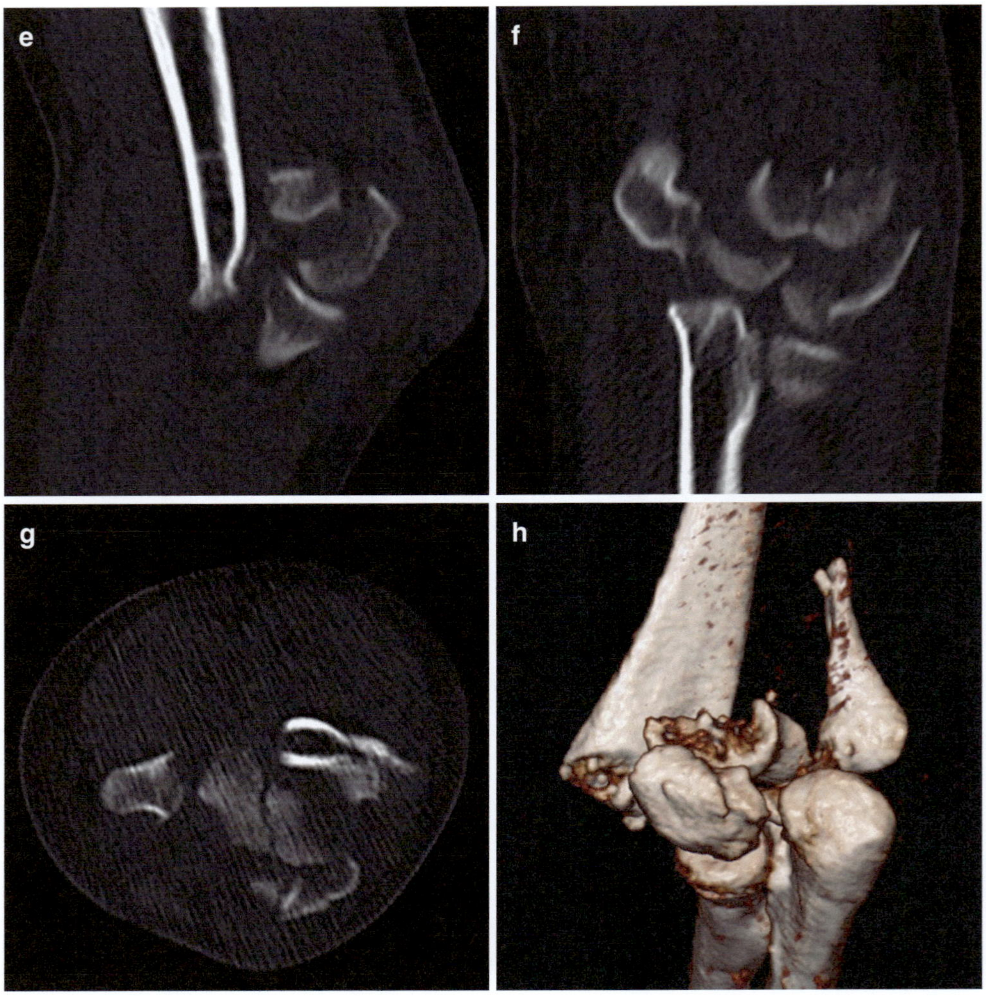

Fig. 3.24 (**e**–**h**) CT coronal reconstruction, coronal reconstruction, and cross-sectional and three-dimensional reconstruction showed humeral supracondylar fracture, displaced at the end of the fracture, bone fracture at the lower end of the humerus, and dislocation

3.2 Proximal Ulnar Fracture

The proximal ulnar bone structure includes the olecranon and the ulnar coronoid process. The two forms of an ulnar forceps articulate with the humeral trochlea; and at the olecranon medial side the ulnar nerve ran along into the ulnar groove. According to the fracture classification of AO principle, the proximal end of the ulnar and the related radial head is classified as a whole. The most commonly used is the Schatzker classification of the olecranon fracture and the Regan and Morrey classification of the ulnar coronoid process. Schatzker classification of olecranon fractures is divided into simple transverse fracture, transverse compression fracture, oblique fracture, comminuted fracture, distal oblique fracture, and fracture-dislocation type. The Regan and Morrey classification of the ulnar coronoid process is divided into the following: avulsion fractures at the top of the coronoid process, <50% of the coronoid process fractures, and more than 50% of the coronoid process fractures.

3.2.1 Identification of Injury Mechanism

The most common cause is direct violence; which acts on the back of the olecranon; which results in a fracture, or followed by a certain altitude fall, outstretched arm in almost full extension, indirectly exerting force onto the elbow, causing an olecranon fracture. When a violent blow acts on the posterior proximal forearm, the proximal ulnar together with the radial head are displaced forward. Due to the blocking effect of the trochlea on the olecranon, the olecranon is comminuted and the humeroradial joint is dislocated. The injury is similar to the Monteggia fracture, so special attention should be given to the restitution of the humeroradial joint during the reduction.

Pathological fracture identification: Given the injury is mild and the fracture occurs trivially, a pathological fracture is highly suspected.

3.2.2 Symptom and Signs Identification

The most common symptoms are pain, swelling, limited mobility, yet lacks specificity, it cannot be used as sole indications for diagnosis. If the fracture end impacted and cause compression, the elbow cannot resist gravity and extent the elbow, it indicates that triceps extension function is lost, and the continuity of the extensor device is helpful. Sometimes fracture associated with ulnar nerve injury, nerve function should be carefully assessed for timely treatment.

3.2.3 Imaging Differential Diagnosis

The most likely cause of misdiagnosis and missed diagnosis is due to the absence of a standard elbow lateral radiograph. In the emergency department, a standard lateral plane X-ray cannot be obtained due to the patient's pain. Subsequently, this cannot fully judge the length of the fracture. The degree of comminution, the range of the articular surface tear at the half-moon notch, and the displacement of the radial head, those are important factors to obtain a standard elbow lateral view.

1. Identification of simple displaced fracture and non-displaced fracture of olecranon
   1.1. X-ray (Fig. 3.25a–d)

Fig. 3.25 Identification of a simple displaced fracture and non-displaced fracture of olecranon. (**a**, **c**) X-ray shows transverse fracture of olecranon ulnar, separation of broken ends; (**b**, **d**) Schematic

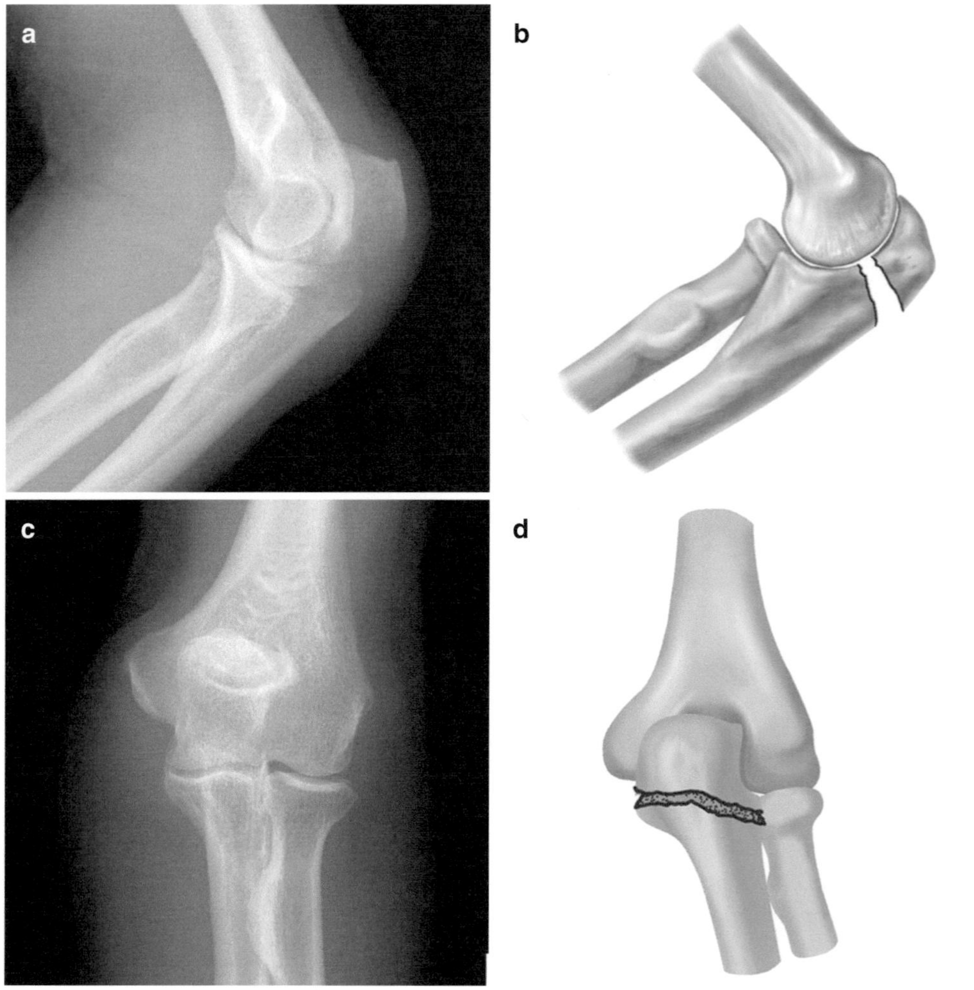

   1.2. CT scan (Fig. 3.25e, f)

Fig. 3.25 (**e**, **f**) CT sagittal reconstruction and coronal reconstruction showed transverse fracture of olecranon, dislocation of joint surface

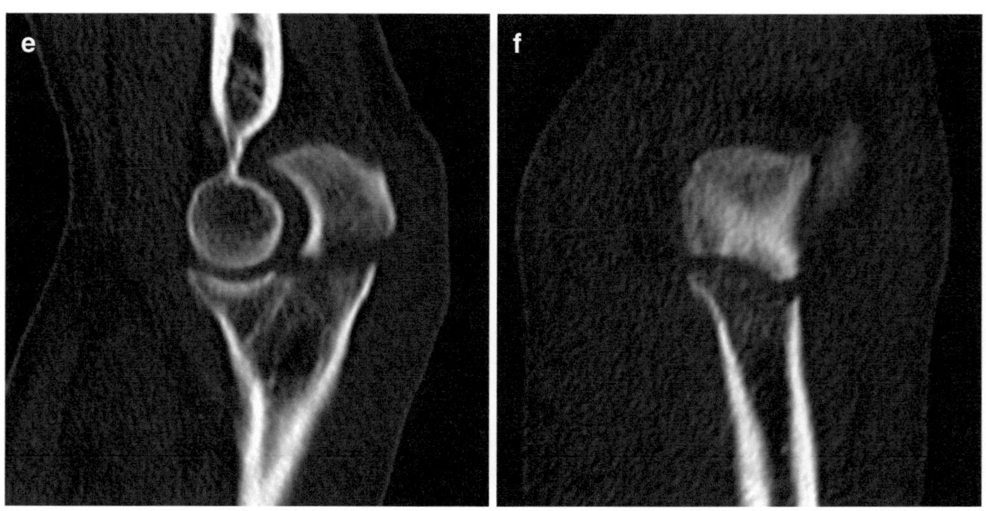

1.3. MR scan (Fig. 3.25g, h)

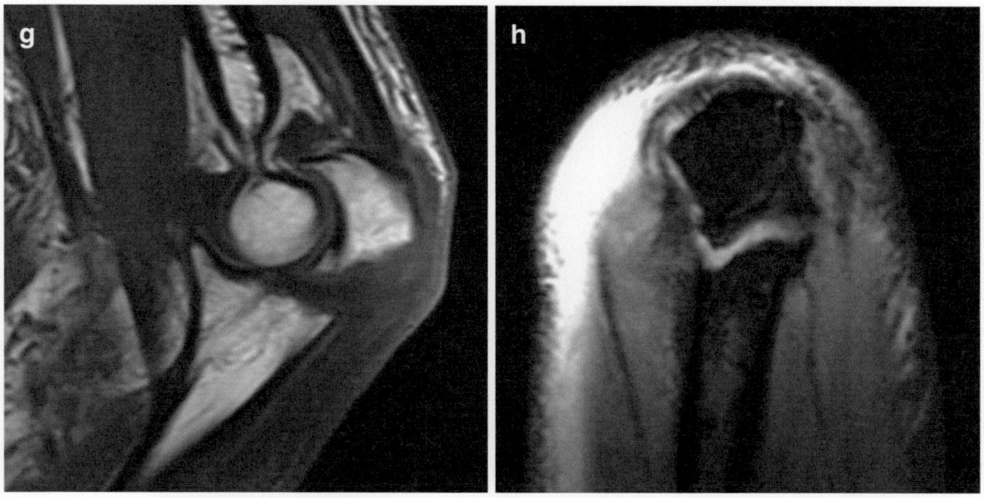

Fig. 3.25 (**g**, **h**) MRI sagittal T1WI and coronal T2WI showed transverse olecranon fracture, dislocation at the fracture end, long T1 long T2 signal at the fracture line, surrounding soft tissue edema

2. Identification of the ulnar olecranon comminuted fracture with the simple fracture
   2.1. X-ray (Fig. 3.26a–d)

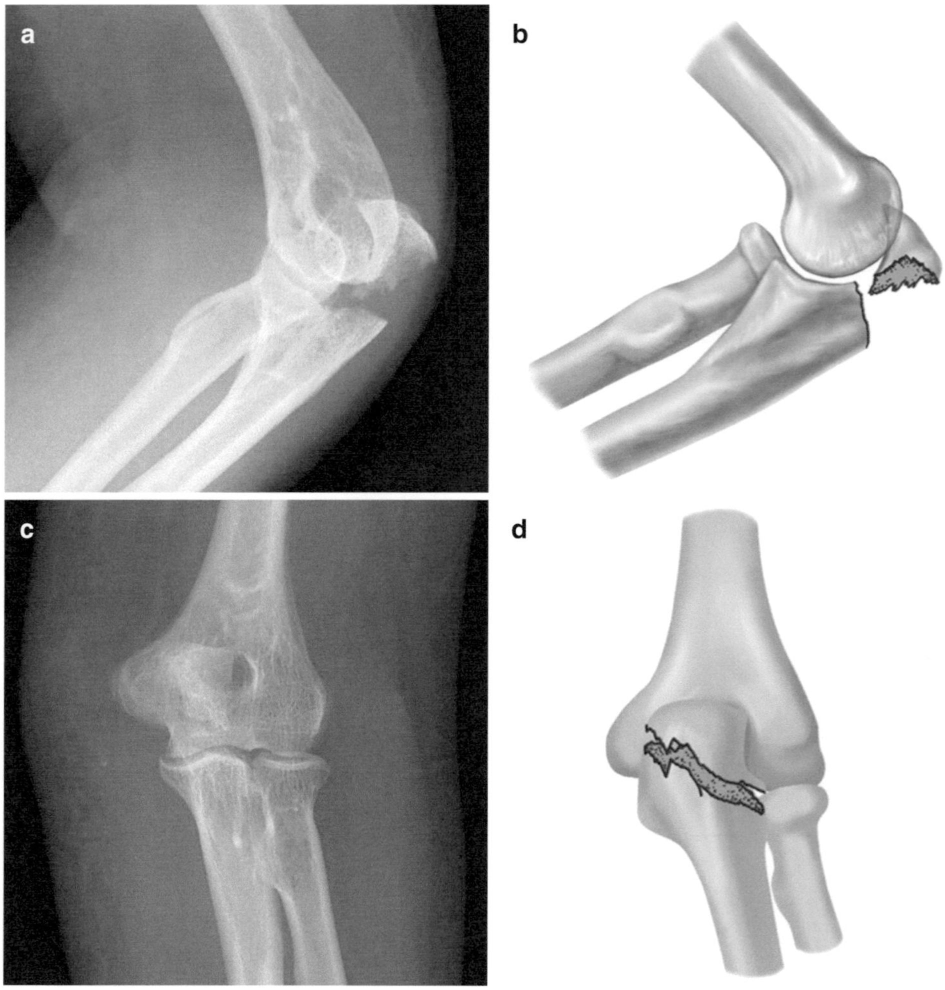

Fig. 3.26 Identification of the ulnar olecranon comminuted fracture with the simple fracture. (**a**, **c**) X-ray shows transverse fracture of olecranon, dislocation of broken end; (**b**, **d**) Schematic

   2.2. CT scan (Fig. 3.26e, f)

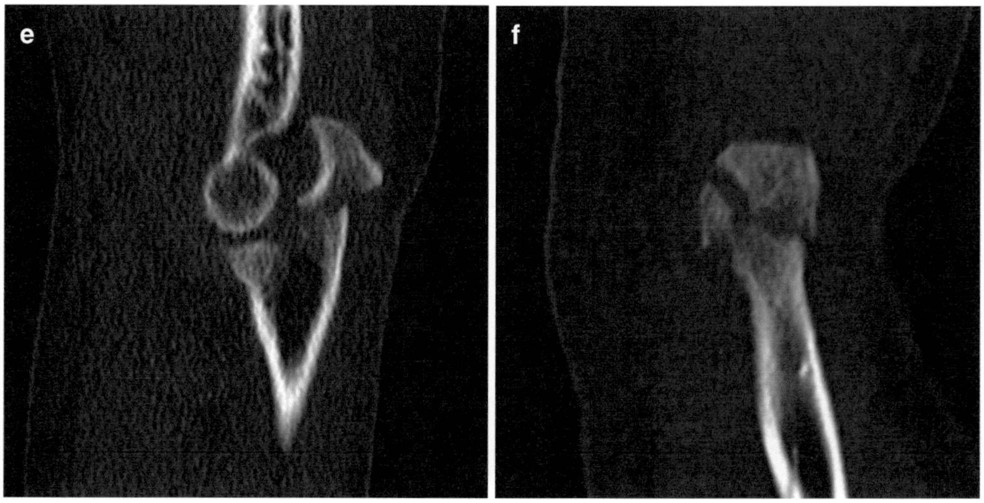

Fig. 3.26 (**e**, **f**) CT sagittal reconstruction and coronal reconstruction showed ulnar olecranon fracture, visible multiple fragments, dislocation of the articular surface

3. Identification of the olecranon transverse compression comminuted fracture with simple fracture.
   3.1. X-ray (Fig. 3.27a–d)

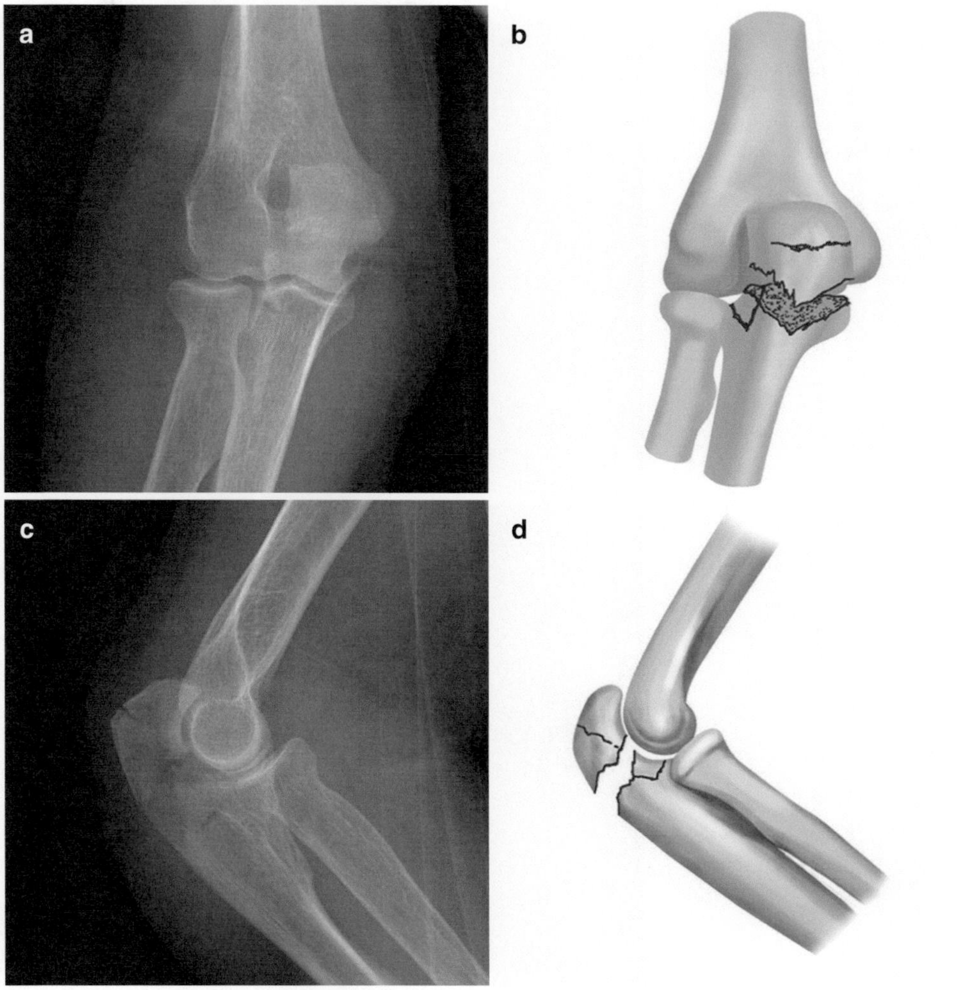

Fig. 3.27 Identification of the olecranon transverse compression comminuted fracture with simple fracture. (**a**, **c**) X-ray shows transverse compression fracture of olecranon, visible multiple bone segments, irregular articular surface; (**b**, **d**) Schematic

   3.2. CT scan (Fig. 3.27e, f)

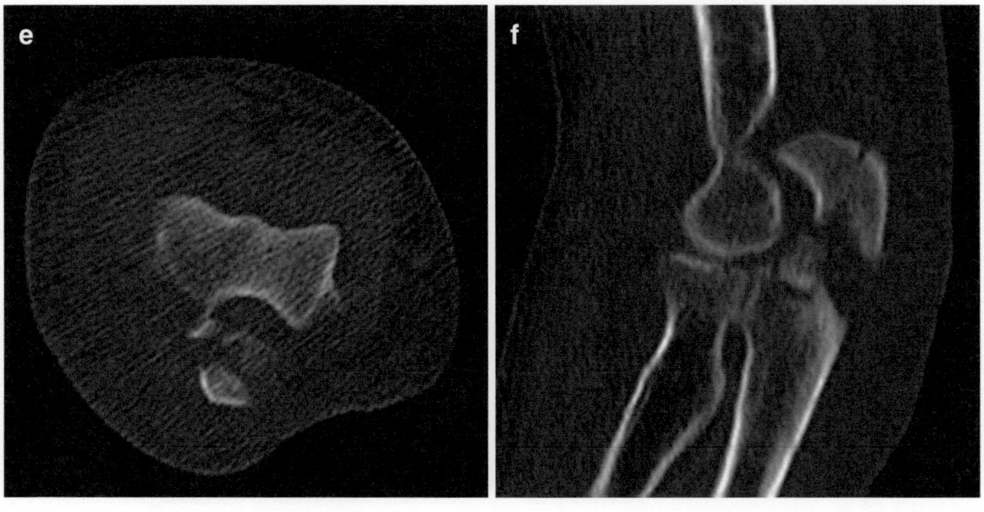

Fig. 3.27 (**e**, **f**) CT cross-section and sagittal reconstruction showed ulnar olecranon fracture cracked, multiple bone segments visible on the articular surface

4. Identification of the ulnar olecranon comminuted fracture with the simple fracture

4.1. X-ray (Fig. 3.28a–d)

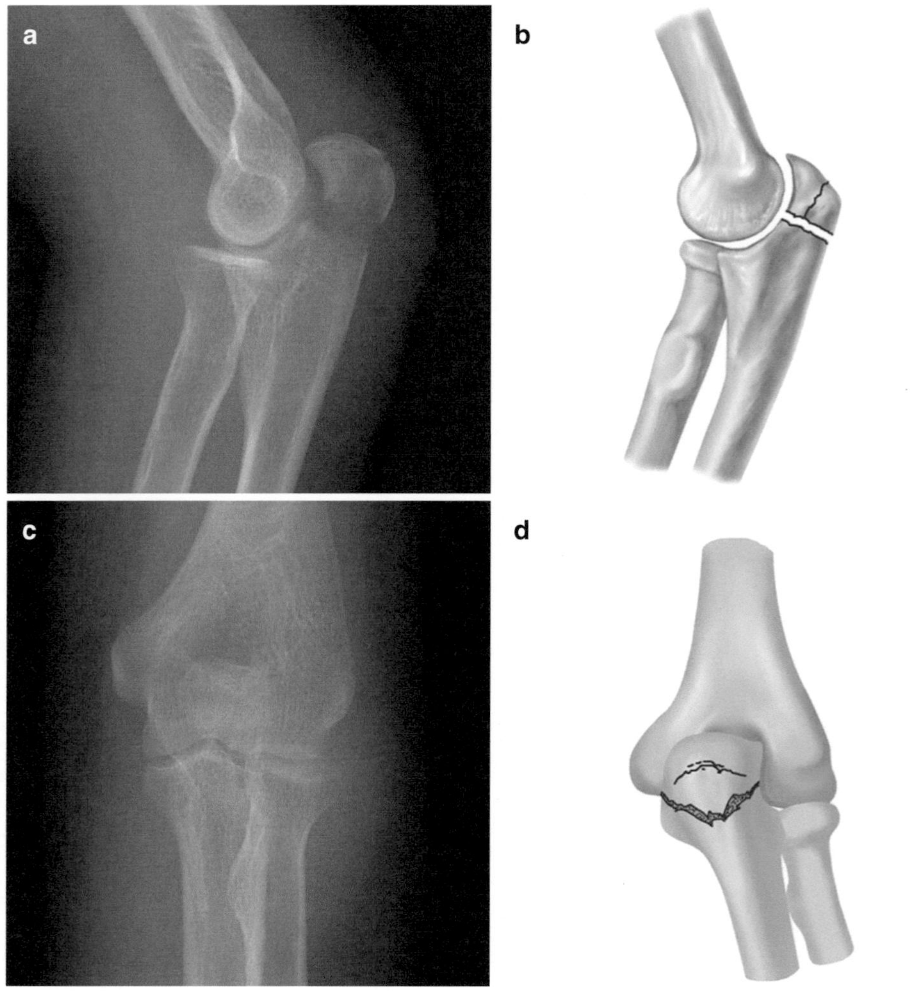

Fig. 3.28 Identification of the ulnar olecranon comminuted fracture with the simple fracture. (**a**, **c**) X-ray shows transverse compression fracture of olecranon, fracture end separated, irregular articular surface; (**b**, **d**) Schematic

4.2. CT scan (Fig. 3.28e, f)

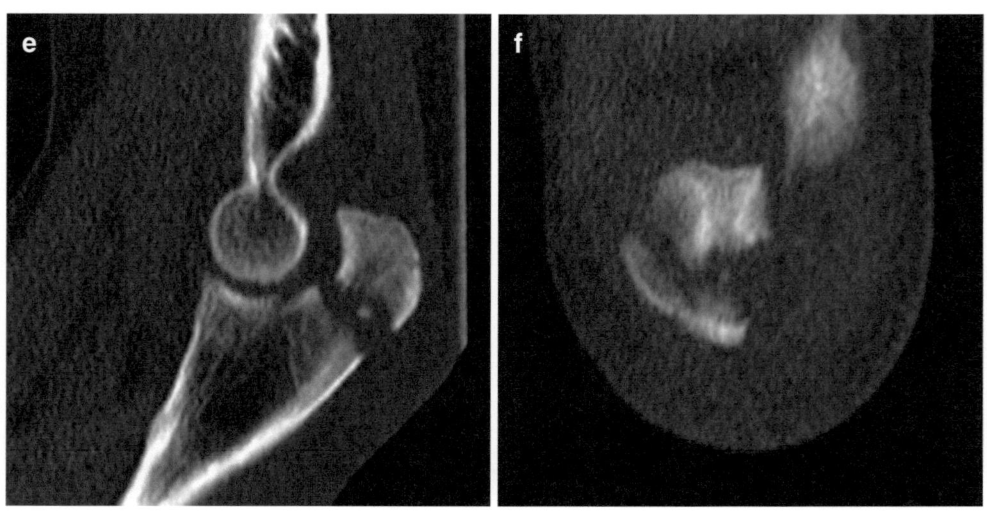

Fig. 3.28 (**e**, **f**) CT sagittal reconstruction and coronal reconstruction showed ulnar olecranon fracture. Multiple bone segments can be seen on the articular surface, with local inlays

5. Identification of the ulnar olecranon compression comminuted fracture with simple fracture
   5.1. X-ray (Fig. 3.29a–d)

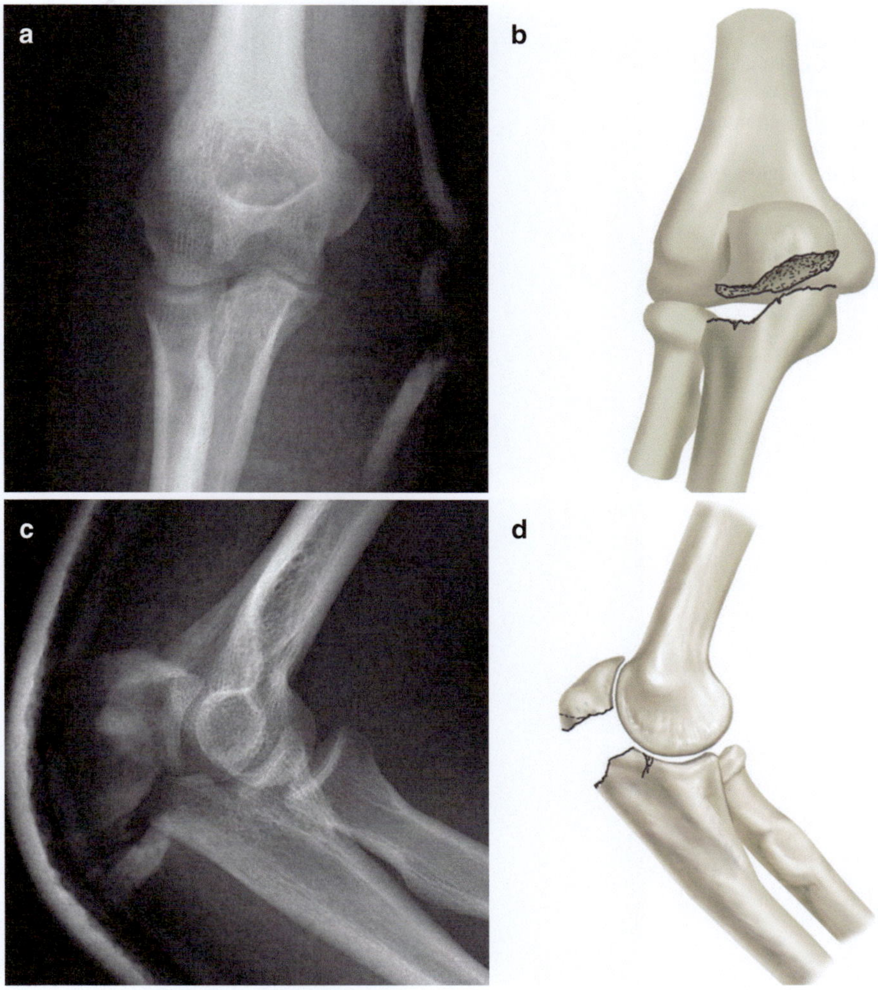

Fig. 3.29 Identification of the ulnar olecranon compression comminuted fracture with simple fracture. (**a**, **c**) X-ray shows transverse compression fracture of olecranon, irregular articular surface; (**b**, **d**) Schematic

   5.2. CT scan (Fig. 3.29e, f)

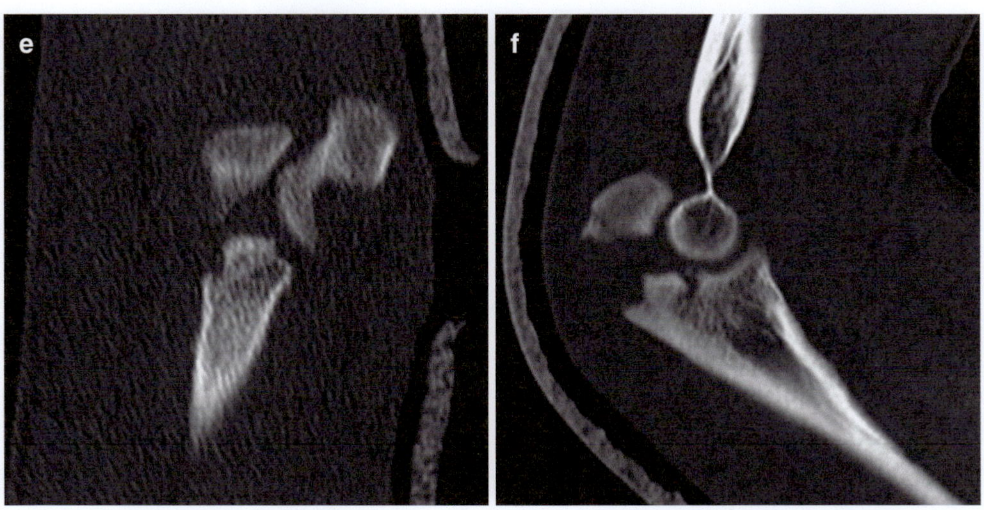

Fig. 3.29 (**e**, **f**) CT coronal reconstruction and sagittal reconstruction showed fracture of ulnar olecranon, visible joint surface bone mass, partially impacted

6. Identification of the ulnar olecranon oblique fracture with the suspicious fracture
   6.1. X-ray (Fig. 3.30a–d)

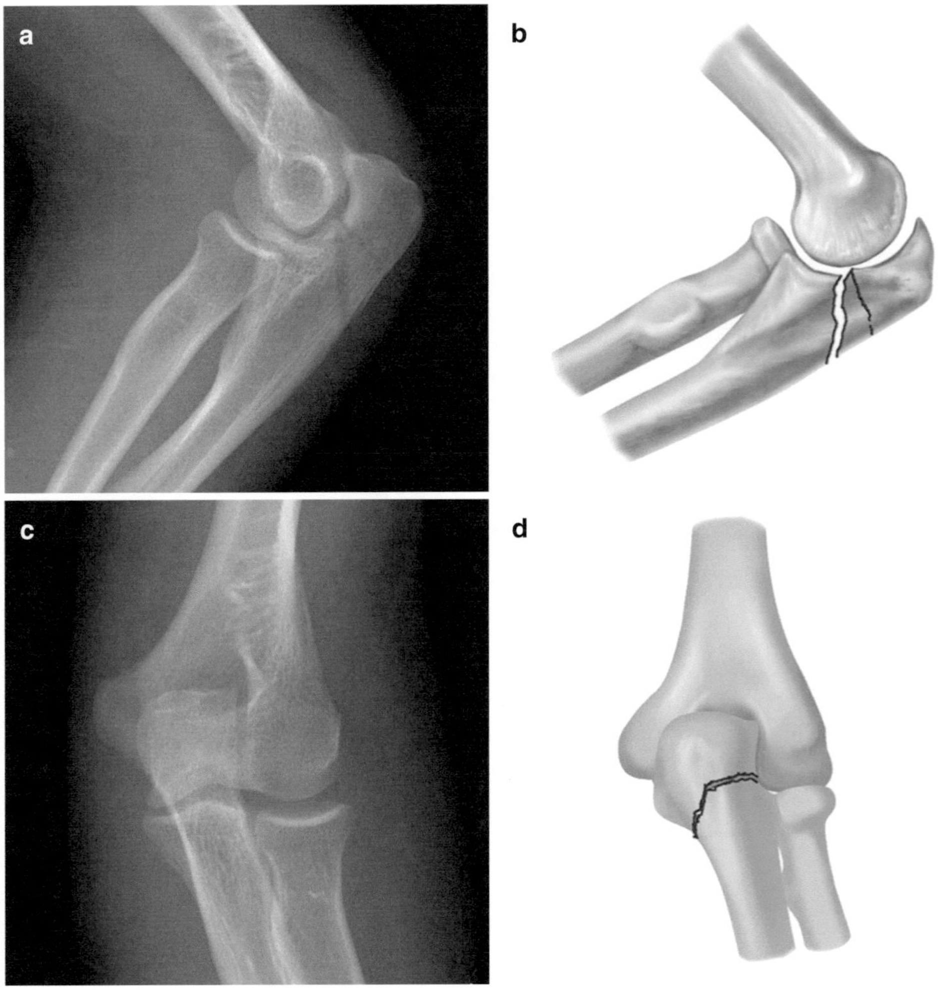

Fig. 3.30 Identification of the ulnar olecranon oblique fracture with the suspicious fracture. (**a**, **c**) X-ray shows oblique fracture of olecranon, the fracture line runs from the joint surface of the olecranon to the midpoint of the half-moon notch, and the displacement of the broken end is not indicated; (**b**, **d**) Schematic

   6.2. CT scan (Fig. 3.30e, f)

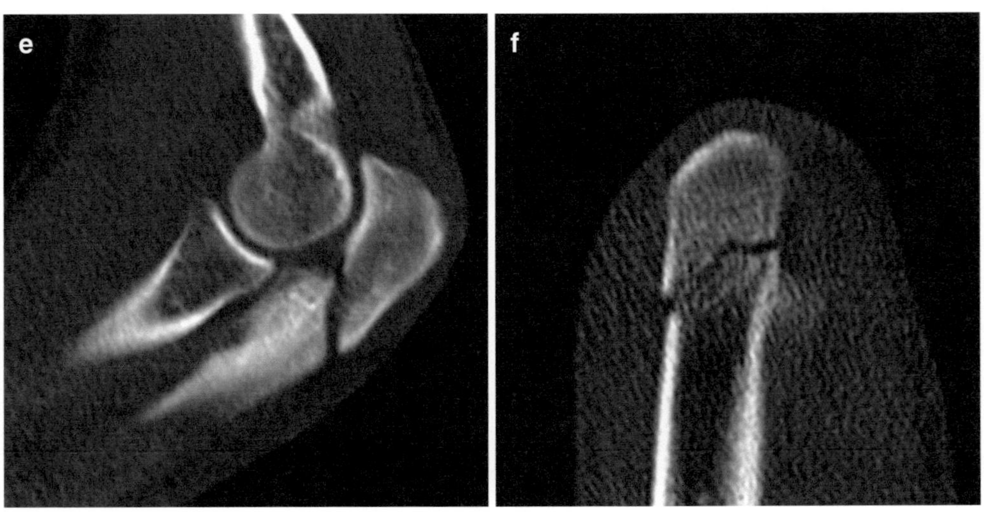

Fig. 3.30 (**e**, **f**) CT sagittal reconstruction and coronal reconstruction showed oblique fracture of the olecranon, no dislocation at the broken end

7. Identification of the ulnar olecranon comminuted fracture with the incomplete fracture
   7.1. X-ray (Fig. 3.31a–d)

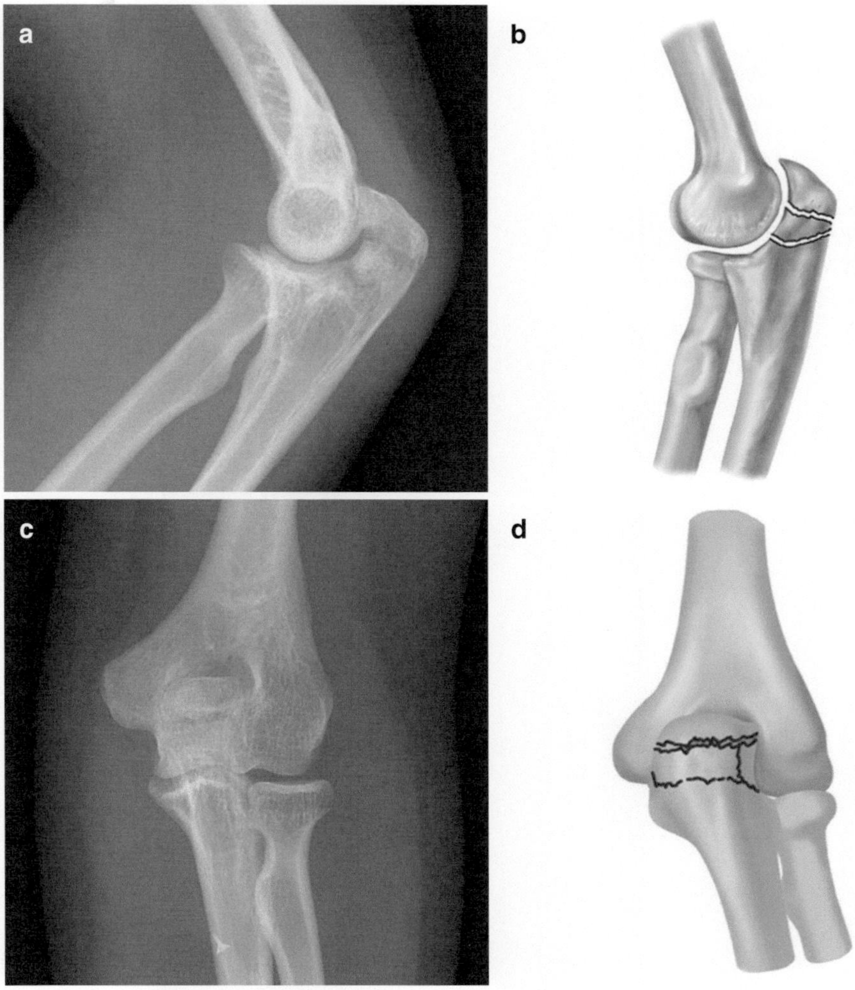

Fig. 3.31 Identification of the ulnar olecranon comminuted fracture with the incomplete fracture. (**a**, **c**) X-ray shows bone fracture at the articular surface of the olecranon, the joint surface is slightly sunken, the cortical bone of the eagle's back is continuous; (**b**, **d**) Schematic

   7.2. CT scan (Fig. 3.31e, f)

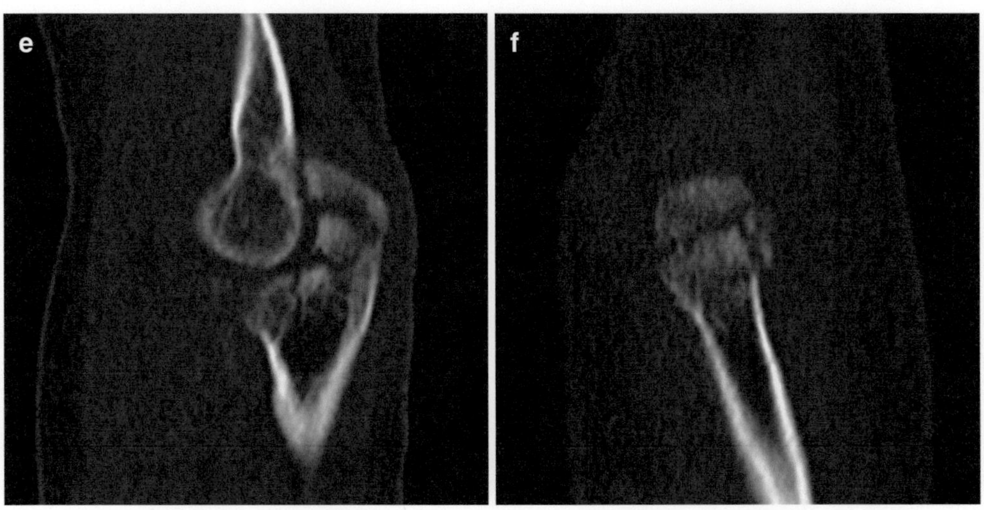

Fig. 3.31 (**e**, **f**) CT sagittal reconstruction and coronal reconstruction ulnar olecranon bone fracture, joint surface dislocation, slightly collapsed, fracture line involving the olecranon posterior edge

8. Identification of the ulnar olecranon comminuted fracture with the fracture dislocation
   8.1. X-ray (Fig. 3.32a–d)

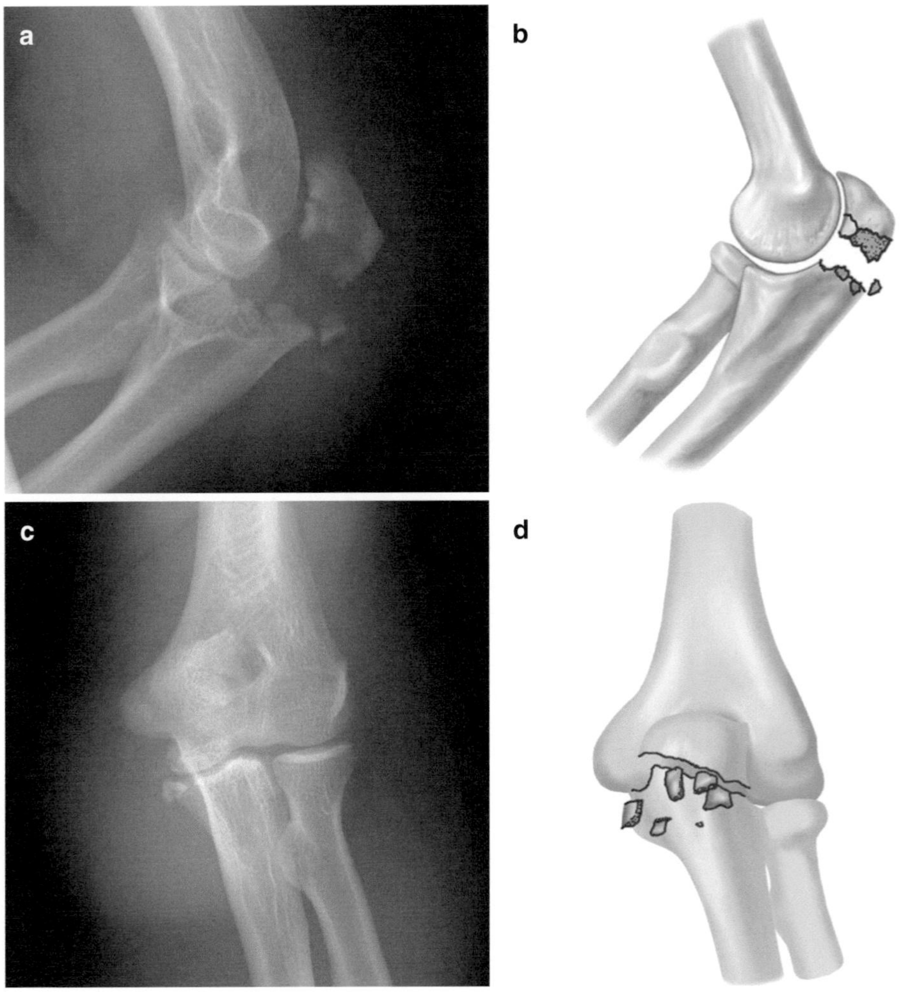

Fig. 3.32 Identification of the ulnar olecranon comminuted fracture with the fracture dislocation. (**a**, **c**) X-ray shows ulnar olecranon comminuted fracture, obvious dislocation of the broken end, fracture end separated, irregular articular surface, and elbow joint alignment; (**b**, **d**) Schematic

8.2. CT scan (Fig. 3.32e–h)

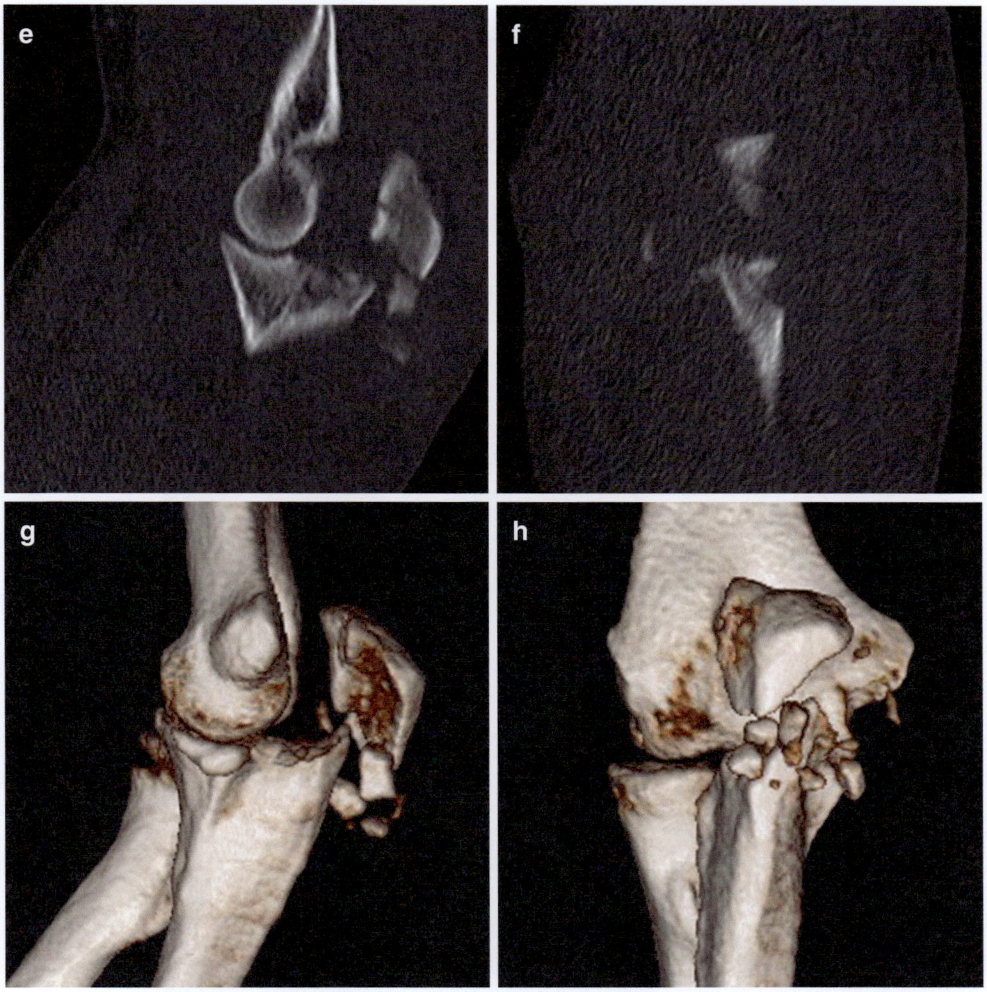

Fig. 3.32 (**e–h**) CT sagittal reconstruction, coronal plane reconstruction, and three-dimensional reconstruction showed the ulnar olecranon bone fractured, multiple bone fragments, obviously backward dislocation, irregular articular surface

9. Identification of the ulnar olecranon distal oblique comminuted fracture with the coronoid process fracture
   9.1. X-ray (Fig. 3.33a–d)

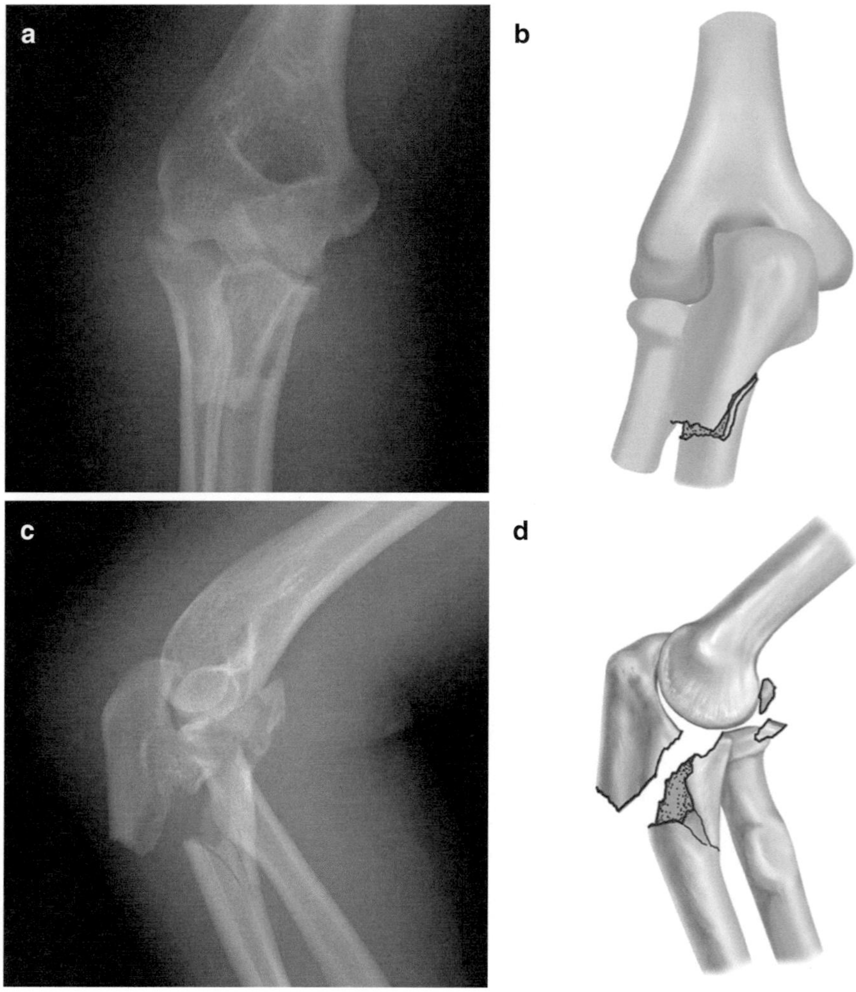

Fig. 3.33 Identification of the ulnar olecranon distal oblique comminuted fracture with the coronoid process fracture. (**a**, **c**) X-ray shows the oblique fracture of the distal end of the olecranon, the fracture line involving the ulnar coronoid, completely displaced, the radial head is irregular; (**b**, **d**) Schematic

9.2. CT scan (Fig. 3.33e–h)

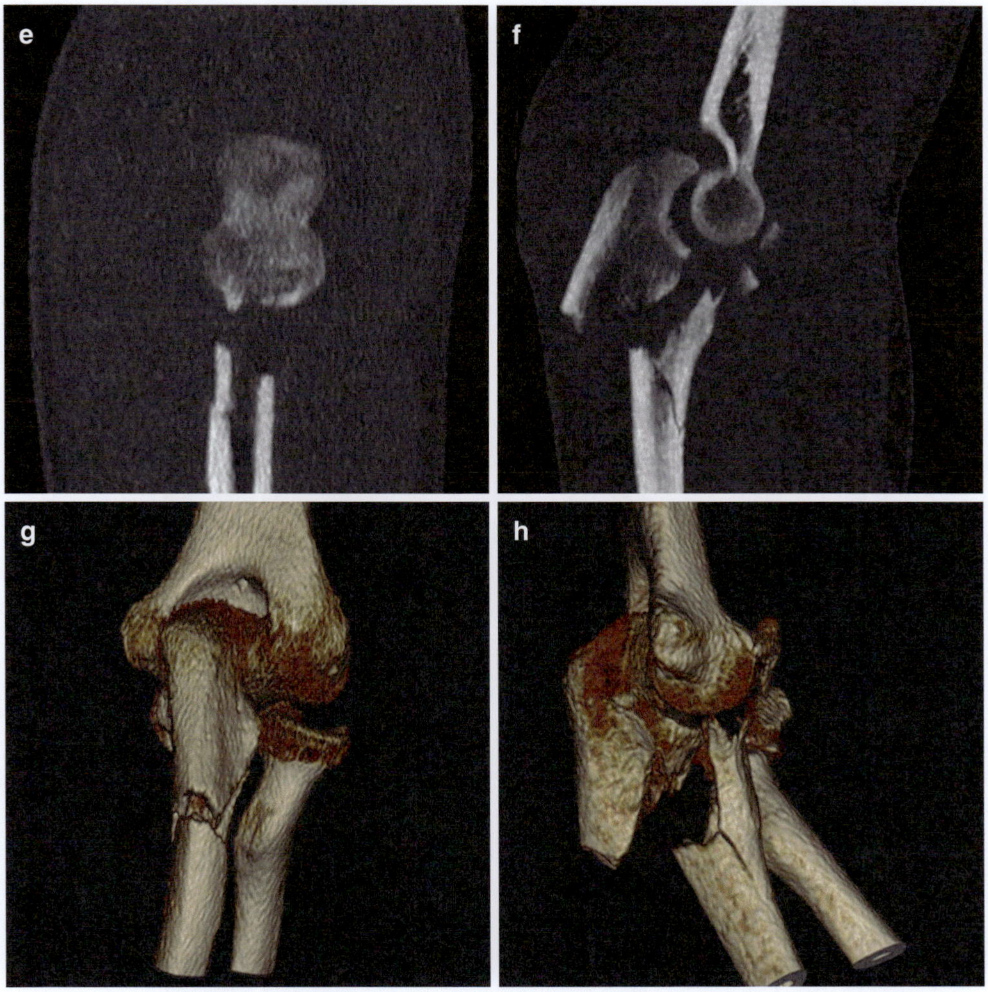

Fig. 3.33 (**e–h**) CT coronal reconstruction, sagittal reconstruction, and three-dimensional reconstruction showed that the distal ulnar olecranon was obliquely fractured, the end of fracture was dislocated, the fracture line reached the coronoid process, and the radial head fracture

10. Identification of the ulnar olecranon dislocation with fracture
    10.1. X-ray (Fig. 3.34a–d)

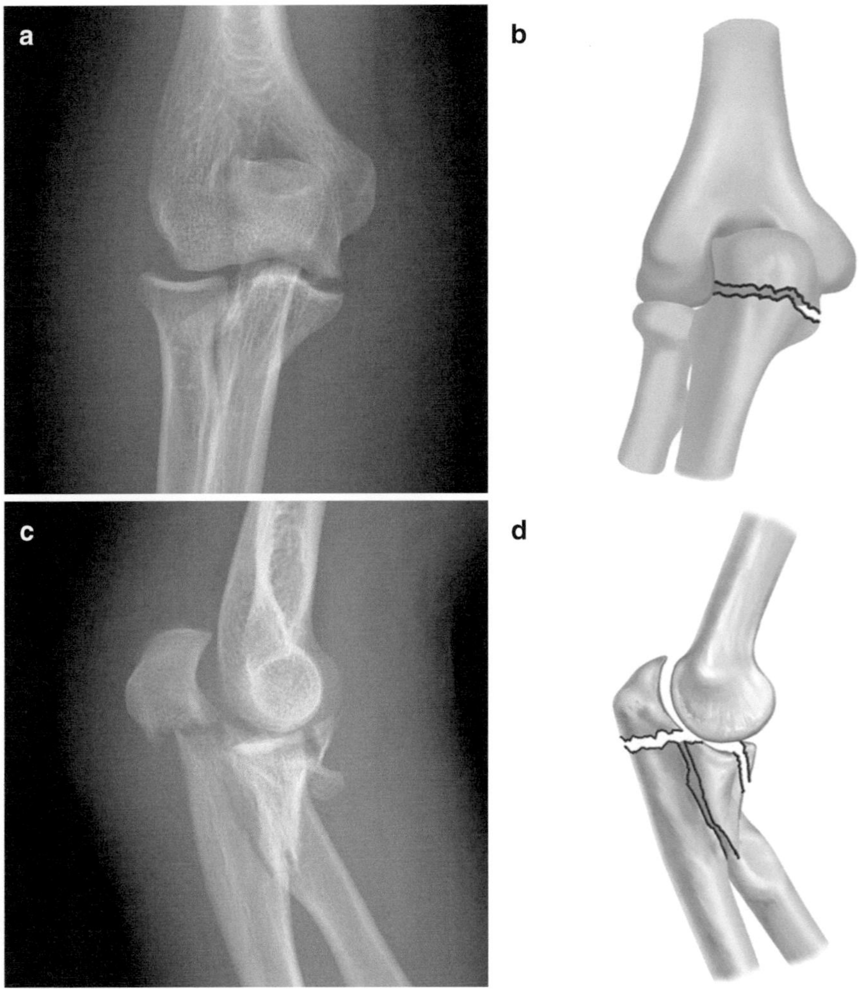

Fig. 3.34 Identification of the ulnar olecranon dislocation with fracture. (**a**, **c**) X-ray shows ulnar olecranon comminuted fracture, ulnar and radial head displaced backwards, ulnar coronoid process irregular, visible bone mass, radial head irregular; (**b**, **d**) Schematic

    10.2. CT scan (Fig. 3.34e, f)

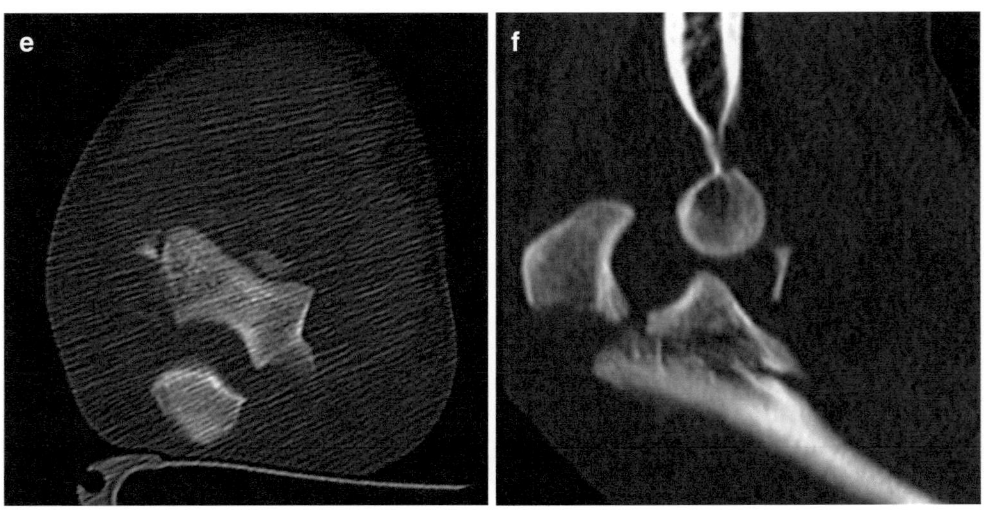

Fig. 3.34 (**e**, **f**) CT cross-section and vector reconstruction of the ulna show that the ulnar olecranon is separated, the fracture is dislocated, the gap between the ulnar joint is widened, the ulna and radial head is dislocated backwards, and the ulnar coronoid process fracture

11. Identification of the ulnar olecranon dislocation fracture with the comminuted fracture
    11.1. X-ray (Fig. 3.35a–d)

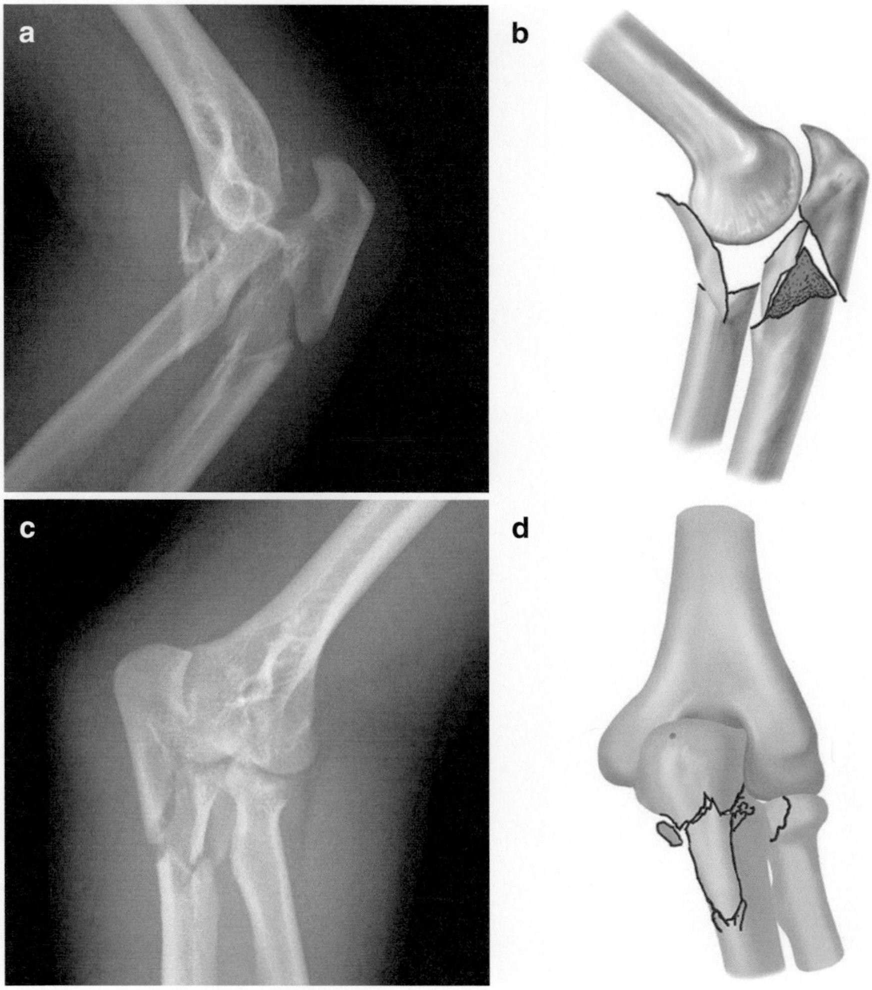

Fig. 3.35 Identification of the ulnar olecranon dislocation fracture with the comminuted fracture. (**a**, **c**) X-ray shows ulnar olecranon comminuted fracture, posterior subluxation of ulnar and radial head, basal bone fracture of ulnar coronoid process, irregular contour of radial head; (**b**, **d**) Schematic

11.2. CT scan (Fig. 3.35e–h)

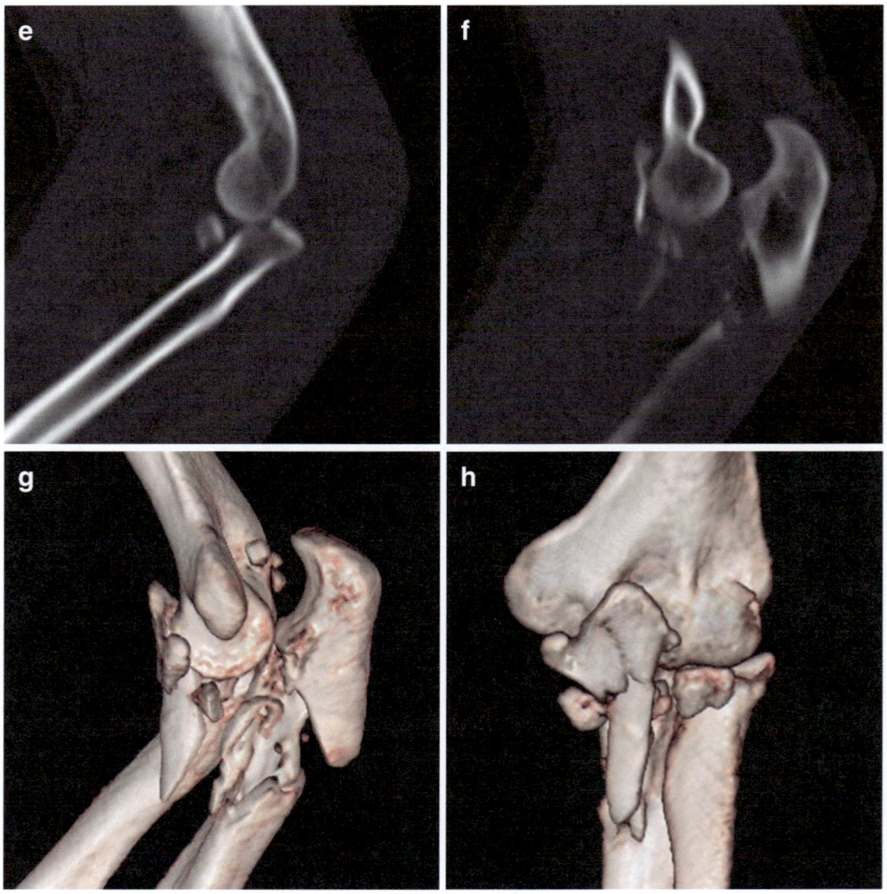

Fig. 3.35 (**e**–**h**) CT sagittal reconstruction and three-dimensional reconstruction showed fracture of the ulnar olecranon, dislocation of the fracture end, fracture of the radial head, and dislocation of the radius and ulna

12. Identification of the tip of coronoid process fracture with non-fracture
    12.1. X-ray (Fig. 3.36a–d)

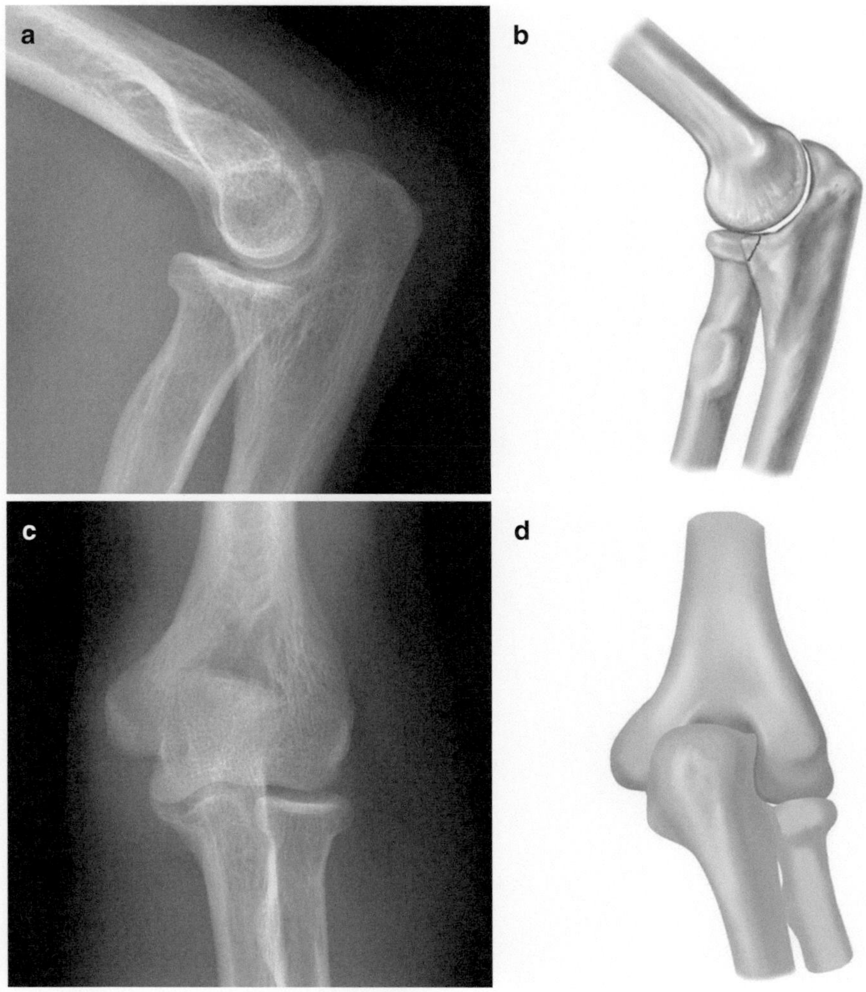

Fig. 3.36 Identification of the tip of coronoid process fracture with non-fracture. (**a**, **c**) X-ray shows no obvious fracture signs in the elbow joint bones; (**b**, **d**) Schematic

    12.2. CT scan (Fig. 3.36e, f)

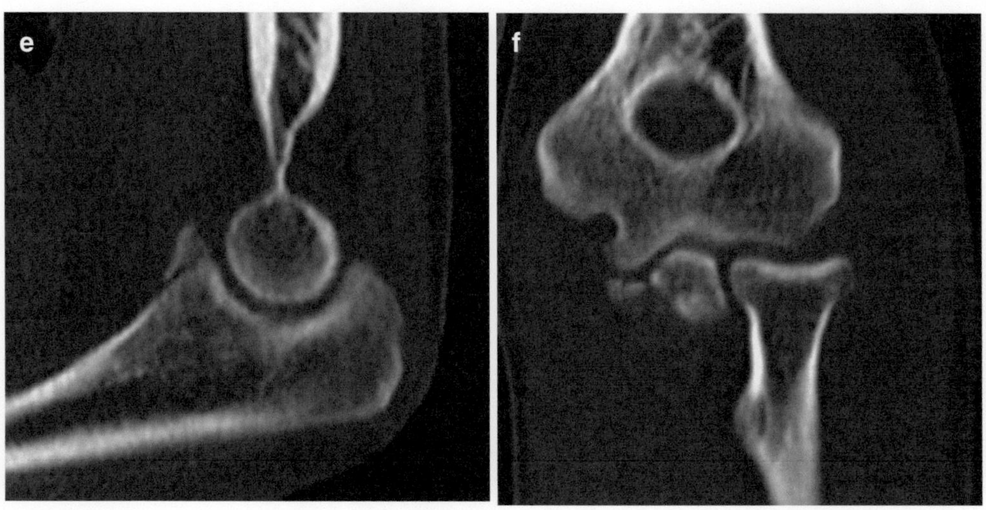

Fig. 3.36 (**e**, **f**) CT sagittal reconstruction and coronal reconstruction showed a linear translucent on the top of the ulnar coronoid process, no dislocation

13. Identification of the top of coronoid process fracture with the suspicious fracture
    13.1. X-ray (Fig. 3.37a–d)

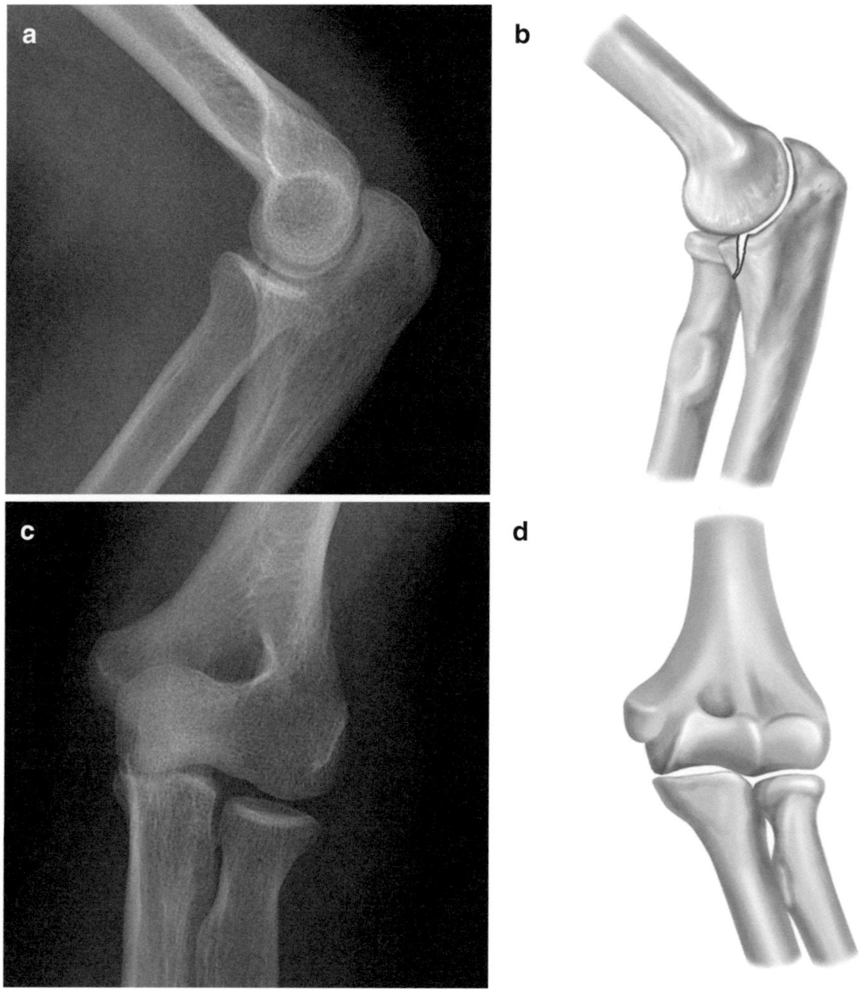

Fig. 3.37 Identification of the top of coronoid process fracture with the suspicious fracture. (**a**, **c**) X-ray shows the linear radiolucent on the top of the ulnar coronoid process, the dislocation is not obvious; (**b**, **d**) Schematic

13.2. CT scan (Fig. 3.37e–h)

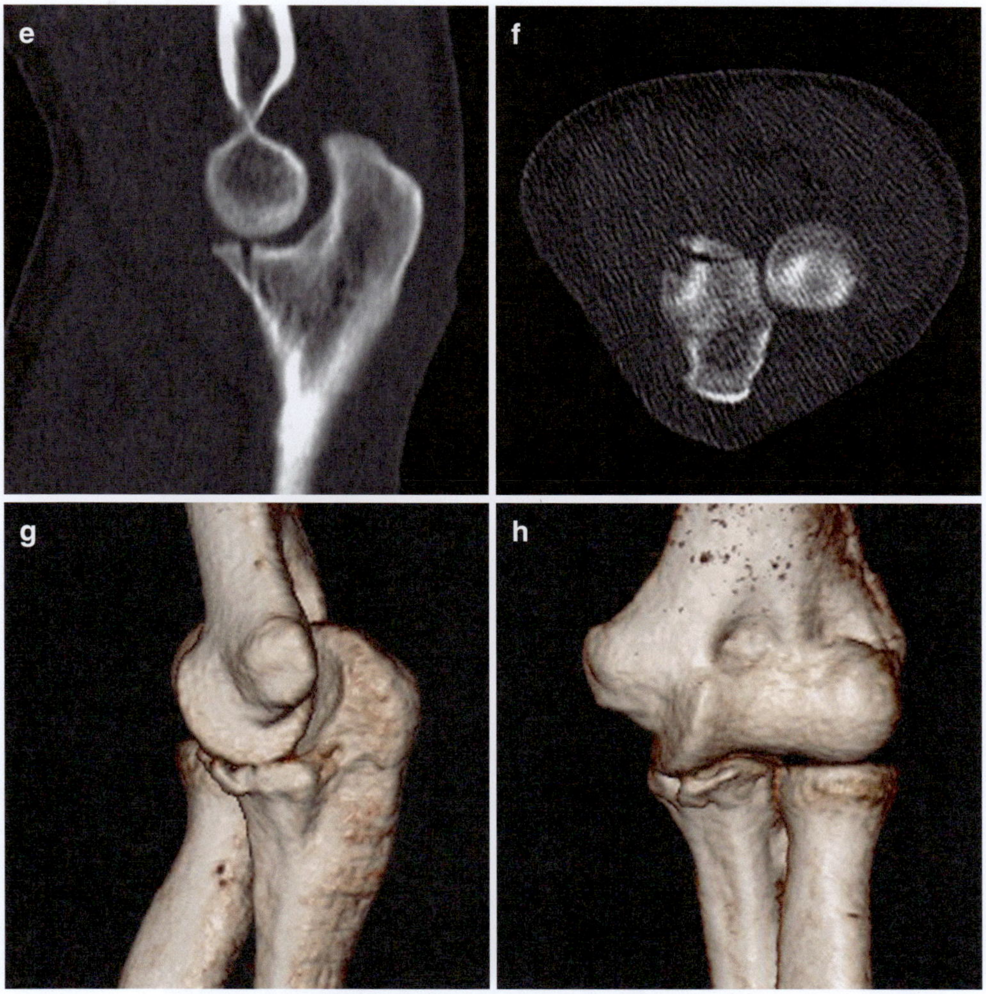

Fig. 3.37 (**e**–**h**) CT sagittal reconstruction, cross-section, and three-dimensional reconstruction show the ulnar coronoid process top fracture, joint slightly separated displacement

14. Identification of the top coronoid process fracture dislocation of the ulnar with the simple fracture
    14.1. X-ray (Fig. 3.38a–d)

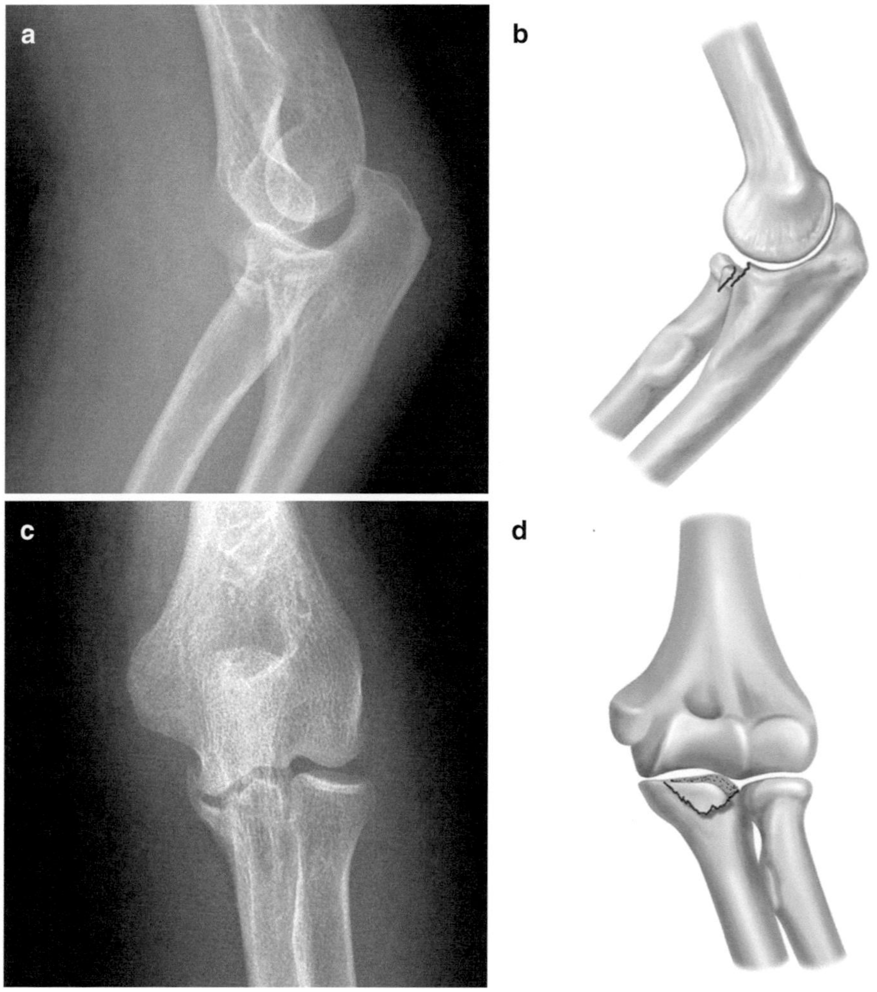

Fig. 3.38 Identification of the top coronoid process fracture dislocation of the ulnar with the simple fracture. (**a**, **c**) X-ray shows the linear radiolucent on the top of the ulnar coronoid process, the dislocation is not obvious; (**b**, **d**) Schematic

    14.2. CT scan (Fig. 3.38e, f)

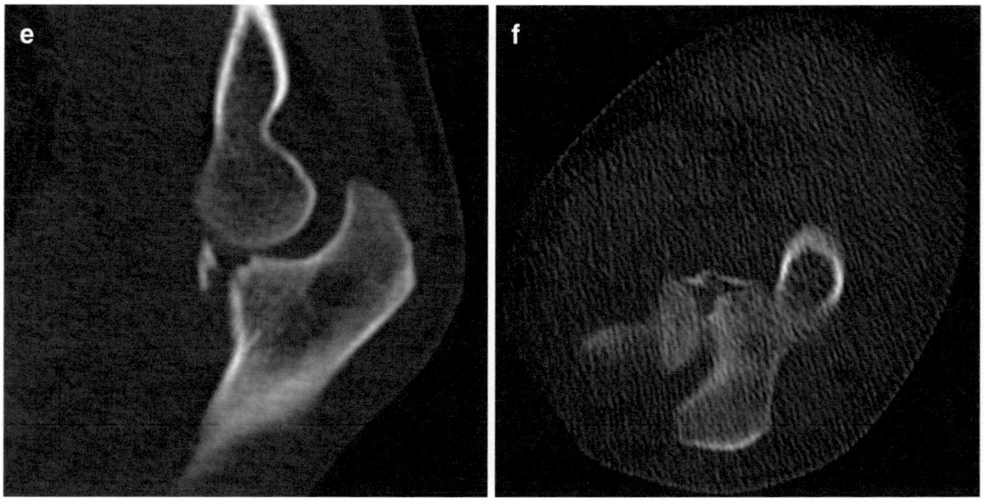

Fig. 3.38 (**e**, **f**) CT sagittal reconstruction, cross-section, and three-dimensional reconstruction show the ulnar coronoid process top fracture, joint slightly separated displacement

15. Identification of the ulnar coronoid process medial comminuted fracture with the simple fracture
    15.1. X-ray (Fig. 3.39a–d)

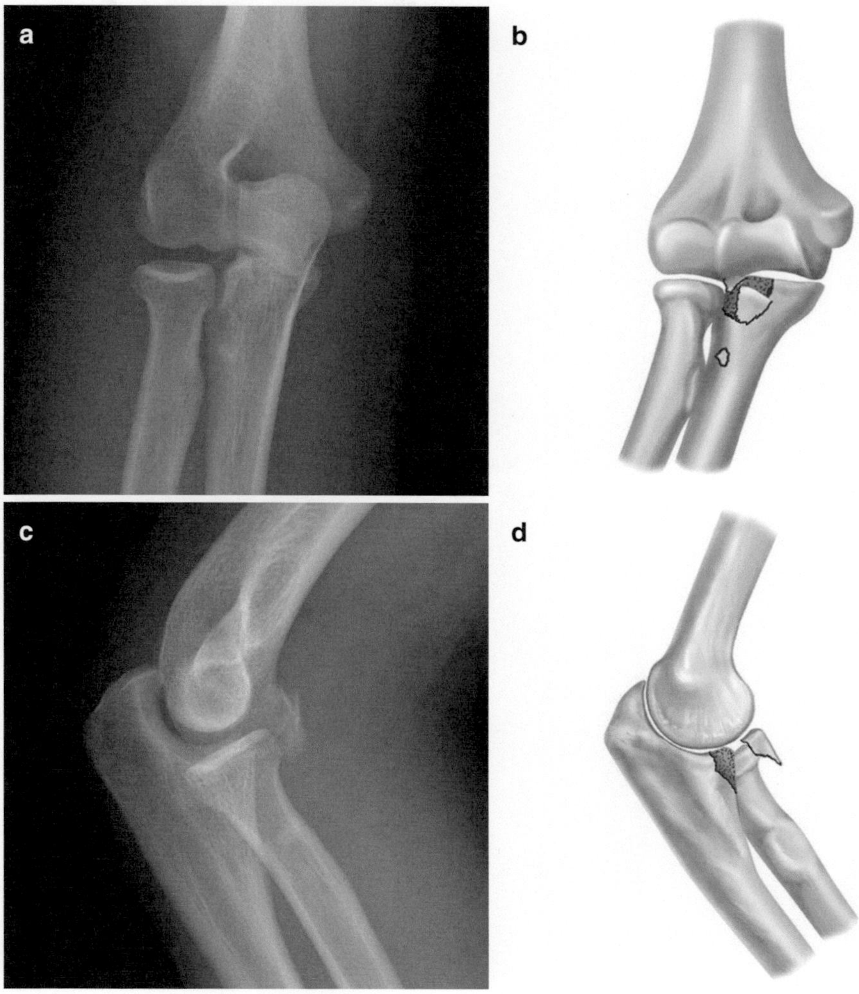

Fig. 3.39 Identification of the ulnar coronoid process medial comminuted fracture with the simple fracture. (**a**, **c**) X-ray films show an ulnar coronoid bone fracture, broken end displacement, fracture separated; (**b**, **d**) Schematic

15.2. CT scan (Fig. 3.39e–h)

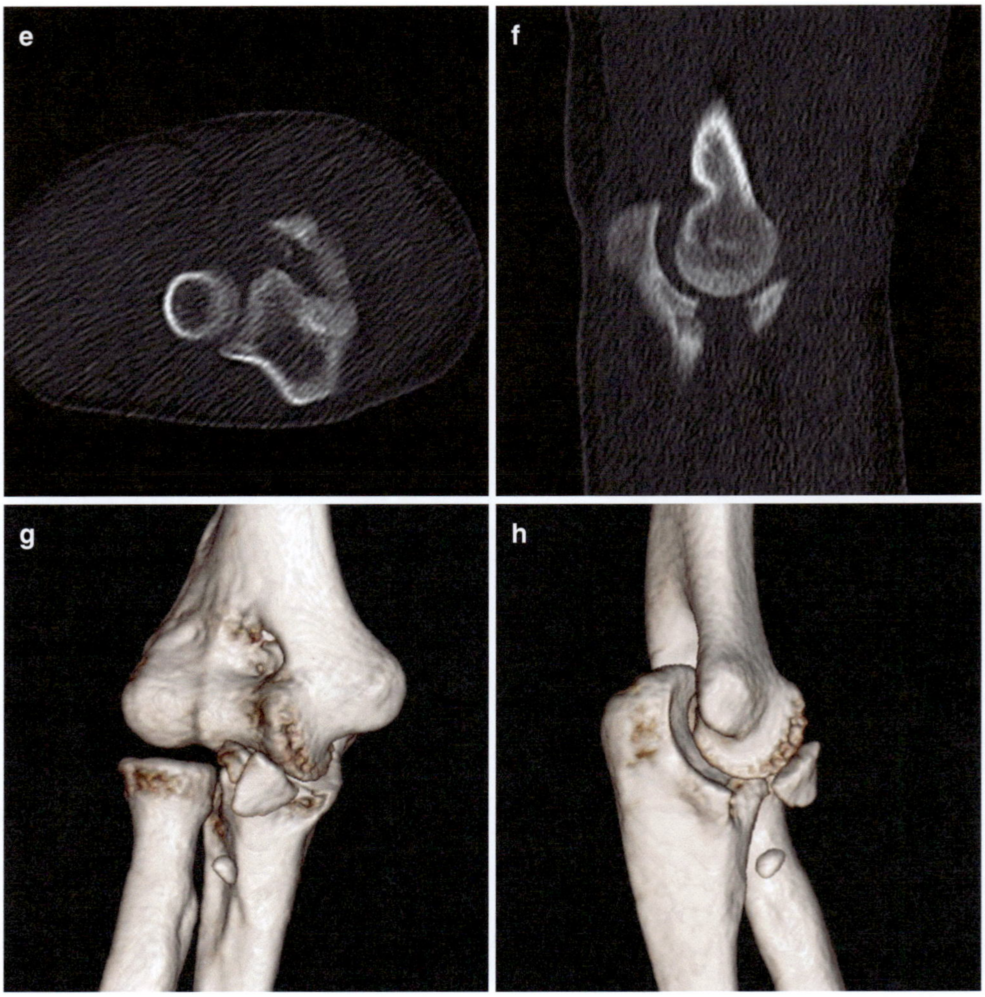

Fig. 3.39 (**e**–**h**) CT cross-section, sagittal reconstruction, and three-dimensional reconstruction showed ulnar coronoid process fracture, complete dislocation

16. Identification of the ulnar coronoid process medial fracture with the suspicious fracture
    16.1. X-ray (Fig. 3.40a–d)

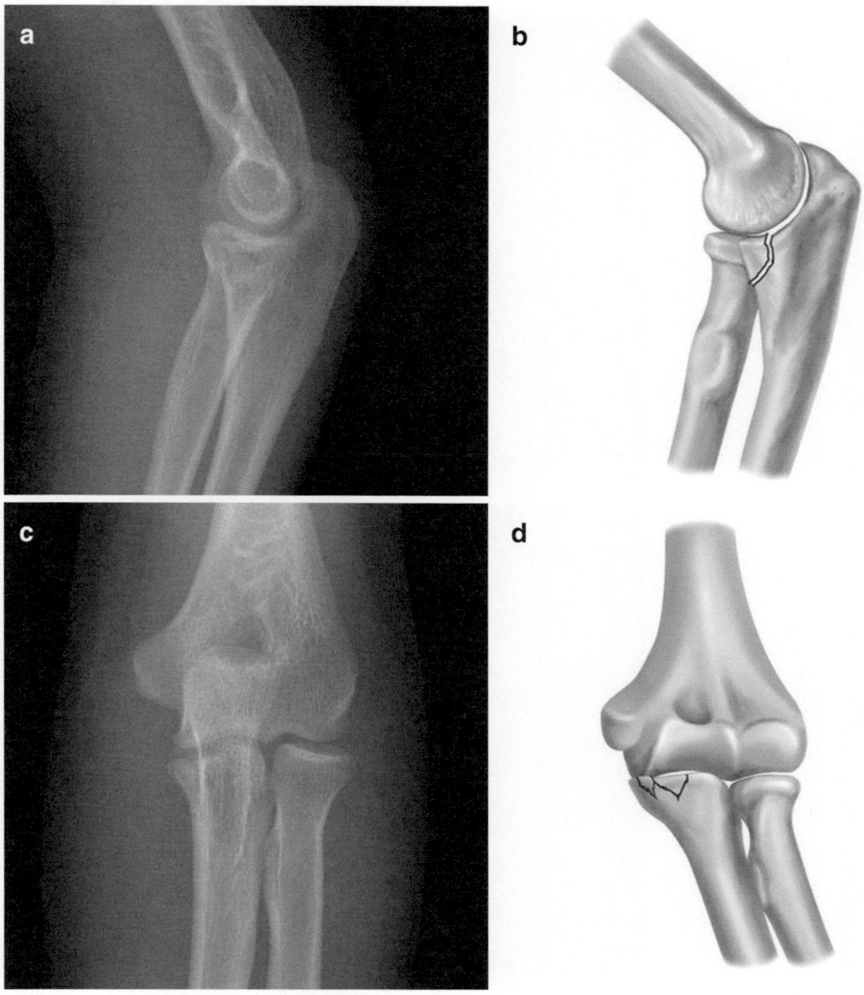

Fig. 3.40 Identification of the ulnar coronoid process medial fracture with the suspicious fracture. (**a**, **c**) X-ray films showed ulnar coronoid bone structure disorder, uneven radial density; (**b**, **d**) Schematic

    16.2. CT scan (Fig. 3.40e, f)

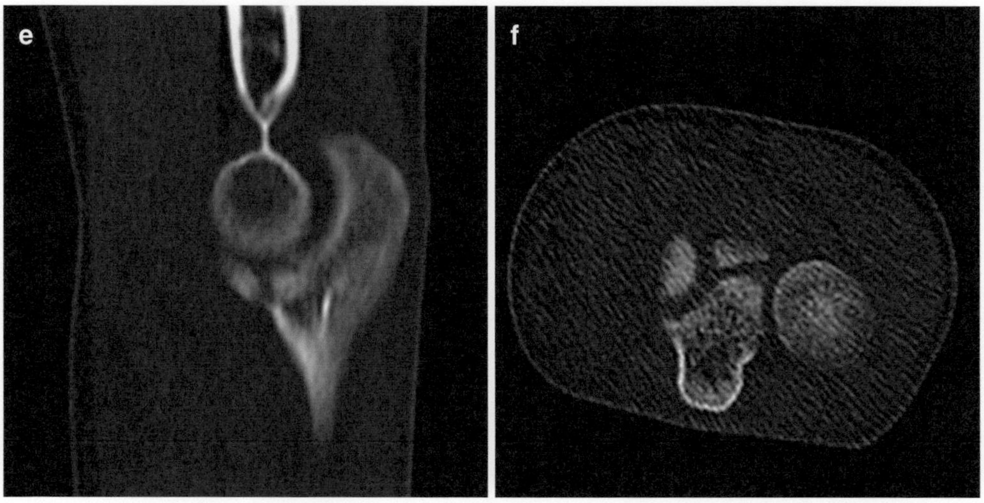

Fig. 3.40 (**e**, **f**) CT sagittal reconstruction and cross-section showing ulnar coronoid bone fracture, slightly displaced joint surface

17. Identification of the base of coronoid process comminuted fracture of the ulnar with the simple fracture
    17.1. X-ray (Fig. 3.41a–d)

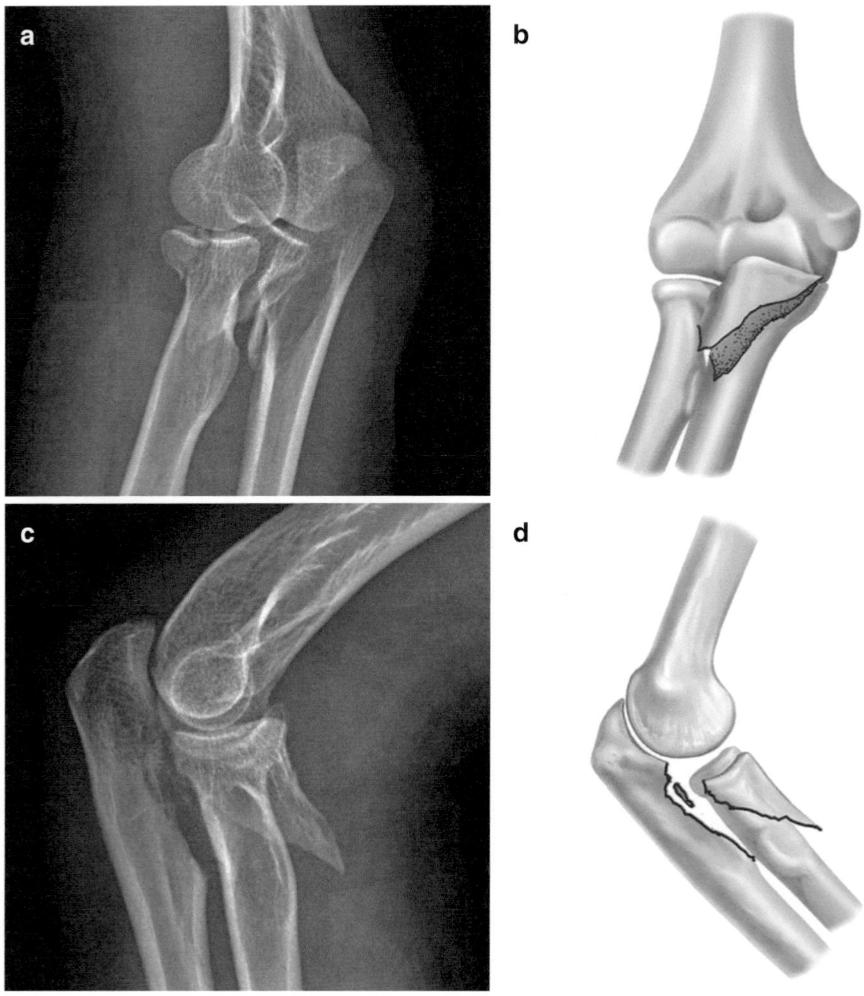

Fig. 3.41 Identification of the base of coronoid process comminuted fracture of the ulnar with the simple fracture. (**a**, **c**) X-ray shows ulnar coronoid base fracture, fracture end dislocation, separation, articular surface dislocation; (**b**, **d**) Schematic

17.2. CT scan (Fig. 3.41e–h)

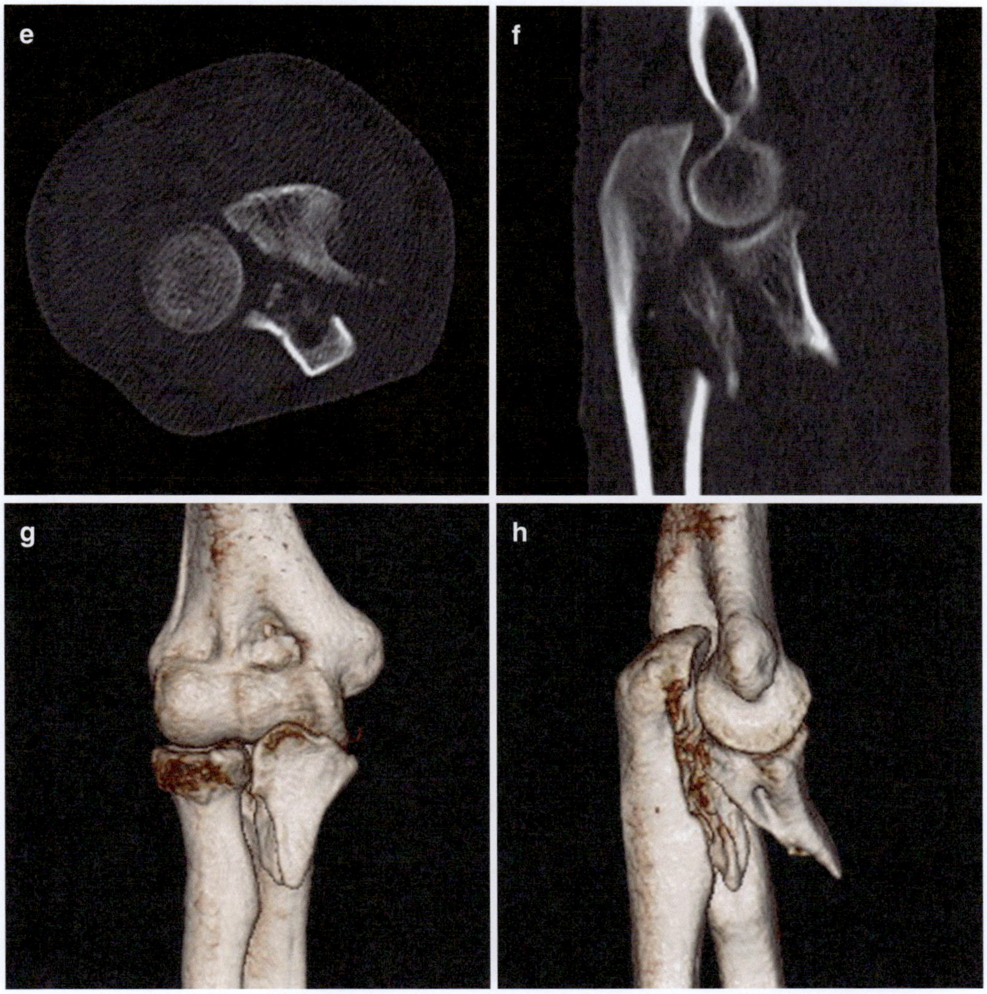

Fig. 3.41 (**e**–**h**) CT cross-section, sagittal reconstruction, and three-dimensional reconstruction showing ulnar coronoid basal bone fracture, visible multiple bone mass, displacement, dislocation of joint surface

3.3 Proximal Radius Fracture

The proximal radius structure includes the radial head and radial neck. The radial head articulate with humeral capitulum as a ball and socket joint, articulate with proximal radial notch of ulnar forms an axle joint. The radial head is surrounded by annular ligament. According to the AO classification, the proximal end of the ulna and radial head is classified as a whole. The Mason classification of the radial head fracture and the Judet classification of the radial neck fracture are the most commonly used in clinical practice.

The Mason classification of radial head fractures is divided into radial head fracture without displacement; radial head fracture with displacement, fracture involving 30–50% of radial head; radial head comminuted fracture involving the entire radial head; and radial head fracture combined with humeroradial joint dislocation. The Judet classification of radial neck fractures is divided into fracture without displacement and inclination; fracture with displacement less than half of the transverse diameter, inclination <30°; fracture with displacement greater than half of the transverse diameter, inclination 30–60°; and complete fracture with dislocation, tilt 60–90°.

3.3.1 Identification of Injury Mechanism

Fractures of the radial neck and the radial head are often caused by indirect violence. The hand pronated with palm hit the ground upon a fall. The elbow joint is in an extension and external rotation position. The thrust force is transmitted along the longitudinal axis, causing an excessive elbow valgus blow, making the lateral side of radial head collide with the humeral capitulum, resulting in a fracture of the radial head or neck. The fracture fragment is often rotated outwards or downwards, and there is slight displacement to the proximal or medial side. If a large fracture block is found in the front and the proximal side of the radial head at the level of the elbow joint, a fracture should be highly suspected. The mass comes from the small head of the radius, not the smashed humeral capitulum.

3.3.2 Symptom and Sign Identification

A proximal radial fracture without displacement or slight displacement has mild local symptoms; thus, it is easily missed.

Displacement fractures often cause pain in the lateral elbow, and the pain is aggravated when the elbow flexes and extends or rotated, its mobility is limited. Occasionally, the bone grinding can be detected on the outside. Subcutaneous bruise on the lateral side of the elbow is rare. The fracture is commonly combined with a medial collateral ligament injury; therefore, special attention should be paid onto identification. A severe injury of the medial collateral ligament reduces the stability of the elbow joint. On examination the medial side of the elbow has severe pain by palpation, swelling, and bruise.

The elbow joint valgus stress test with elbow extension shows a distinct increase in the elbow's valgus angle, thus, a medial collateral ligament injury should be highly suspected. Attention should also be paid to the pain and swelling of the forearm and wrist joints. If the wrist joint is painful, it may be associated with an acute lower ulna-radius joint separation, forearm interosseous ligament and triangular fibrocartilage complex injury.

3.3.3 Imaging Identification

X-ray films of the elbow joint are often able to confirm the fracture diagnosis. However, if there is a "fat pad sign," and the anteroposterior and lateral X-ray film shows no obvious fractures, the radial head X-ray film or CT should be performed to determine whether there is a fracture to avoid a missed diagnosis.

1. Identification of the radial head fracture with the suspicious fracture.
   1.1. X-ray (Fig. 3.42a–d)

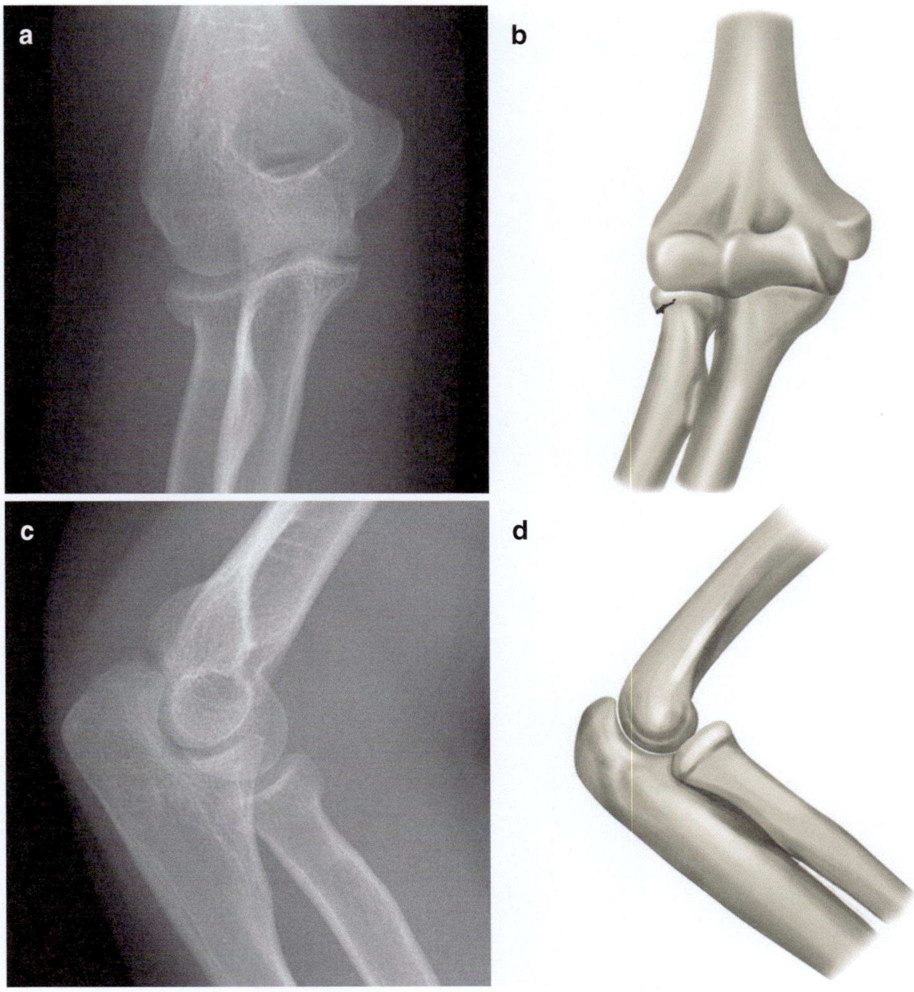

Fig. 3.42 Identification of the radial head fracture with the suspicious fracture. (**a**, **c**) X-ray shows visible folds in the cortical bone of the outer edge of the radial head, no clear fracture signs were seen; (**b**, **d**) Schematic

   1.2. CT scan (Fig. 3.42e, f)

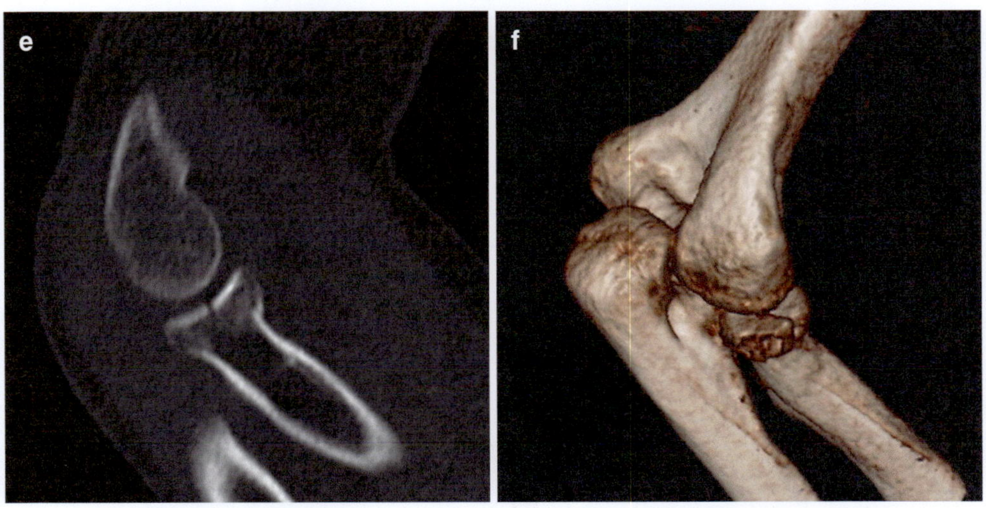

Fig. 3.42 (**e**, **f**) CT sagittal reconstruction and three-dimensional reconstruction showed radial head fracture, fracture line reached the joint. No dislocation

2. Identification of the radial head fracture with the non-fracture.
    2.1. X-ray (Fig. 3.43a–d)

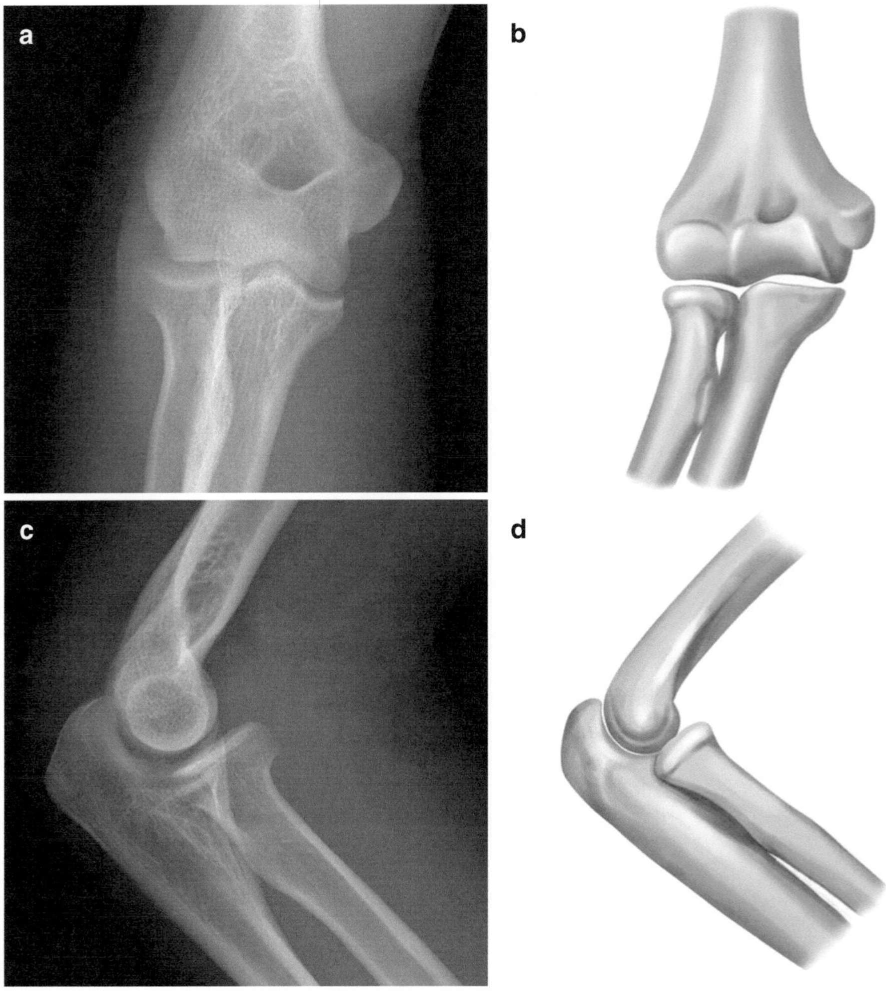

Fig. 3.43 Identification of the radial head fracture with the non-fracture. (**a**, **c**) X-ray shows no obvious fracture signs of the radial head; (**b**, **d**) Schematic

    2.2. CT scan (Fig. 3.43e, f)

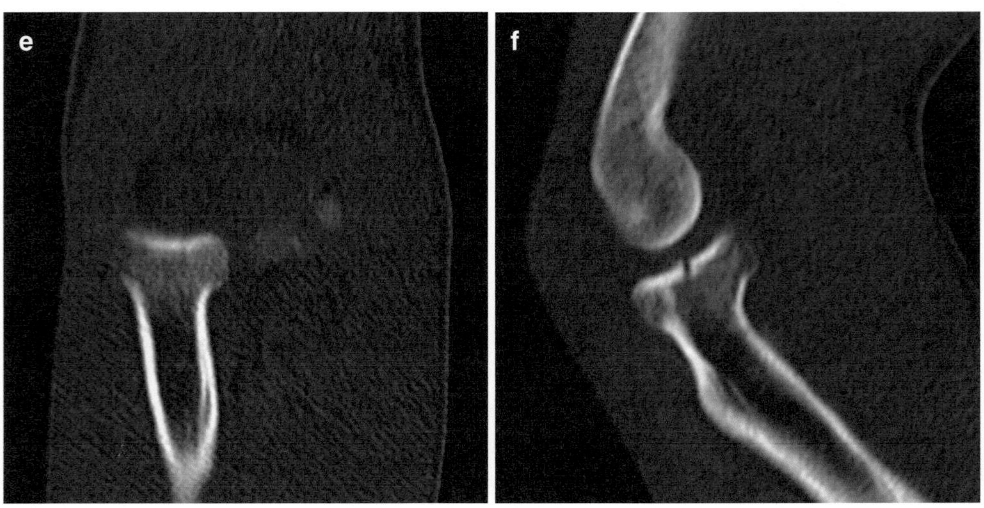

Fig. 3.43 (**e**, **f**) CT coronal reconstruction and sagittal reconstruction showed radial head fracture and articular surface fracture, and dislocation is not detected

3. Identification of the radial head fracture with the suspicious fracture.
    3.1. X-ray (Fig. 3.44a–d)

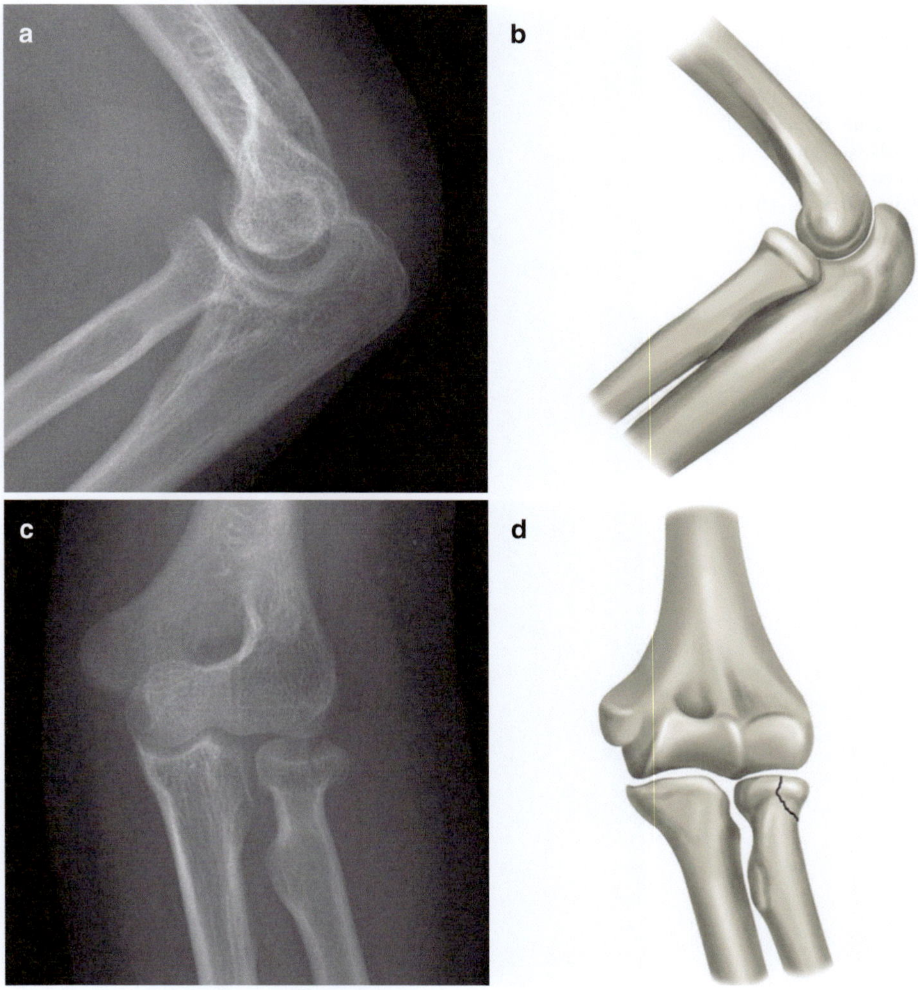

Fig. 3.44 Identification of the radial head fracture with the suspicious fracture. (**a**, **c**) X-ray shows a linear radiolucent on the articular surface of the radial head, no obvious signs of fracture in the radial neck cortex; (**b**, **d**) Schematic

    3.2. CT scan (Fig. 3.44e, f)

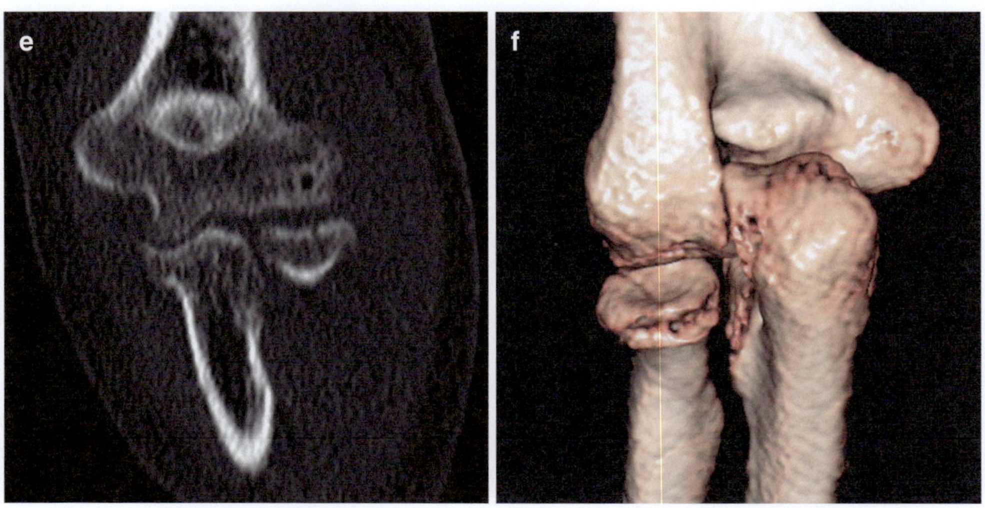

Fig. 3.44 (**e**, **f**) CT coronal reconstruction and three-dimensional reconstruction showed radial head fracture. The fracture line reaches the articular surface, and the dislocation is not present

4. Identification of the radial head comminuted fracture with the simple fracture.
   4.1. X-ray (Fig. 3.45a–d)

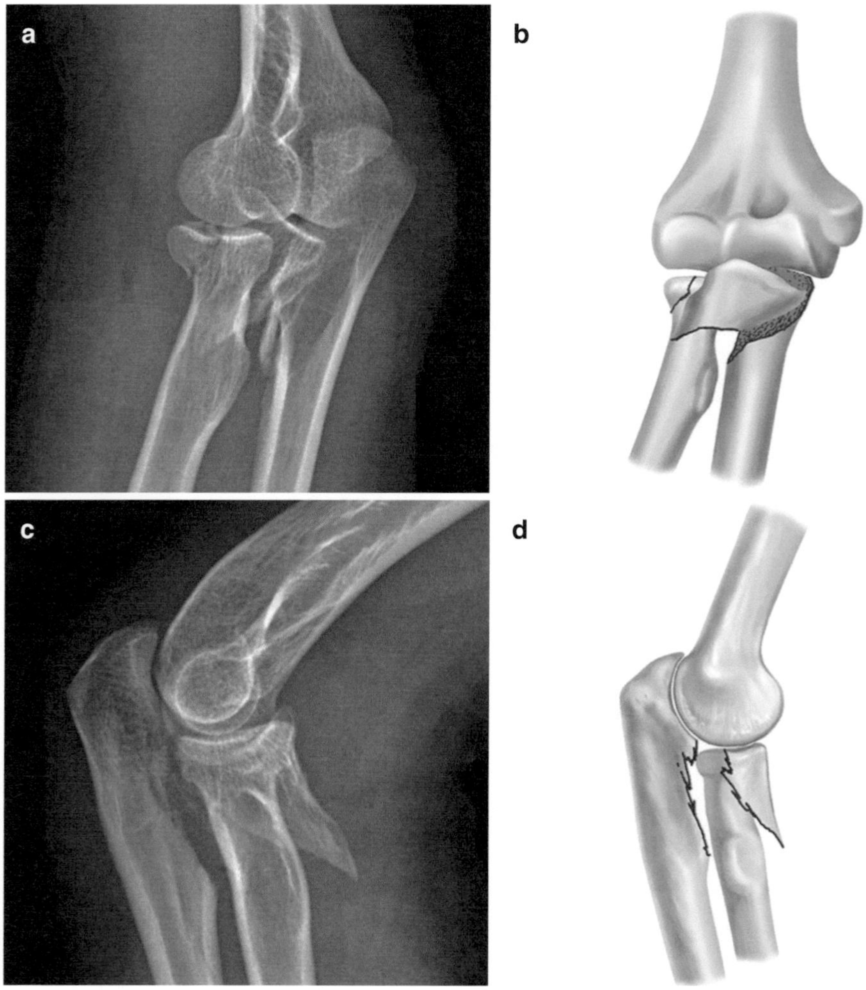

Fig. 3.45 Identification of the radial head comminuted fracture with the simple fracture. (**a**, **c**) X-ray shows oblique fracture of the radial head, no dislocation, ulnar coronoid base fracture, marked displacement; (**b**, **d**) Schematic

   4.2. CT scan (Fig. 3.45e, f)

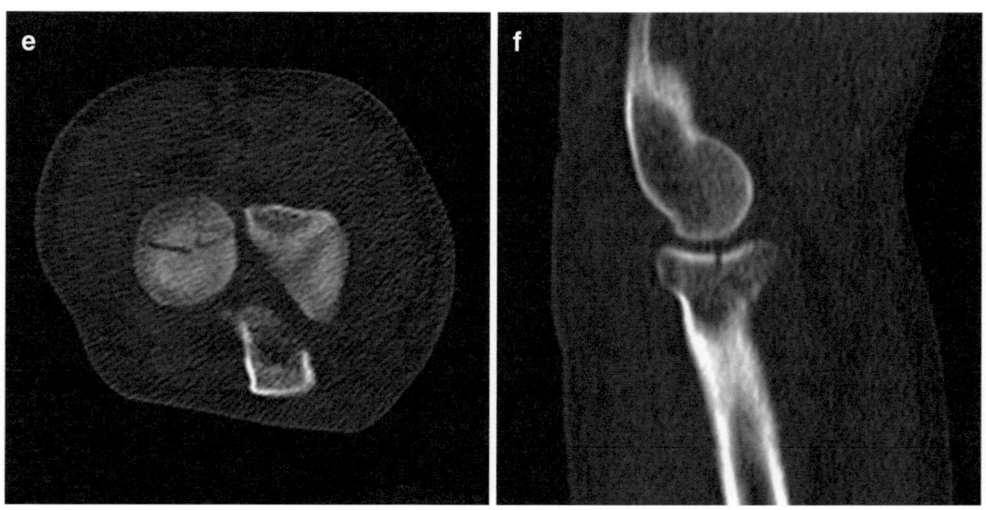

Fig. 3.45 (**e**, **f**) CT cross-section and sagittal reconstruction showed radial head bone fracture, visible multiple bones, no dislocation of the articular surface, proximal ulna fracture

5. Identification of the radial head displacement fracture with the suspicious fracture.
   5.1. X-ray (Fig. 3.46a–d)

Fig. 3.46 Identification of the radial head displacement fracture with the suspicious fracture. (**a**, **c**) X-ray shows irregular shape of the radial head; fracture line is not clear; (**b**, **d**) Schematic

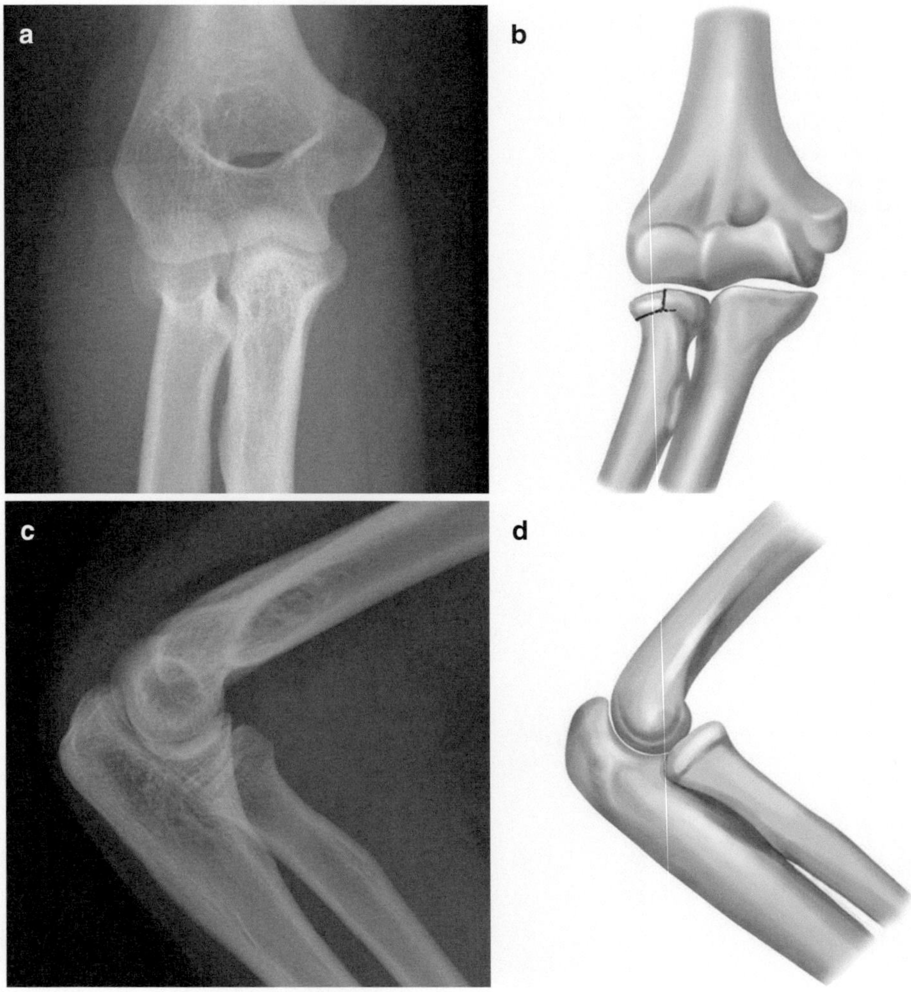

   5.2. CT scan (Fig. 3.46e, f)

Fig. 3.46 (**e**, **f**) CT cross-section and coronal reconstruction showed that the outer edge of the radial head is about 2/5 split, with displacement and joint surface unevenness

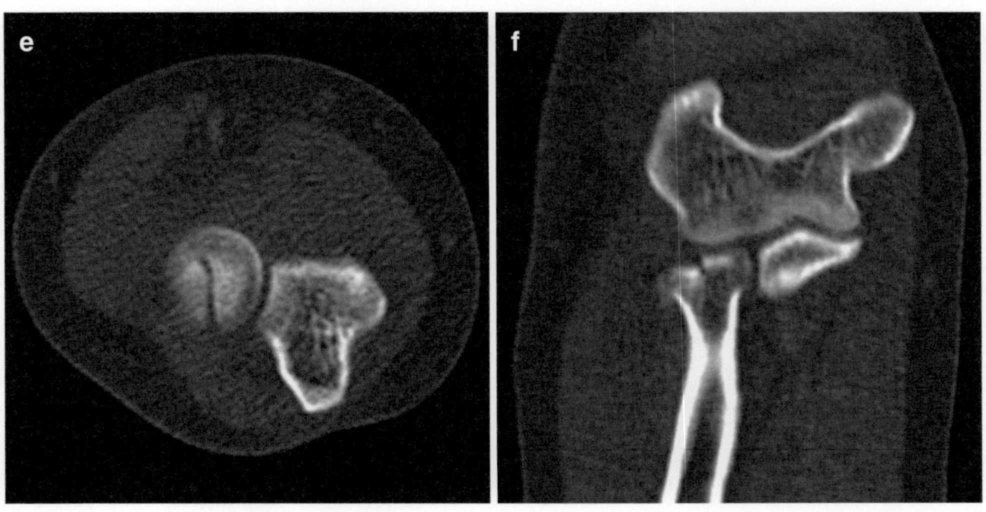

6. Comparison of the radial head displacement X-ray with the CT.
   6.1. X-ray (Fig. 3.47a–d)

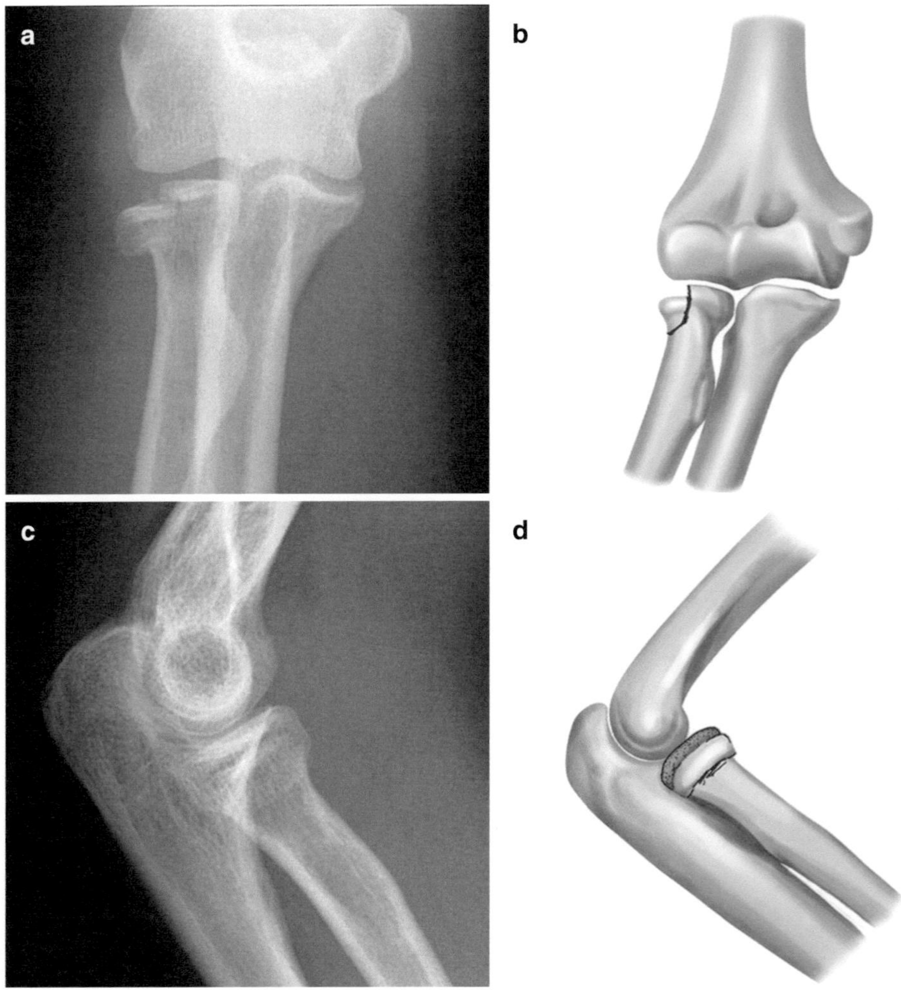

Fig. 3.47 Comparison of the radial head displacement fracture X-ray with the CT. (**a**, **c**) X-ray shows the radial head lateral side split, the bone mass is dislocated, the articular surface is not even; (**b**, **d**) Schematic

   6.2. CT scan (Fig. 3.47e, f)

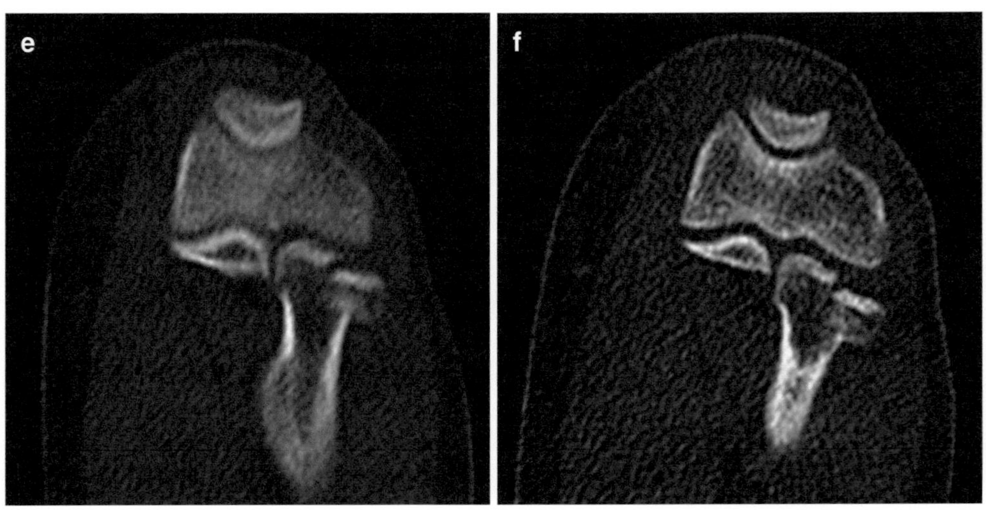

Fig. 3.47 (**e**, **f**) CT coronal reconstruction shows the lateral part of the radial head bone fracture, broken end dislocation, joint surface collapse

7. Identification of the radial head comminuted displacement fracture with the simple fracture.
   7.1. X-ray (Fig. 3.48a–d)

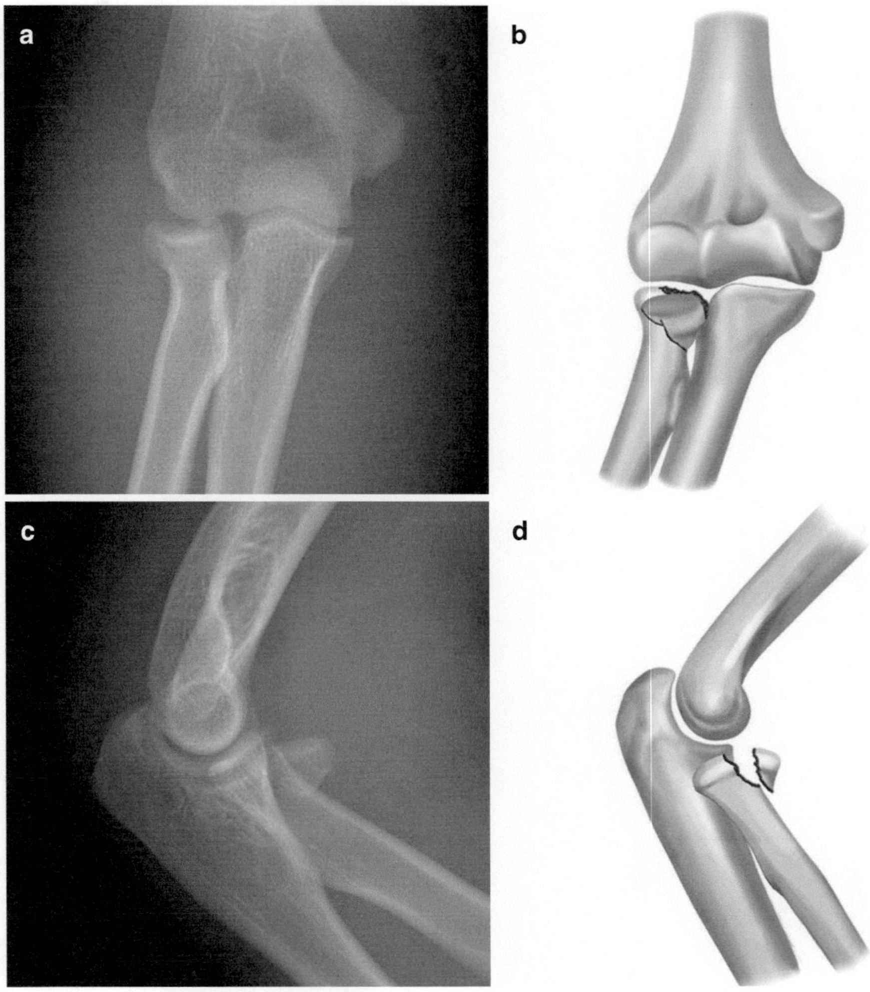

Fig. 3.48 Identification of the radial head comminuted displacement fracture with the simple fracture. (**a**, **c**) X-ray shows the fracture of the radial head chipped edge, the bone mass is completely displaced, the joint surface is uneven; (**b**, **d**) Schematic

   7.2. CT scan (Fig. 3.48e, f)

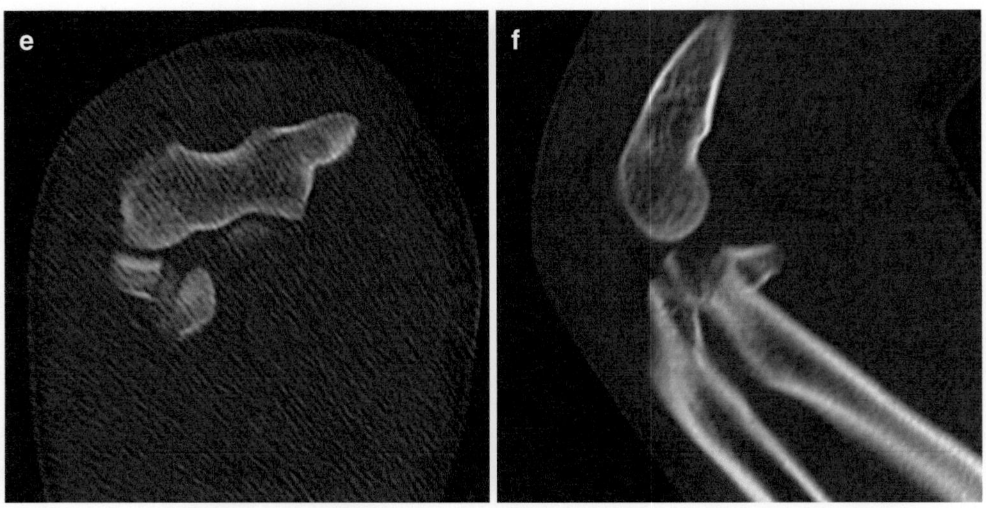

Fig. 3.48 (**e**, **f**) CT coronal reconstruction and sagittal reconstruction showed anterior medial fragmentation of the radial head, complete dislocation, articular surface collapse

8. Identification of the radial head comminuted fracture with the simple fracture.
   8.1. X-ray (Fig. 3.49a–d)

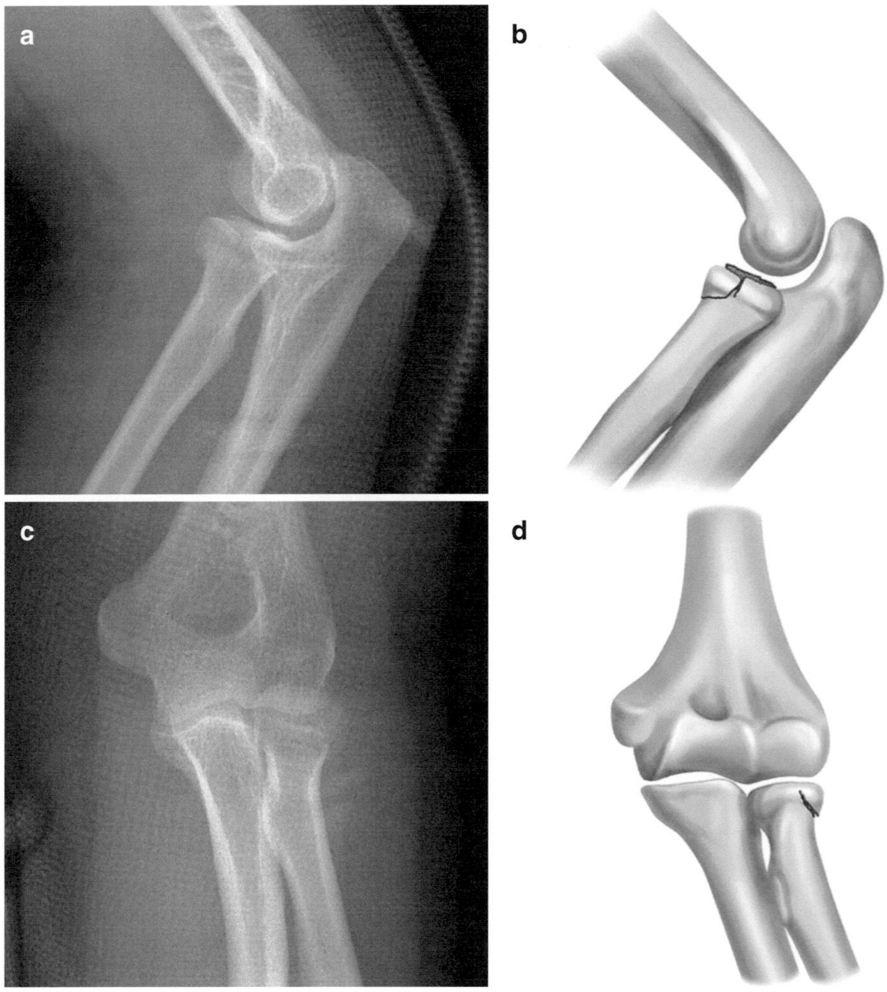

Fig. 3.49 Identification of the radial head comminuted fracture with the simple fracture. (**a**, **c**) The X-ray film shows the linear radiolucent at the radial head, the joint surface is slightly displaced; (**b**, **d**) Schematic

   8.2. CT scan (Fig. 3.49e, f)

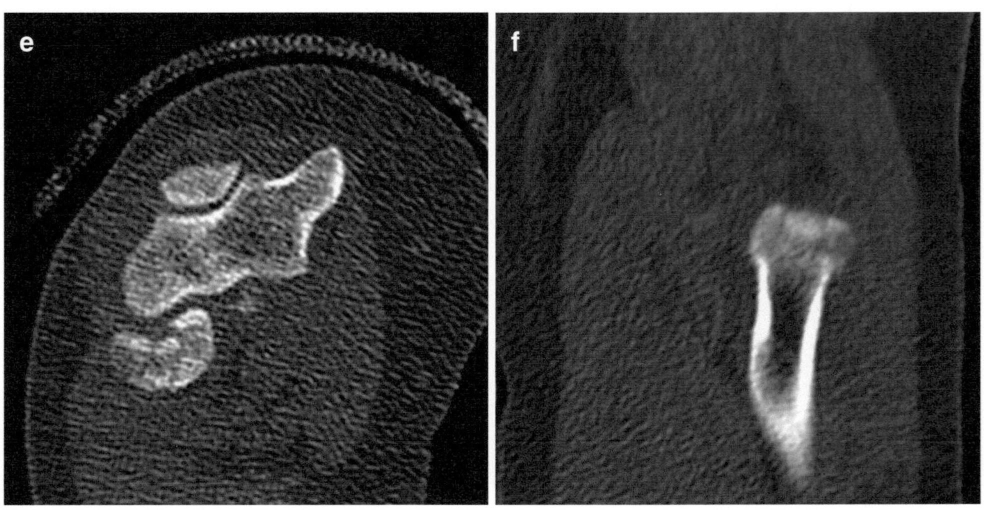

Fig. 3.49 (**e**, **f**) CT cross-section and coronal reconstruction show that the radial head is fragmented, and multiple bone masses can be seen on the articular surface with a slight collapse of the articular surface

9. Identification of the radial head comminuted impaction fracture with the simple fracture.
   9.1. X-ray (Fig. 3.50a–d)

Fig. 3.50 Identification of the radial head comminuted impaction fracture with the simple fracture. (**a**, **c**) X-ray shows that the radial head has visible linear radiolucent, the joint surface is tilted; (**b**, **d**) Schematic

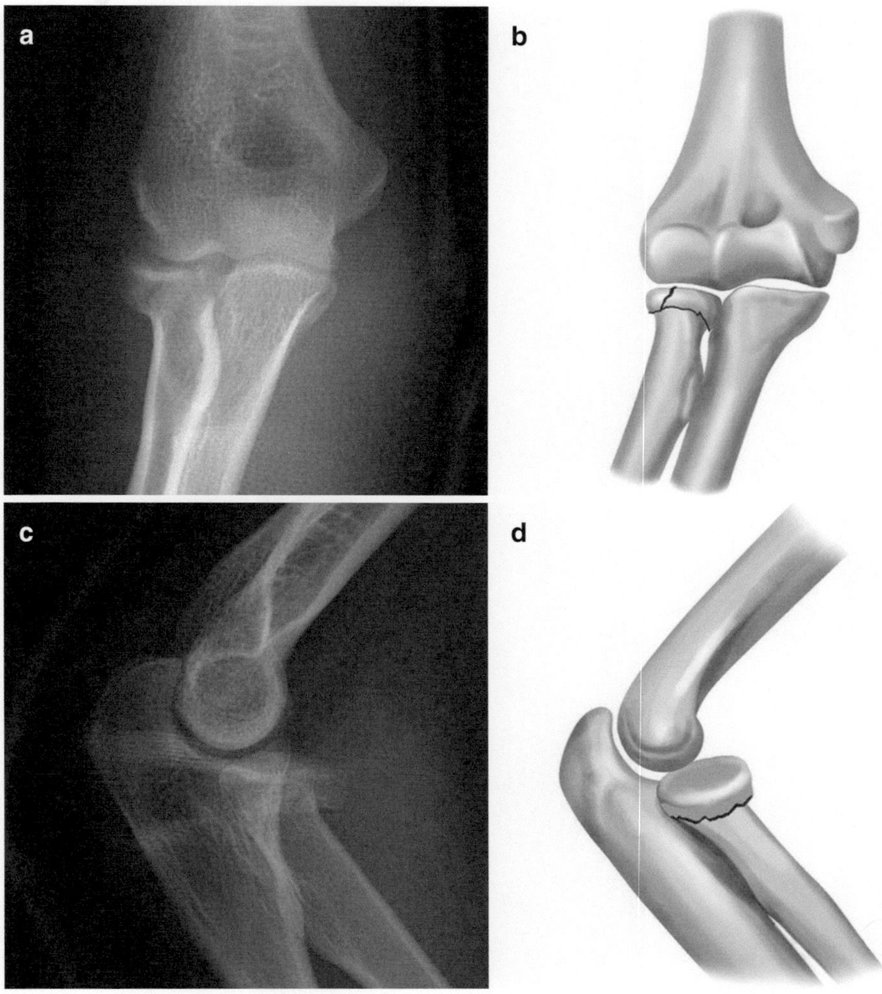

   9.2. CT scan (Fig. 3.50e, f)

Fig. 3.50 (**e**, **f**) CT coronal reconstruction and sagittal reconstruction show that the radial head is fragmented, joint surface presented with few bone masses, the radial head joint surface is tilted forward

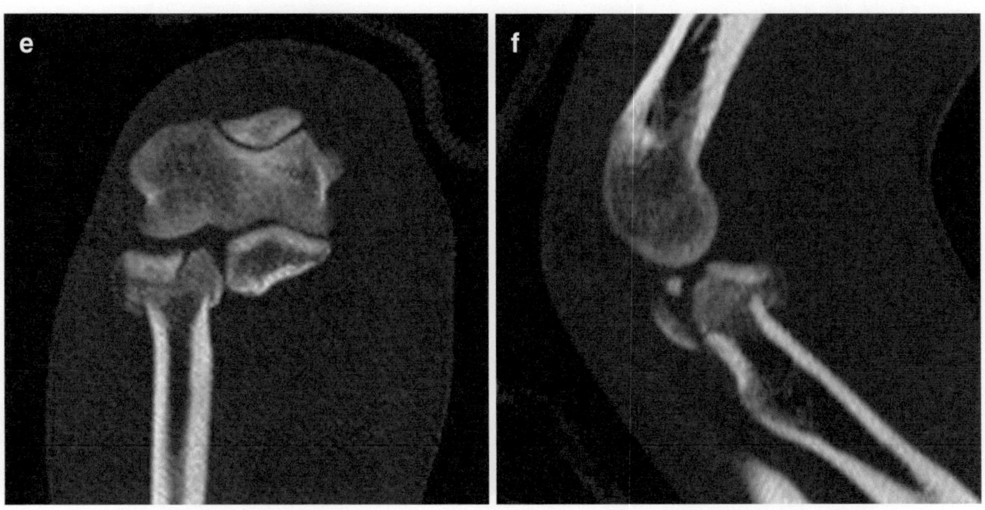

10. Identification of the radial head comminuted impacted fracture with the simple fracture.
    10.1. X-ray (Fig. 3.51a–d)

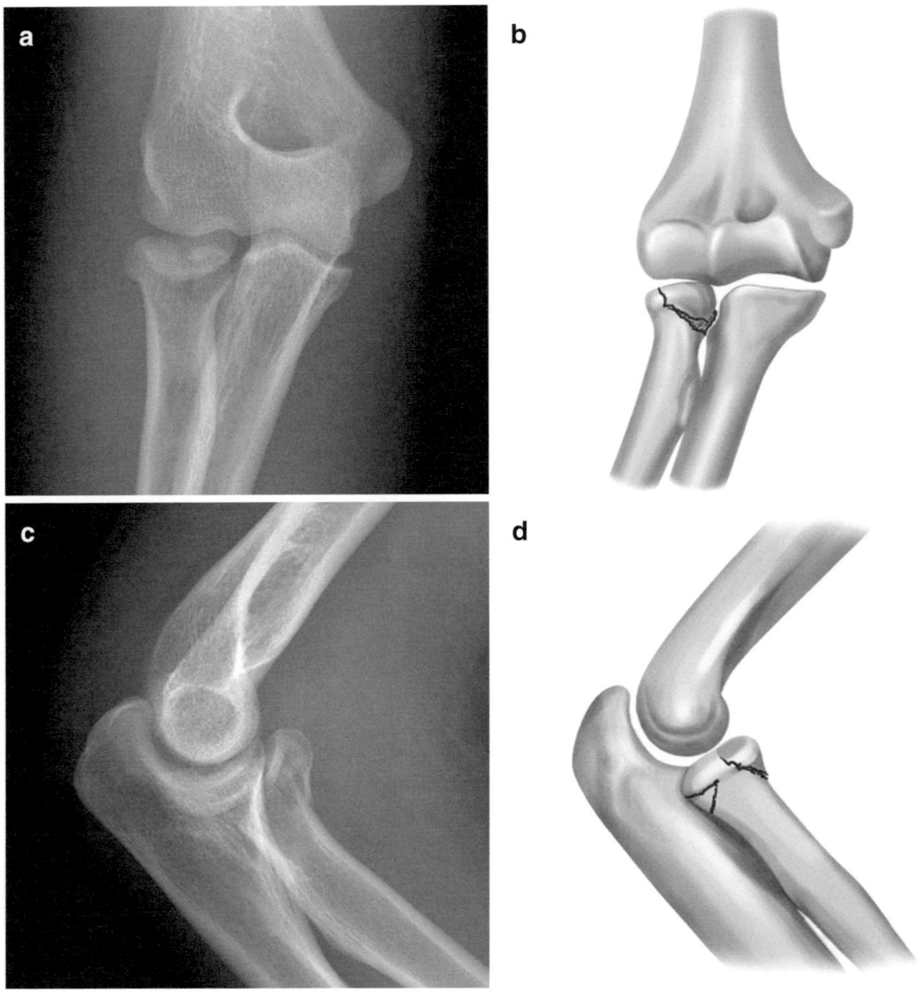

Fig. 3.51 Identification of the radial head comminuted impacted fracture with simple fracture. (**a**, **c**) X-ray shows the anterior rim of the radial head, and the articular surface is impacted; (**b**, **d**) Schematic

    10.2. CT scan (Fig. 3.51e, f)

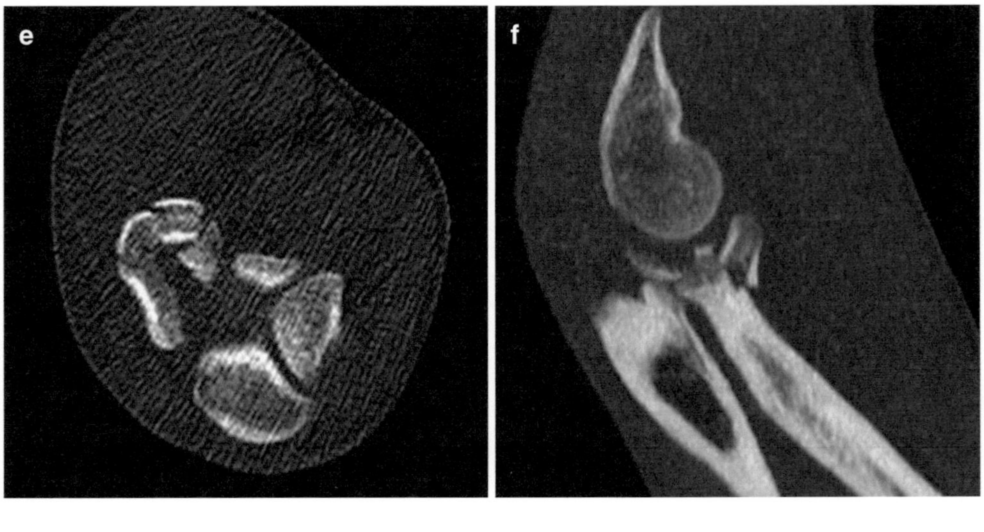

Fig. 3.51 (**e**, **f**) CT cross-section and sagittal reconstruction showed that the radial head was fragmented and the joint surface collapsed and displaced

11. Identification of the radial head fracture dislocation with the simple fracture.
    11.1. X-ray (Fig. 3.52a–d)

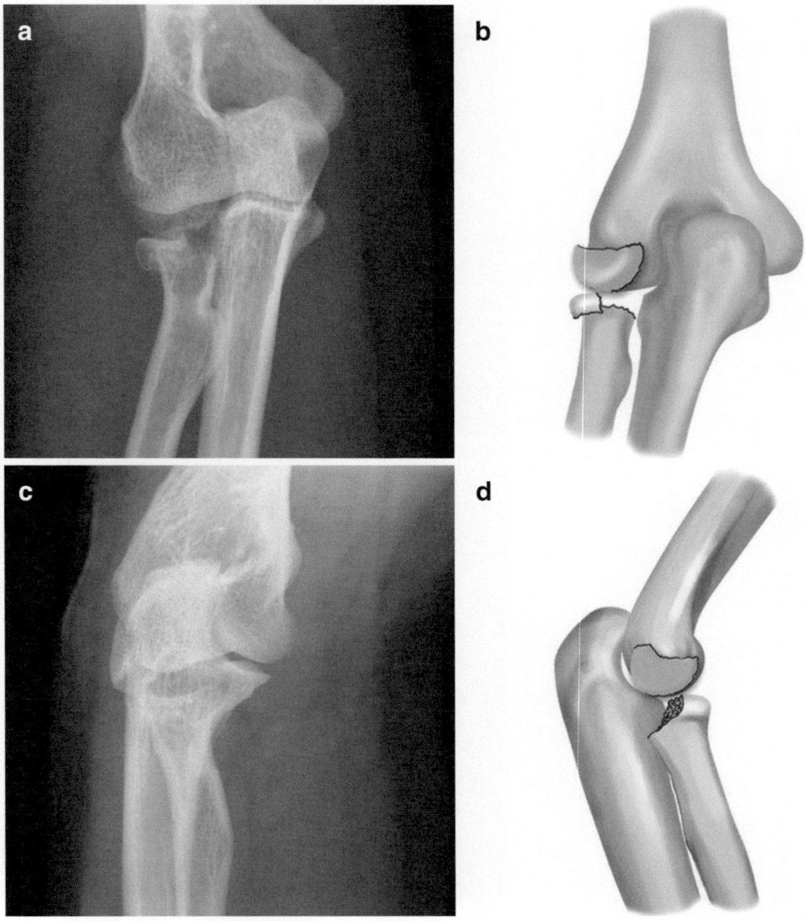

Fig. 3.52 Identification of the radial head fracture dislocation with the simple fracture. (**a**, **c**) X-ray shows the radial head fragmentation, dislocation; (**b**, **d**) Schematic

11.2. CT scan (Fig. 3.52e–h)

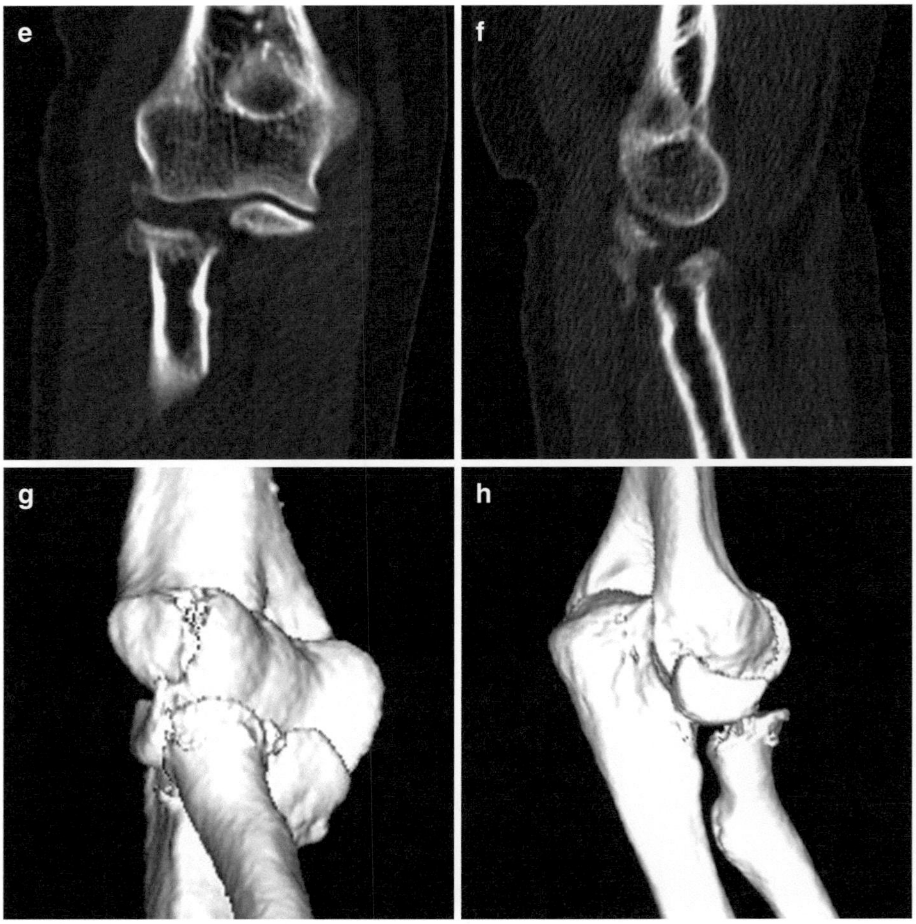

Fig. 3.52 (**e**–**h**) CT coronal reconstruction, sagittal reconstruction, and three-dimensional reconstruction showed the humeral head joint surface fragmentation, the majority of joint lateral surface displacement, loss of normal correspondence with the humeral capitulum

12. Identification of the radial head fracture dislocation with the simple fracture.
    12.1. X-ray (Fig. 3.53a–d)

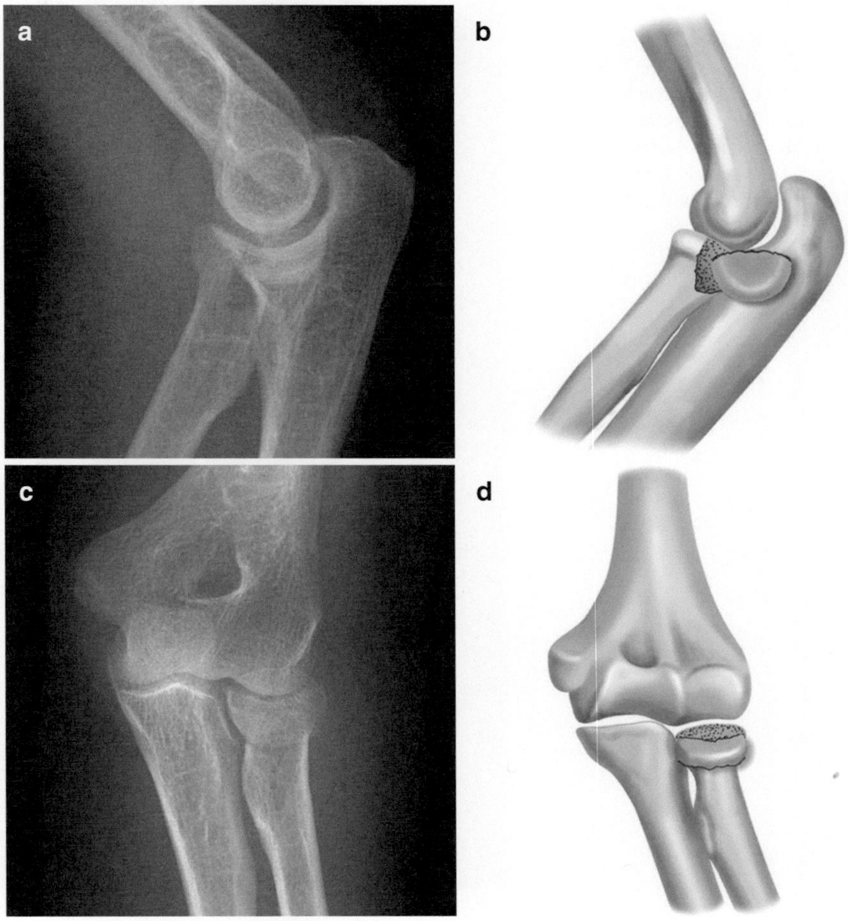

Fig. 3.53 Identification of the radial head fracture dislocation with the simple fracture. (**a**, **c**) X-ray shows the fracture of the radial head, the dislocation of the broken end; (**b**, **d**) Schematic

12.2. CT scan (Fig. 3.53e–h)

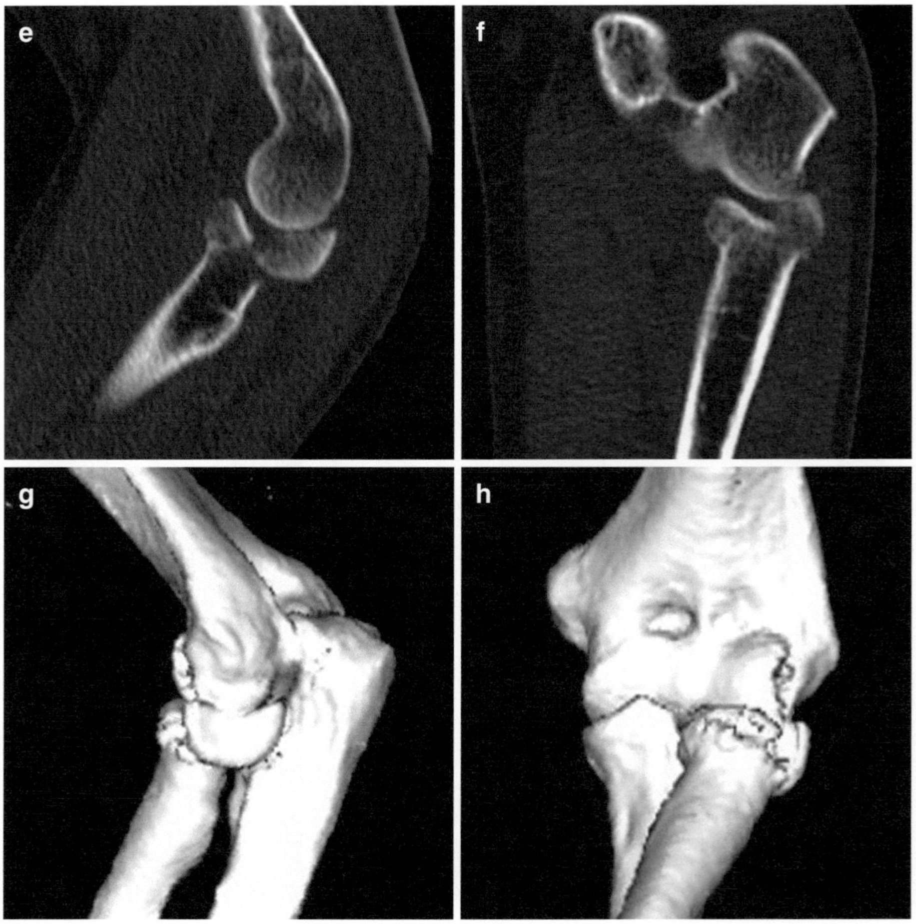

Fig. 3.53 (**e**–**h**) CT sagittal reconstruction, coronal reconstruction, and three-dimensional reconstruction showed that the radial head joint surface is fragmented, most radial head joint fragments displaced to the outside, the joint surface faces outward and loses normal correspondence with the humeral capitulum

13. Identification of the radial head fracture dislocation with the simple fracture.
    13.1. X-ray (Fig. 3.54a–d)

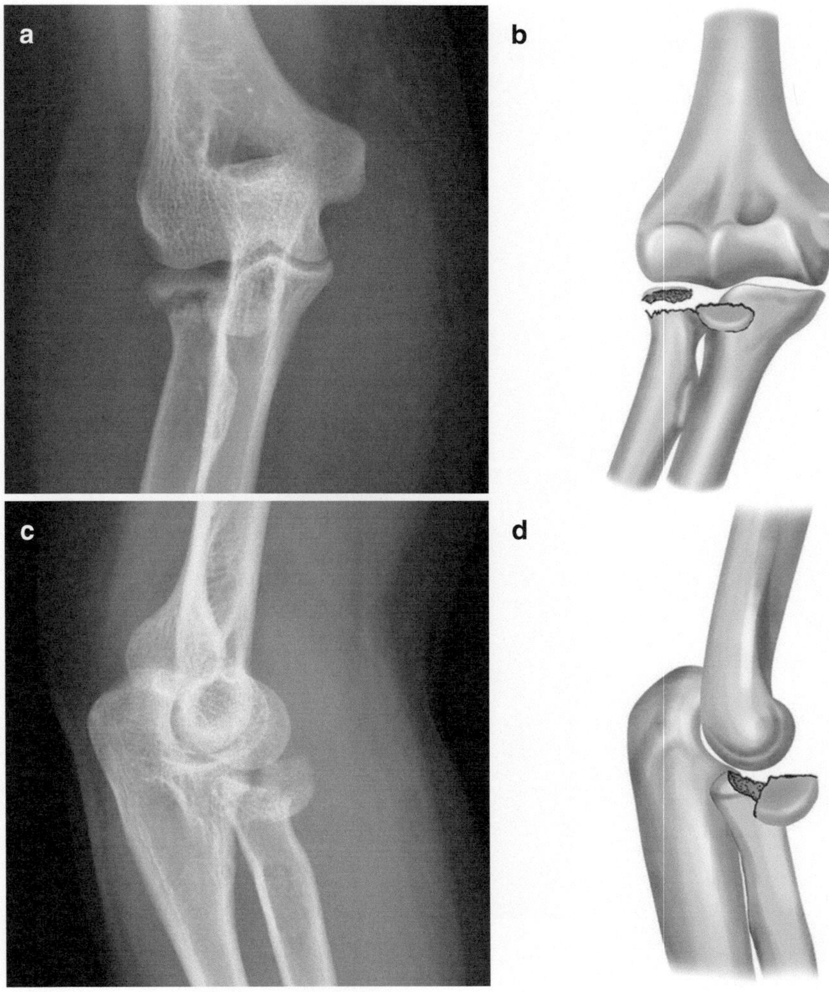

Fig. 3.54 of the radial head fracture dislocation with the simple fracture. (**a**, **c**) X-ray shows the fracture of the radial head, the joint surface is dislocated; (**b**, **d**) Schematic

13.2. CT scan (Fig. 3.54e, f)

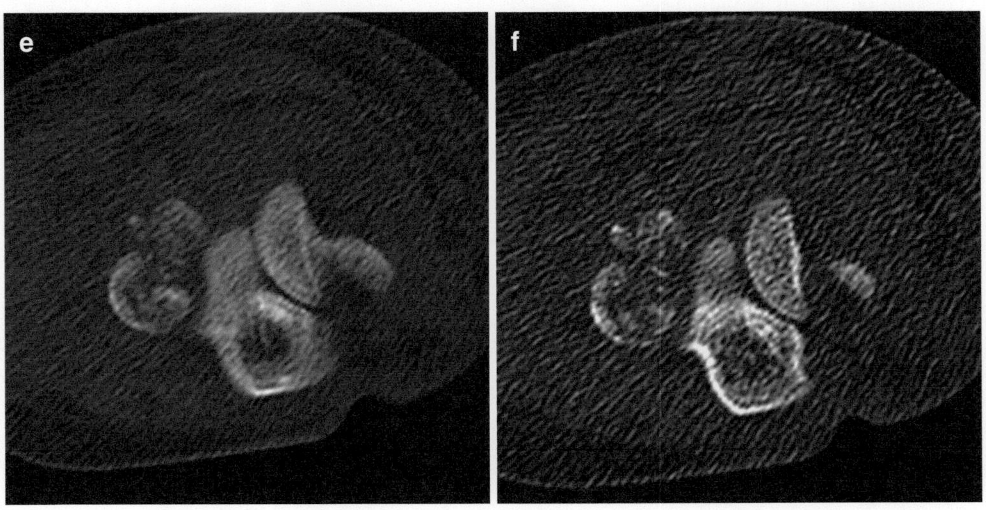

Fig. 3.54 (**e**, **f**) CT cross-section shows the radial head joint surface fragmentation, the majority of the joint surface is displaced forward, and the radial head loses normal correspondence

14. Identification of the radial neck fracture with the non-fracture.
    14.1. X-ray (Fig. 3.55a–d)

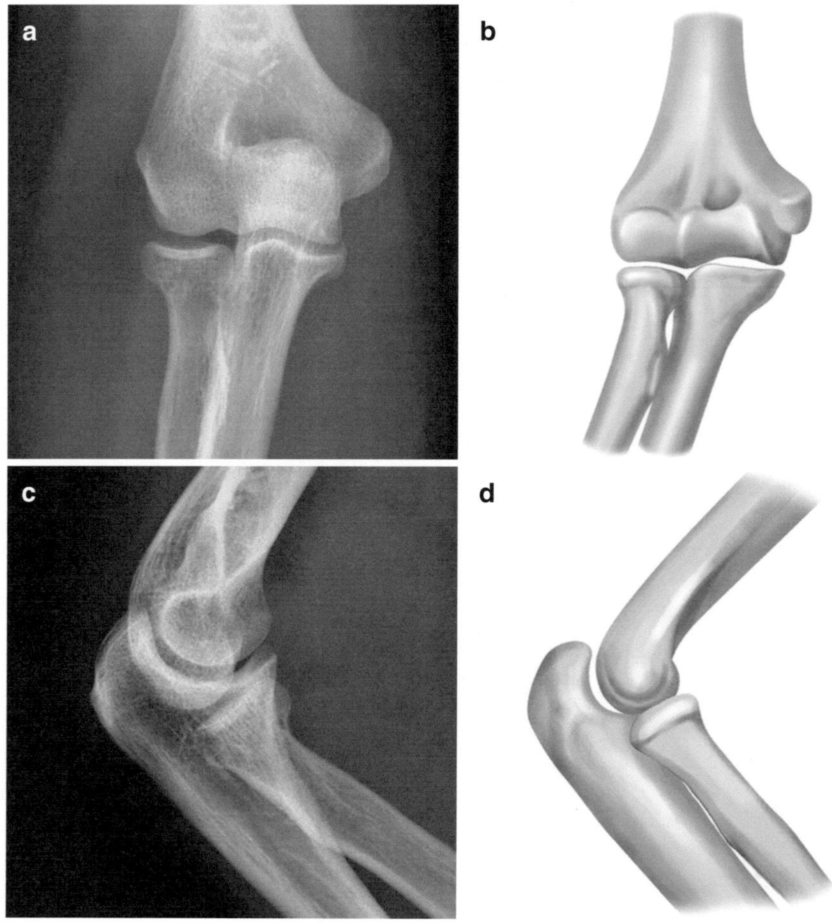

Fig. 3.55 Identification of the radial neck fracture with non-fracture. (**a**, **c**) X-ray shows no obvious fracture signs in the elbow joint bones; (**b**, **d**) Schematic

    14.2. CT scan (Fig. 3.55e, f)

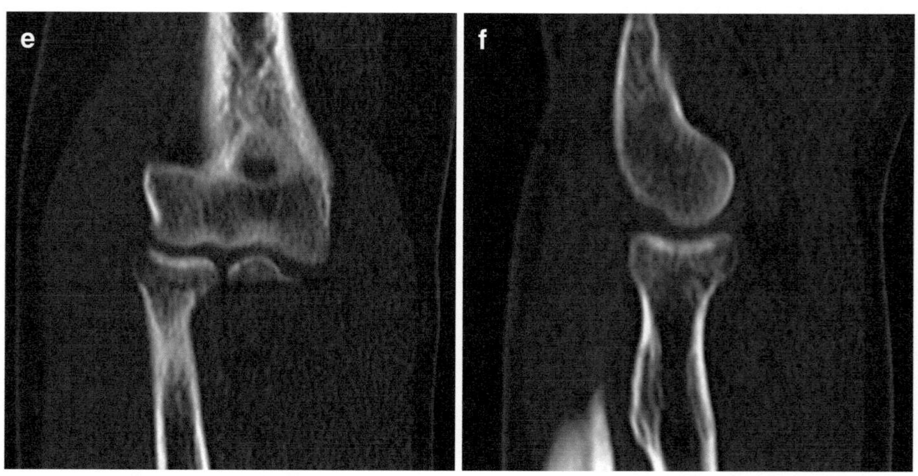

Fig. 3.55 (**e**, **f**) CT coronal reconstruction and sagittal reconstruction showed the radial neck trabecular bone rupture

14.3. MR scan (Fig. 3.55g, h)

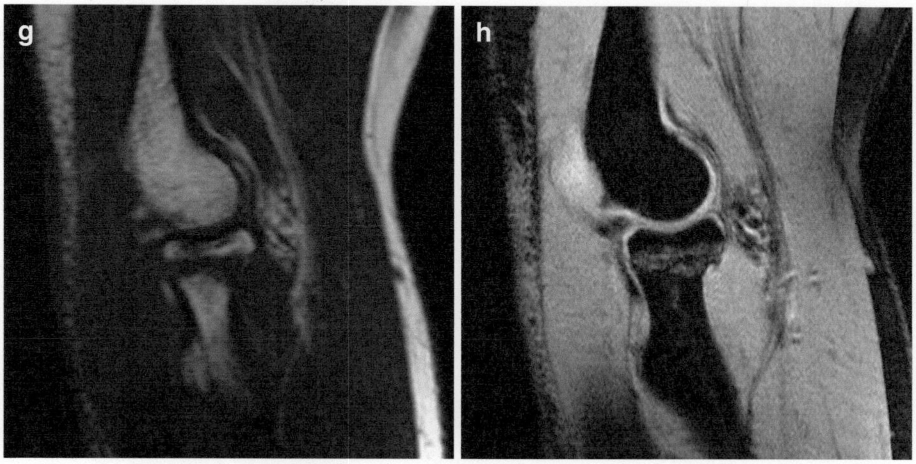

Fig. 3.55 (**g**, **h**) MRI sagittal T1WI and T2WI fat suppression sequence shows radial neck bone fracture, showing long T1 long T2 signal

15. Identification of the radial neck fracture with the non-fracture.
    15.1. X-ray (Fig. 3.56a–d)

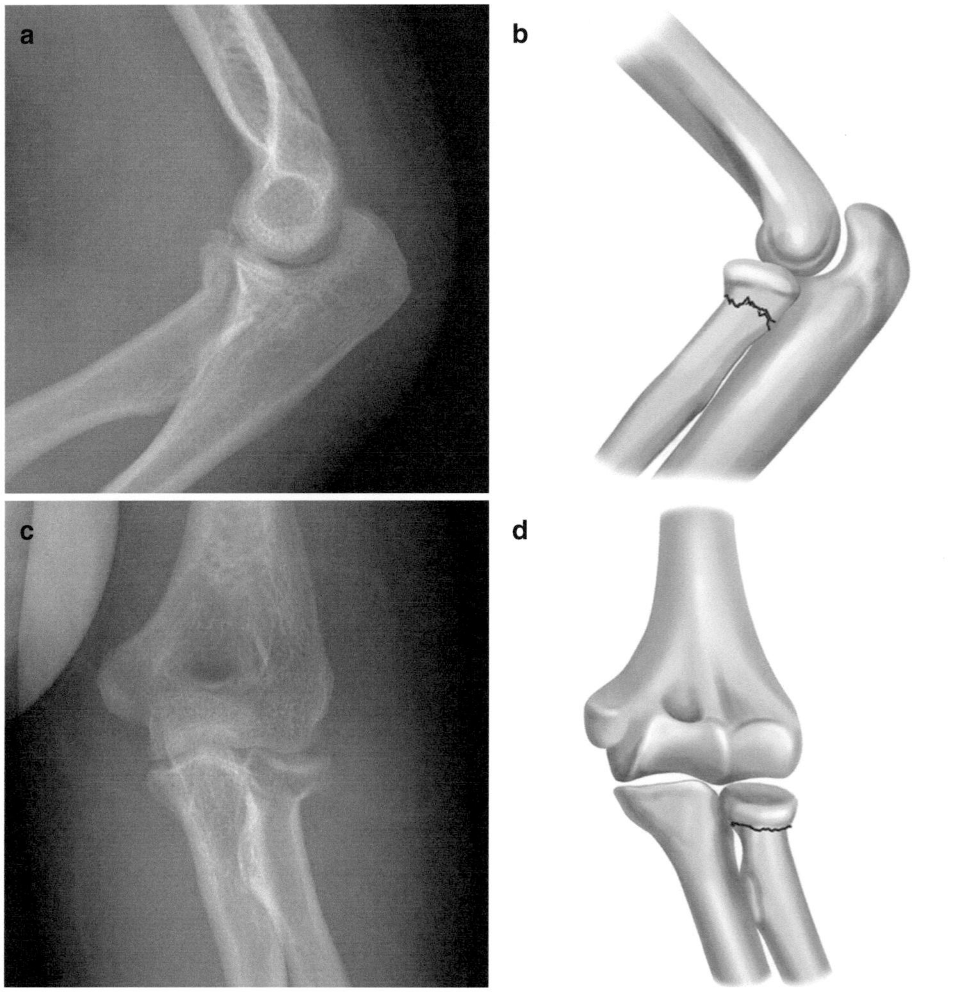

Fig. 3.56 Identification of the radial neck fracture with the non-fracture. (**a**, **c**) X-ray shows radial neck fracture, no dislocation at the end; (**b**, **d**) Schematic

    15.2. CT scan (Fig. 3.56e, f)

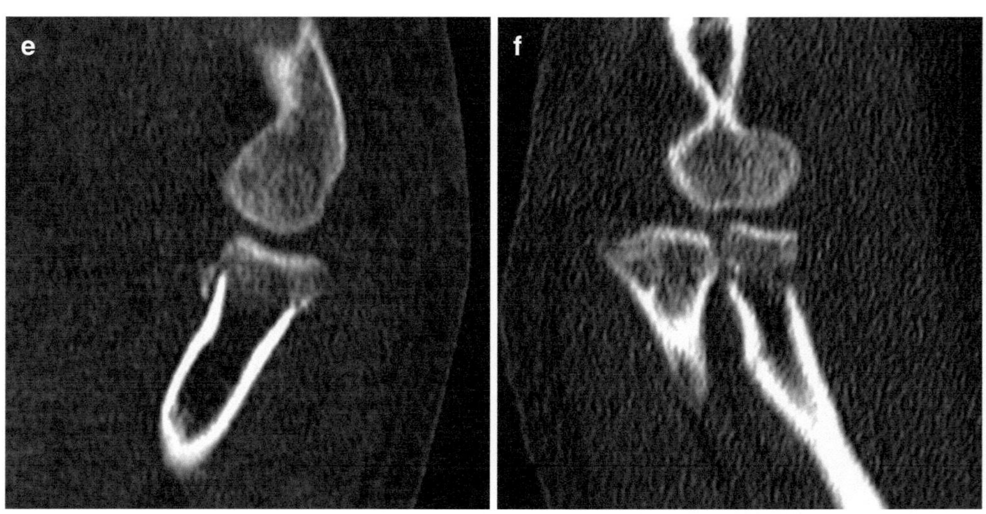

Fig. 3.56 (**e**, **f**) CT sagittal reconstruction and coronal reconstruction showed radial neck fracture, no dislocation

16. Identification of the radial neck oblique comminuted fracture with the simple fracture.
    16.1. X ray (Fig. 3.57a–d)

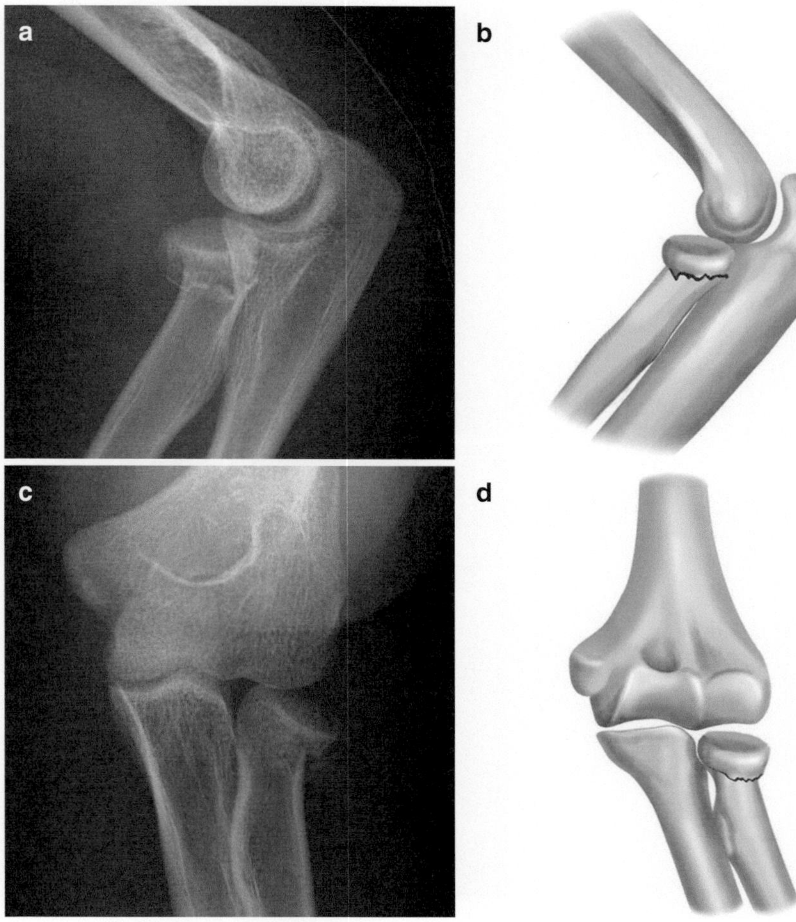

Fig. 3.57 Identification of the radial neck oblique comminuted fracture with simple fracture. (**a**, **c**) X-ray shows radial neck fracture, broken end impaction, displaced, joint surface anterior laterally tilted; (**b**, **d**) Schematic

16.2. CT scan (Fig. 3.57e–h)

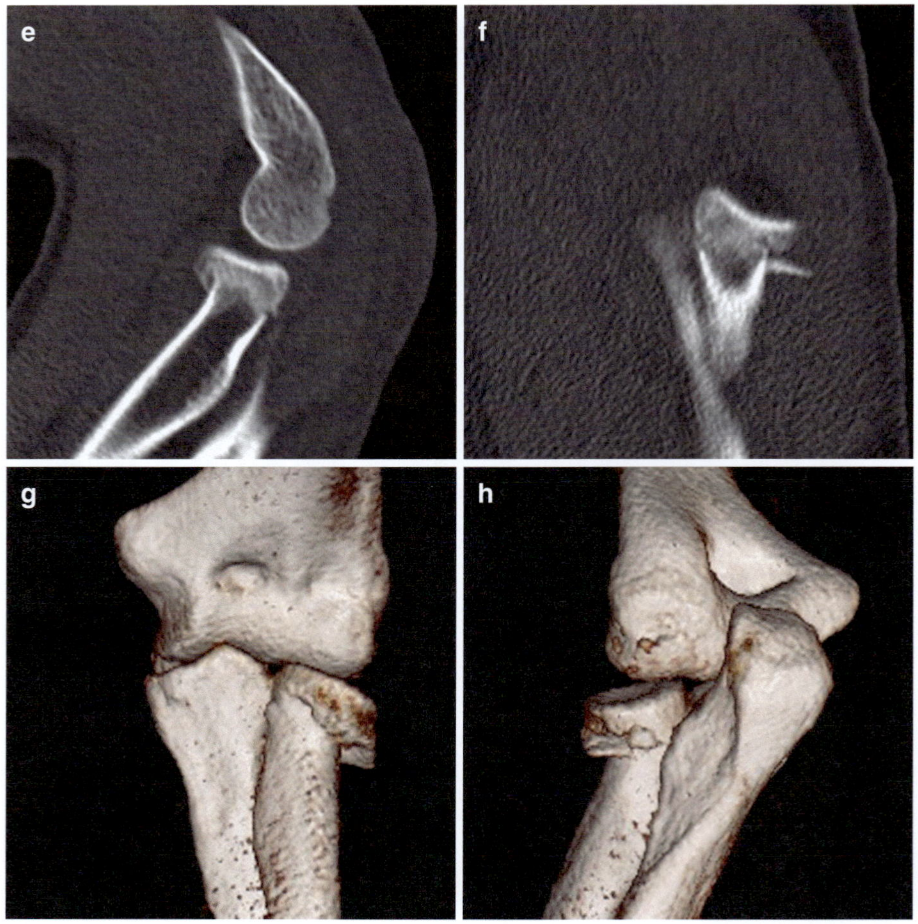

Fig. 3.57 (**e**–**h**) CT sagittal reconstruction, coronal reconstruction, and three-dimensional reconstruction showing radial neck bone fragmentation, broken ends impaction, displacement, multiple small bone fragments visible, articular surface tilted

17. Identification of the radial neck impaction fracture with the suspicious fracture.
    17.1. X-ray (Fig. 3.58a–d)

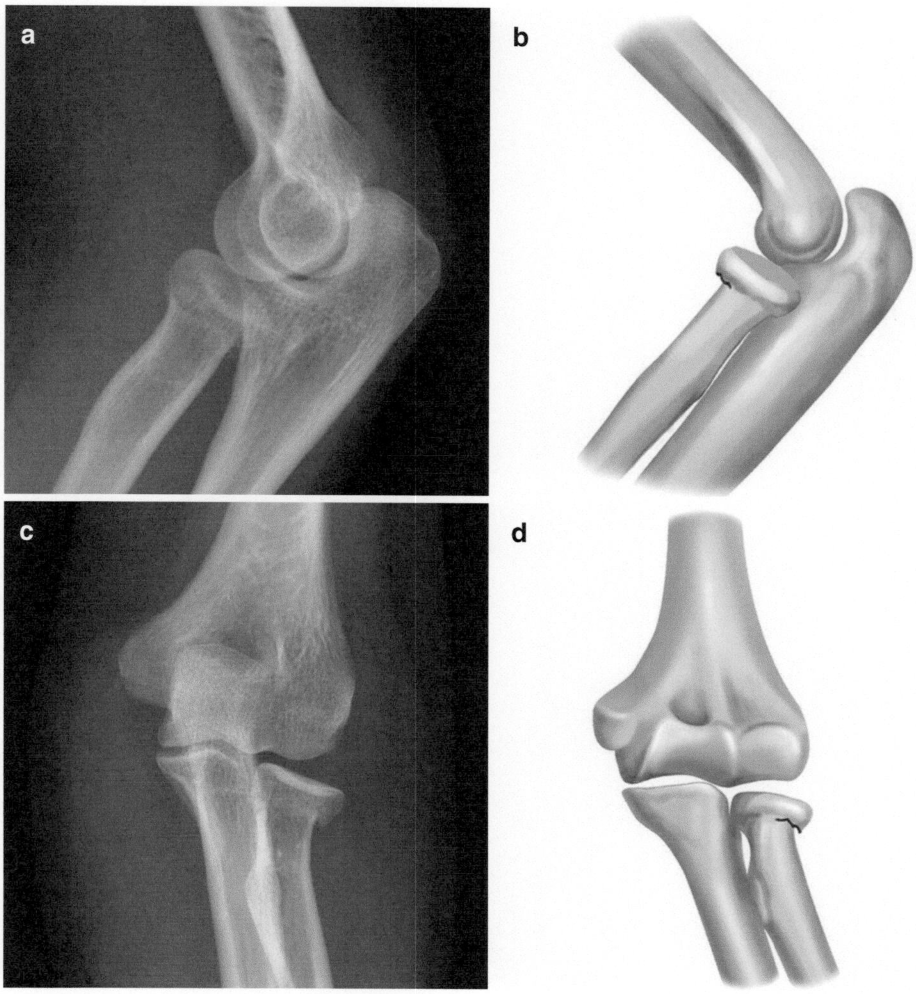

Fig. 3.58 Identification of the radial neck impaction fracture with the suspicious fracture. (**a**, **c**) X-ray shows the disarranged structure of the radial neck, the density is increased, the joint is inclined to the outside; (**b**, **d**) Schematic

    17.2. CT scan (Fig. 3.58e, f)

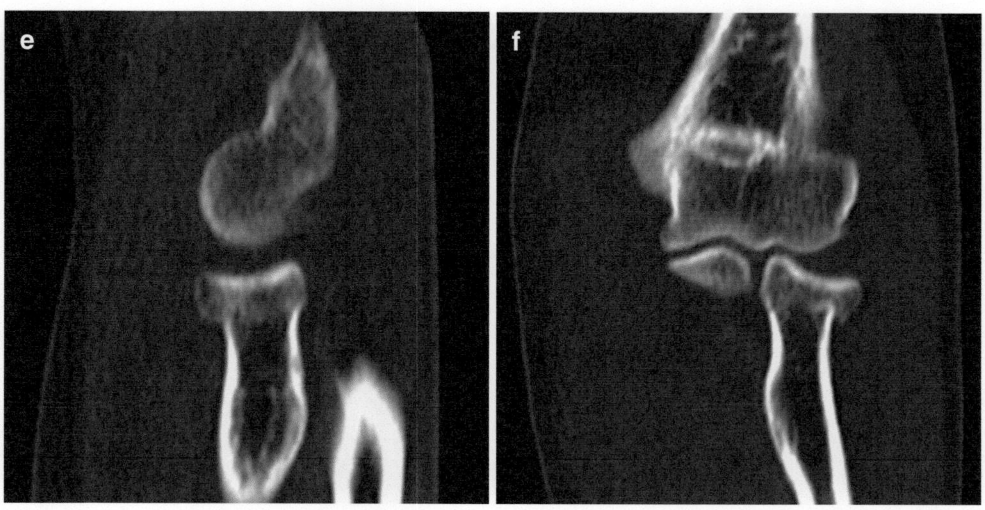

Fig. 3.58 (**e**, **f**) CT sagittal reconstruction and coronal reconstruction show the radial neck fracture, the end of the fracture impacted, displaced, articular surface tilted

18. Identification of the radial neck fracture with radial head fracture.
    18.1. X-ray (Fig. 3.59a–d)

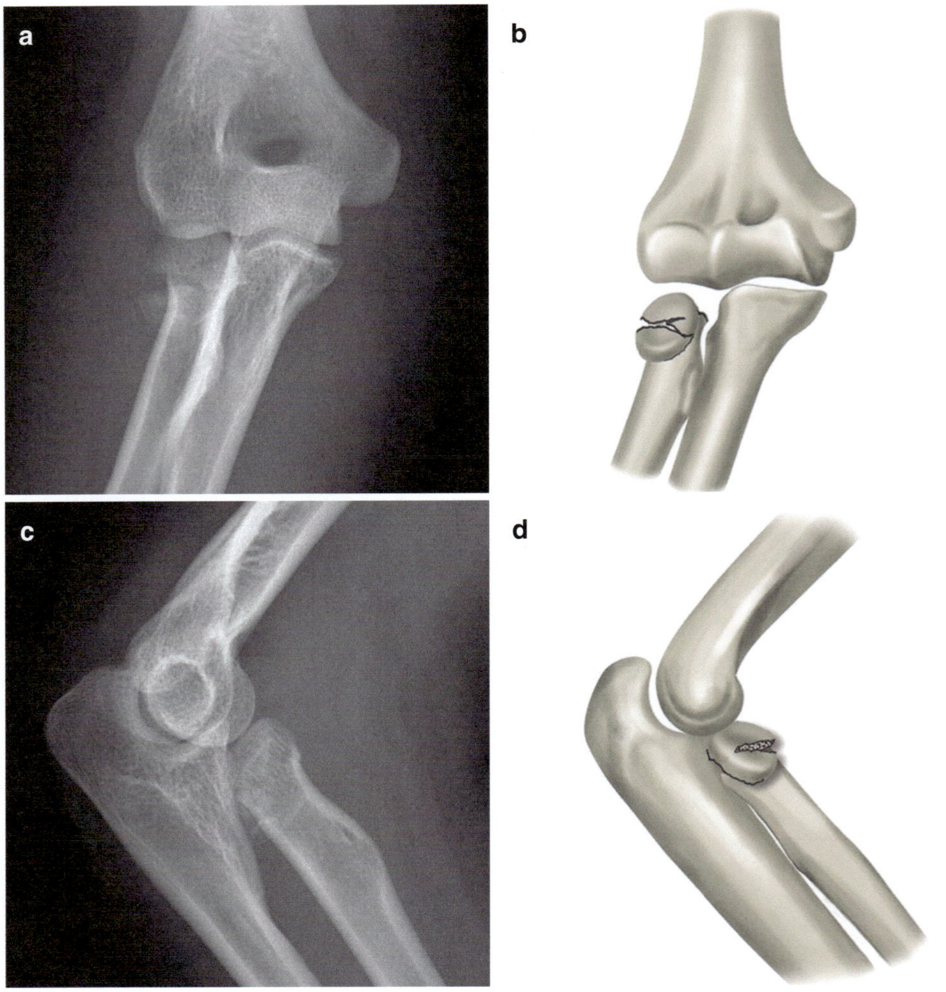

Fig. 3.59 Identification of the radial neck fracture with the radial head fracture. (**a**, **c**) X-ray shows radial neck fracture, broken end impaction, dislocation, partial fracture of joint surface, inclined to the outside; (**b**, **d**) Schematic

    18.2. CT scan (Fig. 3.59e, f)

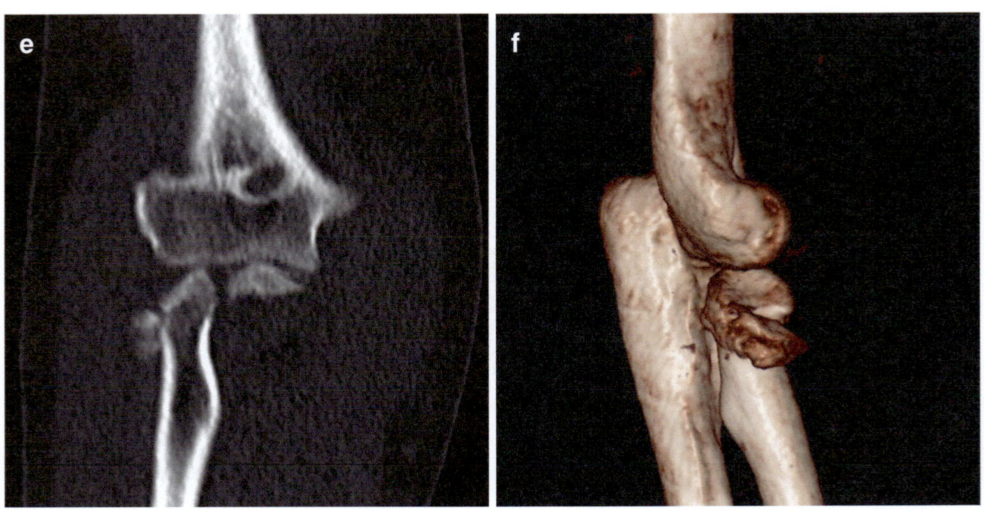

Fig. 3.59 (**e**, **f**) CT coronal reconstruction and three-dimensional reconstruction showing radial neck fracture, the end of the fracture impacted, displaced, the joint surface is lapsed, obviously inclined to the outside

19. Identification of the radial neck impacted fracture with the incomplete fracture.
    19.1. X-ray (Fig. 3.60a–d)

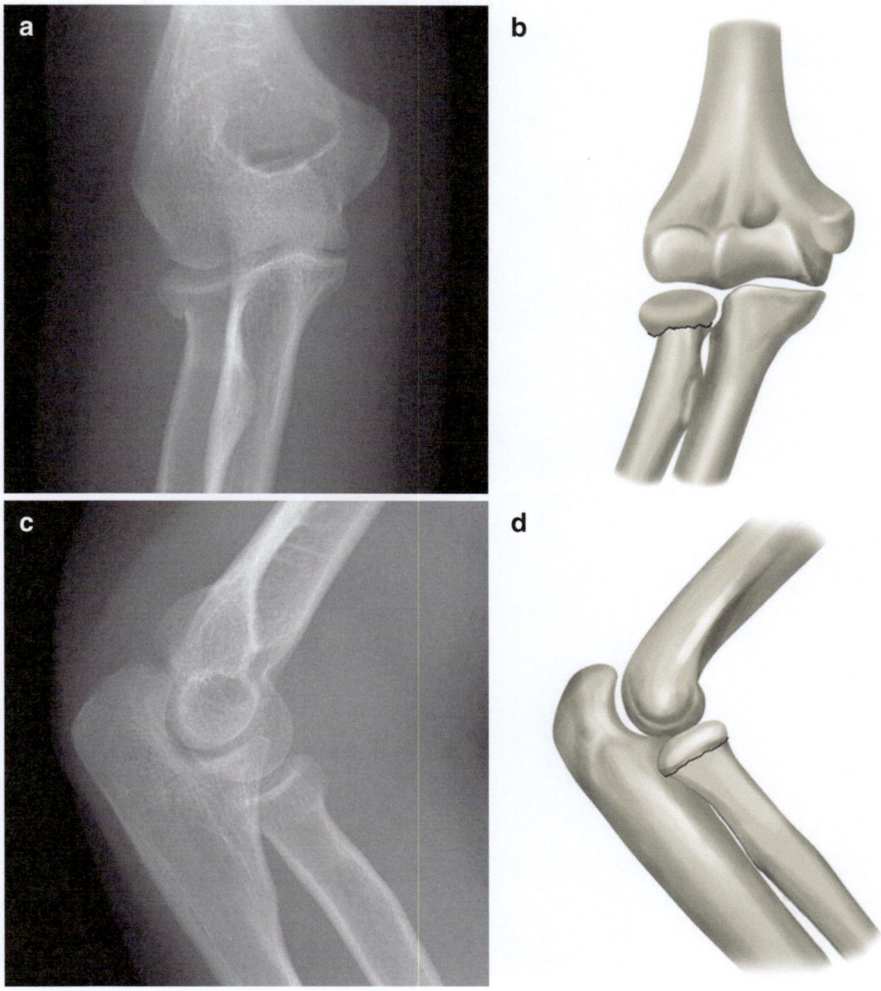

Fig. 3.60 Identification of the radial neck impacted fracture with the incomplete fracture. (**a**, **c**) X-ray shows the radial neck outer edge of bone fracture, the broken end is slightly impacted, the joint surface is inclined to the outside; (**b**, **d**) Schematic

    19.2. CT scan (Fig. 3.60e, f)

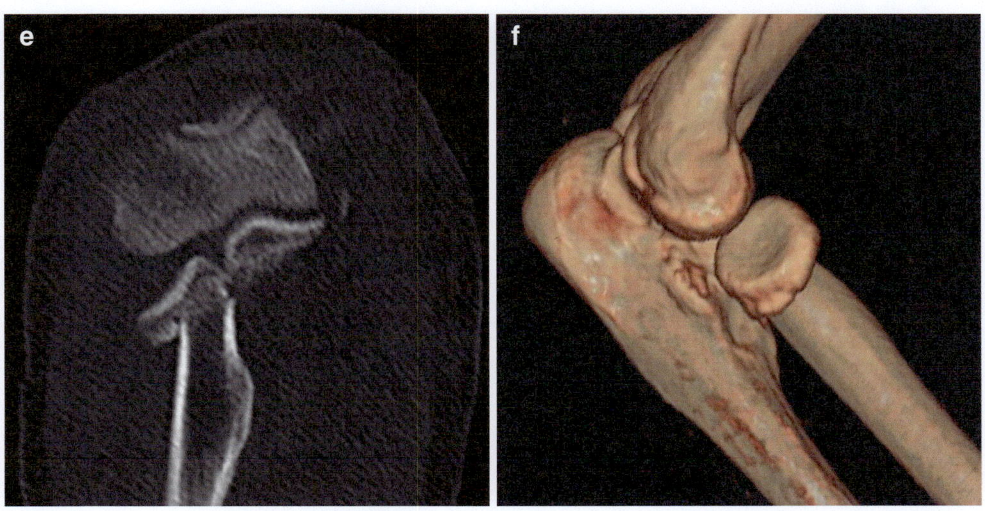

Fig. 3.60 (**e**, **f**) CT coronal reconstruction and three-dimensional reconstruction show the radial neck bone fracture, broken end impaction, displacement, the joint surface is inclined to the outside

20. Identification of the radial neck completed displacement fracture with the radial head fracture.
    20.1. X-ray (Fig. 3.61a–d)

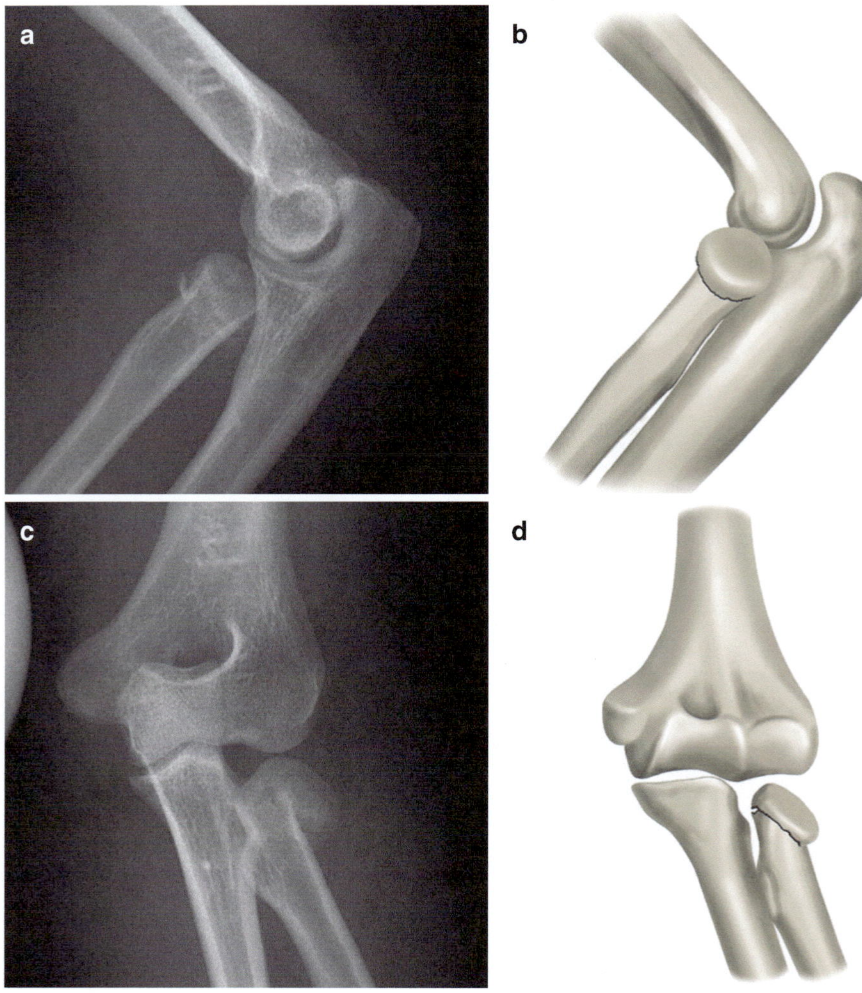

Fig. 3.61 Identification of the radial neck complete displacement fracture with the radial head fracture. (**a**, **c**) X-ray shows a fracture of the radial neck, the staggered dislocation was obvious, slightly impacted, the joint surface was obviously inclined to the outside; (**b**, **d**) Schematic

    20.2. CT scan (Fig. 3.61e, f)

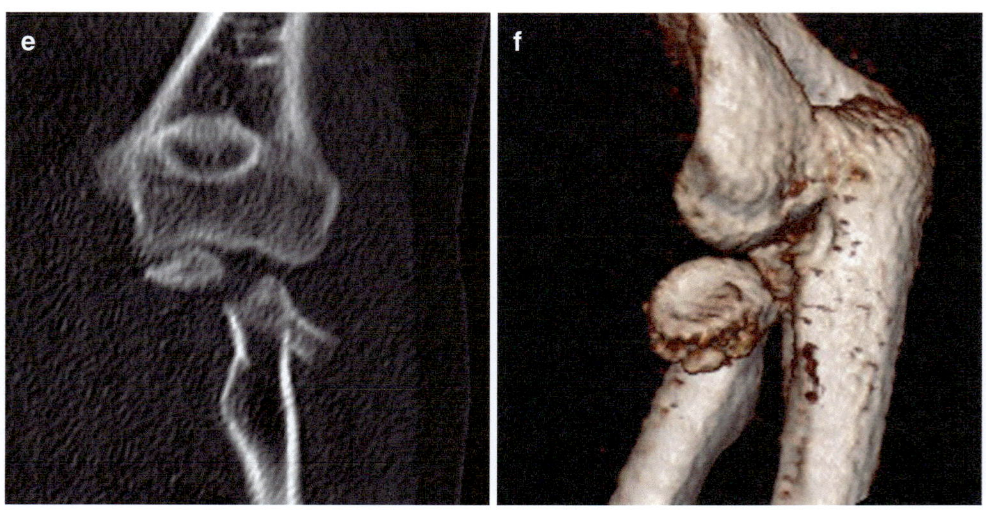

Fig. 3.61 (**e**, **f**) CT coronal reconstruction and three-dimensional reconstruction showed radial neck fracture. The broken end is impacted and dislocated, and the joint surface is obviously inclined to the outside

21. Identification of the radial neck comminuted fracture with the simple fracture.
    21.1. X-ray (Fig. 3.62a–d)

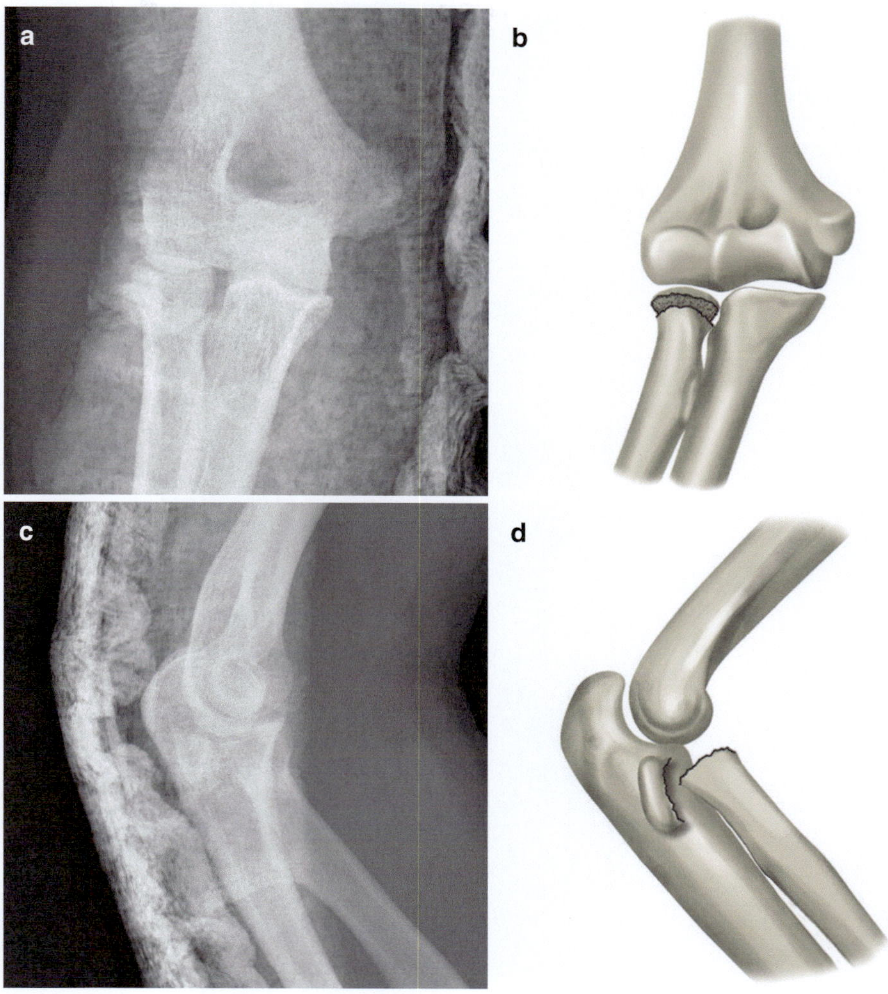

Fig. 3.62 Identification of the radial neck comminuted fracture with the simple fracture. (**a**, **c**) X-ray shows irregular shape of the proximal radius, bone shadow behind the radial neck, plaster of Paris overlap that resulted in partial display which is unclear; (**b**, **d**) Schematic

    21.2. CT scan (Fig. 3.62e, f)

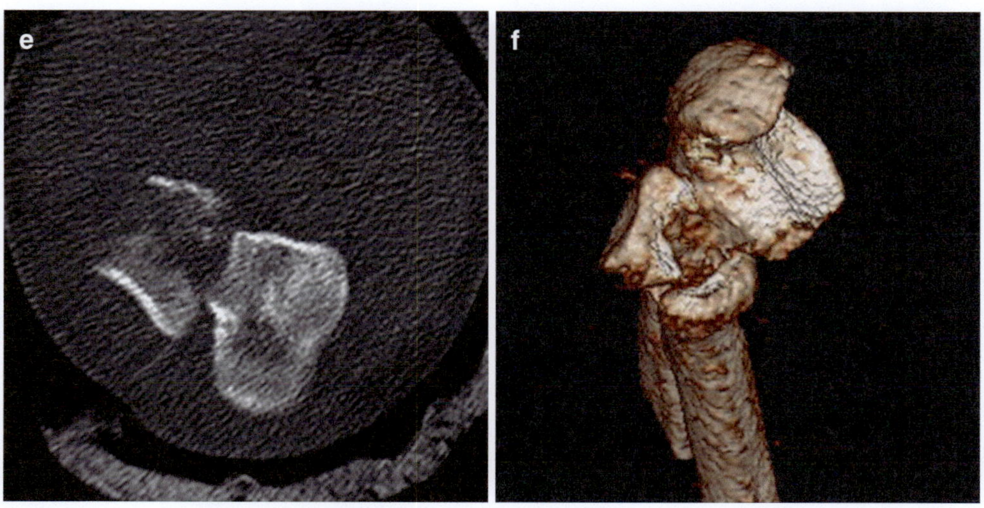

Fig. 3.62 (**e**, **f**) CT cross-section and 3D reconstruction showing radial neck bone fragmentation, the broken end is completely dislocated, the joint is inclined posteriorly, and the rotation is about 90°

22. Identification of the radial neck fracture dislocation with the elbow dislocation.
    22.1. X-ray (Fig. 3.63a, d)

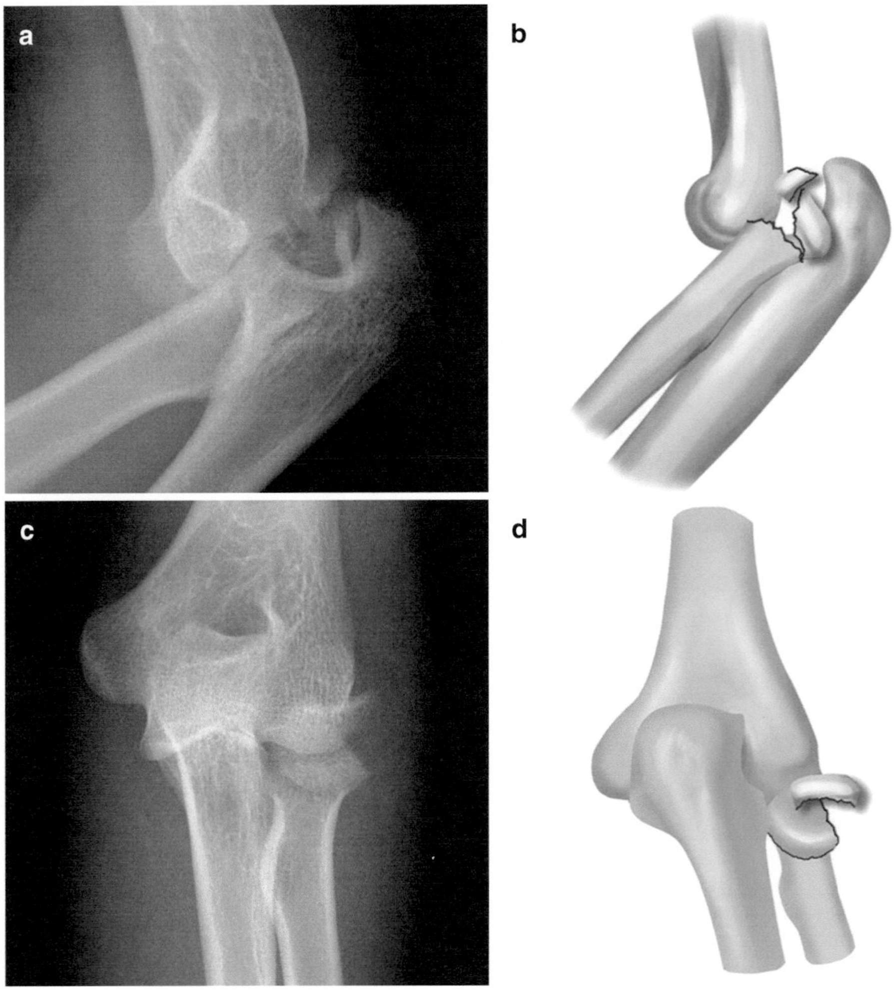

Fig. 3.63 Identification of the radial neck fracture dislocation with the elbow joint dislocation. (**a**, **c**) X-ray shows radial neck fracture, dislocation, posterior elbow dislocation; (**b**, **d**) Schematic

    22.2. CT scan (Fig. 3.63e, f)

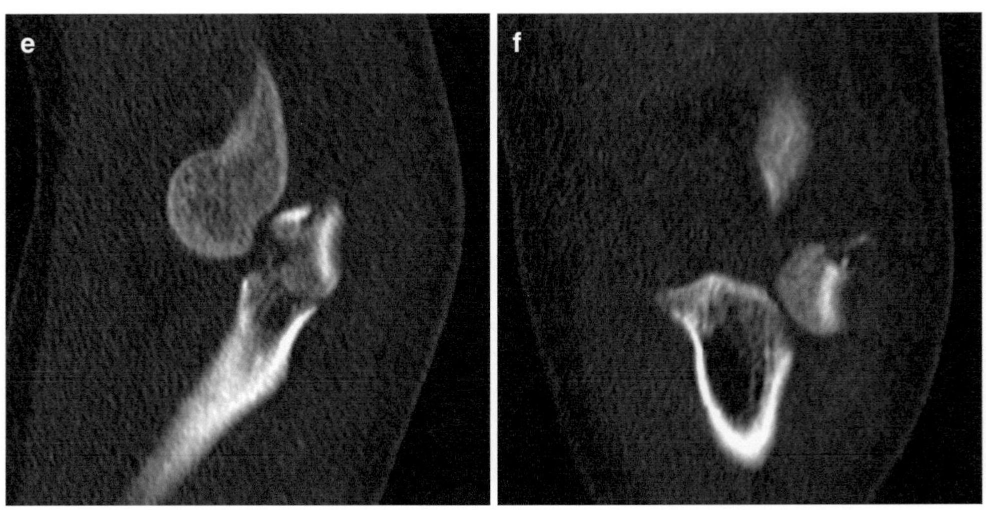

Fig. 3.63 (**e**, **f**) CT sagittal reconstruction and coronal reconstruction showed radial neck fracture, significantly dislocated, joint tilting backwards, rotating about 90°, dislocation of the humeroradial joint

3.4 Summary

1. The elbow joint is formed by the lower end of the humerus and the proximal end of the ulna and the radius. The three joints are wrapped in one joint capsule and are composite joints. The elbow joint is the most common site for fractures in children, and is often accompanied by various other dislocations and subluxations.
2. Elbow joint fractures in children include supracondylar fracture of the humerus, lateral epicondyle fracture, medial epicondyle fracture, radial head and neck fracture, and olecranon fracture. X-ray film should be used to observe the corresponding relationship between bone and bone, the order of ossification center appears, whether there is soft tissue swelling and its parts, whether there is effusion (hemorrhage) in the joint, and pay attention to the small fracture pieces. Contralateral contracts should be used to judge suspicious fractures. For patients with difficult judgments, CT scans should be carried out. A CT plain scan combined with a multiplanar reconstruction and three-dimensional reconstruction has great advantages for identifying fractures and dislocations. An MR scan has great advantages for the evaluation of cartilage osteophytes, cartilage growth plate structure, degree of injury, and injury of other uncalcified tissues.
3. Children and adults with adjacent articular surface fractures can be identified using CT scan and reconstruction; to assess the fracture type, size, and number; and to evaluate whether there is a fracture mass into the joint space.
4. An MR scan is used to evaluate tendon and soft tissue damage around the elbow joint.

Wrist Fracture

4

Wei Chen and Yingze Zhang

4.1 Fracture of Distal Radius/Ulna

The structure of the distal radius and ulna mainly includes the articular surface of the distal radius, distal radio ulnar joint (DRUJ), and styloid process of the radius and ulna. The slope of the dorsal to palmar articular surface of the distal radius and the slope from the distal articular surface of the radius to the radial shaft form a palmar tilt angle and a radial inclination angle, respectively. The distal portion of the radius and the proximal portion of the carpal bone form the radiocarpal joint, and distal radioulnar articulation is formed by the head of the ulna and the ulnar notch on the distal radius. The distal radius is a predilection site of fracture, accounting for 63.38% of all fractures of the radius/ulna in adult. Based on AO classification, it is divided into three types: extra-articular fracture, partial articular fracture, and complex articular fracture. Extra-articular fractures are further divided into distal ulnar fracture, radius simple or impact fracture, and comminuted extra-articular radial fracture, which account for 2.79%, 46.82%, and 2.89% of adult ulnar and radial fractures, respectively. Partial articular fractures of the radius are further divided into sagittal partial fracture of the distal radius, radius dorsal rim frontal fracture, and radius volar rim frontal fracture, which account for 2.85%, 1.31%, and 0.75% of adult ulnar and radial fractures, respectively. Complex articular fractures of the radius are further divided into articular simple fracture, metaphyseal simple fracture, metaphyseal comminuted fracture, and articular comminuted fracture. The articular simple and metaphyseal simple fractures account for 2.44% of adult ulnar and radial fractures, whilst metaphyseal comminuted fracture is 2.26% and articular comminuted fracture accounts for 1.27%.

4.1.1 Injury Mechanism

Fractures of the distal radius or ulna result from force transmitted through the hand and wrist to the distal radius or ulna, which often occurs from a fall on an outstretched hand. Various types of rotational forces result in different fracture variation. For instance, Colles fracture results from a fall on an outstretched pronated hand, with impact on the palm and subsequent forced dorsiflexion and hyperextension. Smith fractures are often caused by a fall onto the hand back, with the hand and carpus in hyperflexion.

4.1.2 Signs and Symptoms

Patients with fractures of the distal radius or ulna may present with pain, swelling, and loss of wrist motion. If fractures are accompanied by significant displacement or angulation, a typical deformity will appear. A "dinner fork" deformity of the wrist is caused by dorsal displacement of the carpal bones (Colles fracture). Reverse deformity could be seen in volar angulation in Smith's fracture.

W. Chen · Y. Zhang (✉)
Department of Orthopaedics, The Third Hospital of Hebei Medical University, Shijiazhuang, Hebei, China

Y. Zhang (ed.), *Differential Diagnosis of Fracture*, https://doi.org/10.1007/978-981-13-8339-7_4

4.1.3 Imaging Differential Diagnosis

Standard X-rays are efficient for the diagnosis of adult distal radius or ulna fracture. A CT scan is performed to further investigate small avulsion fractures, the articular morphology of the fracture site, and other important details, but the radiation is relatively large. MR scanning is critical for the diagnosis of tendon and soft tissue injury around the distal radius or ulna, especially in children with metaphyseal fractures and wrist ligament injuries.

1. Differentiation of distal ulnar styloid fracture with Barton fracture and Colles fracture
   1.1. X-ray (Fig. 4.1a–d)

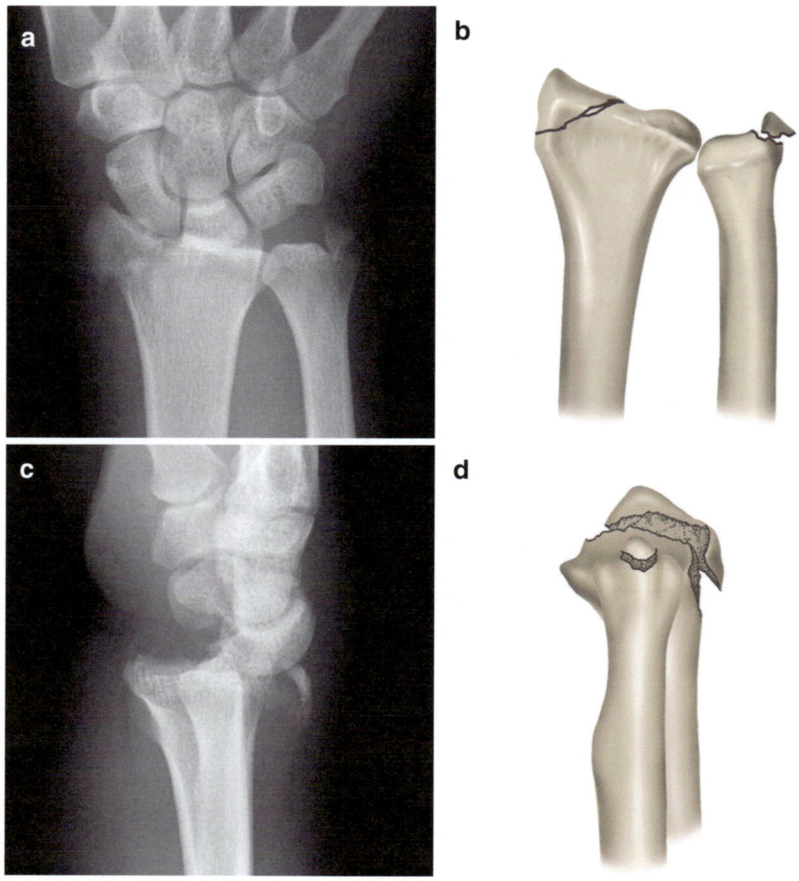

Fig. 4.1 X-rays (**a**, **c**) and illustrations (**b**, **d**) show displaced ulnar styloid process fracture, fractures of radial styloid process, and dorsal rim of the radius. Radial carpal joint is dislocated, and carpal bones *moved towards dorsal surface* of the forearm. After reduction, a CT scan was ordered

1.2. CT scan (Fig. 4.1e–h)

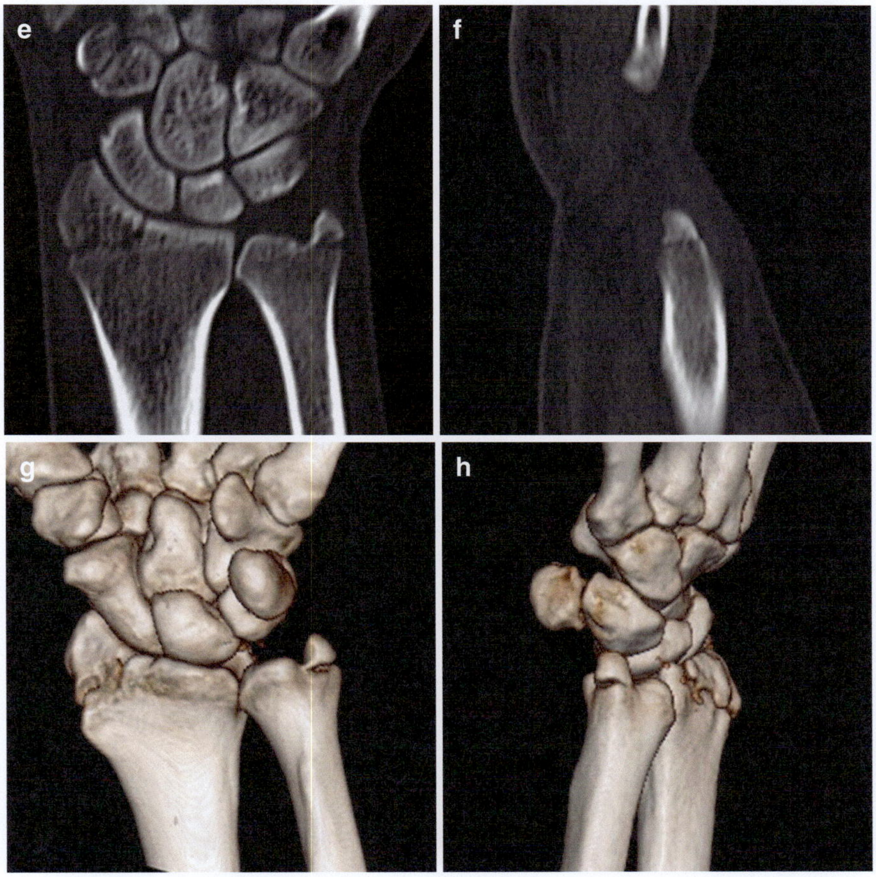

Fig. 4.1 The coronal plane (**e**), sagittal plane (**f**), and three-dimensional reconstruction (**g**, **h**) images show ulnar/radial styloid process fracture and displaced ulnar styloid process, and the radial styloid process is slightly displaced

2. Differentiation of distal ulnar fracture with Colles fracture and Barton fracture
   2.1. X-ray (Fig. 4.2a–d)

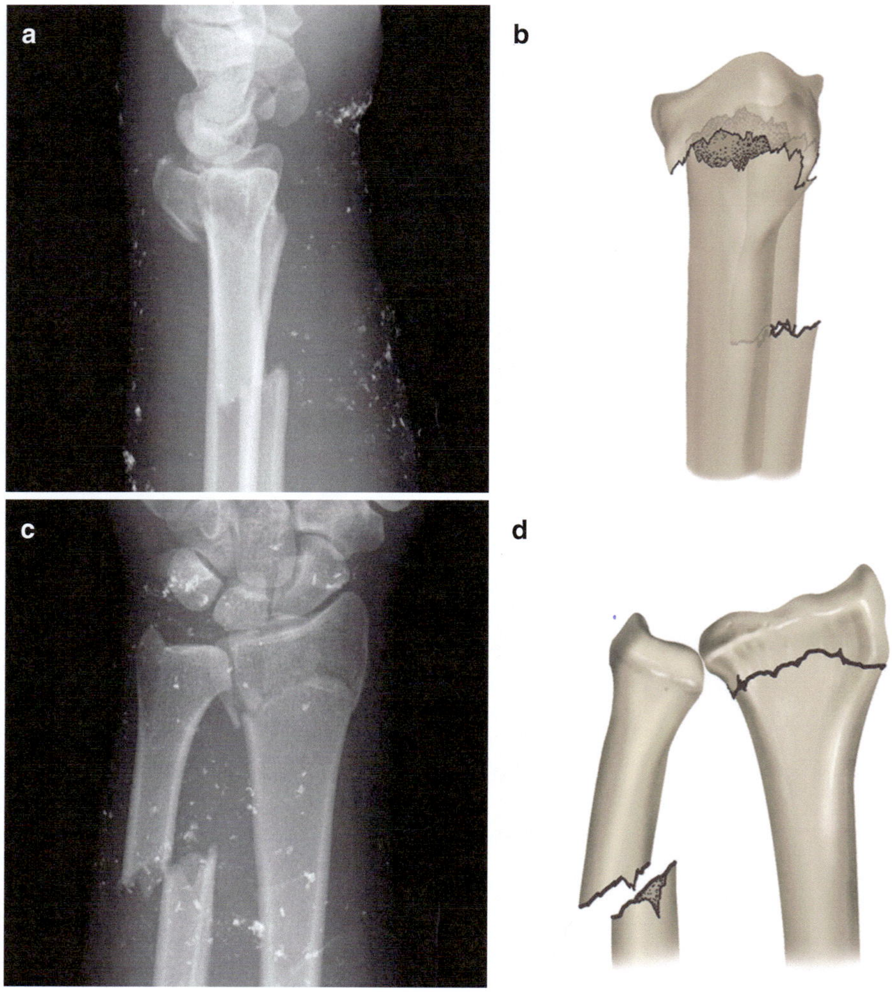

Fig. 4.2 X-rays (**a**, **c**) and illustrations (**b**, **d**) show displaced distal ulnar fracture, fracture of distal radius. The distal end moves backwards and the anteversion angle becomes negative

   2.2. CT scan (Fig. 4.2e, f)

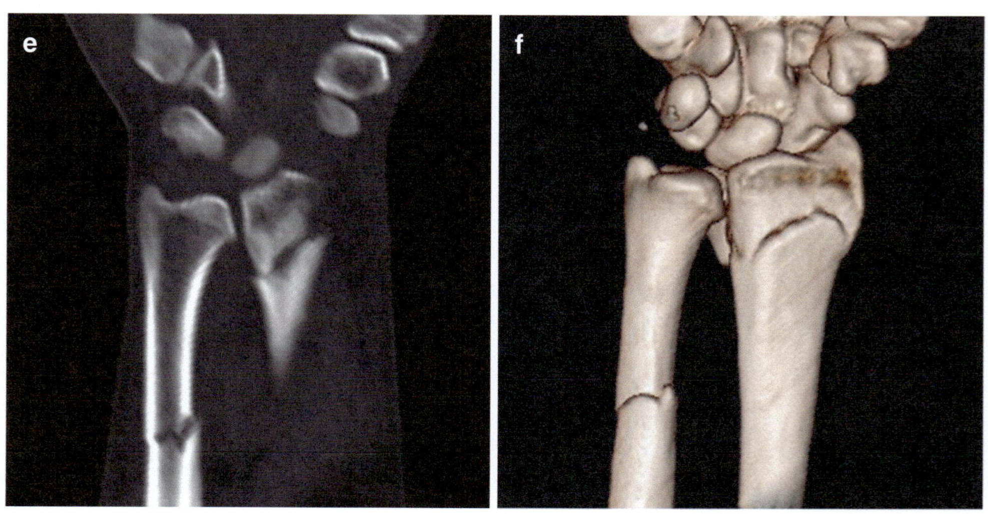

Fig. 4.2 The coronal CT plane (**e**) and three-dimensional reconstruction (**f**) images show distal ulnar and radial fracture. The fracture line extends into the articular surface, and the anteversion angle becomes negative

3. Differentiation of distal radius impact fracture and greenstick fracture
   3.1. X-ray (Fig. 4.3a–d)

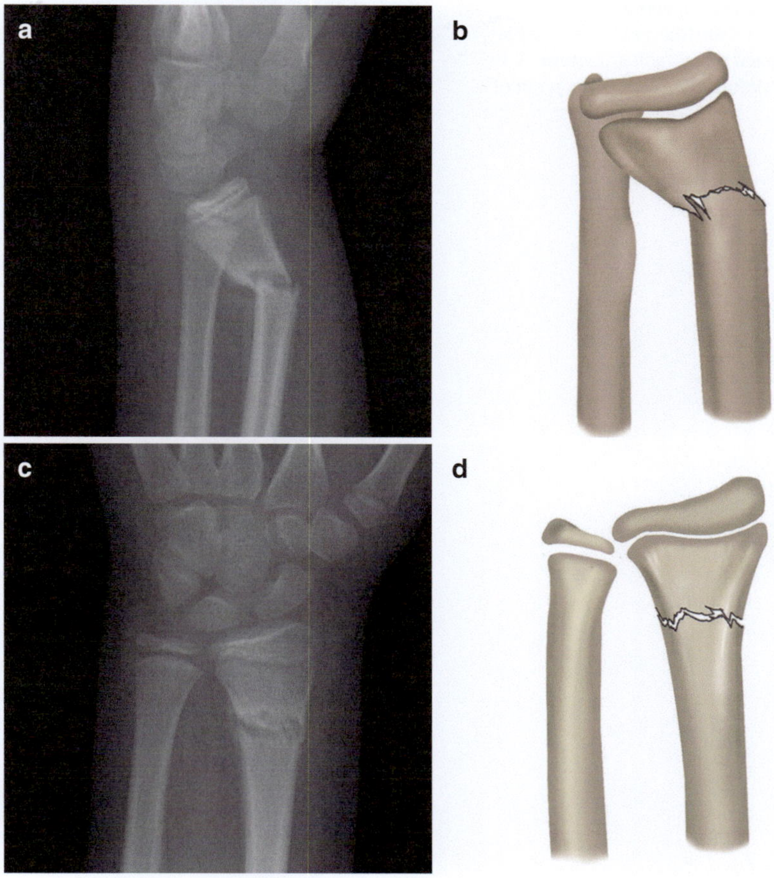

Fig. 4.3 X-rays (**a**, **c**) and illustration (**b**, **d**) show distal radius fracture. The ends are impacted, with angle *towards* the *palm* of the hand. Minor callus can be seen around it

3.2. CT scan (Fig. 4.3e–h)

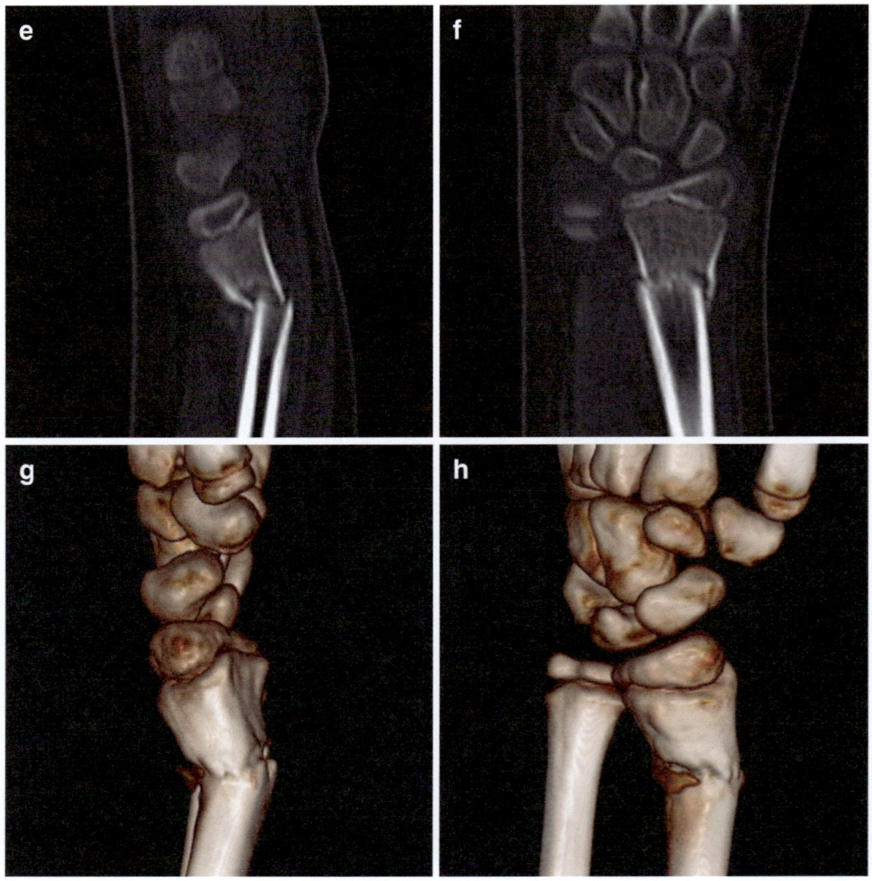

Fig. 4.3 The sagittal CT plane (**e**), coronal CT plane (**f**), and three-dimensional reconstruction (**g**, **h**) images show impacted distal radius fracture, with angulation deformity *towards* the *palm* of the hand

4. Differentiation of distal ulnar impact fracture and greenstick fracture
   4.1. X-ray (Fig. 4.4a–d)

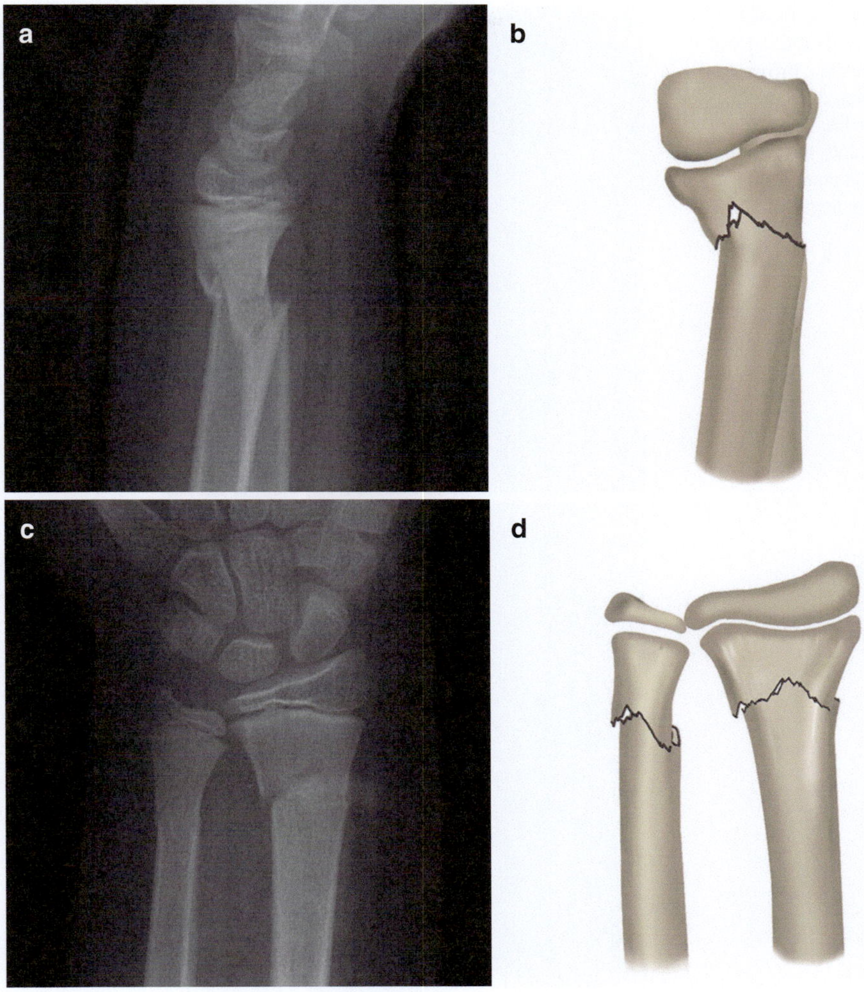

Fig. 4.4 X-rays (**a**, **c**) and illustrations (**b**, **d**) show impacted distal radius fracture and cortical bone of distal ulna is distorted

   4.2. CT scan (Fig. 4.4e, f)

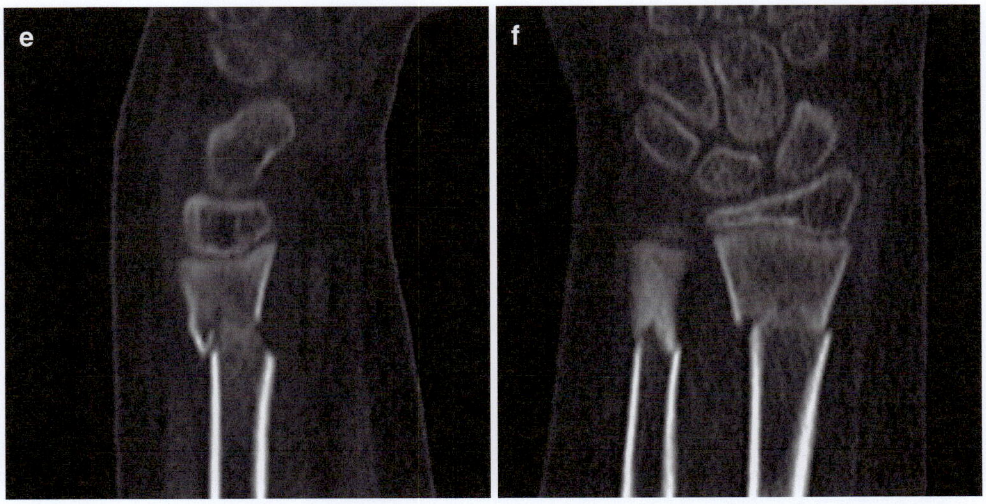

Fig. 4.4 The sagittal CT plane (**e**) and coronal CT plane (**f**) images show impacted distal radius and ulnar fracture, whilst the broken ends are slightly displaced

5. Differentiation of extra-articular comminuted and simple fracture of distal radius
   5.1. X-ray (Fig. 4.5a–d)

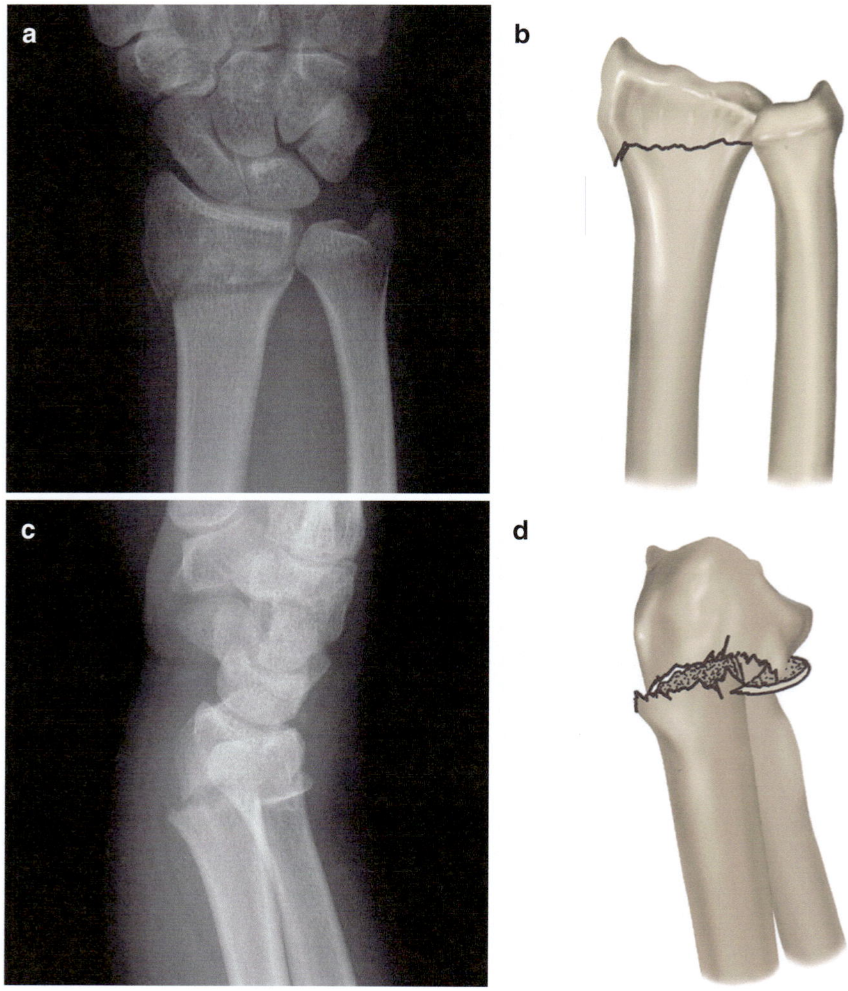

Fig. 4.5 X-rays (**a**, **c**) and illustrations (**b**, **d**) show distal radius fracture. The broken ends are impacted and bent towards the palm. Fracture line extended into the articular surface and the anteversion angle becomes negative

   5.2. CT scan (Fig. 4.5e, f)

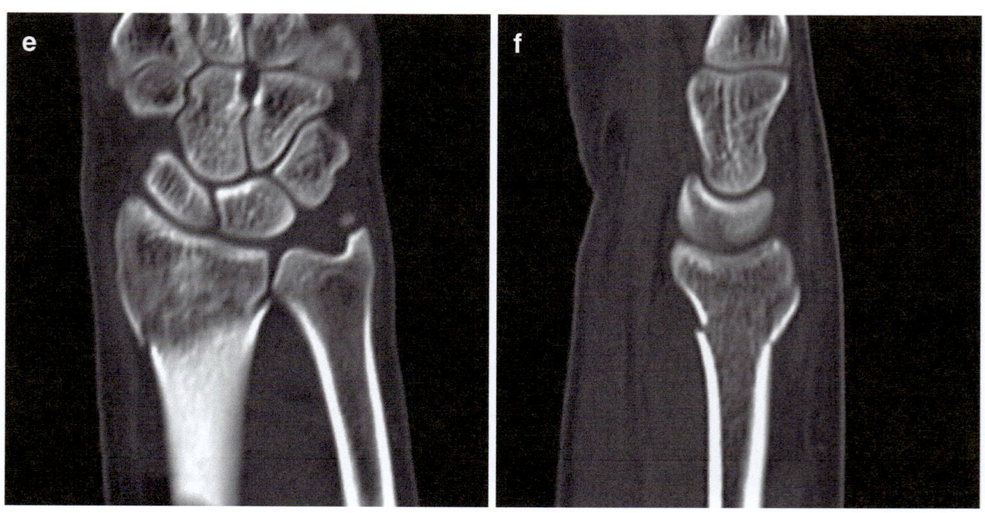

Fig. 4.5 The coronal CT plane (**e**) and sagittal CT plane (**f**) images show distal radius fracture with multi-fragments. Fracture line extends into the articular surface and the anteversion angle becomes flat

6. Differentiation of extra-articular comminuted and partial articular fracture of distal radius
   6.1. X-ray (Fig. 4.6a–d)

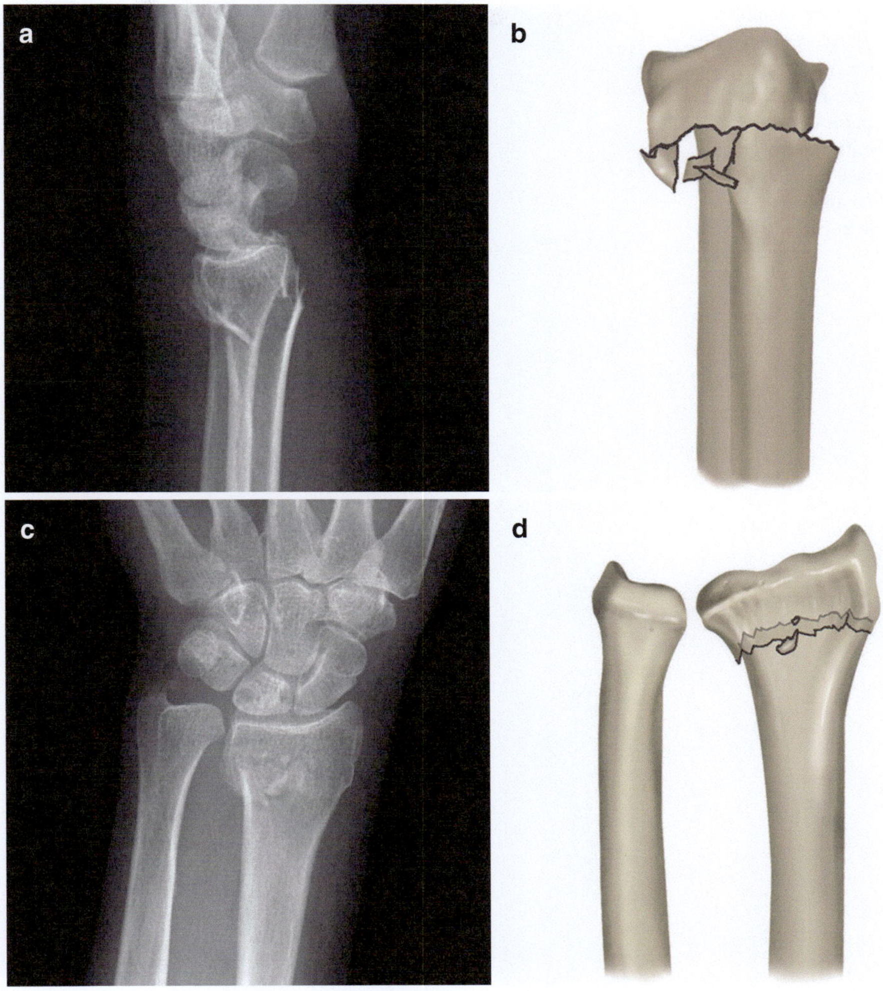

Fig. 4.6 X-rays (**a**, **c**) and illustrations (**b**, **d**) show distal radial fracture. The broken ends are slightly impacted with multiple fragments. The anterior border of the joint is irregular, and the anteversion angle becomes negative. Cysts can be seen in the lunate bone

   6.2. CT scan (Fig. 4.6e, f)

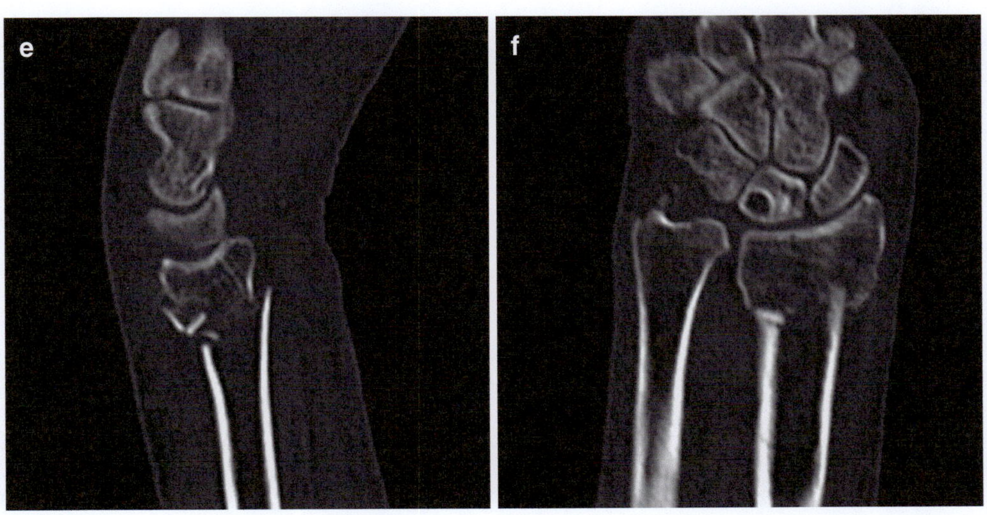

Fig. 4.6 The sagittal CT plane (**e**) and coronal CT plane (**f**) images show distal radial fracture with multi-fragments. The fracture line extends into the articular surface and the anteversion angle becomes negative

7. Differentiation of extra-articular comminuted and partial articular fracture of distal radius
   7.1. X-ray(Fig. 4.7a–d)

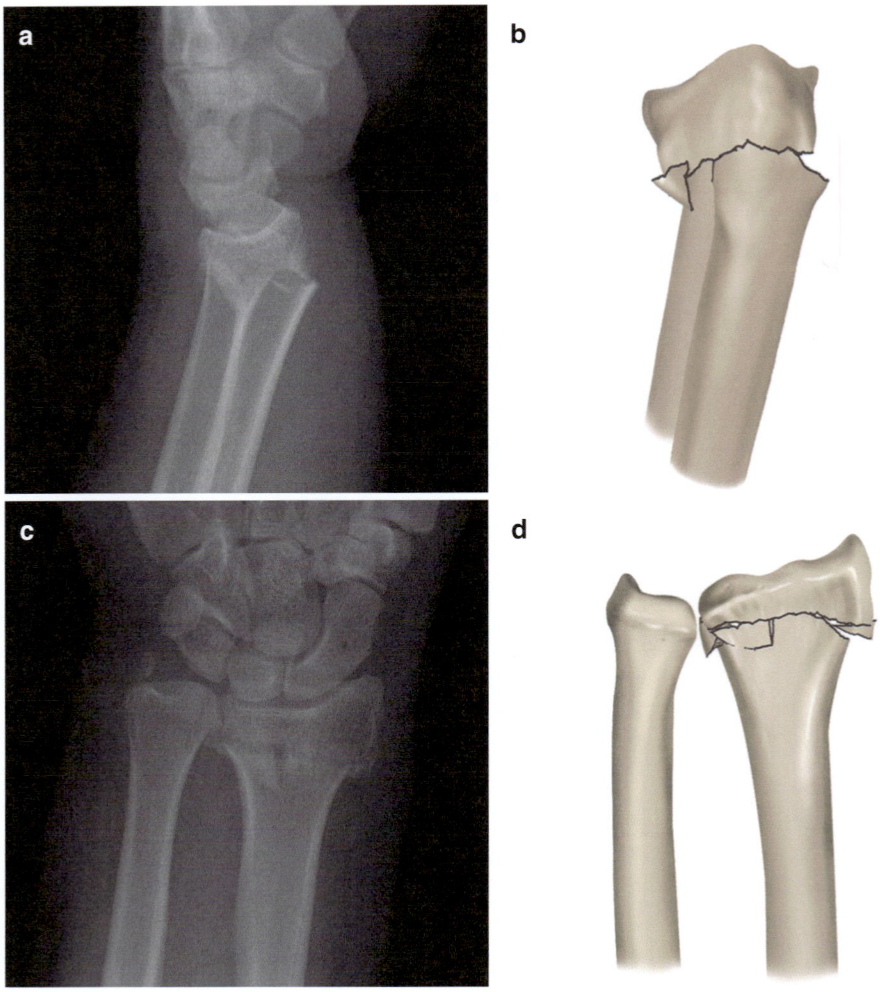

Fig. 4.7 X-rays (**a**, **c**) and illustrations (**b**, **d**) show distal radius fracture. The ends are slightly displaced and bent towards the palm with multi-fragments and irregular articular surface on the medial border and the anteversion angle became negative

   7.2. CT scan(Fig. 4.7e, f)

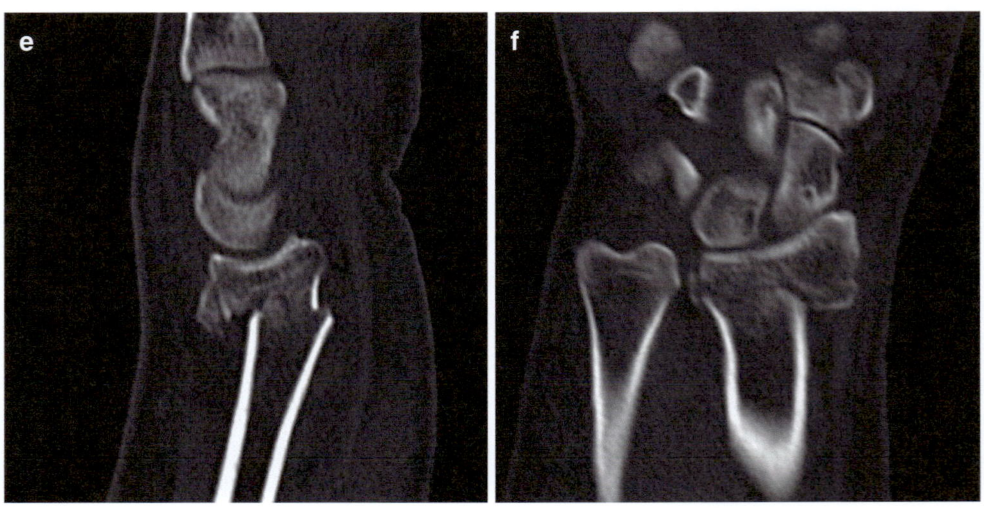

Fig. 4.7 The sagittal CT plane (**e**) and coronal CT plane (**f**) images show distal radius fracture with multi-fragments. The fracture line extends into the articular surface, and the anteversion angle becomes negative

8. Differentiation of distal radius sagittal fracture and non-fracture
   8.1. X-ray (Fig. 4.8a–d)

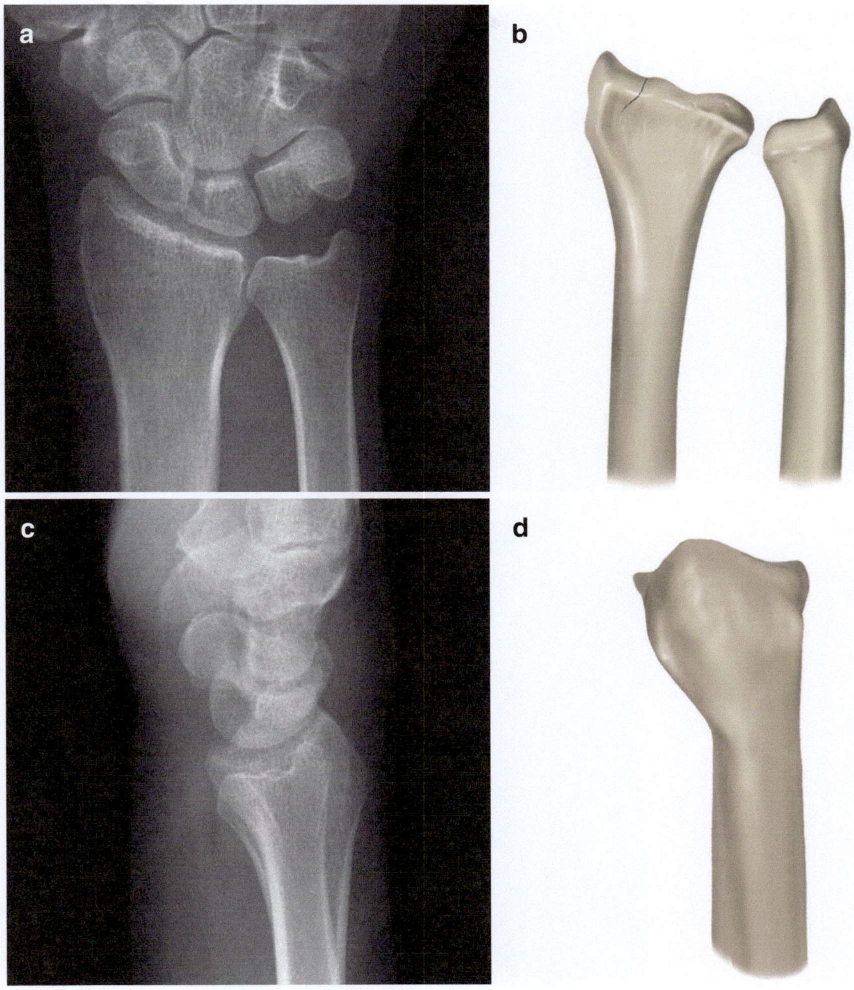

Fig. 4.8 X-rays (**a**, **c**) and illustrations (**b**, **d**) show the trabecular bone disorder of the radial styloid process, which is an ambiguous fracture

   8.2. CT scan (Fig. 4.8e, f)

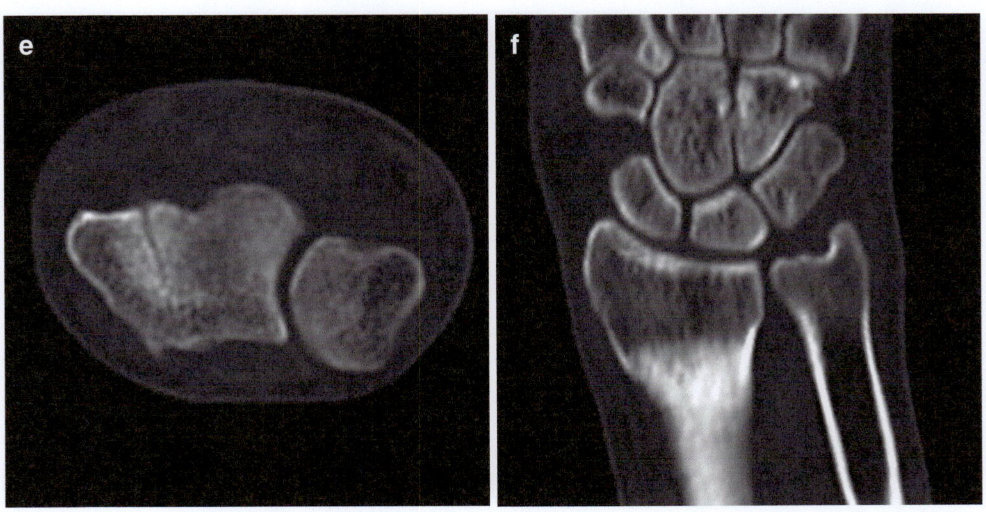

Fig. 4.8 The cross-section (**e**) and coronal CT plane (**f**) images show distal radius fracture. The fracture line runs through the sagittal plane and did not reach the articular surface, without obvious displacement

9. Differentiation of distal radius sagittal displaced fracture and simple fracture
   9.1. X-ray(Fig. 4.9a–d)

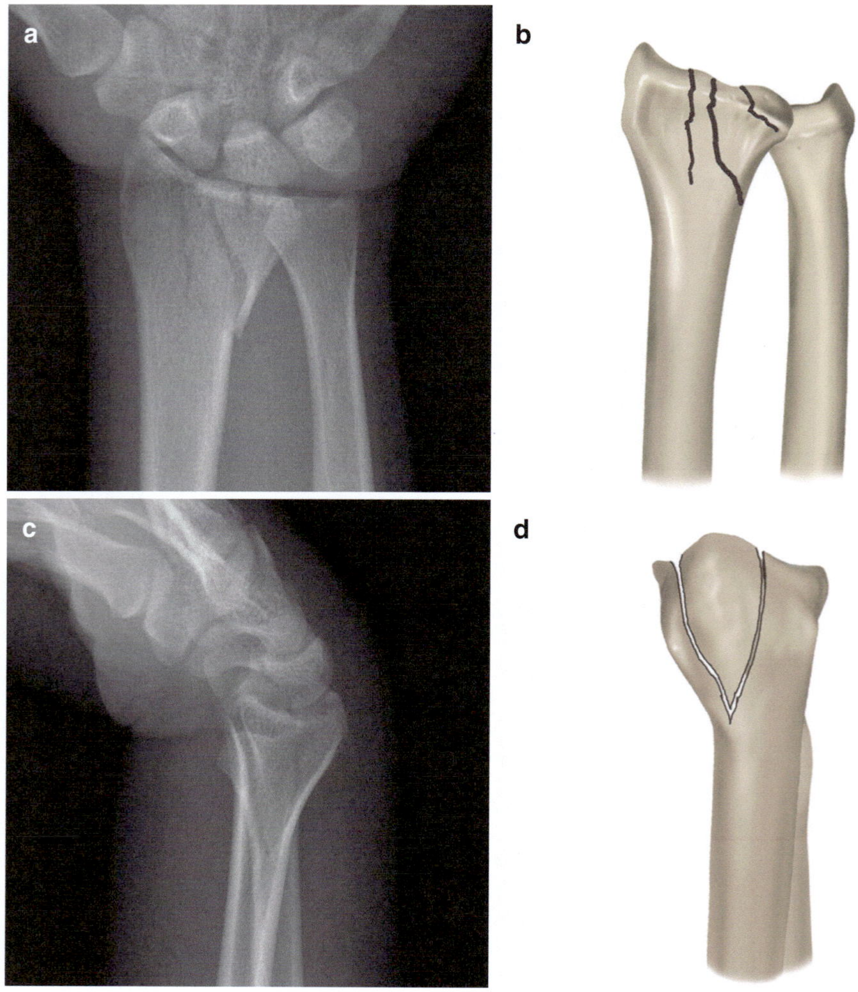

Fig. 4.9 X-rays (**a**, **c**) and illustrations (**b**, **d**) show distal radius fracture; fracture line runs longitudinally and extends into the articular surface, and the alignment is almost anatomic

   9.2. CT scan (Fig. 4.9e, f)

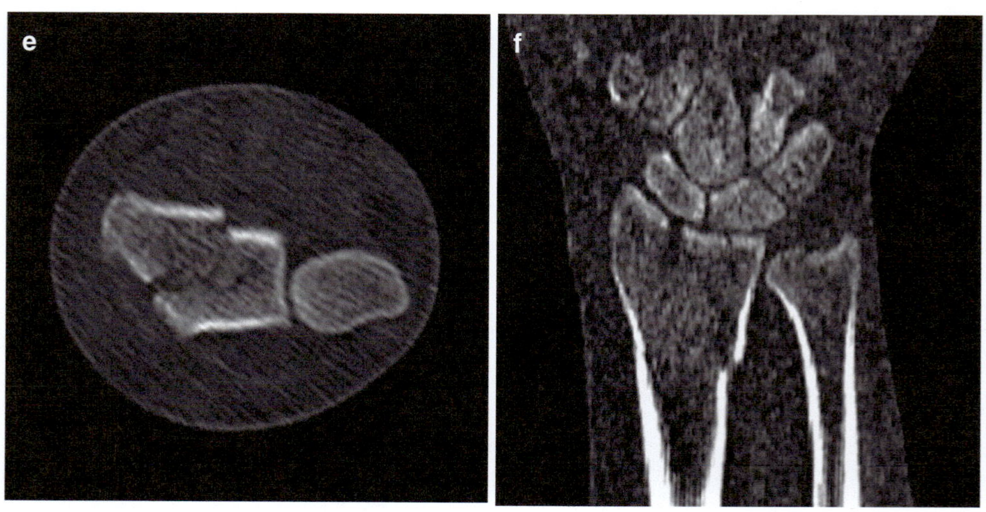

Fig. 4.9 The cross-section (**e**) and coronal CT plane (**f**) images show distal radius fracture, and the fracture line runs through the sagittal plane and extended to the articular surface. The broken ends are displaced and articular surfaces are separated

10. Differentiation of distal radius partial articular fracture and non-fracture
    10.1. X-ray (Fig. 4.10a–d)

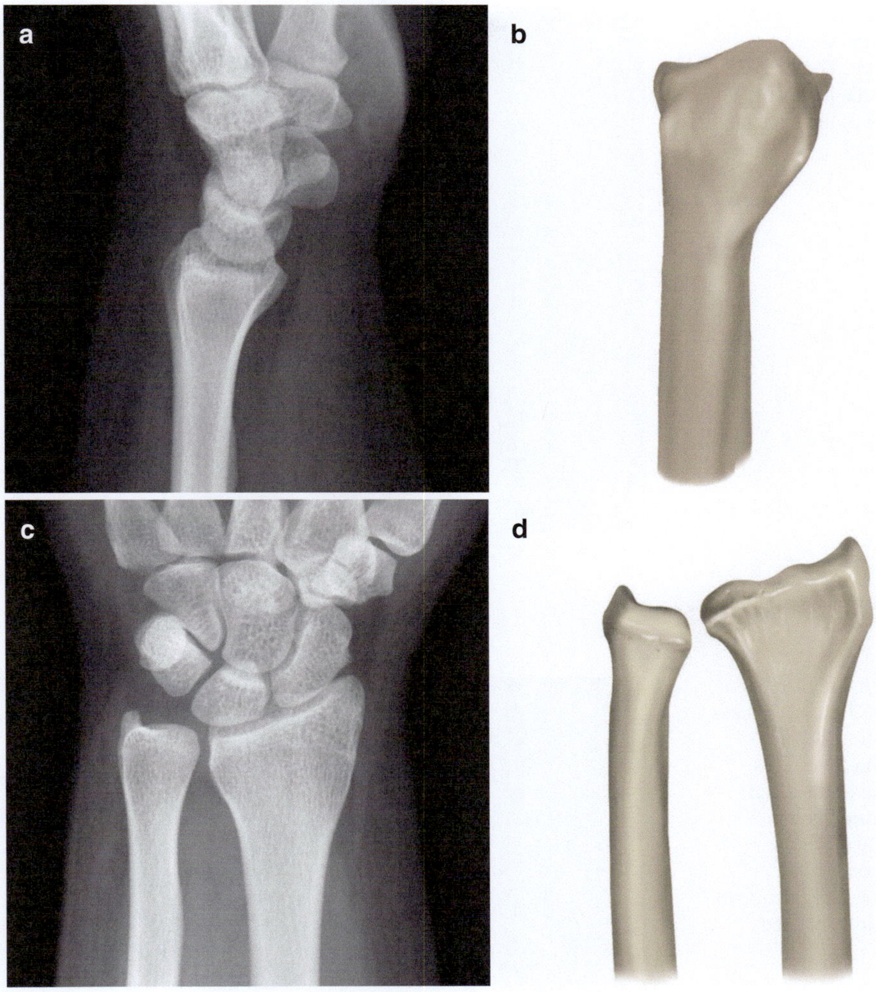

Fig. 4.10 X-rays (**a**, **c**) and illustrations (**b**, **d**) show no definite sign of distal radius fracture

    10.2. CT scan (Fig. 4.10e, f)

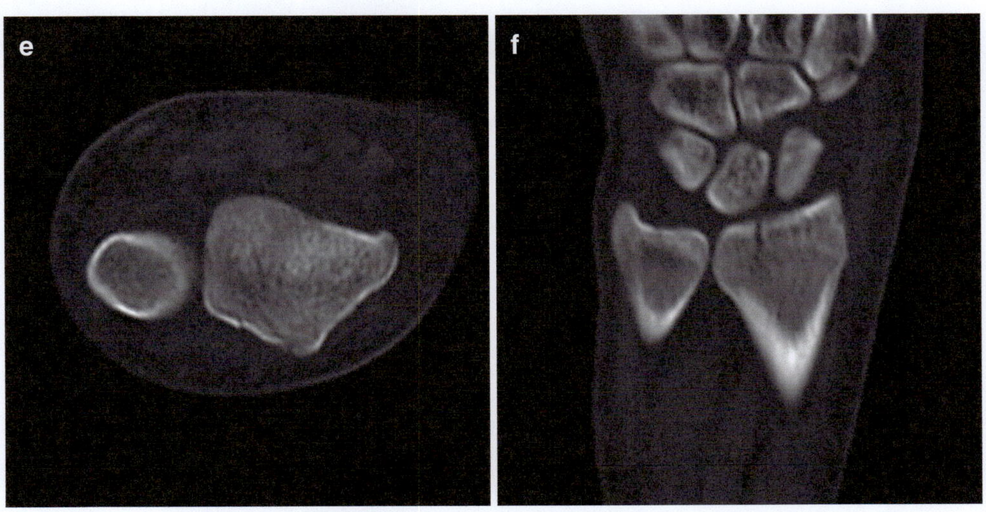

Fig. 4.10 The cross-section (**e**) and coronal CT plane (**f**) images show distal radius fracture. The fracture line runs through the sagittal plane and extends to the articular surface. The broken ends are slightly displaced

11. Differentiation of distal radius partially comminuted articular fracture and simple fracture
    11.1. X-ray (Fig. 4.11a, b)

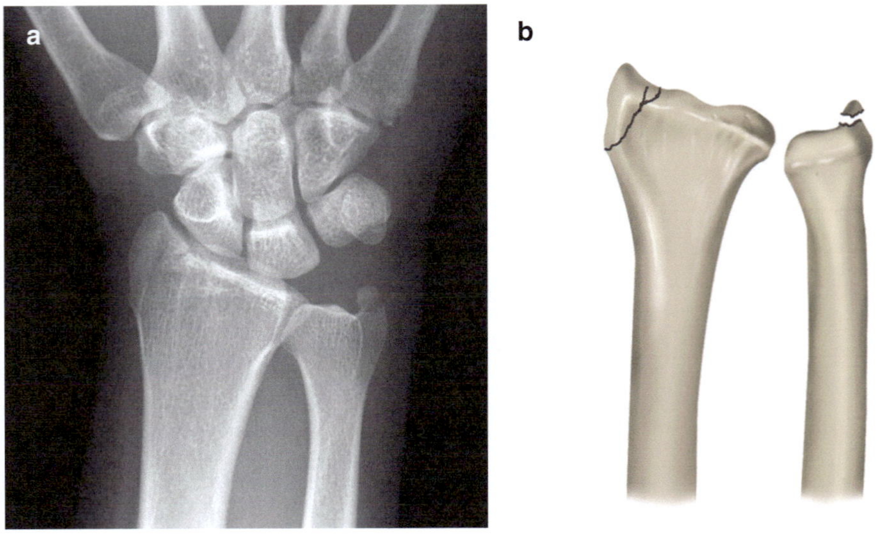

Fig. 4.11 X-rays (**a**) and illustrations (**b**) show distal radius fracture. The fracture line reaches the joint surface with fracture of the ulnar styloid process

    11.2. CT scan (Fig. 4.11c–e)

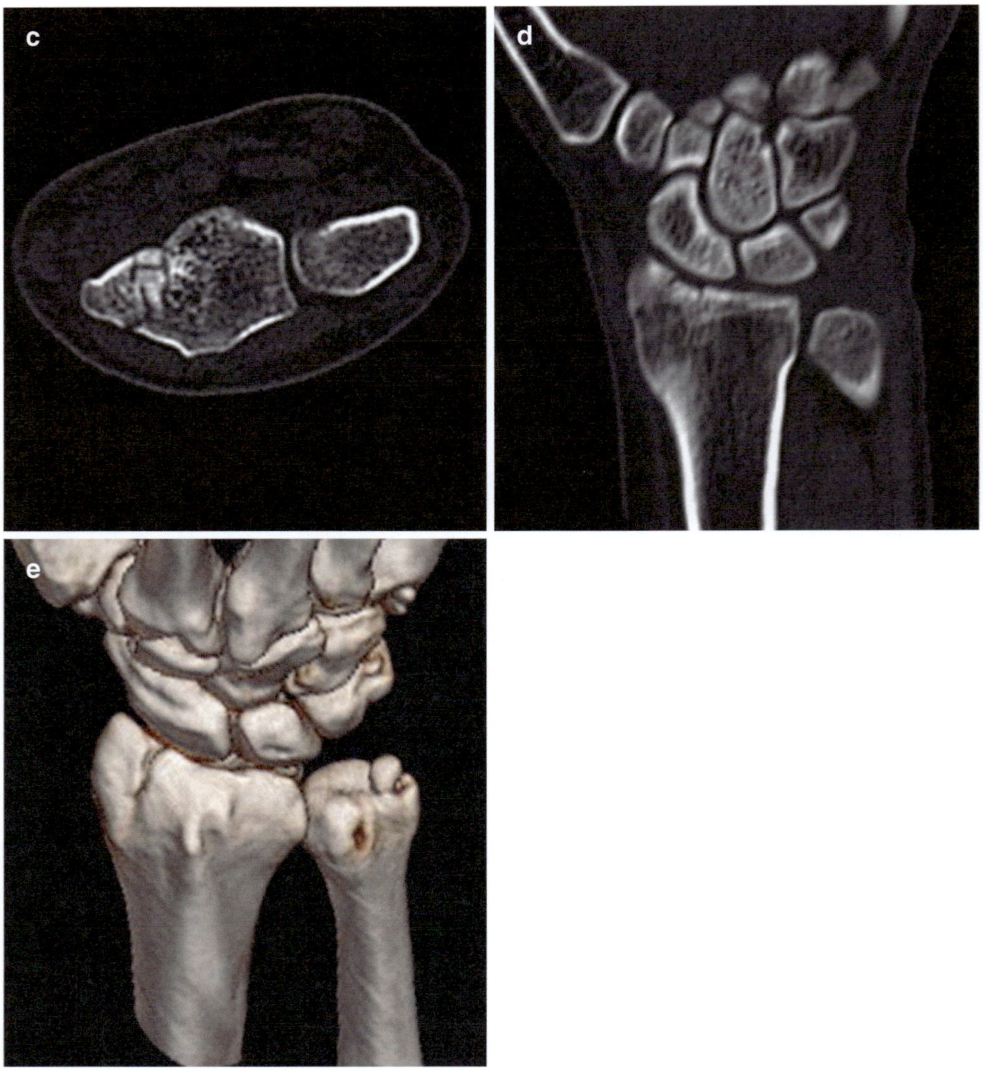

Fig. 4.11 The cross-section (**c**), coronal CT plane (**d**), and three-dimensional reconstruction (**e**) images show fracture of the distal radius. Fracture line runs longitudinally. Articular surface is smashed and slightly depressed; fracture of the ulnar styloid is noted

12. Differentiation of dorsal Barton fracture and Colles fracture of distal radius
    12.1. X-ray (Fig. 4.12a–d)

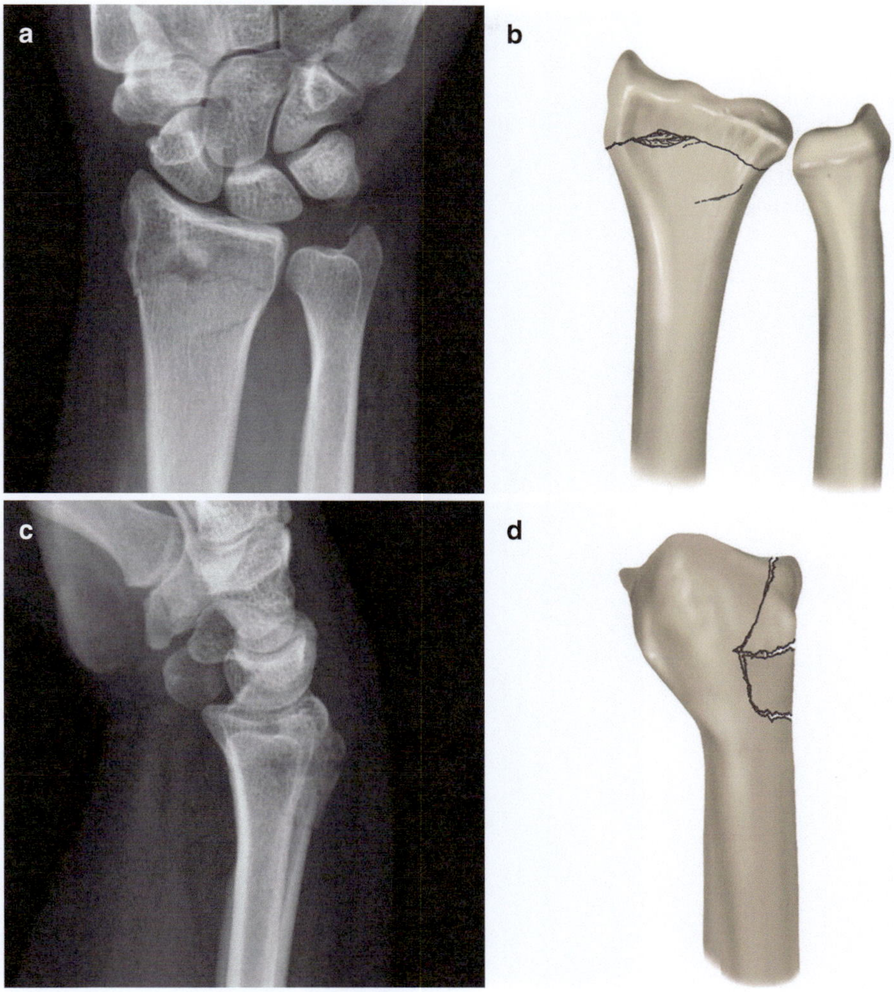

Fig. 4.12 X-rays (**a**, **c**) and illustrations (**b**, **d**) show fracture of the posterior rim of the distal radius. Fracture line extends to the joint surface, whilst the fragments line up almost anatomically. A tiny fragment can be seen at the styloid process

    12.2. CT scan (Fig. 4.12e, f)

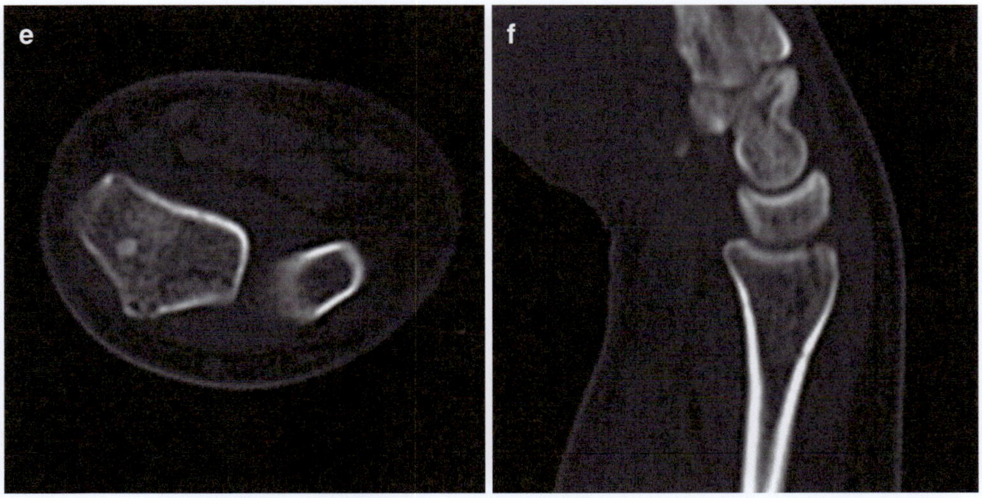

Fig. 4.12 The cross-section (**e**) and sagittal CT plane (**f**) images show slightly displaced fracture of posterior distal radius. Fracture line runs through the coronal plane and extended to the articular surface

13. Differentiation of Colles and Barton fracture

13.1. X-ray (Fig. 4.13a–d)

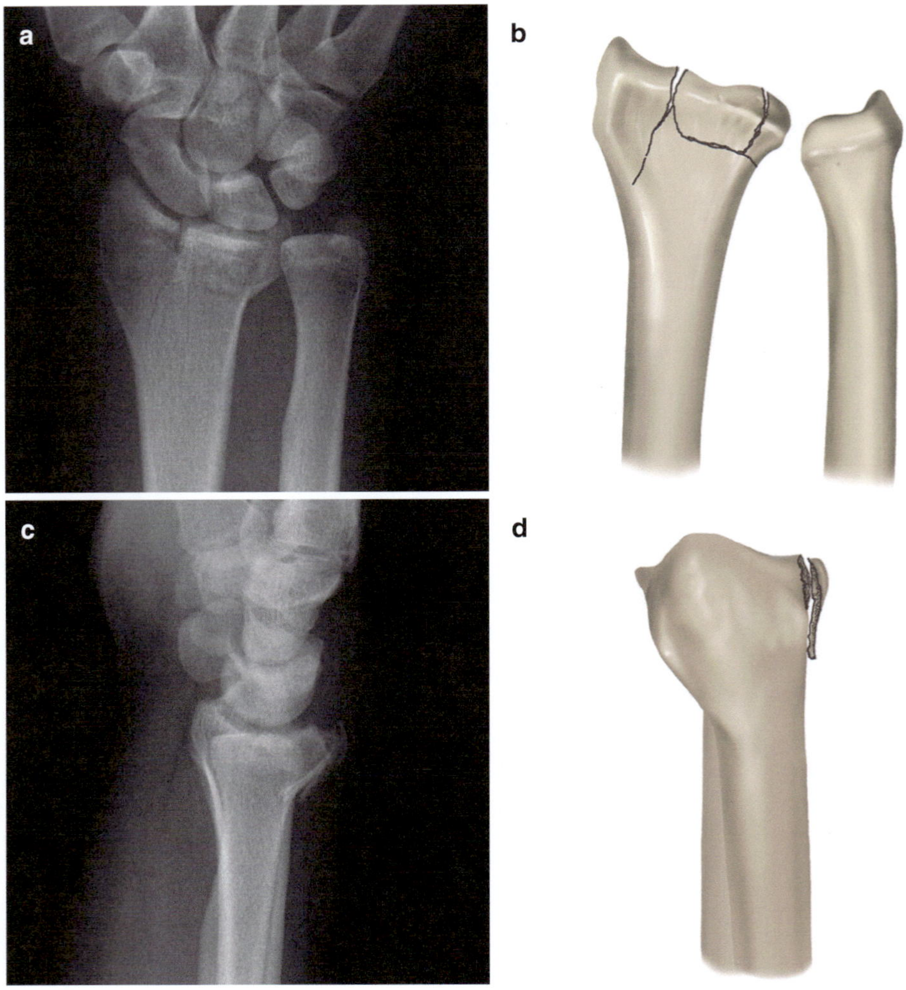

Fig. 4.13 X-rays (**a**, **c**) and illustrations (**b**, **d**) show fracture of the distal radius, the dorsal fragment is split longitudinally. The fracture line extends to the articular surface with displaced broken ends. The anteversion angle becomes negative

13.2. CT scan (Fig. 4.13e, f)

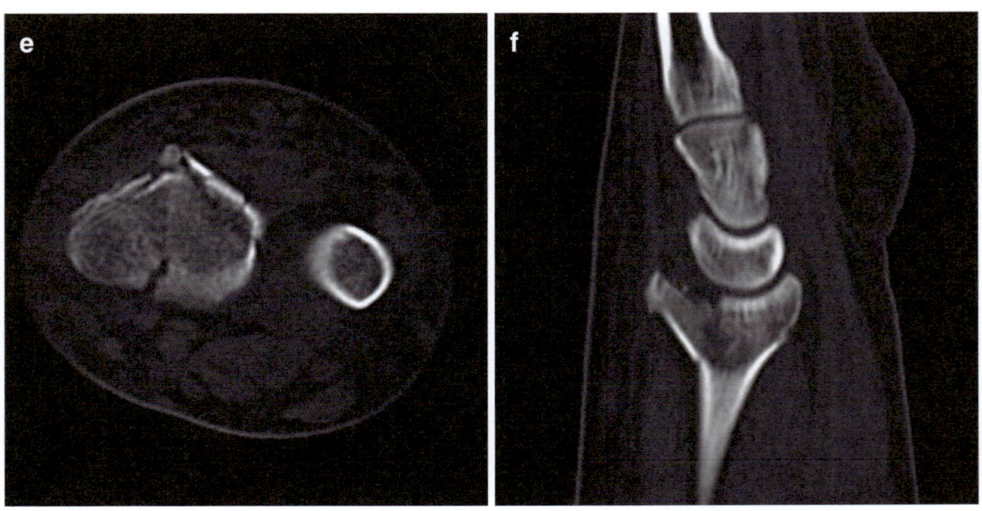

Fig. 4.13 The cross-section (**e**) and sagittal CT plane (**f**) images show fracture of the distal radius. The fracture line comes across the dorsal radius and ran through the coronal plane and extends to the anterior rim of radius and articular surface. The anteversion angle becomes negative

14. Differentiation of Barton fracture and Smith fracture
    14.1. X-ray (Fig. 4.14a–d)

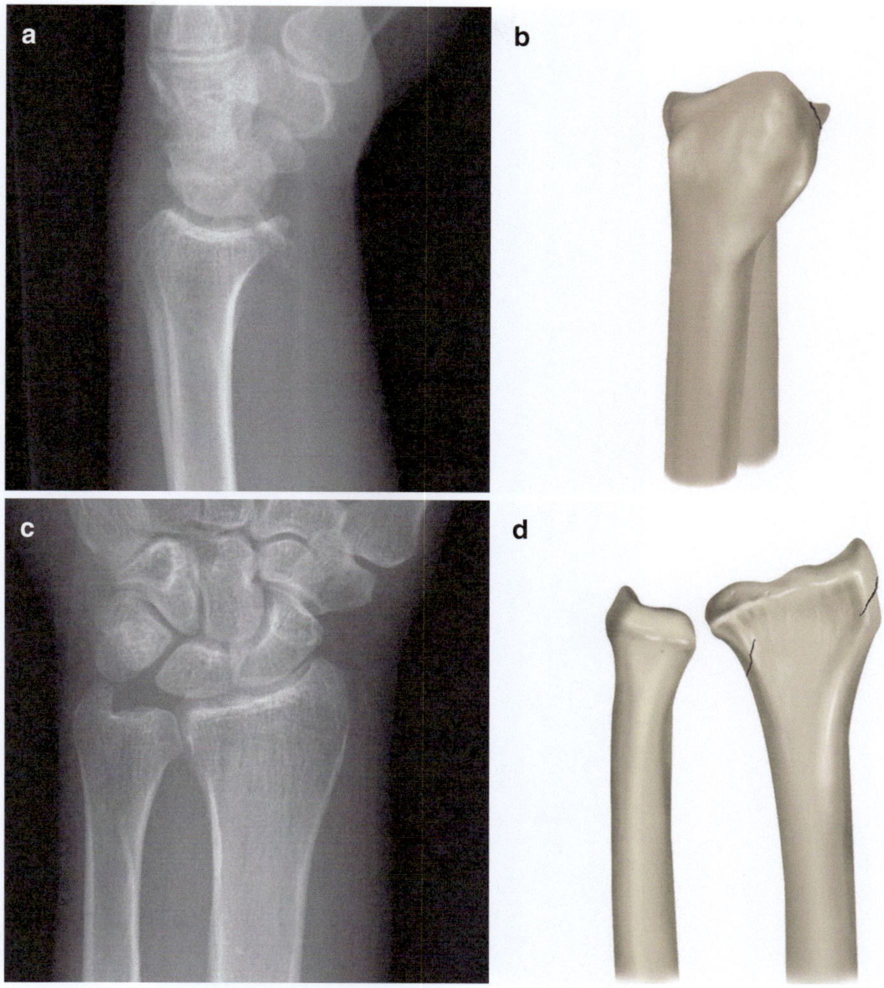

Fig. 4.14 X-rays (**a**, **c**) and illustrations (**b**, **d**) show fracture of anterior border of distal radius. The fracture line extends to the articular surface and the broken ends are slightly displaced

    14.2. CT scan (Fig. 4.14e, f)

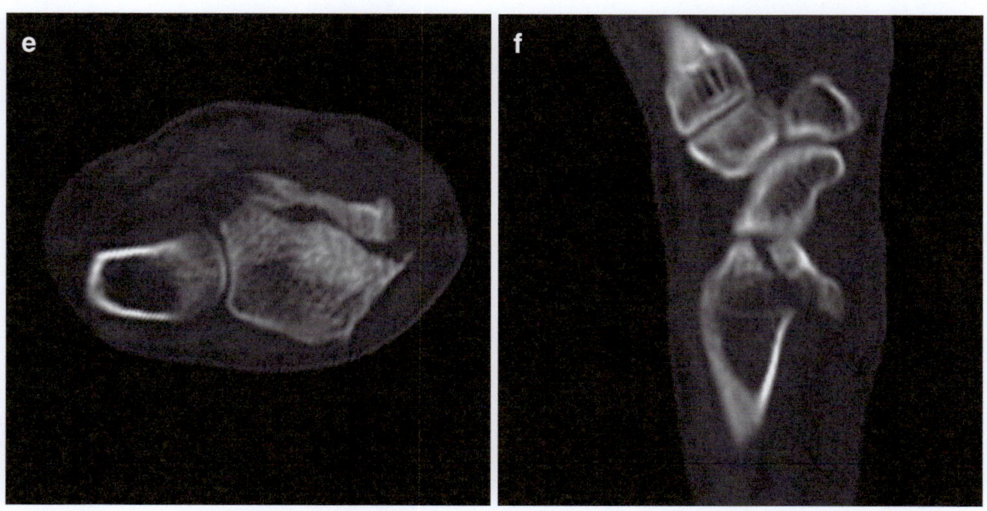

Fig. 4.14 The cross-section (**e**) and sagittal CT plane (**f**) images show fracture of anterior distal radius. The fracture line runs through the coronal plane and reaches the articular surface

15. Differentiation of Barton fracture and suspected fracture
    15.1. X-ray (Fig. 4.15a–d)

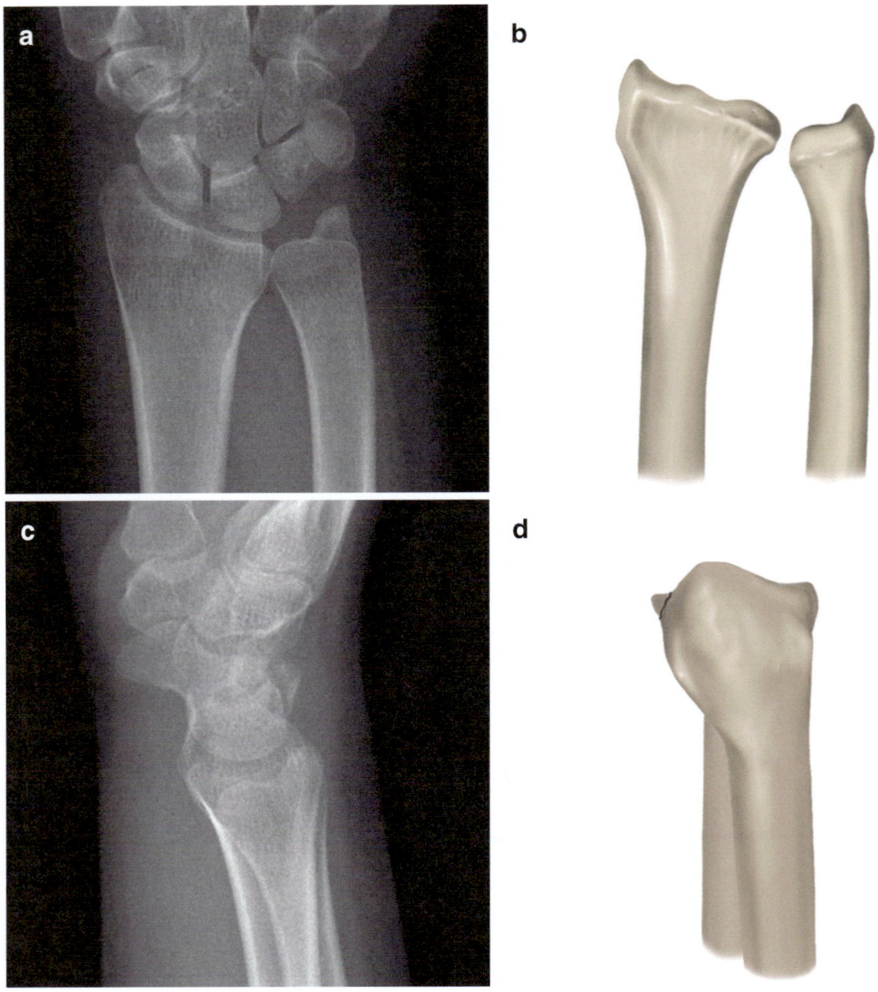

Fig. 4.15 X-rays (**a**, **c**) and illustrations (**b**, **d**) show irregular anterior border of distal radius

    15.2. CT scan (Fig. 4.15e, f)

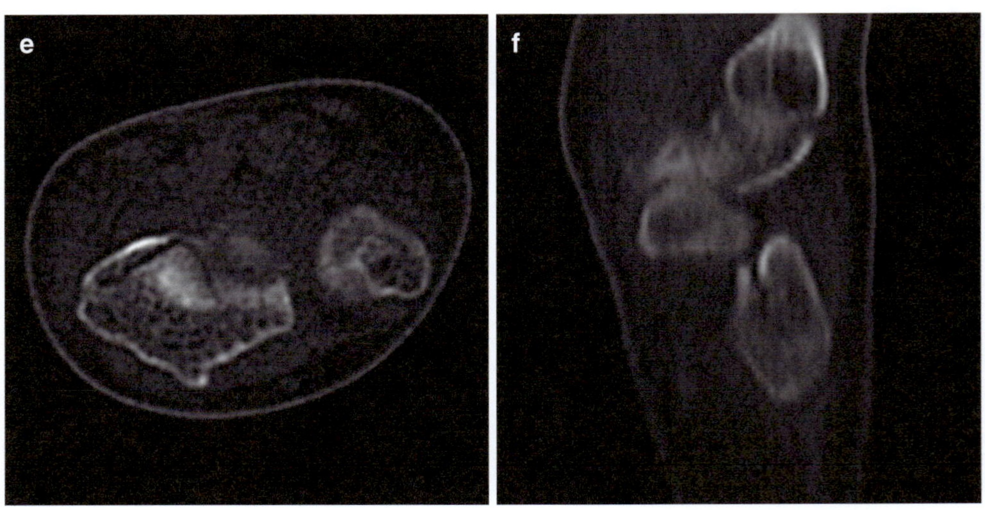

Fig. 4.15 The cross-section (**e**) and sagittal CT plane (**f**) images show fracture of the anterior distal radius. The fracture line runs in the coronal plane and reaches the articular surface

16. Differentiation of articular and extra-articular fracture of distal radius
    16.1. X-ray(Fig. 4.16a–d)

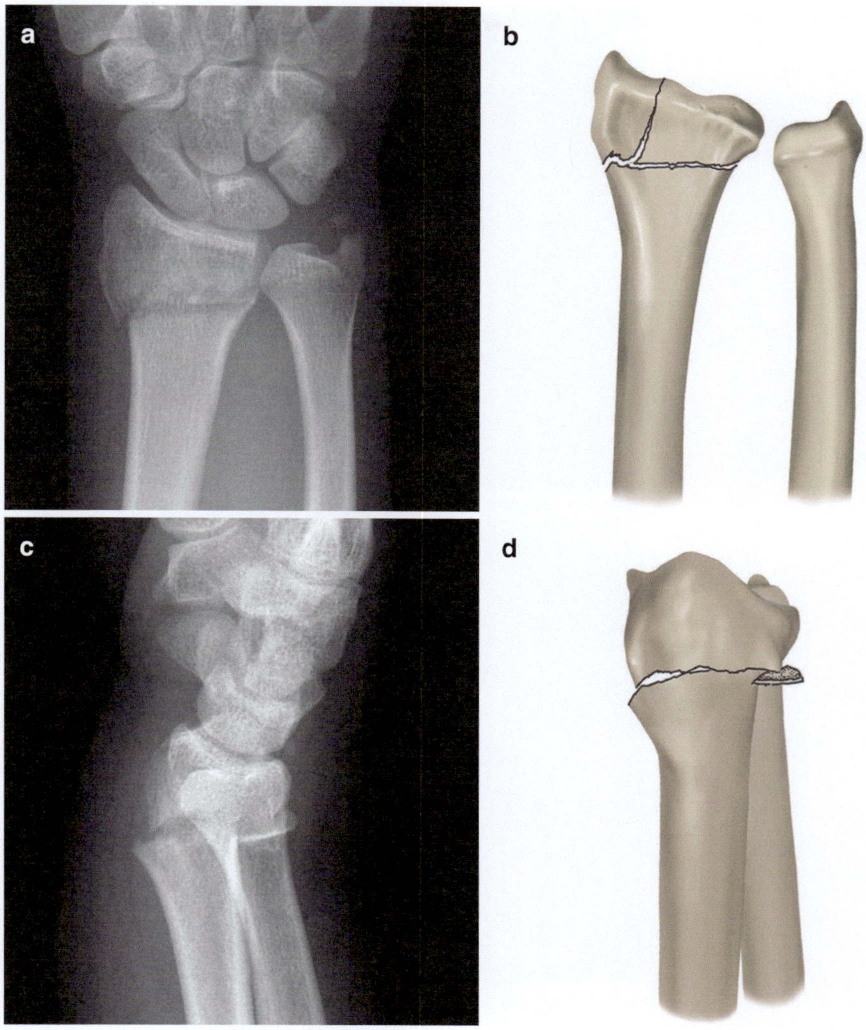

Fig. 4.16 X-rays (**a**, **c**) and illustrations (**b**, **d**) show displaced distal radius fracture

    16.2. CT scan(Fig. 4.16e, f)

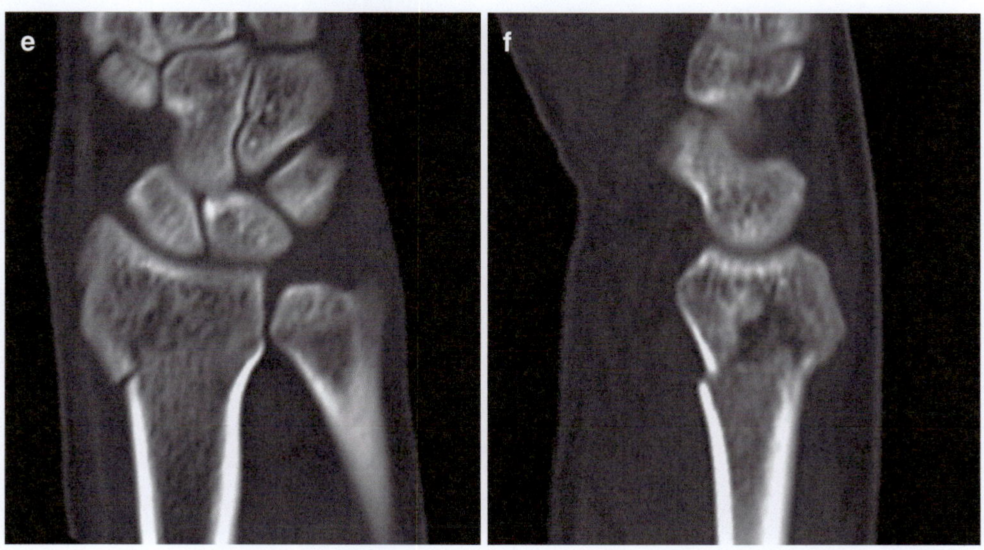

Fig. 4.16 The anteversion angle becomes negative. The coronal CT plane (**e**) and sagittal CT plane (**f**) images show displaced distal radius fracture. The fracture line extends to the articular surface

17. Differentiation of articular and extra-articular fracture of distal radius
    17.1. X-ray (Fig. 4.17a–d)

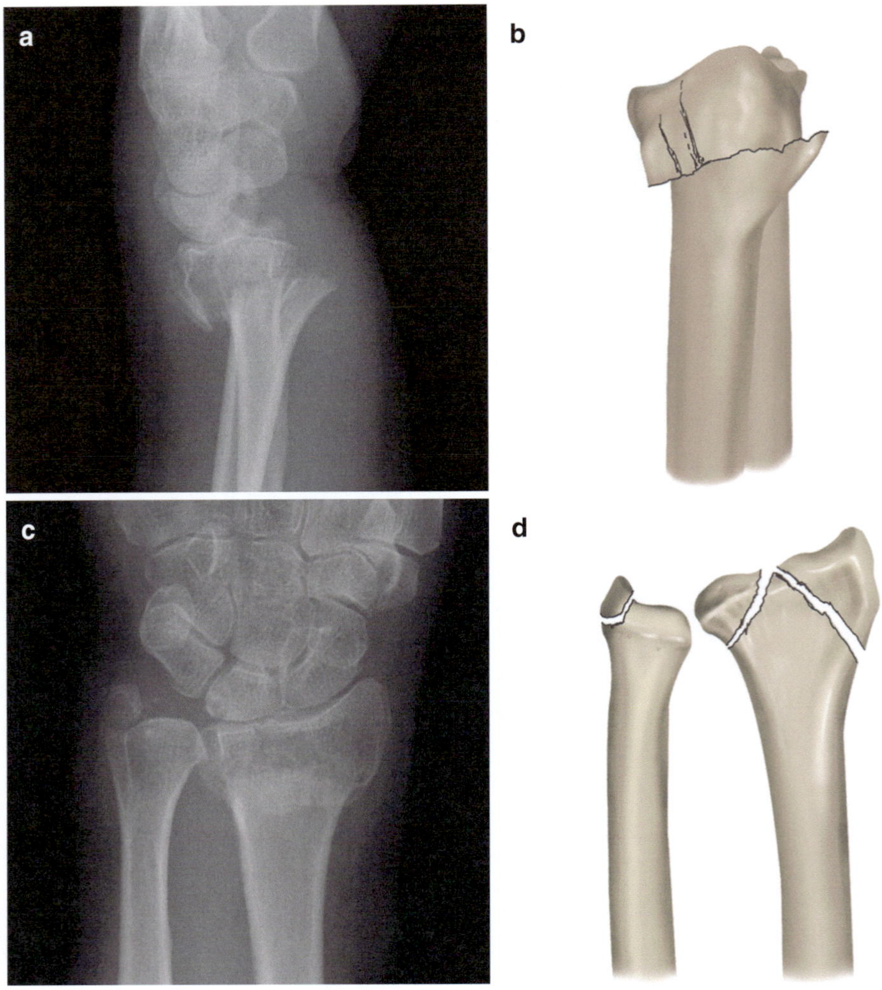

Fig. 4.17 X-rays (**a**, **c**) and illustrations (**b**, **d**) show displaced distal radius fracture. The anteversion angle becomes negative, and the fracture line extends to the articular surface

    17.2. CT scan (Fig. 4.17e, f)

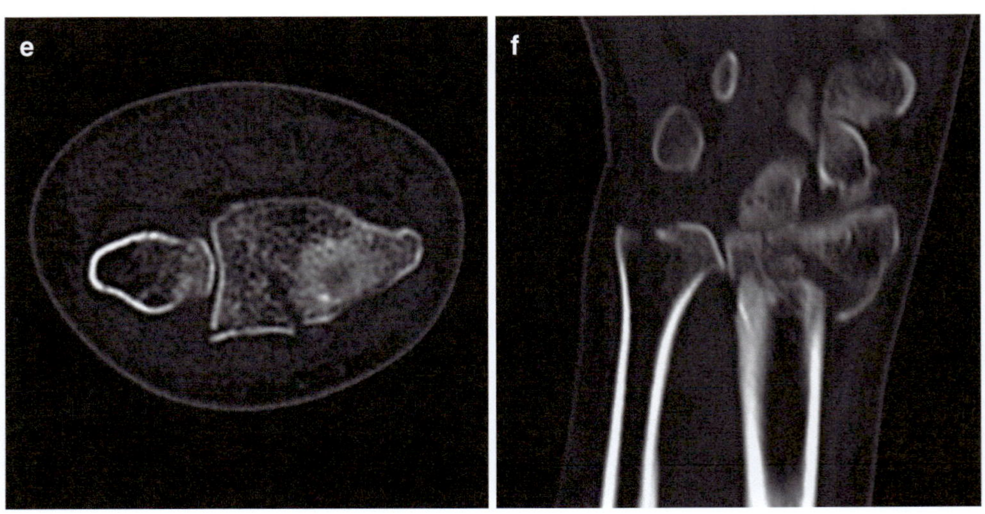

Fig. 4.17 The cross-section (**e**) and coronal CT plane (**f**) images show displaced distal radial fracture with fracture line reaching the articular surface

18. Differentiation of complete and partial articular fracture of distal radius
    18.1. X-ray (Fig. 4.18a–d)

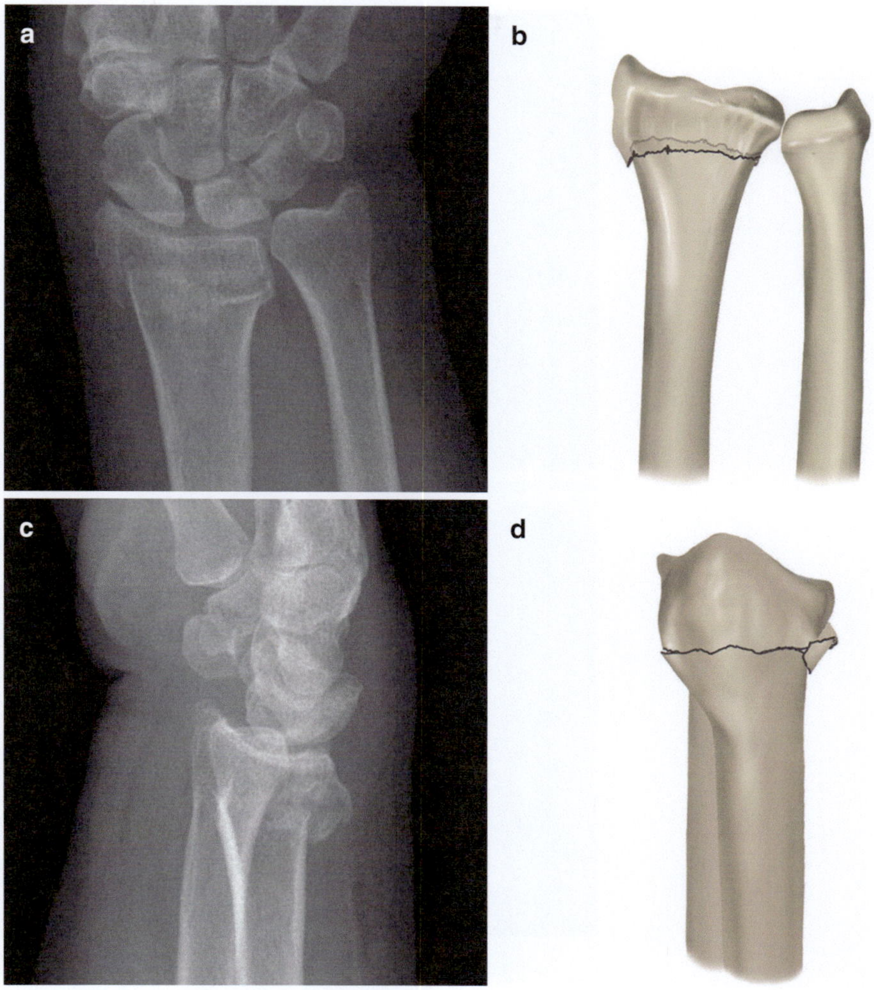

Fig. 4.18 X-rays (**a**, **c**) and illustration (**b**, **d**) show displaced distal radius fracture. Multiple fragments shadow can be seen, and the anteversion angle becomes negative

18.2. CT scan (Fig. 4.18e, f)

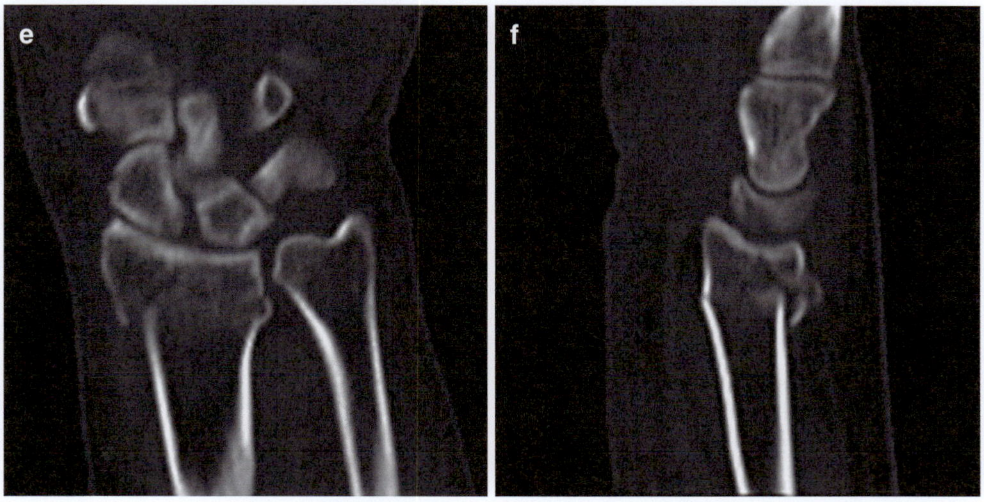

Fig. 4.18 The coronal CT plane (**e**) and sagittal CT plane (**f**) images show displaced distal radius fracture. Multiple fragments shadow can be seen in the metaphysis area, and the fracture line extends to the articular surface

19. Differentiation of simple and comminuted articular fracture of distal radius
    19.1. X-ray (Fig. 4.19a–d)

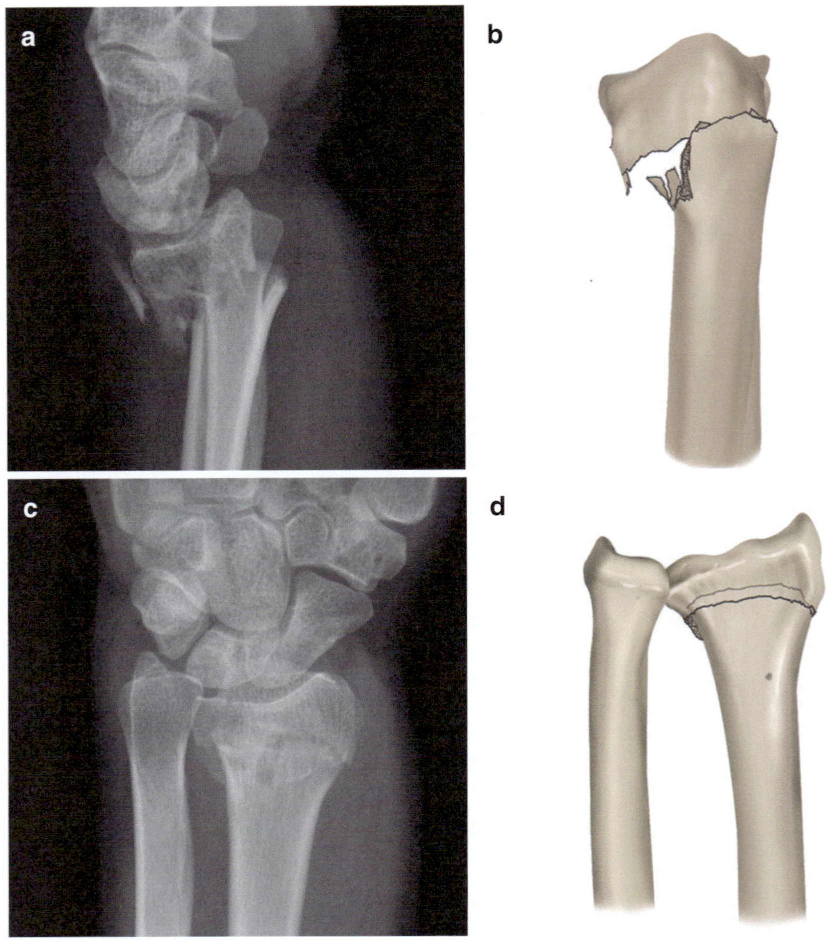

Fig. 4.19 X-rays (**a**, **c**) and illustration (**b**, **d**) images show comminuted fracture of distal radius, broken ends are displaced, and the anteversion angle becomes negative. Multiple fragments shadow can be seen

    19.2. CT scan (Fig. 4.19e, f)

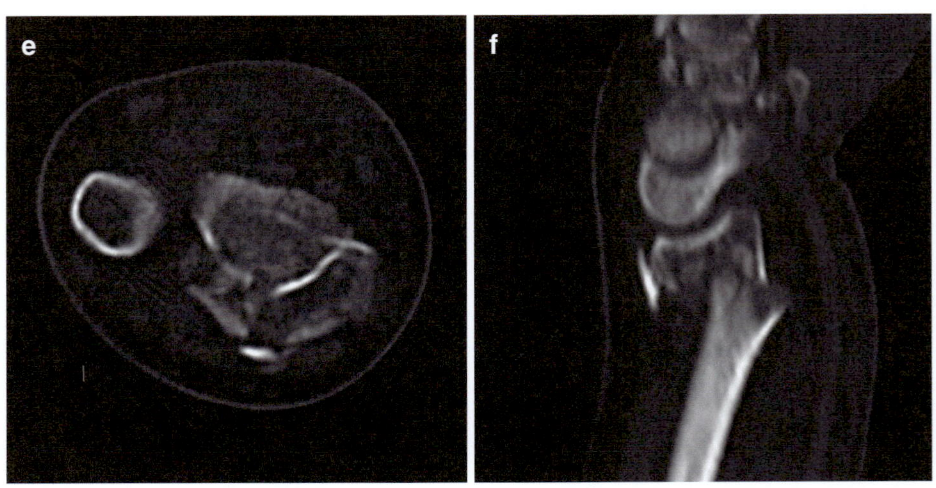

Fig. 4.19 The cross-section (**e**) and coronal CT plane (**f**) images show displaced distal radius fracture. Multiple fragments shadow can be seen in the metaphysis area. The fracture line extends to the articular surface

20. Differentiation of simple and comminuted articular fracture of distal radius
    20.1. X-ray (Fig. 4.20a–d)

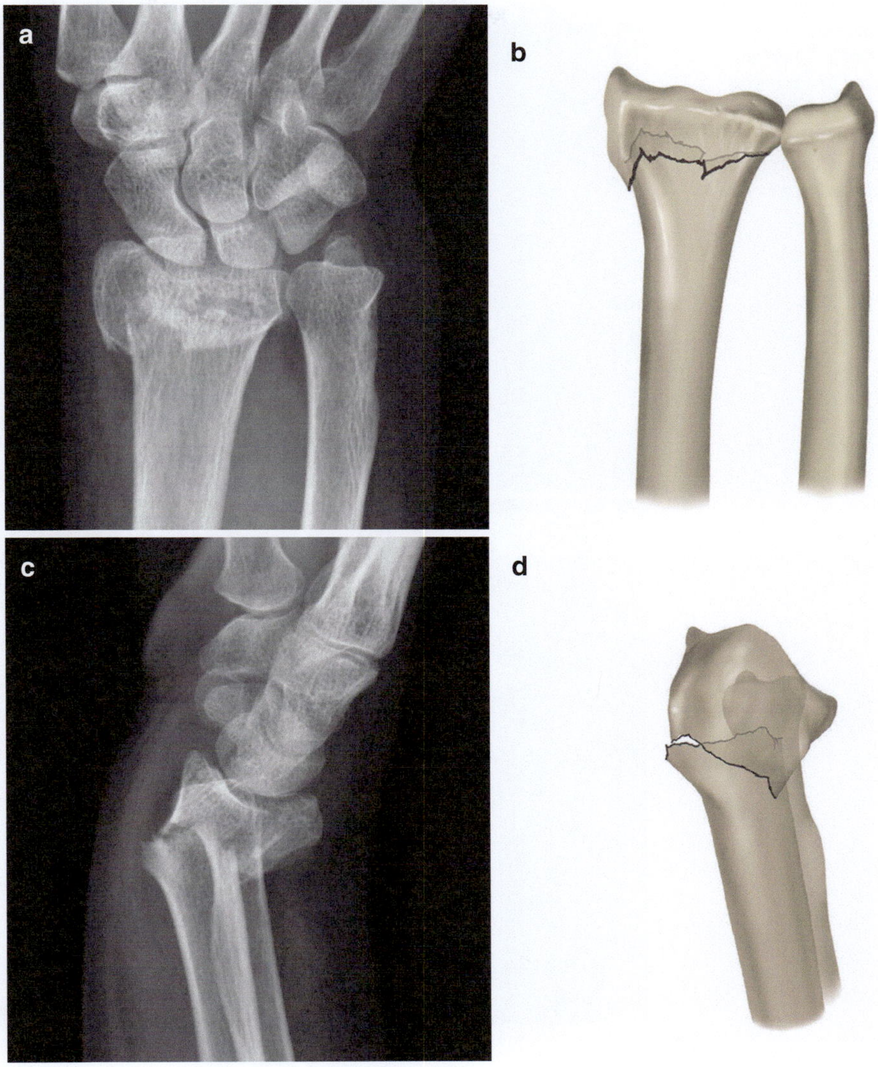

Fig. 4.20 X-rays (**a**, **c**) and illustrations (**b**, **d**) show distal radius fracture; broken ends are impacted and displaced. The anteversion angle becomes negative and multiple fragments shadow can be seen

20.2. CT scan (Fig. 4.20e–h)

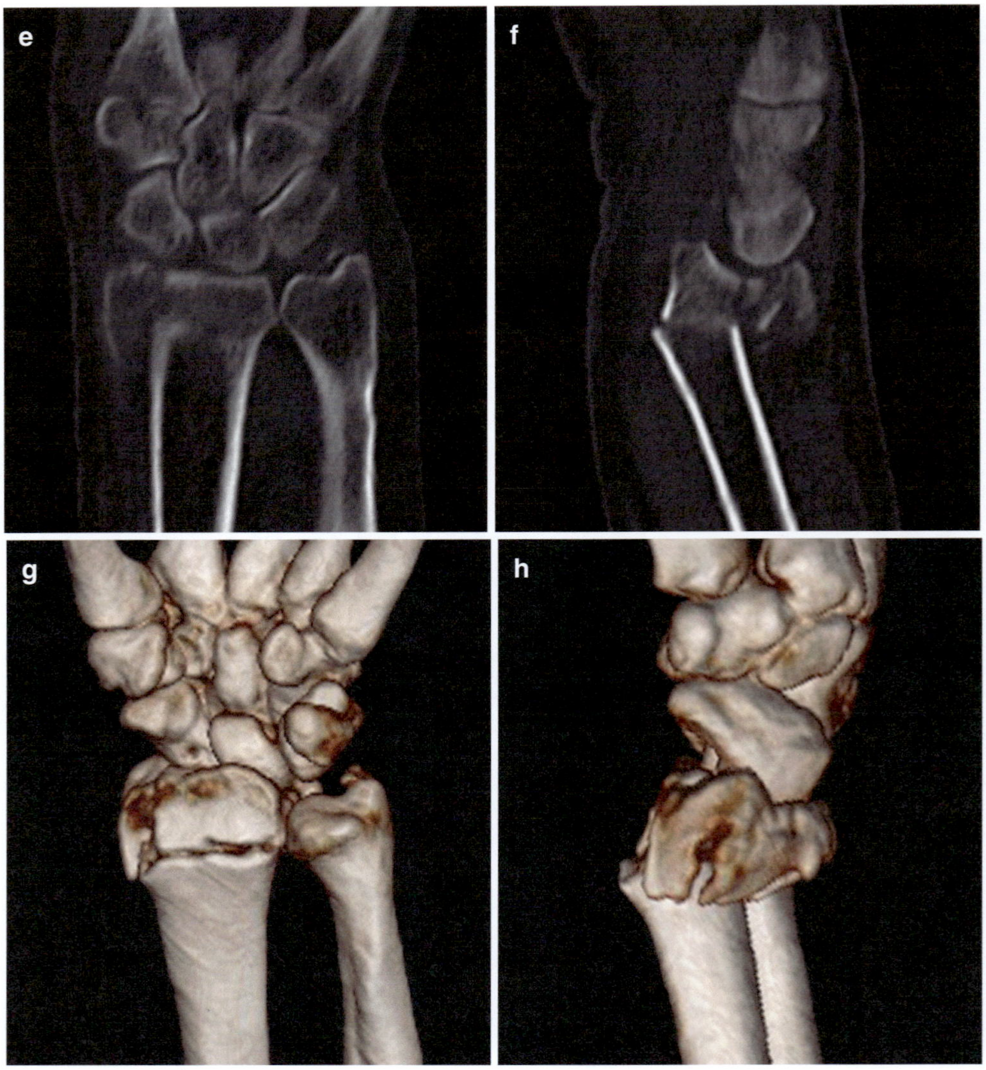

Fig. 4.20 The cross-section (**e**), coronal CT plane (**f**), and three-dimensional reconstruction (**g**, **h**) images show displaced distal radius fracture. Multiple fragments and uneven articular surface can be seen. The anteversion angle becomes negative

21. Differentiation of comminuted and simple articular fracture of distal radius
    21.1. X-ray (Fig. 4.21a–d)

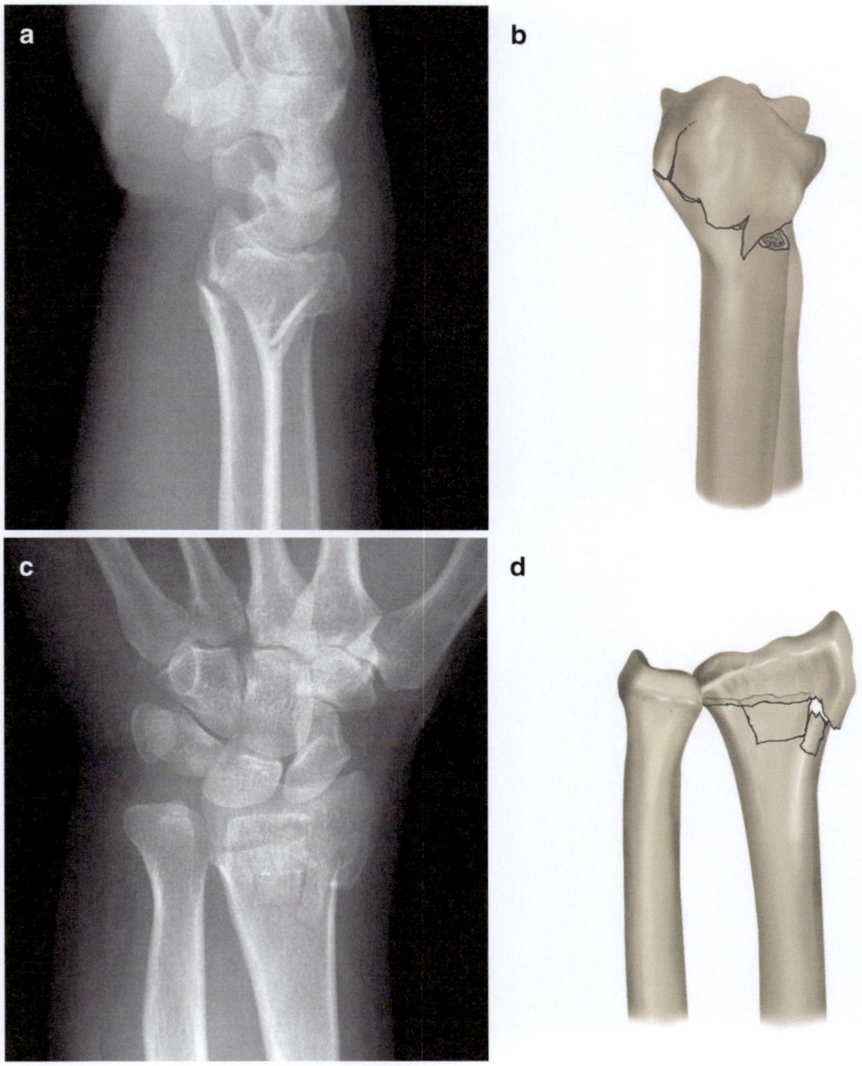

Fig. 4.21 X-rays (**a**, **c**) and illustrations (**b**, **d**) show distal radius fracture with displaced broken ends. The fracture line extends to the articular surface and the anteversion angle is negative

21.2. CT scan (Fig. 4.21e–h)

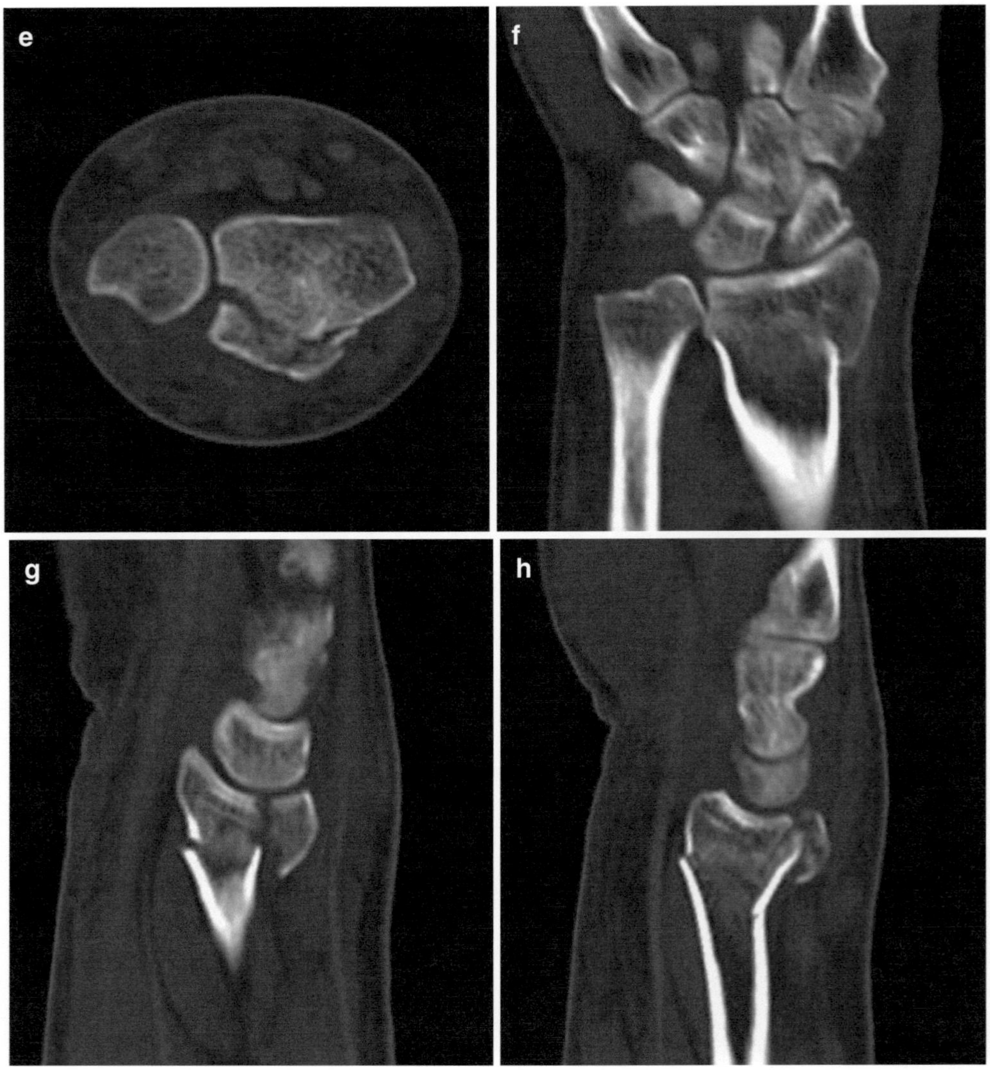

Fig. 4.21 The cross-section (**e**), coronal CT plane (**f**), and three-dimensional reconstruction (**g**, **h**) images show displaced distal radius fracture. Multiple fragments and uneven articular surface can be seen. The anteversion angle becomes negative

22. X-ray and CT of comminuted articular distal radius fracture
    22.1. X-ray (Fig. 4.22a–d)

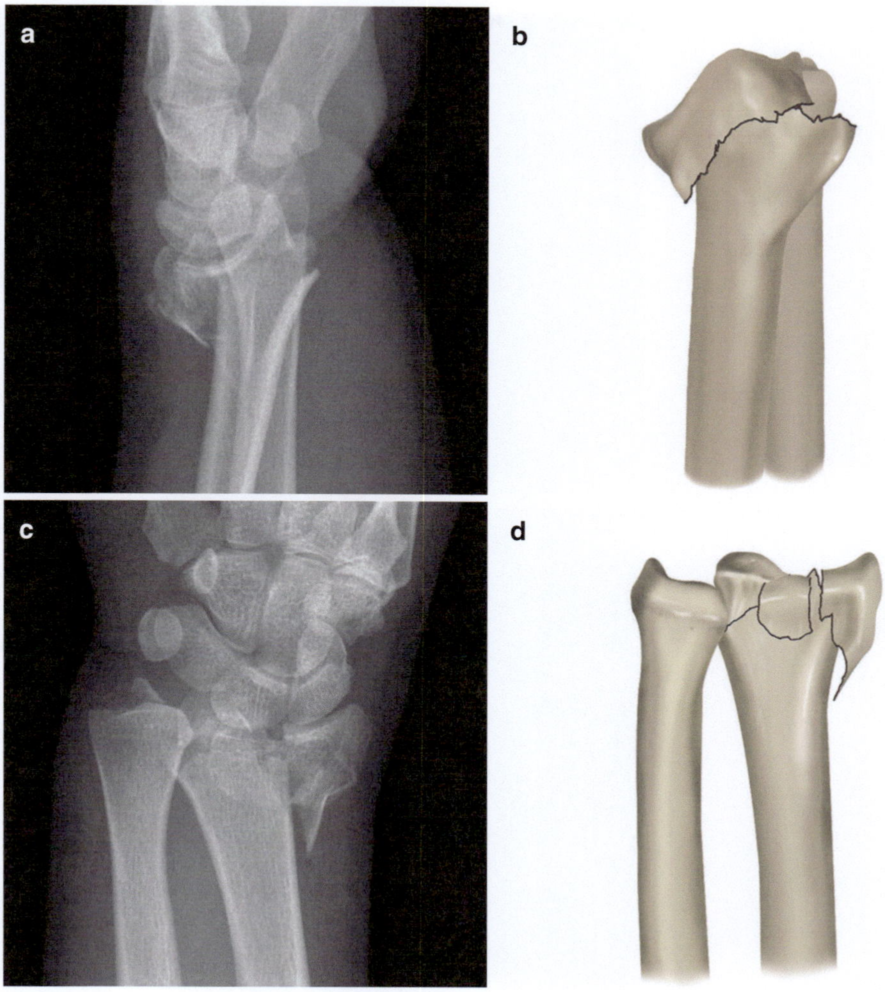

Fig. 4.22 X-rays (**a**, **c**) and illustration (**b**, **d**) show displaced distal radius fracture, fracture line extends to the articular surface and the anteversion angle becomes negative

    22.2. CT scan (Fig. 4.22e–h)

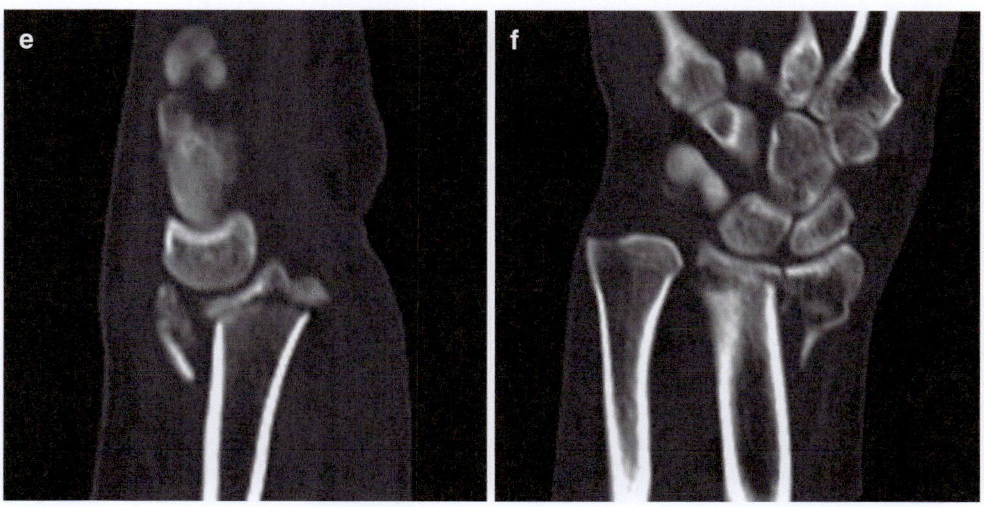

Fig. 4.22 The sagittal CT plane (**e**) and coronal CT plane (**f**) images show displaced distal radius fracture. Multiple fragments, uneven surface, and negative anteversion angle can be seen

23. Differentiation of comminuted and simple articular fracture of distal radius
    23.1. X-ray (Fig. 4.23a–d)

Fig. 4.23 X-rays (**a**, **c**) and illustrations (**b**, **d**) show displaced distal radius fracture. The fracture line runs through the articular surface and the anteversion angle becomes negative

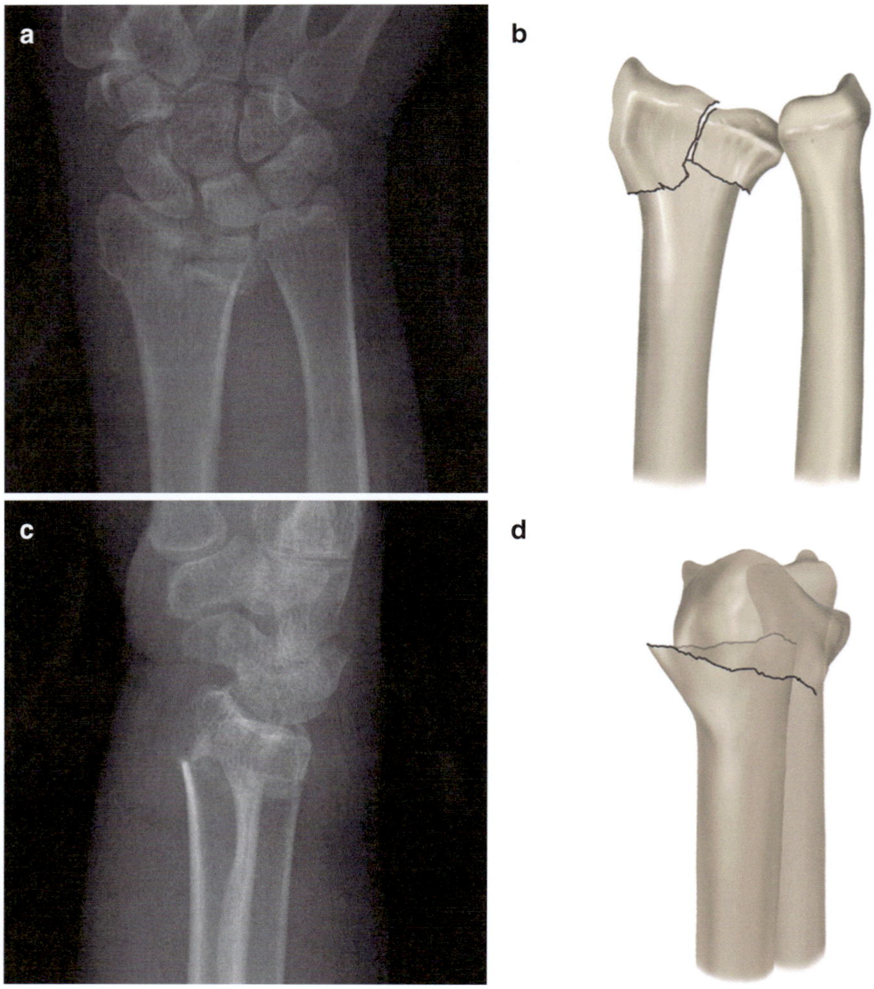

    23.2. CT scan (Fig. 4.23e–h)

Fig. 4.23 The coronal CT plane (**e**) and sagittal CT plane (**f**) images show displaced distal radius fracture. Multiple fragments, uneven surface, and negative anteversion angle can be seen

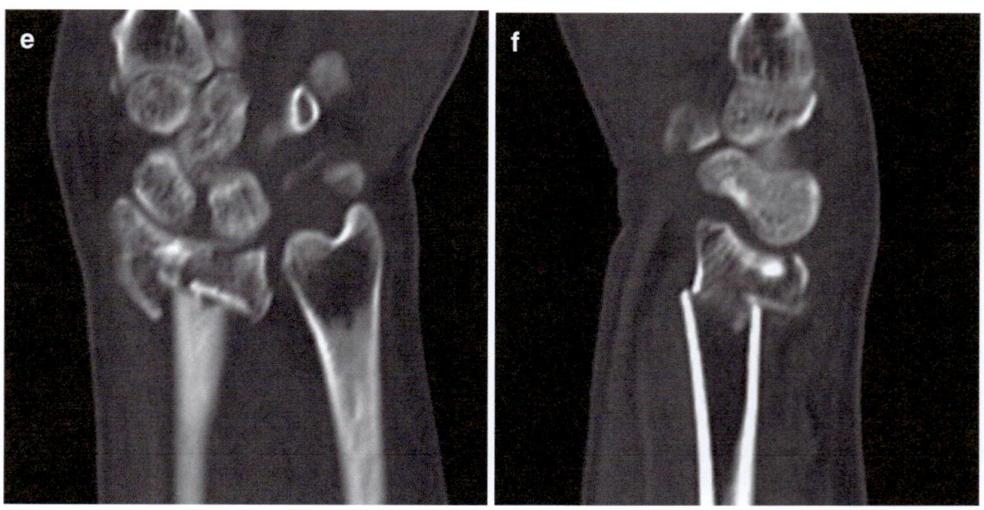

24. X-ray and CT of articular comminuted distal radius fracture
    24.1. X-ray (Fig. 4.24a–h)

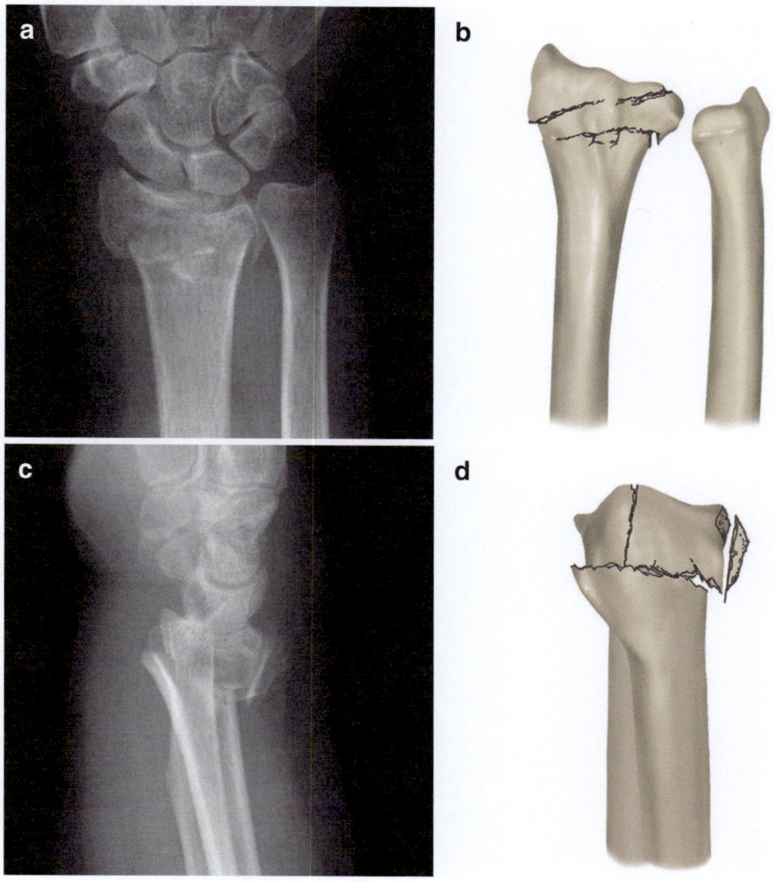

Fig. 4.24 X-rays (**a**, **c**) and illustrations (**b**, **d**) images show displaced distal radius fracture, fracture line runs through the articular surface, and the anteversion angle becomes negative. The cross-section (**e**), coronal CT plane (**f**), and sagittal reconstruction (**g**, **h**) images show displaced fracture of the distal radius. Multiple fragments and uneven articular surface can be seen with negative anteversion angle

24.2. CT scan (Fig. 4.24e–h)

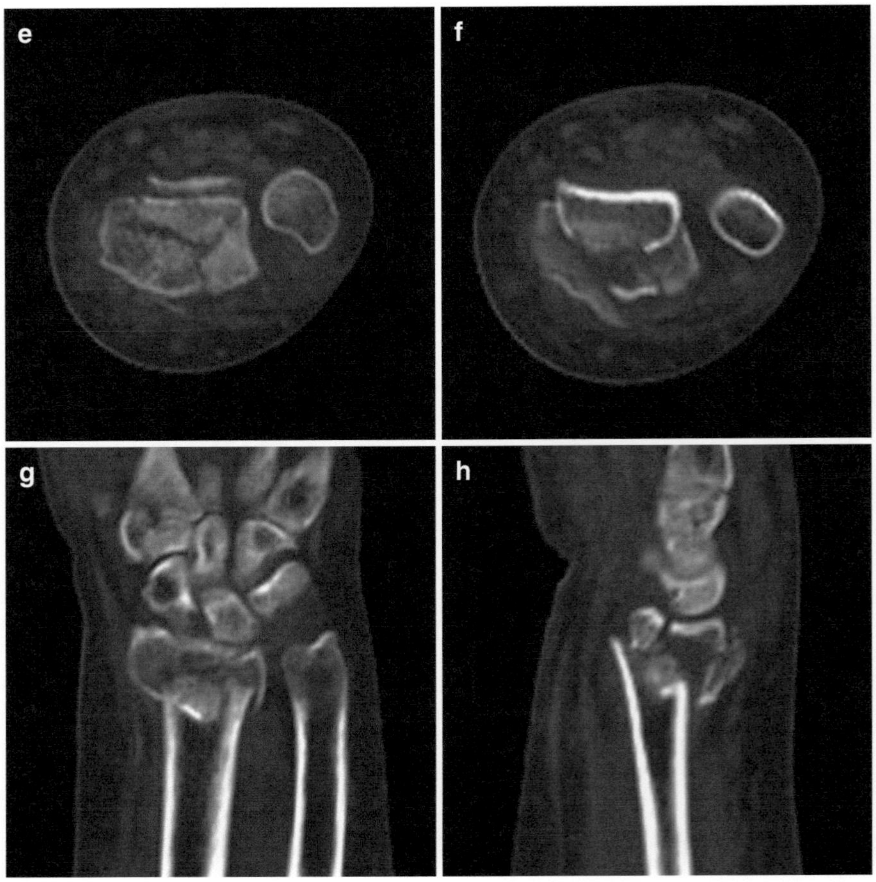

Fig. 4.24 (**e**), coronal CT plane (**f**), and sagittal reconstruction (**g**, **h**) images show displaced fracture of the distal radius. Multiple fragments and uneven articular surface can be seen with negative anteversion angle

25. X-ray and CT of articular comminuted distal radius fracture
 25.1. X-ray (Fig. 4.25a–h)

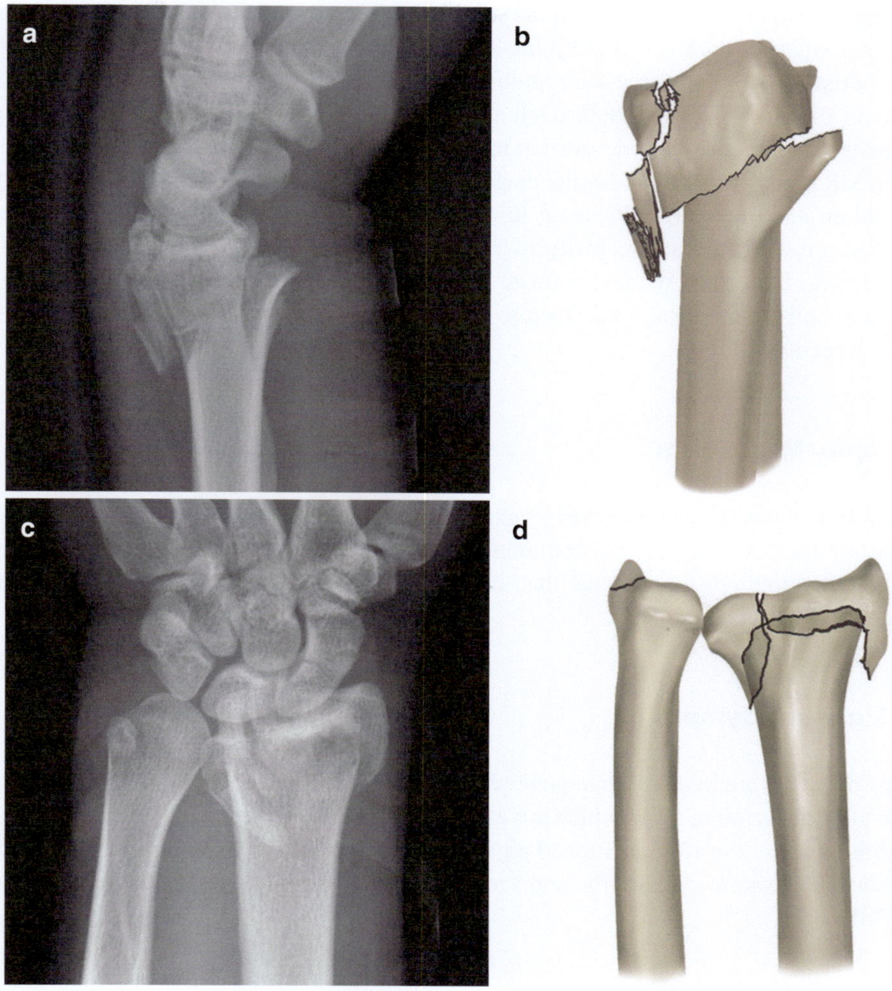

Fig. 4.25 X-rays (**a**, **c**) and illustrations (**b**, **d**) show distal radius fracture. The articular surface is affected. Multiple bone shadows on the dorsal edge and ulnar styloid fracture can be seen

 25.2. CT scan (Fig. 4.25e, f)

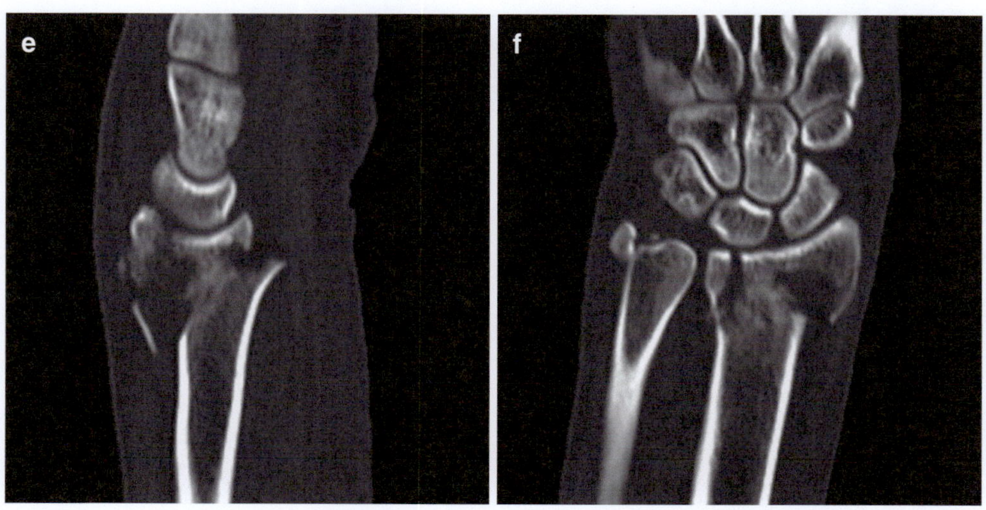

Fig. 4.25 Displaced distal radius fracture, uneven surface, multiple fragments at metaphysis, and articular area can be seen on the sagittal CT plane (**e**) and coronal CT plane (**f**) images

4.2 Carpal Fracture

Carpal bones are a complex of eight bones, roughly arranged in two rows across the wrist. Beginning with the thumb-side of the wrist, the proximal row is made up of the scaphoid, lunate, triquetrum, and pisiform. Except for the pisiform, the remaining bones are a part of the radiocarpal joint. The distal row is made up of the trapezium, trapezoid, capitates, and hamate bone. The wrist is a complex area with multiple bones within proximity of one another, and in some case, they are overlapped. Thus, diagnosing a fracture through an X-ray film is difficult, which risks misdiagnosis and missed diagnosis. CT can eliminate the influence of bone overlap in the plain film, and depict the carpal bones and the origin of fragment more accurately. MR scans are essential for the diagnosis of peripheral tendon and soft tissue injury, especially in epiphyseal injuries in children and inter-carpal ligament injuries. The AO/OTA classification of carpal fractures include lunate fracture, scaphoid fracture, capitate fracture, pisiform fracture, ulnar carpal bones (triquetrum and pisiform) fracture, and radial carpal bone (trapezium, trapezoid) fracture. Lunate fracture, scaphoid fracture, capitate fracture, pisiform fracture, ulnar carpal bone fracture, and radial carpal bone fracture account for 1.78%, 84.45%,, 0.44%,,1.78%,, 9.11%, and 2.44% of all carpal fractures, respectively.

4.2.1 Injury Mechanism

The most common mechanism is caused by axial trauma onto the outstretched hand, as well as from flexion trauma. Reversal and direct trauma, however, are less common. In addition, the type of injury is also correlated to the time of the violence lasting. For example, if the trauma that causes scaphoid fracture persists, it may cause trans-scaphoid perilunate dislocation.

4.2.2 Signs and Symptoms

Symptoms of a fractured carpal bone generally include sudden pain, rapid swelling, limitations in mobility, and obvious deformity after dislocation, all of which are easily identified. However, there are many cases of slightly displaced fractures which exhibit none of the aforementioned physical symptoms, subsequently could be missed. Therefore, patients with wrist trauma should be examined carefully, and suspicious cases should be examined by a series of hand and wrist X-rays, CT scans, or MRI.

4.2.3 Imaging Differential Diagnosis

Standard X-rays continue to be the first choice of detection for displacement scaphoid fractures. Other high quality views of the wrist from different angles may also be obtained: scaphoid position, carpal tunnel position, post-anterior tangential position, wrist bridge position, and random tangential position. CT scans may be conducted to identify small avulsion fractures and contrapositions of the joint surface in fracture site; however, the ionizing radiation is relatively higher. An MR imaging is beneficial for surrounding soft tissue injuries connected to the wrist, especially for children with epiphyseal injury and wrist ligament injuries.

4.2.3.1 Lunate Fracture

1. Differentiation of lunate fracture and non-fracture
   1.1. X-ray (Fig. 4.26a–d)

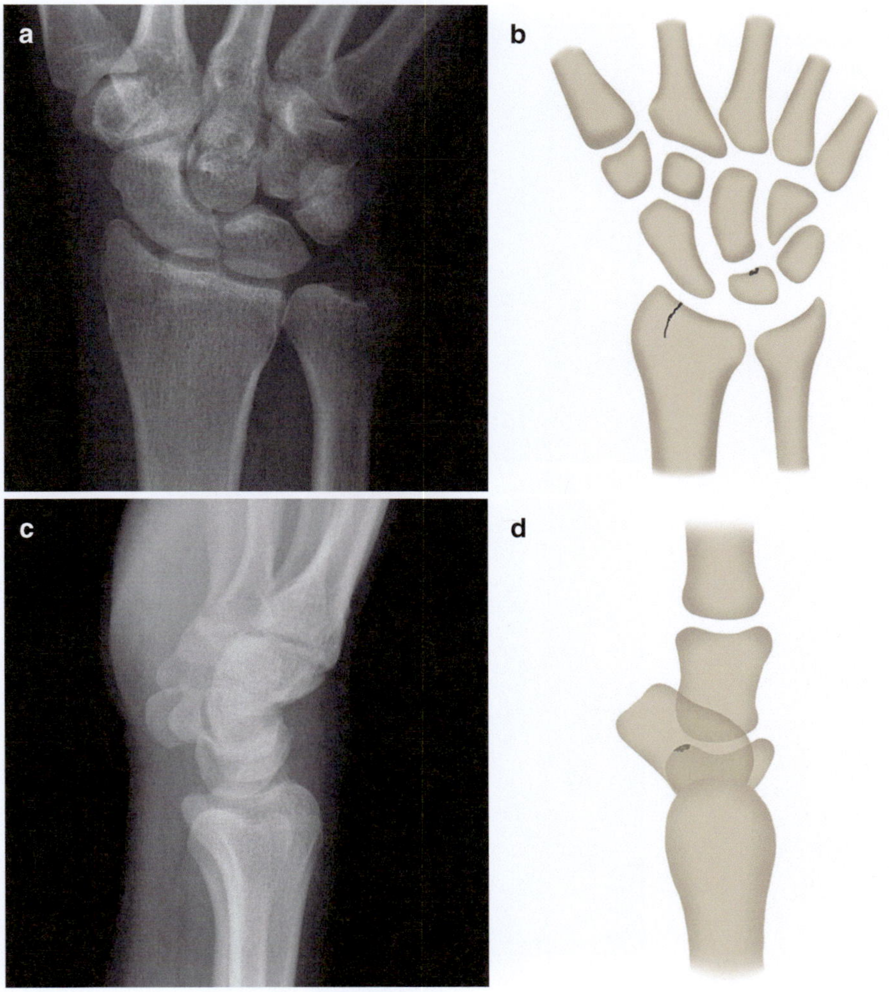

Fig. 4.26 X-rays (**a**, **c**) and illustrations (**b**, **d**) indicate trabecular bone disruption at distal radius area without definite fracture of lunate bone

   1.2. CT scan (Fig. 4.26e, f)

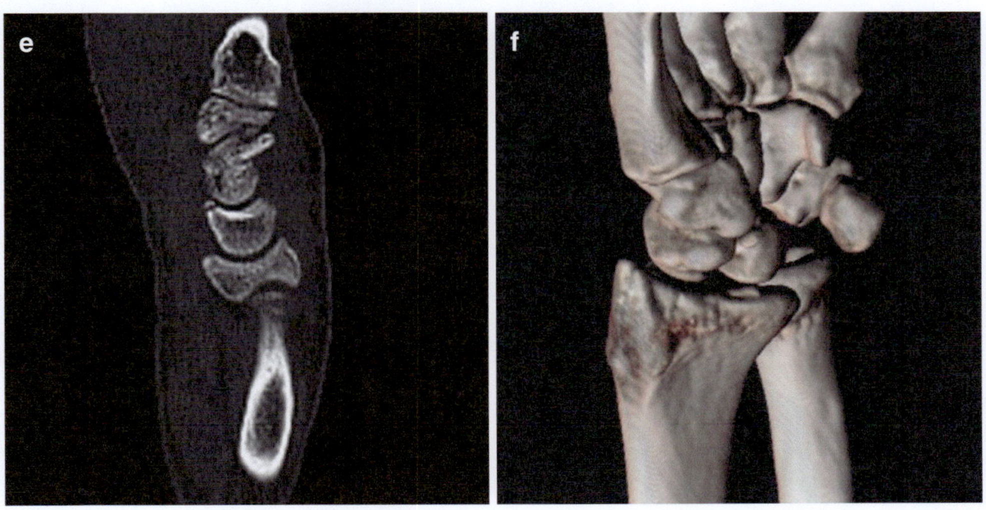

Fig. 4.26 Sagittal computed tomography (CT) scan (**e**) and three-dimensional CT reconstruction image (**f**) show a frontal fracture of lunate with visible small bone shadow

2. Differentiation of lunate fracture and non-fracture
   2.1. X-ray (Fig. 4.27a–d)

Fig. 4.27 X-rays (**a**, **c**) and illustration (**b**, **d**) show trabecular bone disruption on distal radius area without definite fracture of lunate bone

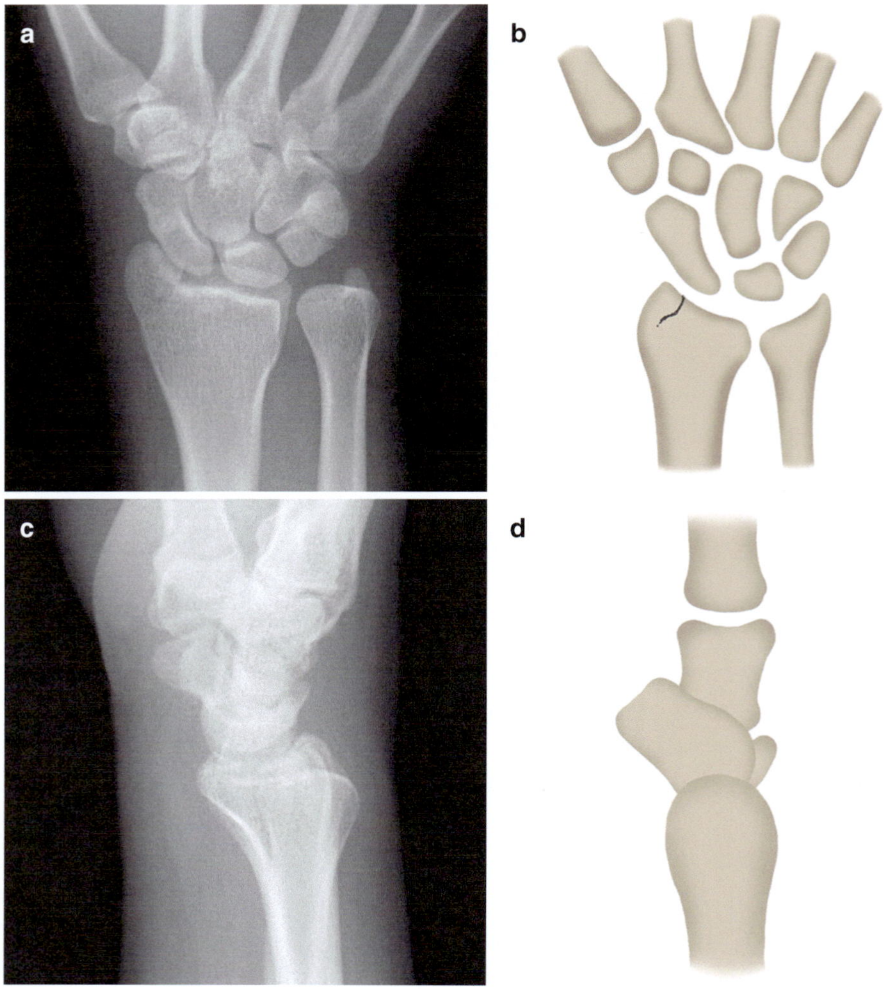

   2.2. CT scan (Fig. 4.27e, f)

Fig. 4.27 Cross-section CT scans (**e**, **f**) show an ulnar fracture of the body of the lunate with visible small bone shadow

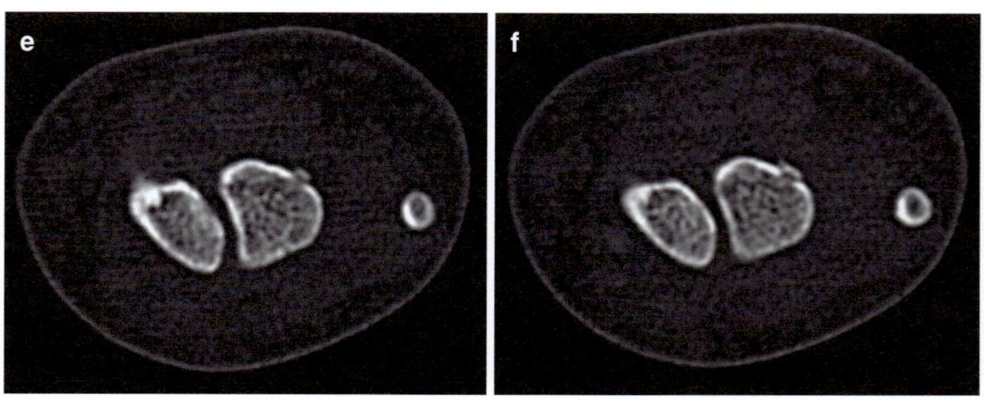

3. X-ray and CT scan of proximal scaphoid fracture
   3.1. X-ray (Fig. 4.28a–d)

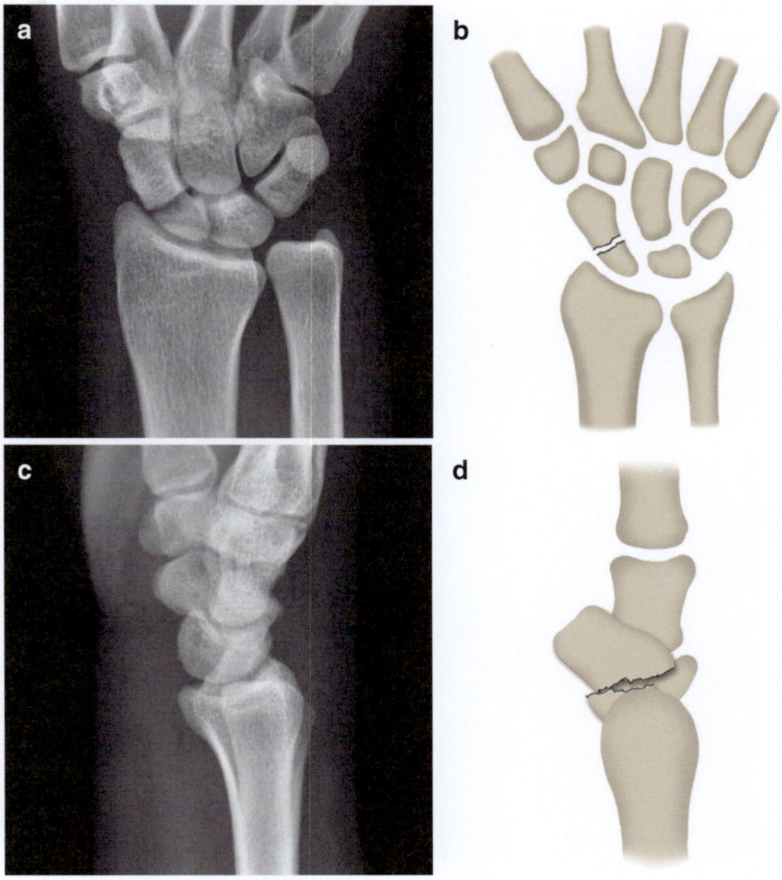

Fig. 4.28 X-rays (**a**, **c**) and illustrations (**b**, **d**) reveal proximal scaphoid fracture. The gap is slightly wider and fragments are slightly displaced

3.2. CT scan (Fig. 4.28e–h)

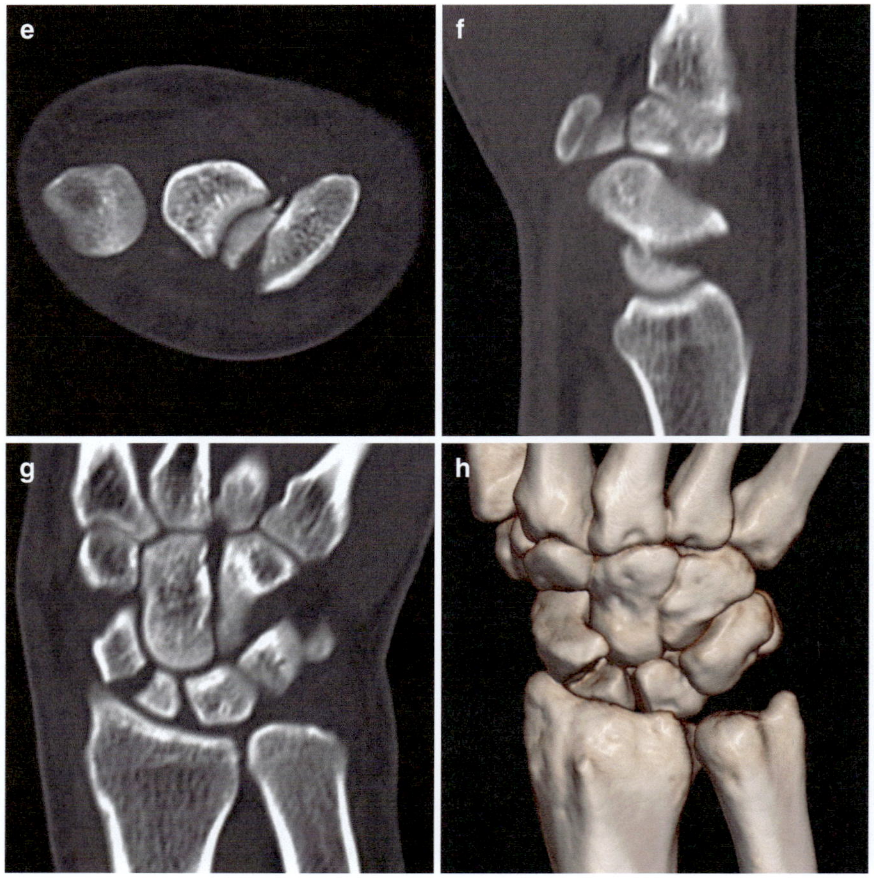

Fig. 4.28 The cross-section (**e**), sagittal CT plane (**f**), coronal plane (**g**), and three-dimensional reconstruction CT (**h**) images show proximal scaphoid fracture. Fragments are separated and displaced, and a small fragment is found in the anterior pole

4. Differentiation of scaphoid waist fracture and suspicious fracture
    4.1. X-ray (Fig. 4.29a–d)

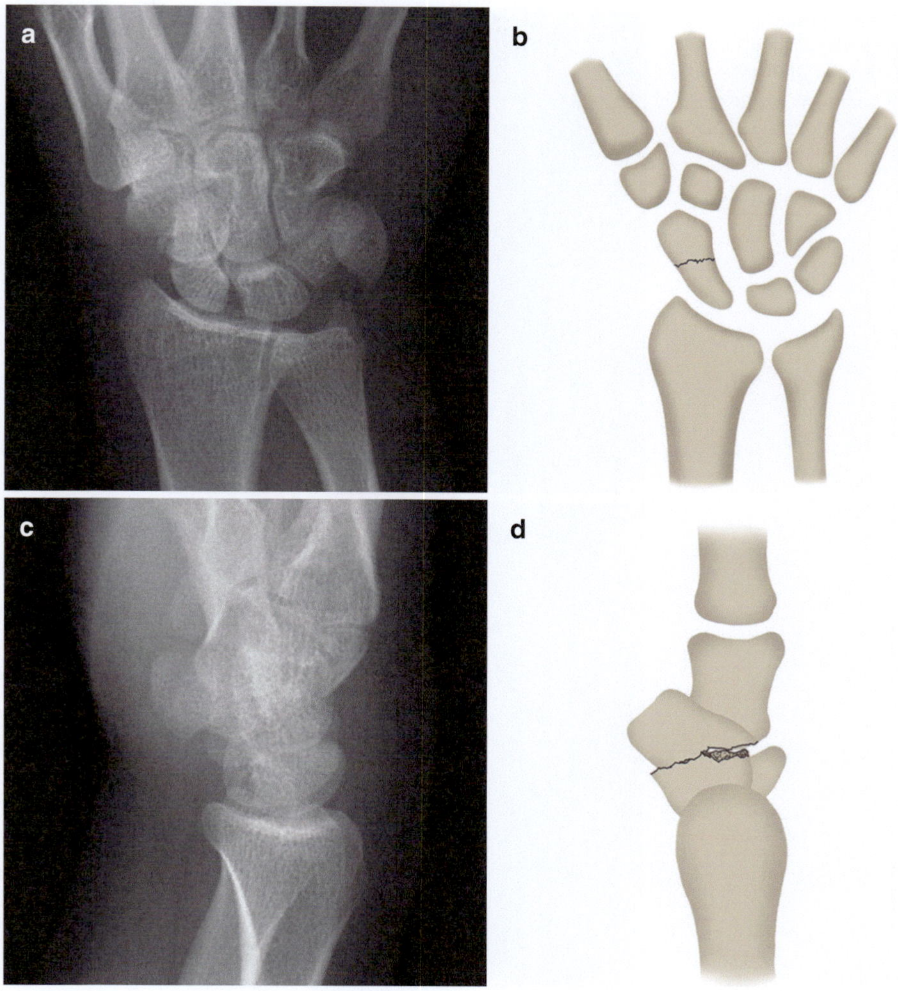

Fig. 4.29 X-rays (**a**, **c**) and illustration (**b**, **d**) show scaphoid waist fracture, irregular profile of scaphoid, and disordered structure. Additional scaphoid position X-ray should be ordered

    4.2. CT scan (Fig. 4.29e, f)

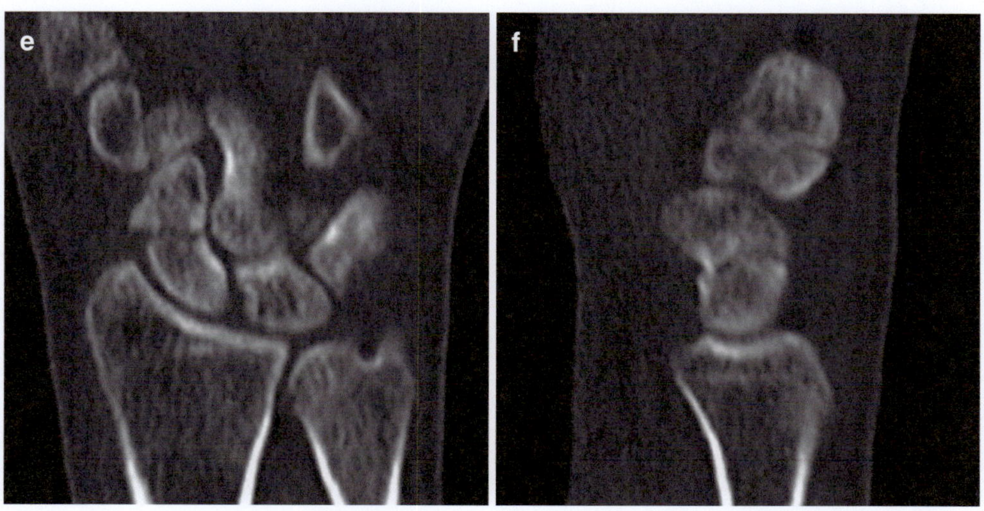

Fig. 4.29 The coronal plane (**e**) and sagittal plane (**f**) CT scans show a break in the "waist" of the scaphoid with slightly displaced fragments

5. Differentiation of distal scaphoid fracture and suspected fracture
   5.1. X-ray (Fig. 4.30a–d)

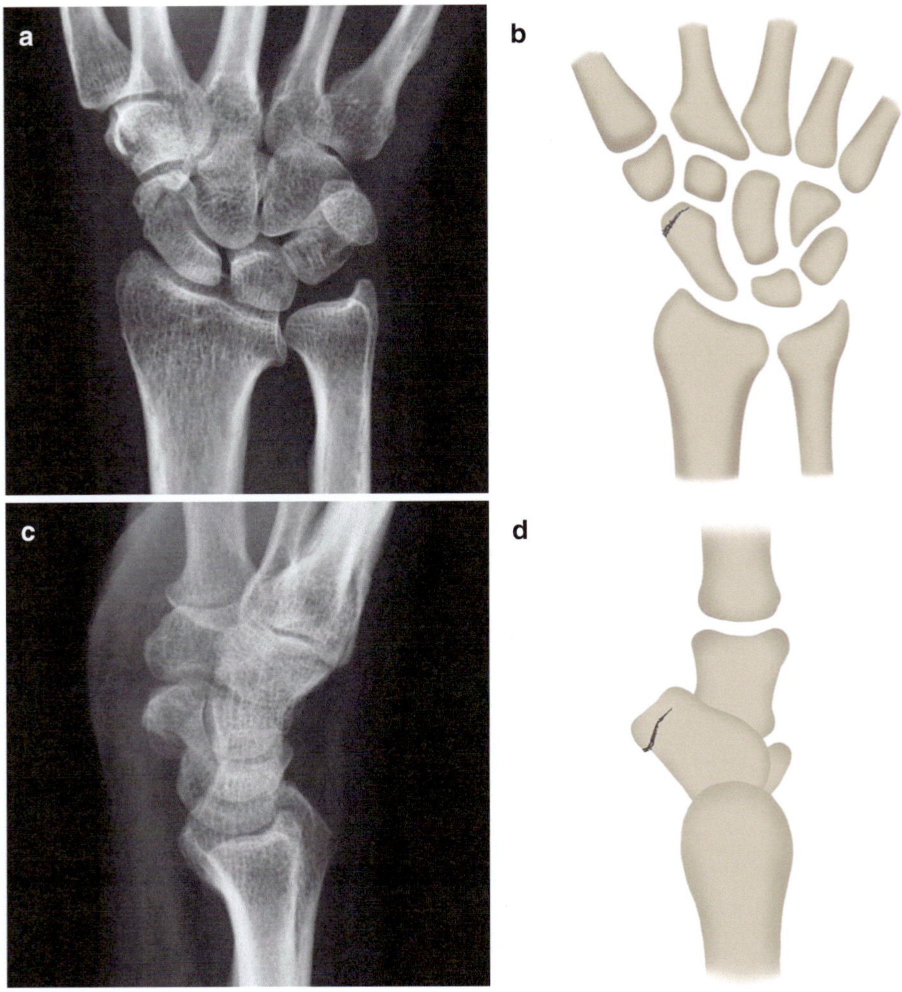

Fig. 4.30 X-rays (**a**, **c**) and illustration (**b**, **d**) indicate trabecular disorder of distal scaphoid. Fracture at this area is ambiguous

   5.2. CT scan (Fig. 4.30e, f)

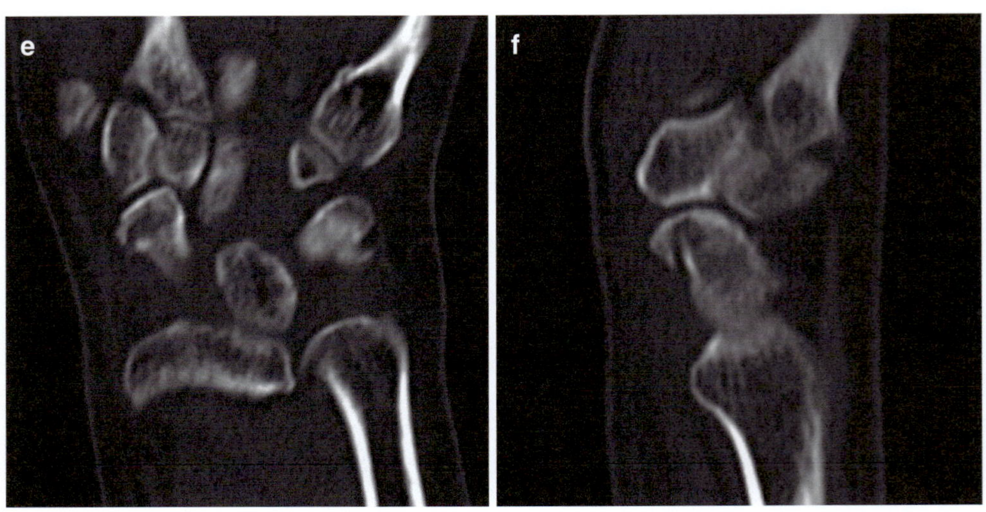

Fig. 4.30 The coronal plane (**e**) and sagittal plane (**f**) CT scans show displaced distal scaphoid fracture with slightly displaced fragments

6. Differentiation of scaphoid nodule fracture and suspected fracture
   6.1. X-ray (Fig. 4.31a–d)

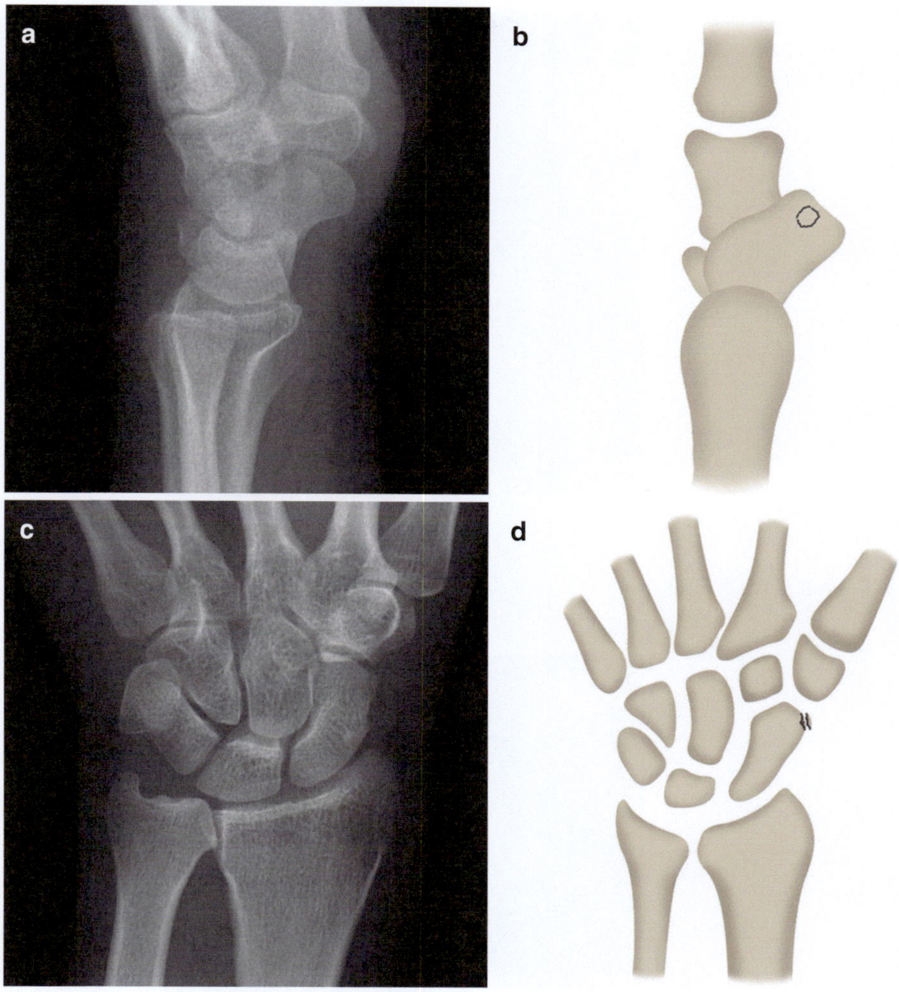

Fig. 4.31 X-rays (**a**, **c**) and illustrations (**b**, **d**) show irregular profile of scaphoid nodule

   6.2. CT scan (Fig. 4.31e, f)

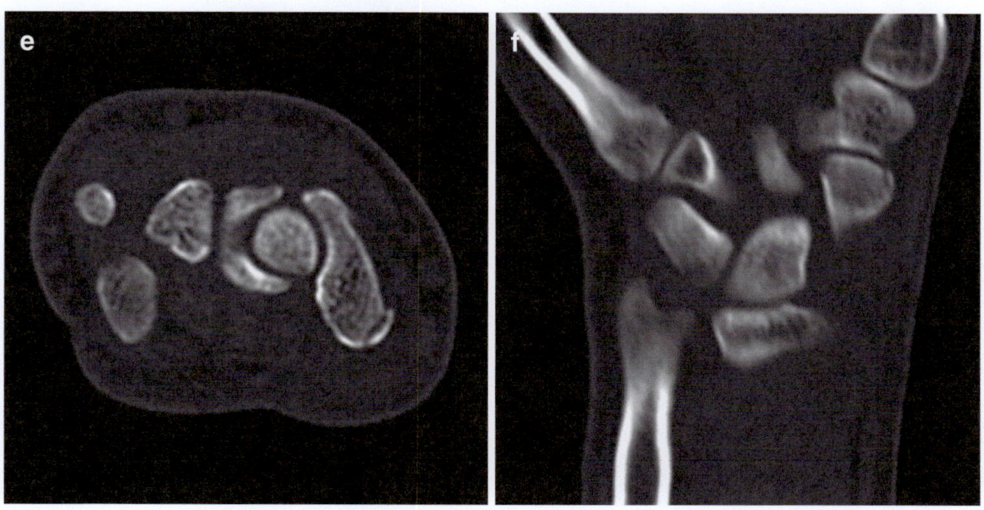

Fig. 4.31 The cross-section (**e**) and coronal plane (**f**) CT scans show scaphoid nodule fracture with slightly displaced fragments

7. Differentiation of scaphoid incomplete fracture and suspicious fracture
   7.1. X-ray (Fig. 4.32a, b)

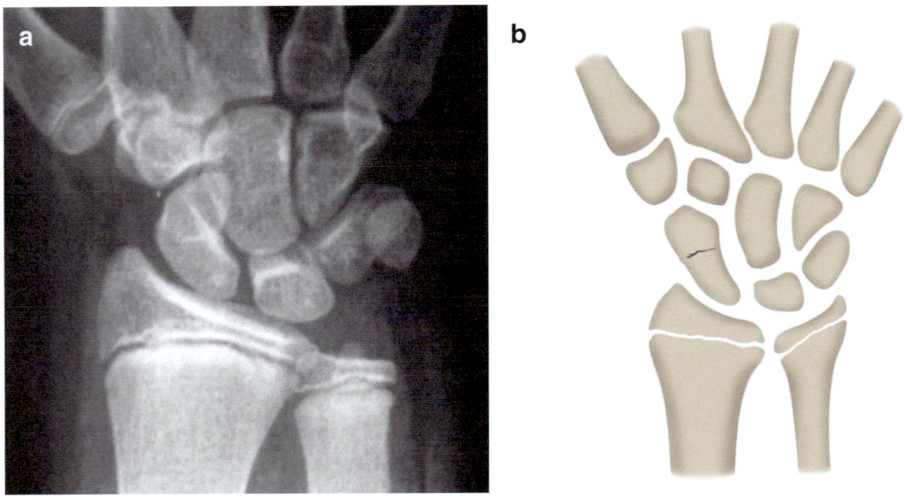

Fig. 4.32 X-rays (**a**) and illustrations (**b**) show an irregular profile of the waist of scaphoid bone

   7.2. MR scan (Fig. 4.32c)

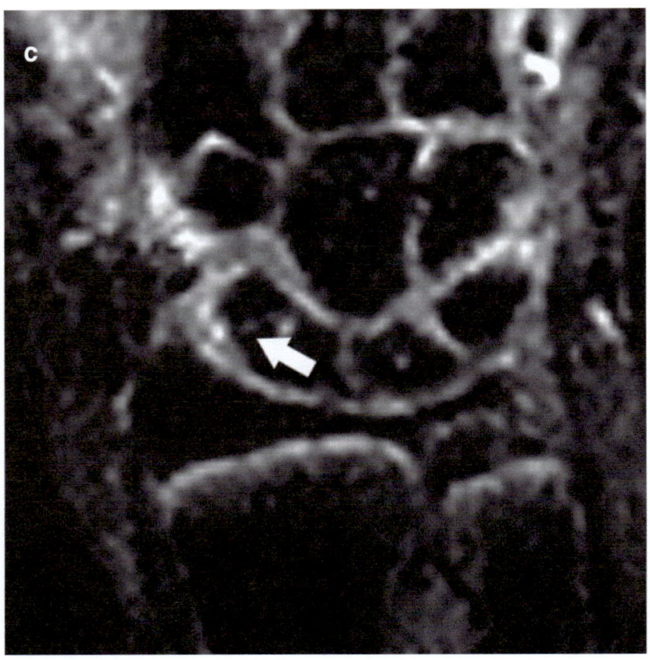

Fig. 4.32 T2WI coronal image (**c**) shows a line-like high signal at the waist of scaphoid bone

8. Differentiation of incomplete waist fracture of scaphoid and non-fracture
   8.1. X-ray (Fig. 4.33a–d)

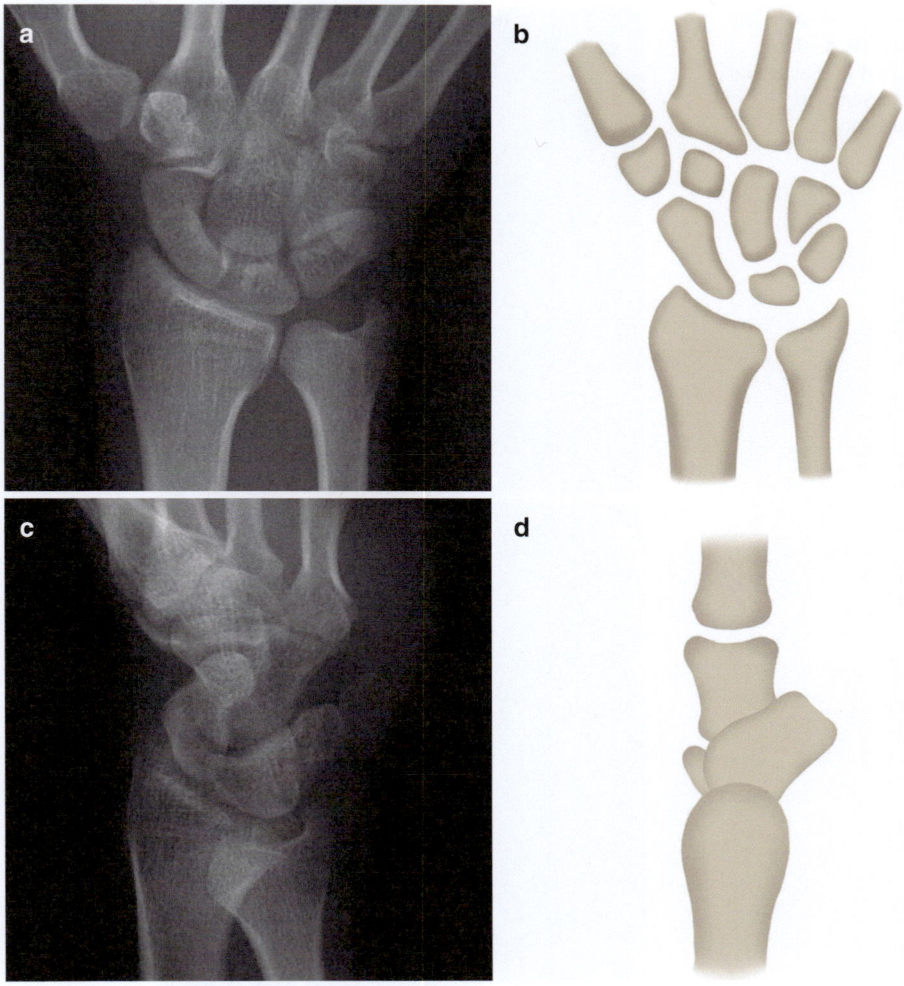

Fig. 4.33 X-rays (**a**, **c**) and illustrations (**b**, **d**) show no *visible* scaphoid fracture

   8.2. CT scan (Fig. 4.33e, f)

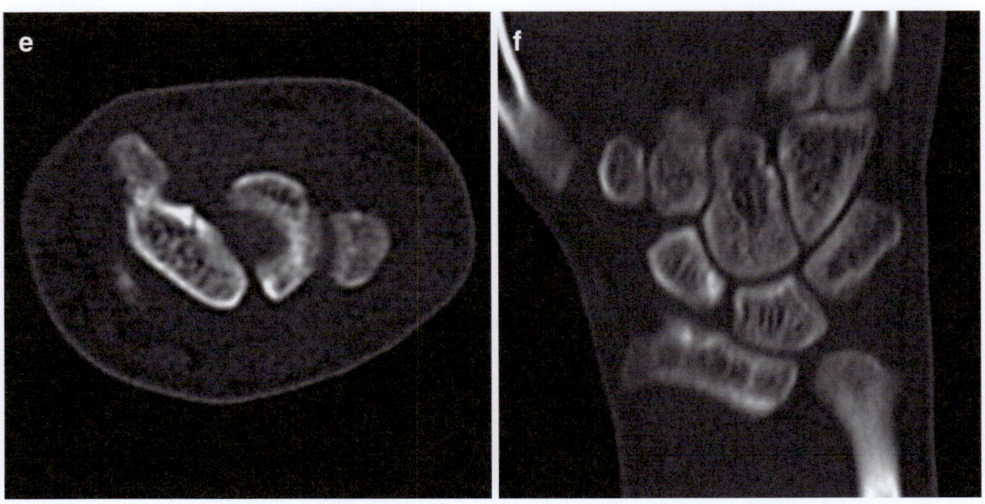

Fig. 4.33 The cross-section (**e**) and coronal plane (**f**) CT scans show anterior-superior waist fracture of scaphoid with slightly displaced fragments

9. Comparison of dynamic plain film and CT of after ischemic necrosis scaphoid waist fracture
   9.1. X-ray (Fig. 4.34a–d)

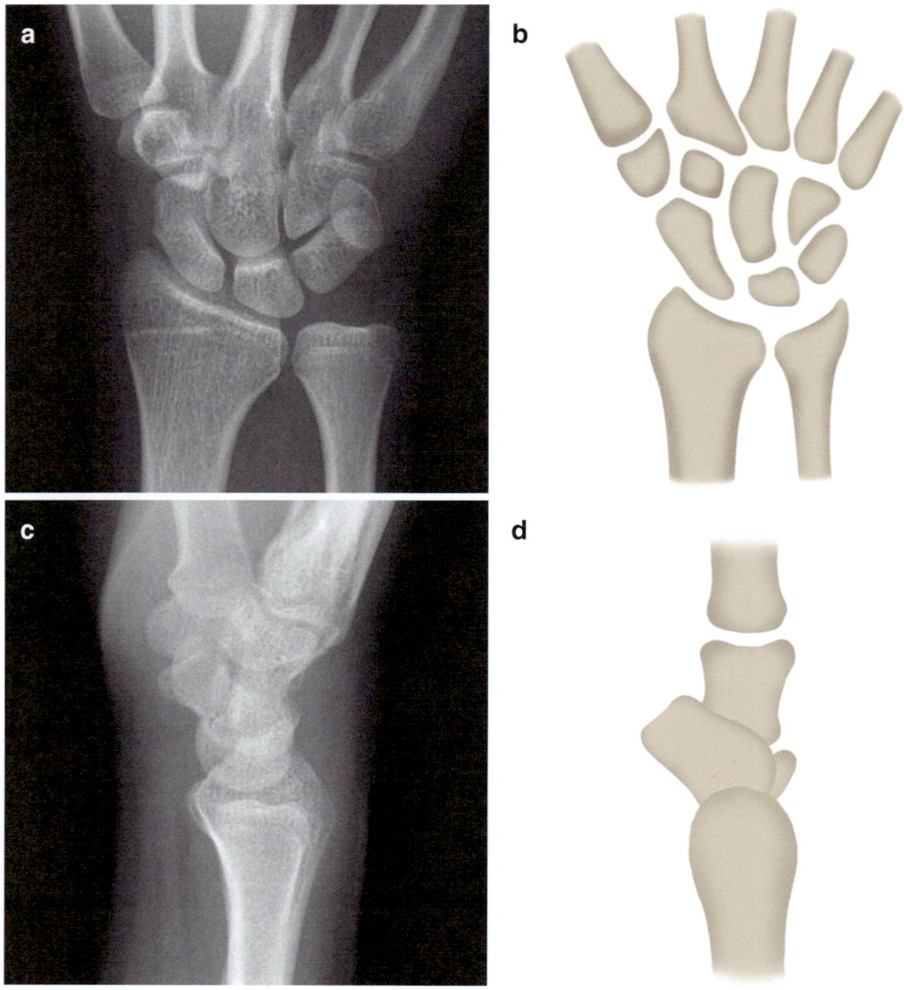

Fig. 4.34 X-rays (**a**, **c**) and illustrations (**b**, **d**) show irregular profile of scaphoid waist and disordered trabecular bone

   9.2. CT scan (Fig. 4.34e, f)

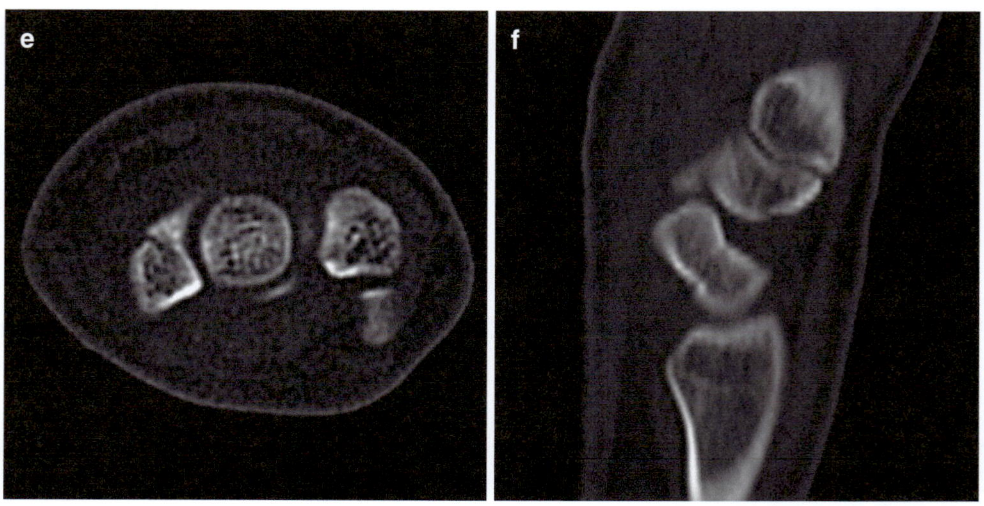

Fig. 4.34 The cross-section (**e**) and sagittal plane (**f**) CT scans show scaphoid waist fracture, which is slightly displaced. Patient should be re-examined in 3 months after initial examination

9.3. X-ray (Fig. 4.34g, h)

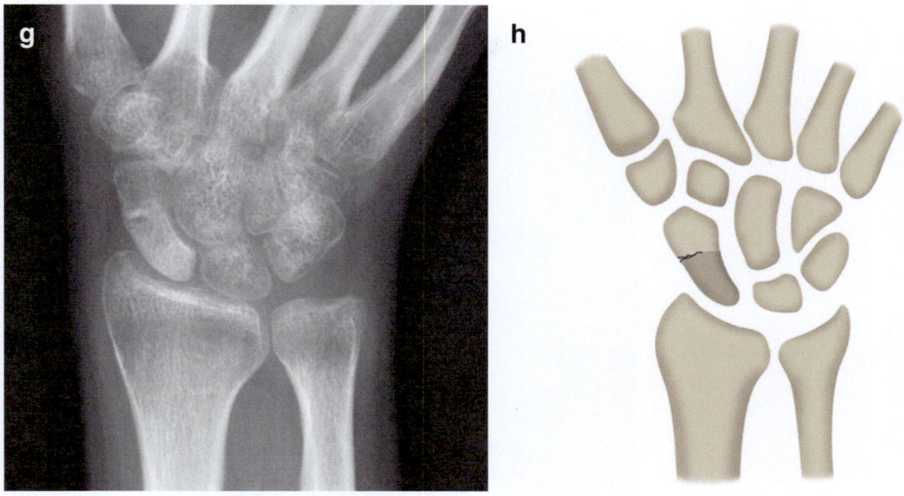

Fig. 4.34 The X-rays (**g**) and illustrations (**h**), taken at 3 months after injury, show sclerosis and increased density on proximal scaphoid

9.4. CT scan (Fig. 4.34i–k)

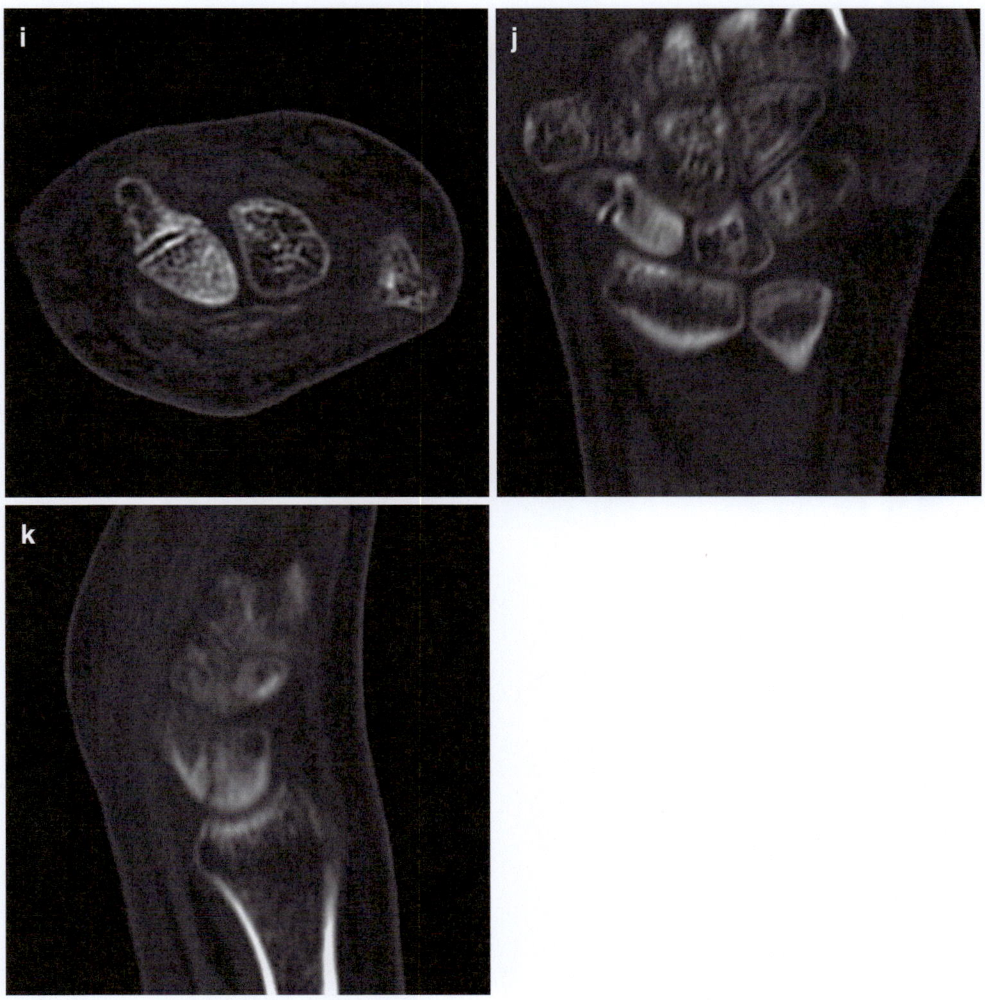

Fig. 4.34 The cross-section (**i**), coronal CT plane (**j**), and sagittal CT plane images (**k**) show clear fracture line, sclerosis, and increased bone density of the proximal scaphoid

10. Differentiation of occult hamate fracture and non-fracture
    10.1. X-ray (Fig. 4.35a, b)

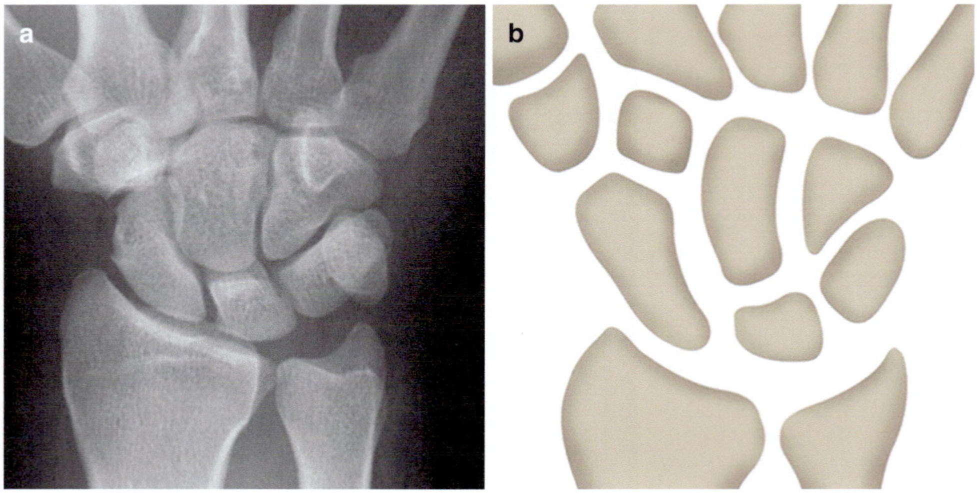

Fig. 4.35 X-rays (**a**) and illustrations (**b**) show no definite fracture sign of hamate bone

    10.2. MR imaging (Fig. 4.35c, d)

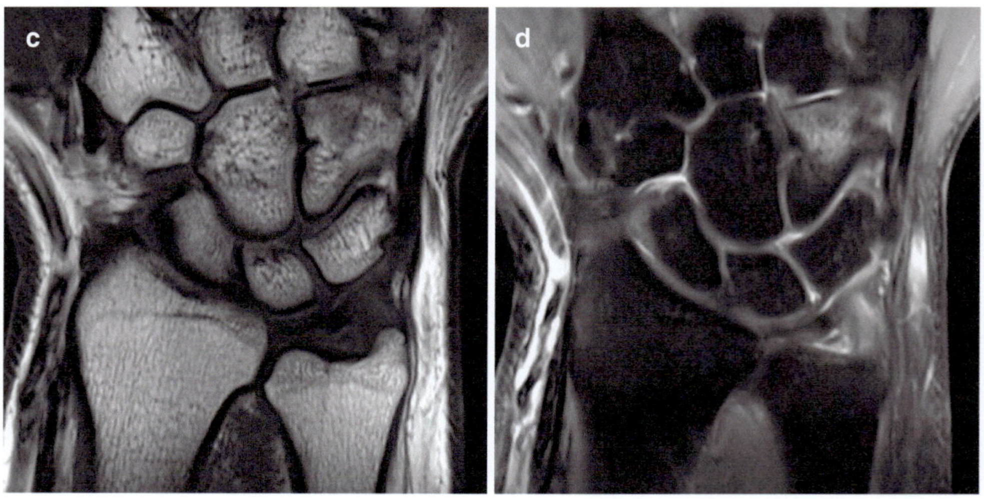

Fig. 4.35 The coronal T1WI (**c**) and coronal T2WI images (**d**) show a line-like oblique low signal on hamate bone with adjacent edematous area having long *T1 and* long *T2* signal

11. Differentiation of comminuted hamate fracture and non-fracture
    11.1. X-ray (Fig. 4.36a–d)

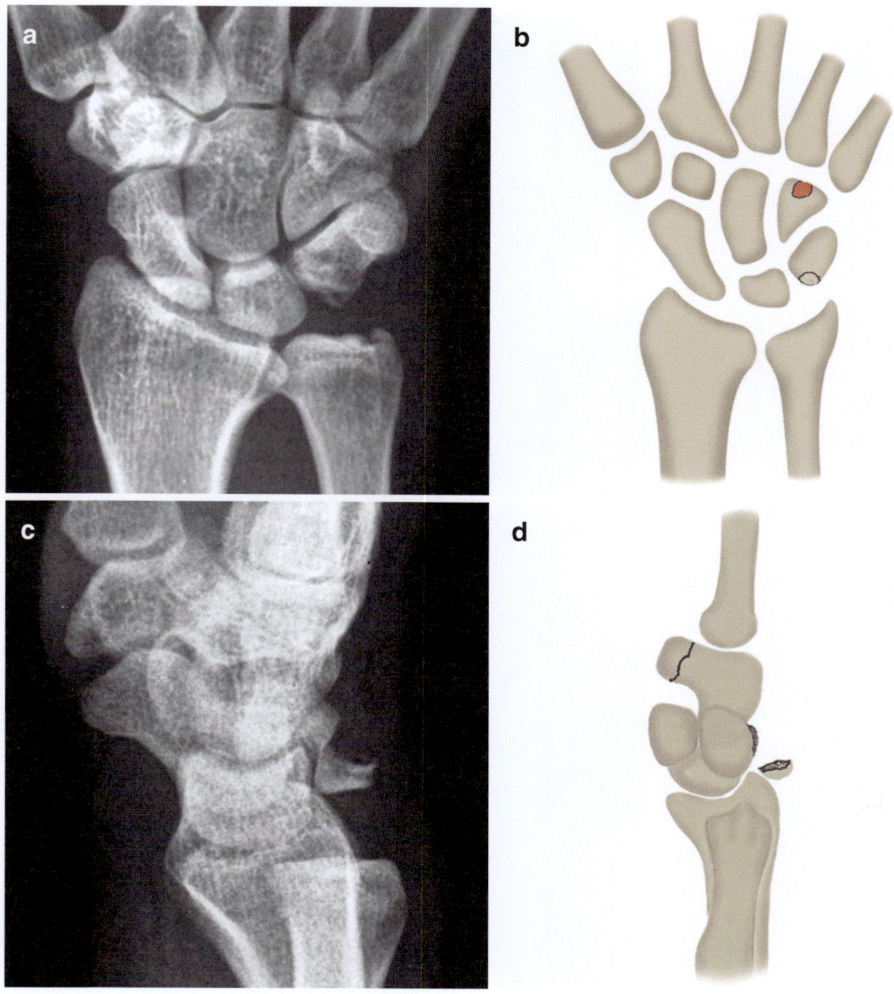

Fig. 4.36 X-rays (**a**, **c**) and illustrations (**b**, **d**) show triquetral fracture, broken ends moving dorsally, without definite sign of hamate fracture

    11.2. CT scan (Fig. 4.36e, f)

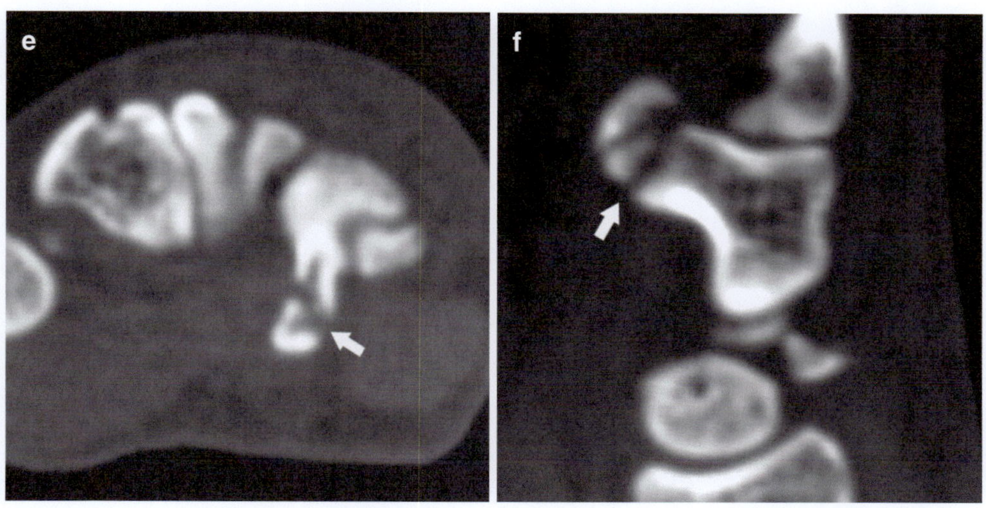

Fig. 4.36 The cross-section (**e**) and coronal CT plane (**f**) images show triquetral fracture, with multi-fragments, and with slightly displaced broken ends

12. Differentiation of hamate hook fracture and non-fracture
    12.1. X-ray (Fig. 4.37a–d)

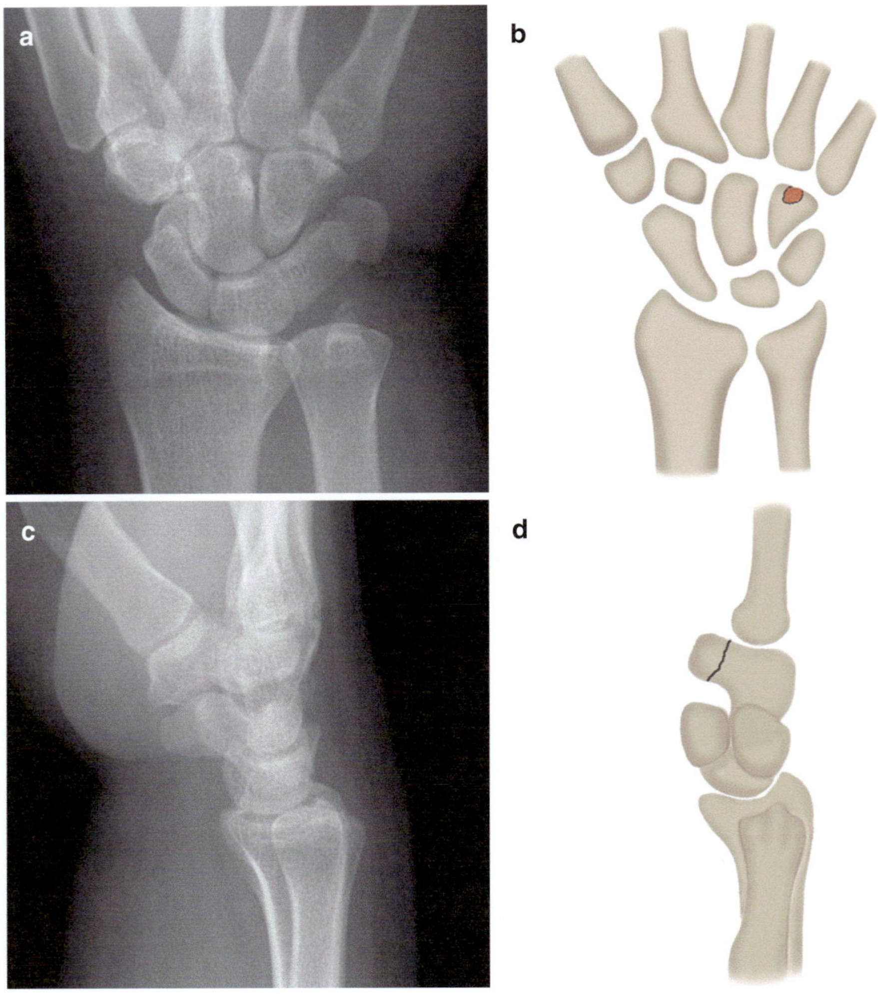

Fig. 4.37 X-rays (**a**, **c**) and illustrations (**b**, **d**) show no definite sign of hamate fracture

    12.2. CT scan (Fig. 4.37e, f)

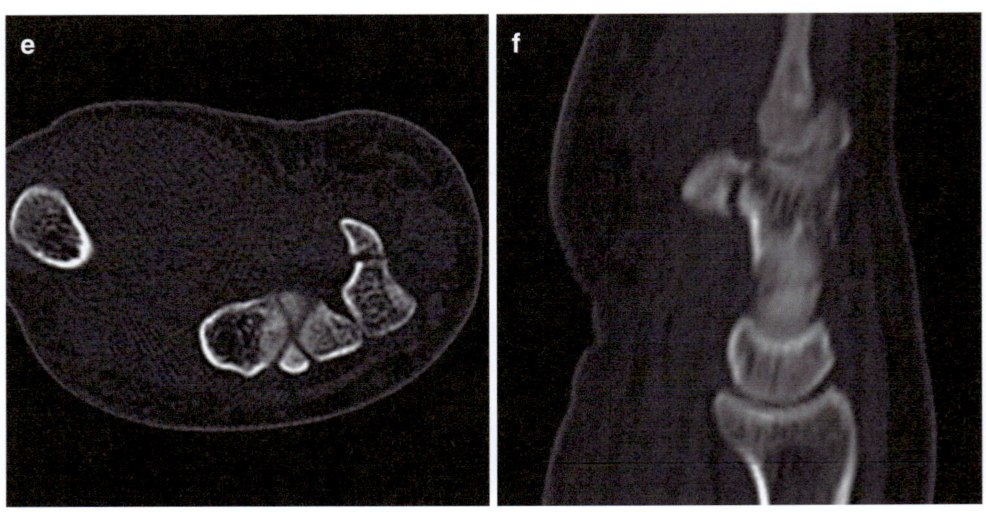

Fig. 4.37 The cross-section (**e**) and sagittal CT plane (**f**) images show hamate hook fracture with slightly displaced broken ends

13. Differentiation of comminuted triquetral fracture and simple fracture
    13.1. X-ray (Fig. 4.38a–d)

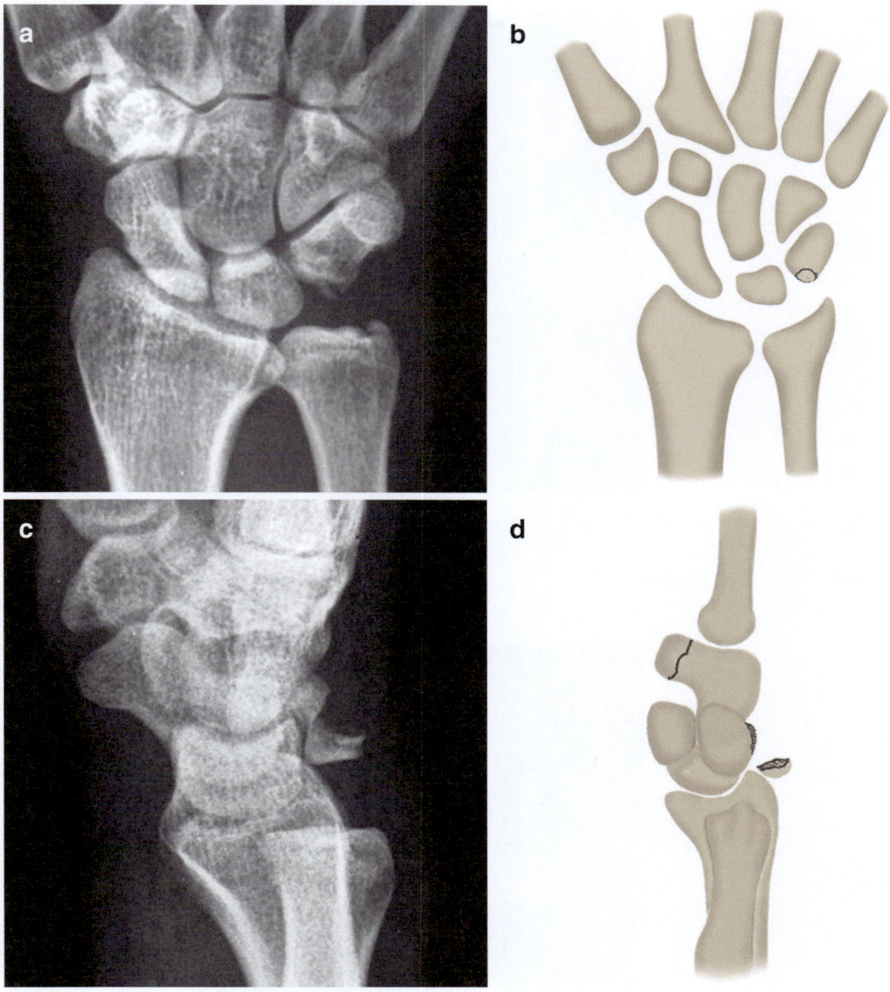

Fig. 4.38 X-rays (**a**, **c**) and illustrations (**b**, **d**) show fracture of triquetral, with dorsally displaced fragments

    13.2. CT scan (Fig. 4.38e, f)

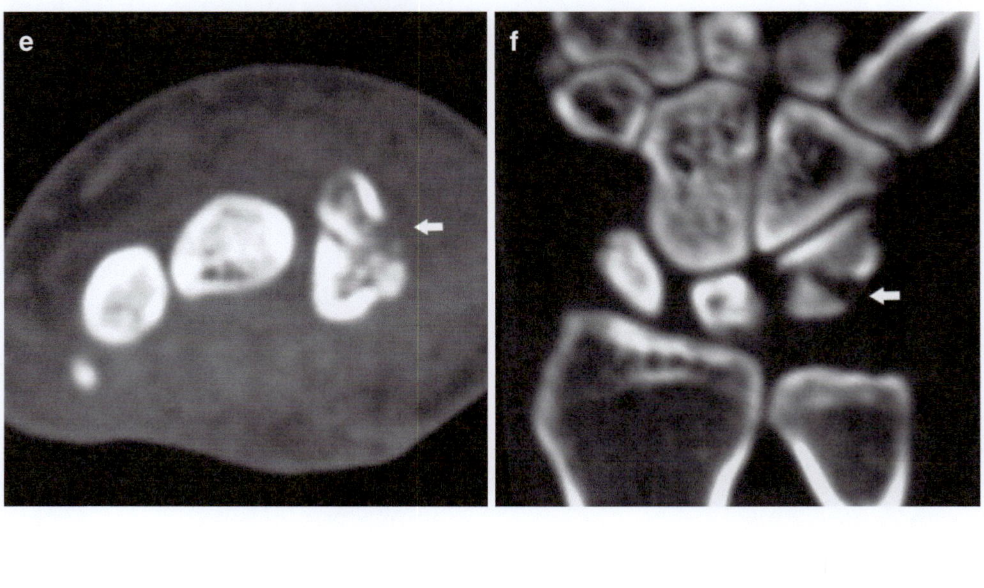

Fig. 4.38 The cross-section (**e**) and coronal CT plane (**f**) images show displaced fracture of triquetral with tiny fragments around

14. Differentiation of triquetral fracture and suspected fracture
    14.1. X-ray (Fig. 4.39a, b)

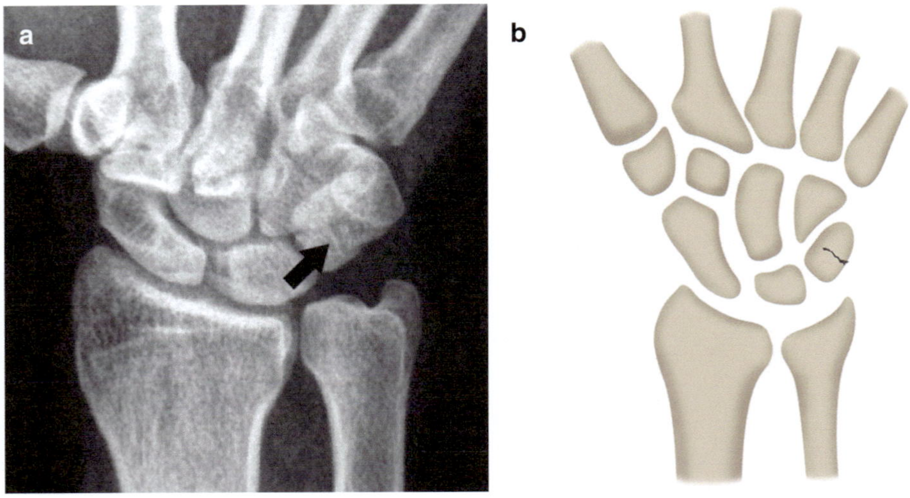

Fig. 4.39 X-rays (**a**) and illustrations (**b**) images show line-like low density shadow on triquetral bone with slightly displaced fragments

    14.2. MR scan (Fig. 4.39c)

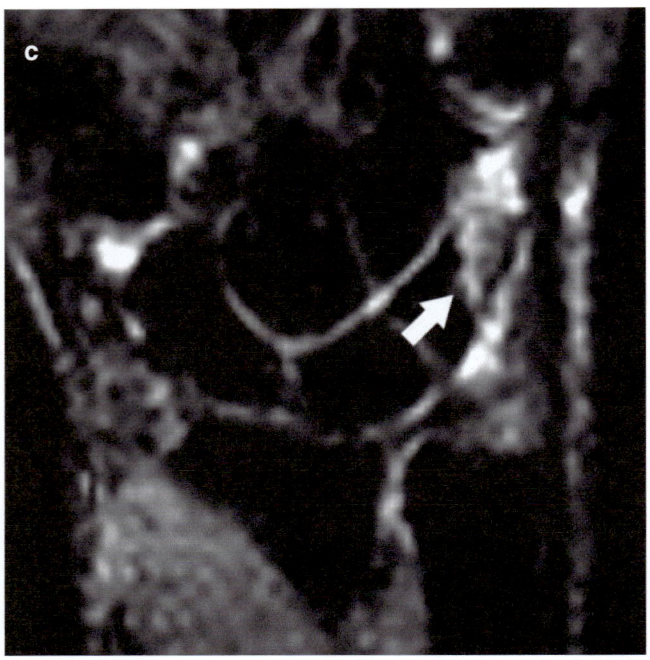

Fig. 4.39 The coronal T2WI (**c**) shows fracture of triquetral bone, fracture line, and adjacent area edema in high signal

15. Differentiation of triquetral fracture, pisiform fracture, and suspected fracture
    15.1. X-ray (Fig. 4.40a–d)

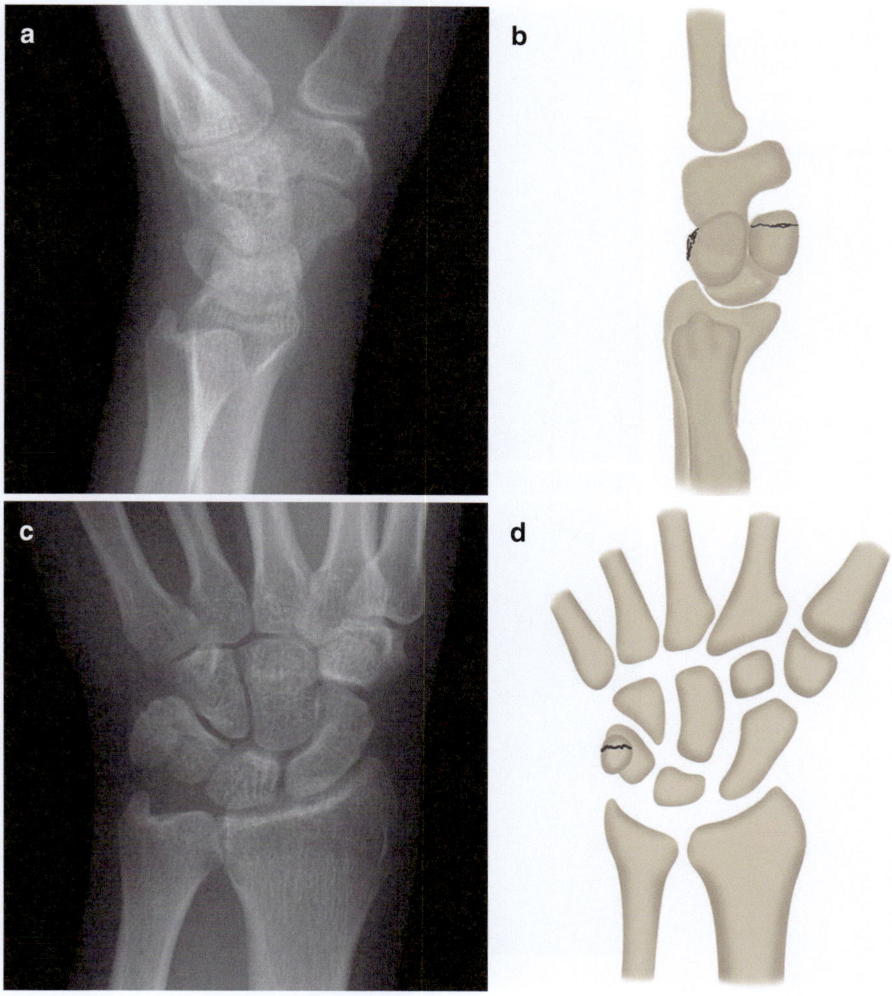

Fig. 4.40 X-rays (**a**, **c**) and illustrations (**b**, **d**) images show irregular profile of triquetral and pisiform

15.2. CT scan (Fig. 4.40e–h)

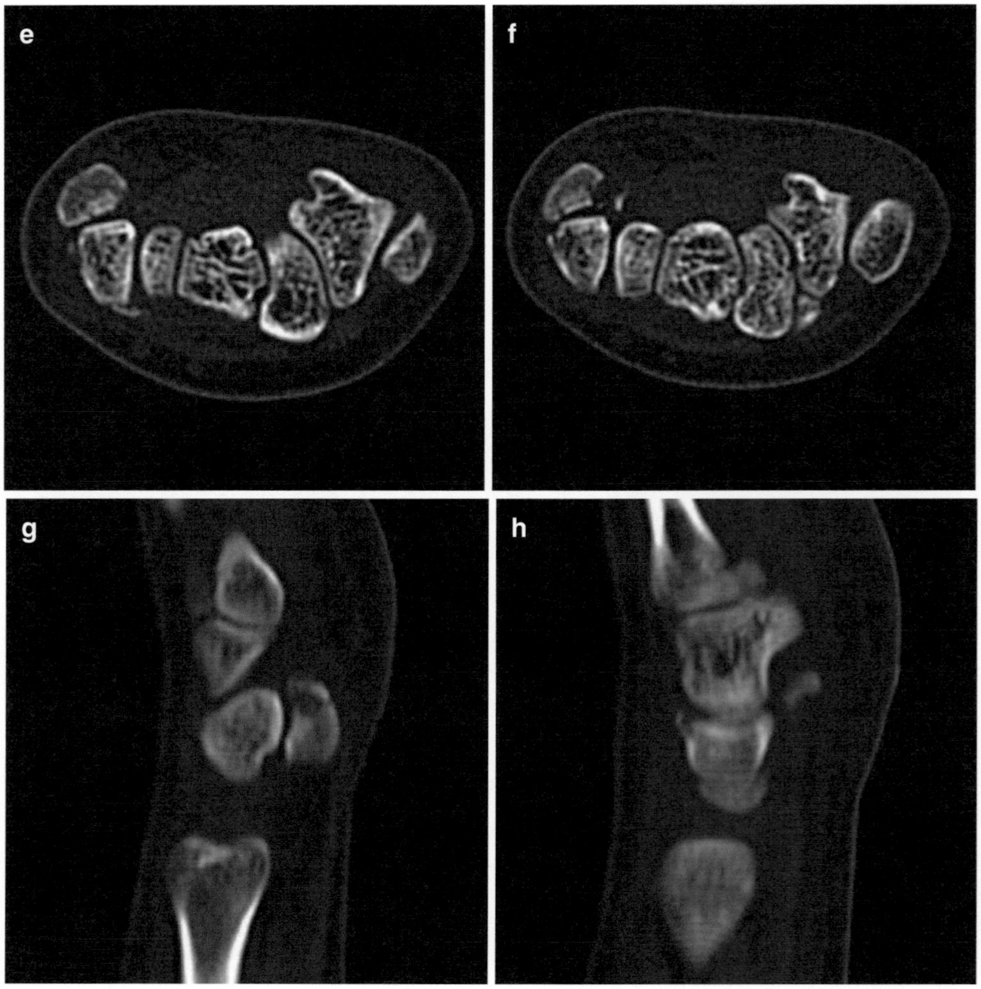

Fig. 4.40 The cross-section (**e**, **f**) and coronal CT plane (**g**, **h**) scan show displaced dorsal fracture of triquetral with visible fragment shadow. Pisiform fracture and the radial fragment displaced distinctively

16. Differentiation of comminuted trapezium fracture and simple fracture
    16.1. X-ray (Fig. 4.41a–d)

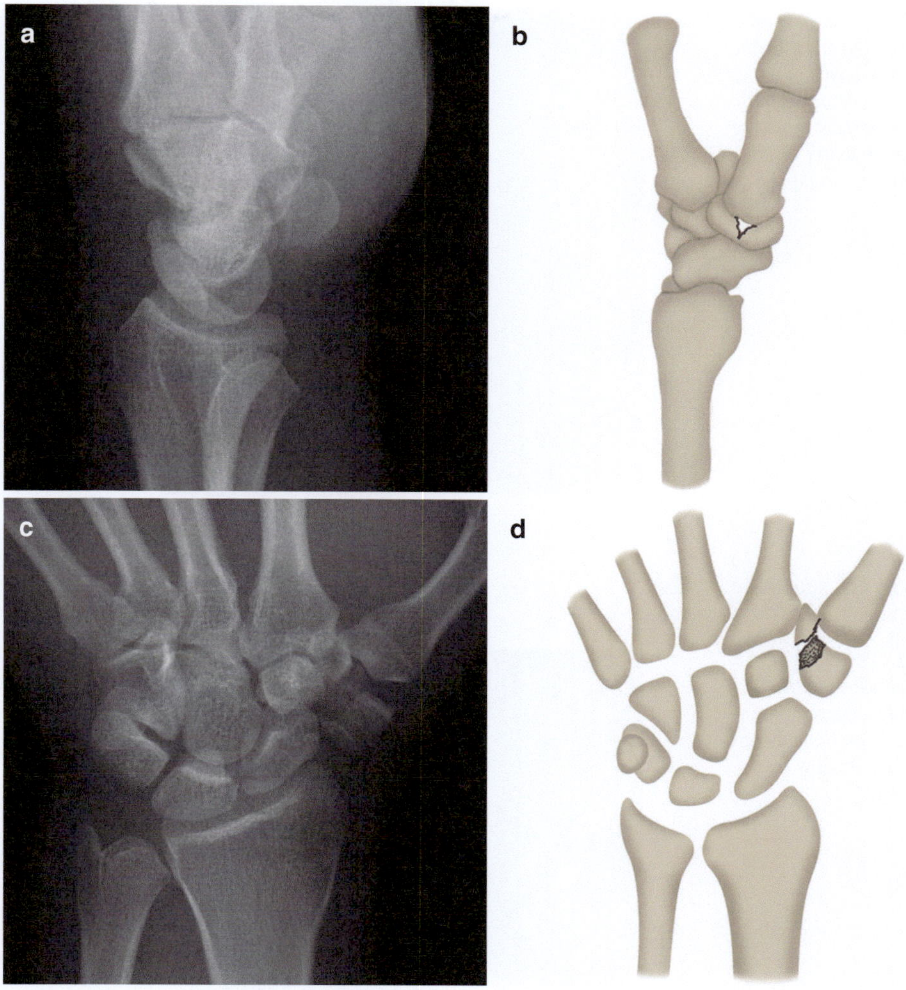

Fig. 4.41 X-rays (**a**, **c**) and illustrations (**b**, **d**) show fracture of trapezium with broken ends being displaced distinctively

    16.2. CT scan (Fig. 4.41e, f)

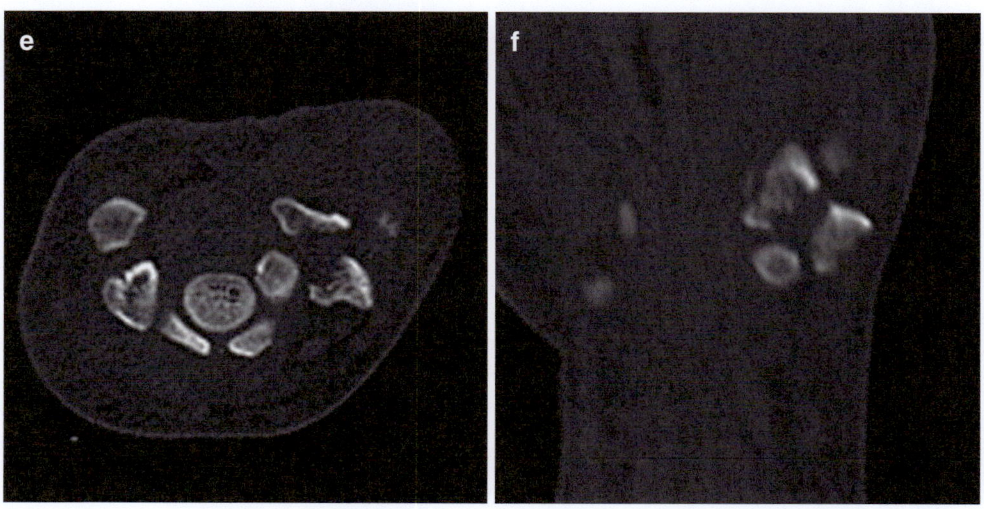

Fig. 4.41 The cross-section (**e**) and coronal CT plane (**f**) scan show fracture of trapezium, with multi-fragments. The broken ends displaced distinctively

17. Differentiation of trapezium fracture, trapezoid fracture, and non-fracture
    17.1. X-ray (Fig. 4.42a, b)

Fig. 4.42 X-rays (**a**) and illustrations (**b**) show distal scaphoid fracture and no definite signs of trapezoid fracture. The local structure displayed unclearly as the plaster image overlapped

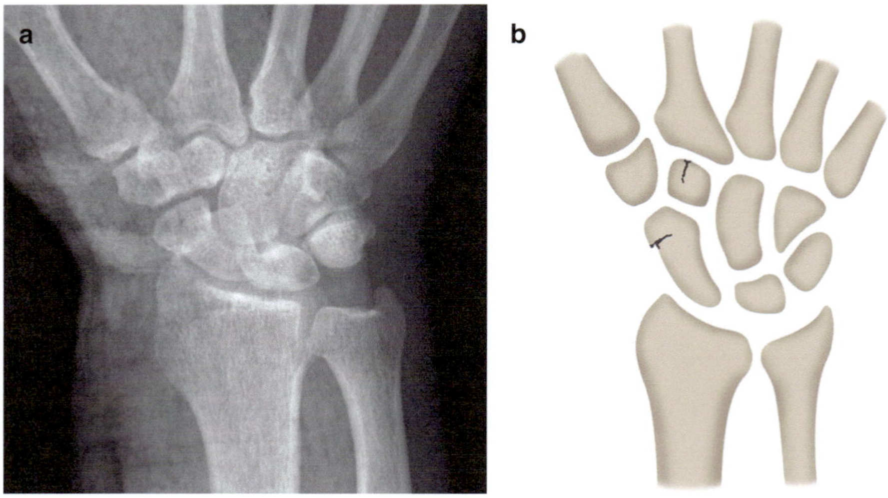

17.2. CT scan (Fig. 4.42c, d)

Fig. 4.42 The cross-section (**c**, **d**) scan shows distal scaphoid fracture and trapezoid fracture, and the Micro-osteo shadow on fracture site

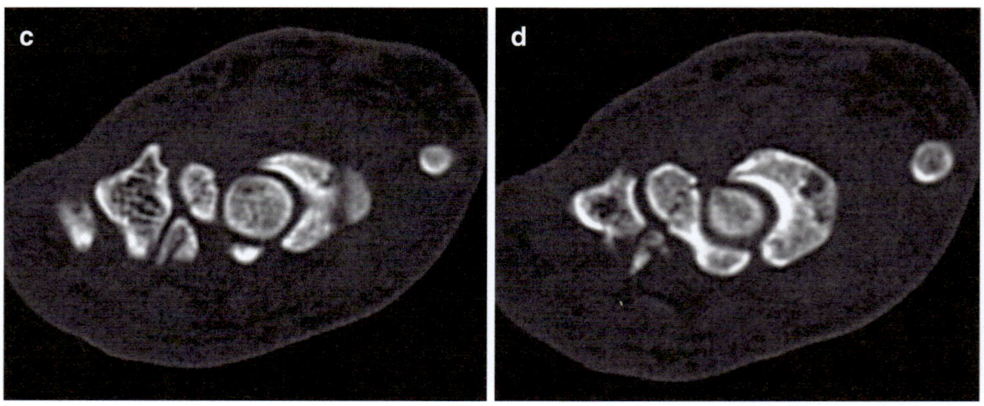

18. Differentiation of comminuted trapezium fracture, trapezoid fracture, and other fracture
    18.1. X-ray (Fig. 4.43a–d)

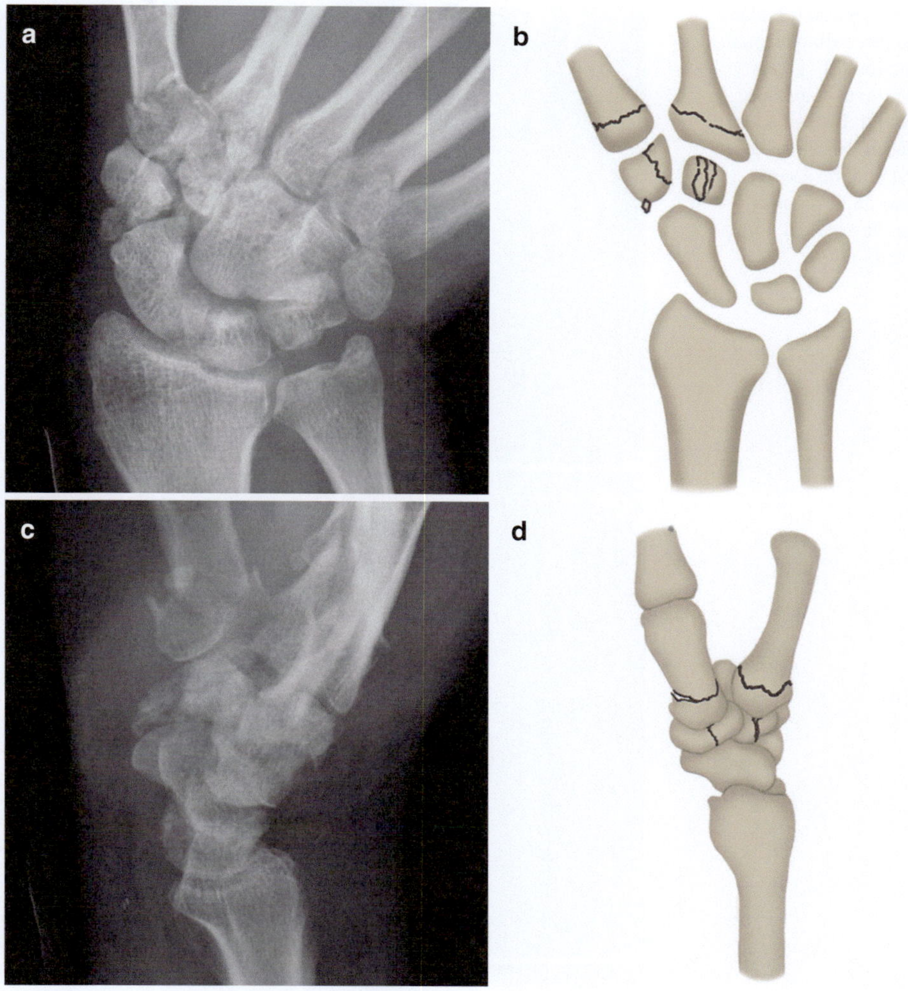

Fig. 4.43 X-rays (**a**, **c**) and illustrations (**b**, **d**) show fracture of trapezium, trapezoid, and the basal part of the first and the second metacarpus. Bone structure is disordered

18.2. CT scan (Fig. 4.43e–j)

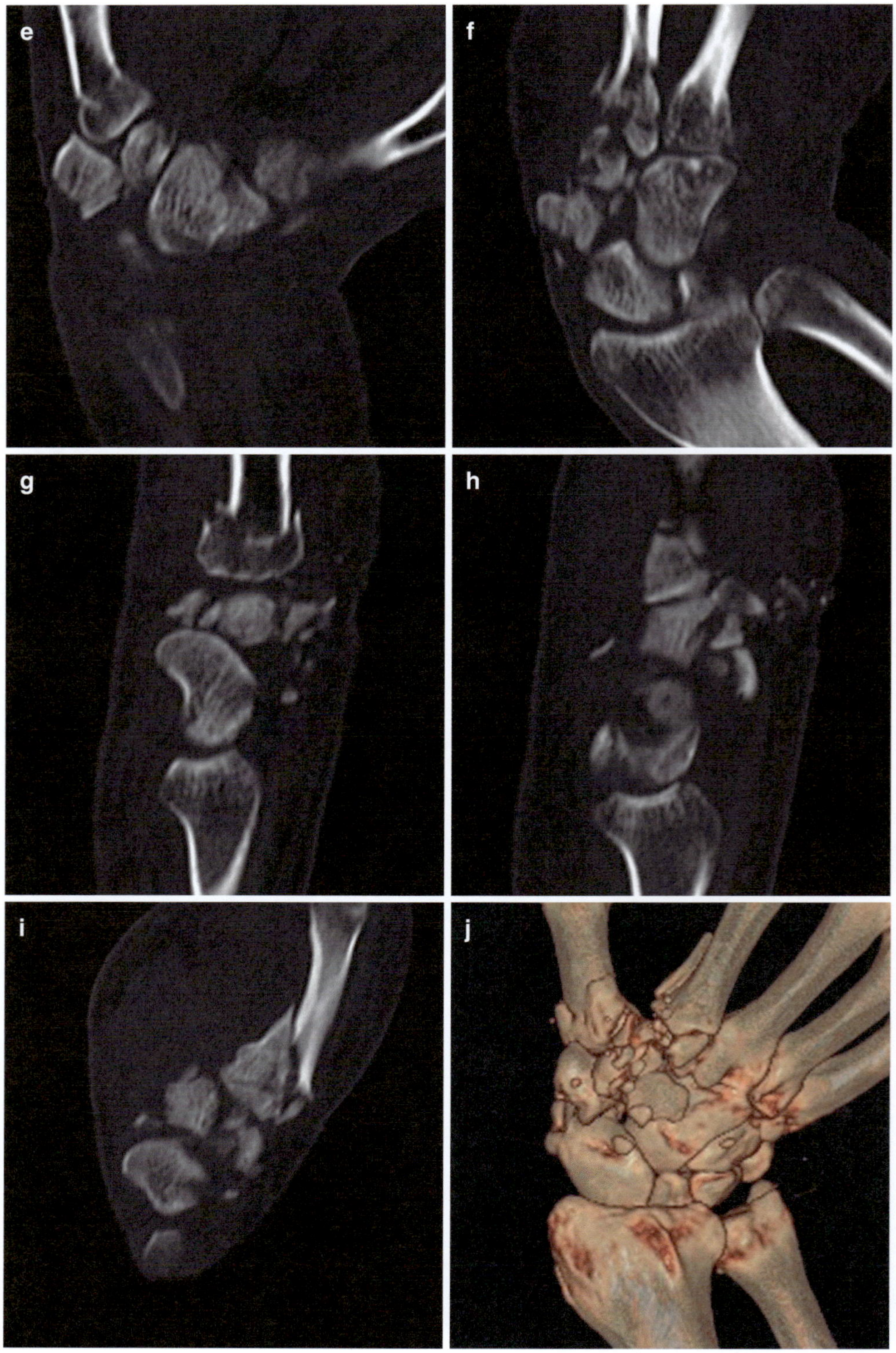

Fig. 4.43 The coronal CT plane (**e**, **f**), sagittal CT plane (**g**–**i**), and three-dimensional reconstruction CT (**j**) scans show fracture of trapezium and trapezoid. Broken ends are displaced. Basal fracture of the first and the second metacarpus and irregular defects in the articular cortex are detected

4.3 Summary

The wrist is made up of eight small carpal bones, which connects with the radius and ulna. There are three joints in this area: radiocarpal joint, intercarpal joint, and the carpometacarpal joint. Distal radius fracture, also known as wrist fracture, typically occurs in the elderly, while most of scaphoid fractures are present in younger patients.

Standard X-ray has its limitation in depicting fragment shape and type of fracture of adjacent joints. So additional CT scan, multi-plane and three-dimensional reconstructions are needed.

There are many bones in the region of the wrist, all within proximity of one another, and in some case overlapped. Therefore, the diagnosis of such fractures using an X-ray film is sometimes deemed difficult, resulting in misdiagnosis or missing diagnosis. CT can eliminate the influence of bone overlap, and depict the carpal bones and the origin of fragment more accurately. MR scan is essential for the diagnosis of peripheral tendon and soft tissue injury, especially in epiphyseal injury in children and inter-carpal ligament injuries.

5 Hand Fracture

Bing Zhang and Yingze Zhang

5.1 Metacarpal Fracture

Each metacarpus consists of three parts: a body, head, and base. The base articulates with the carpus and with the adjoining metacarpal bones. The body is curved in the form of a prismoid; thus convex in the longitudinal direction posteriorly. There is a tubercle on either side of the head for the attachment of the collateral ligaments of the metacarpophalangeal joint. Based on the OTA classification, metacarpal fractures are classified as the following: metacarpal proximal (16.73% of all metacarpal fractures) and distal (15.93% of all metacarpal fractures) extra-articular fracture, diaphysis non-comminuted fracture (43.33% of all metacarpal fractures), metacarpal proximal (8.24% of all metacarpal fractures), distal (2.48% of all metacarpal fractures), partial articular fracture and diaphysis wedge comminuted fracture (6.12% of all metacarpal fractures), metacarpal proximal (2.78% of all metacarpal fractures) and distal (1.42% of all metacarpal fractures), complete articular fracture and diaphysis comminuted fracture (2.78% of all metacarpal fractures).

5.1.1 Injury Mechanism

Metacarpal fractures are mostly caused by a straightforward force when the hand is held in a fist position. Injury to the metacarpal diaphysis occurs when an axial or torsional force is transmitted through a partially flexed thumb metacarpal, and the basilar fracture of the metacarpals is often after an axial force attack.

5.1.2 Signs and Symptoms

Pain, swelling, and loss of motion are the main manifestations of any fracture. Yet clinically, many non-displaced or slightly displaced fractures do not exhibit the above physical signs, therefore they are easily misdiagnosed. Doctors are therefore encouraged to carry out a comprehensive physical examination when presented with patients suffering injuries in this area. Nonetheless, once suspected, an X-ray or CT scan needs to be ordered.

5.1.3 Imaging Differential Diagnosis

CT scans should be ordered if there are uncertainties in an X-ray outcome, but normally a standard X-ray of the hand can well define the nature of the displaced fracture, as well as the degree of the displacement.

B. Zhang · Y. Zhang (✉)
Department of Orthopaedics, The Third Hospital of Hebei Medical University, Shijiazhuang, Hebei, China

Y. Zhang (ed.), *Differential Diagnosis of Fracture*, https://doi.org/10.1007/978-981-13-8339-7_5

1. Differentiation of Winterstein and Rolando fracture
   1.1 X-ray (Fig. 5.1a–d)

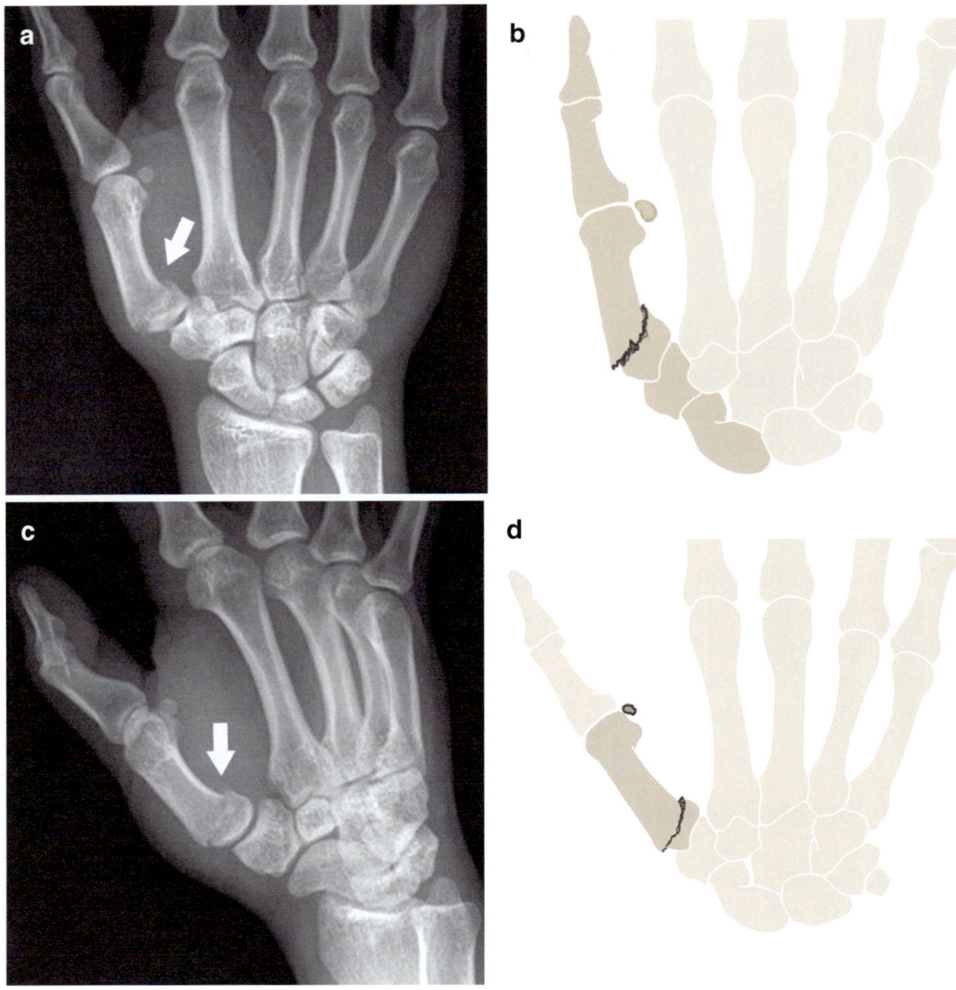

Fig. 5.1 X-ray (**a**, **c**) and illustration (**b**, **d**) show a transverse basilar part fracture of the first metacarpal, the distal end slightly moved to the radial side, and the articular surface was not affected

1.2 CT scan (Fig. 5.1e–h)

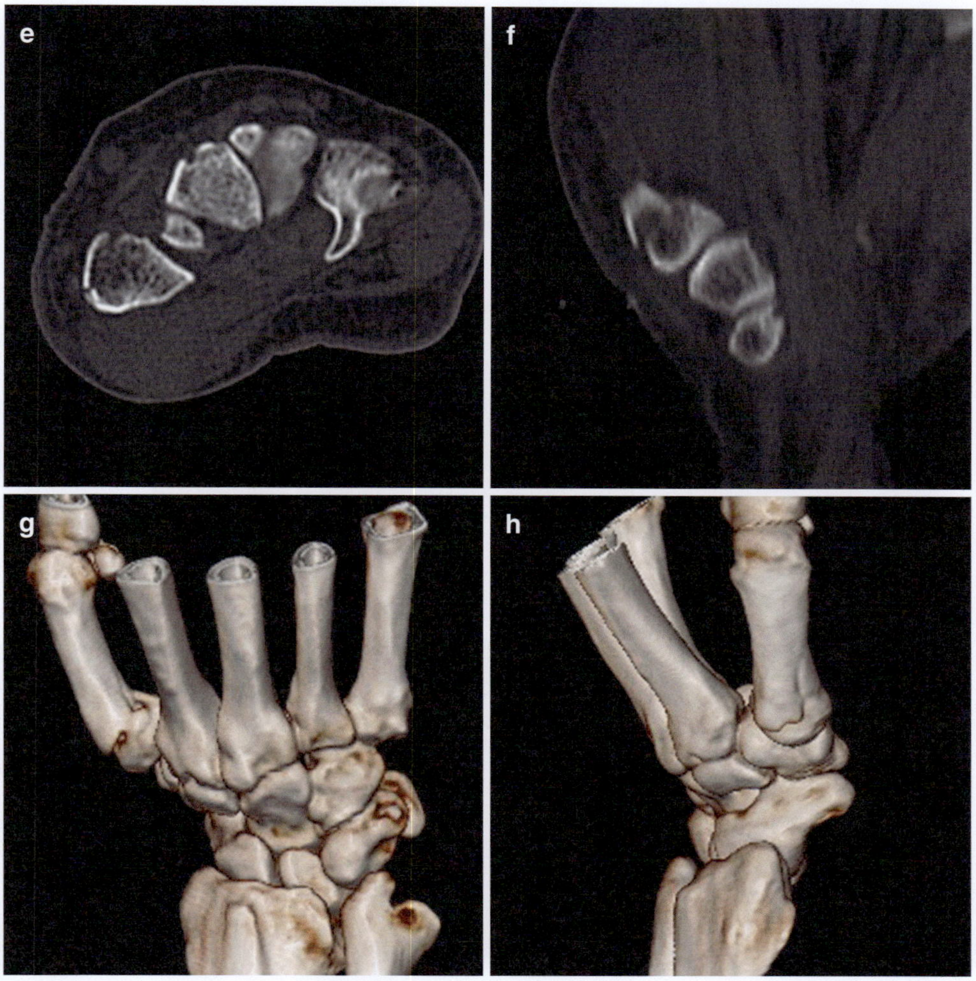

Fig. 5.1 The cross-section (**e**), coronal CT plane (**f**), and three-dimensional reconstruction (**g**, **h**) show transverse basilar part fracture of metaphysis, slight angular deformity, the distal end slightly moved to the radial side, and the articular surface was not affected

2. Differentiation of Winterstein fracture and Bennett fracture
   2.1 X-ray (Fig. 5.2a, b)

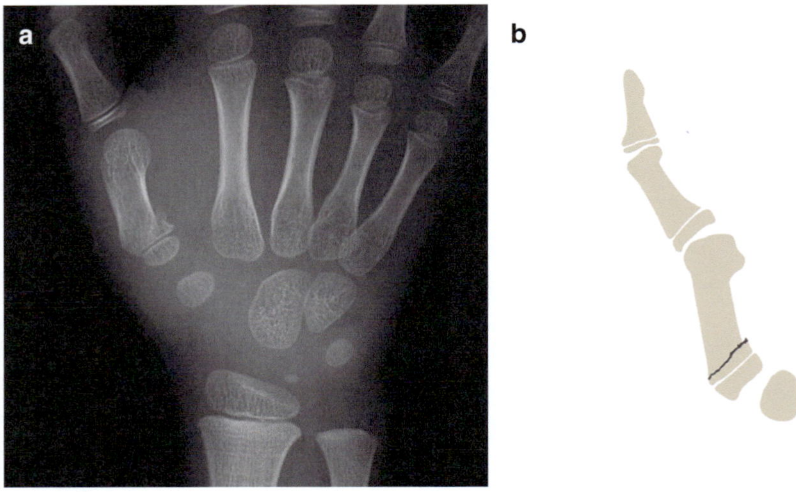

Fig. 5.2 X-ray (**a**) and illustration (**b**) show separated proximal epiphysis from metaphyseal cleavage of the first metacarpal, fracture displaced, and the articular surface was not affected

   2.2 CT scan (Fig. 5.2c–f)

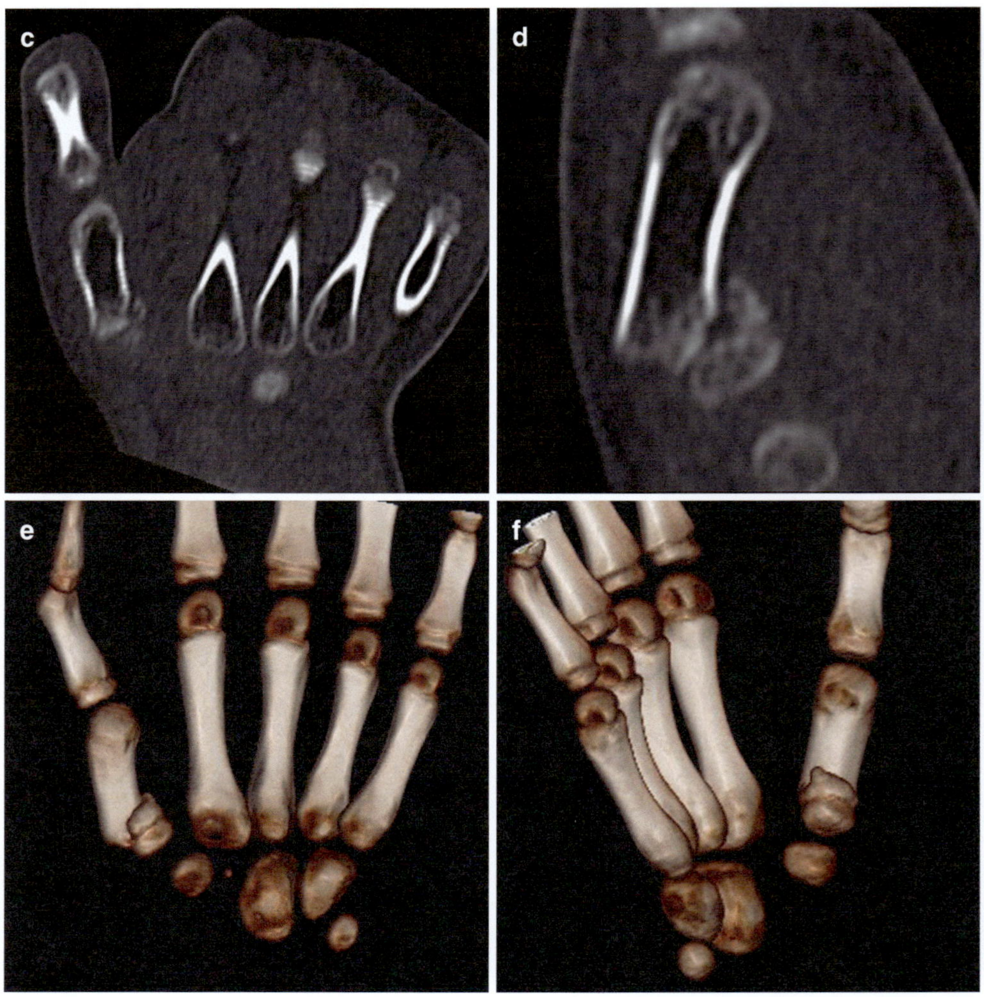

Fig. 5.2 The cross-section (**c**), coronal CT plane (**d**), and three-dimensional reconstruction (**e**, **f**) show separated proximal epiphysis from metaphyseal cleavage of the first metacarpal, distinct fracture displacement and angular deformity, articular surface was not affected

3. Differentiation of metacarpal diaphysis impacted fracture and simple fracture
   3.1 X-ray (Fig. 5.3a, b)

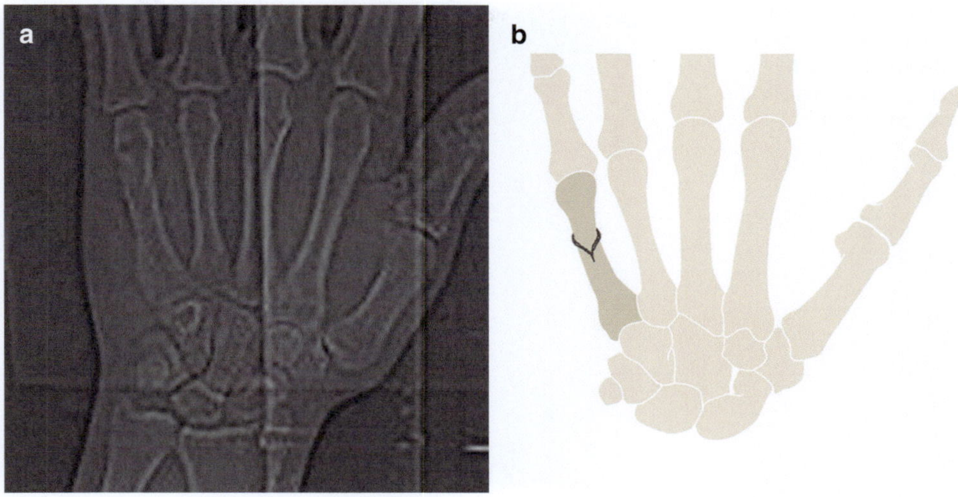

Fig. 5.3 X-ray (**a**) and illustration (**b**) show the fifth metacarpal fracture, no significant displacement and angulation

   3.2 CT scan (Fig. 5.3c–e)

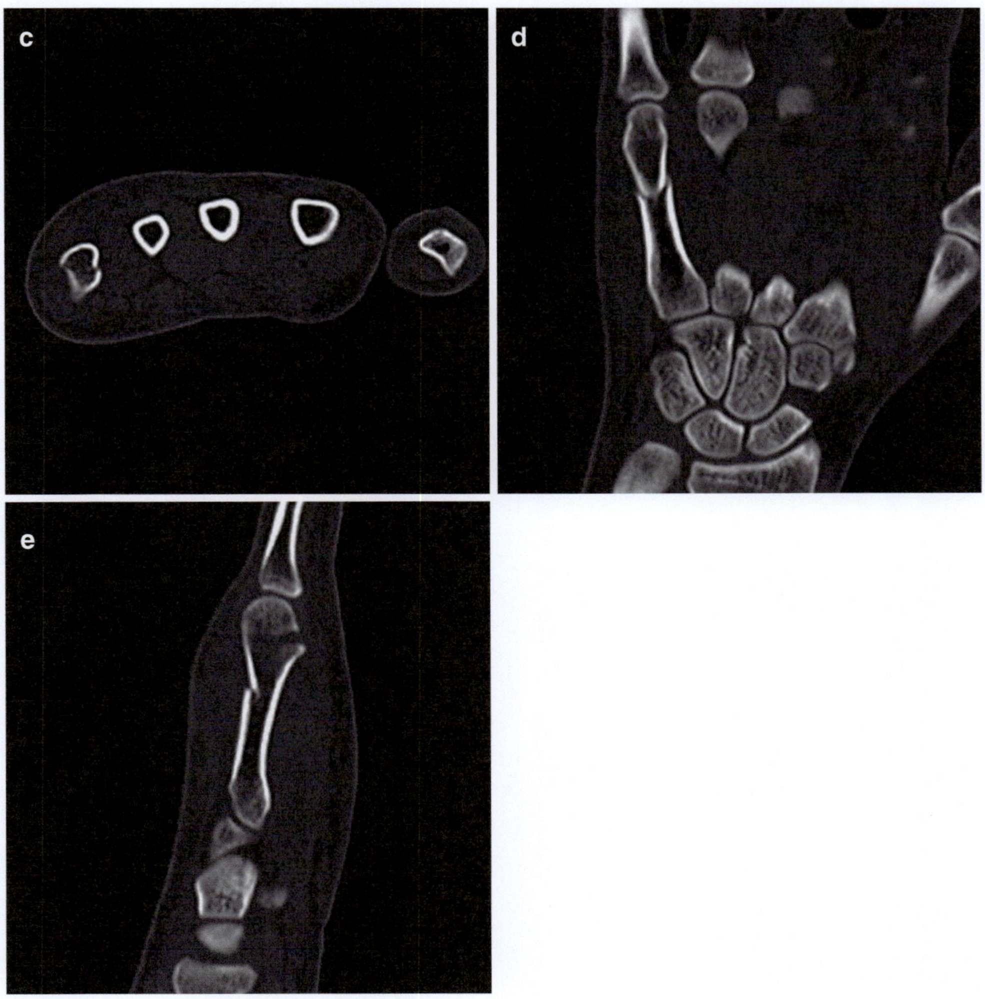

Fig. 5.3 The cross-section (**c**), coronal CT plane (**d**), and sagittal CT plane (**e**) show the fifth metacarpal fracture, broken ends were impacted and displaced

4. Differentiation of the fourth metacarpal head impacted fracture and suspected fracture
   4.1 X-ray (Fig. 5.4a, b)

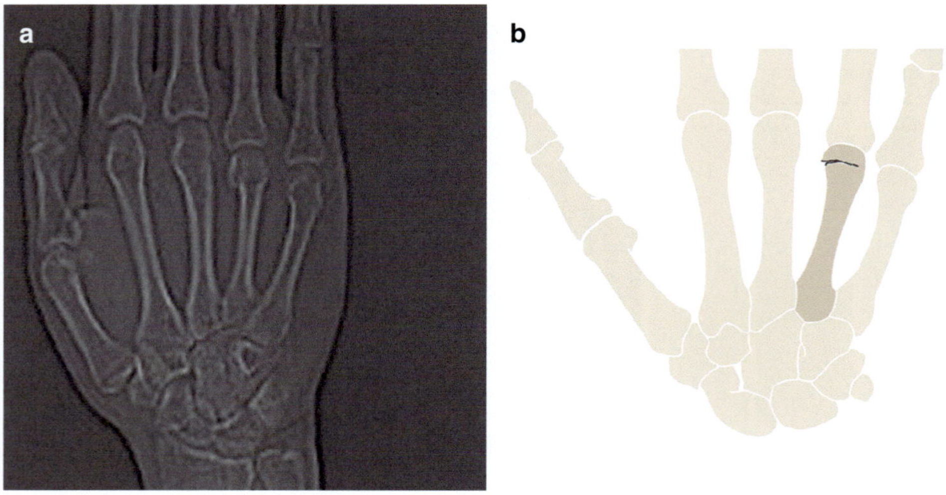

Fig. 5.4 X-ray (**a**) and illustration (**b**) show bone disorder of the fourth metaphysis and intercalation of trabecular bone

4.2 CT scan (Fig. 5.4c–g)

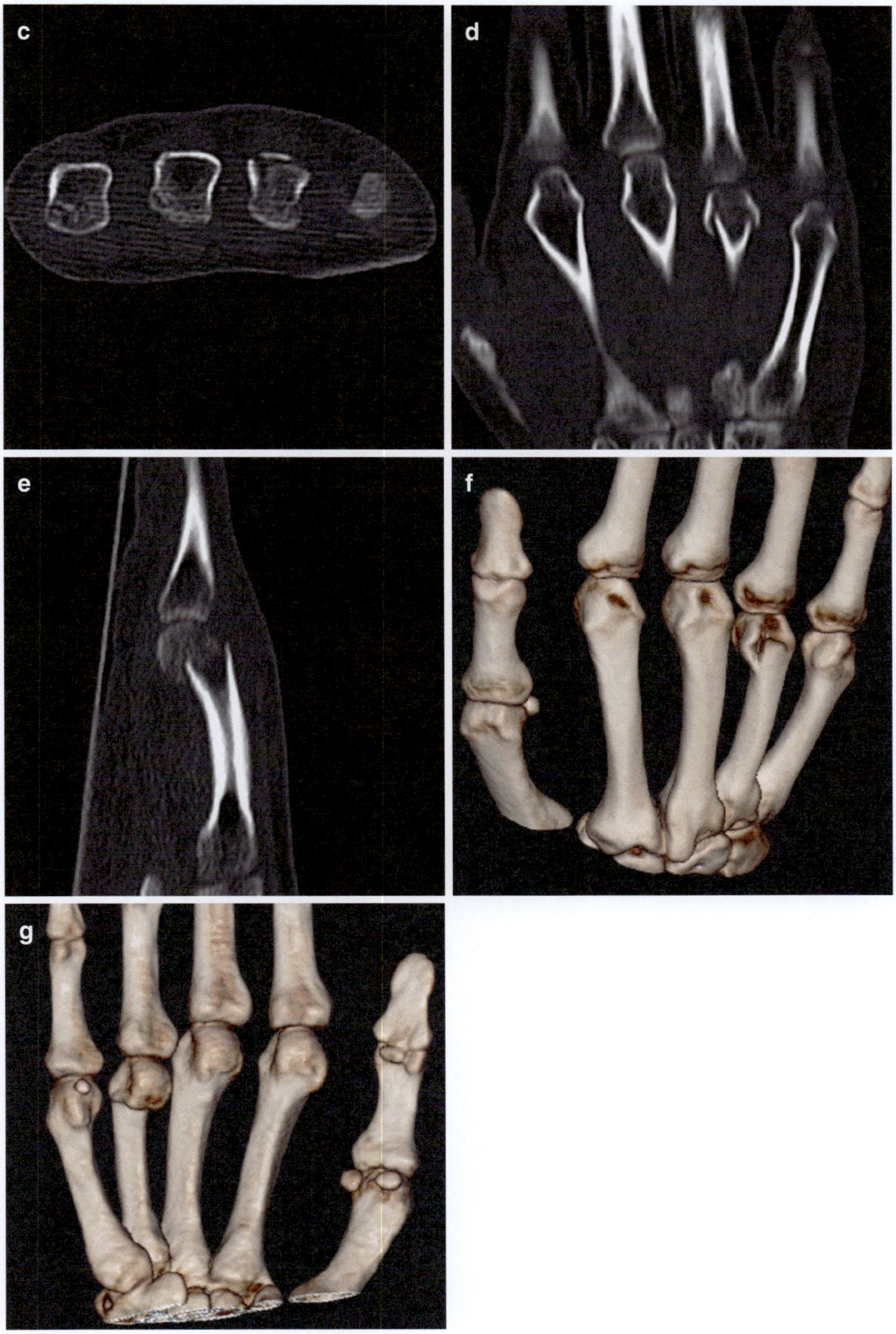

Fig. 5.4 The cross-section (**c**), coronal CT plane (**d**), sagittal CT plane (**e**), and three-dimensional reconstruction (**f**, **g**) show the fourth metacarpal fracture, the broken ends were slightly impacted and displaced

5. Differentiation of Bennett fracture and suspected fracture
   5.1 X-ray (Fig. 5.5a–d)

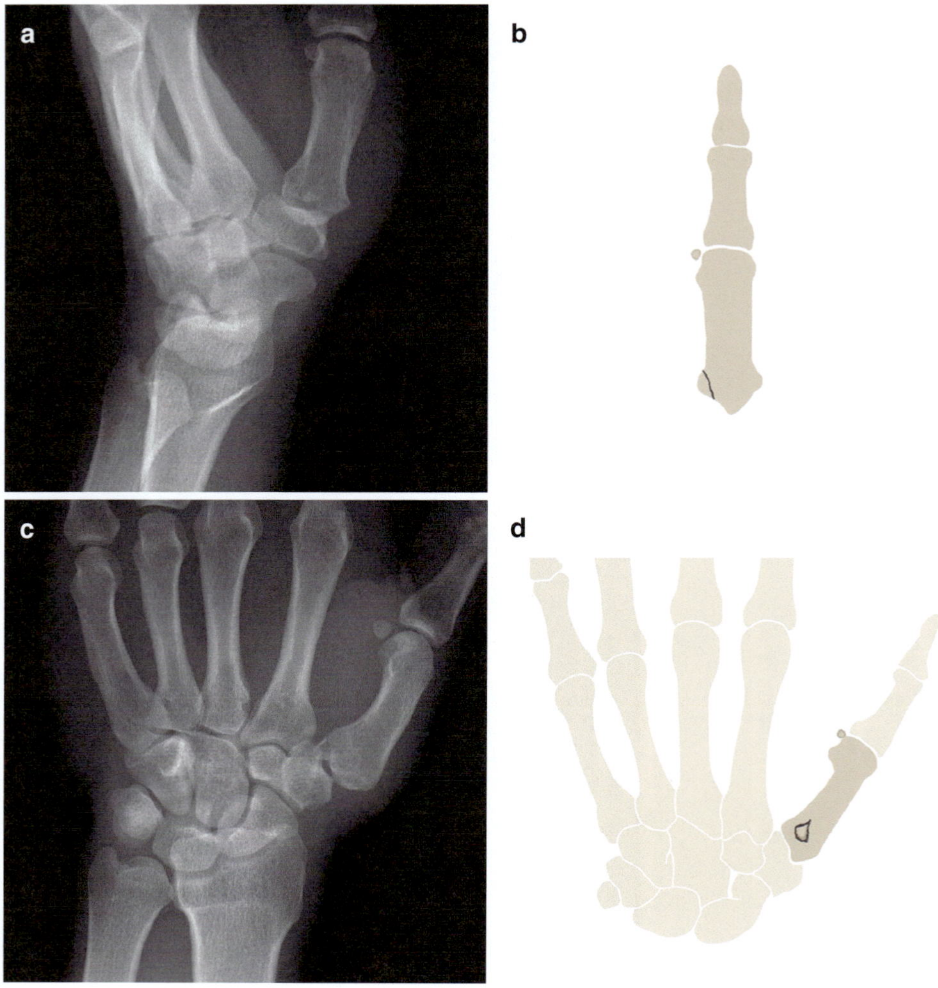

Fig. 5.5 X-ray (**a**, **c**) and illustration (**b**, **d**) show irregular ulnar margin of the basal metaphysis, a tiny fragment shadow seemingly, and the basilar part moved to the radius side

5.2 CT scan (Fig. 5.5e–h)

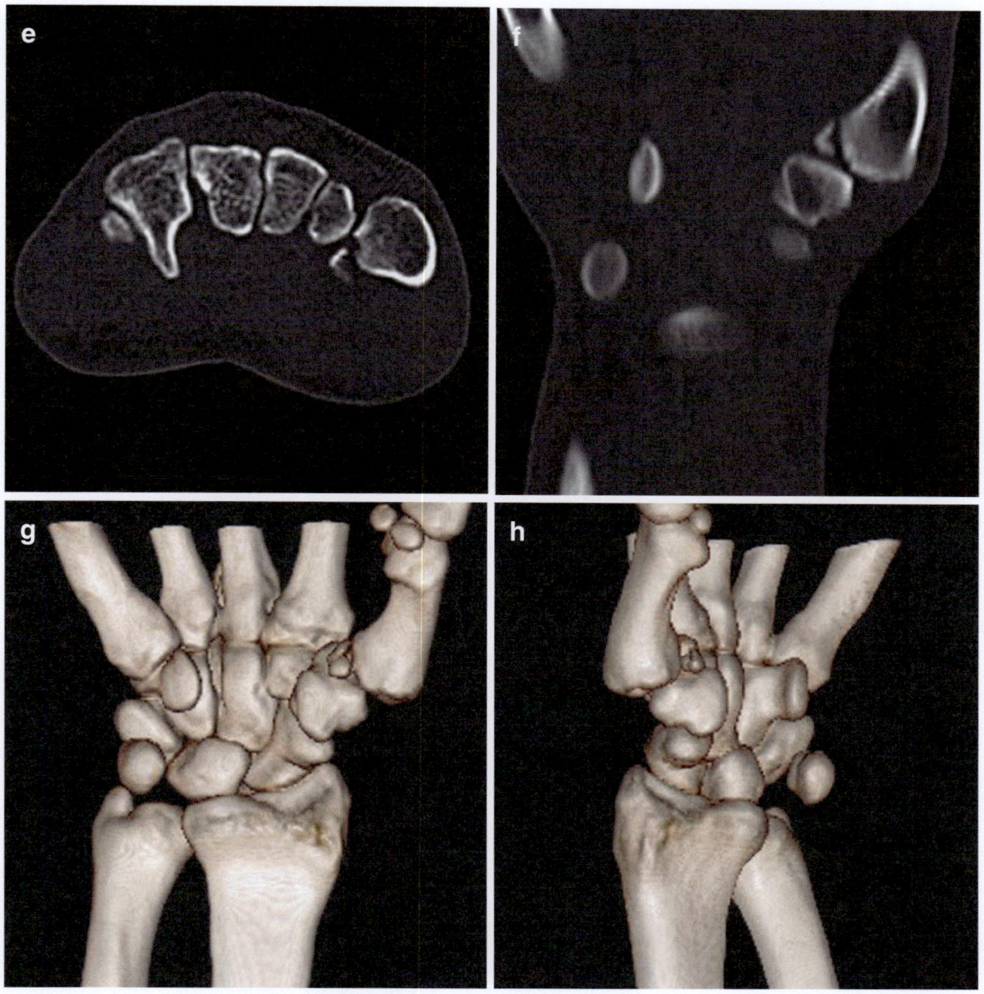

Fig. 5.5 The CT coronal plane (**e**), sagittal CT plane (**f**), and three-dimensional reconstruction (**g**, **h**) show fracture through the base of first metaphysis on the ulnar aspect, fracture line extended into the articular surface, blocks located in situ, while subluxation of the basilar part moved to the radial side

6. Differentiation of the fifth metacarpal basal fracture and suspected fracture
   6.1 X-ray (Fig. 5.6a, b)

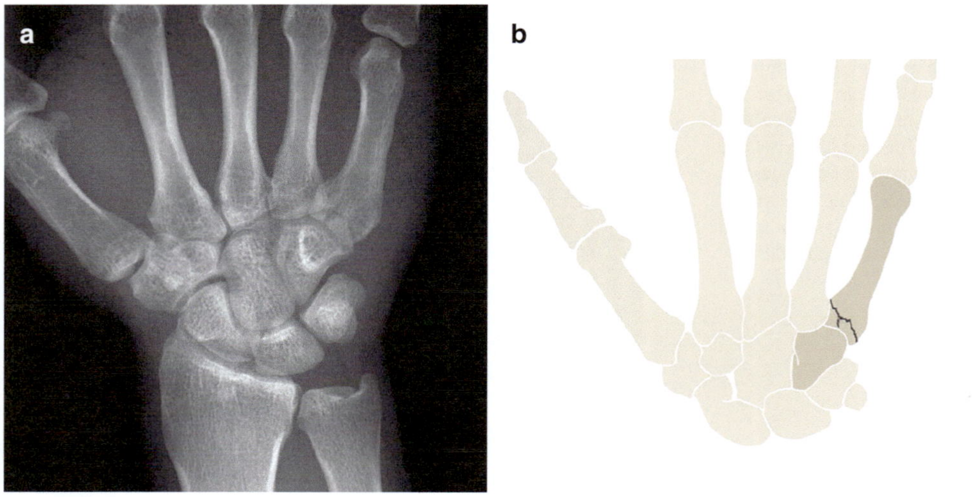

Fig. 5.6 X-ray (**a**) and illustration (**b**) show disordered structure of metacarpal base, longitudinally line-like low density shadow on this area

   6.2 CT scan (Fig. 5.6c–e)

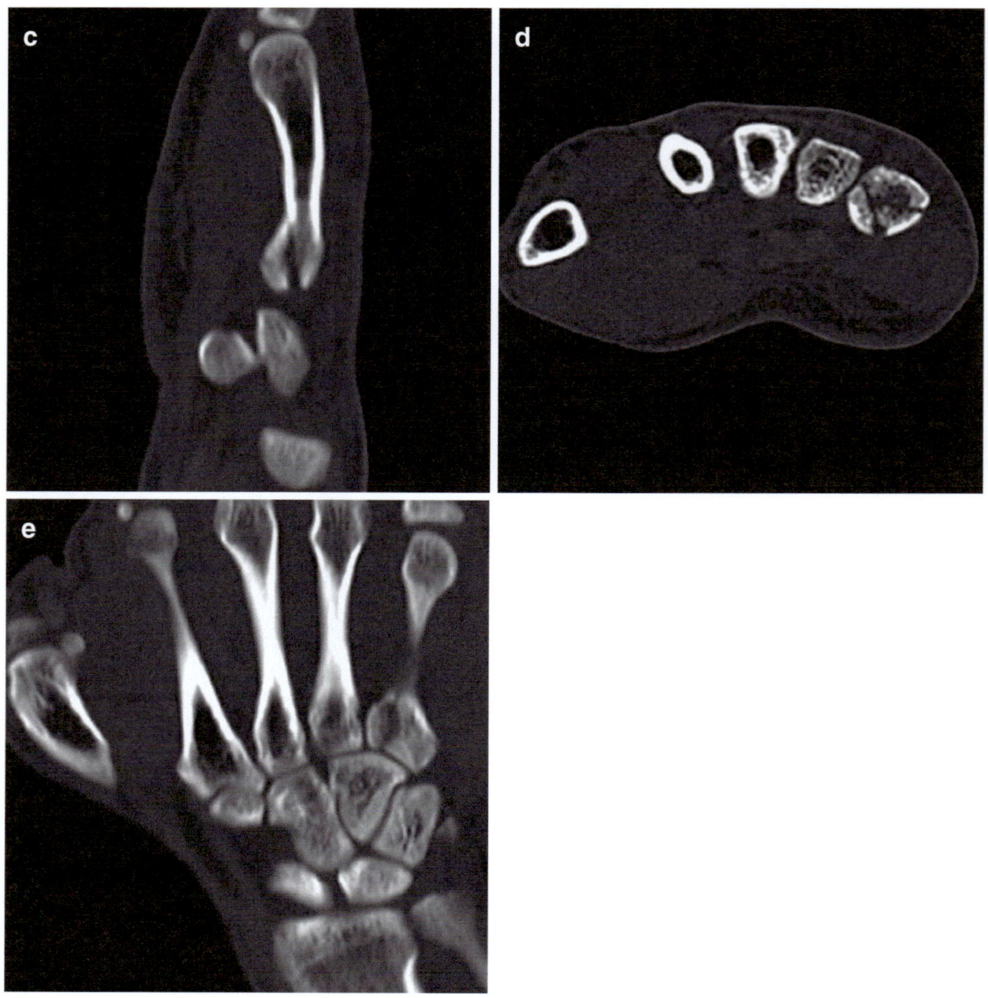

Fig. 5.6 The cross-section (**c**), coronal CT plane (**d**), and sagittal CT plane (**e**) show the fifth metacarpal fracture, broken ends were slightly displaced and the fracture line extended into the articular surface

7. Differentiation of the fifth metacarpal base fracture and non-fracture
   7.1 X-ray (Fig. 5.7a–d)

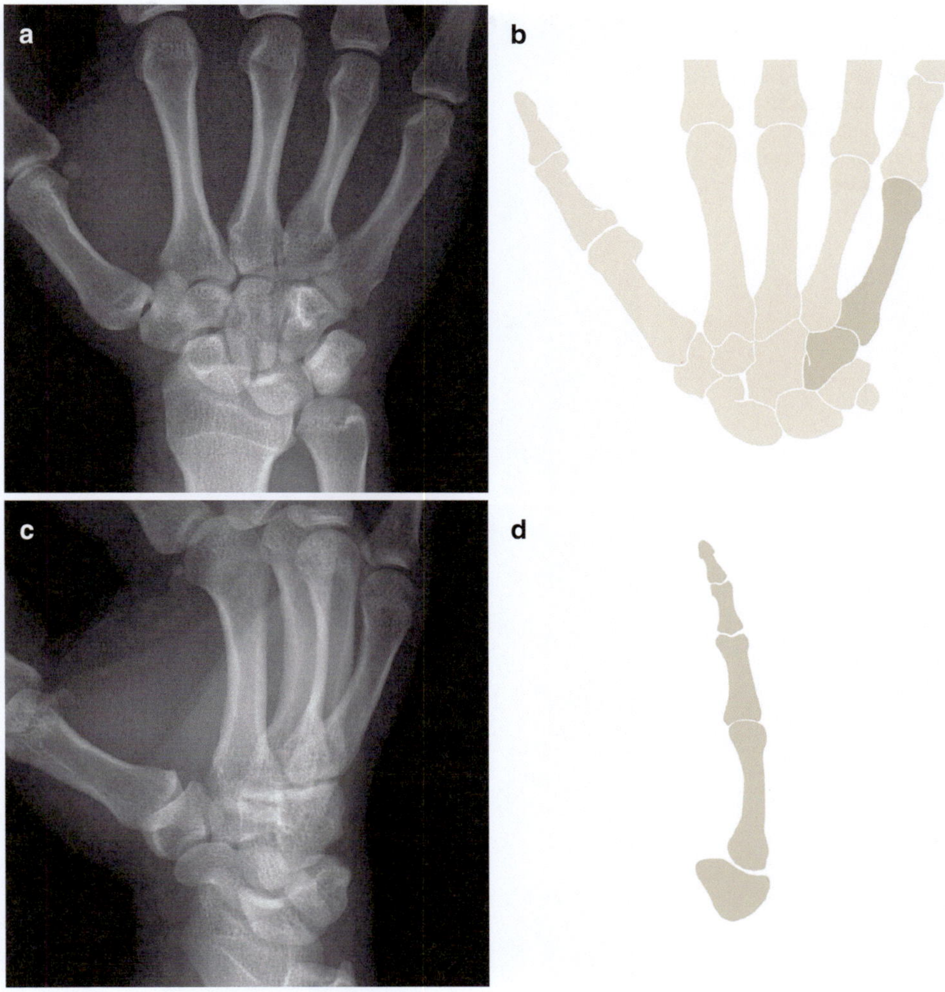

Fig. 5.7 X-ray (**a**, **c**) and illustration (**b**, **d**) show no sign of the fifth metacarpal base fracture

   7.2 CT scan (Fig. 5.7e, f)

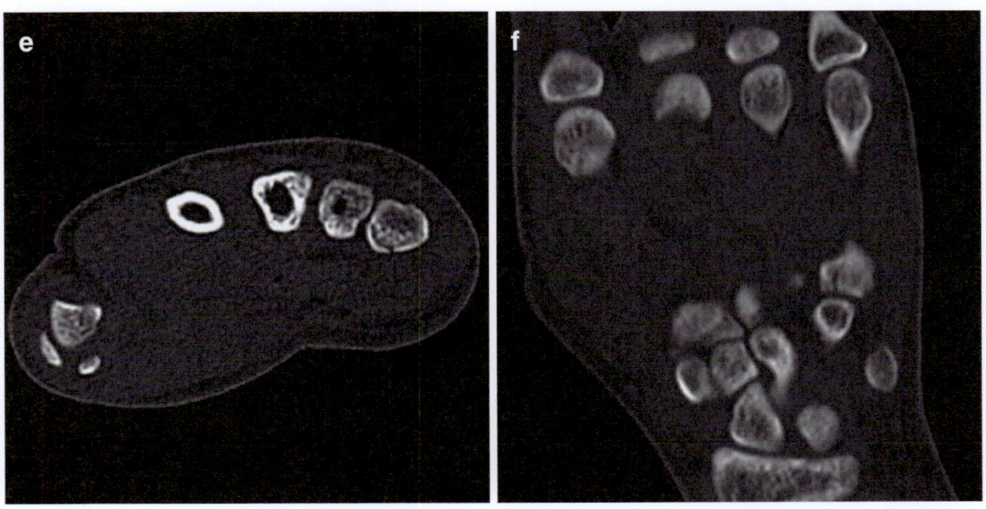

Fig. 5.7 The cross-section (**e**) and coronal CT plane (**f**) show fracture of volar margin of the fifth metacarpal base, broken ends were slightly displaced and the fracture line extended into the articular surface

8. Displaced wedge fracture of the fifth metacarpal diaphysis
   8.1 X-ray (Fig. 5.8a–d)

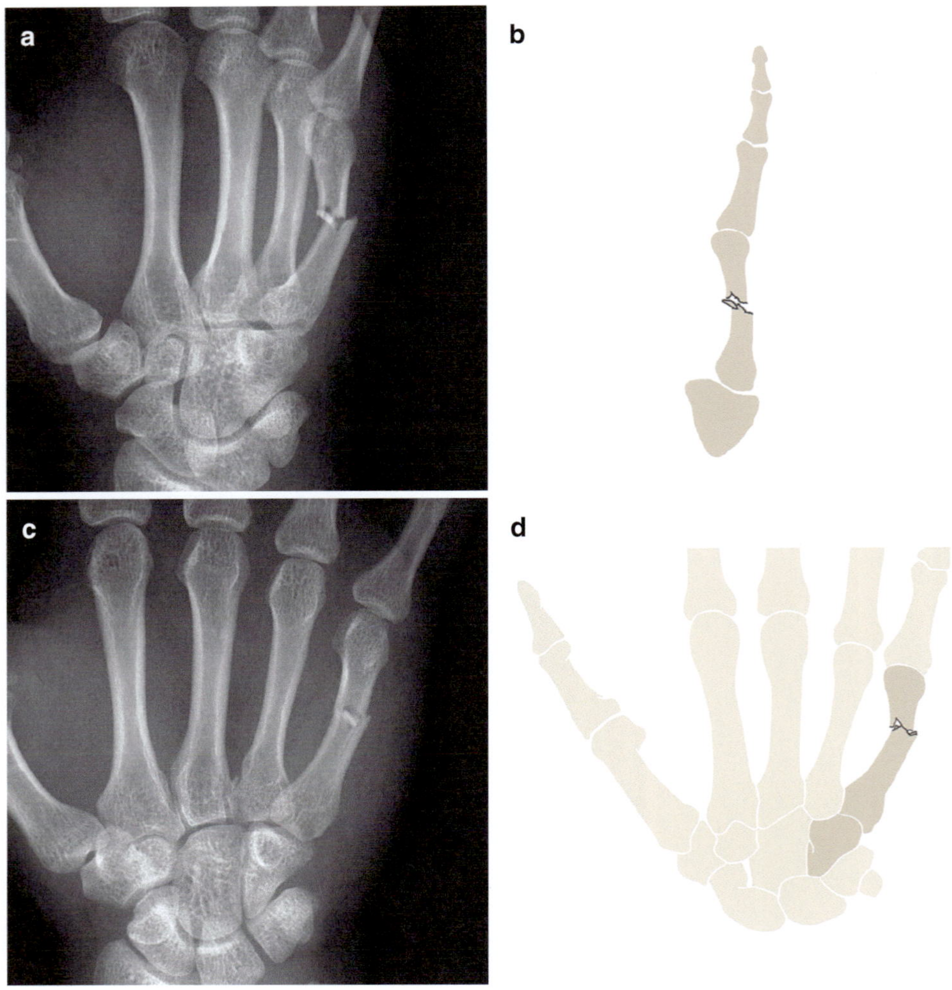

Fig. 5.8 X-ray (**a**, **c**) and illustration (**b**, **d**) show fifth metacarpal diaphysis fracture, broken ends were displaced and slightly angulated, cuneiform fragment can be seen in this area

9. Partially displaced fracture of the fourth metacarpal head
   9.1 CT scan (Fig. 5.9a–d)

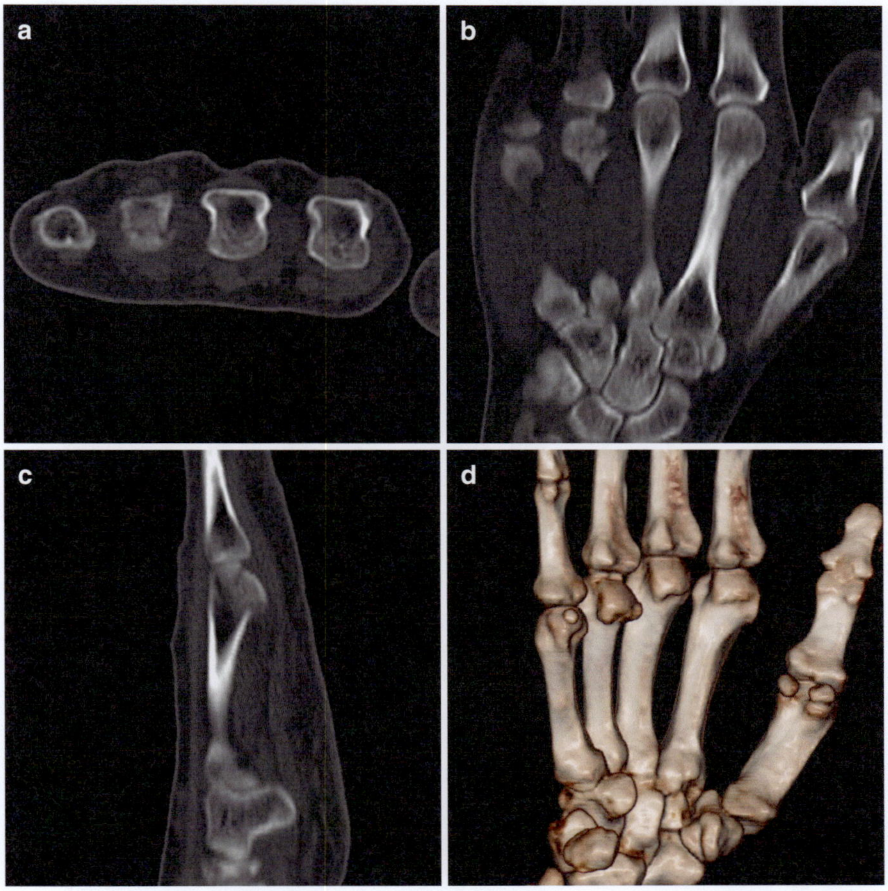

Fig. 5.9 The cross-section (**a**), coronal CT plane (**b**), sagittal CT plane (**c**), and three-dimensional reconstruction (**d**) show fracture of the fourth metacarpal head, fracture line extended into the articular surface, and articular surface of the volar side was displaced

10. Differentiation of impacted comminuted and simple fracture of the fifth intra-articular metacarpal base fracture
    10.1 X-ray (Fig. 5.10a–d)

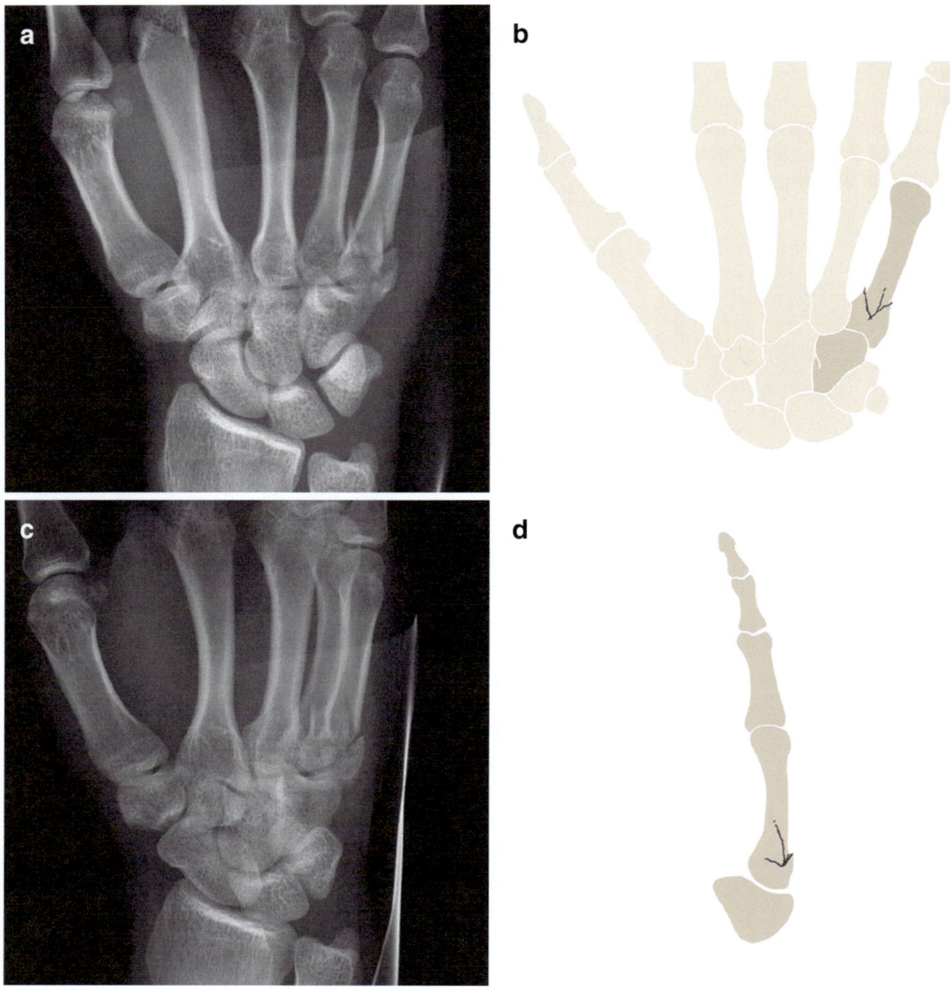

Fig. 5.10 X-ray (**a**, **c**) and illustration (**b**, **d**) show comminuted fracture of the fifth metacarpal base, broken ends were displaced, and articular surface was affected

10.2 CT scan (Fig. 5.10e–h)

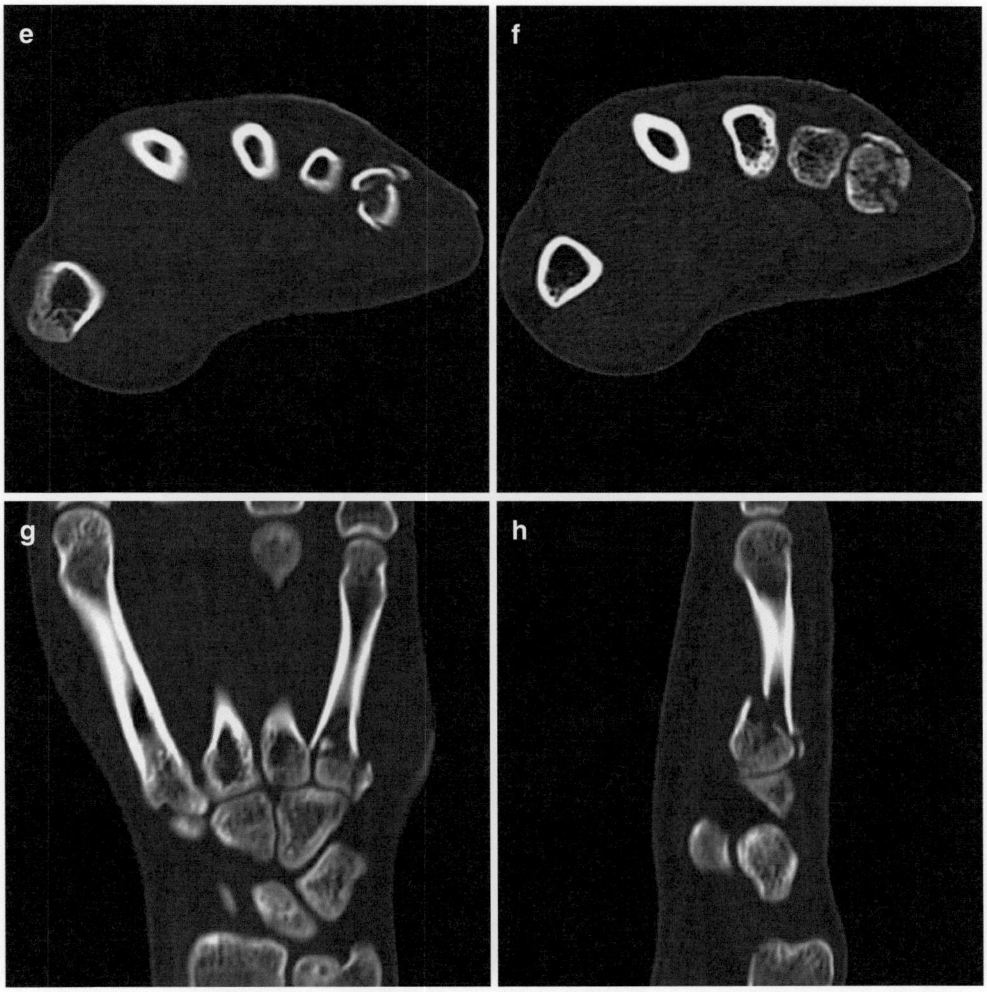

Fig. 5.10 The cross-section (**e**, **f**), coronal CT plane (**g**), and sagittal CT plane (**h**) show fracture of the fifth metacarpal basilar fracture, broken ends were slightly displaced, and fracture line extended into the articular surface

11. Differentiation of the first metacarpal basilar comminuted intra-articular fracture and Winterstein fracture
    11.1 X-ray (Fig. 5.11a–d)

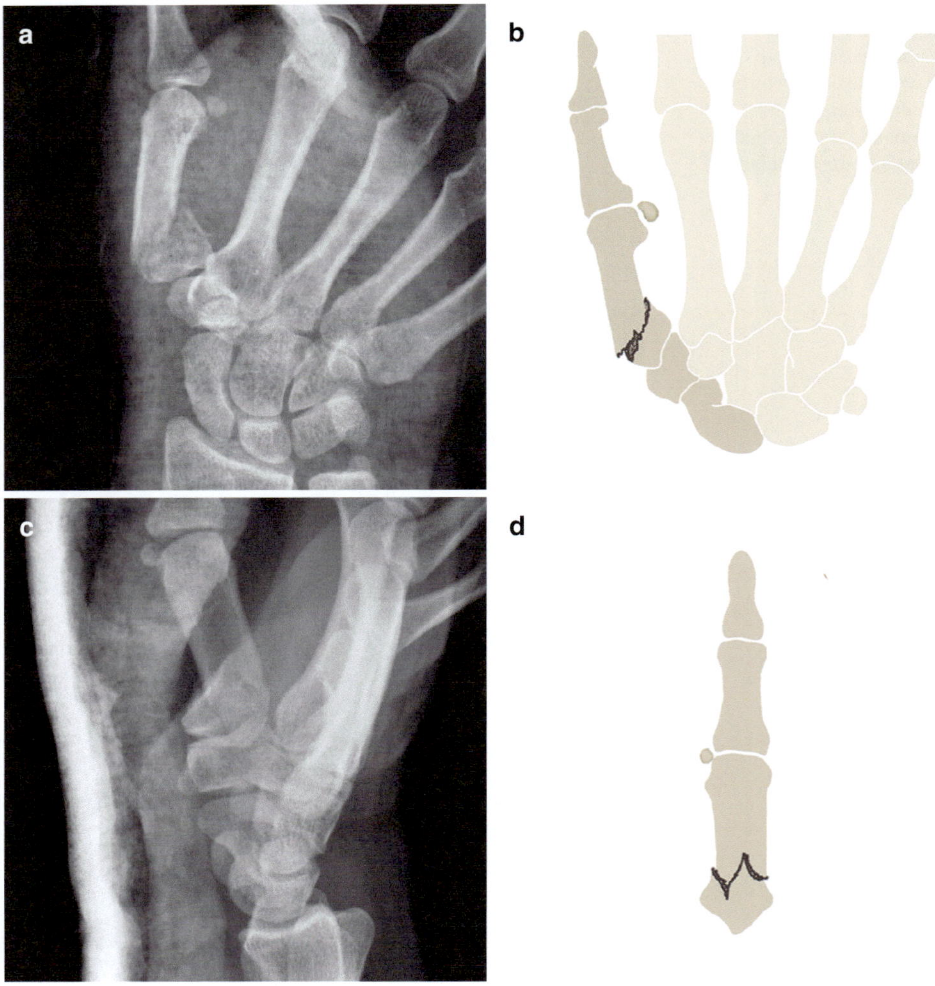

Fig. 5.11 X-ray (**a**, **c**) and illustration (**b**, **d**) show the first metacarpal basilar oblique fracture, broken ends were displaced and angulated

11.2 CT scan (Fig. 5.11e–h)

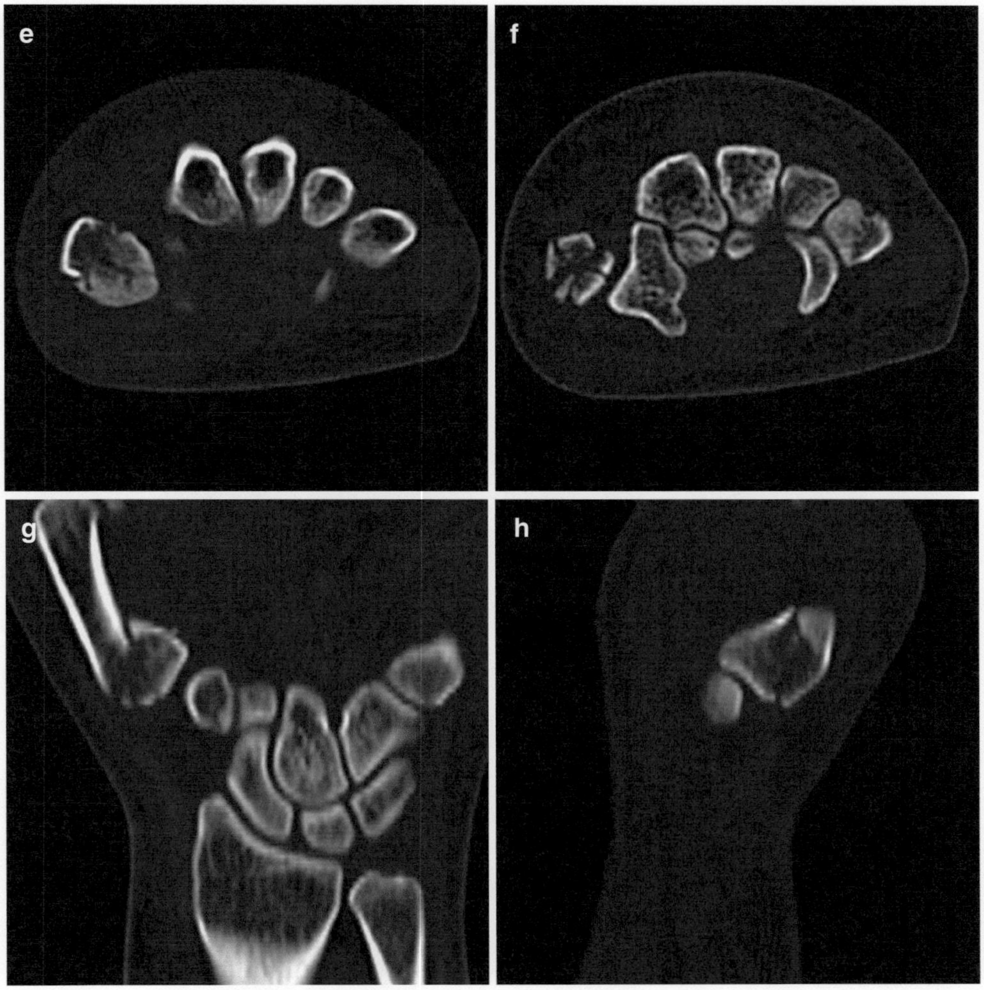

Fig. 5.11 The cross-section (**e**, **f**), coronal CT plane (**g**), and sagittal CT plane (**h**) show a basilar part fracture at ulnar side of the first metaphysis. The broken ends were slightly displaced, and the fracture line extended into the articular surface. Blocks located in situ, while subluxation of the basilar part moved to the radial side

12. Differentiation of simple and comminuted intra-articular basilar fracture of the fifth metaphysis
    12.1 X-ray (Fig. 5.12a–d)

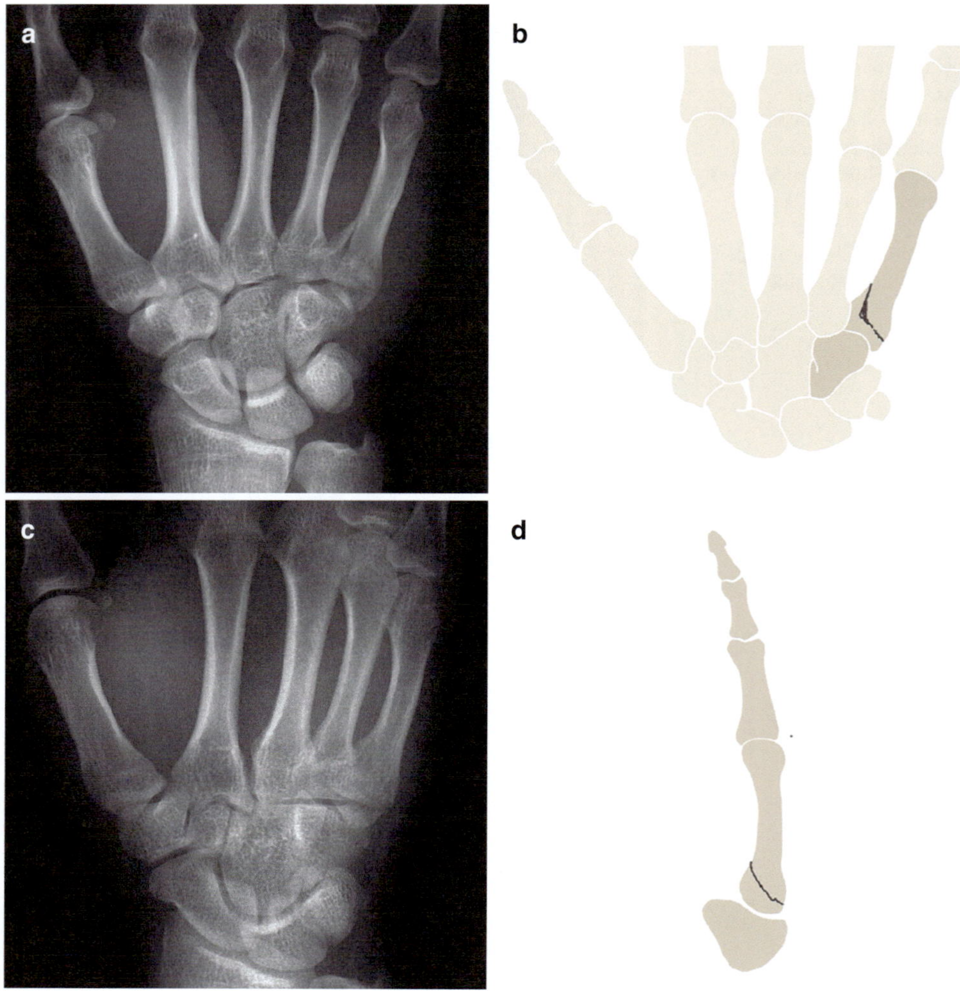

Fig. 5.12 X-ray (**a**, **c**) and illustration (**b**, **d**) show the fifth metacarpal basilar fracture, broken ends were displaced

12.2 CT scan (Fig. 5.12e, f)

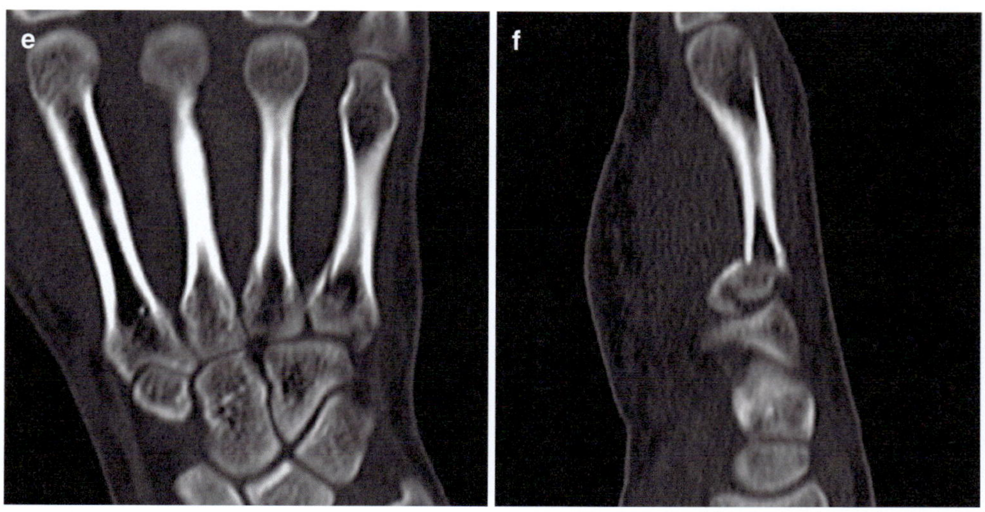

Fig. 5.12 The cross-section (**e**) and sagittal CT plane (**f**) show fracture of the fifth metacarpal basilar fracture, broken ends were displaced, and fracture line extended into the articular surface

13. The fifth metacarpal diaphysis comminuted fracture
    13.1 X-ray (Fig. 5.13a–d)

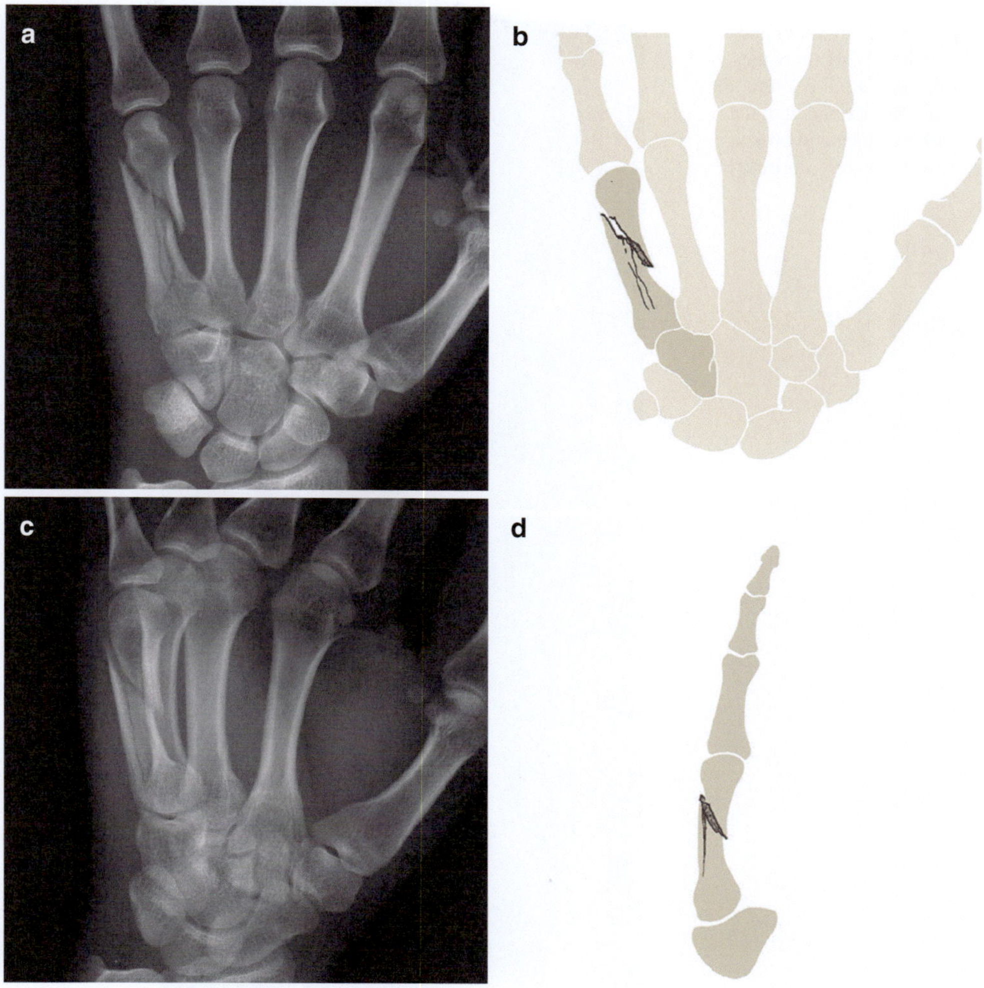

Fig. 5.13 X-ray (**a**, **c**) and illustration (**b**, **d**) show the fifth metacarpal diaphysis fracture, broken ends were slightly displaced and angular deformity was relatively small

14. Differentiation of comminuted and partially intra-articular head fractures of the fifth metaphysis
    14.1 X-ray (Fig. 5.14a–d)

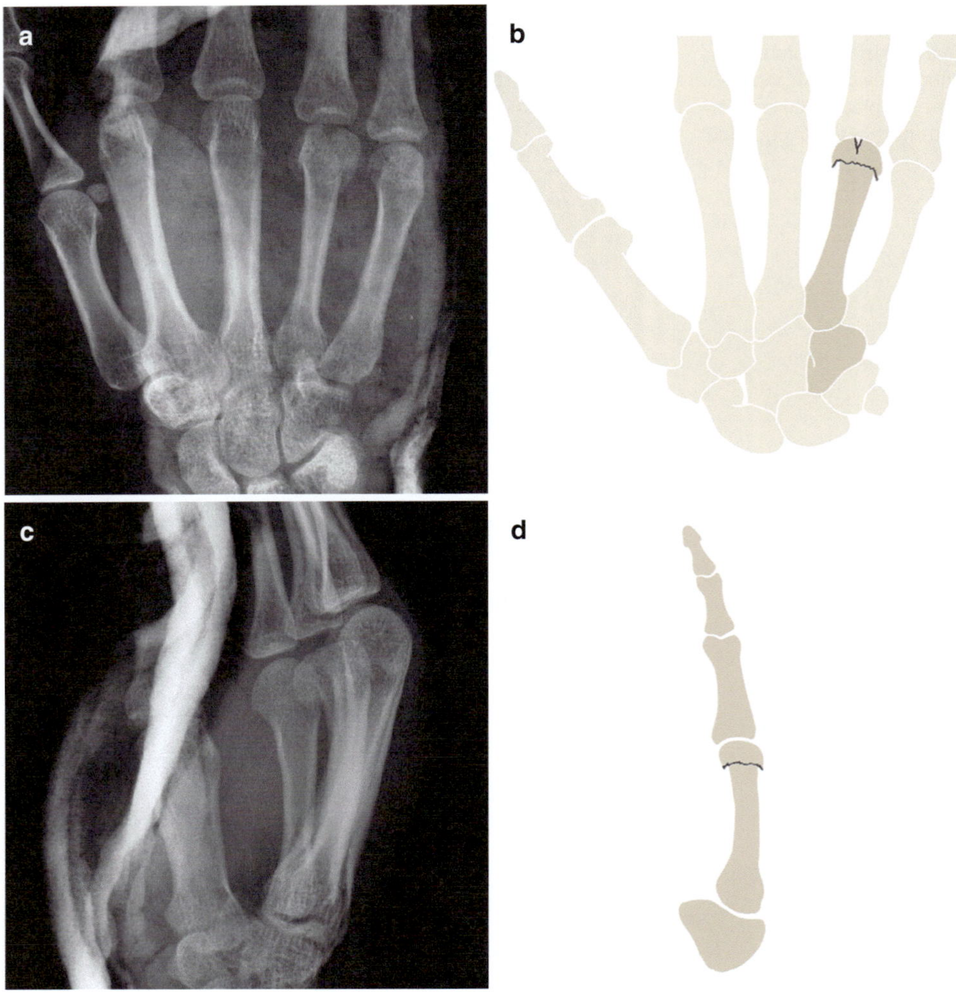

Fig. 5.14 X-ray (**a**, **c**) and illustration (**b**, **d**) show the fourth metacarpal fracture, the fracture line extended to the articular surface and broken ends were slightly impacted

    14.2 CT scan (Fig. 5.14e, f)

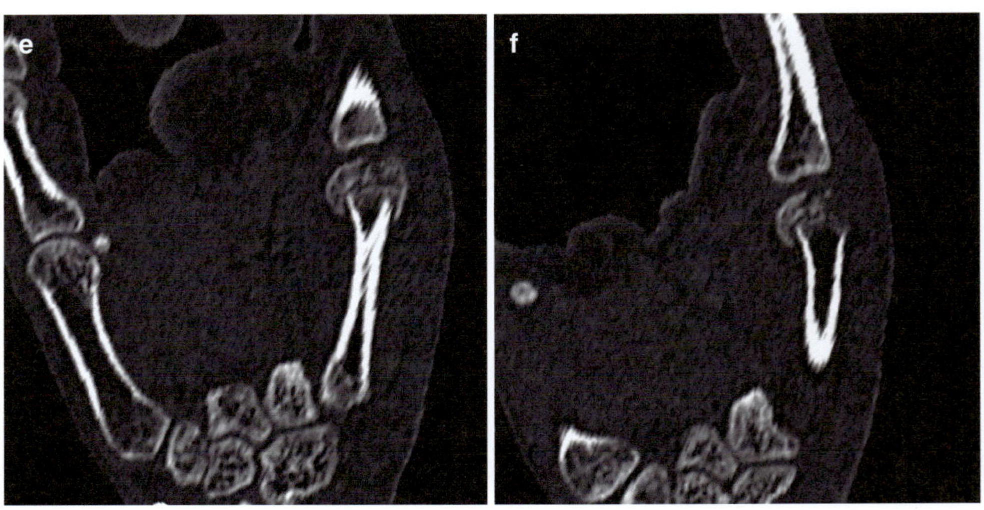

Fig. 5.14 The coronal (**e**) and sagittal CT plane (**f**) showed fracture of the fourth metacarpal head fracture, the broken ends were impacted and the articular surface fell apart

5.2 Phalangeal Fracture

The phalanges are all long tubular bones, and can be roughly divided into three kinds of phalanges according to its location: the proximal phalanx, the middle phalanx, and the distal phalanx, except for the thumb that contains only two phalanges. Each phalange has a base, shaft, and head (also called the trochlea of the phalanx). The Orthopedic Trauma Association (OTA) classified phalangeal fractures into nine types as follows: phalangeal proximal (8.81% of all phalangeal fractures) and distal extra-articular fracture (22.98% of all phalangeal fractures), phalangeal diaphysis non-comminuted fracture (35.18% of all phalangeal fractures), phalangeal proximal (5.76% of all phalangeal fractures) and distal partial articular fracture (5.07% of all phalangeal fractures), phalangeal diaphysis wedge comminuted fracture (11.78% of all phalangeal fractures), phalangeal proximal (2.08% of all phalangeal fracture) and distal complete articular fracture (4.79% of all phalangeal fractures), phalangeal diaphysis comminuted fracture (3.55% of all phalange fractures).

5.2.1 Injury Mechanism

Phalangeal tuberosity and epiphysis fractures are mostly seen in crush injury and the phalanx basal fracture is mostly avulsion.

5.2.2 Signs and Symptoms

Common indications of a fracture include pain, swelling, and abnormality of motion, but these clinical features may occur in many slightly displaced fractures and easily misdiagnosed. Therefore, a comprehensive physical examination should be done meticulously. If there is a suspicion, X-ray, CT, or MRI radiographs need to be ordered.

5.2.3 Imaging Differential Diagnosis

CT scans should be ordered if there are uncertainties of the X-ray outcome, but normally a standard X-ray of the hand can well define the nature of displaced fracture, and the degree of the displacement of the phalangeal fracture.

1. Diagnosis of transverse fracture of proximal phalange of the little finger on an X-ray
   1.1 X-ray (Fig. 5.15a–d)

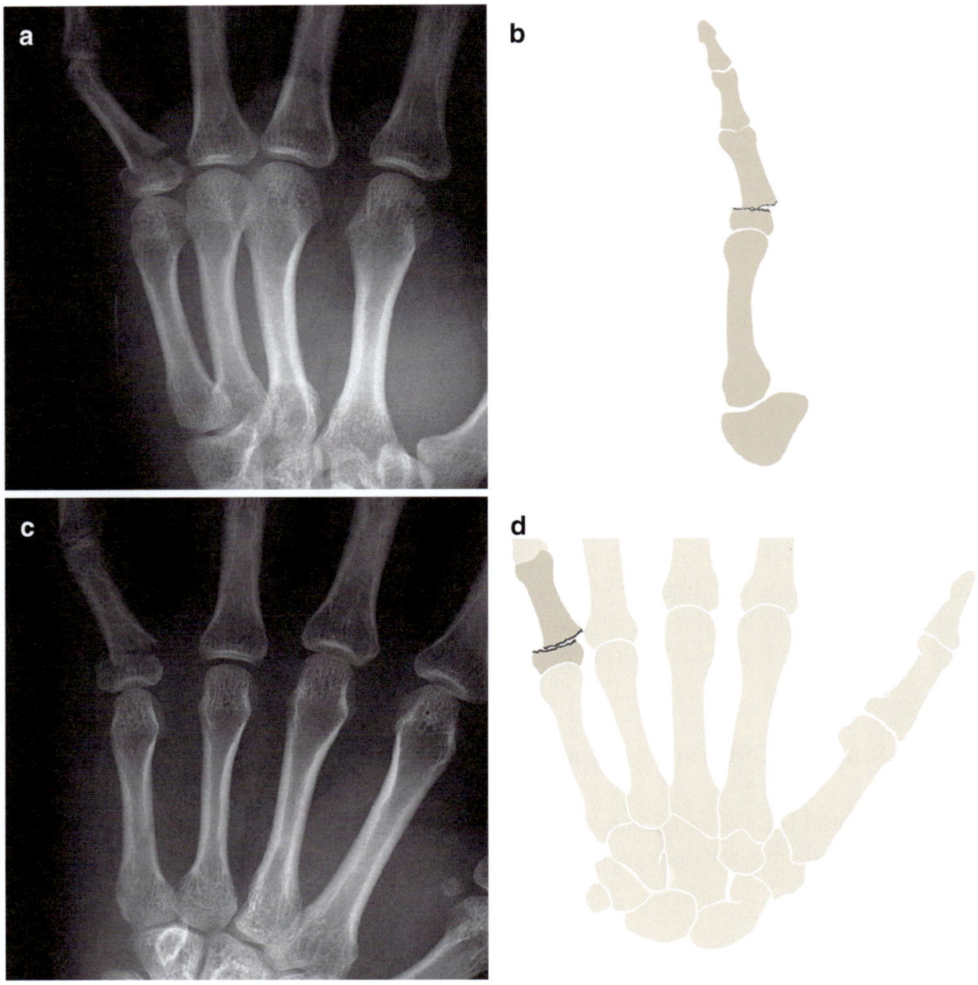

Fig. 5.15 X-ray (**a**, **c**) and illustration (**b**, **d**) show transverse fracture of proximal phalange of the little finger, broken ends were displaced and angulated. Fracture line was not extended to the articular surface

2. Diagnosis of transverse fracture of proximal phalange diaphysis of the index finger on an X-ray
   2.1 X-ray (Fig. 5.16a–d)

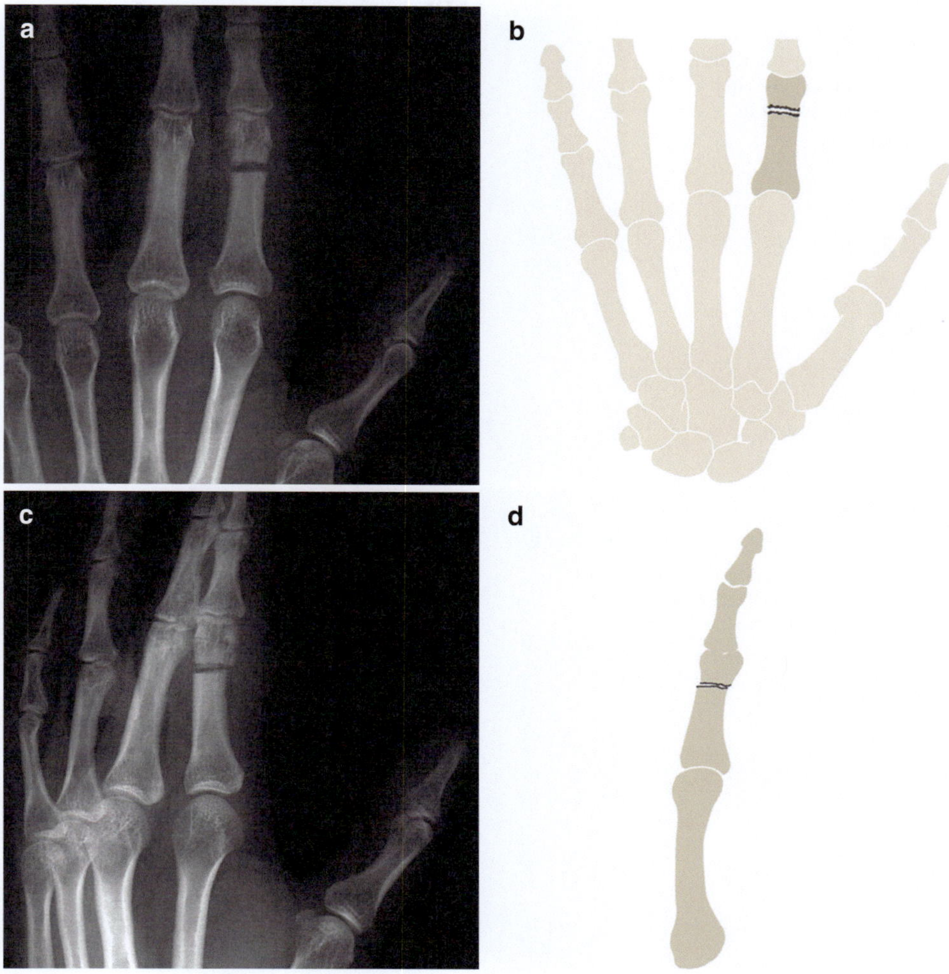

Fig. 5.16 X-ray (**a**, **c**) and illustration (**b**, **d**) show transverse fracture of proximal phalange diaphysis of the index finger, broken ends were slightly displaced and angulated

3. Diagnosis of distal transverse fracture of middle phalange of the middle finger on an X-ray
   3.1 X-ray (Fig. 5.17a–d)

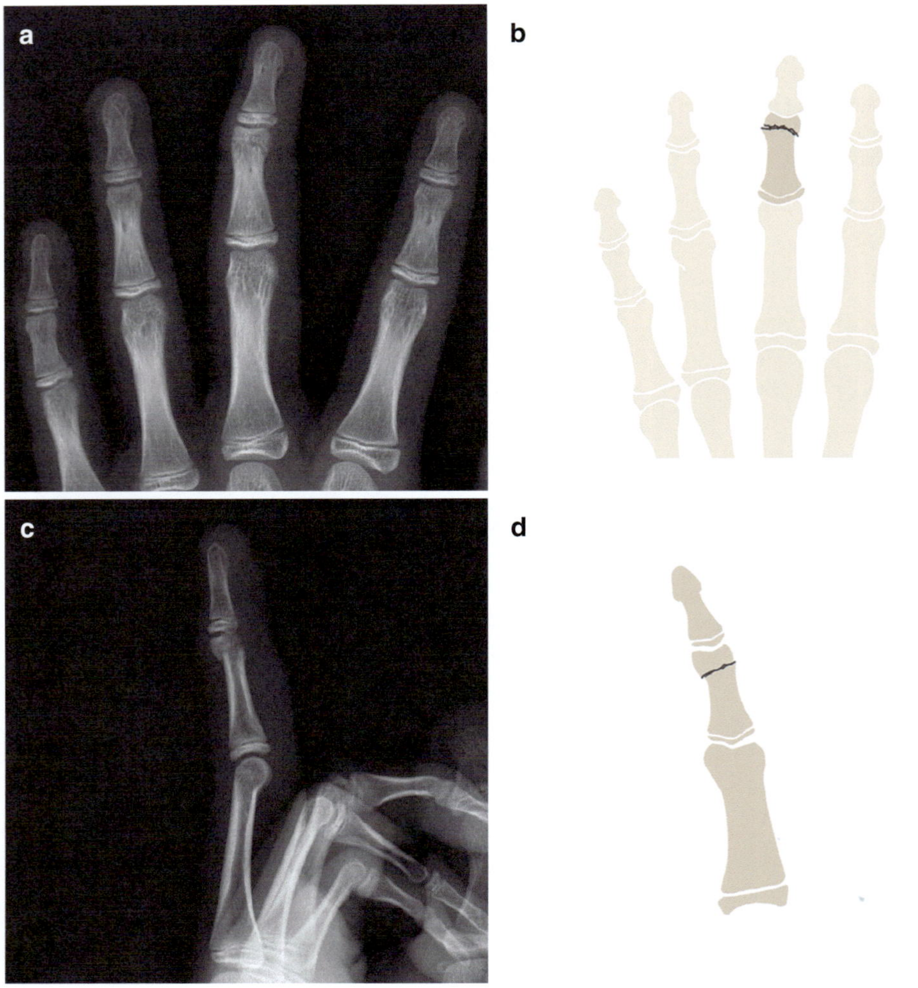

Fig. 5.17 X-ray (**a**, **c**) and illustration (**b**, **d**) show distal transverse fracture of middle phalange of the middle finger, broken ends were slightly displaced

4. Differentiation of proximal intra-articular partial fracture and suspected fracture of distal phalange of thumb
   4.1 X-ray (Fig. 5.18a–d)

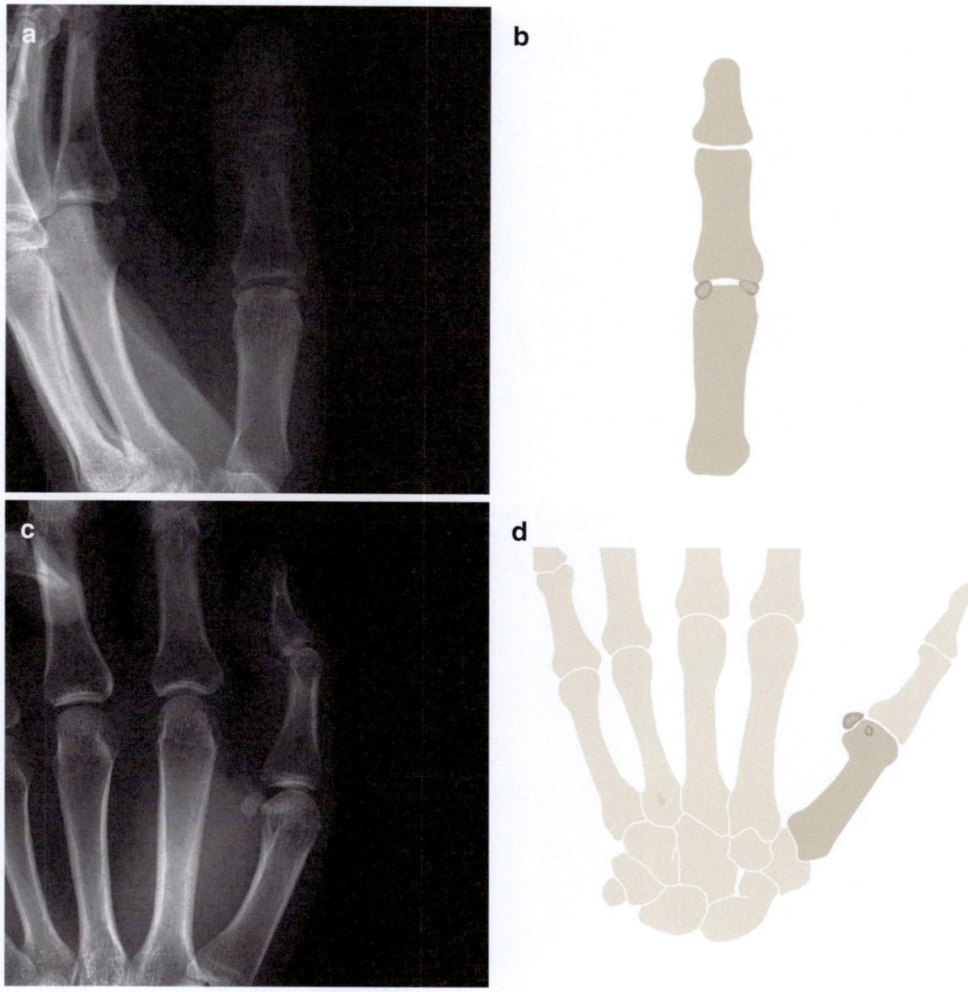

Fig. 5.18 X-ray (**a**, **c**) and illustration (**b**, **d**) show no fracture sign of thumb, only disordered structure at the basal part of the distal phalange can be observed

   4.2 CT scan (Fig. 5.18e, f)

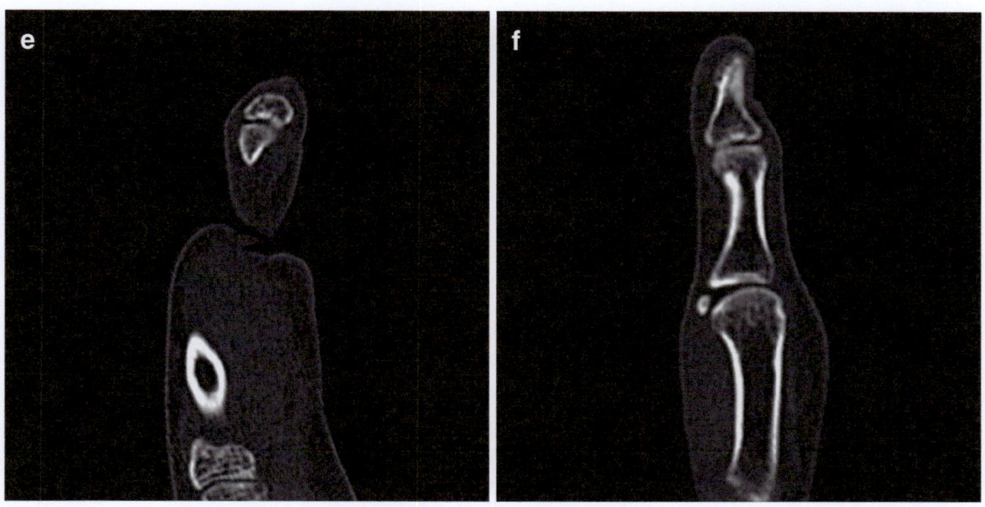

Fig. 5.18 The coronal CT plane (**e**) and sagittal CT plane (**f**) show partially collapse at the basal part of distal phalange of thumb, bone was broken

5. Differentiation of proximal intra-articular partial fracture and suspected fracture of proximal phalange of thumb
   5.1 X-ray (Fig. 5.19a–d)

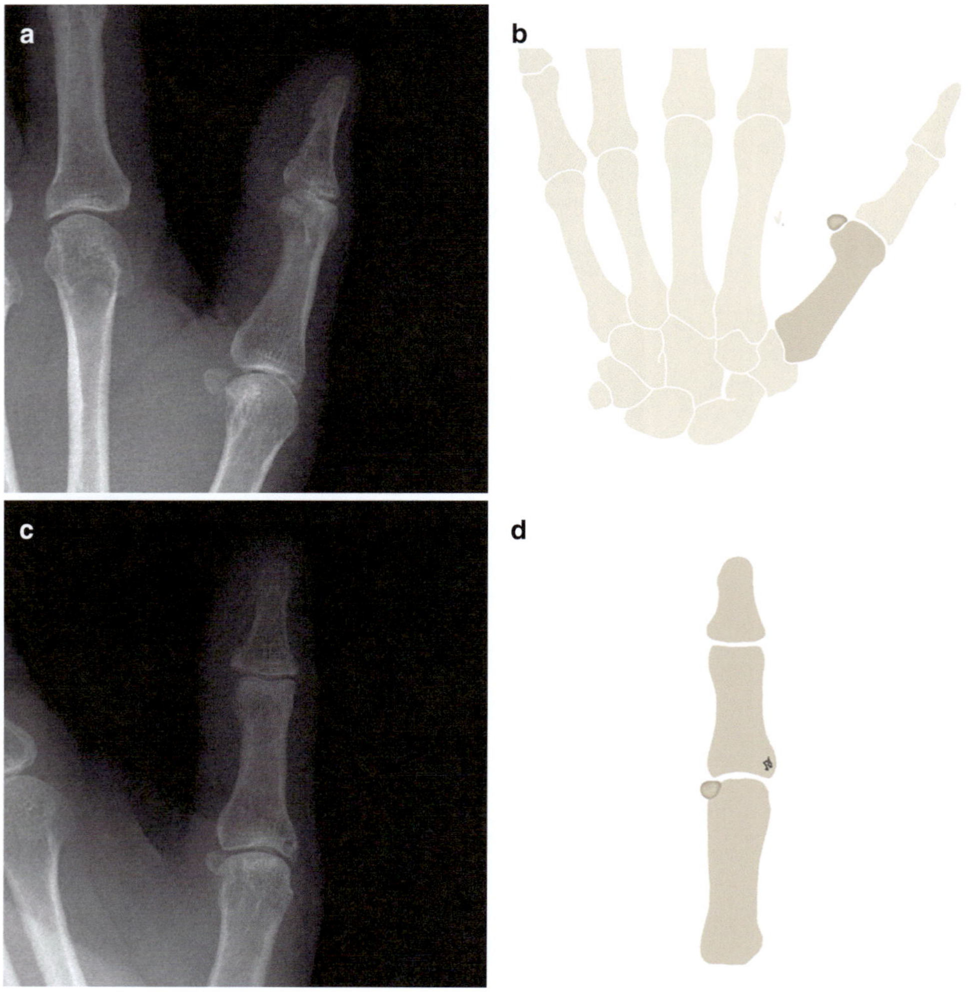

Fig. 5.19 X-ray (**a**, **c**) and illustration (**b**, **d**) show irregular radial border of the proximal phalange of thumb, some punctiform bone shadow can be identified

   5.2 CT scan (Fig. 5.19e, f)

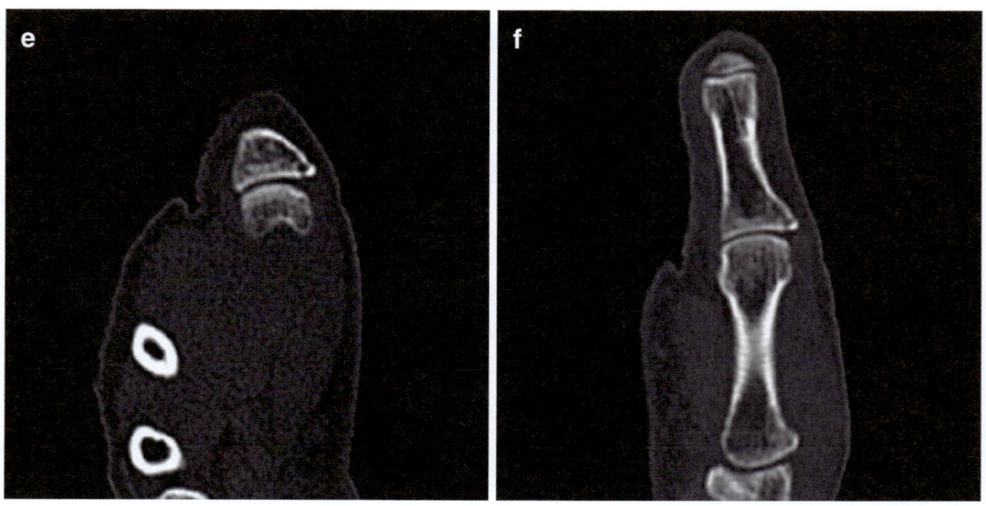

Fig. 5.19 The sagittal CT plane (**e**) and coronal CT plane (**f**) show articular surface fracture of the metacarpophalangeal joint of thumb on radial side, small bone shadow can be identified

6. Differentiation of proximal intra-articular comminuted fracture of proximal phalange of thumb and other fracture
   6.1 X-ray (Fig. 5.20a–d)

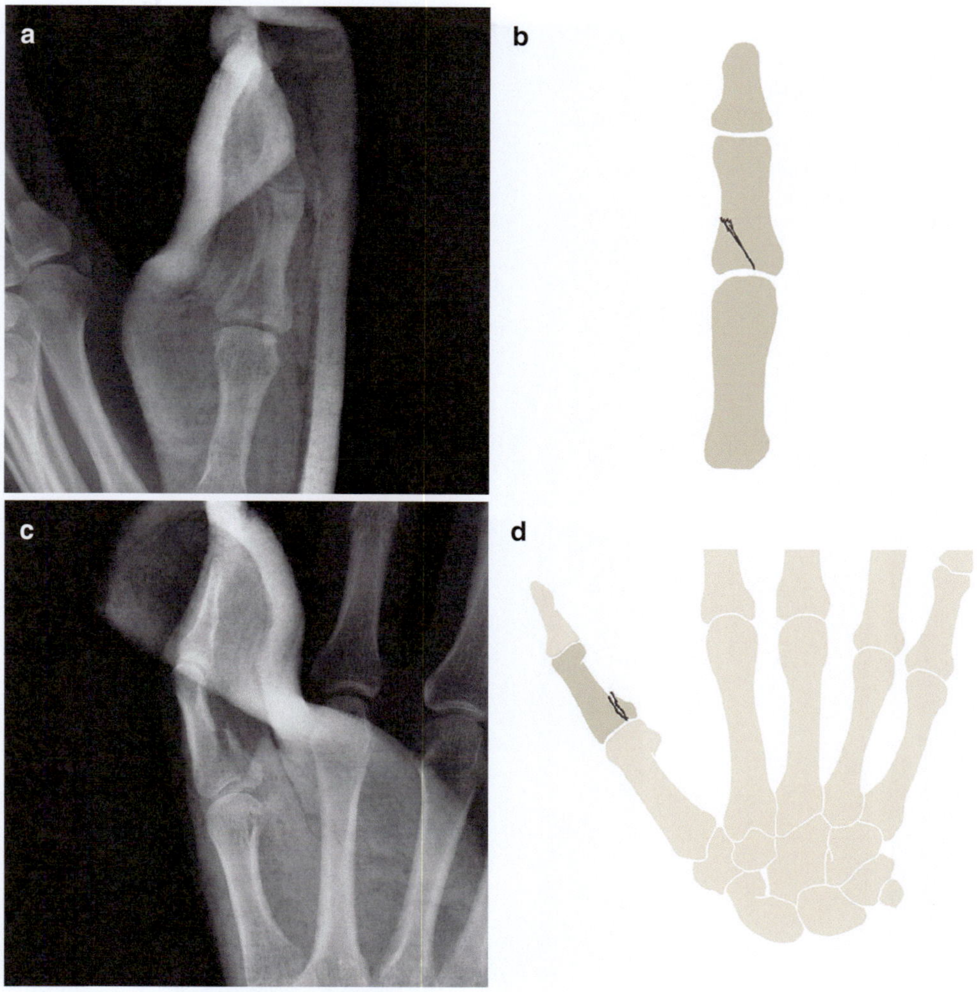

Fig. 5.20 X-ray (**a**, **c**) and illustration (**b**, **d**) show longitudinal basal fracture of the proximal phalange of thumb, fracture line extended to the articular surface and broken ends were slightly displaced

   6.2 CT scan (Fig. 5.20e, f)

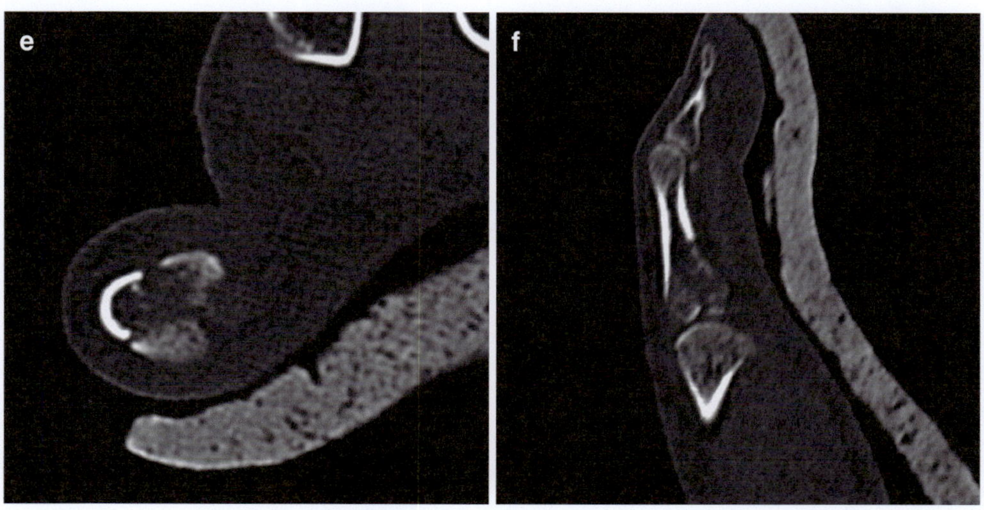

Fig. 5.20 The cross-section (**e**) and sagittal CT plane (**f**) showed multi-fragments and basal fracture of the proximal phalange of thumb, fracture line extended to the articular surface

7. Diagnosis of wedge fracture of proximal phalange diaphysis of the index finger on an X-ray
   7.1 X-ray (Fig. 5.21a–d)

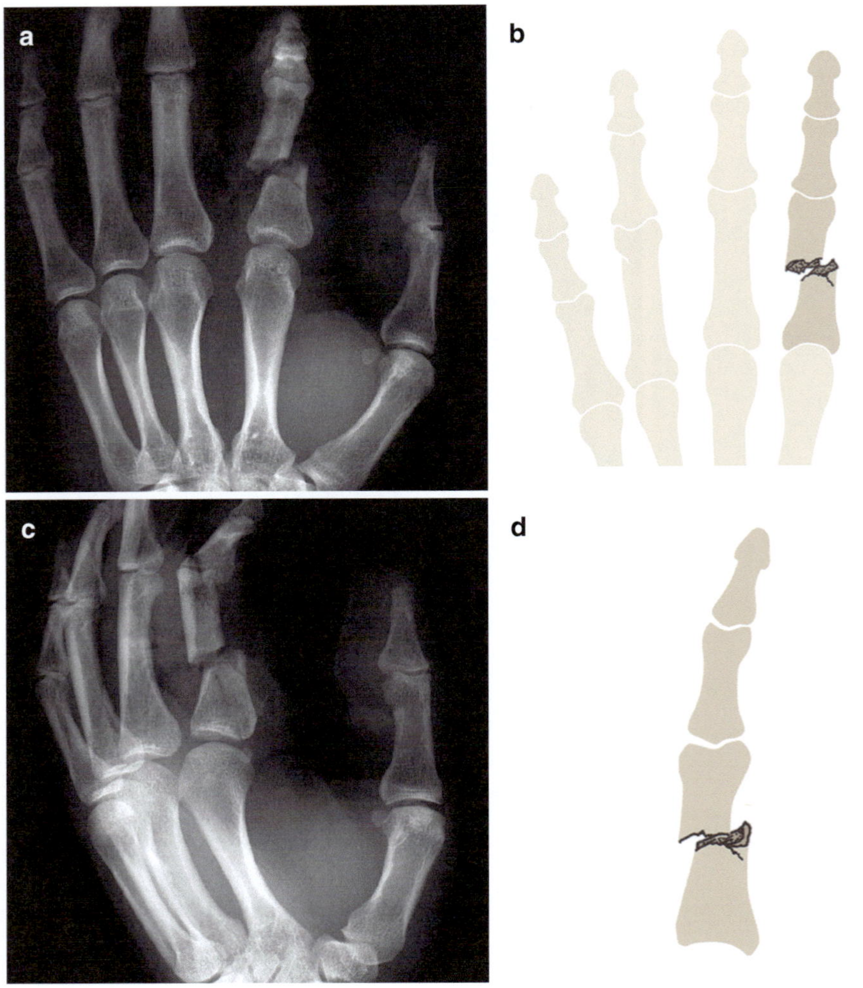

Fig. 5.21 X-ray (**a**, **c**) and illustration (**b**, **d**) show fracture of the proximal phalange of the index finger, cuneiform fragments on the radial side, broken ends were displaced and slightly angulated

8. Diagnosis of distal articular fracture of the middle phalange of middle finger on an X-ray
   8.1 X-ray (Fig. 5.22a–d)

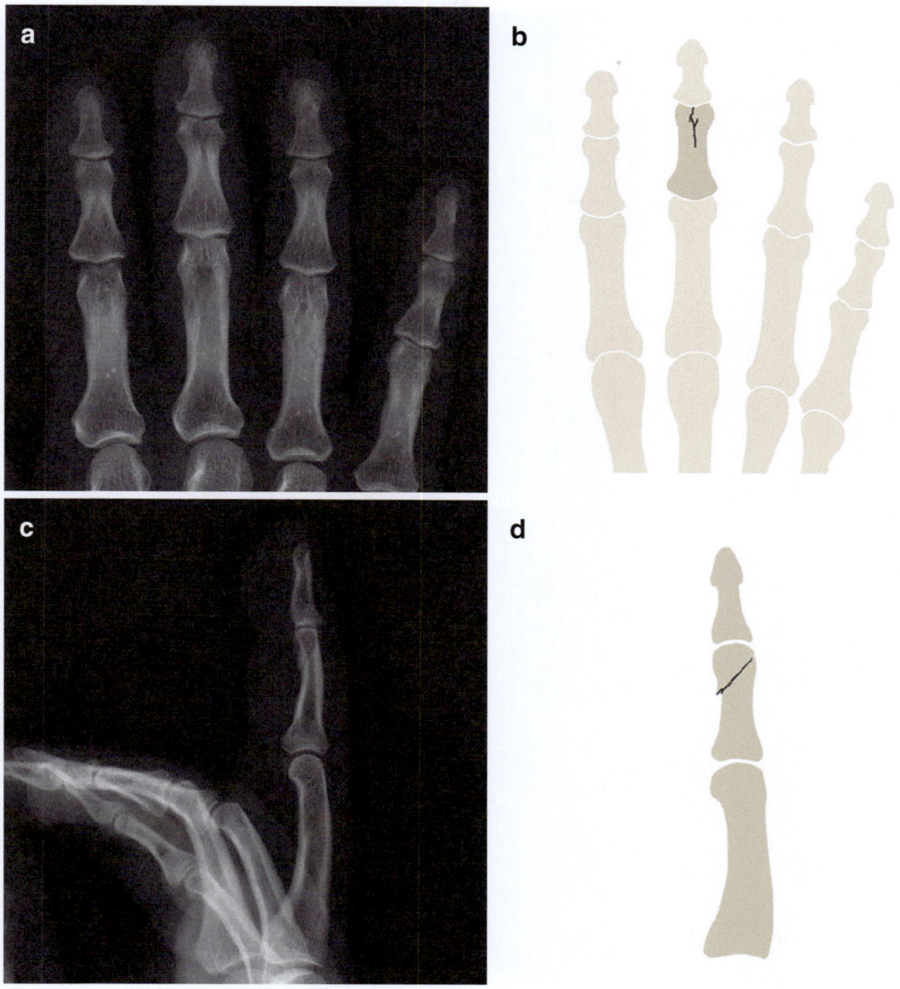

Fig. 5.22 X-ray (**a**, **c**) and illustration (**b**, **d**) show distal fracture of the middle phalange of the middle finger, fragments split longitudinally, articular surface on the ulnar side was slightly dislocated

9. Differentiation of basal comminuted fracture of the proximal phalange of index finger and the fracture
   9.1 X-ray (Fig. 5.23a–d)

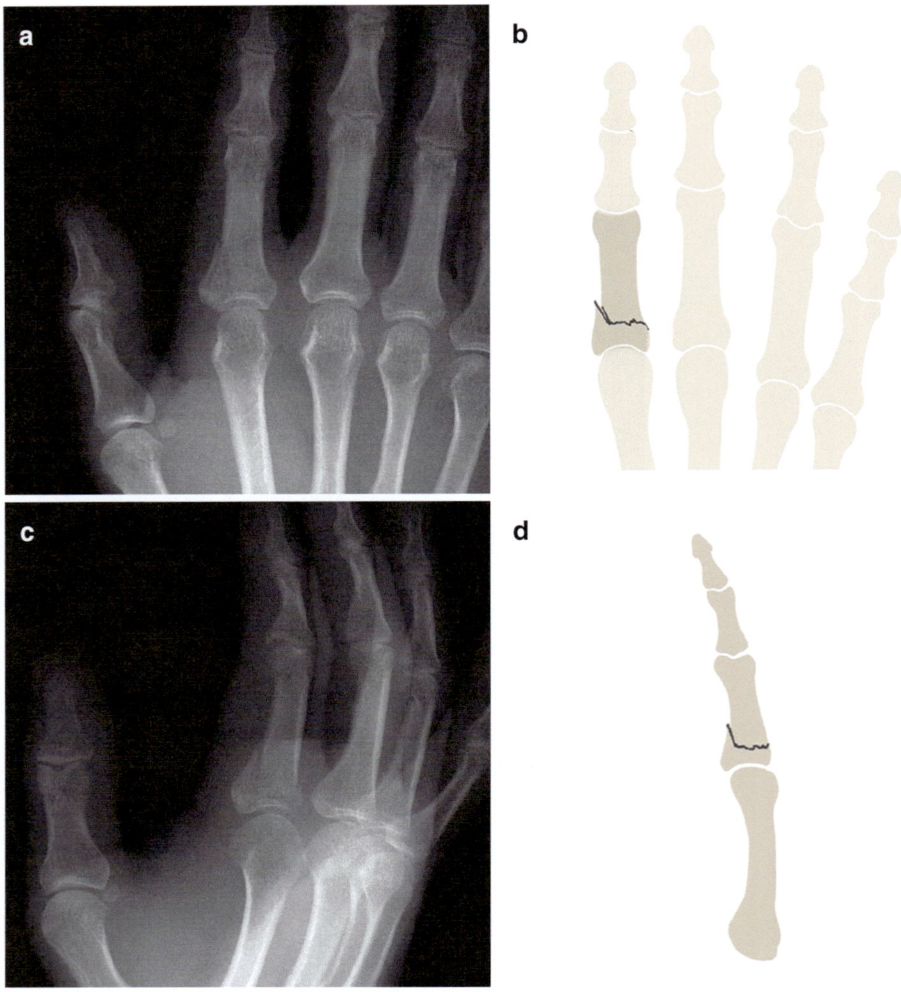

Fig. 5.23 X-ray (**a**, **c**) and illustration (**b**, **d**) show basal fracture of the proximal phalange of the index finger, broken ends were slightly displaced

9.2 CT scan (Fig. 5.23e–h)

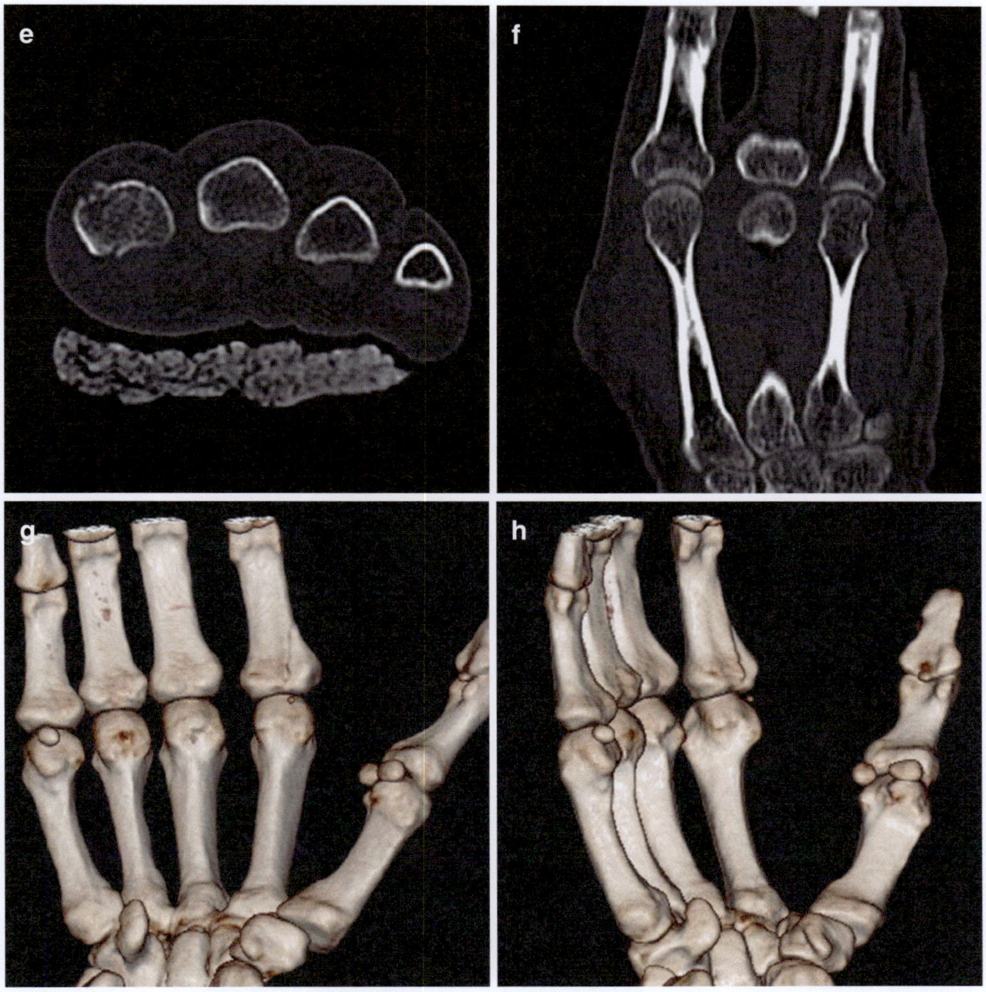

Fig. 5.23 The cross-section (**e**), coronal CT plane (**f**), and three-dimensional reconstruction (**g**, **h**) show basal fracture of the proximal phalange of the index finger, broken ends were slightly displaced

10. Basal comminuted fracture of the middle phalange of the ring finger
    10.1 CT scan (Fig. 5.24a–d)

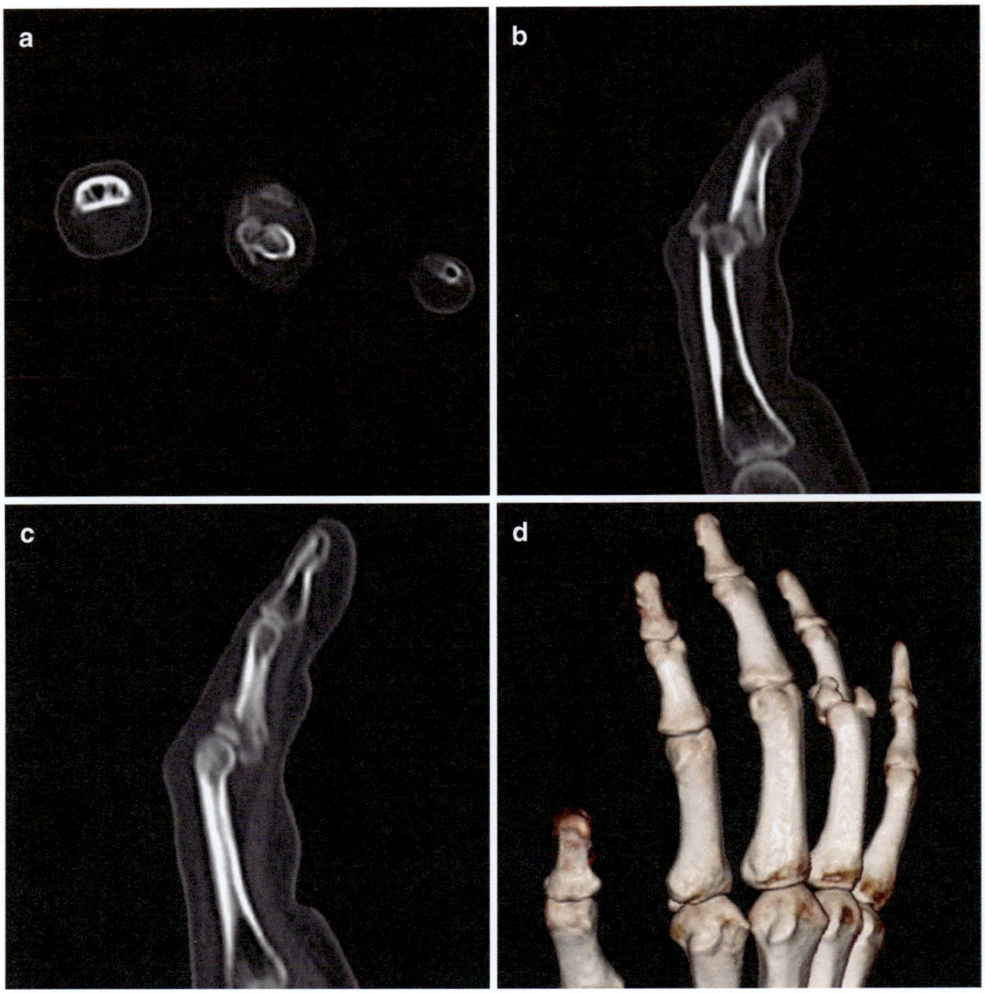

Fig. 5.24 The cross-section (**a**), sagittal CT plane (**b**, **c**), and three-dimensional reconstruction (**d**) show displaced basal fracture of the middle phalange of the ring finger and irregular defects in the articular cortex

11. Comminuted fracture of the proximal phalangeal diaphysis of ring finger
    11.1 X-ray (Fig. 5.25a–d)

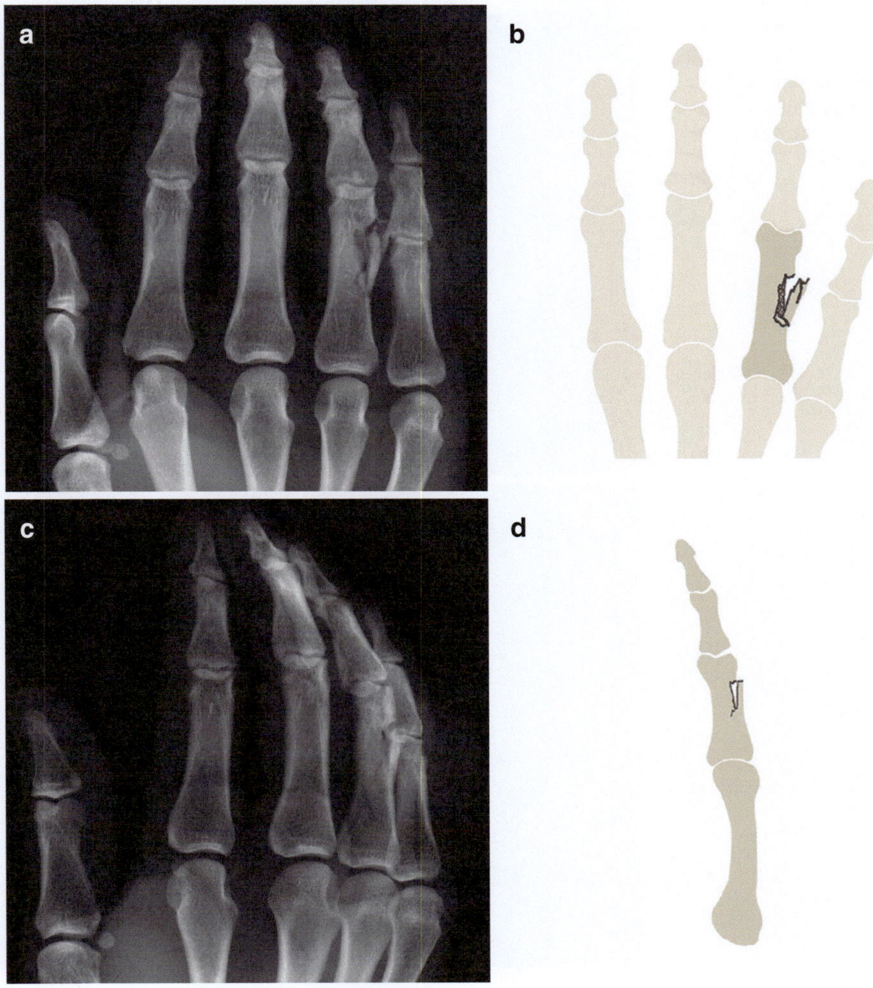

Fig. 5.25 X-ray (**a**, **c**) and illustration (**b**, **d**) show fracture of proximal phalange diaphysis of the ring finger, multi-fragments and the ulnar part were moved

11.2 CT scan (Fig. 5.25e–h)

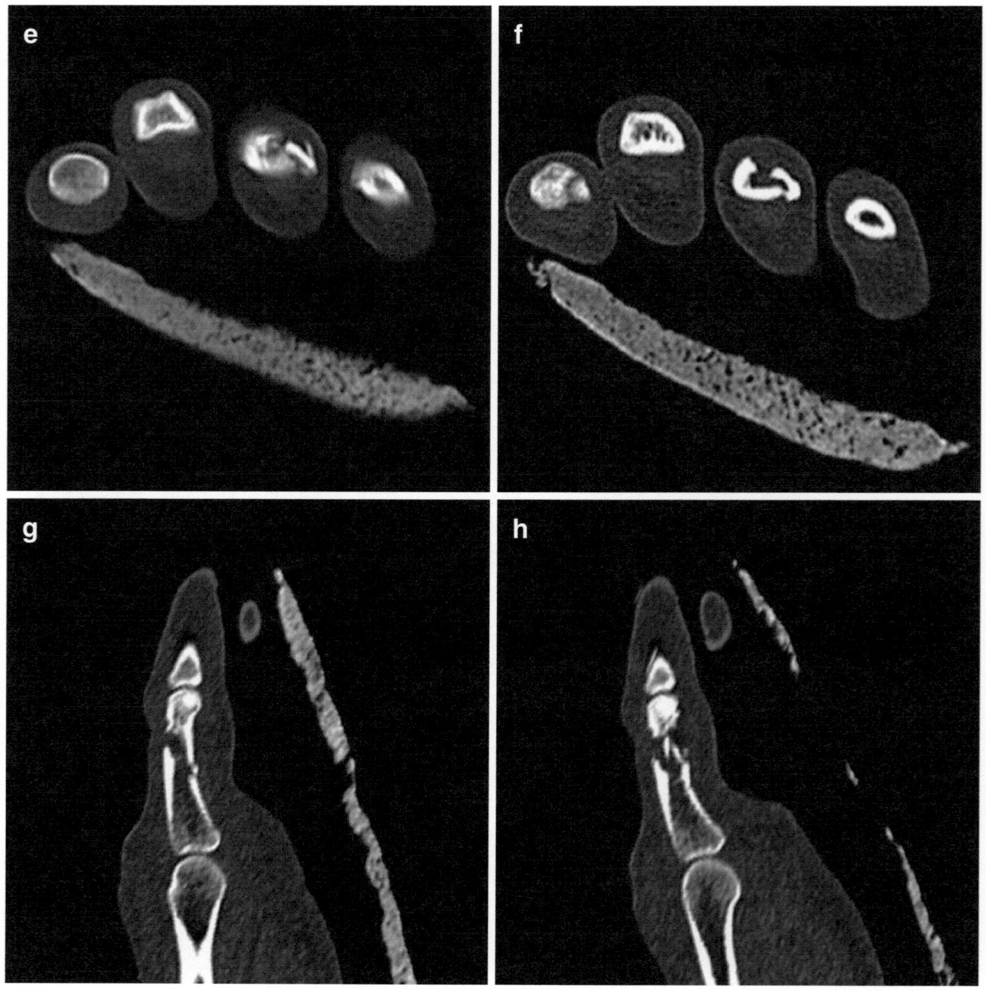

Fig. 5.25 The cross-section (**e**, **f**) and sagittal CT plane (**g**, **h**) show fracture of the proximal phalange diaphysis of the ring finger, multi-fragments and the broken ends were moved

12. Distal articular fracture of the middle phalange of ring finger
    12.1 X-ray (Fig. 5.26a–d)

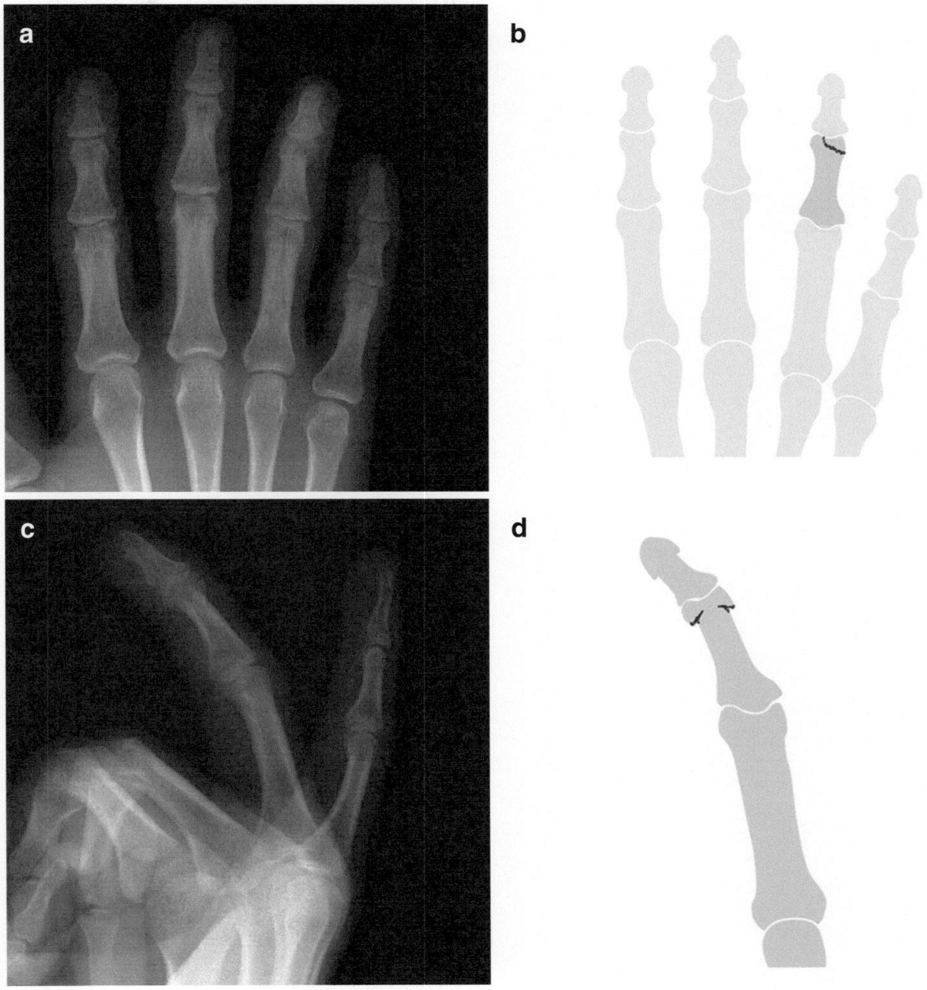

Fig. 5.26 X-ray (**a**, **c**) and illustration (**b**, **d**) show distal fracture of the middle phalange of ring finger, broken ends were slightly displaced

12.2 CT scan (Fig. 5.26e, f)

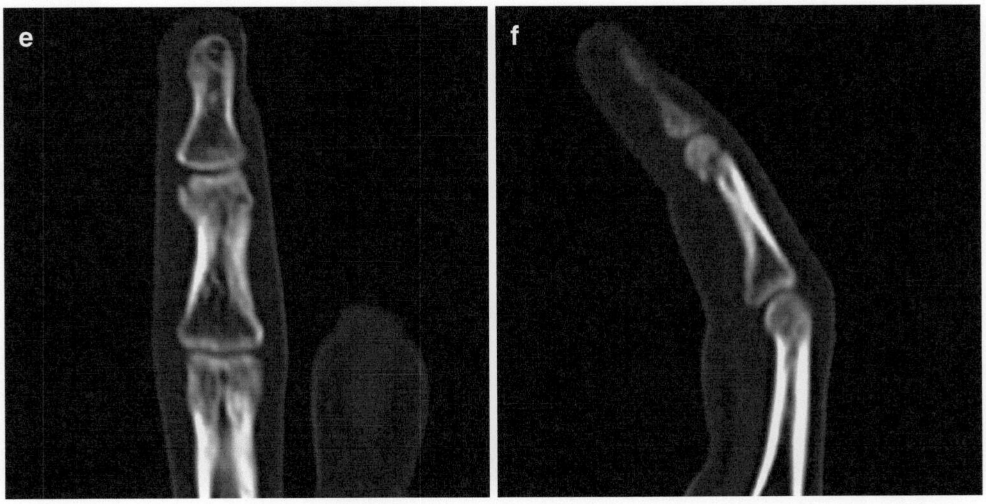

Fig. 5.26 The coronal (**e**) and sagittal CT plane (**f**) show distal fracture of the middle phalange of the ring finger, broken ends were slightly displaced

5.3 Summary

1. A standard AP and lateral view radiographs of the hand can confirm the diagnosis of most displaced fracture, while a post contrast CT scan and 3D reconstruction are better for identifying little avulsion fragments.
2. A fracture type is tied to its injury mechanism. Phalangeal fracture may occur when someone is orientated in a boxing position, whereby the phalanges are directly attacked by force. The diaphysis fractures most likely occur by rotational or longitudinal forces transmitted to the phalanges, while the basal articular fractures are caused by the axial forces.

Upper Limb Shaft Fracture

6

Yake Liu and Yingze Zhang

6.1 Humeral Shaft Fracture

The humeral shaft extends from the upper border of the pectoralis major insertion site to the supracondylar ridge distally. The proximal aspect of the humeral shaft is cylindrical on cross-section; distally, its anteroposterior diameter narrows. The radial nerve is subjected to injury when there is a fracture at the distal thirds of the humeral shaft. The humeral fractures accounted for 37.09% in adult humeral fractures.

6.1.1 Injury Mechanism

The humeral fracture can be caused by direct and indirect trauma. The mechanism can conclude in a fall from height, traffic accident, and tractive injury by machines. Abruptly contracted muscle, such as wrestling, also results in this type of fracture.

6.1.2 Signs and Symptoms

The most common clinical features are pain, swelling, limited mobility, and deformities.

6.1.3 Imaging

Basic radiography can provide sufficient recognition of the humeral fractures. However, one kind of a linear radiolucency formed by a humeral nutrient artery called vascular channel is easily mistaken as fracture; in addition, the Pediatric green-stick fracture also deserves more scrutiny.

Y. Liu · Y. Zhang (✉)
Department of Orthopaedics, The Third Hospital of Hebei Medical University, Shijiazhuang, Hebei, China

Y. Zhang (ed.), *Differential Diagnosis of Fracture*, https://doi.org/10.1007/978-981-13-8339-7_6

1. The comparison of radiography and CT in relation to spiral fracture in the upper middle part of humerus
   1.1 Radiography (Fig. 6.1a–d)

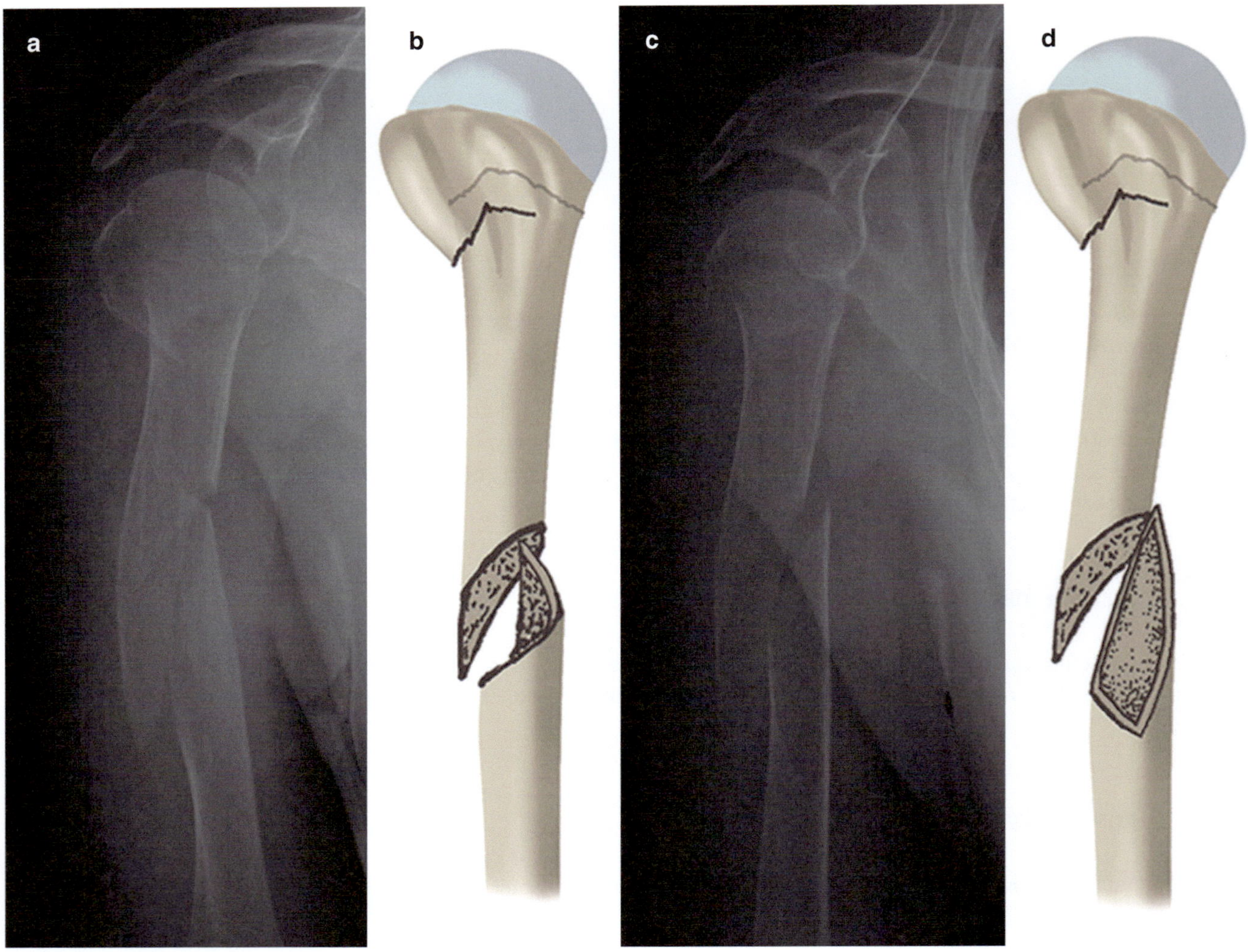

Fig. 6.1 Radiography (**a**, **c**) demonstrated spiral fracture in upper middle part of the humerus with displacement and angulation, humeral surgical neck fracture, displaced, compacted in broken end (**b**, **d**)

1.2 CT (Fig. 6.1e, f)

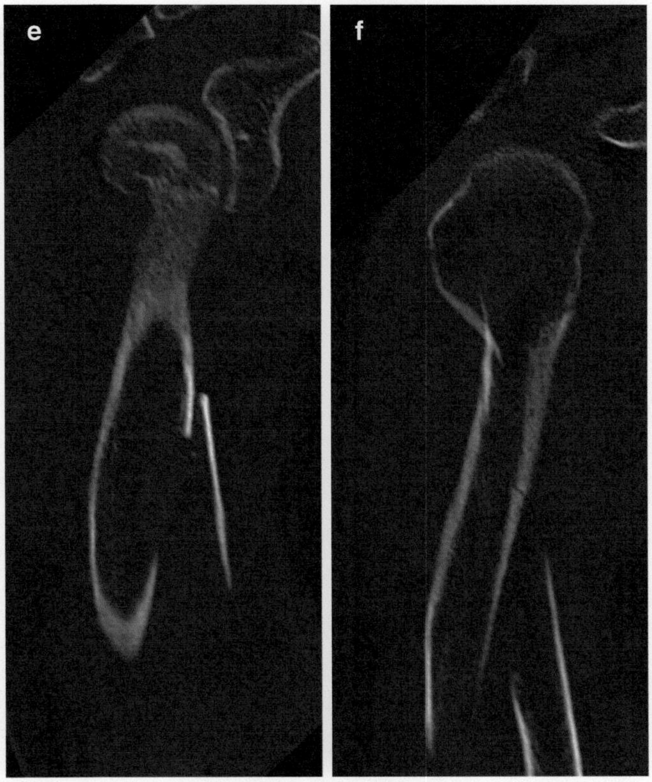

Fig. 6.1 CT in coronal (**e**) and sagittal view (**f**) demonstrates a spiral fracture in the upper middle part of humerus, displaced and angulation, and impacted humeral neck fracture

2. The comparison of a radiography and CT for a spiral fracture in the middle and lower part of humerus
   2.1 Radiography (Fig. 6.2a–d)

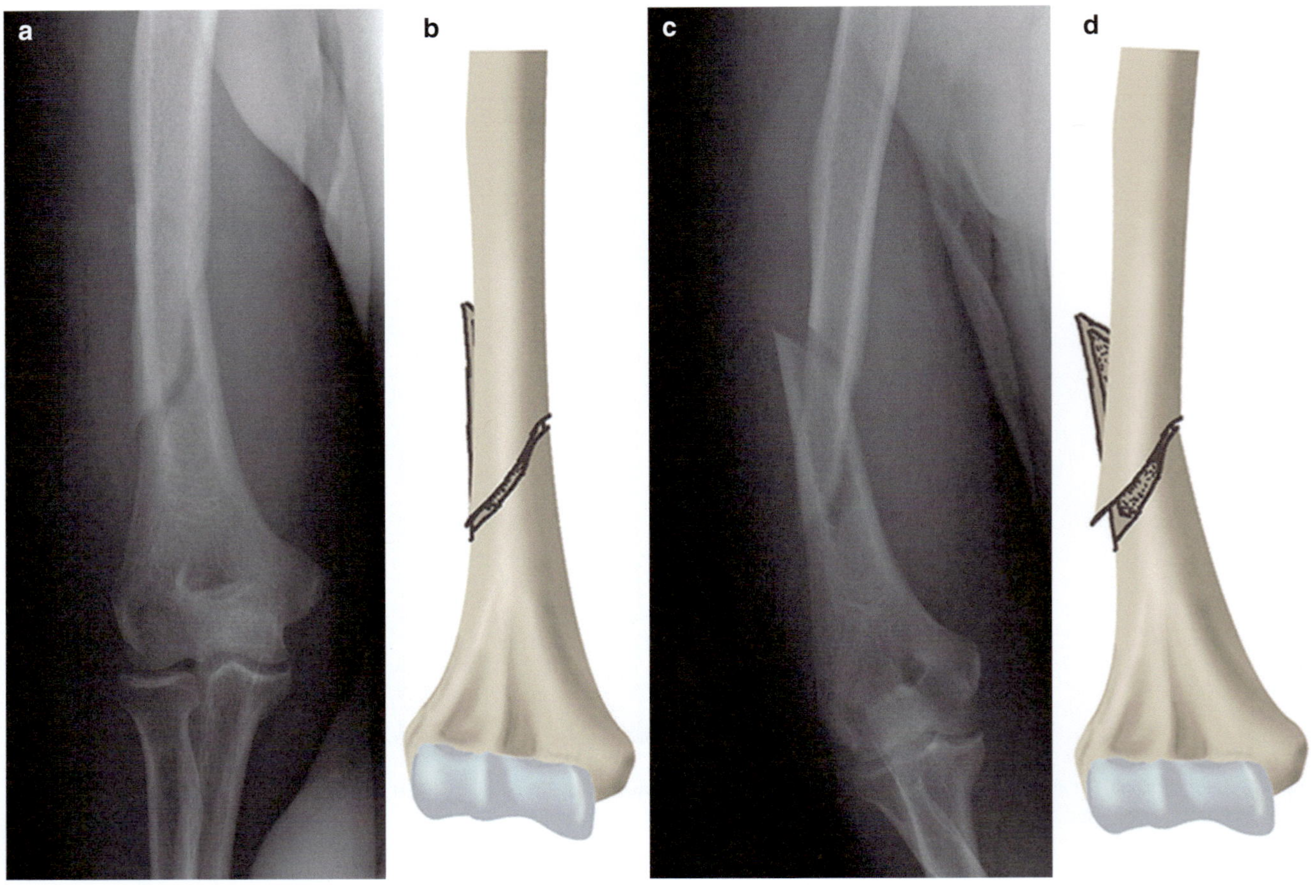

Fig. 6.2 The radiography (**a**, **c**) demonstrates a spiral fracture in middle and lower part of humerus, displaced and angulation, sketch (**b**, **d**)

2.2 CT (Fig. 6.2e–h)

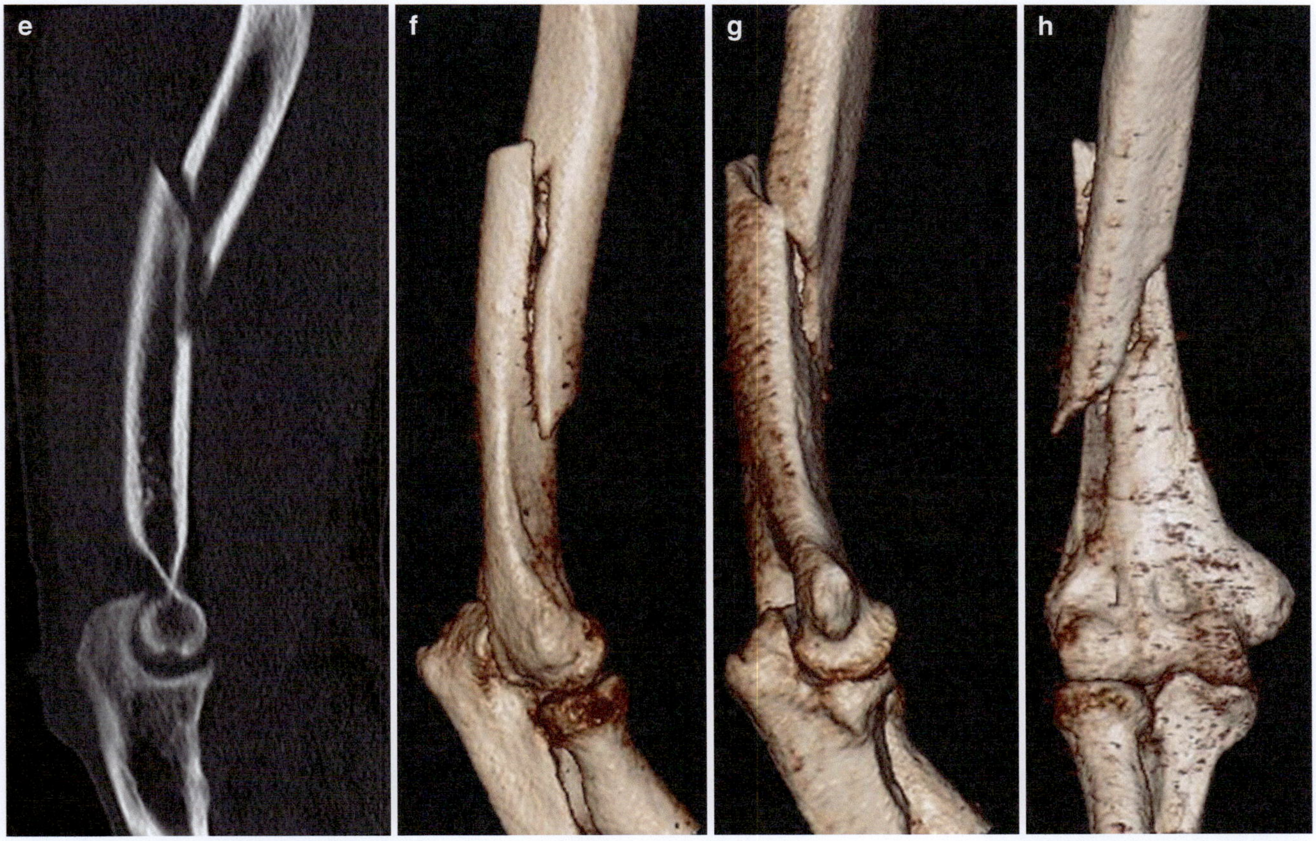

Fig. 6.2 CT in sagittal (**e**) and 3D reconstructions (**f–h**) demonstrates spiral fracture in middle and lower part of humerus, displaced and angulation

3. The comparison of radiography and CT for an oblique fracture in upper end of humerus
   3.1 Radiography (Fig. 6.3a–d)

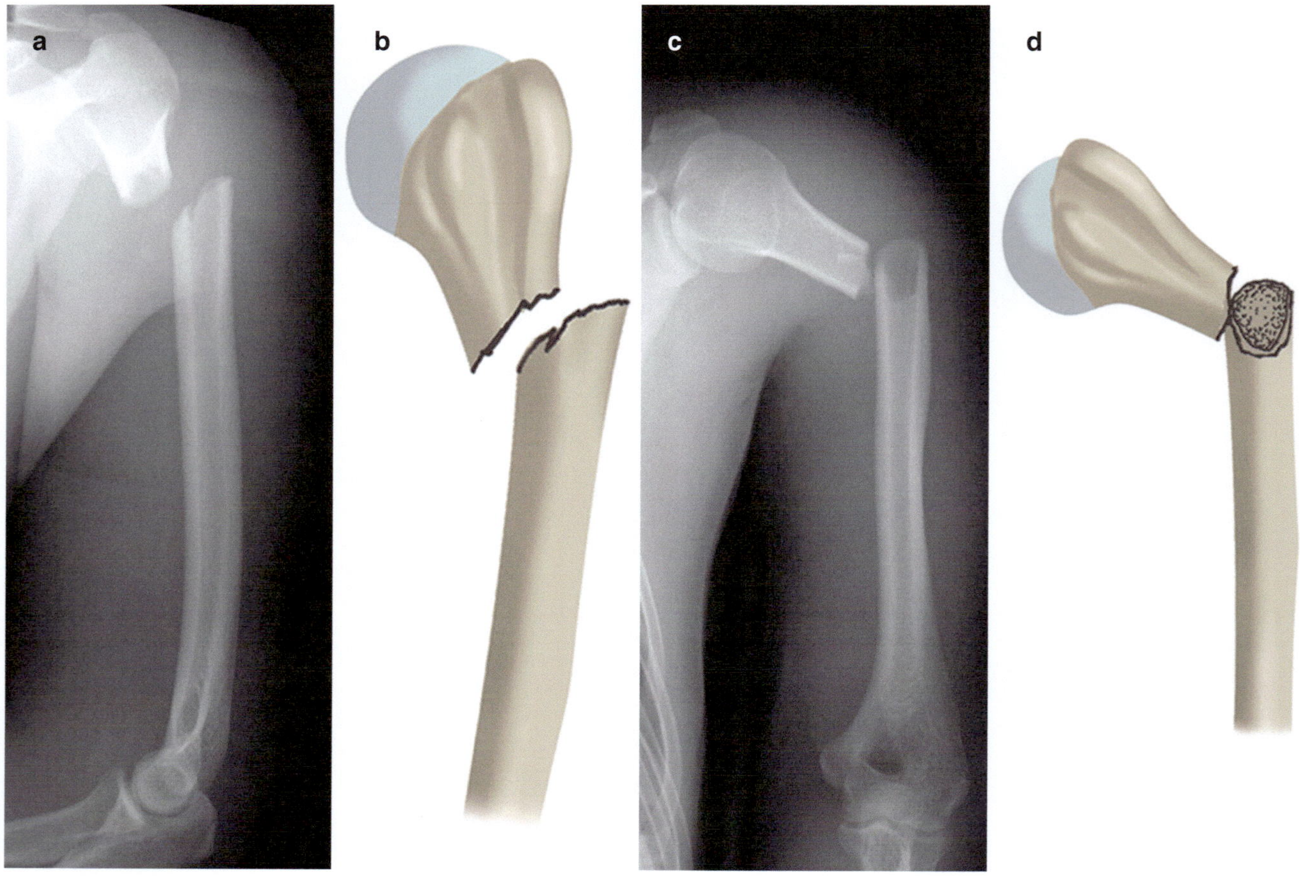

Fig. 6.3 Radiography (**a, c**) demonstrates oblique fracture in upper end of humerus, displaced and angulation, sketch (**b**, **d**)

3.2 CT (Fig. 6.3e, f)

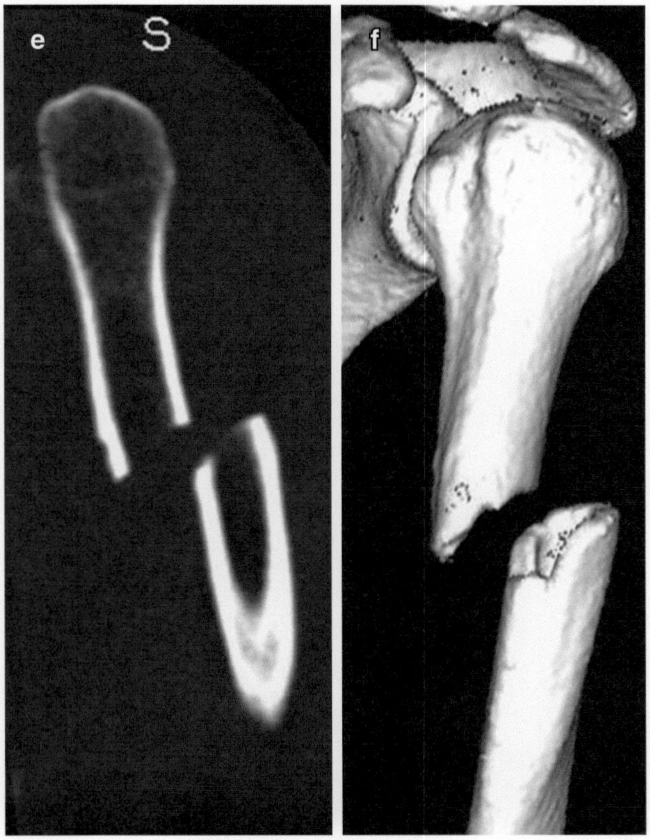

Fig. 6.3 CT in sagittal (**e**) and 3D reconstructions (**f**) demonstrates oblique fracture in upper end of humerus, displaced

4. The comparison of radiography and CT in oblique fracture in upper end of humerus
   4.1 Radiography (Fig. 6.4a–d)

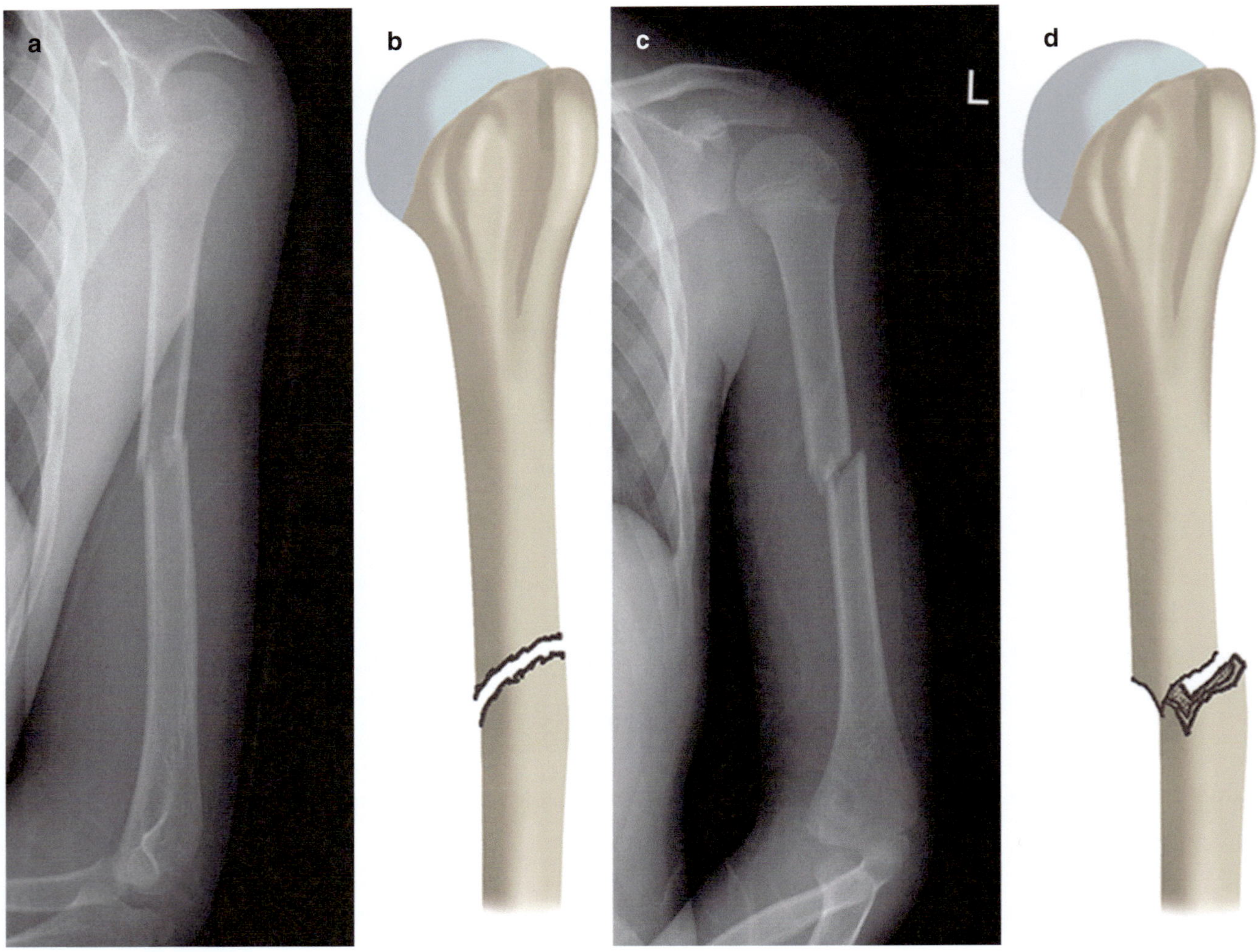

Fig. 6.4 Radiography (**a**, **c**) demonstrates oblique fracture in middle part of humerus, displaced and angulation, sketch (**b**, **d**)

4.2 CT (Fig. 6.4e, f)

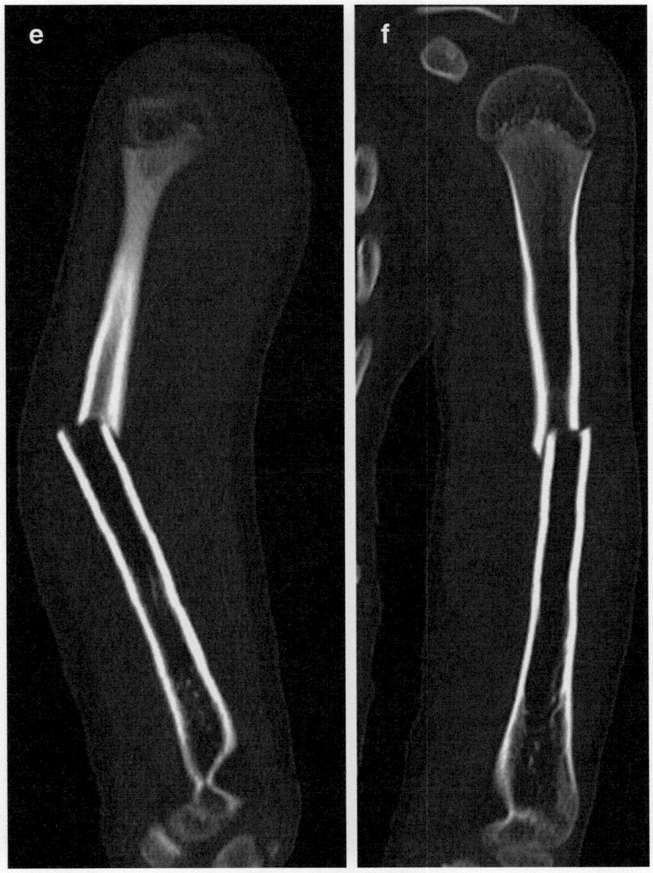

Fig. 6.4 CT in sagittal (**e**) and coronal view (**f**) demonstrates displaced, oblique fracture in middle part of humerus

5. The comparison of radiography and CT of a spiral oblique fracture in the middle part of the humerus
   5.1 Radiography (Fig. 6.5a–d)

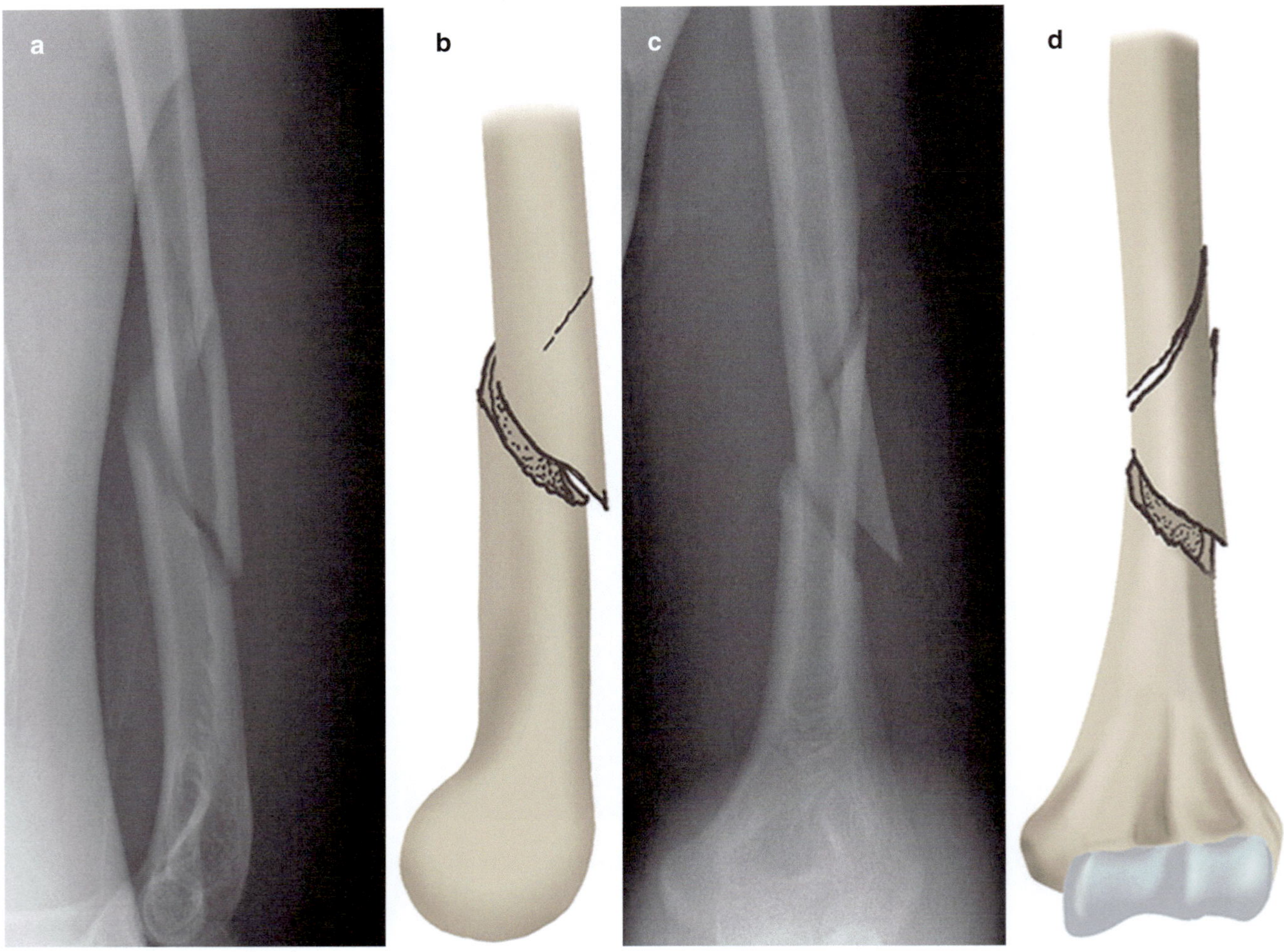

Fig. 6.5 Radiography (**a**, **c**) spiral oblique fracture with displaced and angulation in the middle part of the humerus, sketch (**b**, **d**)

5.2 CT (Fig. 6.5e, f)

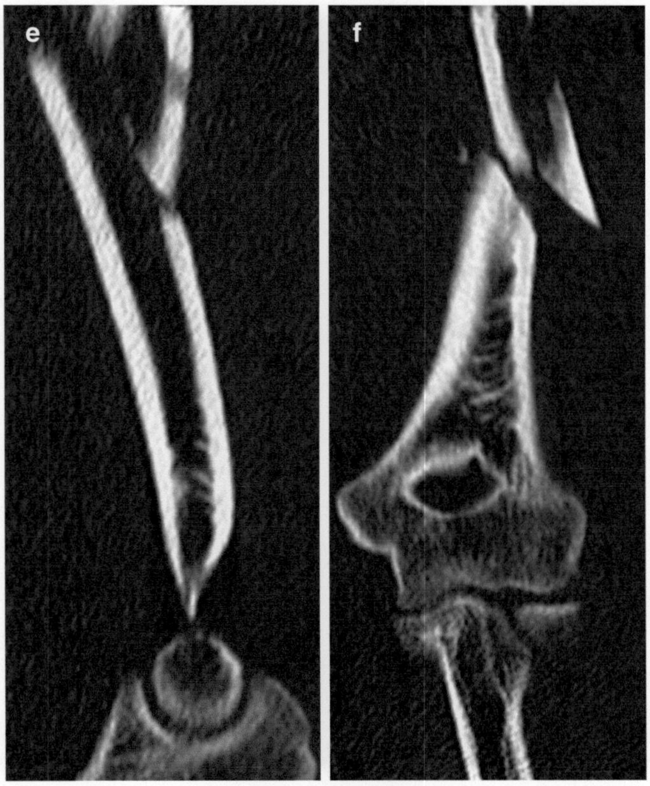

Fig. 6.5 CT in sagittal (**e**) and coronal (**f**) demonstrates displaced and angled spiral fracture in middle part of the humerus

6. The comparison of radiography and CT for oblique fracture in the middle part of the humerus
   6.1 Radiography (Fig. 6.6a–d)

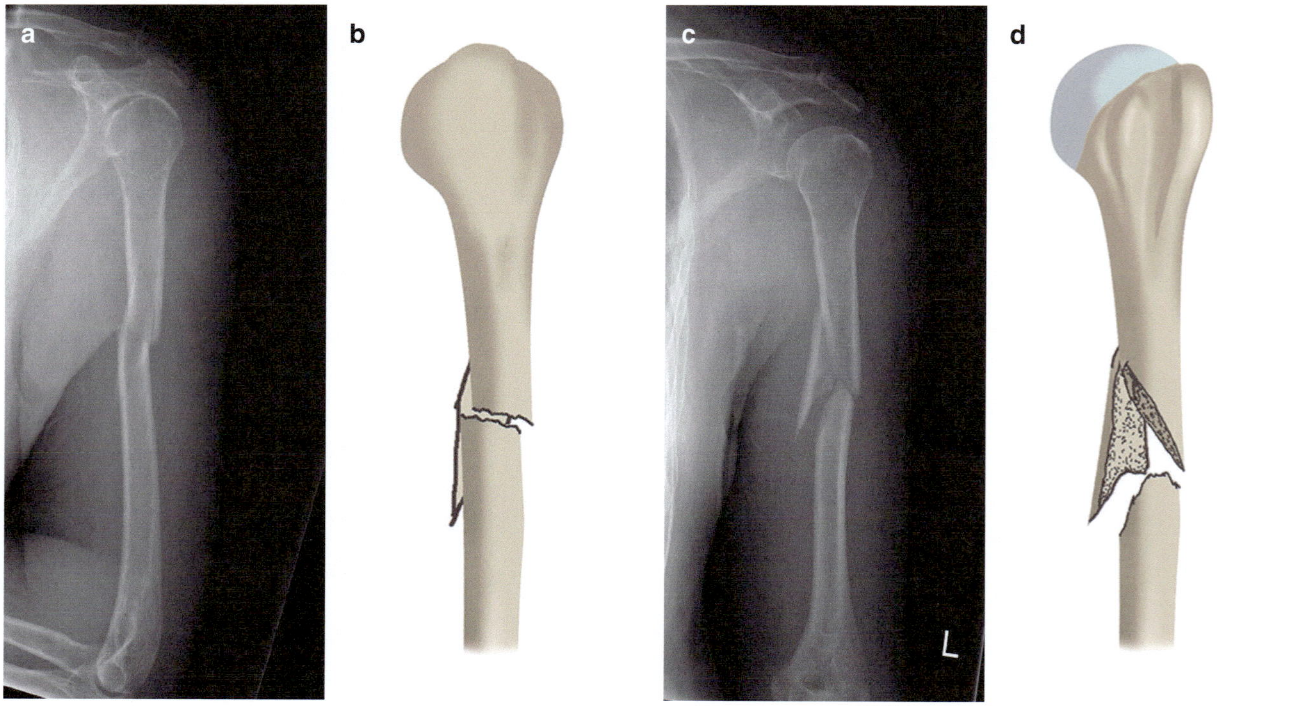

Fig. 6.6 Radiography (**a**, **c**) demonstrates curled and wedge shaped fracture in middle part of the humerus with displacement and angulation, sketch (**b**, **d**)

   6.2 CT (Fig. 6.6e–h)

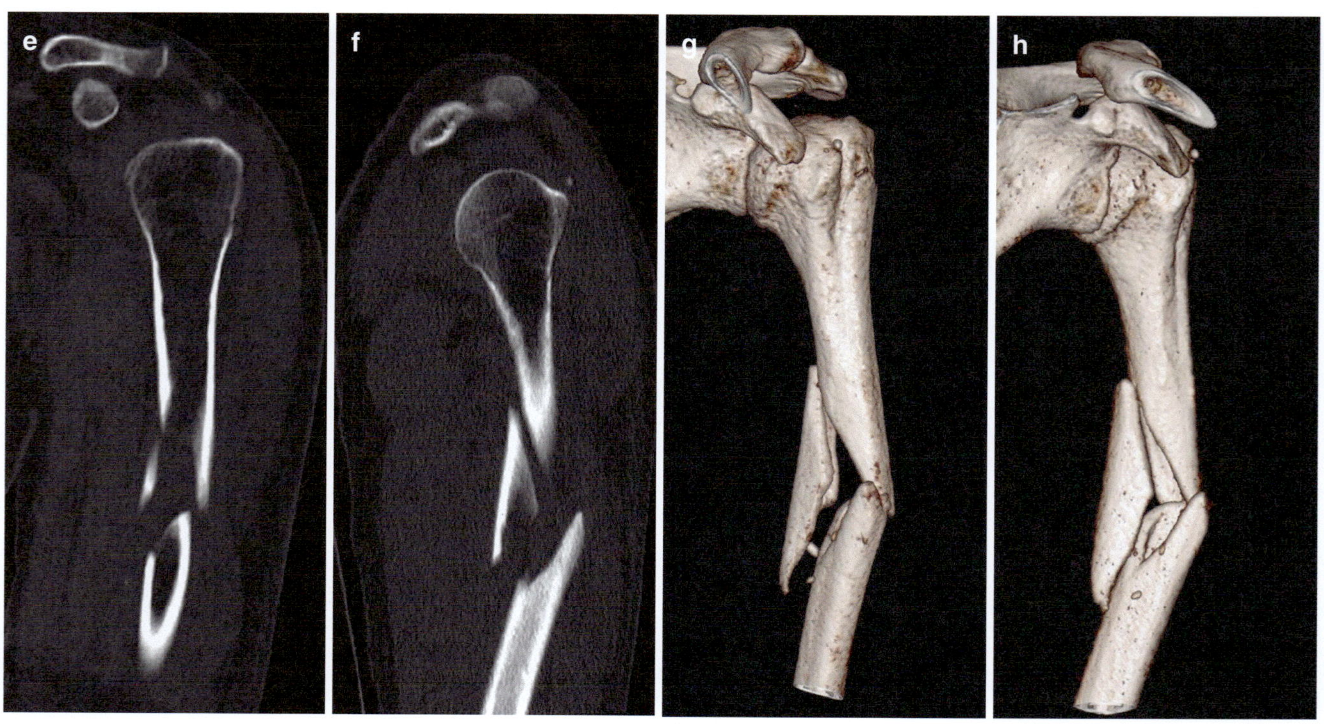

Fig. 6.6 CT in sagittal (**e**), coronal (**f**), and 3D reconstructed view (**g**, **h**) demonstrates spiral fracture in middle part of the humerus with displacement and angulation

7. The comparison of radiography and CT for humeral shaft comminuted fracture
   7.1 Radiography (Fig. 6.7a–d)

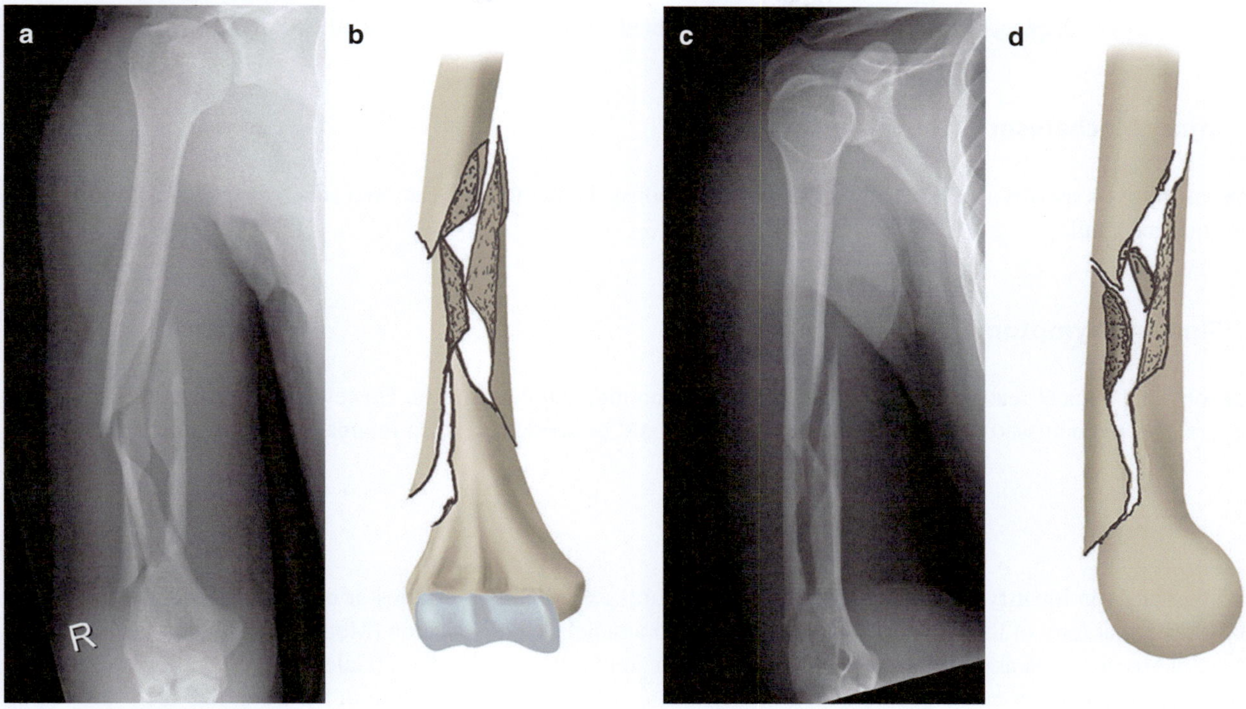

Fig. 6.7 Radiography (**a**, **c**) demonstrates comminuted fracture in middle and lower part of humerus, with some fragments presented and displacement, sketch (**b**, **d**)

   7.2 CT (Fig. 6.7e–h)

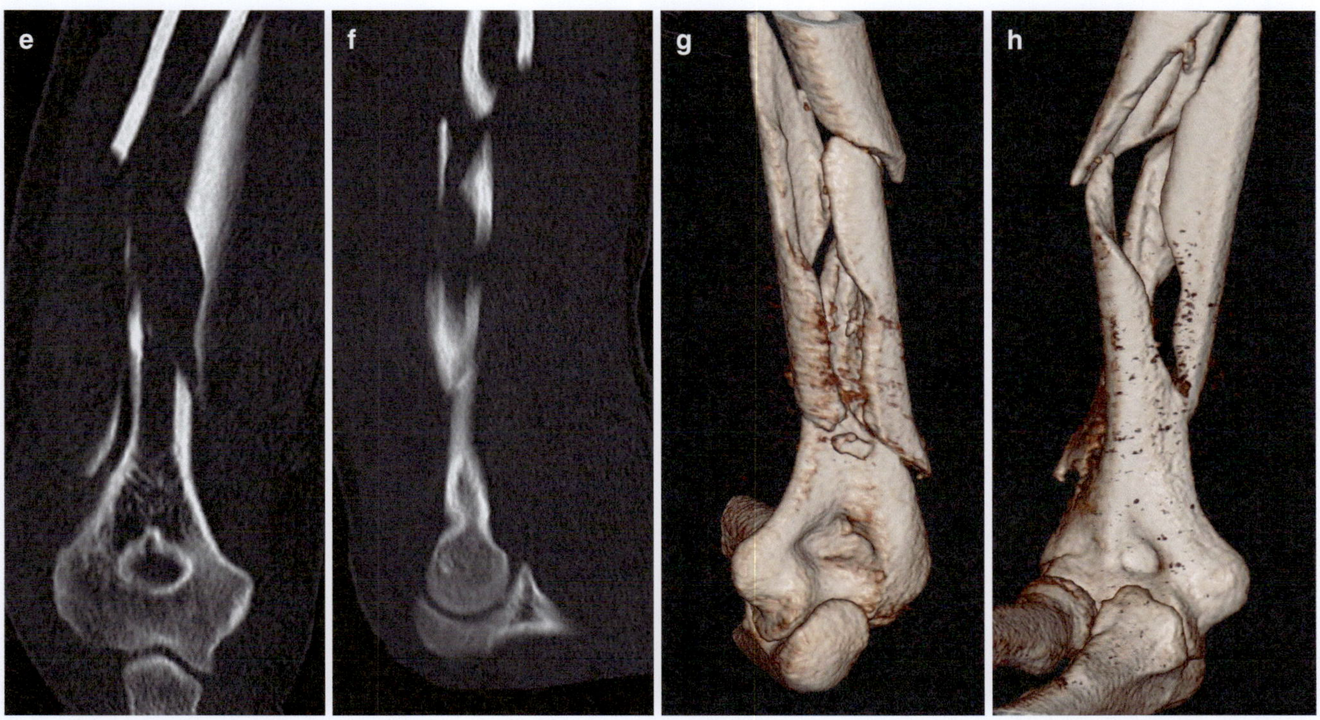

Fig. 6.7 CT in sagittal (**e**), coronal (**f**), and 3D reconstructed view (**g**, **h**) demonstrates humeral comminuted fracture in middle and lower part with displacement and angulation

6.2 Ulnar and Radial Shaft Fracture

The ulna and radius are the bony structures of the forearm, joined by the proximal and distal radioulnar joints, as well as the interosseous membrane (IOM). If one bone shows a fracture with displacement or angulation, usually the other bone will also have a fracture or displacement. The shaft fracture accounted 23.31% in ulnar and radial fractures.

6.2.1 Injury Mechanism

This type of injury is usually caused by direct or indirect trauma. Direct trauma can be a strike or collision; and indirect violence could be a fall.

6.2.2 Sign and Symptoms

The most obvious clinical feature is pain, swelling, limited motion, and deformities. However, many un-displaced simple fractures are easy to be missed. Imagological investigation should be conducted when trauma is present in the forearms

6.2.3 Imaging

Basic radiography can identify humeral fractures. Most fractures exhibited two injuries or dislocations, for instance, fractures of the proximal third of the ulna, often accompanied with a radial head dislocation (Monteggia). Fractures of the distal third of the radius are often associated with a distal radioulnar joint (DRU) dislocation (Galeazzi). In addition, the fracture in the proximal ulna is often accompanied with a humeroradial dislocation. The fracture in the distal radius is likely to be accompanied by a distal radioulnar joint dislocation. However, a few of them were simple fractures. Furthermore, a linear radiolucency formed by a humeral nutrient artery—called a vascular channel—should be ruled out for fractures. It is not unusual that Pediatric greenstick fractures bear the same risk of pitfalls for the unwary.

1. The comparison of radiography and CT about Monteggia fracture
   1.1 Radiography (Fig. 6.8a–d)

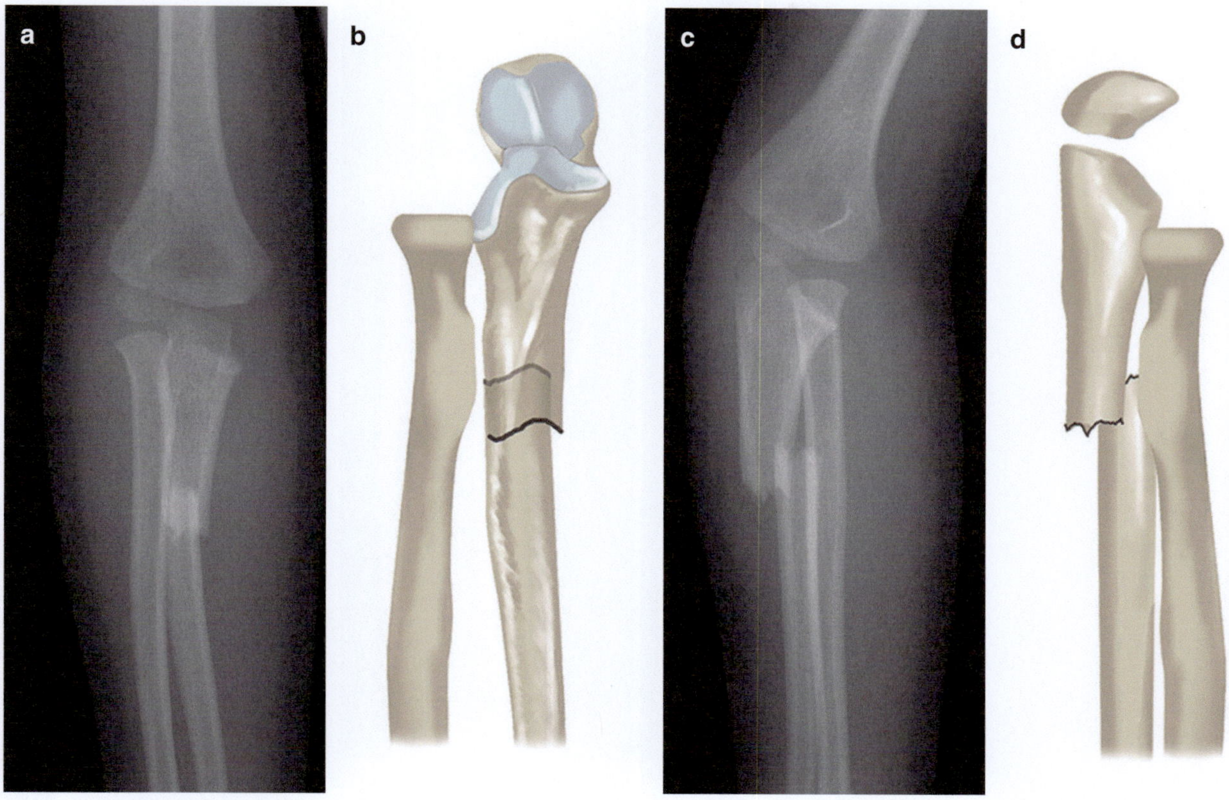

Fig. 6.8 Radiography (**a**, **c**) demonstrates ulna transverse fracture in upper part with displacement and humeroradial joint dislocation, sketch (**b**, **d**)

1.2 CT (Fig. 6.8e, f)

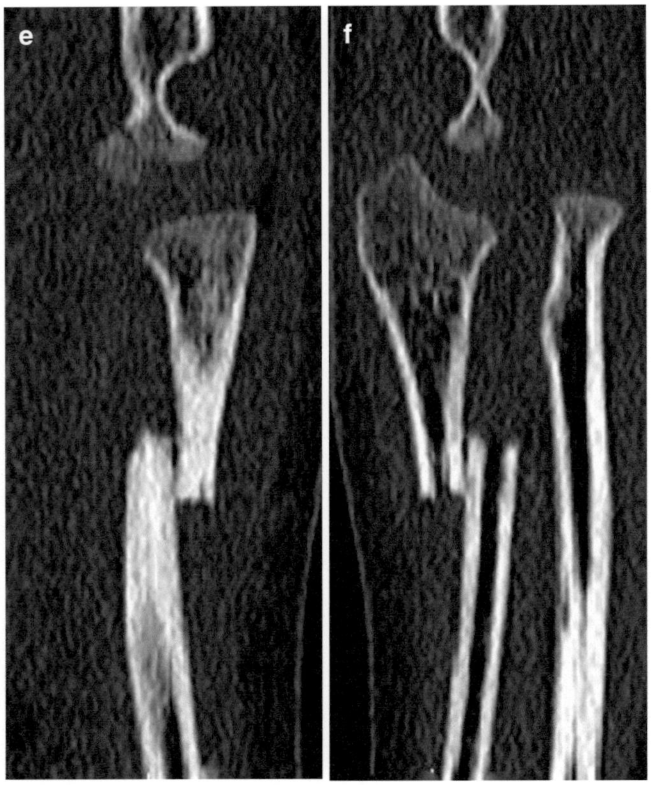

Fig. 6.8 CT in coronal (**e**), sagittal (**f**) view demonstrates ulnar transverse fracture in upper part with displacement, angulation and anterior dislocation of radial head

2. The comparison of radiography and CT about spiral fracture in lower radial part
   2.1 Radiography (Fig. 6.9a, b)

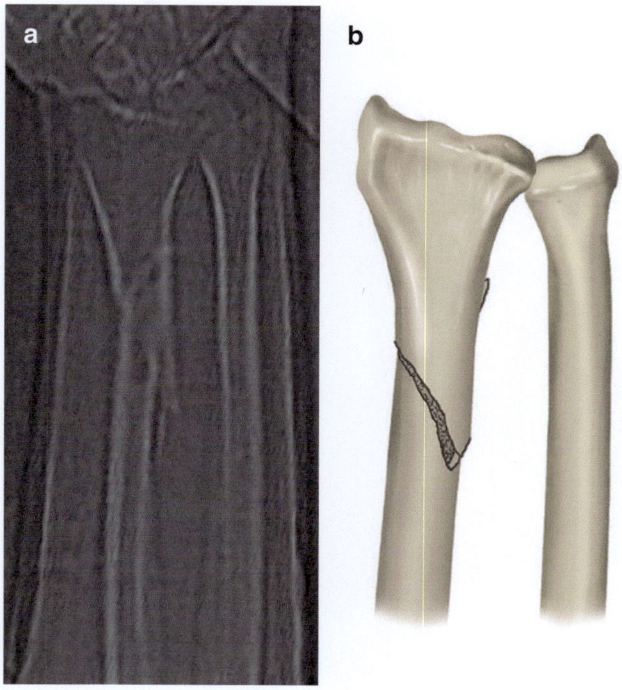

Fig. 6.9 Radiography (**a**) demonstrated oblique fracture in lower part of radius with displacement and angulation, sketch (**b**)

   2.2 CT (Fig. 6.9c–e)

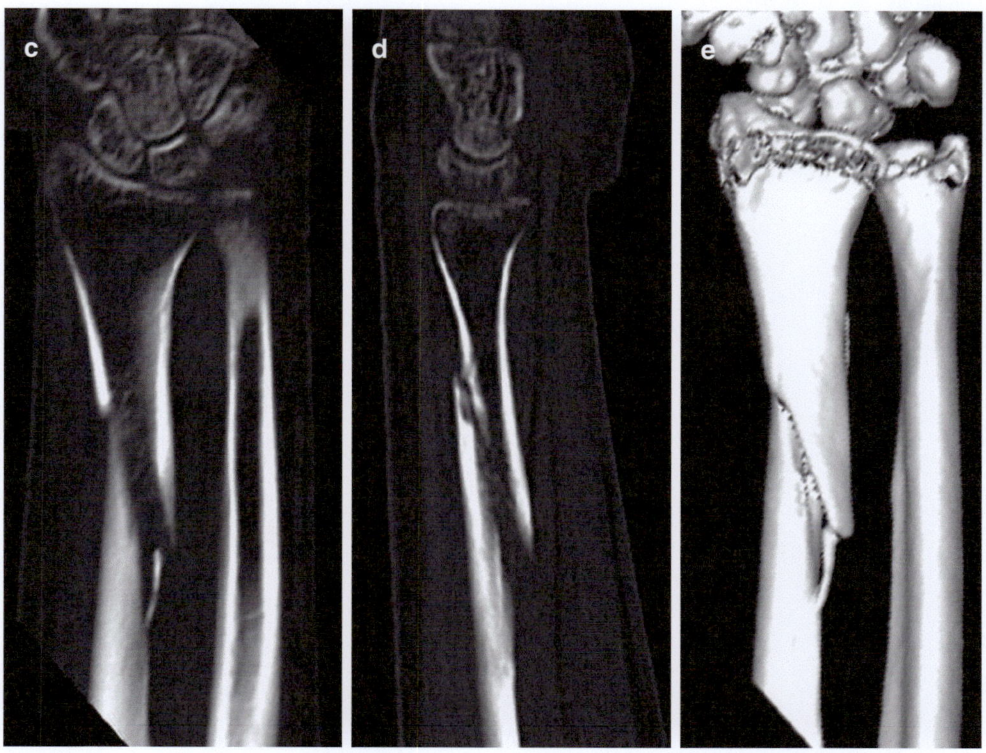

Fig. 6.9 CT in coronal (**c**), sagittal (**d**), and 3D reconstructions view (**e**) demonstrated radial fracture in distal part displacement, wedge shaped bone fragment and angulation

3. The comparison of radiography and CT for transverse fracture of ulna and radius in the lower part
   3.1 Radiography (Fig. 6.10a–d)

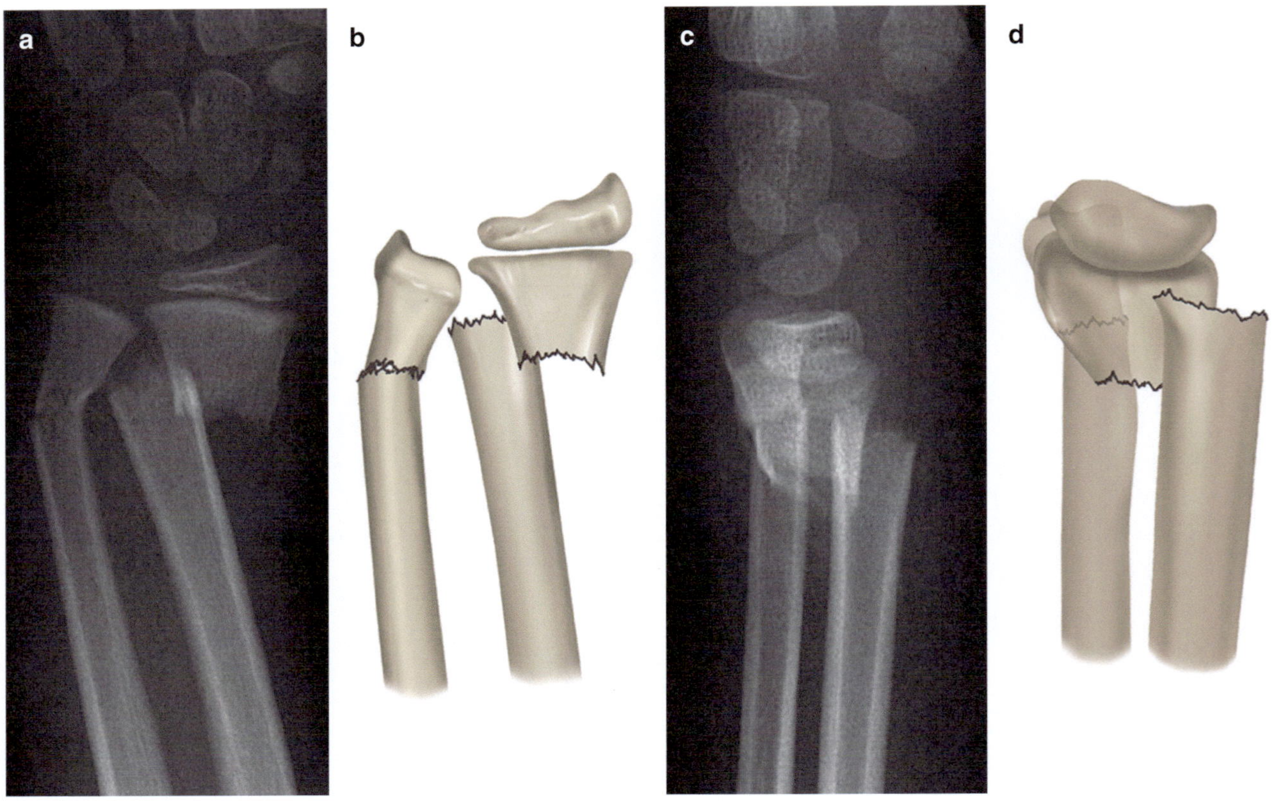

Fig. 6.10 Radiography (**a**, **c**) demonstrates transverse fracture in lower part of the ulna and radius, displacement and angulation in radius, angulation in ulna, sketch (**b**, **d**)

3.2 CT (Fig. 6.10e, f)

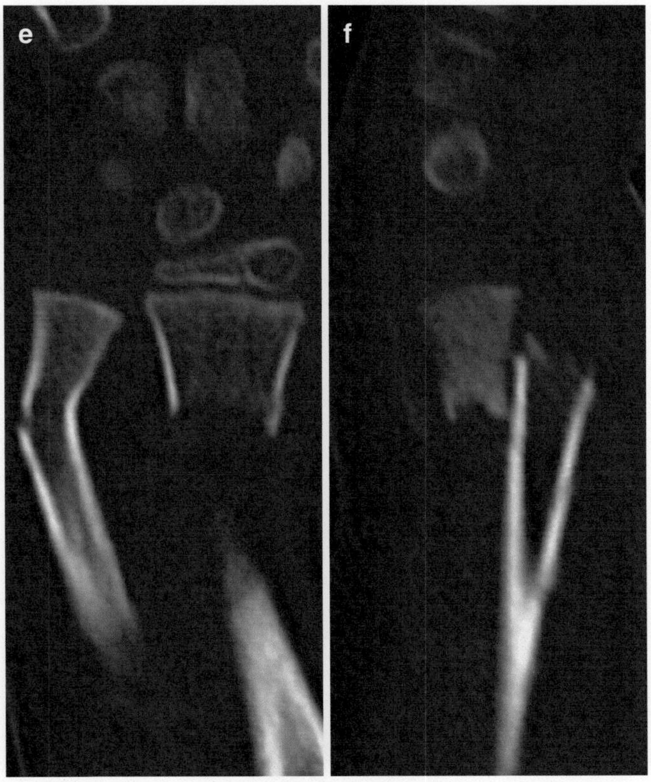

Fig. 6.10 CT in coronal (**e**) and sagittal (**f**) view demonstrates transverse fracture in upper part of ulna and radius with overlap and displacement in radius, angulation in ulna

4. The comparison of radiography and CT about transverse fracture in the upper middle part of the ulna
   4.1 Radiography (Fig. 6.11a–d)

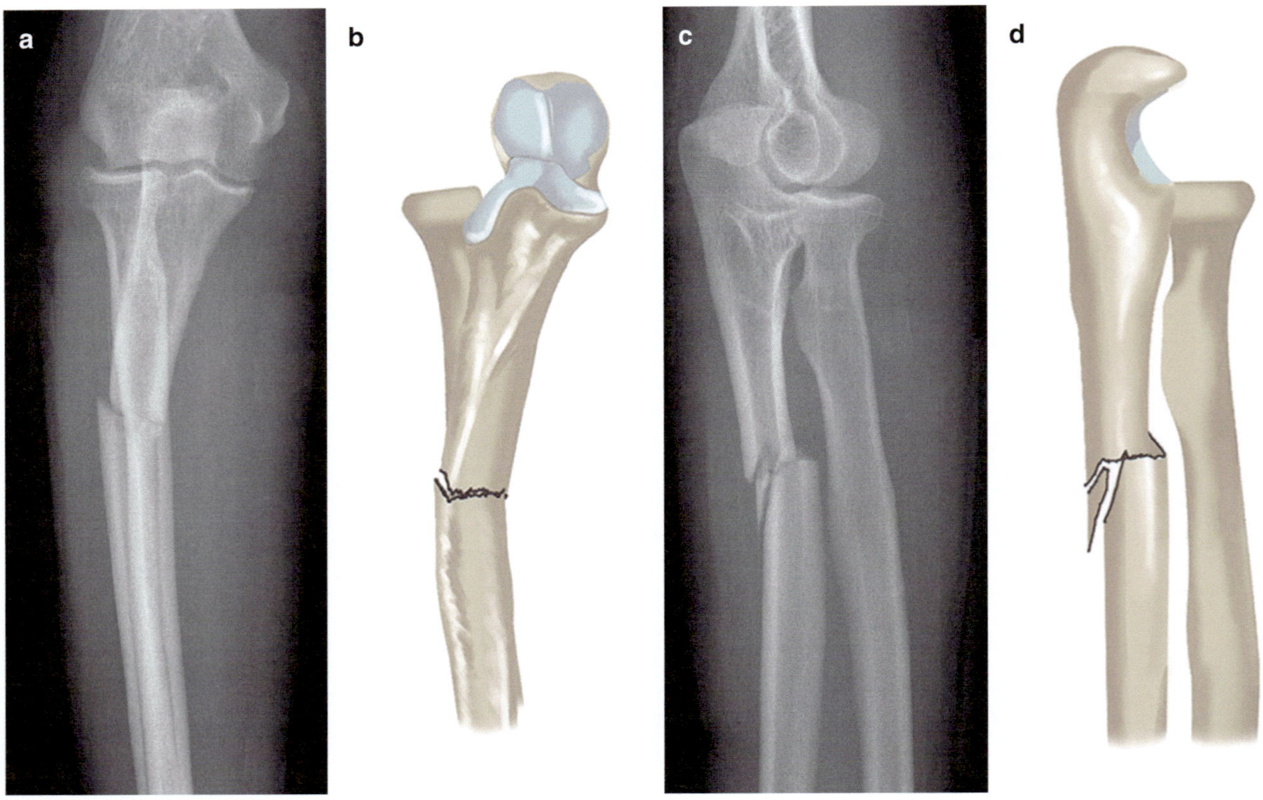

Fig. 6.11 Radiography (**a**, **c**) demonstrates wedge shaped fracture in the upper part of the ulna, displacement and wedge shaped bone fragment, sketch (**b**, **d**)

4.2 CT (Fig. 6.11e, f)

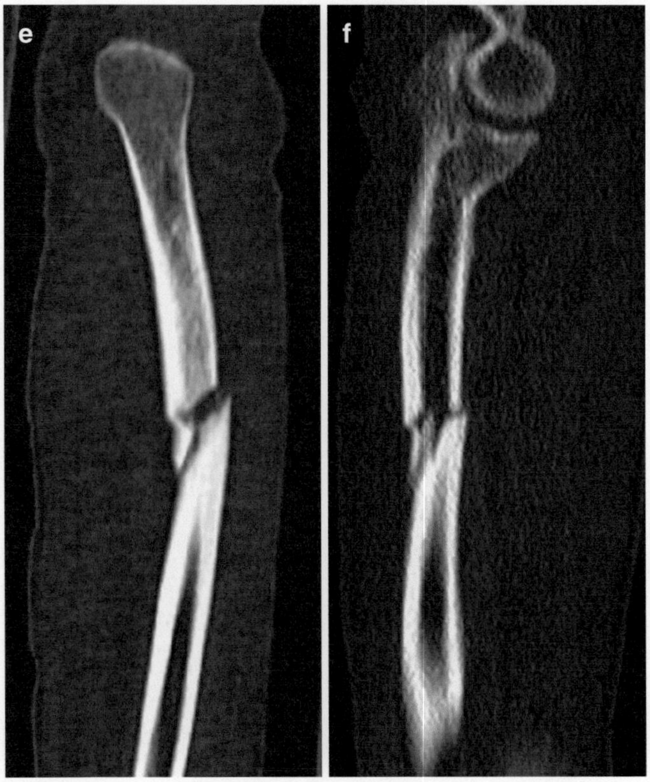

Fig. 6.11 CT in coronal (**e**) and sagittal (**f**) view demonstrates transverse fracture in the upper part of the ulna, displacement and wedge shaped fragment presented

5. The comparison of radiography and CT in wedge shaped fracture in upper middle part of ulna with anterior displacement of radial head
   5.1 Radiography (Fig. 6.12a–d)

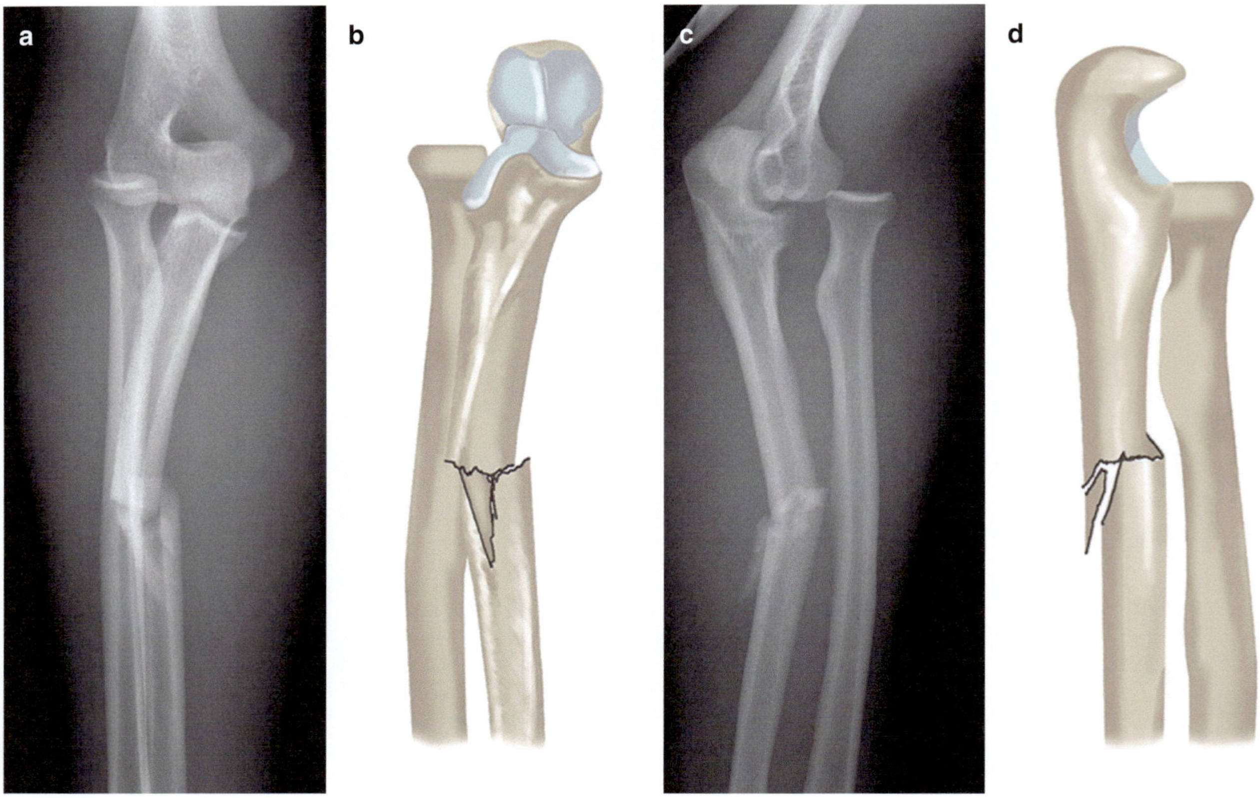

Fig. 6.12 Radiography (**a**, **c**) demonstrates wedge shaped fracture in the upper part of the ulna with displacement and angulation, wedge shaped fragment humeroradial joint dislocation, anterolateral displacement of radial head, sketch (**b**, **d**)

5.2 CT (Fig. 6.12e, f)

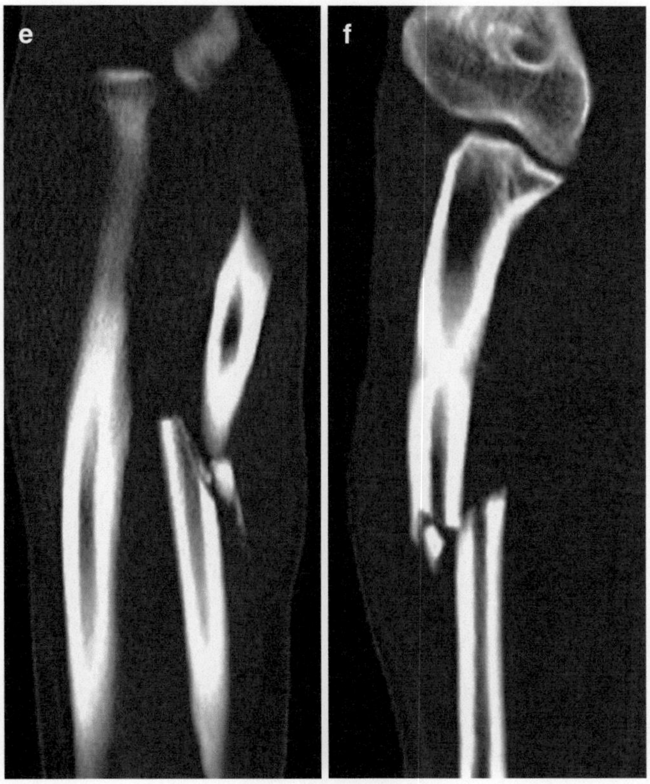

Fig. 6.12 CT in sagittal (**e**) and coronal view (**f**) demonstrates wedge shaped fracture in the upper part of the ulna with fracture displaced and wedge shaped bone fragment, humeroradial joint dislocation, anterolateral displacement of radial head

6. The character of comminuted fracture in upper part of radius
   6.1 CT (Fig. 6.13a–d)

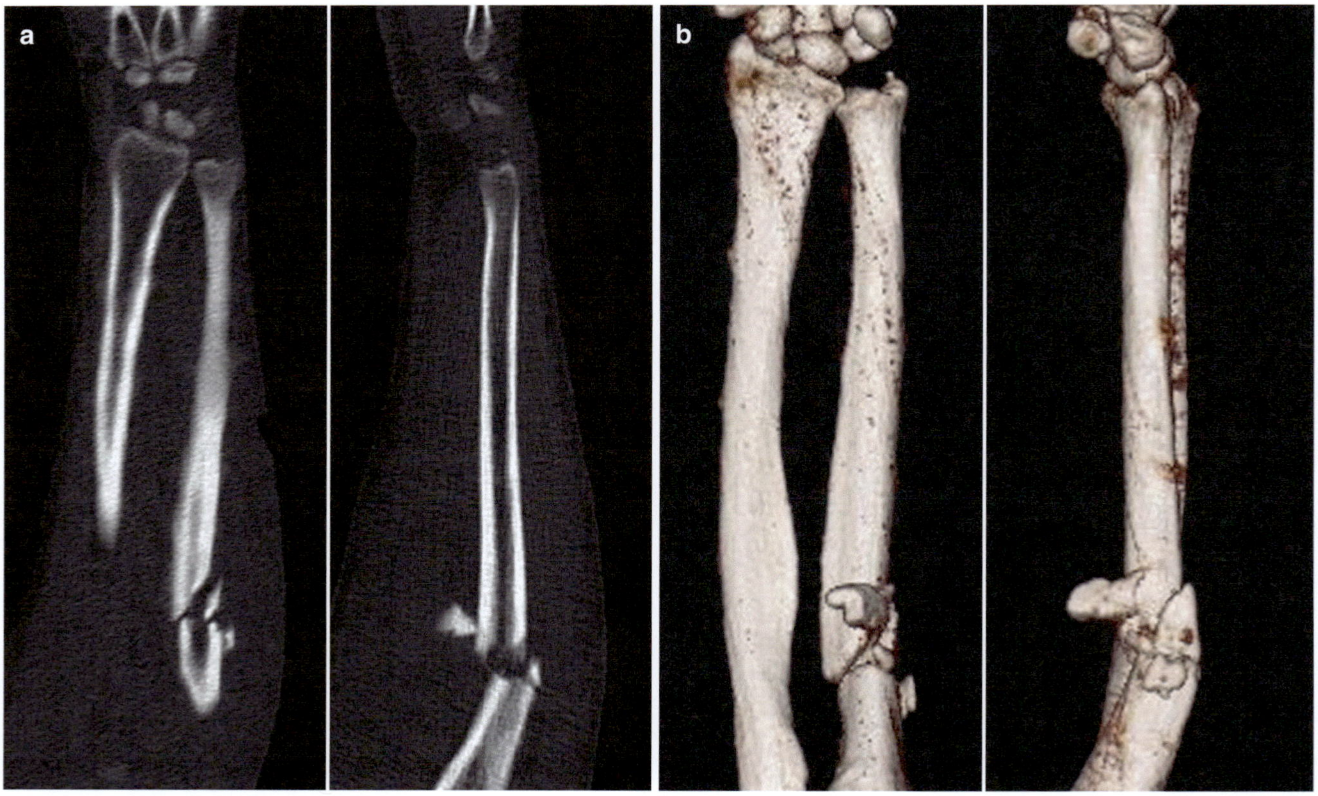

Fig. 6.13 CT in coronal (**a**) and sagittal view (**b**) demonstrates wedge shaped fracture in upper part of radius with displacement and angulation

7. The comparison of radiography and CT about comminuted fracture in the upper middle part of the ulna and radius; with anterior displacement of radial head
   7.1 Radiography (Fig. 6.14a–d)

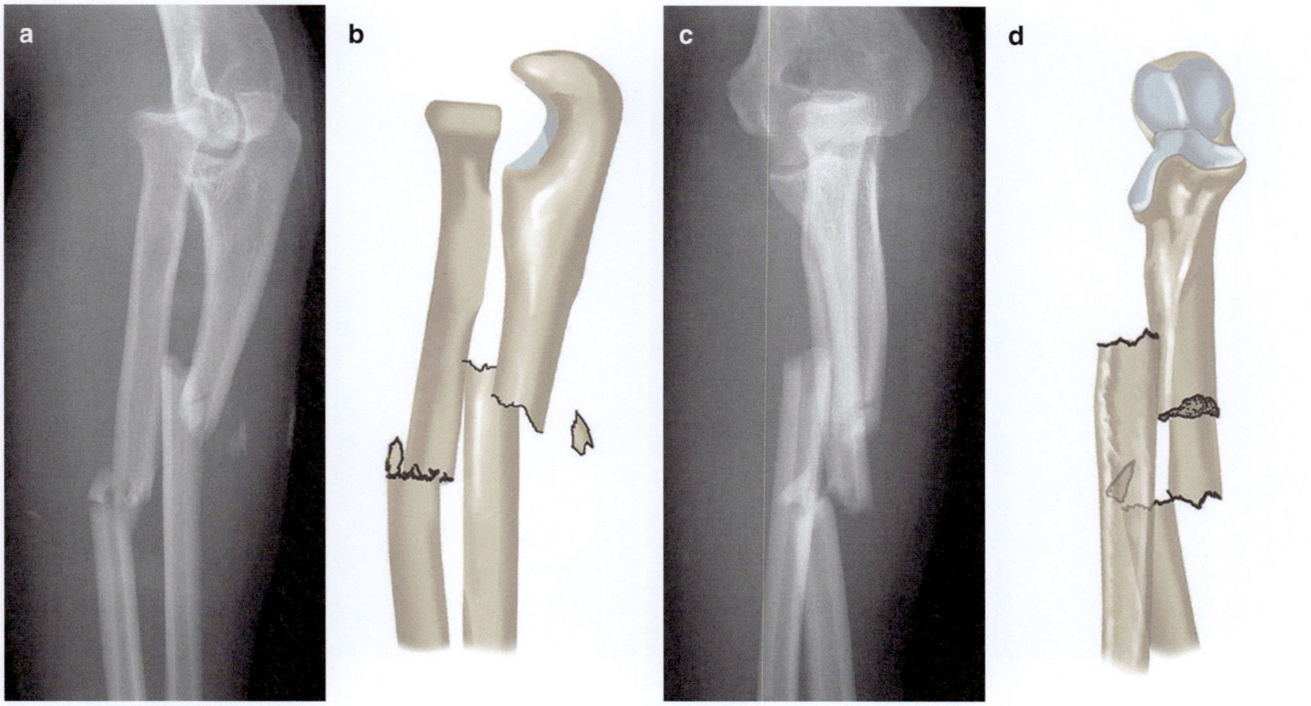

Fig. 6.14 Radiography (**a**, **c**) demonstrates comminuted fracture in the upper middle part of the ulna and radius with displacement and angulation, dislocation of humeroradial joint presented, sketch (**b**, **d**)

   7.2 CT (Fig. 6.14e–h)

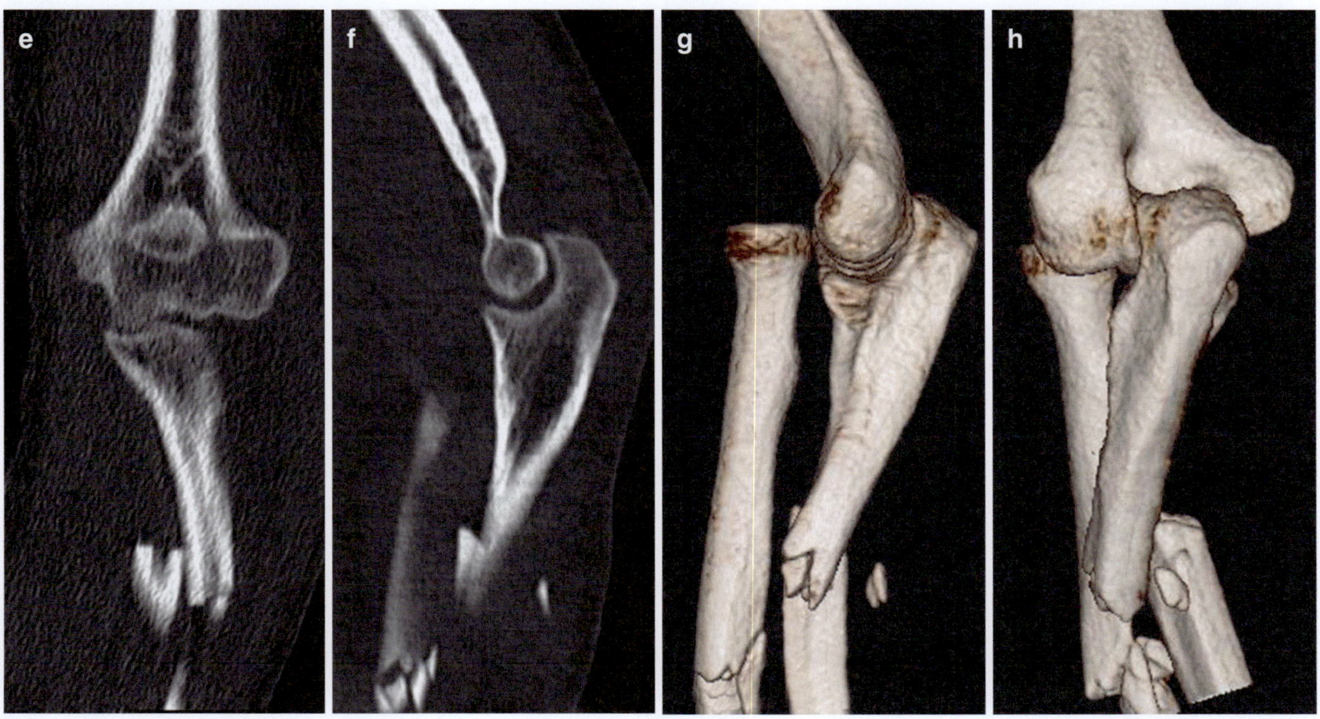

Fig. 6.14 CT in sagittal (**e**), coronal (**f**), and 3D reconstruction (**g**, **h**) view demonstrates comminuted fracture in the upper middle part of ulna and radius with displacement and angulation, dislocation of humeroradial joint, and anterior displacement of radial head

8. The comparison of radiography and CT in pediatric Monteggia fracture
   8.1 Radiography (Fig. 6.15a–d)

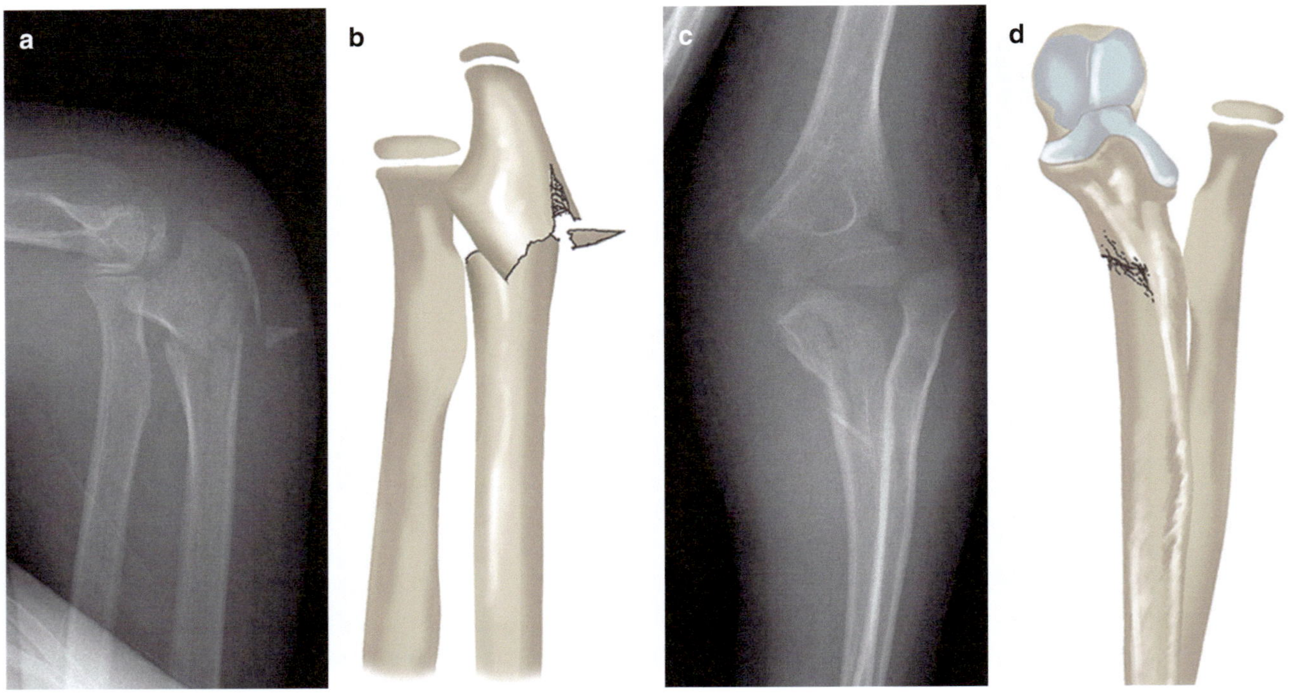

Fig. 6.15 Radiography (**a**, **c**) demonstrates a comminuted fracture in upper part of the ulna with displacement and angulation, dislocation of humeroradial joint and radial displacement of radial head, sketch (**b**, **d**)

   8.2 CT (Fig. 6.15e–h)

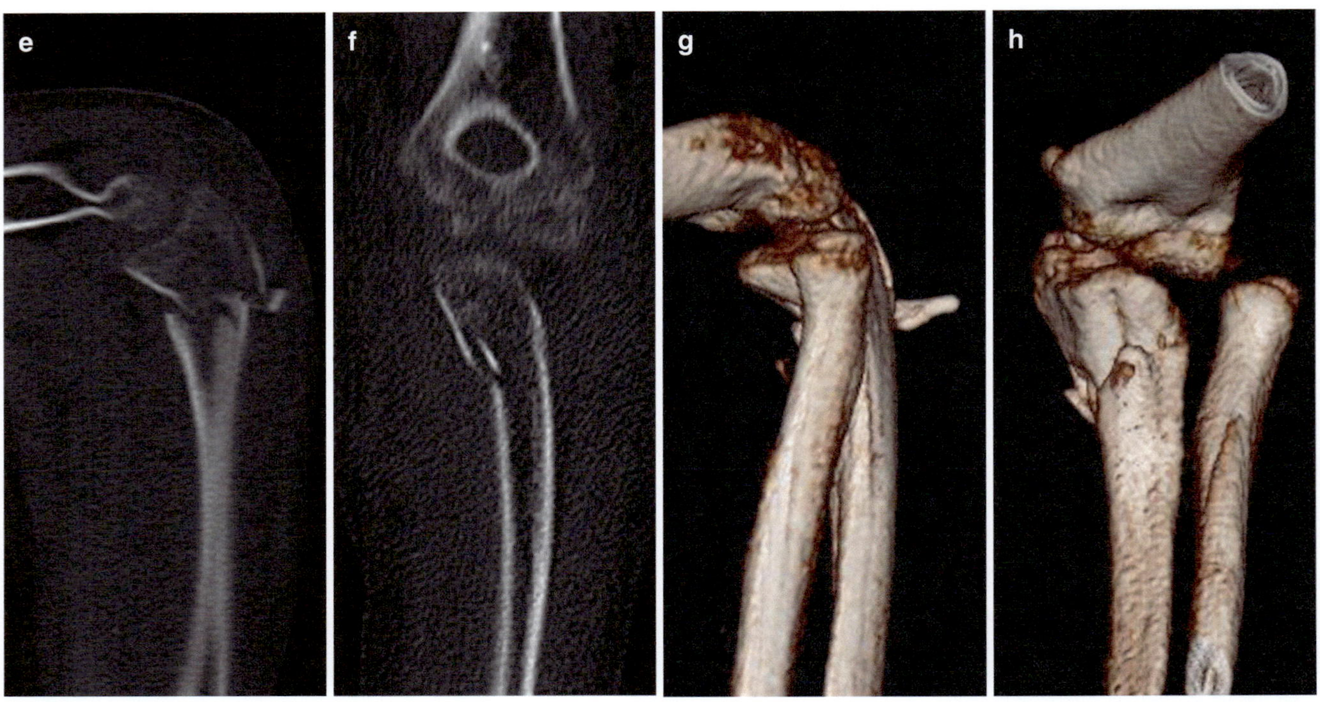

Fig. 6.15 CT in sagittal (**e**), coronal (**f**), and 3D reconstruction (**g**, **h**) view demonstrates fracture in the upper part of the ulna with displacement and angulation, dislocation of humeroradial joint, and radial displacement of radial head

9. The comparison of radiography and CT in adult Monteggia fracture
   9.1 Radiography (Fig. 6.16a–d)

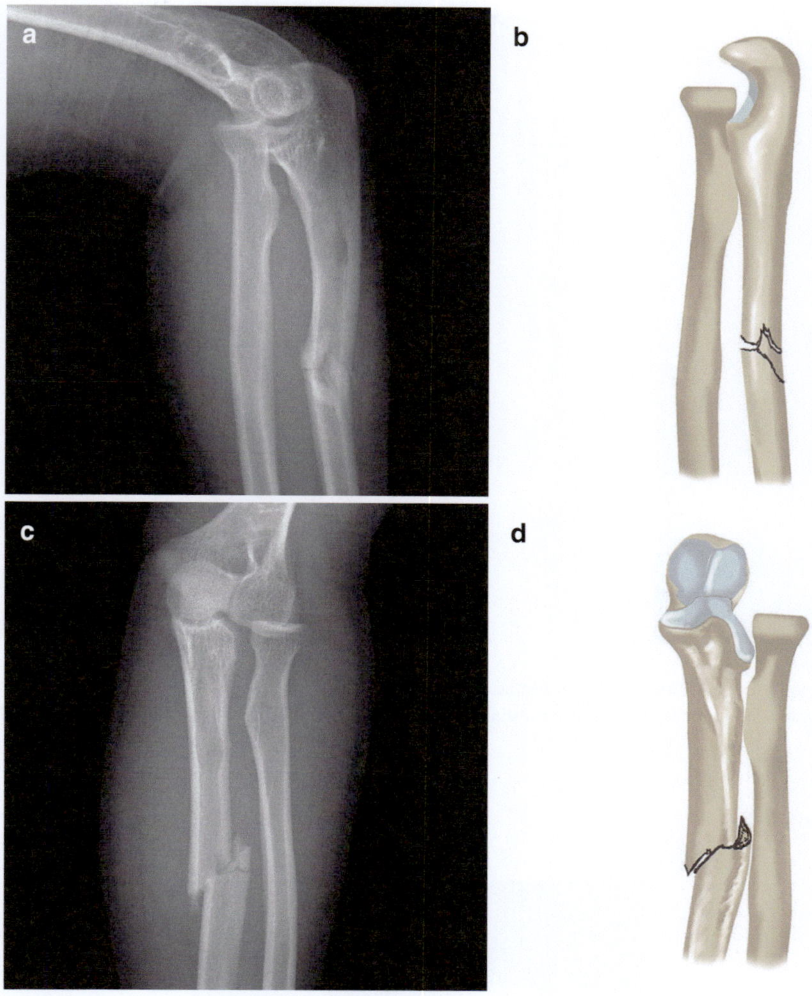

Fig. 6.16 Radiography (**a**, **c**) demonstrates comminuted fracture in the upper part of the ulna with displacement and angulation, wedge block, dislocation of the humeroradial joint, and lateral anterior displacement of radial head sketch (**b**, **d**)

   9.2 CT (Fig. 6.16e, f)

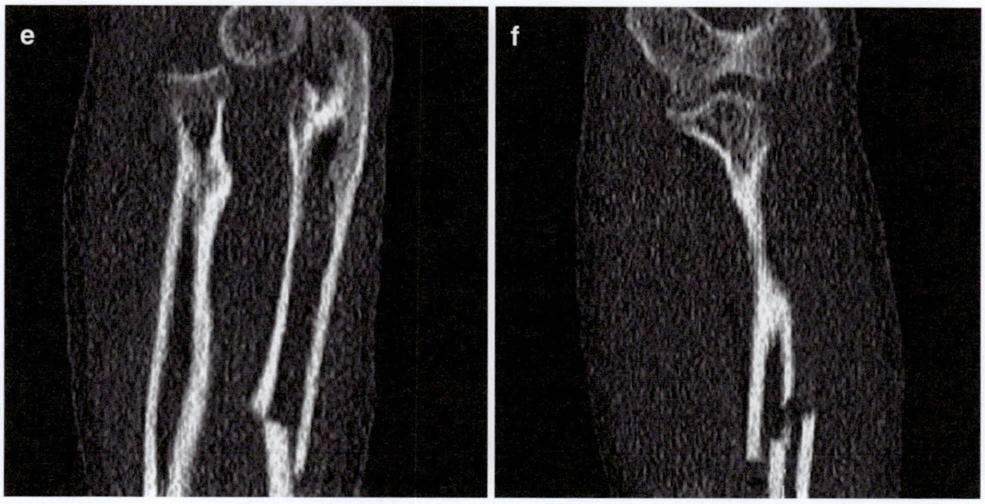

Fig. 6.16 CT in sagittal (**e**), coronal (**f**) view demonstrates comminuted fracture in the upper part of the ulna with displacement and angulation, dislocation of humeroradial joint, and lateral anterior displacement of radial head

10. The comparison of radiography and CT in adult Monteggia fracture
    10.1 Radiography (Fig. 6.17a–d)

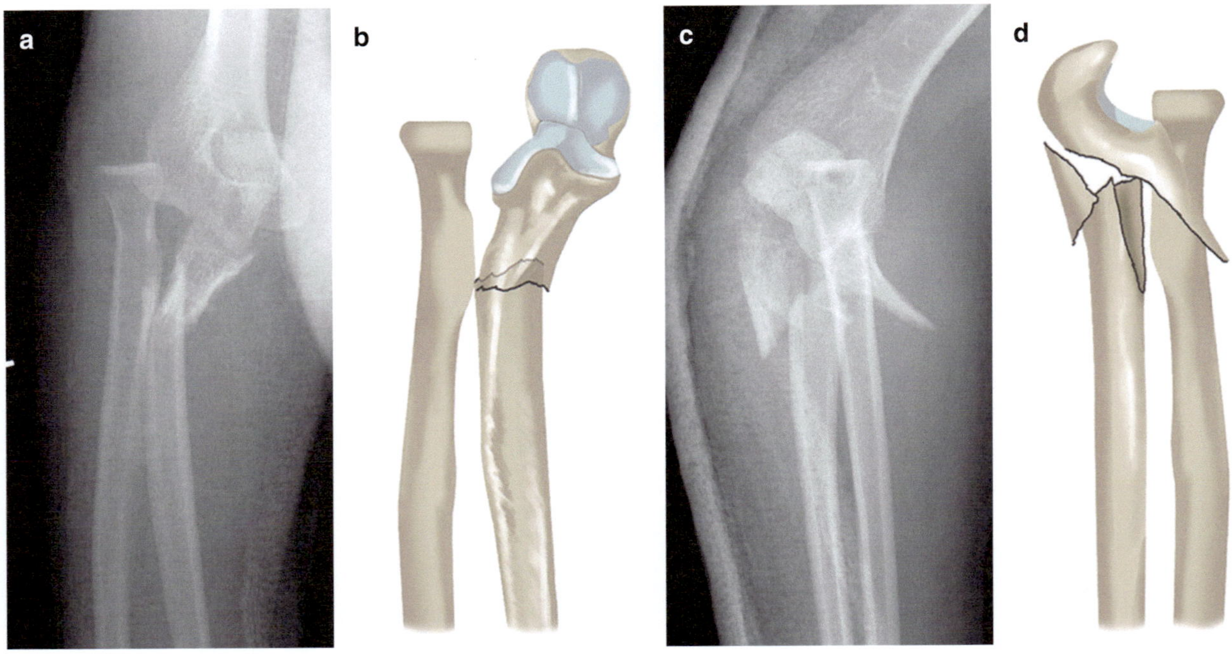

Fig. 6.17 Radiography (**a**, **c**) demonstrated comminuted fracture in the upper part of the ulna with displacement and angulation, fracture lines extend to articular surface, dislocation of humeroradial joint, and lateral anterior displacement of head of radius, sketch (**b**, **d**)

10.2 CT (Fig. 6.17e, f)

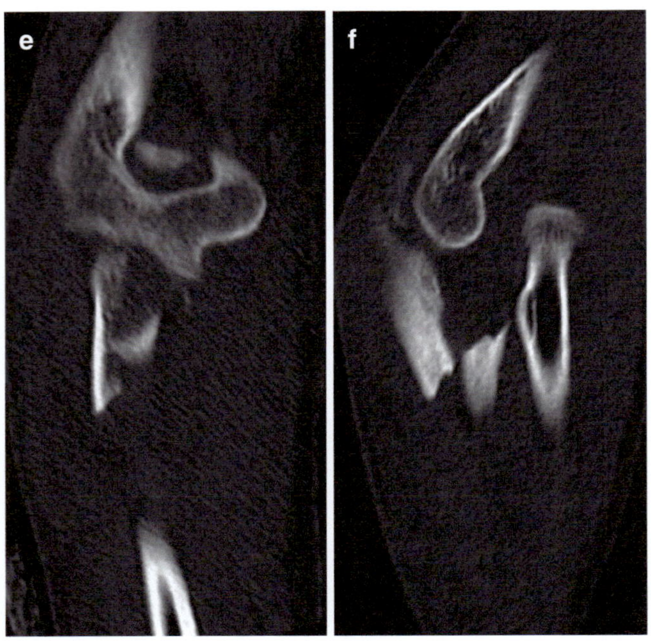

Fig. 6.17 CT in sagittal (**e**) and coronal (**f**) view demonstrates comminuted fracture in upper part of ulna with displacement and angulation, fracture lines extend to articular surface, dislocation of humeroradial joint, and anterior displacement of head of radius

11. The comparison of radiography and CT in adult Monteggia fracture
    11.1 Radiography (Fig. 6.18a–d)

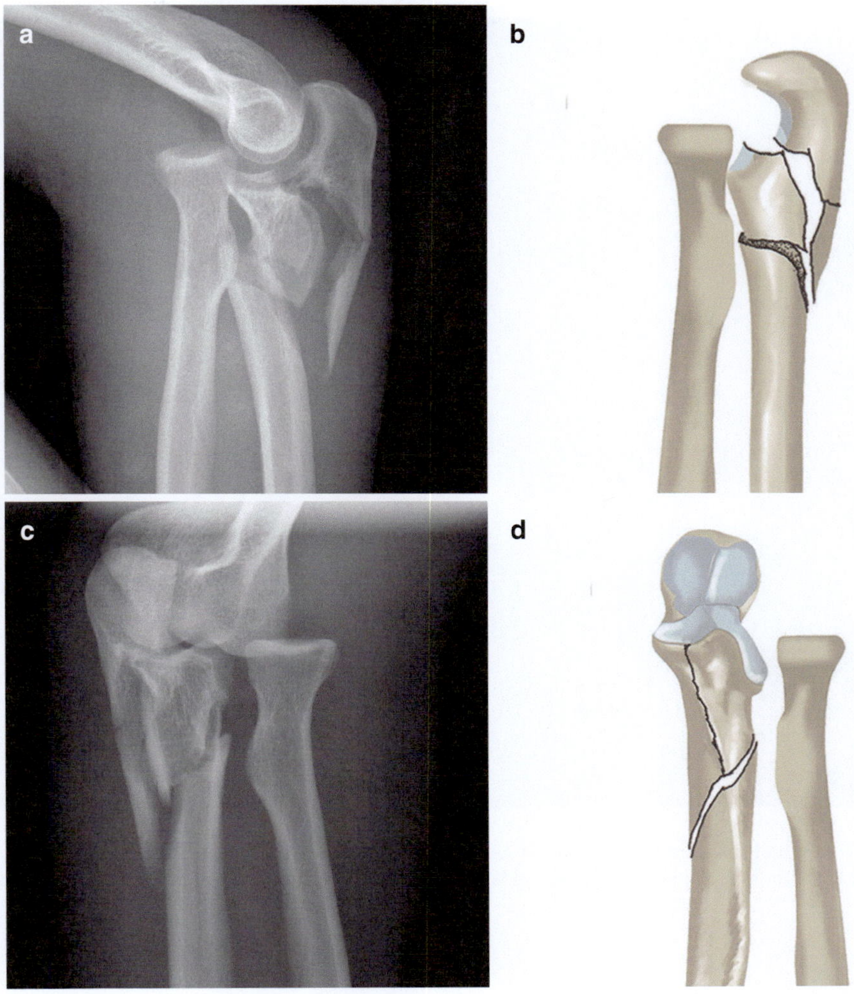

Fig. 6.18 Radiography (**a**, **c**) demonstrates comminuted fracture in the upper part of the ulna with displacement and angulation, fracture lines intend to articular surface, dislocation of humeroradial joint, and anterior displacement of head of radius, sketch (**b**, **d**)

    11.2 CT (Fig. 6.18e, f)

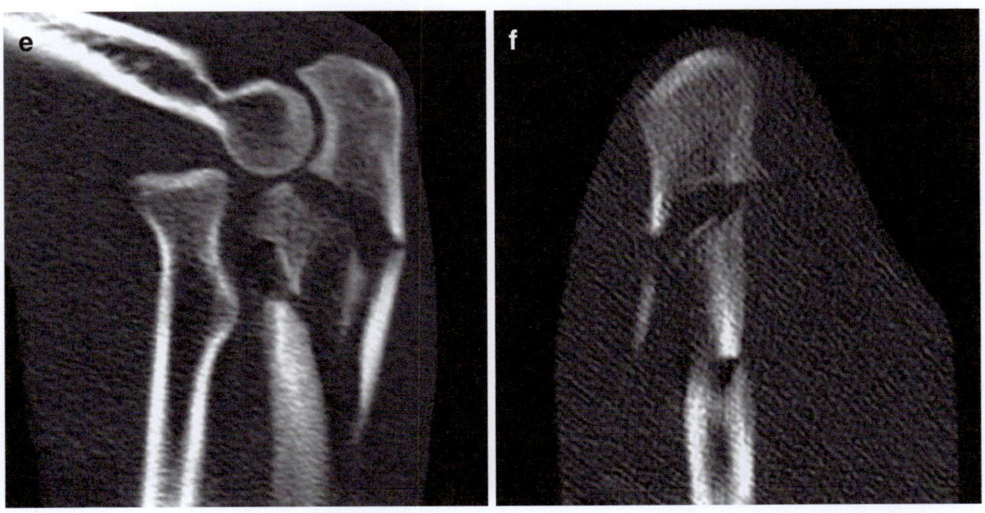

Fig. 6.18 CT in sagittal (**e**) and coronal (**f**) view demonstrates a comminuted fracture in the upper part of the ulna with displacement and angulation, fracture lines involve articular surface, dislocation of humeroradial joint, and anterior displacement of head of radius

12. The character of CT about Galeazzi fracture
    12.1 CT (Fig. 6.19a–d)

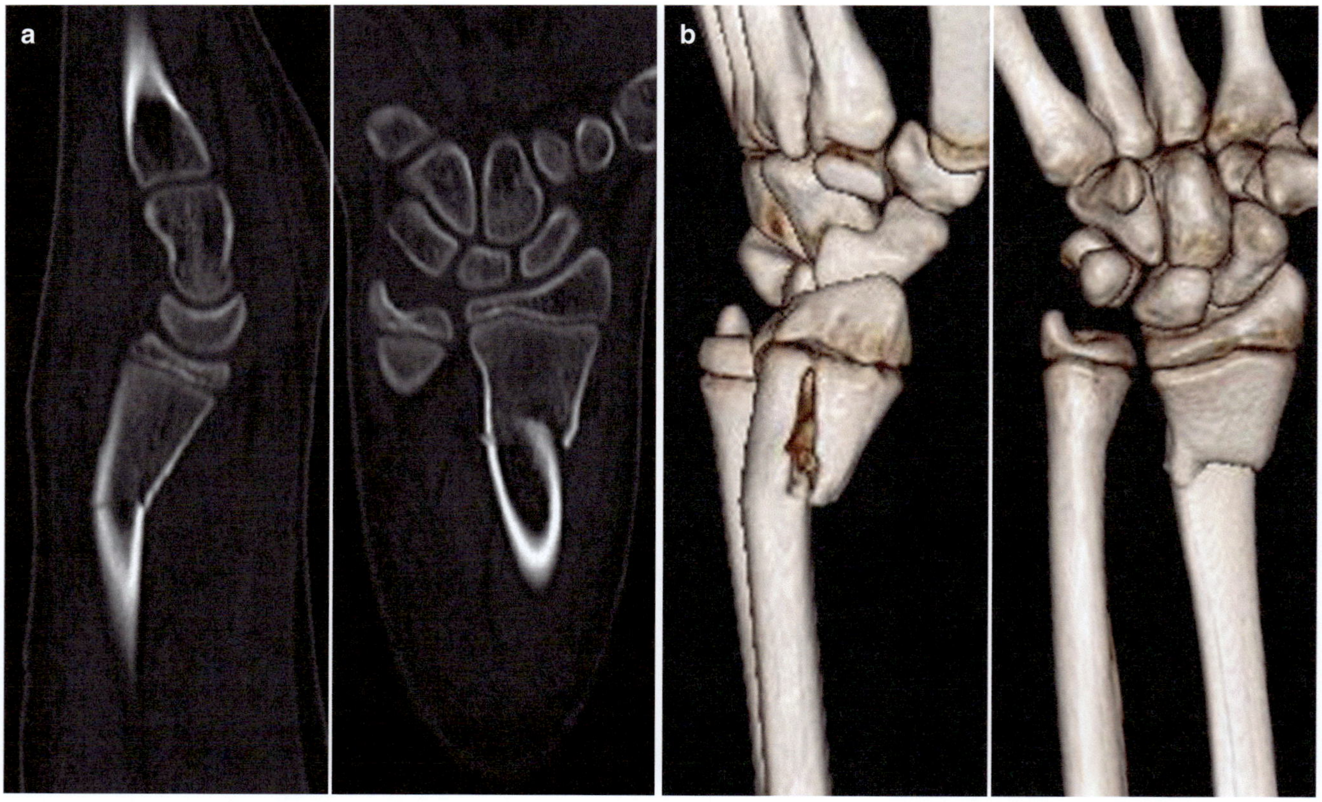

Fig. 6.19 CT in sagittal (**a**), coronal (**b**), and 3D reconstructions view demonstrates a fracture in lower part of radius with displacement and angulation, the distal radioulnar joint separation can be observed, head of ulna located at the dorsal side of the distal radius

13. The comparison of radiography and CT for comminuted fracture in the distal part of the radius and the distal radioulnar joint separated

    13.1 Radiography (Fig. 6.20a–d)

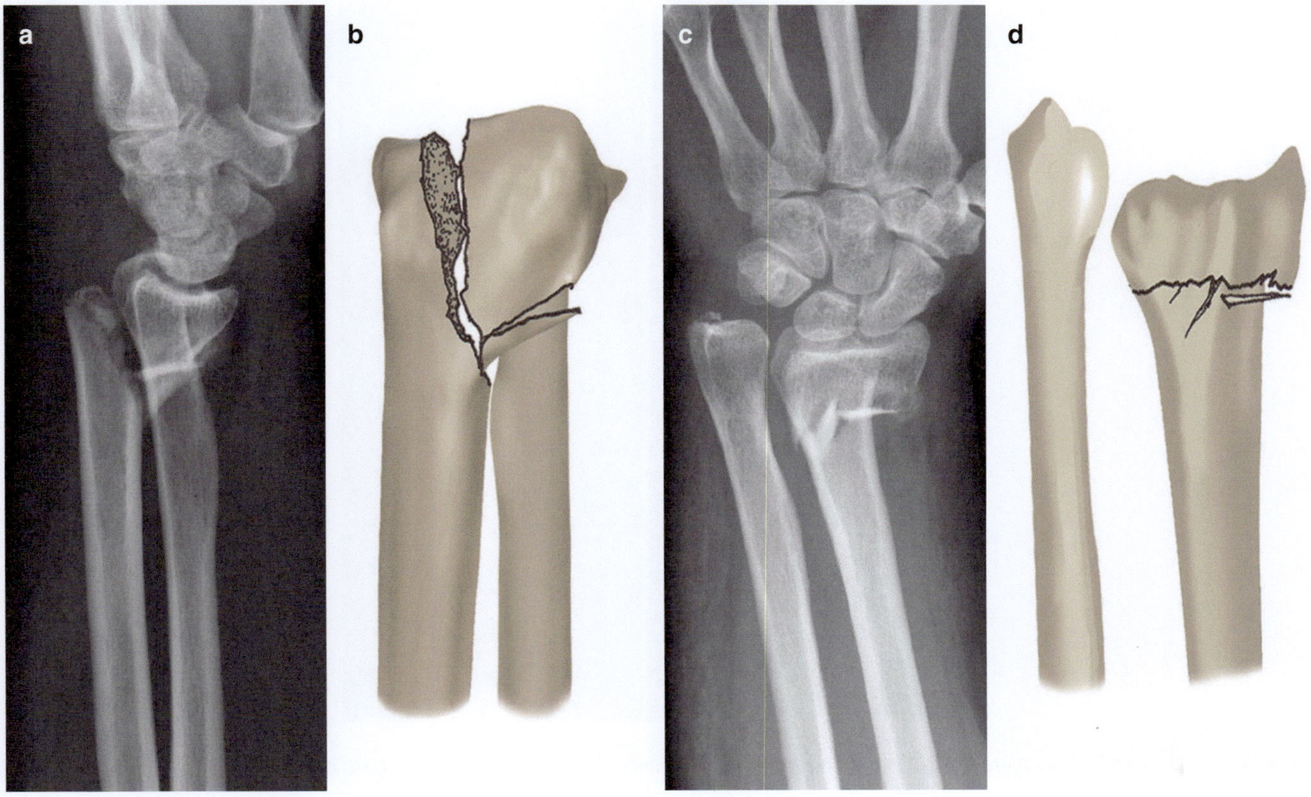

Fig. 6.20 Radiography (**a**, **c**) demonstrates comminuted fracture in the distal part of the radius with displaced fracture, the distal radioulnar joint space widened, sketch (**b**, **d**)

13.2 CT (Fig. 6.20e, f)

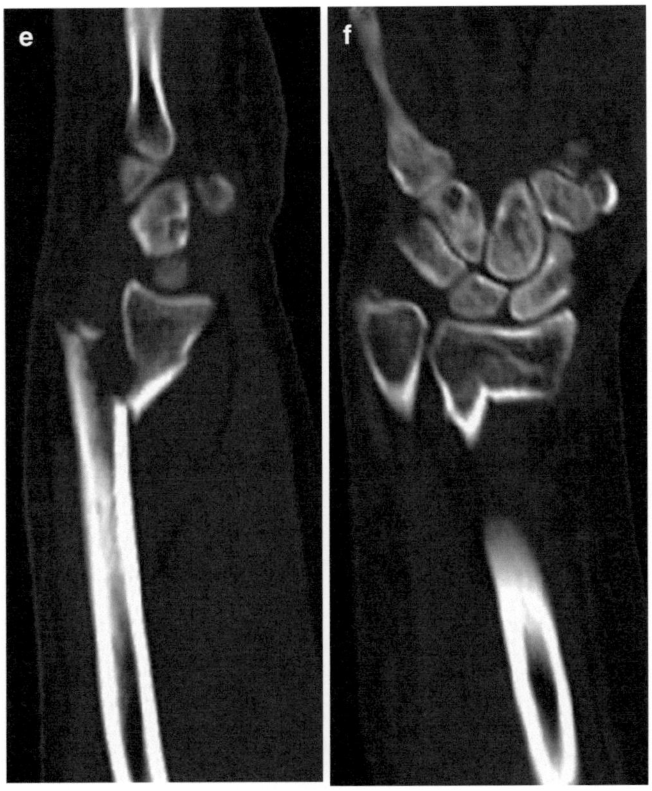

Fig. 6.20 CT in sagittal (**e**) and coronal (**f**) view demonstrates comminuted, displaced fracture in distal part of radius

14. The comparison of radiography and CT about greenstick fracture in the upper part of the ulna with dislocation of head of radius
    14.1 Radiography (Fig. 6.21a–d)

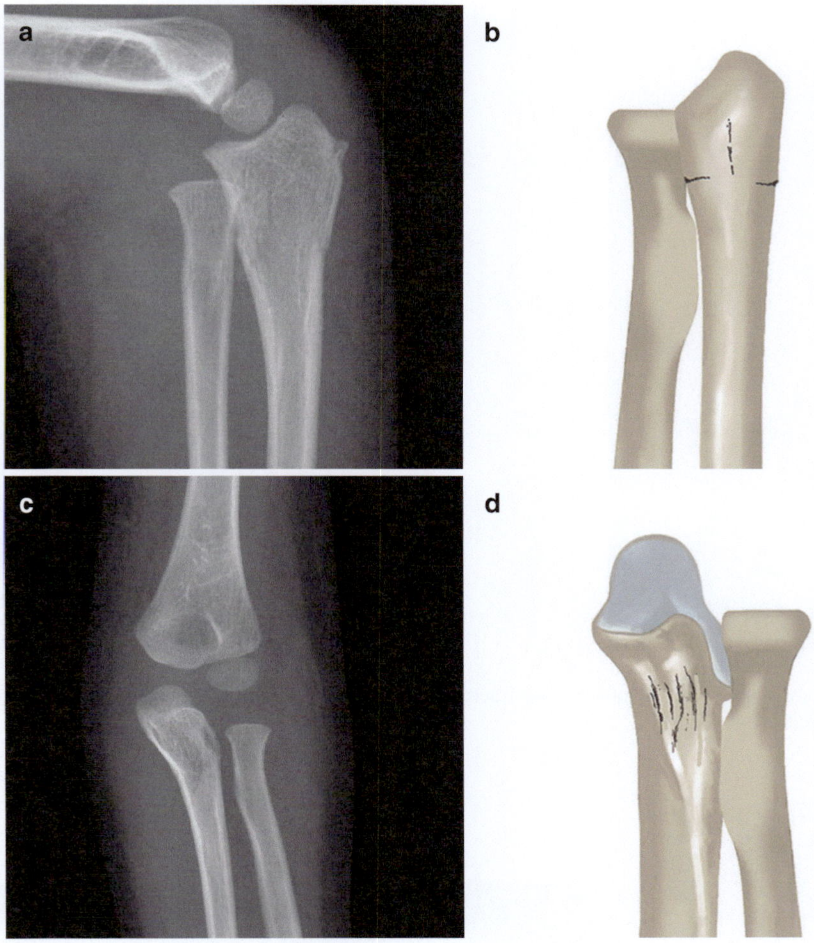

Fig. 6.21 Radiography (**a**, **c**) demonstrates contorted cortical bone in the upper part of the ulna, rugae, and irregular bone trabecula, anterolateral displacement of head of radius, sketch (**b**, **d**)

    14.2 CT (Fig. 6.21e, f)

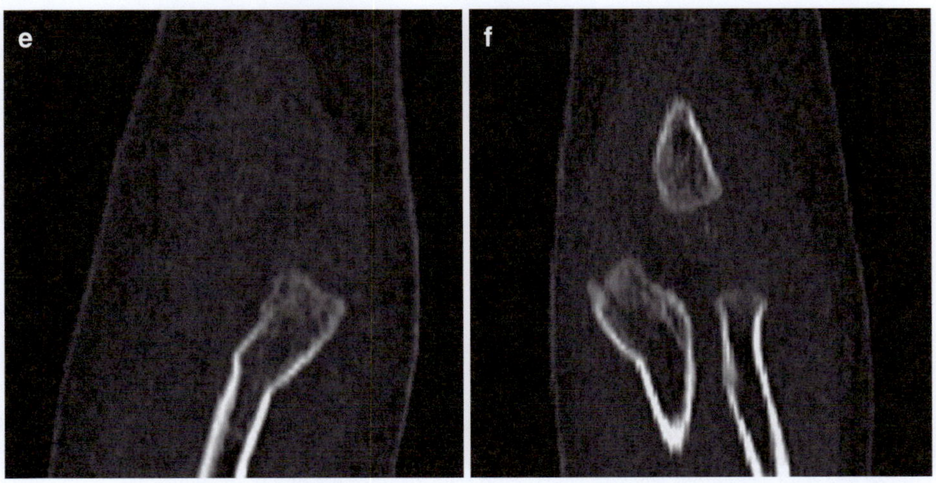

Fig. 6.21 CT in sagittal (**e**) and coronal (**f**) view demonstrates a contorted cortical bone in the upper part of the ulna, rugae, and irregular bone trabecula, anterolateral displacement of head of radius

15. The comparison of radiography and CT for fractures in the middle part of ulna with greenstick fracture in middle part of radius

    15.1 Radiography (Fig. 6.22a–d)

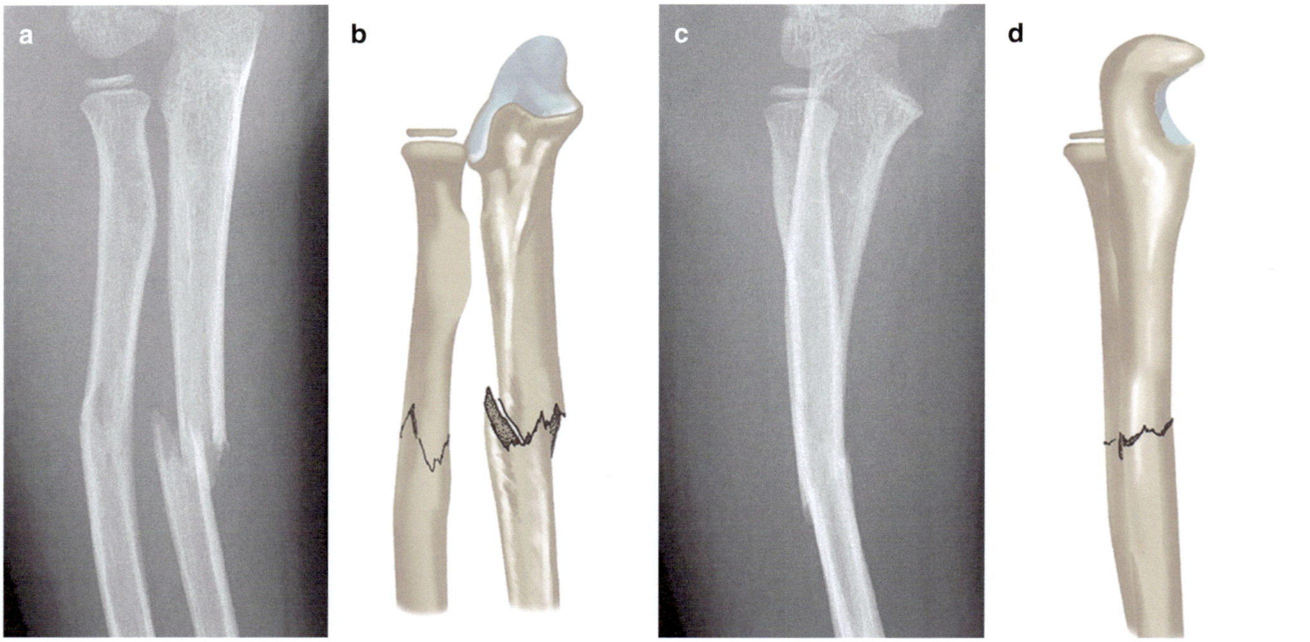

Fig. 6.22 Radiography (**a**, **c**) demonstrates a fracture in the upper part of the ulna, contorted cortical bone in the middle part of radius and rugae can be observed, sketch (**b**, **d**)

    15.2 CT (Fig. 6.22e, f)

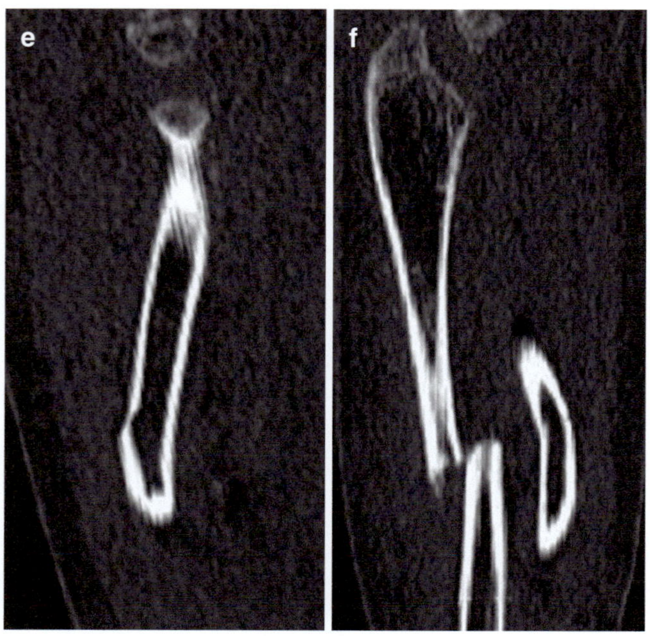

Fig. 6.22 CT in sagittal (**e**) and coronal (**f**) view demonstrates fracture in the upper part of the ulna, contorted cortical bone, and rugae in the middle part of radius can be observed

6.3 Summary

1. Standard radiography can identify the shaft fractures; however, a linear radiolucency—formed by a humeral nutrient artery known as the vascular channel—should be excluded from fracture line. Pediatric greenstick or bending fracture should be brought to attention.
2. Most ulnar and radius fractures have two injuries or dislocation, yet a few of them were simple fractures. Fractures of the ulna or radius should be paid attention to, as well as any accompanied upper or lower ulnar radial joint dislocations. Fractures of the proximal third of the ulna are often accompanied by a radial head dislocation (Monteggia), while fractures of the distal third of the radius are often associated with a distal radioulnar joint (DRU) dislocation (Galeazzi).

7 Pathological Fracture in Upper Limb

Tao Sun and Yingze Zhang

Pathological fractures are caused by many reasons such as osteomyelitis, bone tumors, and osteoporosis. They are common in clinics; however, misdiagnosis can often occur especially with bone tumors. If they are treated as an ordinary fracture, the best treatment time may be delayed. Malignant bone tumor cells could be potentially disseminated through blood circulation, resulting in local recurrence and a failure in limb salvage.

A pathological fracture means the bone tissue has a lesser mechanical strength and viscoelasticity, as well as decreased bone strength. Therefore, a pathological fracture is not a result of a force. Rates of pathological induced fractures are not low, though should be noted reports are rare. Pathological fractures caused by bone tumors or neoplasia are called pathological fracture in a narrow sense, given there are many types of bone tumors. For example, most of them are metastatic tumor, which account for 37.85%, myeloma (14.64%), and fibrous dysplasia (13.81%).

There are different pathological fractures for different age groups and at sites. The humerus is the second most common site where pathological fractures occur. Bone tumors contain bone cyst, metastatic tumor, myeloma, and fibrous dysplasia. The phalanx is the seventh common place to find bone tumor, whereby there is enchondrosis.

For a neoplastic pathological fracture; especially malignancy one; erosion rate succeeds the rate of callus formation. Following a pathological fracture, there may be limited activity, fracture nonunion, and a deteriorating lesion. Overall, to make an accurate diagnosis, the sex, age, site, and imaging manifestations should be considered to provide reliable data for the clinic.

7.1 Mechanism

The force which causes pathological fracture is mild, yet unlikely to cause it, such as a spontaneous fracture when do heavy lifting.

7.2 Signs and Symptoms

Pain, swelling, limited activity are the commonest complaints in an orthopedic clinic. But those are of specificity.

7.3 Imaging Investigation

Fracture which is caused by a trivial trauma should be suspected as a pathological fracture. A CT and MRI are necessary to identify the cause of fracture. If fracture is obscurity and there is a disorder affecting the bone structure, a radiography, CT, and MRI scan should be ordered to rule out the pathological fracture.

T. Sun · Y. Zhang (✉)
Department of Orthopaedics, The Third Hospital of Hebei Medical University, Shijiazhuang, Hebei, China

Y. Zhang (ed.), *Differential Diagnosis of Fracture*, https://doi.org/10.1007/978-981-13-8339-7_7

1. The comparison of radiography, CT, and MRI for pathological fractures caused by plasmocytoma in proximal end of clavicle

   1.1 Radiography (Fig. 7.1a, b)

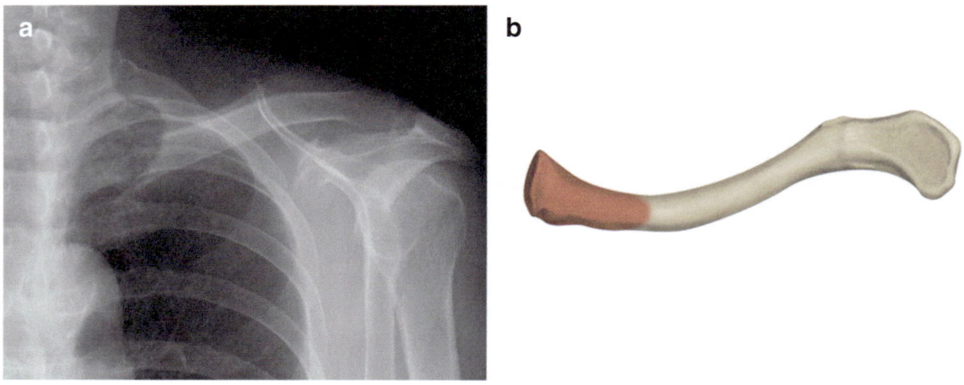

Fig. 7.1 Radiography (**a**) demonstrated discontinuity of cortical bone in proximal end of clavicle, with overlapped tissue and obscure microstructure, sketch (**b**)

   1.2 CT (Fig. 7.1c, d)

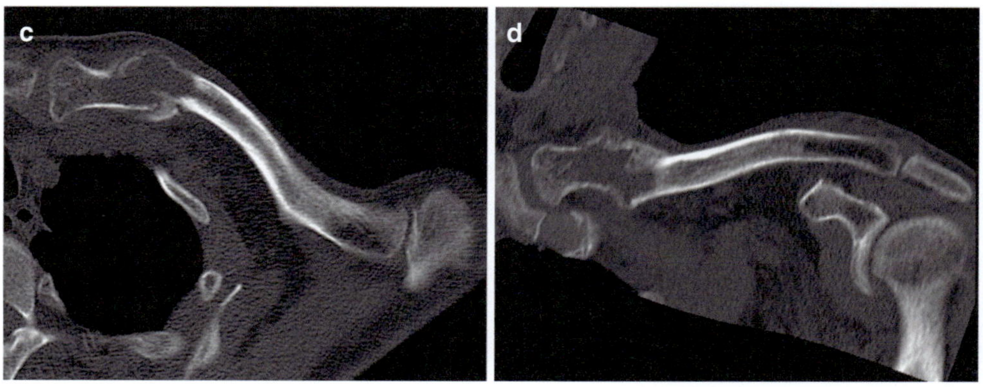

Fig. 7.1 CT in axial (**c**) and coronal view (**d**) demonstrated distensible bone destruction in proximal end of clavicle with pathological fracture and mild displacement

   1.3 MR (Fig. 7.1e, f)

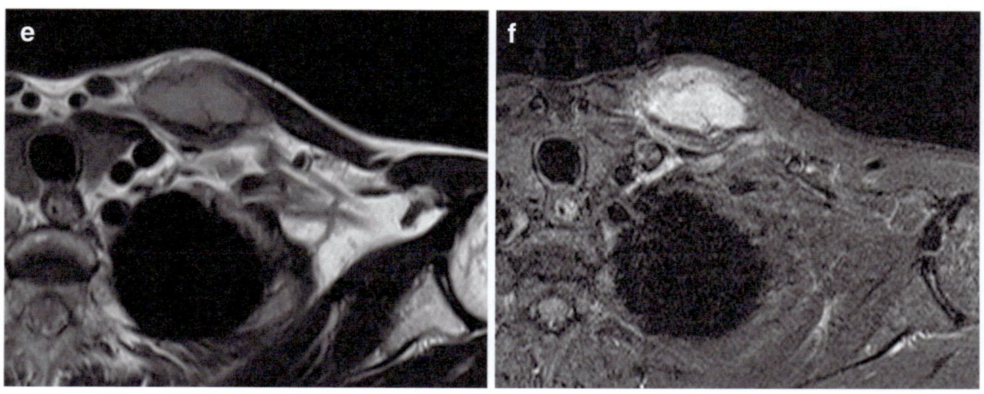

Fig. 7.1 MRI images in axial T1WI (**e**) and T2WI with STIR (**f**) demonstrate distensible bone destruction in proximal end of clavicle, with a long T1 and T2, and pathological fracture is observed

2. The comparison of radiography and CT for a pathological fracture caused by metastatic tumor in proximal end of clavicle

   2.1 Radiography (Fig. 7.2a, b)

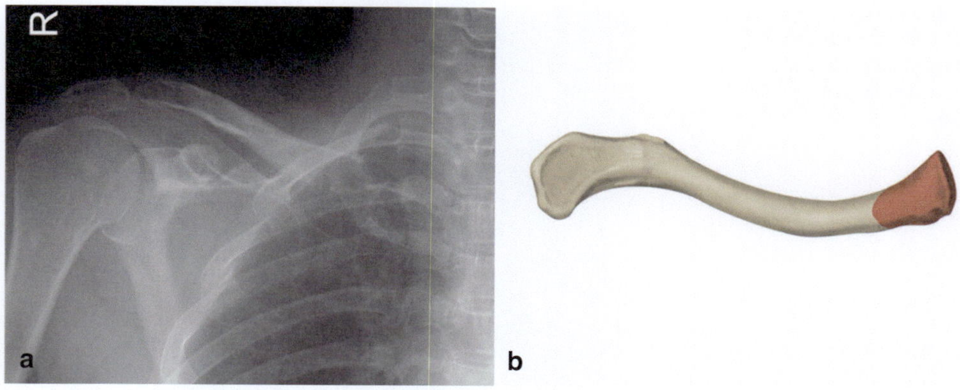

Fig. 7.2 Radiography (**a**) demonstrates discontinuity of cortical bone in proximal end of clavicle, with overlapped tissue and obscure microstructure, sketch (**b**)

   2.2 CT (Fig. 7.2c, d)

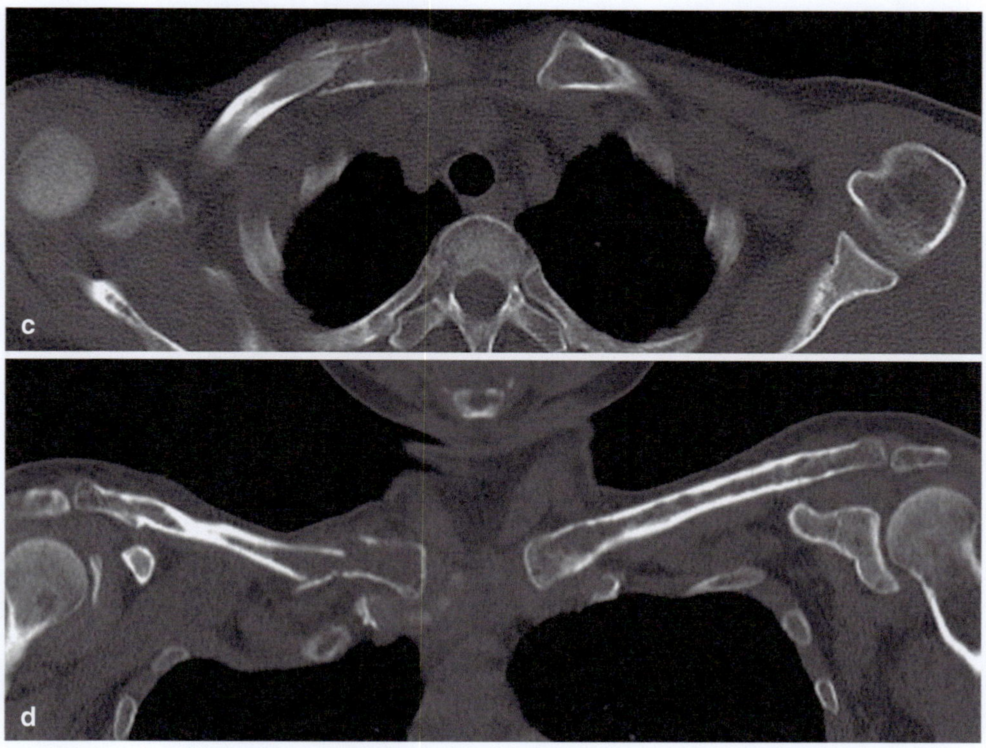

Fig. 7.2 CT in axial (**c**) and coronal view (**d**) demonstrated multiple small mottled bone destruction in proximal end of clavicle, with pathological fracture and mild displacement. Bone mass can be observed

3. The comparison of radiography, CT, and MRI for a pathological fracture in glenoid cavity of scapula
   3.1 Radiography (Fig. 7.3a–d)

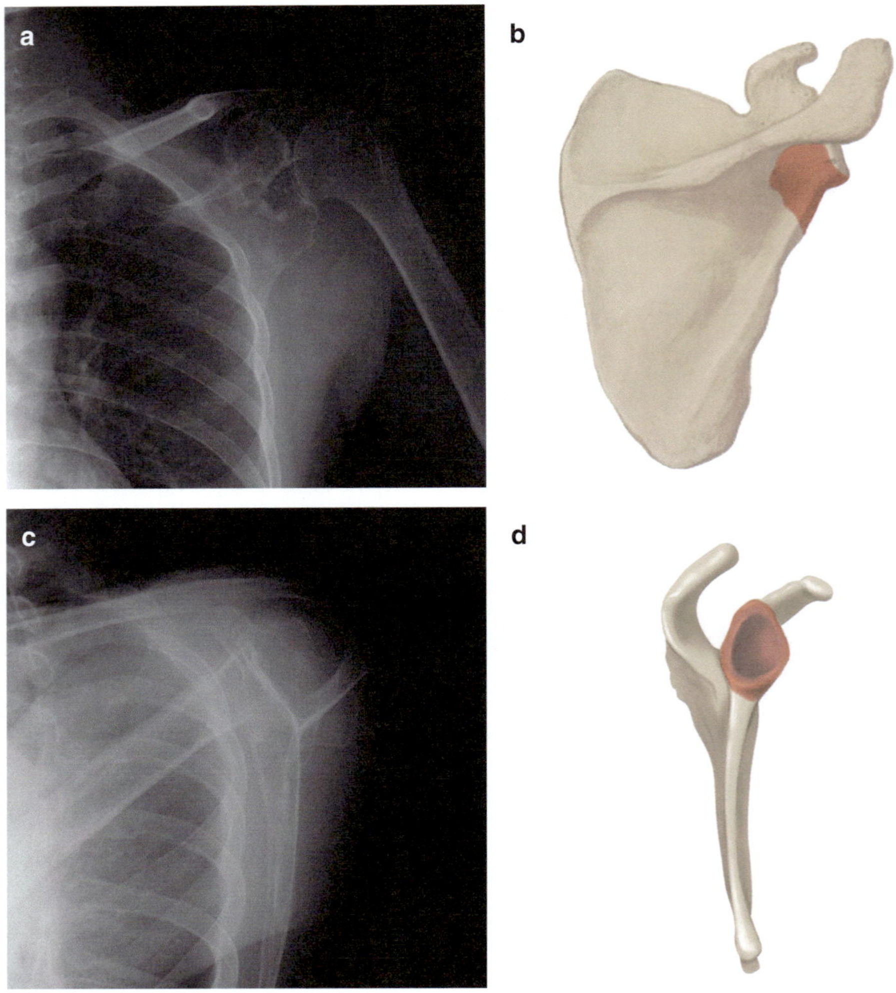

Fig. 7.3 Radiography (**a**, **c**) demonstrated distensible bone destruction in left glenoid cavity of scapula, with heterogenetic density, sketch (**b**, **d**)

   3.2 CT (Fig. 7.3e, f)

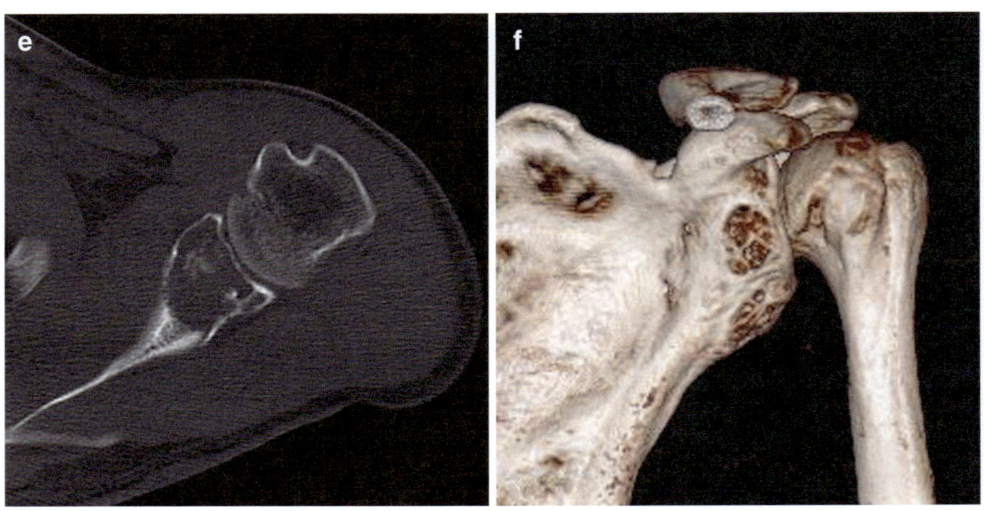

Fig. 7.3 CT in axial (**e**) and coronal view (**f**) demonstrated distensible bone destruction and broken cortical bone at neck in left glenoid cavity of scapula, with heterogenetic density with mild displacement, and mottled high density can be observed

3.3 MR (Fig. 7.3g–j)

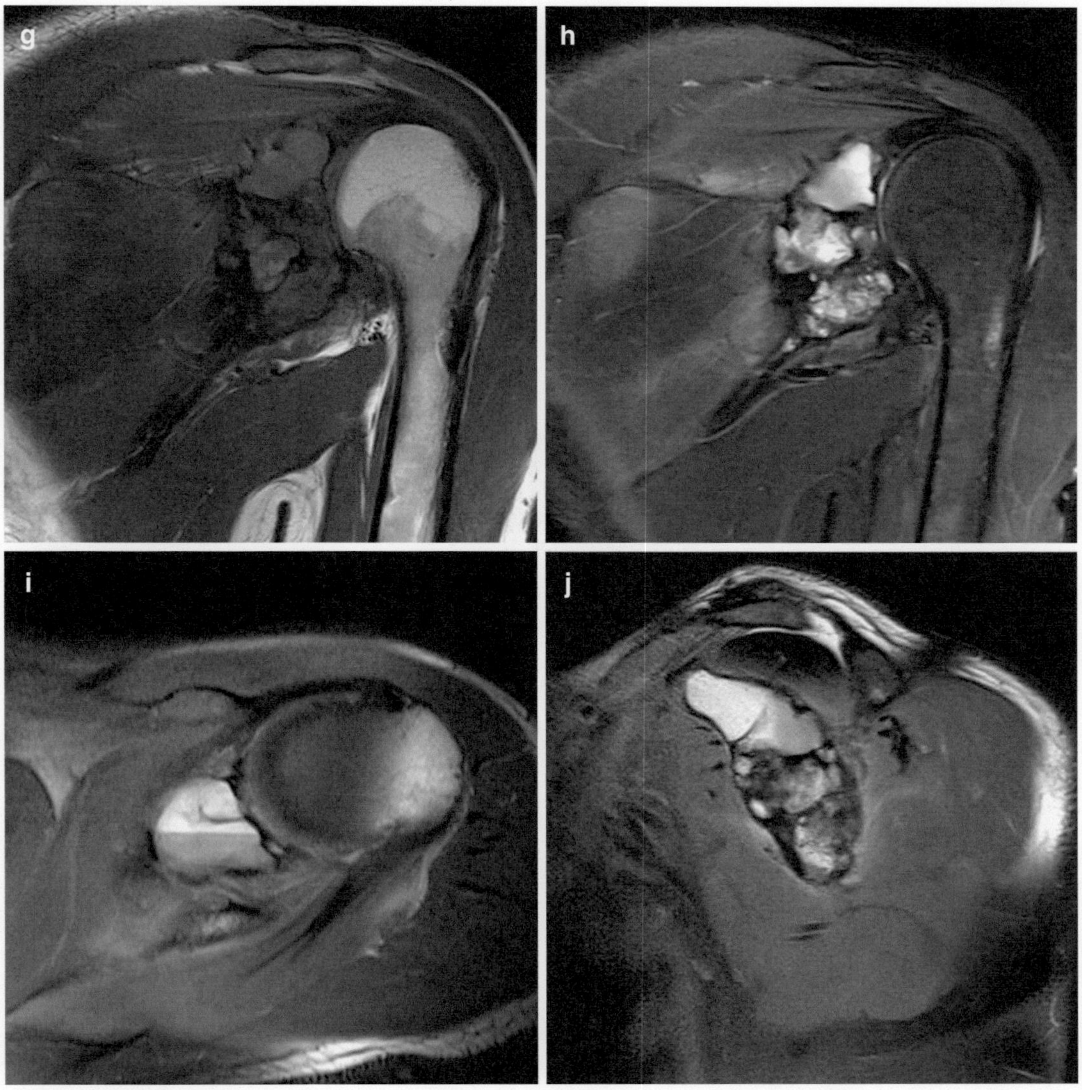

Fig. 7.3 MRI images in coronal T1WI (**g**), T2WI with STIR (**h**), axial and sagittal T2WI (**i**, **j**) demonstrate distensible bone destruction in glenoid cavity of scapula, with a long T1 and T2, scapula neck was not continued, liquid–liquid level and pathological fracture are observed

4. The comparison of radiography and MRI for a pathological fracture caused by myeloma in glenoid cavity of scapula
    4.1 Radiography (Fig. 7.4a–d)

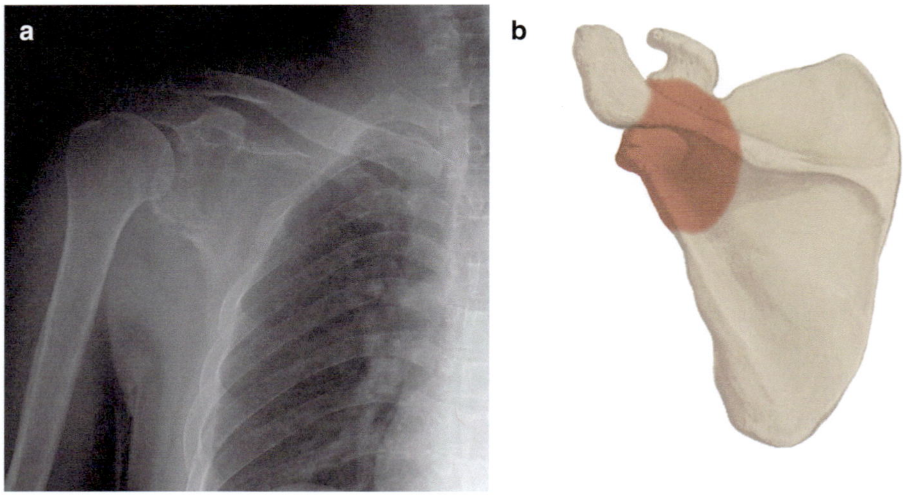

Fig. 7.4 Radiography (**a**, **c**) demonstrates distensible bone destruction in right glenoid cavity of scapula with obscure boundary, and discontinued inferior glenoid cavity is observed (**b**, **d**)

    4.2 MR (Fig. 7.4e–h)

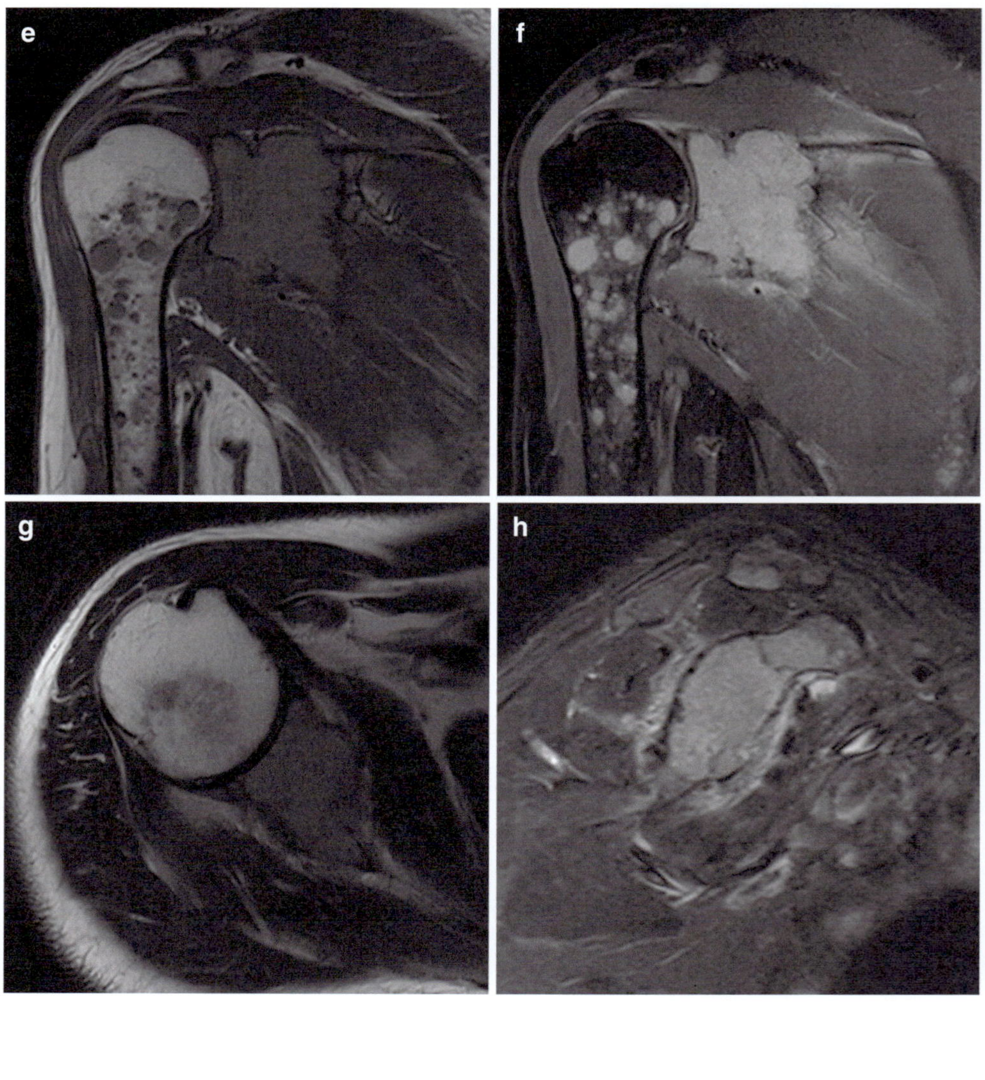

Fig. 7.4 MRI images in coronal T1WI (**e**), T2WI with STIR (**f**), axial T1WI (**g**), and sagittal T2WI (**h**) demonstrate distensible bone destruction in glenoid cavity of scapula, with a long T1 and T2, scapula neck was not continued, a mottle long T1 and T2 in proximal humerus are observed

5. The comparison of radiography, CT demonstrating a pathological fracture in superior angle of scapula
   5.1 Radiography (Fig. 7.5a, b)

Fig. 7.5 Radiography (**a**) demonstrates an uneven density in superior angle of scapula, sketch (**b**)

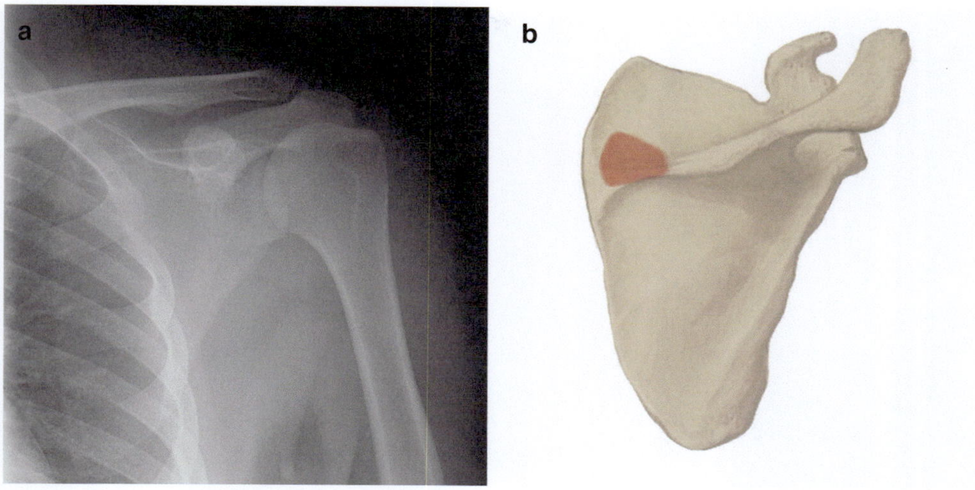

5.2 CT (Fig. 7.5c–e)

Fig. 7.5 CT in axial (**c**), coronal (**d**), and sagittal view (**e**) demonstrates a distensible bone destruction and broken cortical bone at neck in superior angle of scapula with heterogenetic density, and mottled high density can be observed

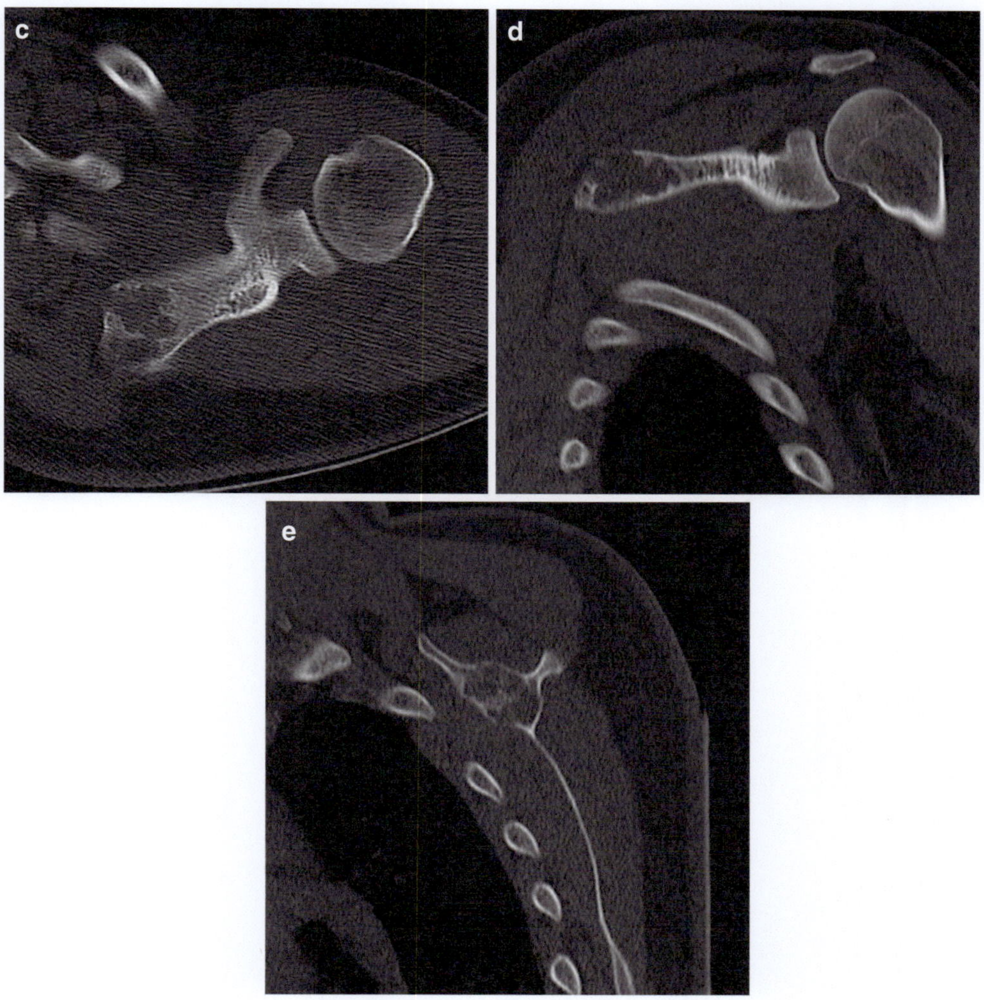

6. The comparison of radiography, CT, and MRI demonstrating a pathological fracture in the proximal humerus
   6.1 Radiography (Fig. 7.6a–d)

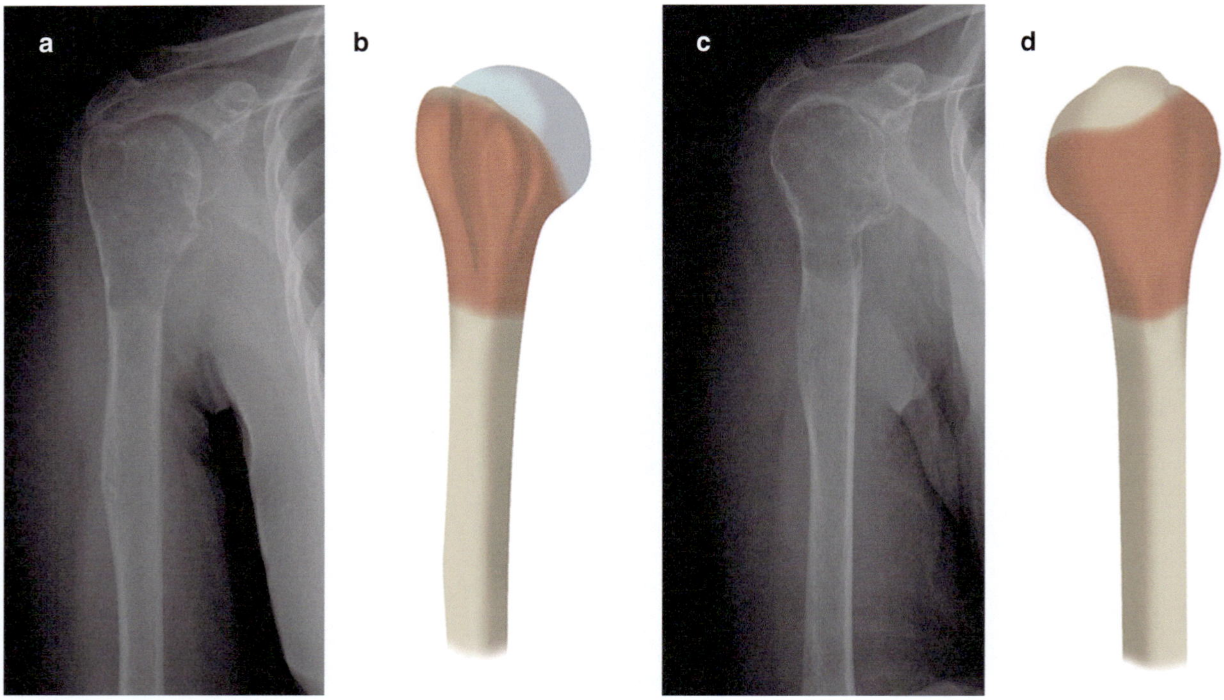

Fig. 7.6 Radiography (**a**, **c**) demonstrates a distensible bone destruction in proximal humerus, sketch (**b**, **d**)

6.2 CT (Fig. 7.6e, f)

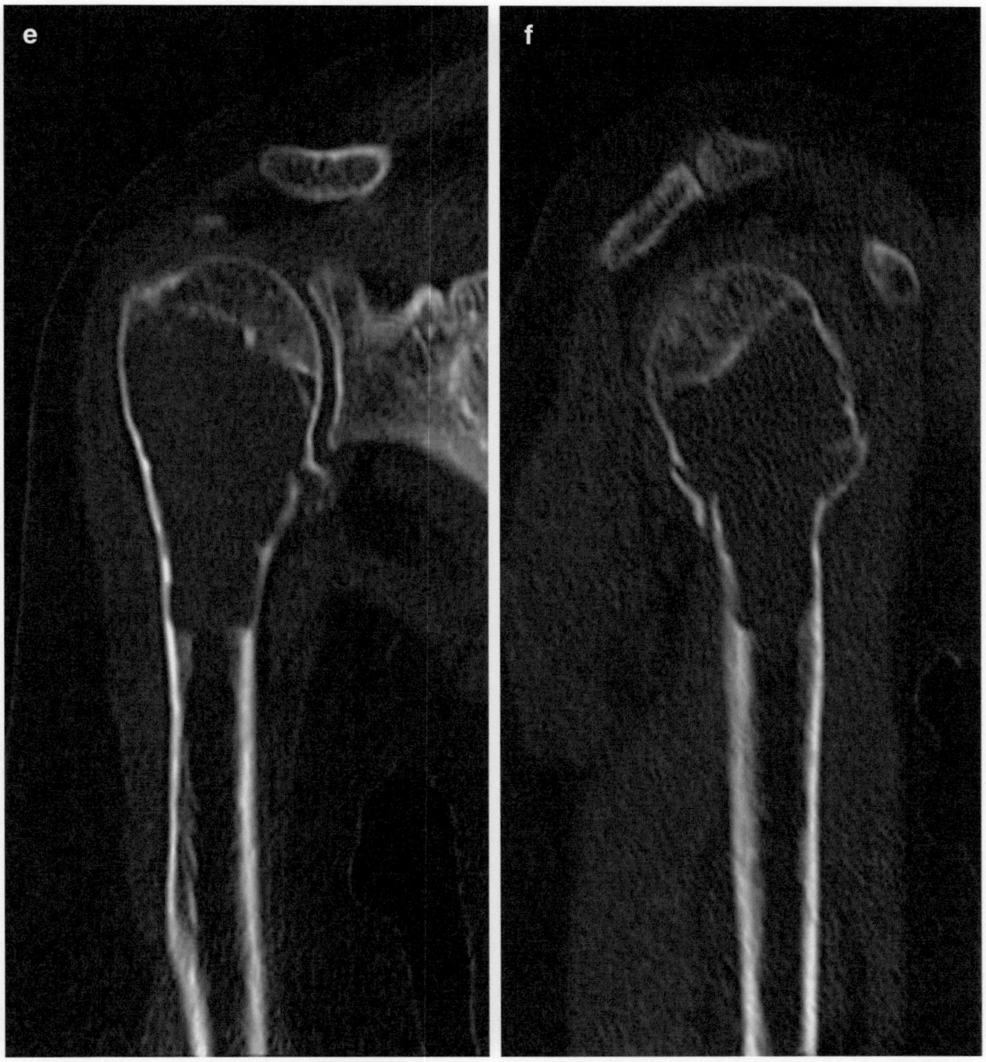

Fig. 7.6 CT in coronal (**e**), sagittal (**f**) view demonstrates a distensible bone destruction in proximal humerus, with homogeneous density and clear boundary, and mottled high density can be observed

6.3 MR (Fig. 7.6g, h)

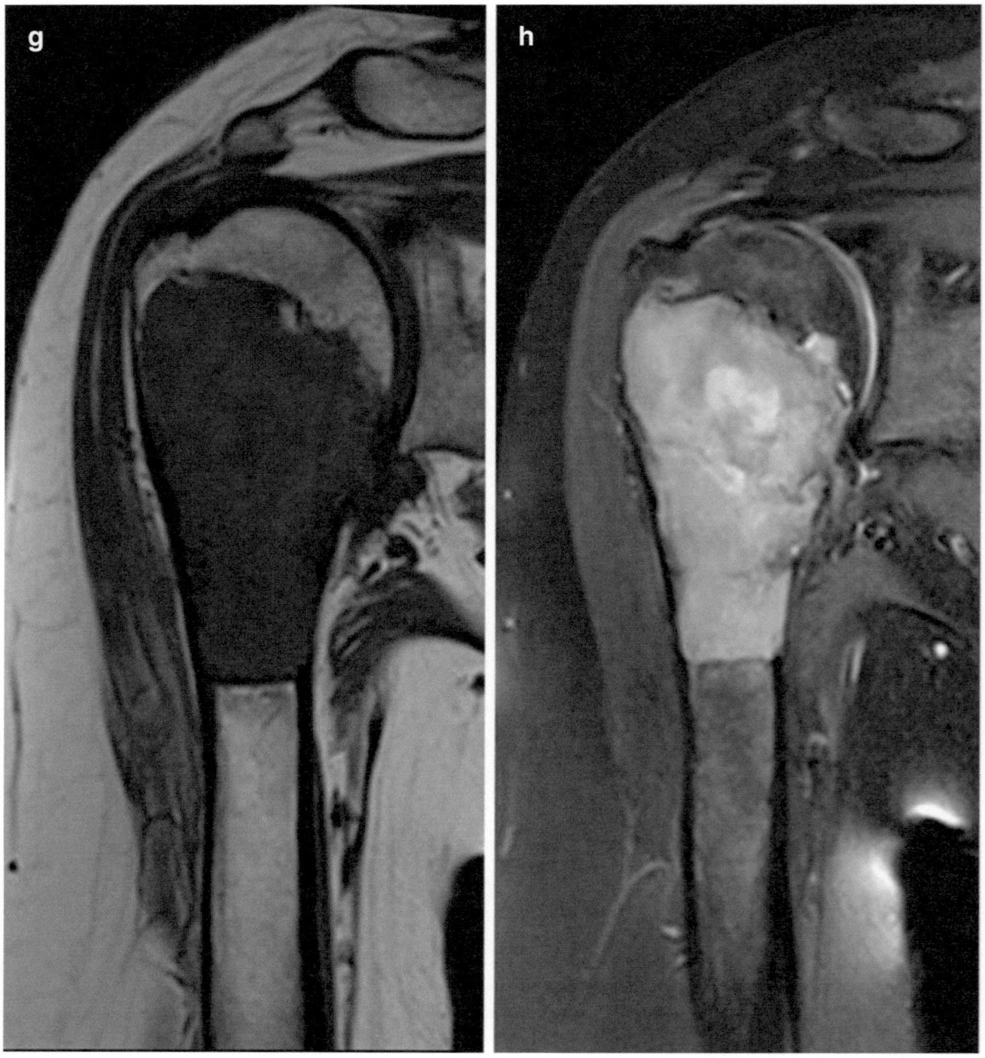

Fig. 7.6 MRI images in coronal T1WI (**g**), T2WI with STIR (**h**) demonstrate a distensible bone destruction in the proximal humerus, with a long T1 and T2. Mottled high density in T2 and pathological fracture can be observed

7. The comparison of radiography, CT, and MRI about pathological fracture in upper part of humerus
   7.1 Radiography (Fig. 7.7a–d)

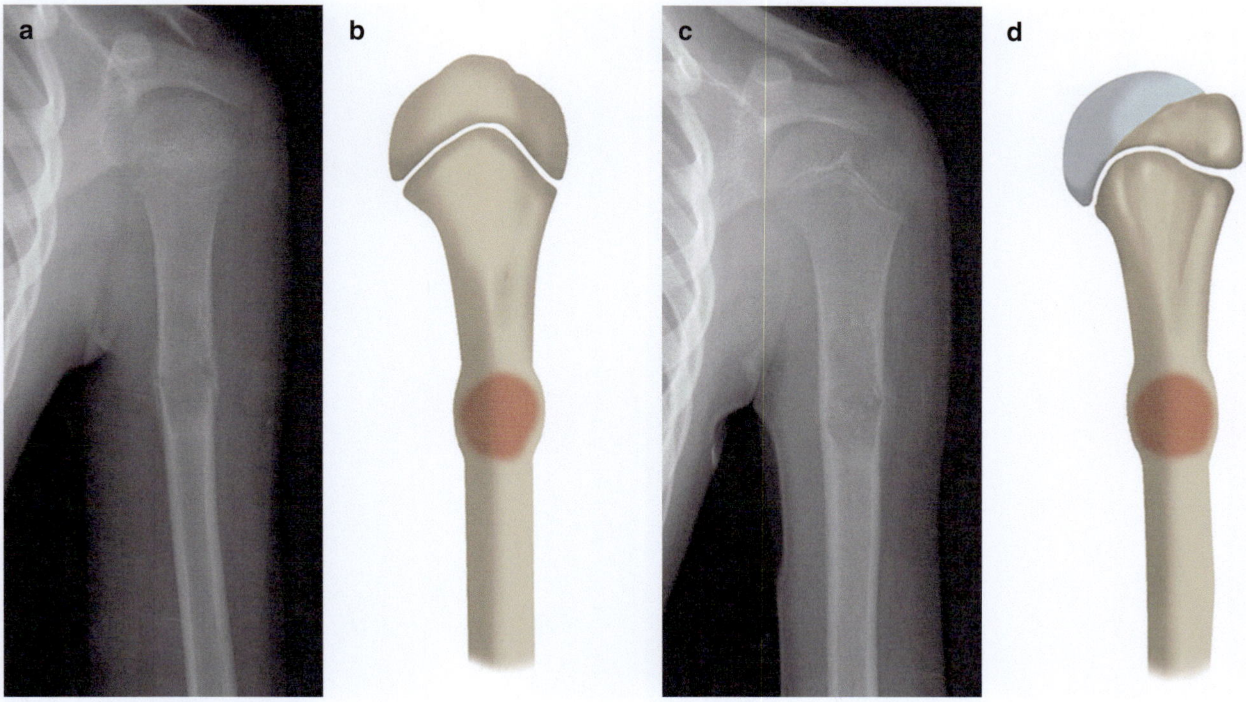

Fig. 7.7 Radiography (**a**, **c**) demonstrates distensible bone destruction in the upper part of the humerus with a pathological fracture, homogeneous density and callus can be observed, sketch (**b**, **d**)

7.2 CT (Fig. 7.7e, f)

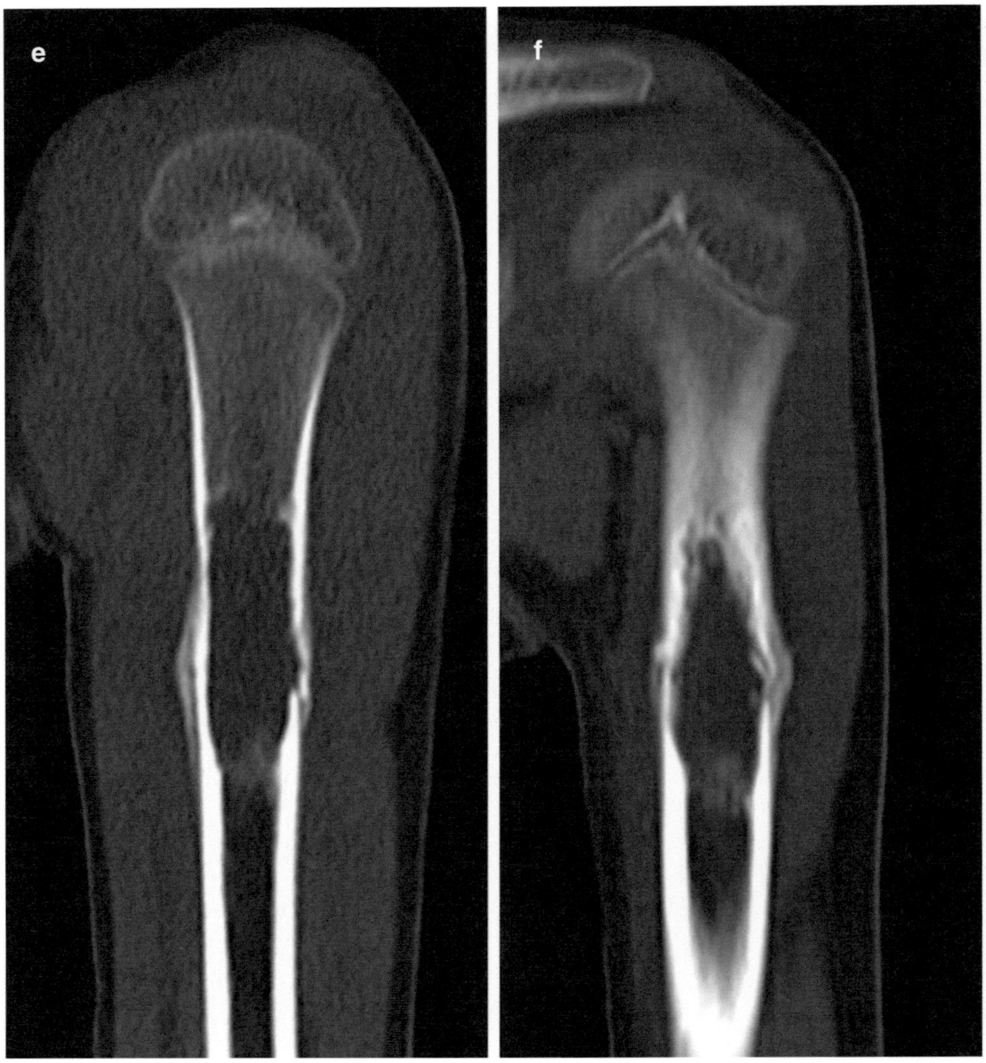

Fig. 7.7 CT in sagittal (**e**), coronal (**f**) view demonstrated distensible bone destruction in the upper part of the humerus, with homogeneous density and a pathological fracture, clear boundary and callus can be observed

7.3 MR (Fig. 7.7g, h)

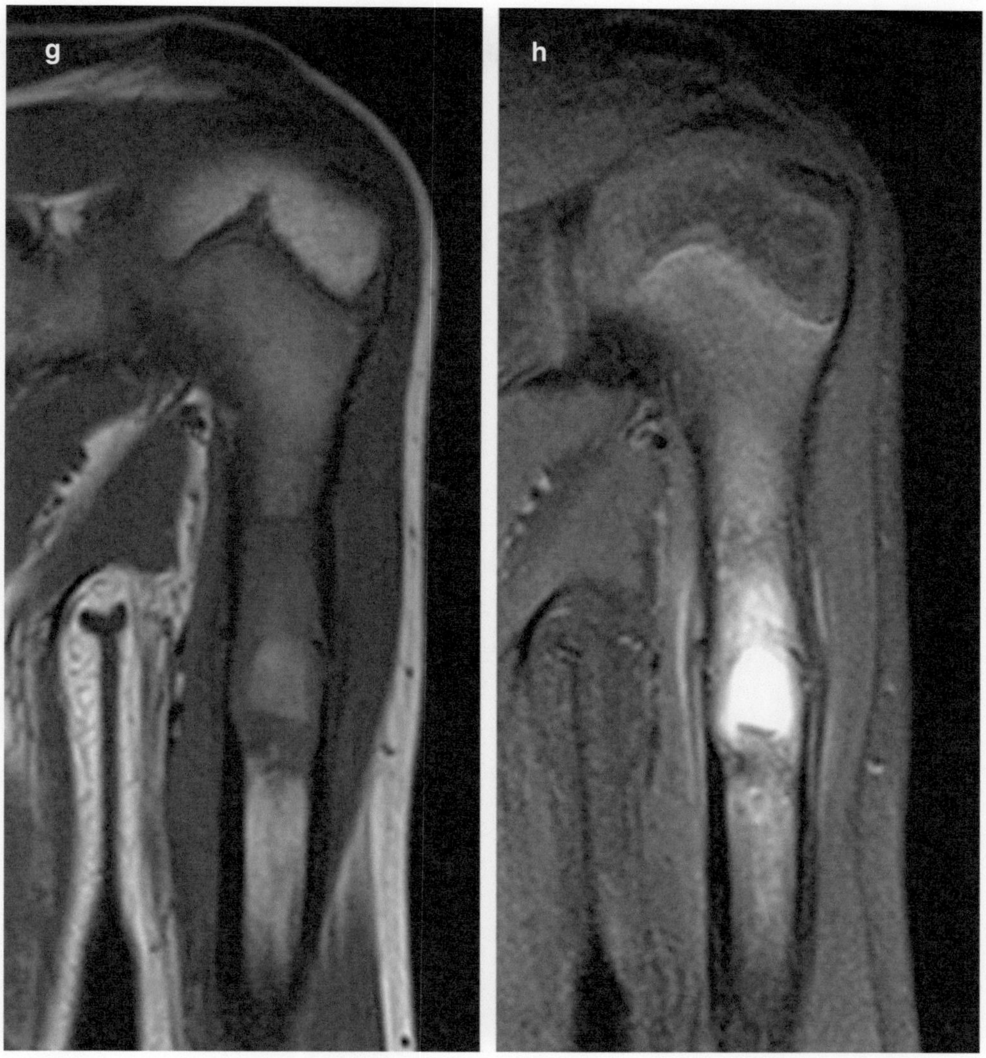

Fig. 7.7 MRI images in coronal T1WI (**g**), T2WI with STIR (**h**) demonstrate a distensible bone destruction in the upper part of the humerus, with a long T1 and T2. Mottled high density in T1W1, broken cortical bone, and pathological fracture can be observed

8. The comparison of radiography, CT, and MRI detailing a pathological fracture in the upper part of the humerus
   8.1 Radiography (Fig. 7.8a–d)

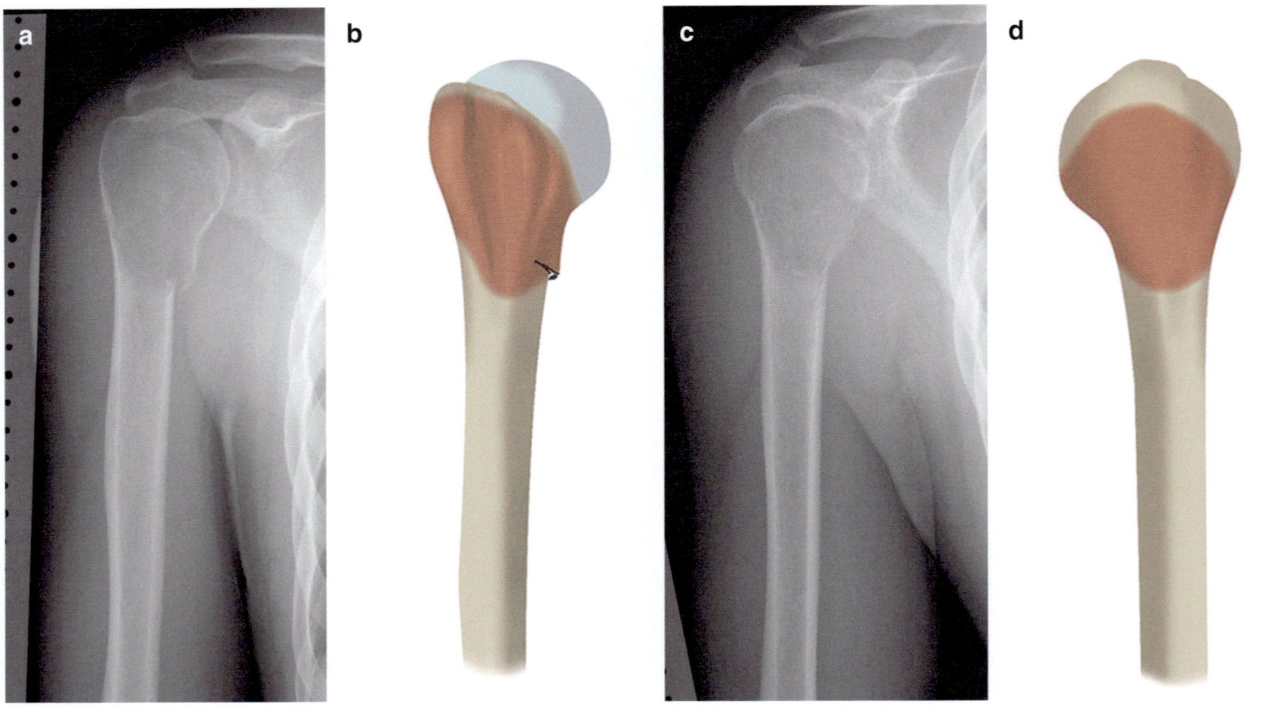

Fig. 7.8 Radiography (**a**, **c**) demonstrates distensible bone destruction in the upper part of right humerus with pathological fracture, homogeneous density and callus can be observed, sketch (**b**, **d**)

8.2 CT (Fig. 7.8e, f)

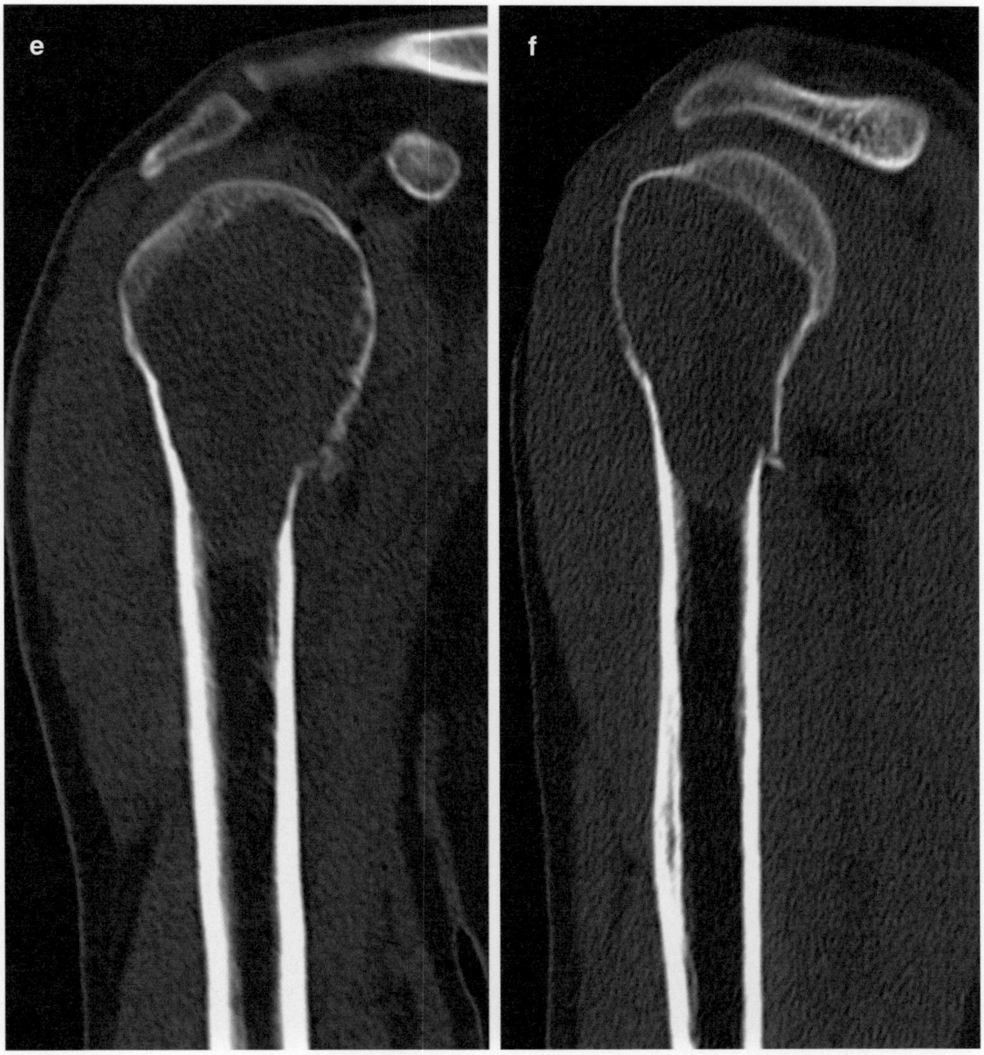

Fig. 7.8 CT in coronal (**e**, **f**) view demonstrates distensible bone destruction in the upper part of the humerus, with homogeneous density and pathological fracture, clear boundary and callus can be observed

8.3 MR (Fig. 7.8g–j)

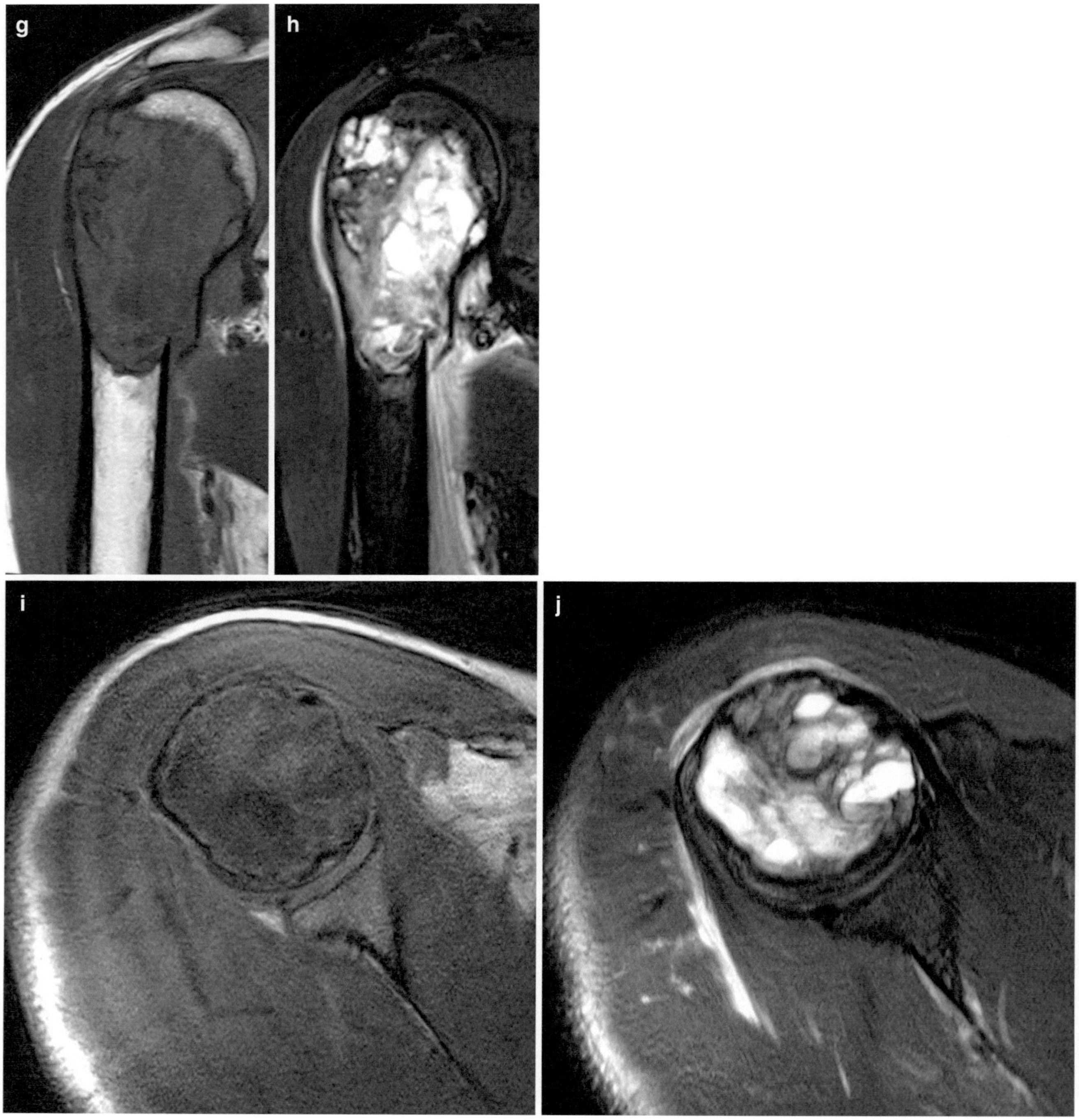

Fig. 7.8 MRI images in coronal T1WI (**g**), T2WI with STIR (**h**), axial T1WI (**i**) and T2WI (**j**) with STIR demonstrate distensible bone destruction in the upper part of the humerus, with a sophistication which is short in T1WI, long in T2WI. Liquid-liquid level, broken cortical bone, and a pathological fracture can be observed

9. The comparison of radiography and MRI showing a pathological fracture in humeral shaft fracture
   9.1 Radiography (Fig. 7.9a–d)

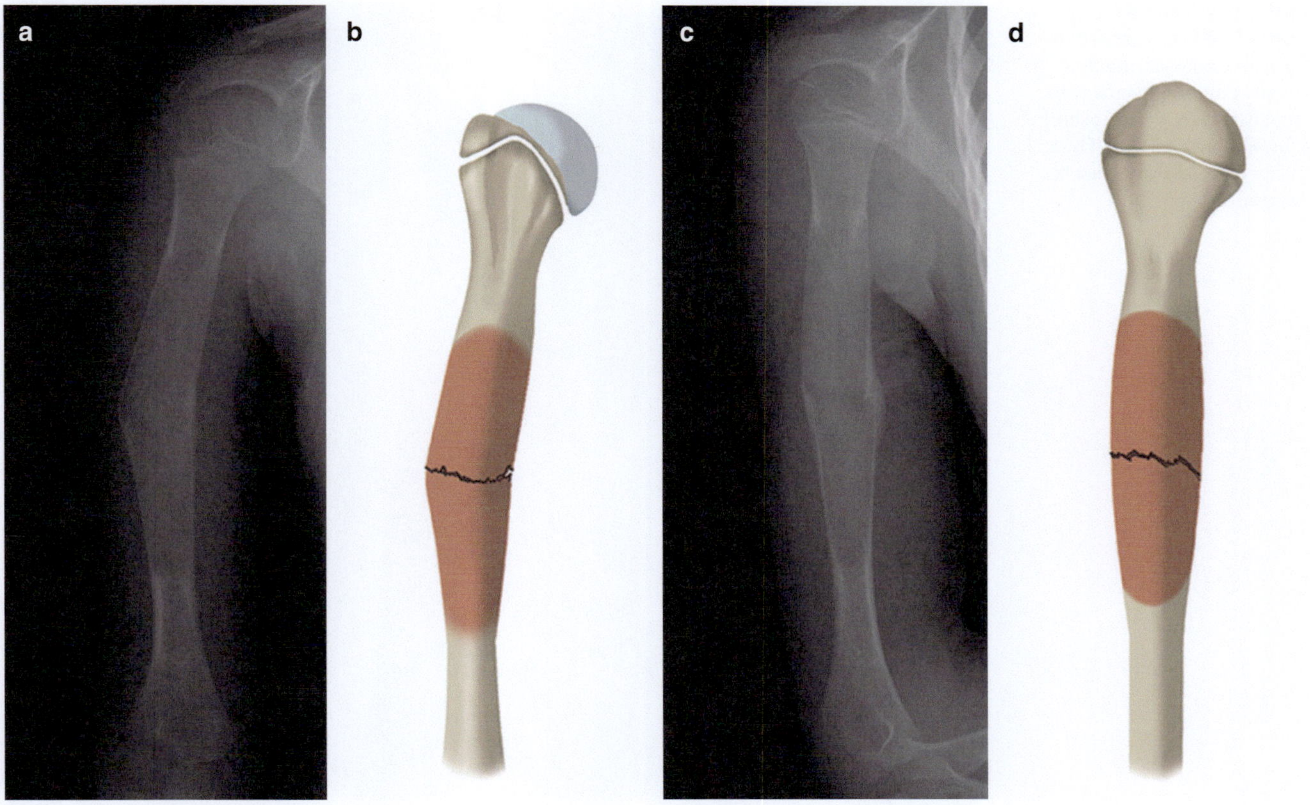

Fig. 7.9 Radiography (**a**, **c**) demonstrates a distensible bone destruction in humeral shaft fracture, with ground-glass opacity, displacement, and angulation which is identified as pathological fracture, obscure boundary can be observed, sketch (**b**, **d**)

9.2 MR (Fig. 7.9e, f)

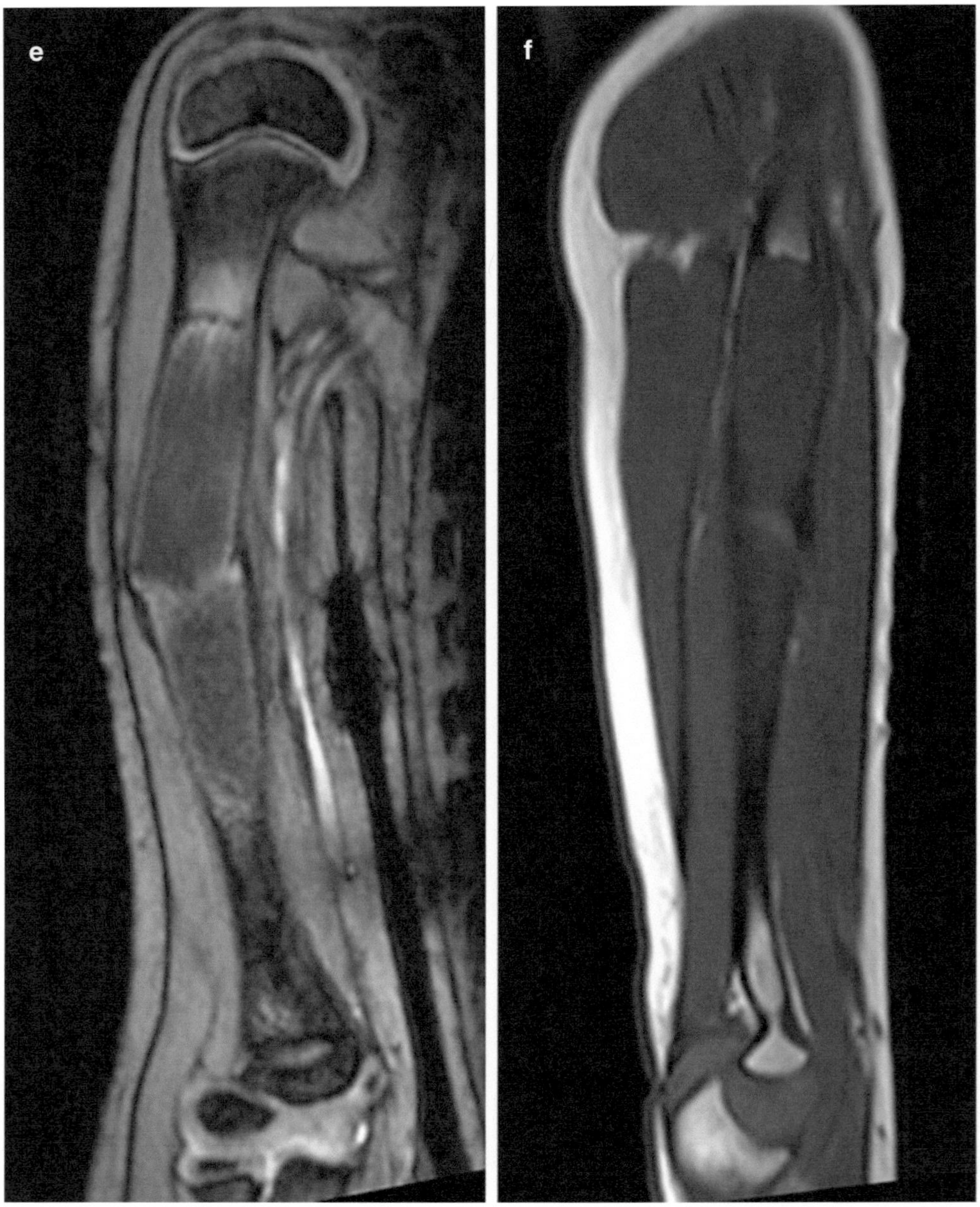

Fig. 7.9 MRI images in coronal T2WI with STIR (**e**), sagittal T1WI (**f**) demonstrate distensible bone destruction in upper part of humerus with a sophistication which is short in T1WI, long in T2WI. High density and angulation can be observed

10. The comparison of a radiography and CT about pathological fracture in upper part of humerus
    10.1 Radiography (Fig. 7.10a–d)

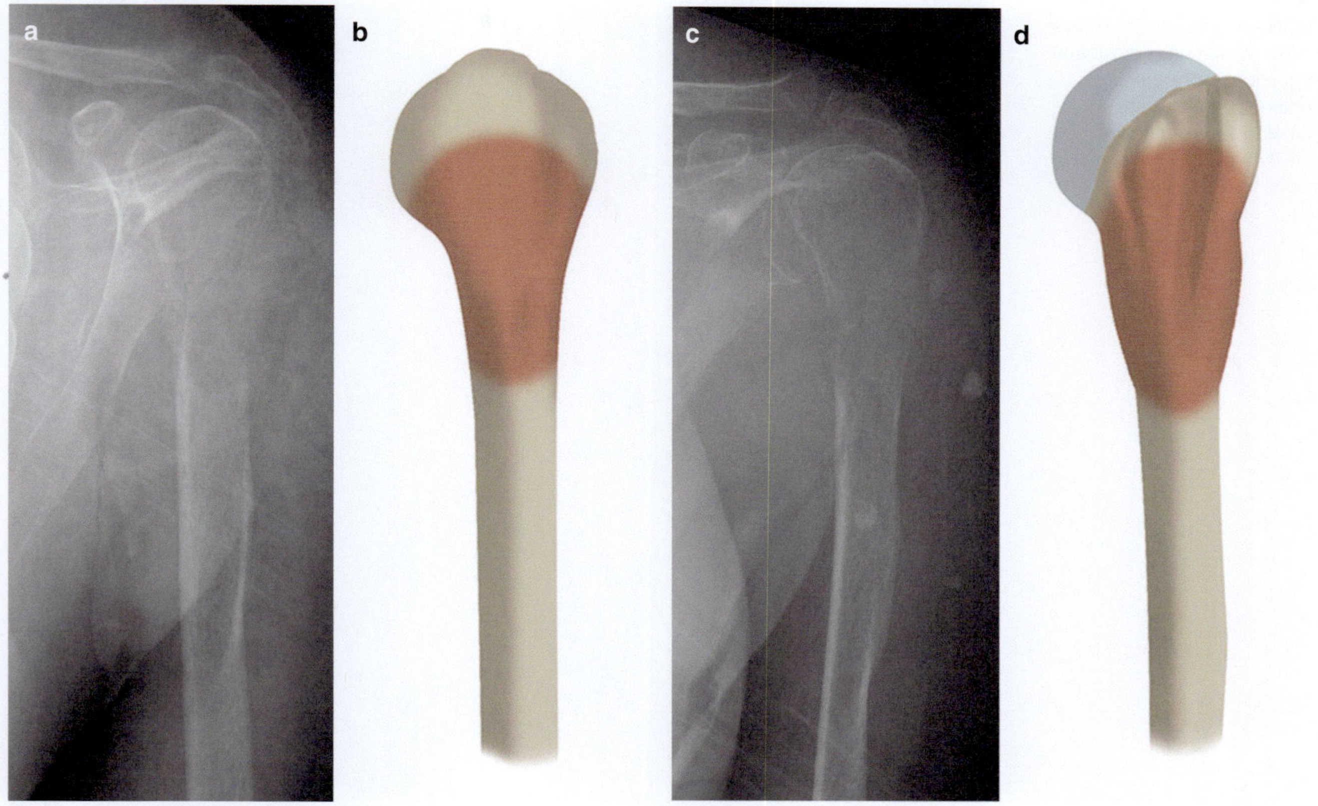

Fig. 7.10 Radiography (**a**, **c**) demonstrates an osteolytic bone destruction in upper part of right humerus with obscure boundary, homogeneous density and cortical deficiency can be observed, sketch (**b**, **d**)

10.2 CT (Fig. 7.10e, f)

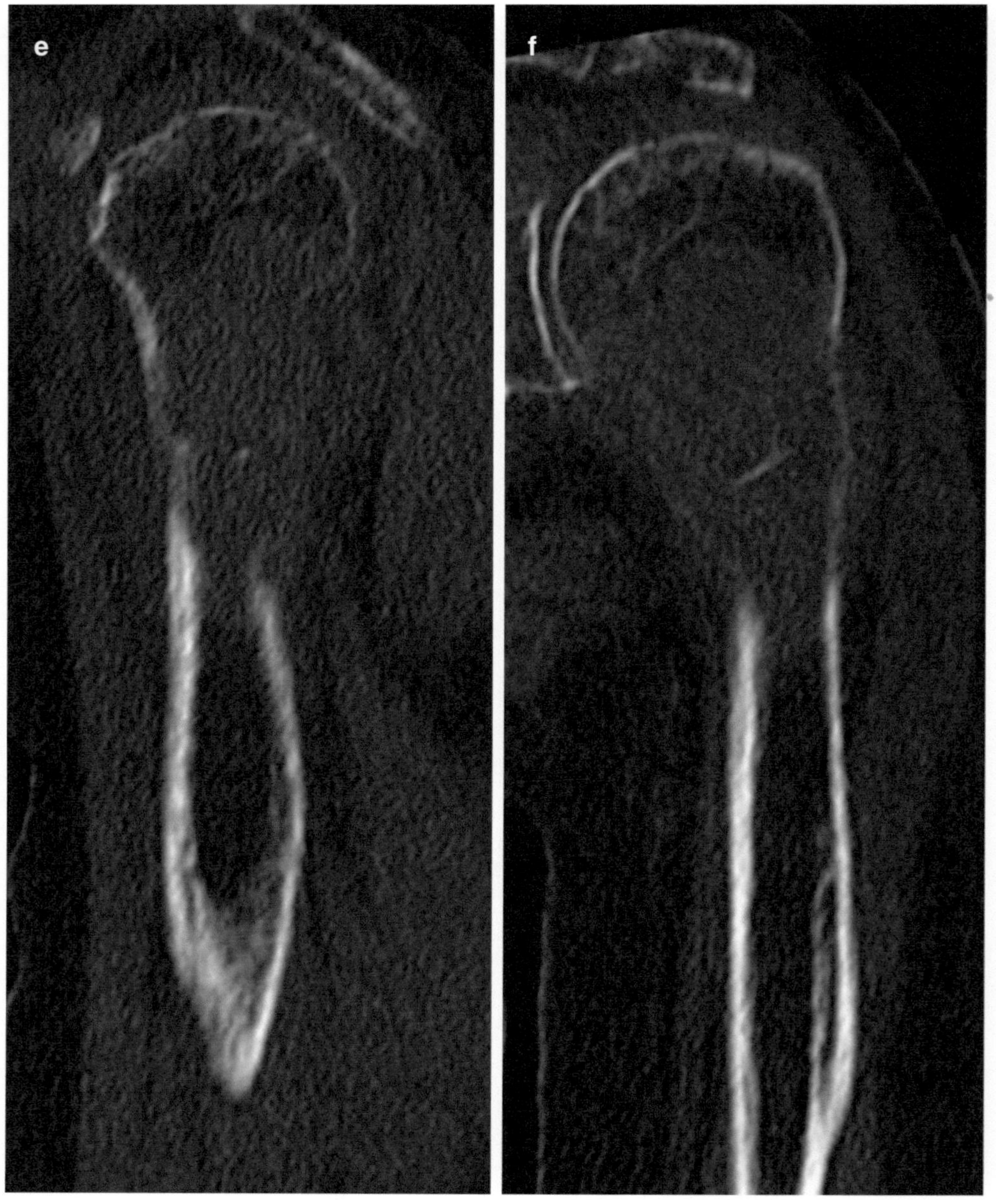

Fig. 7.10 CT in sagittal (**e**), coronal (**f**) view demonstrates an osteolytic bone destruction in upper part of right humerus, with obscure boundary, homogeneous density and cortical deficiency can be observed

11. The comparison of CT and MRI detailing a pathological fracture caused by a metastatic tumor in middle and lower part of radius
    11.1 CT (Fig. 7.11a, b)

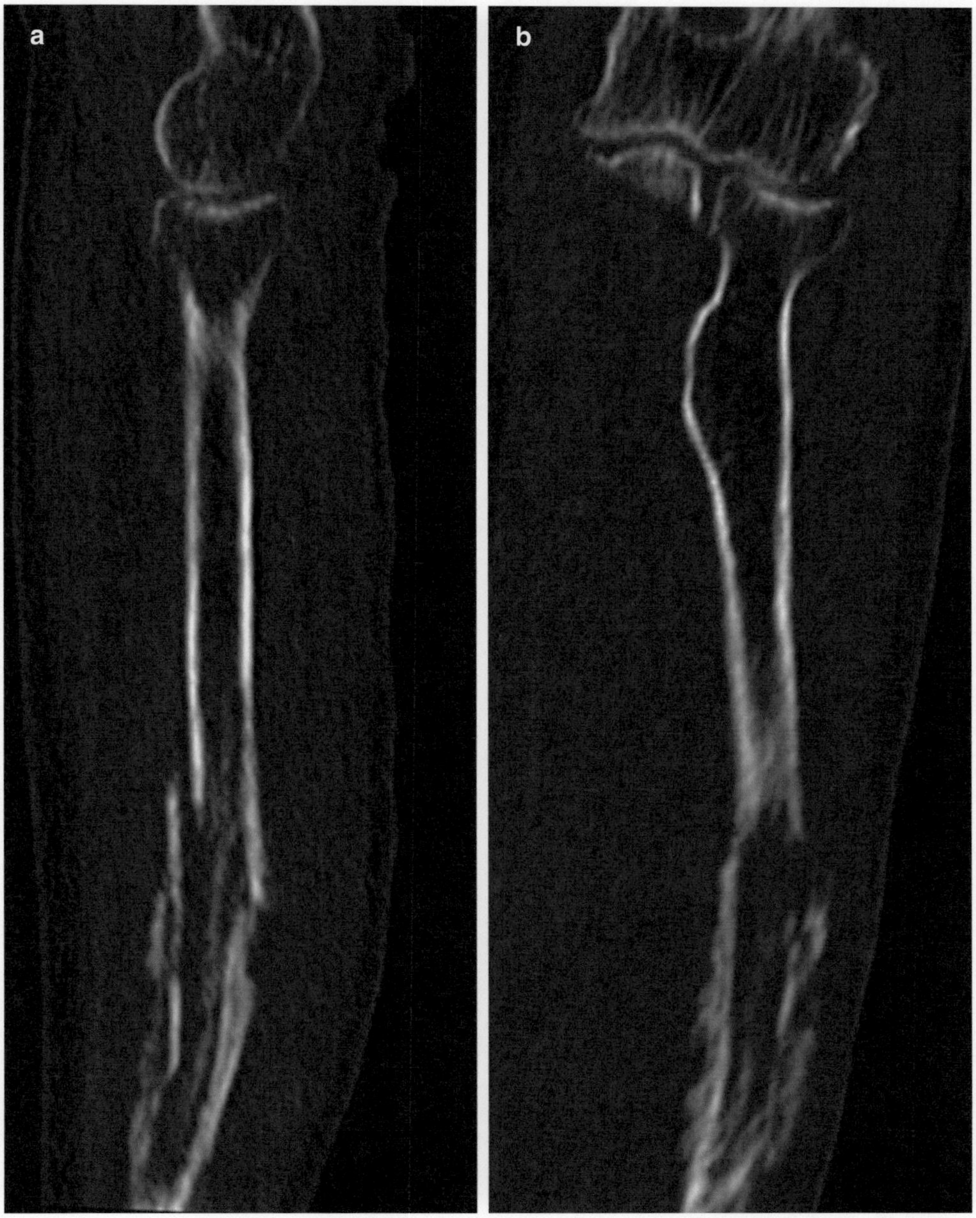

Fig. 7.11 CT in sagittal (**a**), coronal (**b**) view demonstrates a bone destruction in the middle or lower part of the radius with obscure boundary, heterogeneous density and cortical broken can be observed

11.2 MR (Fig. 7.11c, d)

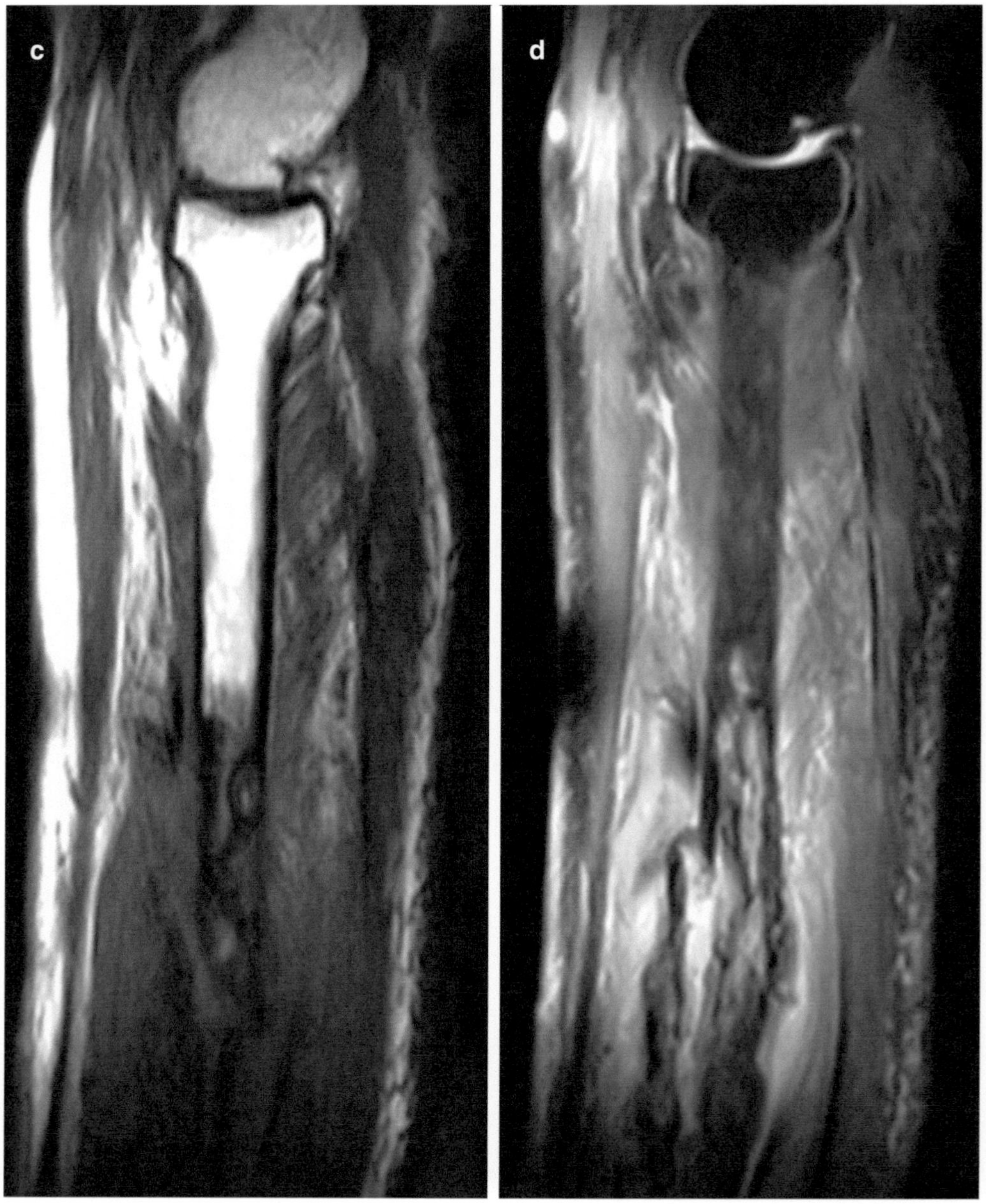

Fig. 7.11 MRI images in sagittal T1WI (**c**), coronal T2WI with STIR (**d**) view demonstrate osteolytic bone destruction in middle or lower part of the radius which is short in T1WI, long in T2WI, and soft tissue swelling can be observed

12. The comparison of radiography and CT showing a pathological fracture caused by a metastatic tumor in middle part of the radius
    12.1 Radiography (Fig. 7.12a–d)

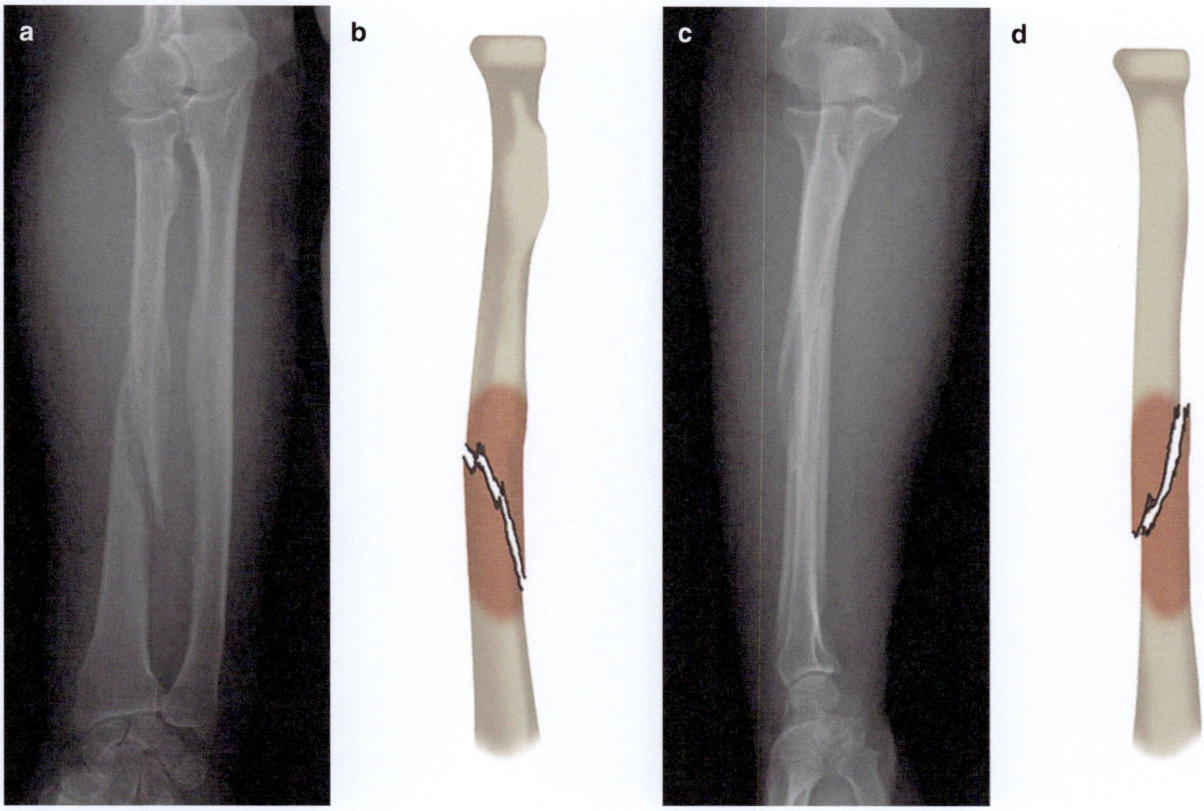

Fig. 7.12 Radiography (**a**, **c**) demonstrated oblique fracture in middle part of the radius with displacement, low density can be observed, sketch (**b**, **d**)

12.2 CT (Fig. 7.12e, f)

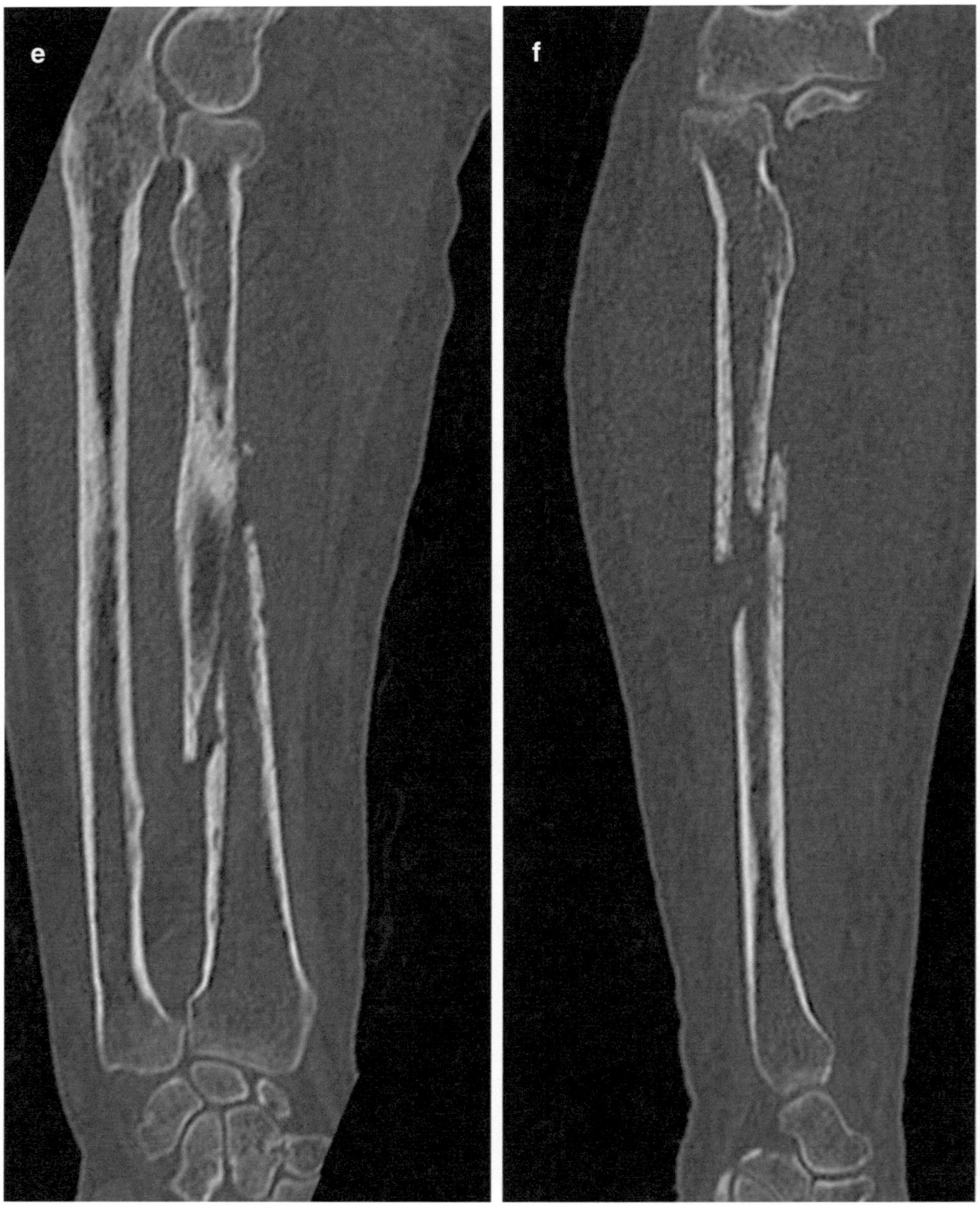

Fig. 7.12 CT in coronal (**e**), sagittal (**f**) view demonstrates an infiltrative bone destruction in the middle part of the radius with a pathological fracture, low bone density and mild displacement can be observed

13. The comparison of radiography, CT, and MRI detailing a pathological fracture caused by a metastatic tumor in middle part of radius
    13.1 Radiography (Fig. 7.13a–d)

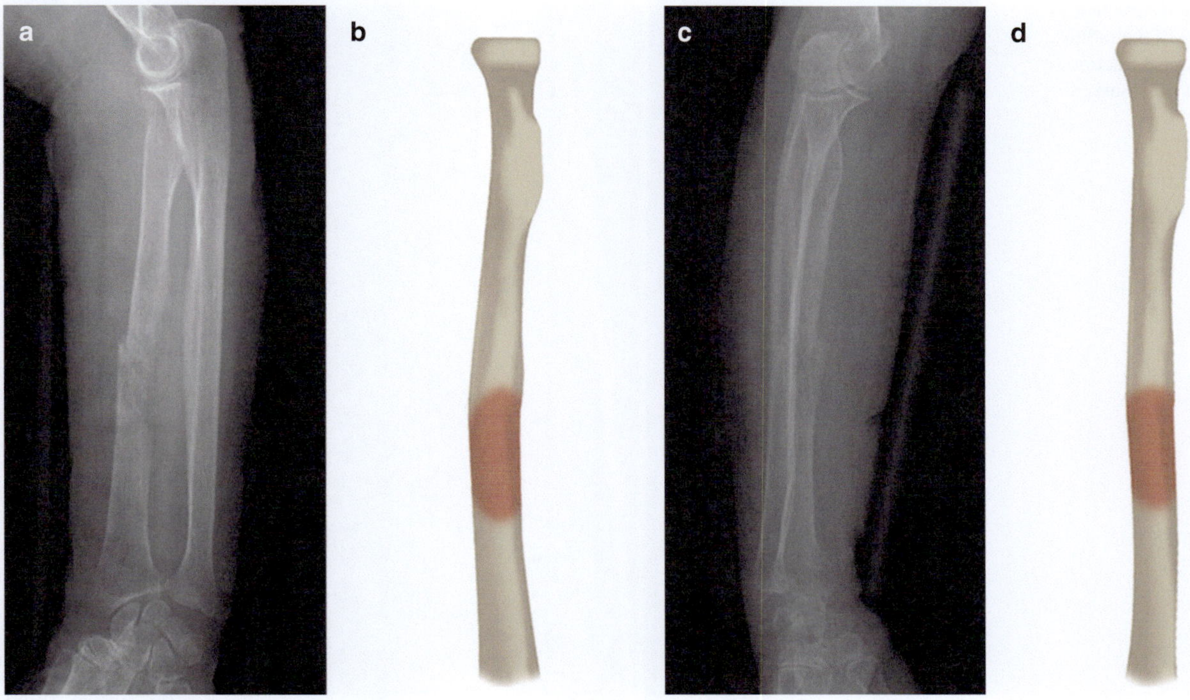

Fig. 7.13 Radiography (**a**, **c**) demonstrates an osteolytic bone destruction in the middle part of the radius with a pathological fracture, low density and medial cortical bone deficiency can be observed, sketch (**b**, **d**)

13.2 CT (Fig. 7.13e, f)

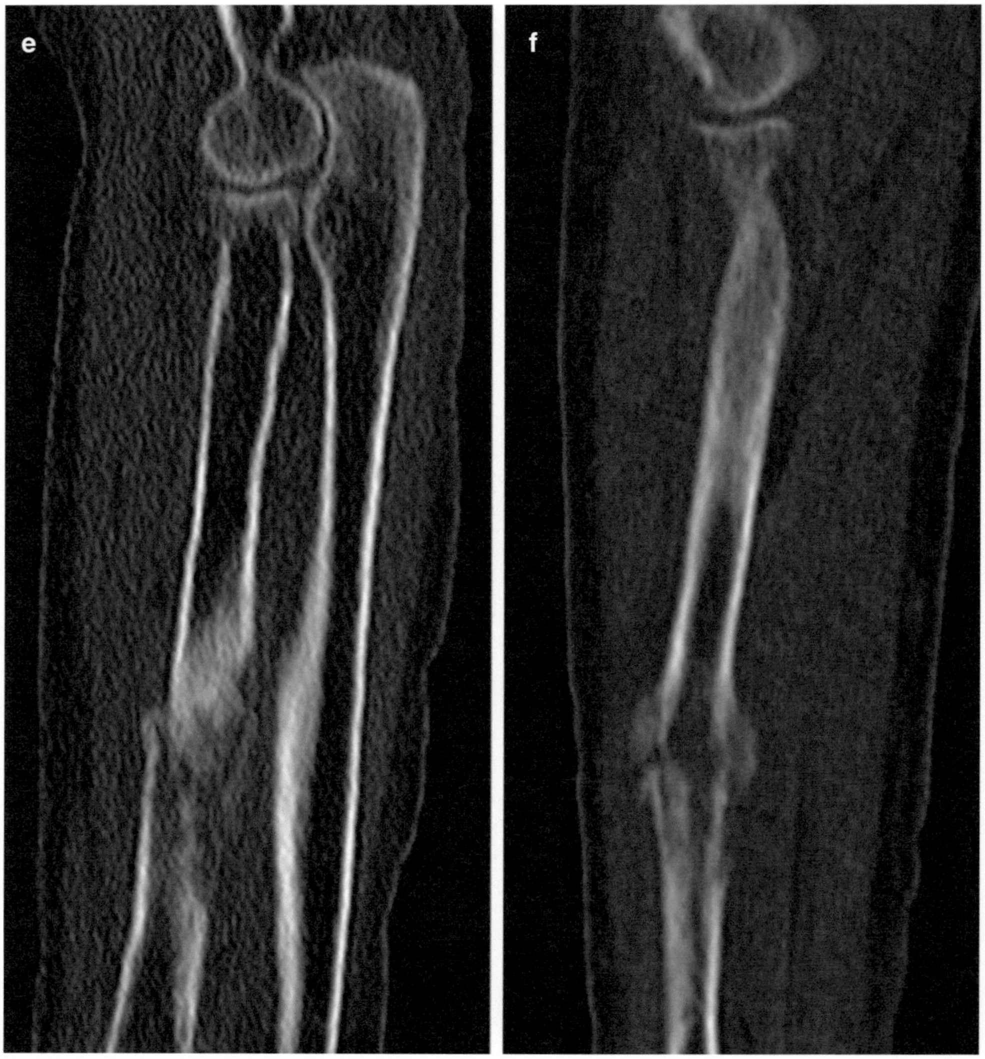

Fig. 7.13 CT in sagittal (**e**, **f**) view demonstrates an osteolytic bone destruction in the middle part of the radius with a pathological fracture, new callus can be observed

13.3 MR (Fig. 7.13g, h)

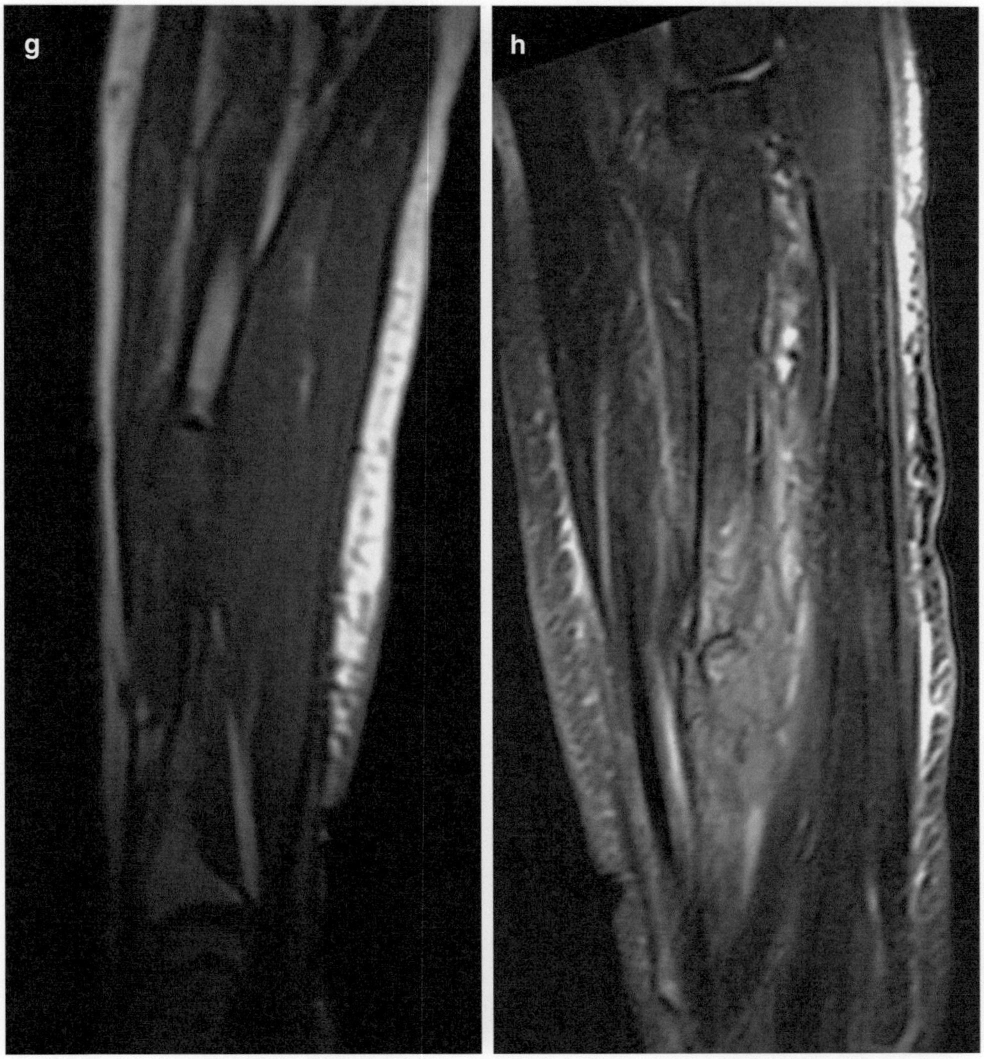

Fig. 7.13 MRI images in sagittal T1WI (**g**), T2WI (**h**) view demonstrate an osteolytic bone destruction in the middle part of the radius with a long T1 and T2, where soft tissue swelling can be observed

14. The comparison of radiography and CT showing a pathological fracture caused by enchondrosis in the middle part of the metacarpal bones
    14.1 Radiography (Fig. 7.14a–d)

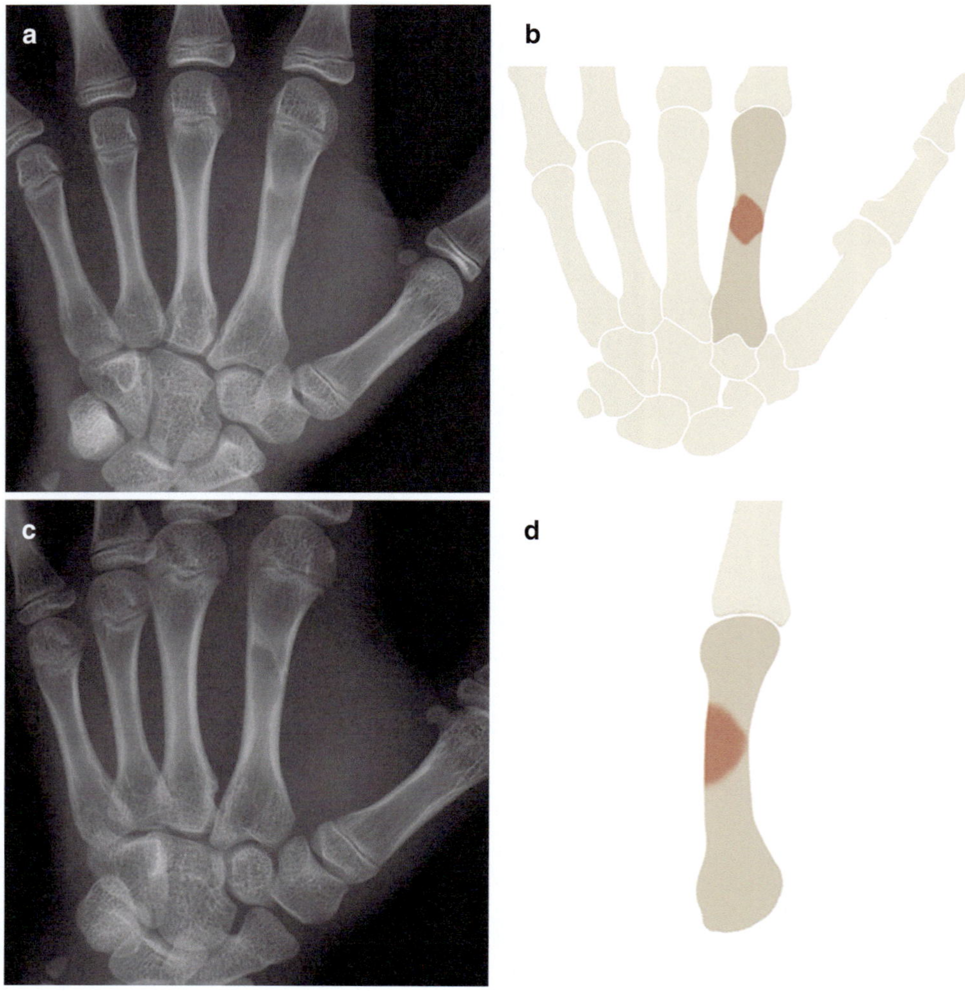

Fig. 7.14 Radiography (**a**, **c**) demonstrated distensible bone destruction in the middle part of the metacarpal bones with a pathological fracture, osteosclerosis and discontinued cortical bone in radius can be observed, sketch (**b**, **d**)

14.2 CT (Fig. 7.14e, f)

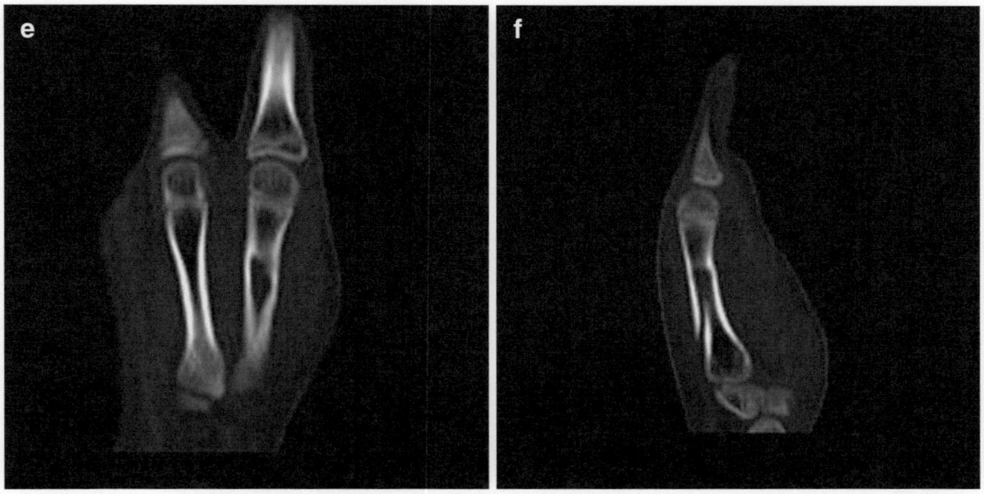

Fig. 7.14 CT in coronal (**e**), sagittal (**f**) view demonstrates a distensible bone destruction in the middle part of the metacarpal bones with a pathological fracture, osteosclerosis can be observed

15. The comparison of a radiography and CT showing a pathological fracture caused by enchondrosis in the phalanx
    15.1 Radiography (Fig. 7.15a–d)

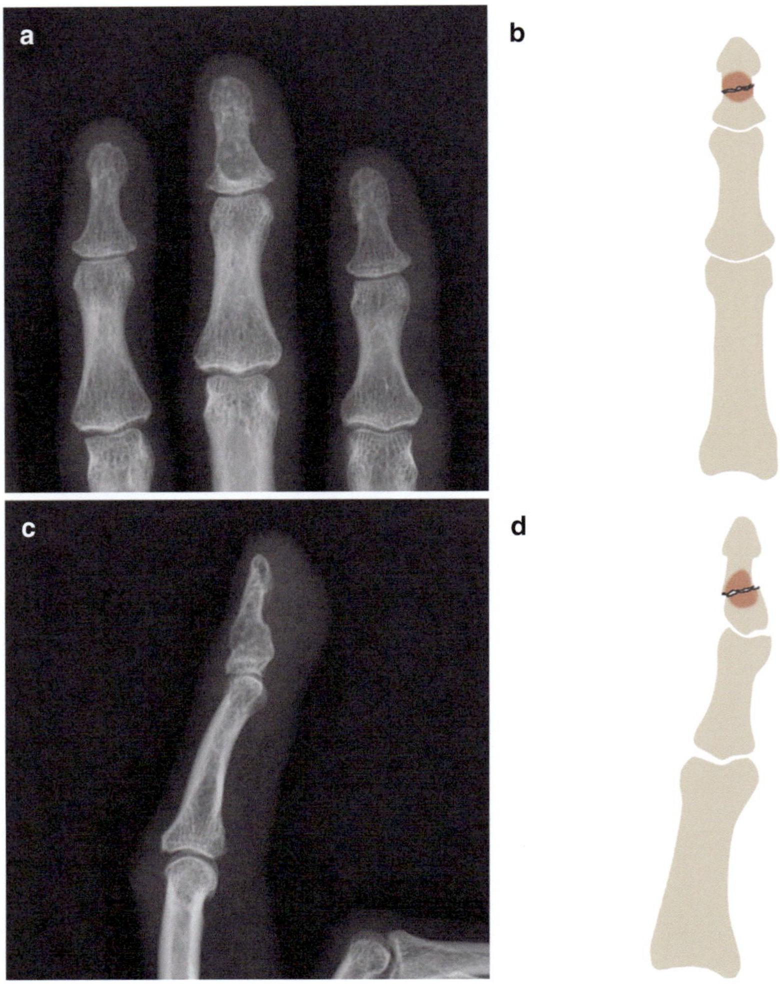

Fig. 7.15 Radiography (**a**, **c**) demonstrates distensible bone destruction in distal phalanx of middle phalanx with clear boundary, mottled calcification and discontinued cortical bone can be observed, sketch (**b**, **d**)

15.2 CT (Fig. 7.15e, f)

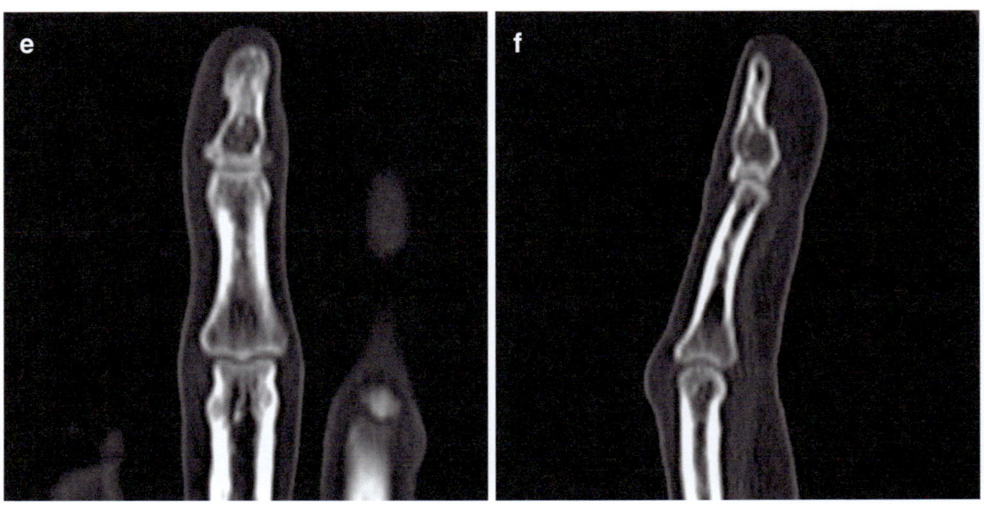

Fig. 7.15 CT in coronal (**e**), sagittal (**f**) view demonstrates distensible bone destruction in distal phalanx of middle phalanx with clear boundary, mottled calcification and discontinued cortical bone can be observed

7.4 Summary

1. The management for a trauma fracture differs from the management when dealing with a pathological fracture. A preoperative surgery is to identify the disease which is essential for a surgical plan. CT and MRI scans are important methods to reveal the lesion, range, and qualitative analysis.
2. Pathologic fractures occur in different age groups and at different sites. For instance, bone cyst is common in pediatric humerus. Metastatic tumor and myeloma occur in old patients. Fibrous dysplasia occurs in young and middle-aged patients. Most logical fracture characterized by enchondrosis happens in the phalanx.
3. A traumatic clavicle fracture occurs in the middle or lateral part. A fracture located in the medial part is prone to be a pathological fracture.

Part III

Fracture of Lower Extremity

Hip Fracture

8

Zhiyong Hou and Yingze Zhang

8.1 Fracture of Acetabulum

The hip bone is composed of three bones: the ilium, ischium, and the pubis. The acetabulum, a large cup-shaped articular cavity, is situated near the middle of the outer surface of the bone, together with the femoral head from the hip joint. The acetabulum is an important part of the hip joint, which is prone to suffer damage because it is a major weight-bearing and flexible joint. An acetabular fracture can be indirectly caused by an ilium, ischium, and pubis fracture, or directly by central dislocation of the hip joint.

The acetabulum is divided into the iliopectineal column and ilioischial column. The Letournel and Judet classification method is the most widely used classification of acetabular fractures in clinical practice and research. It classifies acetabular fractures into two basic types: simple fracture patterns and complex fracture patterns. Simple fracture patterns [1]: A: Posterior wall fractures; B: Posterior column fractures; C: Anterior wall fractures; D: Anterior column fractures; E: Transverse acetabular fracture. Complex fracture patterns: F: Posterior column and posterior wall; G: Transverse and posterior wall; H: T-type fracture; I: Anterior column and posterior hemi transverse fracture, both- column fracture.

8.1.1 Injury Mechanism

Most acetabular fractures occur because of high-energy trauma injuries, which could be indirect and/or a forceful exertion. Most injuries occur when force is exerted onto the femur (greater tuberosity, neck, or head), which then passes through the femoral head, and is transferred to the acetabulum. Axial compression injuries along the femur can also lead to acetabular fractures. The position of the femoral head at the time of the injury, as well as the direction and magnitude of the force determines the pattern of acetabular injury. Flexion and internal rotation of the hip predisposes the patient to posterior column injuries, while extension and external rotation of the hip is a preamble to anterior column injuries.

8.1.2 Signs and Symptoms

Acetabular fractures typically present as groin and hip pain, exacerbated by passive hip motion. Mobility is limited because of the pain. Dislocation of the femoral head corresponds with a lower limb deformity. When there is central dislocation of the hip, the degree of pain and dysfunction is not as serious as an anterior and posterior dislocation; therefore, the signs are not obvious. A severe dislocation may lead to the affected limb to become shortened. An acetabular fracture may be associated with a pelvic hemorrhage, urethral or nerve damage, a rupture of the pelvic ring, and an ipsilateral lower extremity fracture.

Z. Hou · Y. Zhang (✉)
Department of Orthopaedics, The Third Hospital of Hebei Medical University, Shijiazhuang, Hebei, China

Y. Zhang (ed.), *Differential Diagnosis of Fracture*, https://doi.org/10.1007/978-981-13-8339-7_8

8.1.3 Radiographic Diagnosis

Radiographic evaluations include a flat film and CT. An X-ray includes an anteroposterior view and acetabular oblique view. An obturator oblique photographing method is as follows: the ipsilateral hip is raised, crown surface of the body and the bed is at about 45°, X center line is aligned perpendicularly on the film at 5 cm within the ipsilateral iliac spine. An obturator oblique view shows the iliopectineal line (anterior column) of the pelvis and posterior wall. Iliac oblique photographing method is as follows: ipsilateral iliac is near the bed, crown surface of the contralateral side and the bed is at about 45°, X center line is aligned perpendicularly on the film at 5 cm front ipsilateral iliac spine. Iliac oblique views illustrate the ilioischial line (posterior column) and anterior wall. While CT scans of the pelvis, including 3-dimensional reformatted images, may be required to conceptualize the fracture pattern, an orthopedic surgeon can visually observe the fracture which X-rays cannot display, by the reconstruction of CT, and thereby help to decide the best course of treatment of an acetabulum fracture.

The classification of acetabular fractures is often difficult for inexperienced physicians. According to the ten types of fractures in Judet–Letournel, 90% of fractures are the five most common ones (Fig. 8.1). According to whether the fracture involves the obturator ring, it is divided into double-column fractures, T-shaped fractures, transverse fractures, transverse and posterior wall fractures, and simple posterior wall fractures. According to whether the iliopubic line and the ilioischial line are continuous, the fractures can be divided into transverse fracture, transverse and posterior wall fractures, and simple posterior wall fractures. A fracture of the obturator ring is very subtle, and therefore, easy to miss.

1. Diagnosis of common types of acetabular fractures (Fig. 8.1)

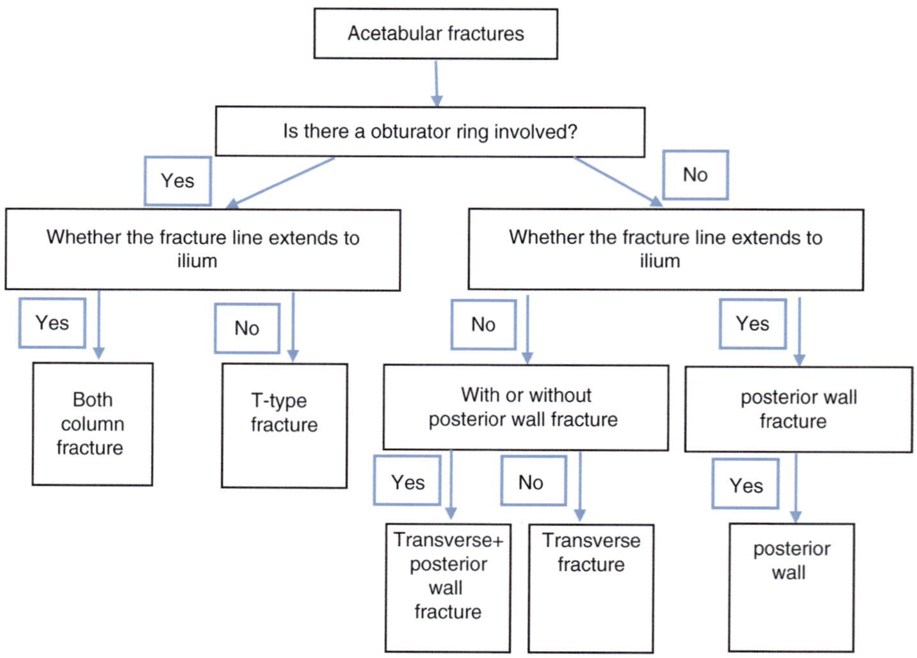

Fig. 8.1 Diagnosis of common types of acetabular fractures

2. Anterior wall acetabular fracture
   2.1 X-ray film (Fig. 8.2a–d)

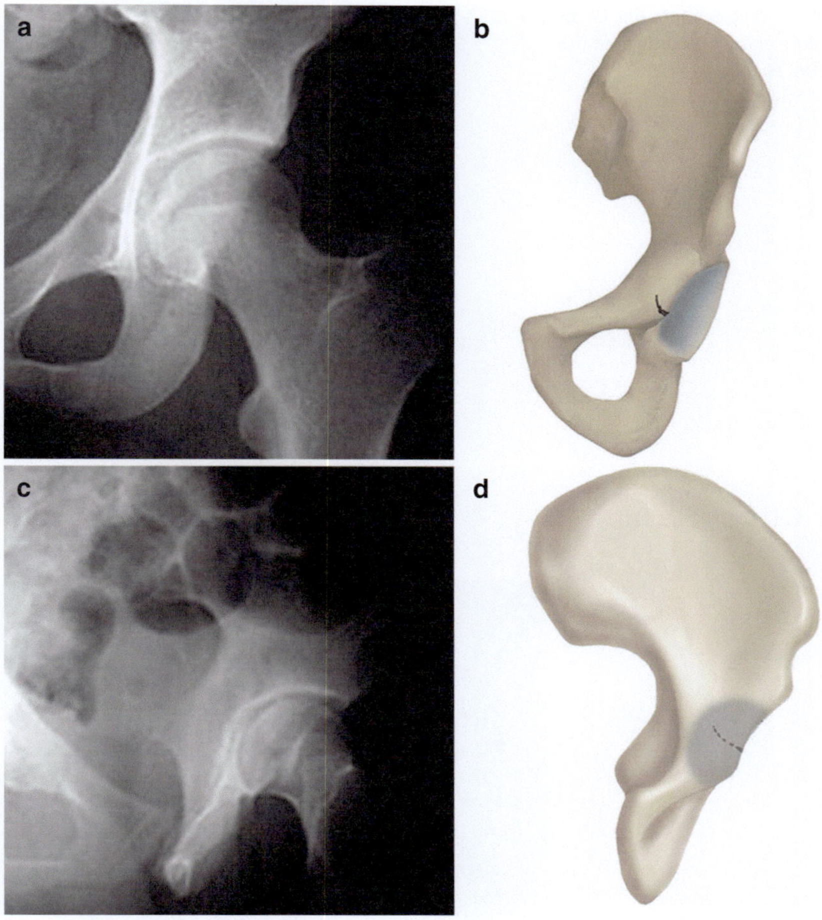

Fig. 8.2 Acetabular anterior wall fracture. (**a**) A horizontal low-density line of acetabulum is shown in the anteroposterior view of hip joint (**b**). (**c**) The acetabular oblique view shows the fracture line at the anterior wall of the acetabulum (**d**). Anterior acetabulum wall fracture: iliopubic line and the ilioischial line are continuous

3. Anterior acetabulum wall fracture
   3.1 X-ray film (Fig. 8.3a, b)

Fig. 8.3 (**a**) The fracture line of the acetabulum cannot be shown on the X-ray film (**b**)

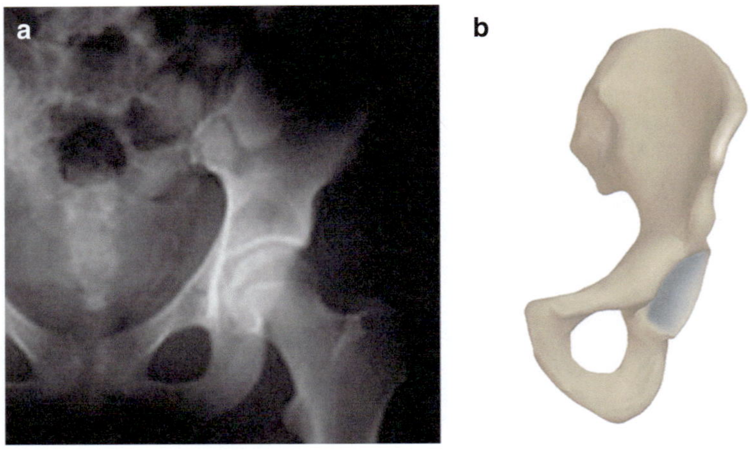

   3.2 CT scan (Fig. 8.3c)

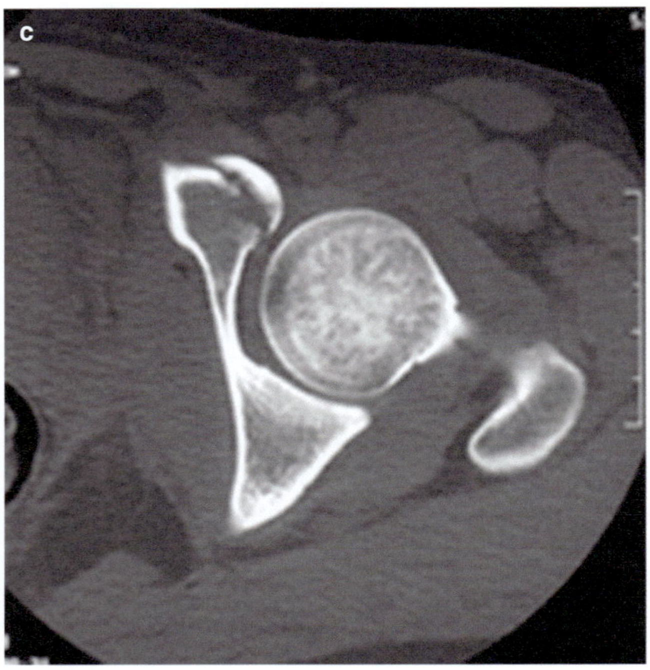

Fig. 8.3 (**c**) Anterior wall fracture-CT shows that the fracture line is located in the anterior wall of the acetabulum

4. Identification of acetabular anterior column fracture and pubic basal fracture
   4.1 X-ray film (Fig. 8.4a, b)

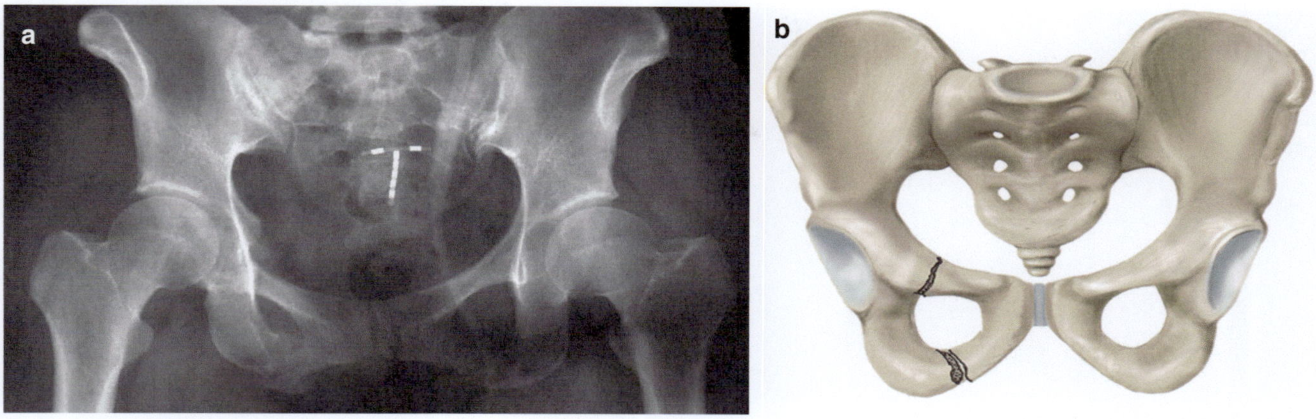

Fig. 8.4 (**a**) X-ray film shows fracture of base of the superior ramus of the right pubis, iliopubic line is not continuous, the fracture involves the inferior ramus of the pubis, and the pelvic ring is deformed (**b**)

   4.2 CT scan (Fig. 8.4c–f)

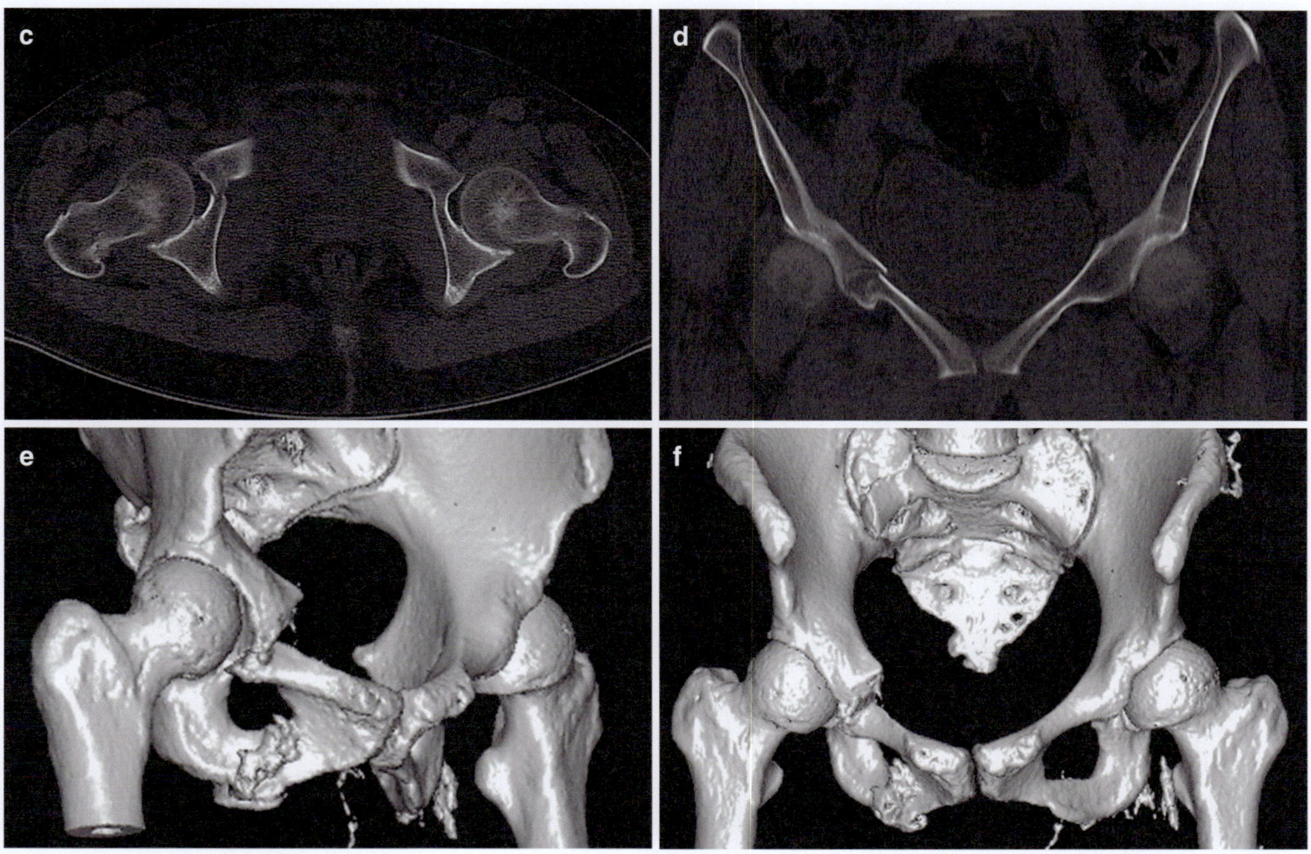

Fig. 8.4 (**c**) (horizontal axis) and (**d**) (coronal reconstruction): CT shows that the fracture involves the anterior column of the acetabulum, and the iliopubic line is discontinuous. (**e, f**) three-dimensional CT reconstruction visually shows fractures of the anterior column and the inferior ramus of the right pubis of right hip, and the iliopubic line is interrupted

5. Posterior wall acetabular fracture
   5.1 X-ray film (Fig. 8.5a, b)

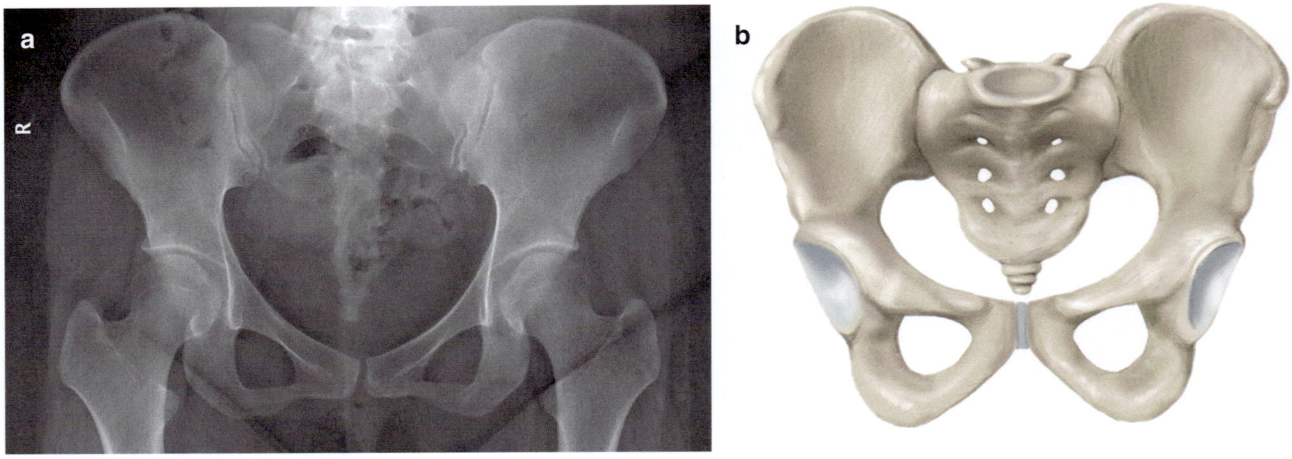

Fig. 8.5 (**a**) The fracture line of the acetabulum cannot be shown on the X-ray film (**b**)

   5.2 CT scan (Fig. 8.5c, d)

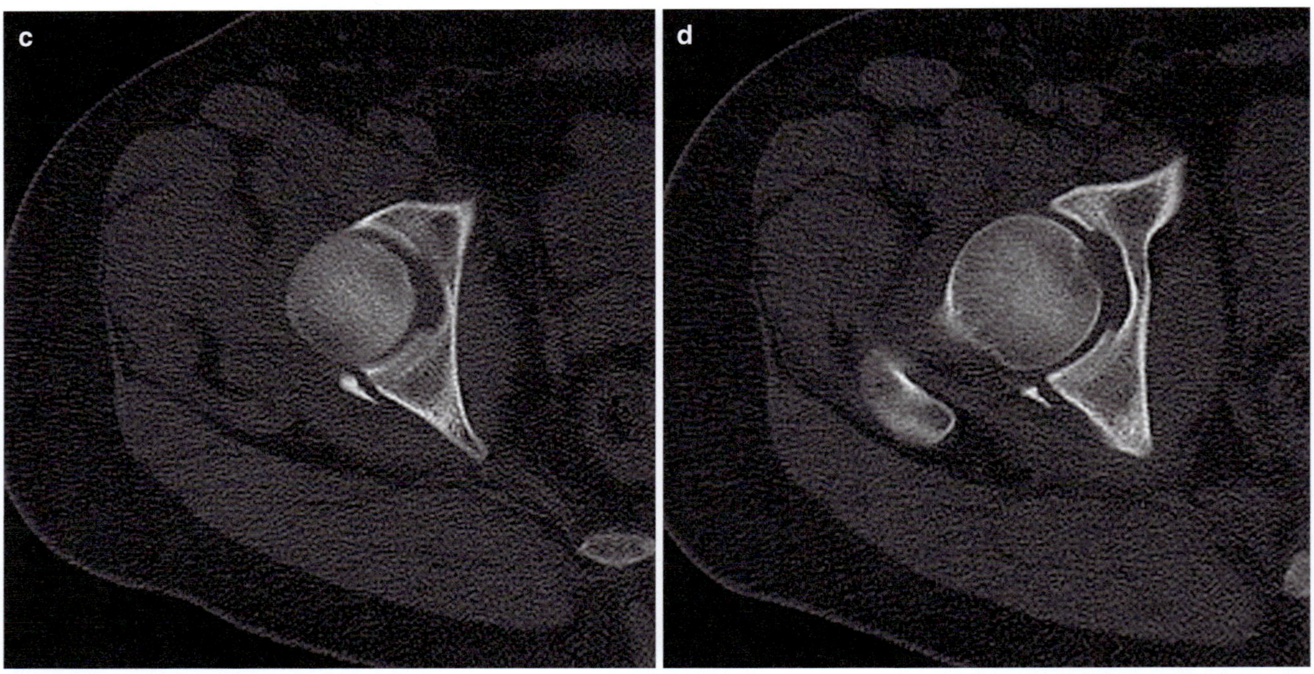

Fig. 8.5 (**c**, **d**) CT shows that the fracture line is located in the posterior wall of the acetabulum. The fracture did not involve the obturator ring, the iliopubic line and the ilioischial line were continuous, and it was a simple posterior acetabular fracture

6. Identification of posterior column of acetabulum fracture and posterior wall acetabular fracture
   6.1 X-ray film (Fig. 8.6a–d)

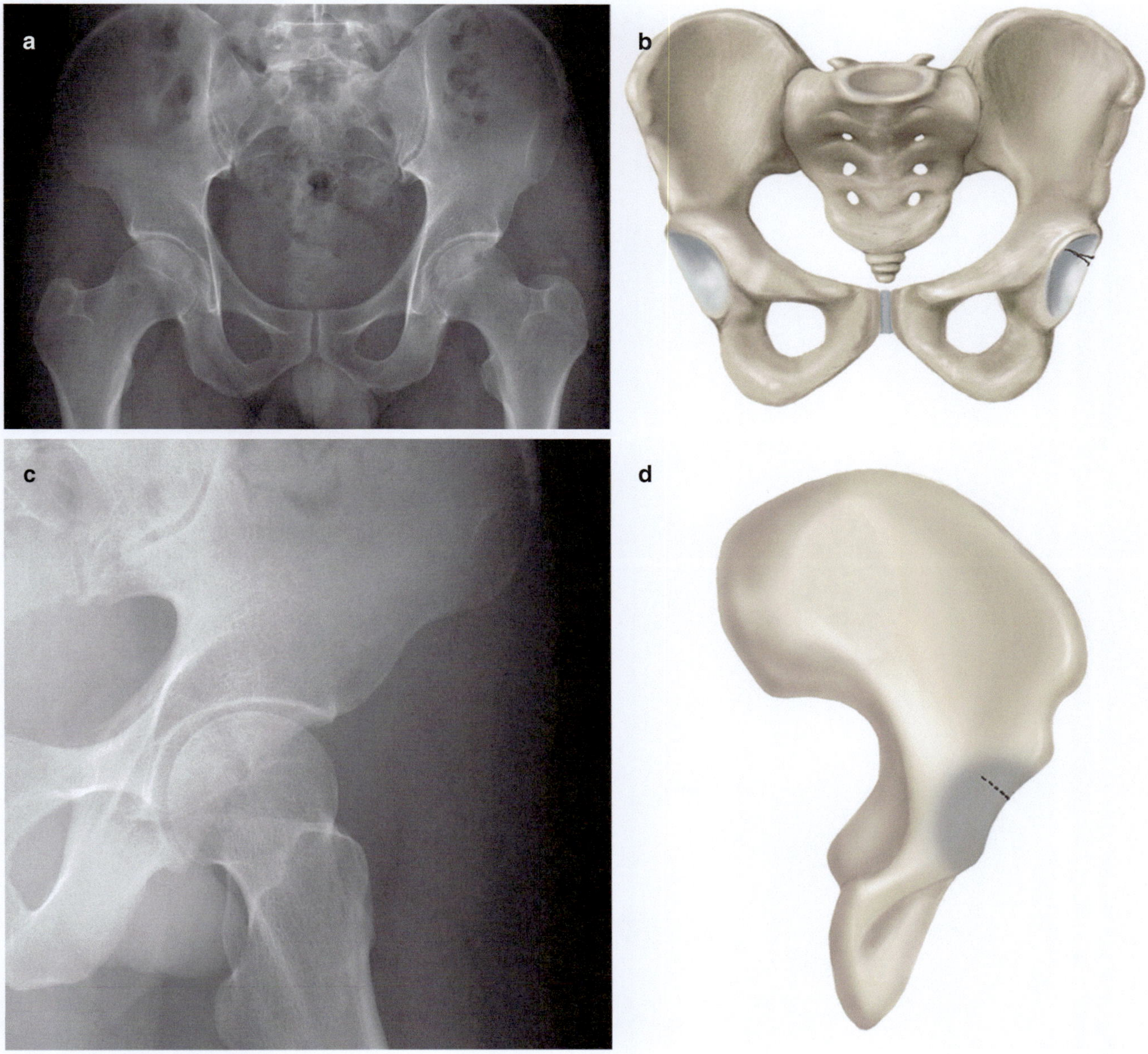

Fig. 8.6 (**a**) X-ray film shows the irregular shape of the posterior lateral margin of the left acetabulum (**b**); (**c**) Iliac oblique views of the left hip clearly show the low-density line of the acetabulum (**d**)

6.2 CT scan (Fig. 8.6e–g)

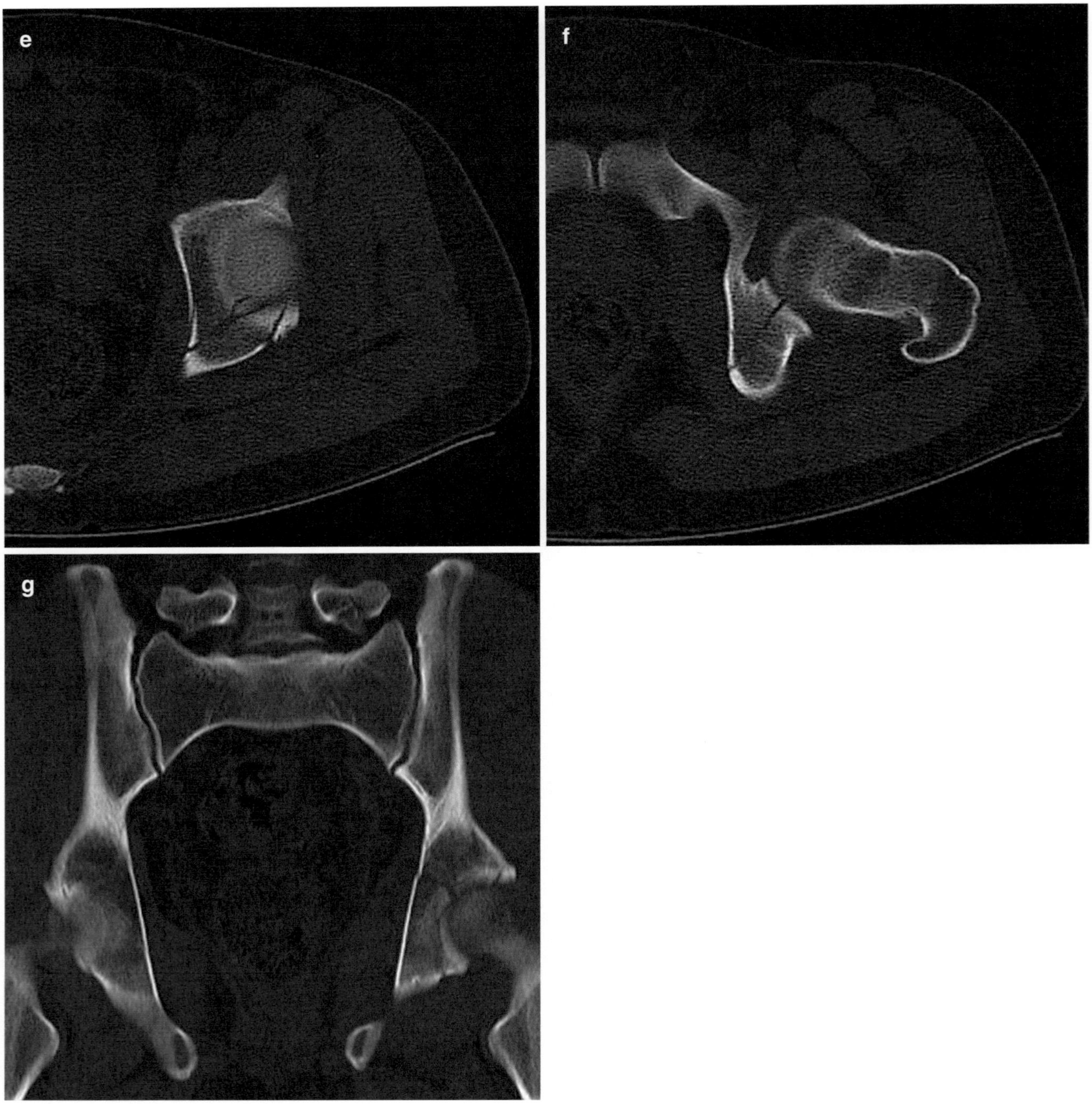

Fig. 8.6 (**e**, **f**) (horizontal axis) and (**g**) (coronal reconstruction): Posterior acetabular fracture— CT shows that the fracture line involves the posterior column of the acetabulum, and the ilioischial line is discontinuous

7. Comparison between X-ray film and CT of acetabular transverse fracture
   7.1 X-ray film (Fig. 8.7a–d)

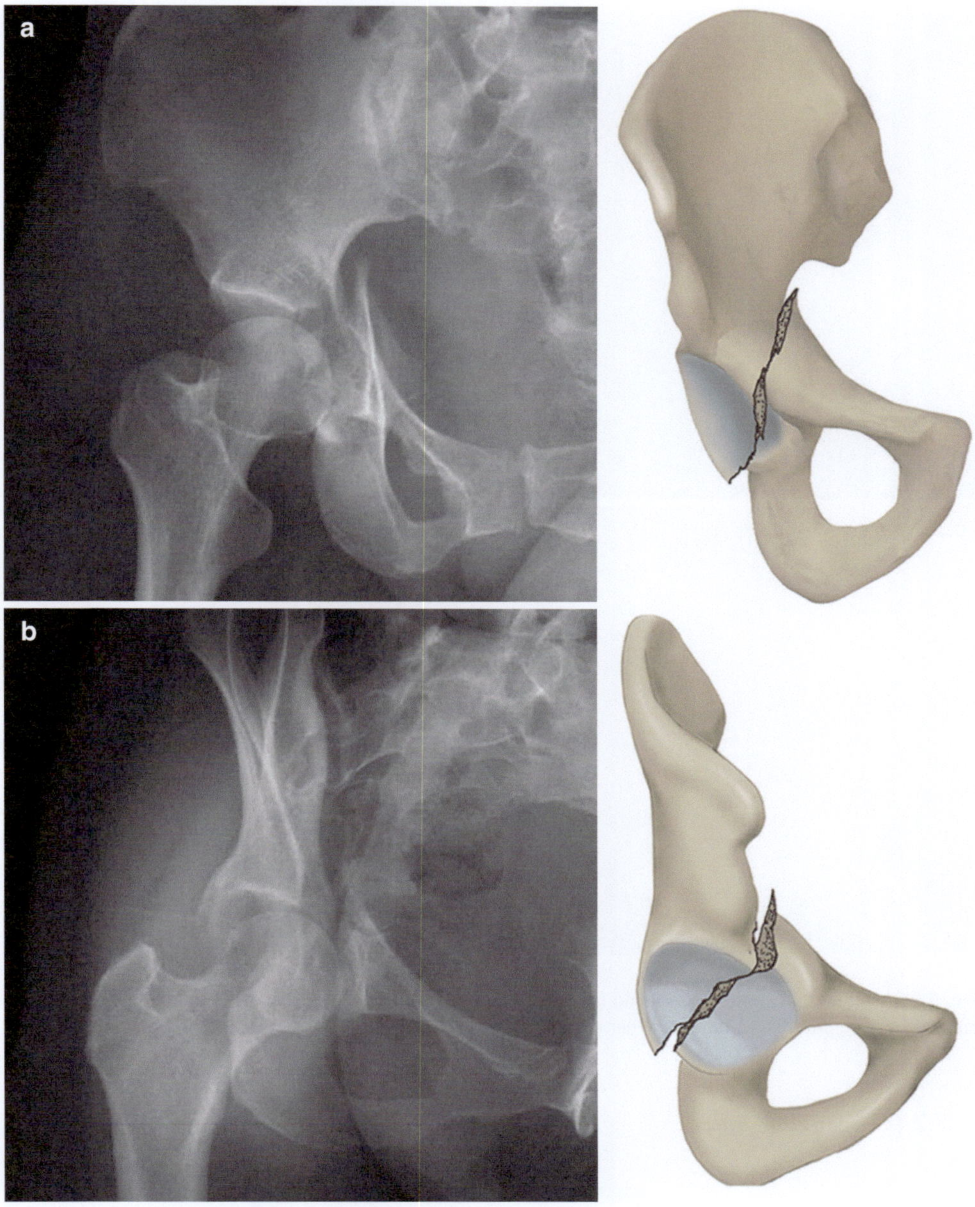

Fig. 8.7 (**a**) (anteroposterior views) and (**c**) (obturator oblique views) show the discontinuity of iliopubic line and ilioischial line (**b**, **d**)

   7.2 CT scan (Fig. 8.7e)

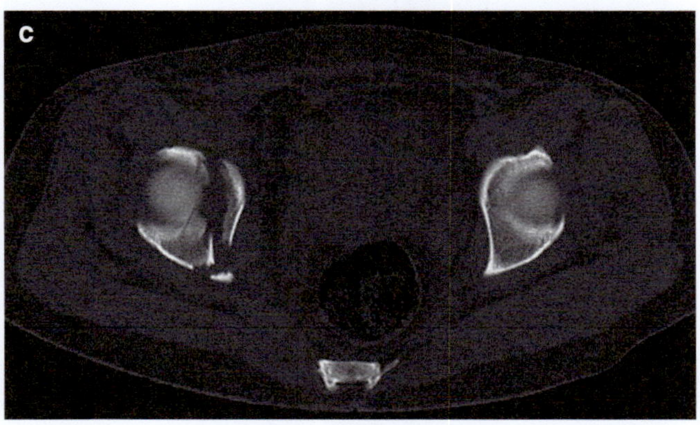

Fig. 8.7 (**e**) CT shows the transverse fractures of the acetabulum line in sagittal views. The fracture does not involve the obturator ring, the iliopubic line and ilioischial line are discontinuous, and there is no fracture of the posterior acetabular wall, so it is a transverse acetabular fracture for this case

8. Comparison of X-ray film and CT of acetabular transverse and posterior wall fractures

8.1 X-ray film (Fig. 8.8a–d)

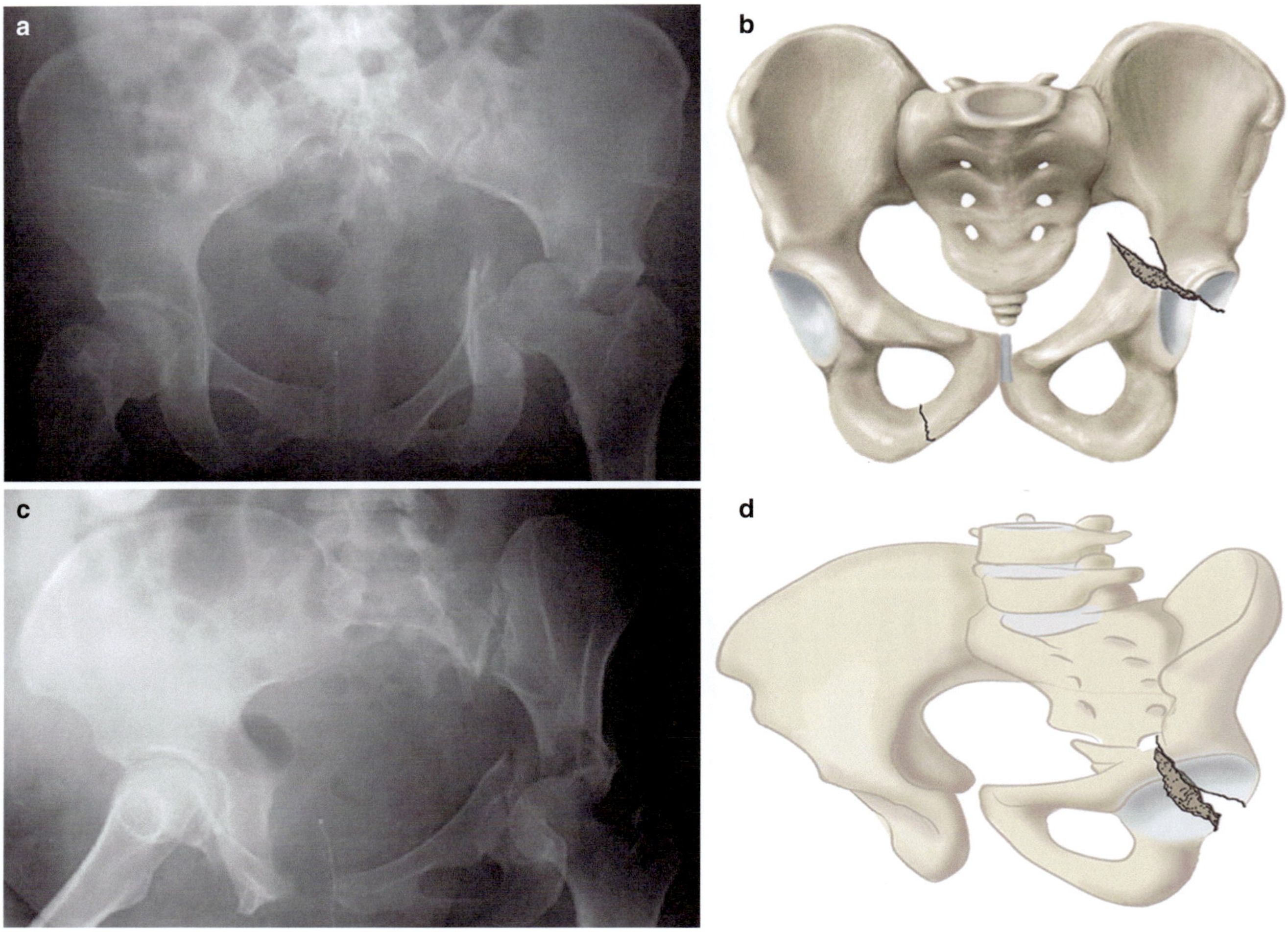

Fig. 8.8 (**a**) (anteroposterior views) and (**c**) (obturator oblique views) show the discontinuity of the iliopubic line and the ilioischial line, the displacement of femoral head, and the separation of symphysis pubis (**b**, **d**)

8.2 CT scan (Fig. 8.8e)

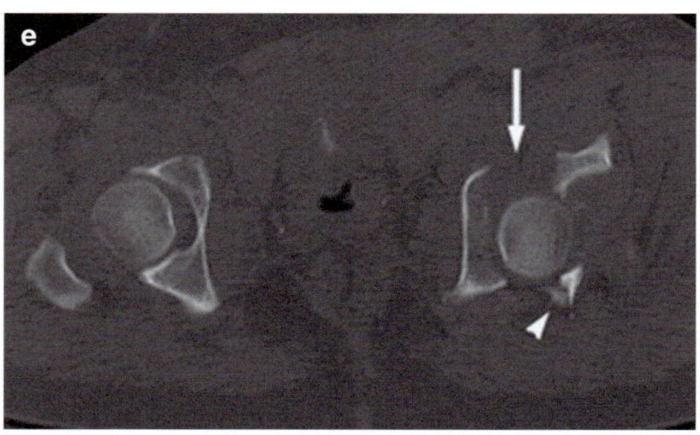

Fig. 8.8 (**e**) CT shows the transverse fracture line of the acetabulum in sagittal plane (arrow) and the fracture line in posterior wall of the acetabulum (arrow). This fracture does not involve the obturator ring, iliopubic line and the ilioischial line are discontinuous, and there is a posterior wall fracture of the acetabulum, so it is a transverse + posterior wall fracture

9. Comparison between X-ray film and CT of acetabular transverse fracture and posterior wall fracture
   9.1 X-ray film (Fig. 8.9a, b)

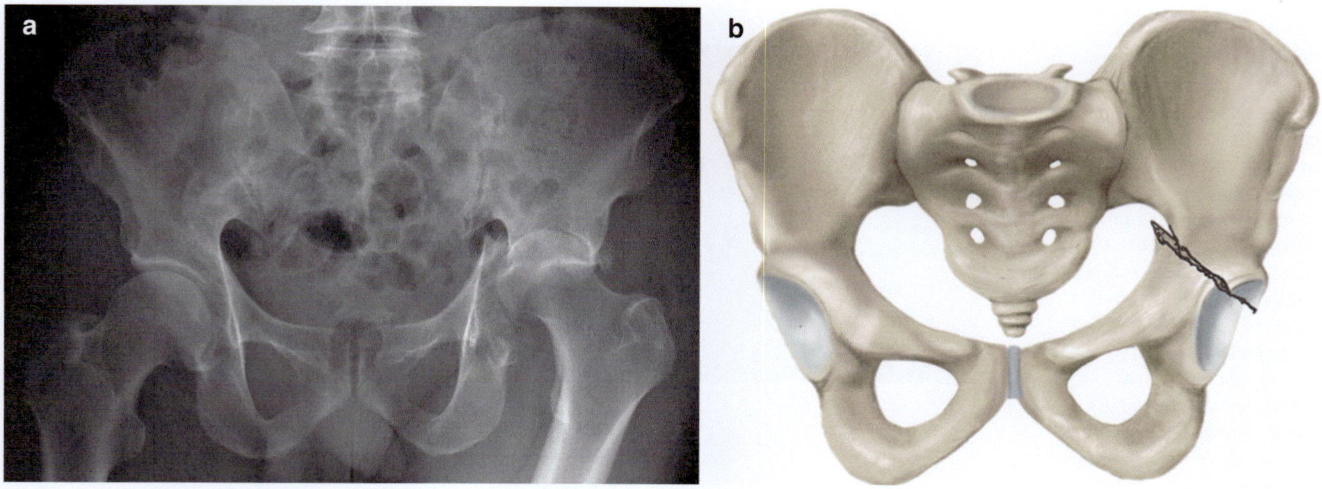

Fig. 8.9 (**a**) (anteroposterior views) shows that the iliopubic line and the ilioischial line are not continuous, the femoral head is displaced to the medial side, and there is separated bone fragment in the upper rim of acetabulum (**b**)

   9.2 CT scan (Fig. 8.9c–e)

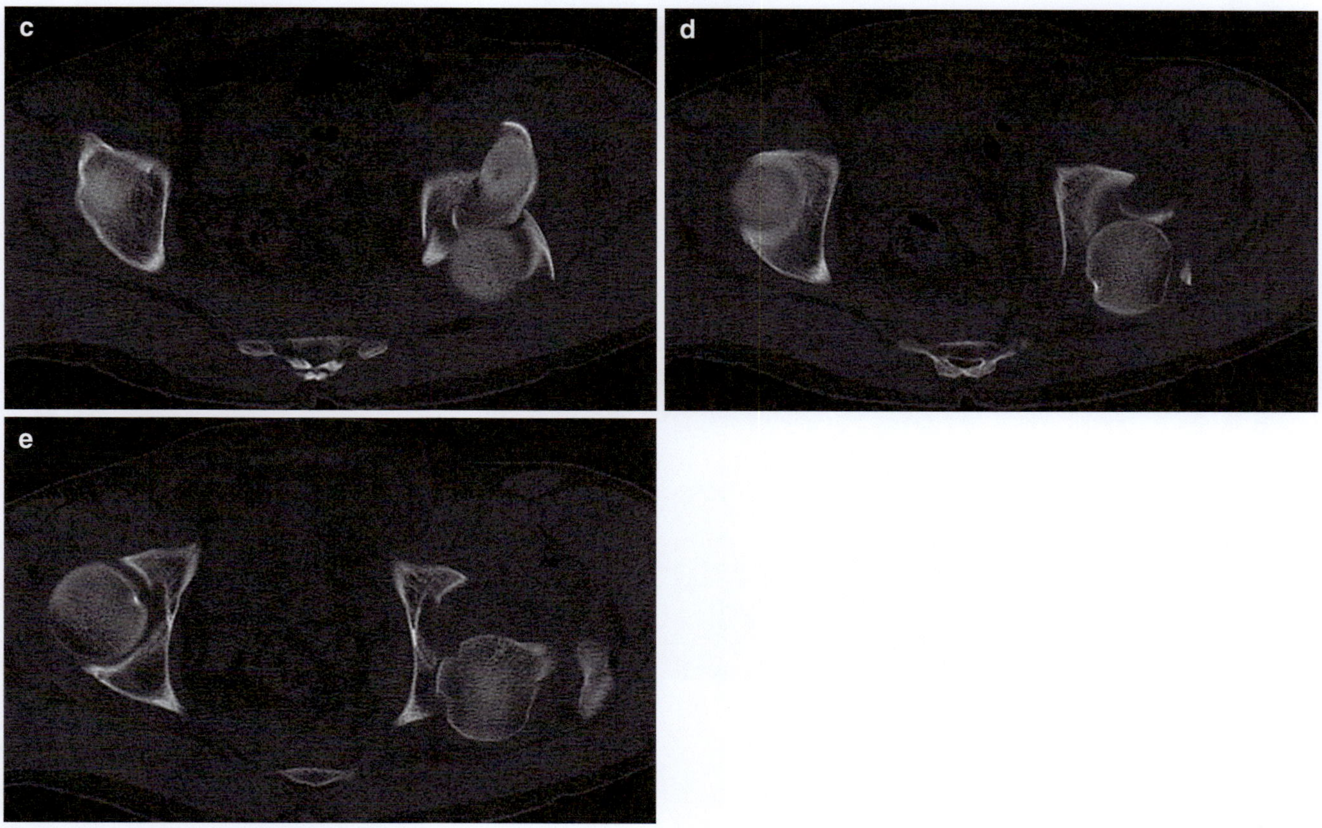

Fig. 8.9 (**c–e**) CT of the transverse axis shows hip joint capsule swelling, acetabular fracture line (arrow), and fragment of bone in the joint capsule, and defect of posterior wall of the acetabulum (arrow). This fracture does not involve the obturator ring, the iliopubic line and ilioischial line are discontinuous, and there is a posterior wall fracture of the acetabulum, so it is a transverse and posterior wall fracture

10. Comparison of X-ray film and CT scan of posterior column and posterior wall fracture combined with posterior dislocation of femoral head
    10.1 X-ray film (Fig. 8.10a–f)

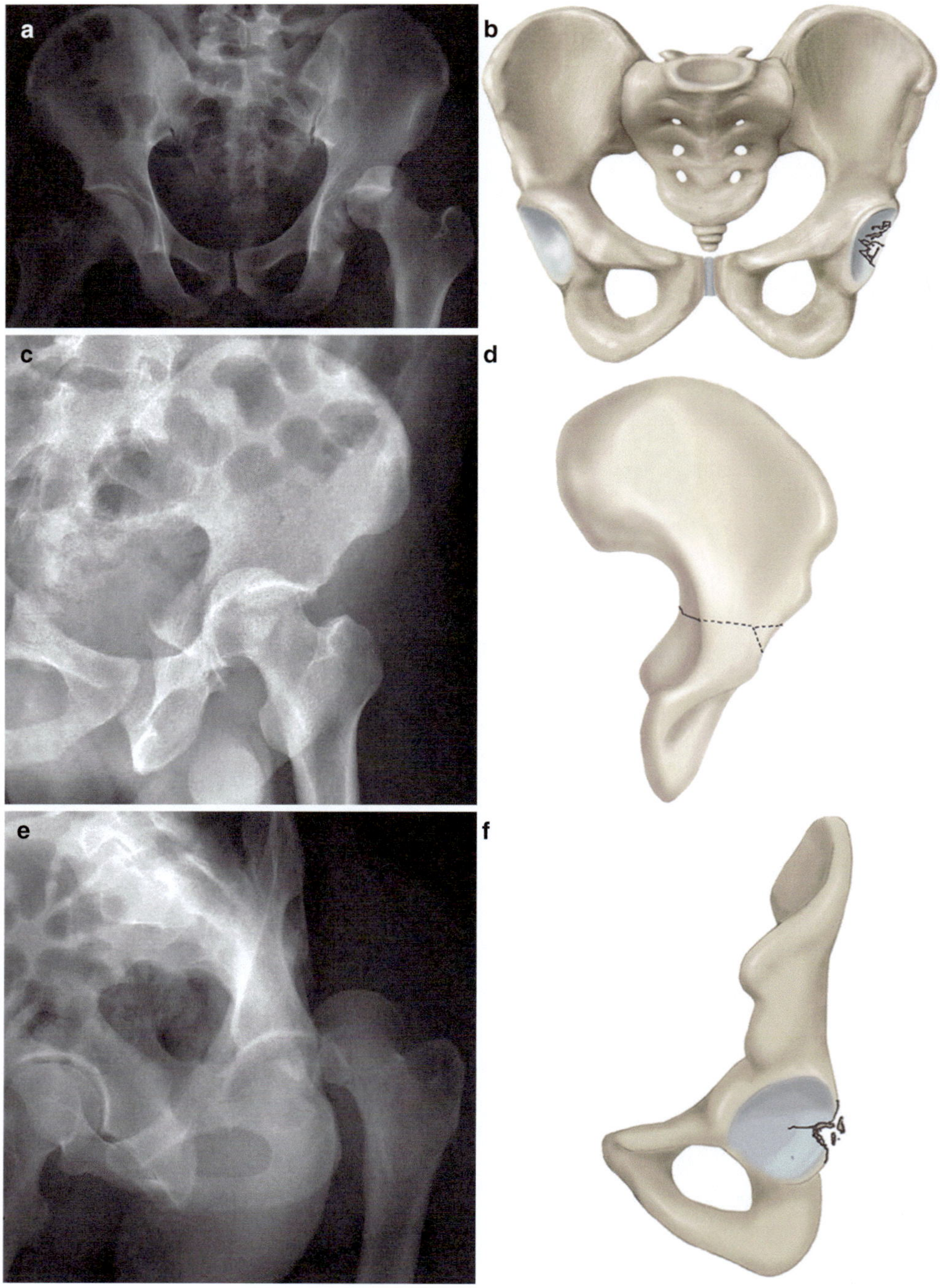

Fig. 8.10 (**a**) (anteroposterior views) X-ray film shows obvious upward displacement of the left femoral head, irregular shape of the acetabulum. Appearance of fracture was unclear due to bone overlapping (**b**). (**c**) (iliac oblique views) shows bone in the acetabulum is ruptured. Iliopubic line and ilioischial line were discontinuous. (**d**). (**e**) (obturator oblique views) clearly shows the backwards dislocation of femoral head, and bone fragment in the posterior margin of the acetabulum (**f**)

10.2 CT scan (Fig. 8.10g)

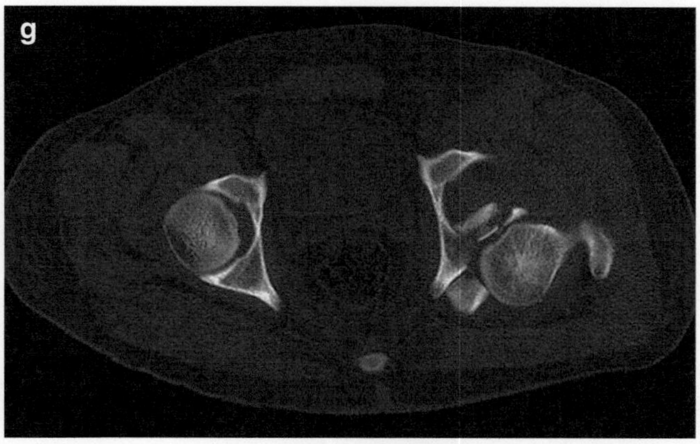

Fig. 8.10 (**g**) Horizontal axis of CT shows fractures involving the posterior column and posterior wall of the acetabulum, displacement of the bone fragment, and dislocation of the femoral head. In this case, the iliopubic line and ilioischial line were discontinuous and the fracture did not involve the obturator ring. This is posterior column and posterior wall fracture combined with posterior dislocation of the femoral head

11. Comparison of X-ray film and CT of posterior column and posterior wall fractures of the acetabulum with posterior dislocation plane of femoral head
    11.1 X-ray film (Fig. 8.11a–f)

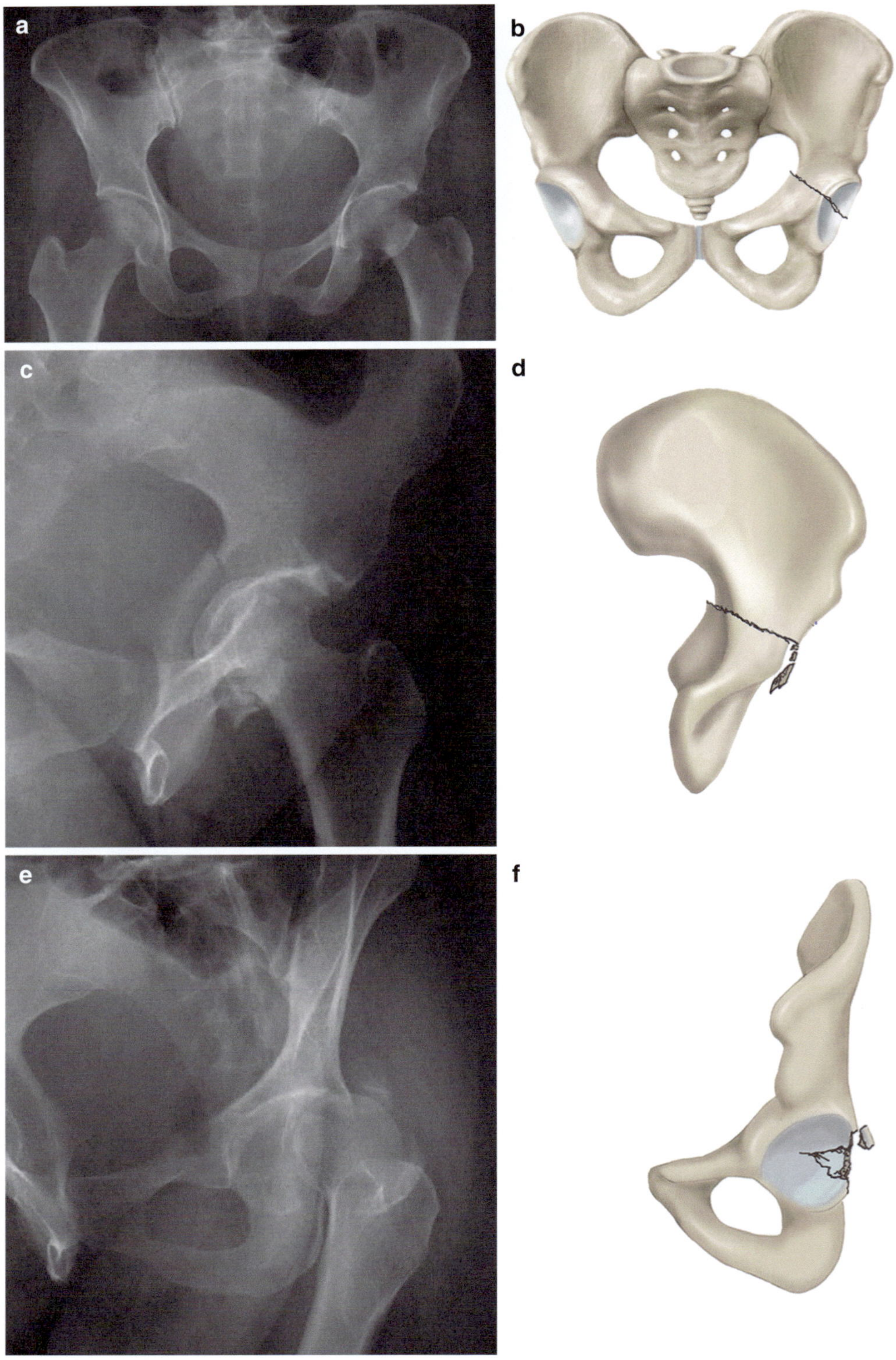

Fig. 8.11 (**a**) (anteroposterior views) X-ray film shows the bone of the left acetabulum is discontinuous. It is difficult to diagnose whether the fracture involves iliopubic line or ilioischial line (**b**). (**c**) (iliac oblique views) shows the bone in acetabulum is ruptured and the ilioischial line is discontinuous (**d**). (**e**) (obturator oblique views) shows iliopubic line is continuous, backward dislocation of femoral head, and bone fragments can be seen on the posterior upper margin of the acetabulum (**f**)

11.2 CT scan (Fig. 8.11g–j)

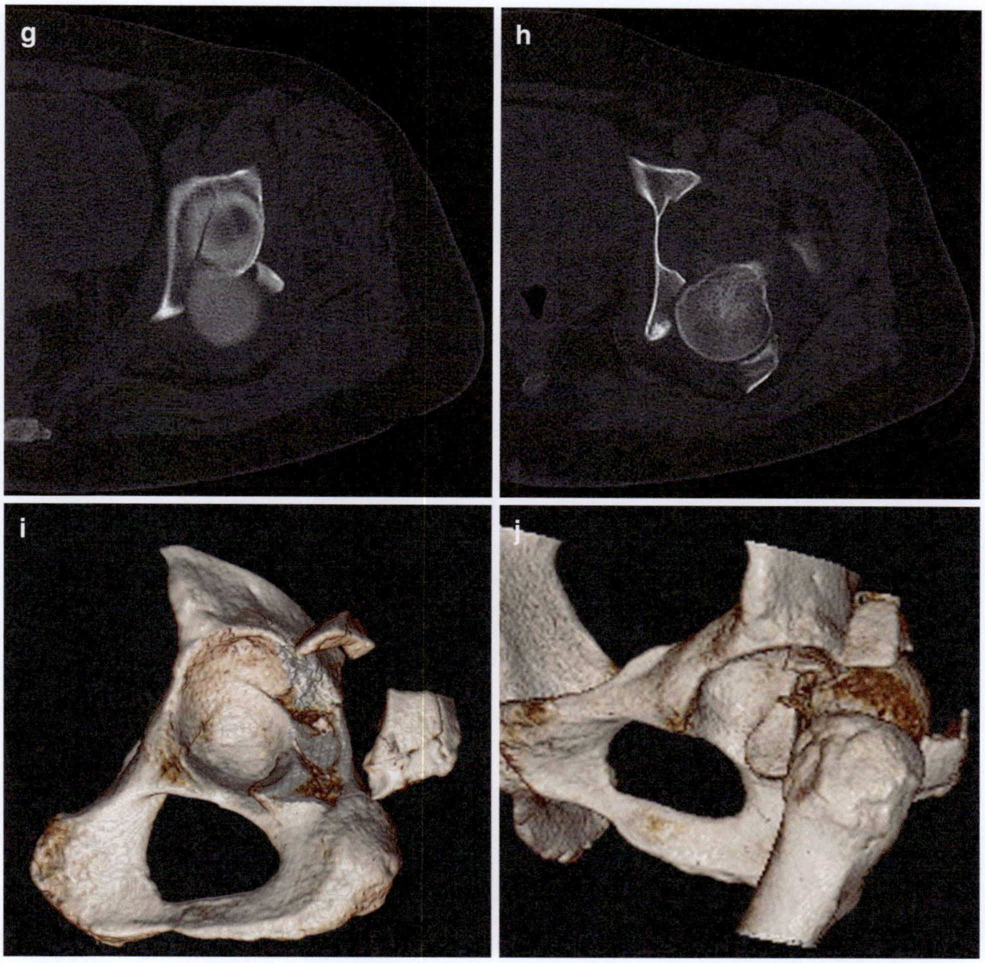

Fig. 8.11 (**g**, **h**) The horizontal axis of CT shows that the fracture involves the posterior column and posterior wall of the acetabulum, the displacement of the bone fragment, and posterior dislocation of the femoral head. (**i**, **j**) 3-dimentional reconstruction shows fracture of left acetabulum. For this case, the iliopubic line is continuous but the ilioischial line is not continuous, the fracture do not involves obturator ring, so it is posterior column and posterior wall fracture combined with posterior dislocation of femoral head

12. Comparison between X-ray film and CT of acetabular T-type fracture
    12.1 X-ray film (Fig. 8.12a, b)

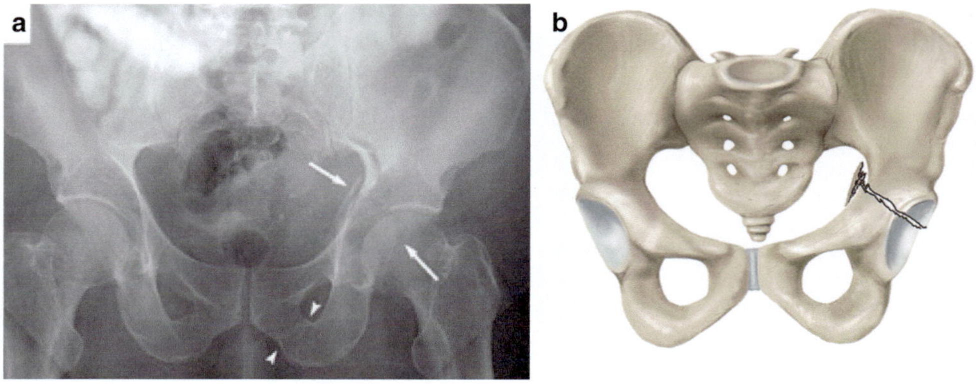

Fig. 8.12 (**a**) X-ray film shows that the iliopubic line and ilioischial line are discontinuous, the fracture involves obturator ring, this fracture is easy to miss (**b**)

    12.2 CT scan (Fig. 8.12c)

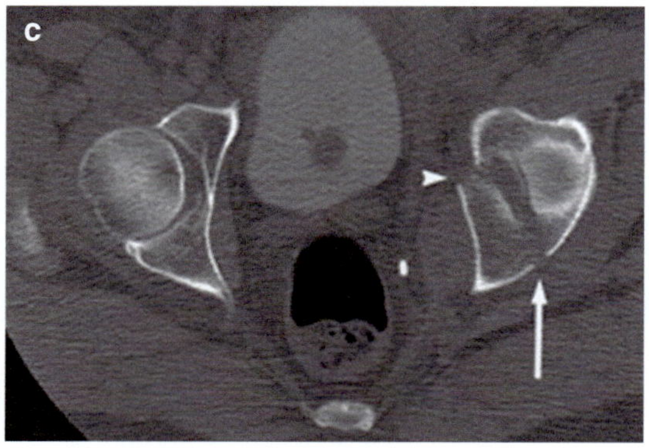

Fig. 8.12 (**c**) CT shows that the fracture line is in the sagittal plane of the acetabulum. It is a transverse fracture, and there is no fracture in the posterior wall. The fracture does not involve the obturator ring, the iliopubic line and ilioischial line are discontinuous but the fracture not extended to the upper iliac, so it is a T-type fracture

13. Comparison between X-ray film and CT for both column fracture of the acetabulum
    13.1 X-ray film (Fig. 8.13a, b)

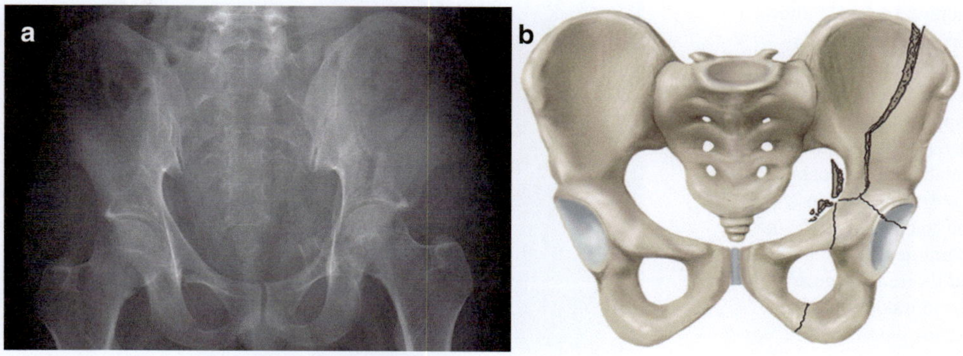

Fig. 8.13 (**a**) (anteroposterior views) shows that the iliopubic line and ilioischial line are discontinuous, the fracture involves the obturator ring (this fracture is not clearly shown on the X-ray film and can easily be ignored) and extends to the upper iliac (**b**)

13.2 CT scan (Fig. 8.13c–i)

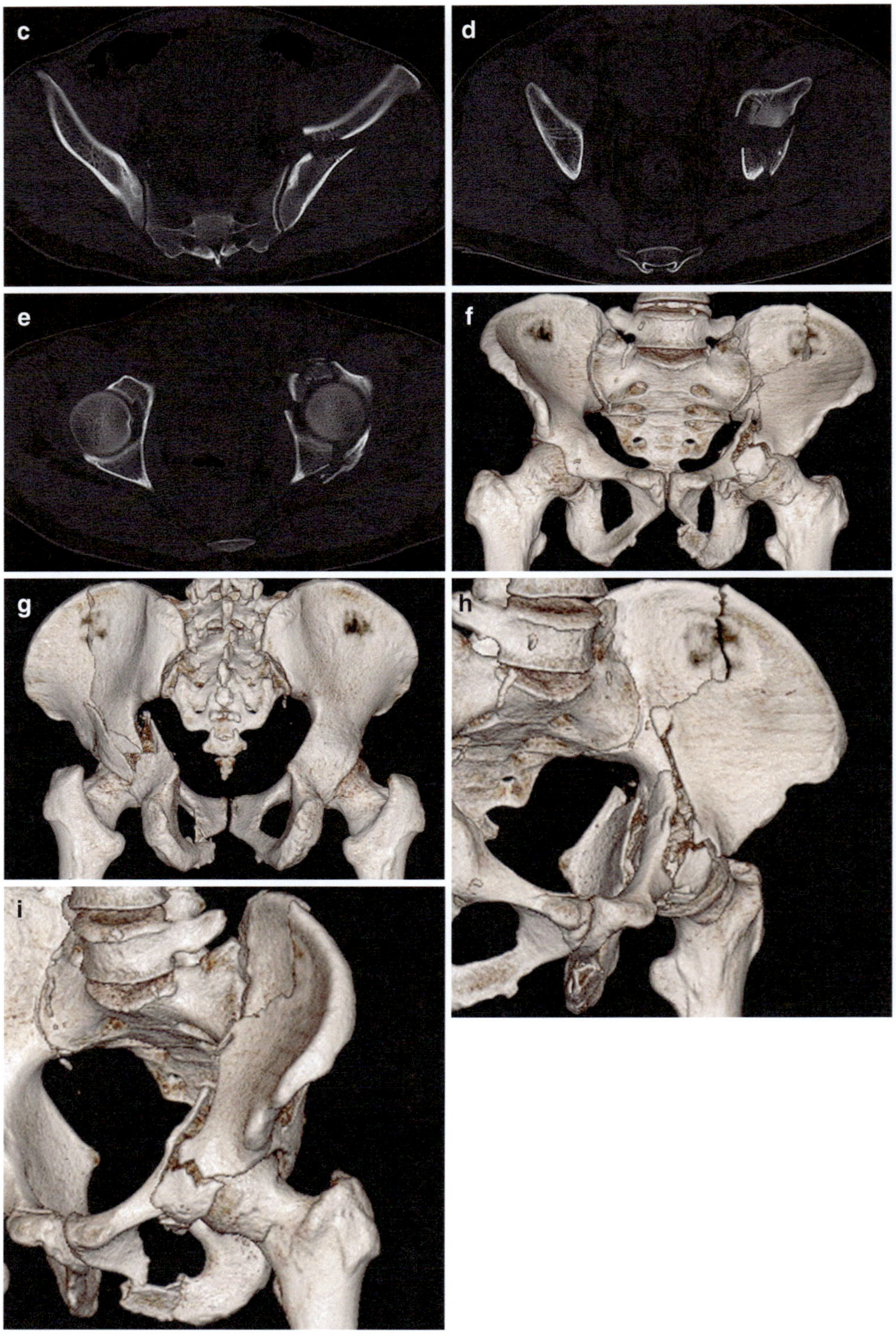

Fig. 8.13 (**c**) CT shows iliac fracture; (**d**, **e**) CT shows a fracture line on the acetabulum; (**f–i**) CT 3-dimentional reconstruction displays anterior column and posterior column of the acetabulum fractures and iliac fracture stereoscopically. The fracture involves the obturator ring, iliopubic line and ilioischial line are discontinuous, and the fracture extends to the upper iliac, so this fracture is classified as both-column fracture

14. Comparison between X-ray film and CT of acetabular fractures of both columns
    14.1 X-ray film (Fig. 8.14a–f)

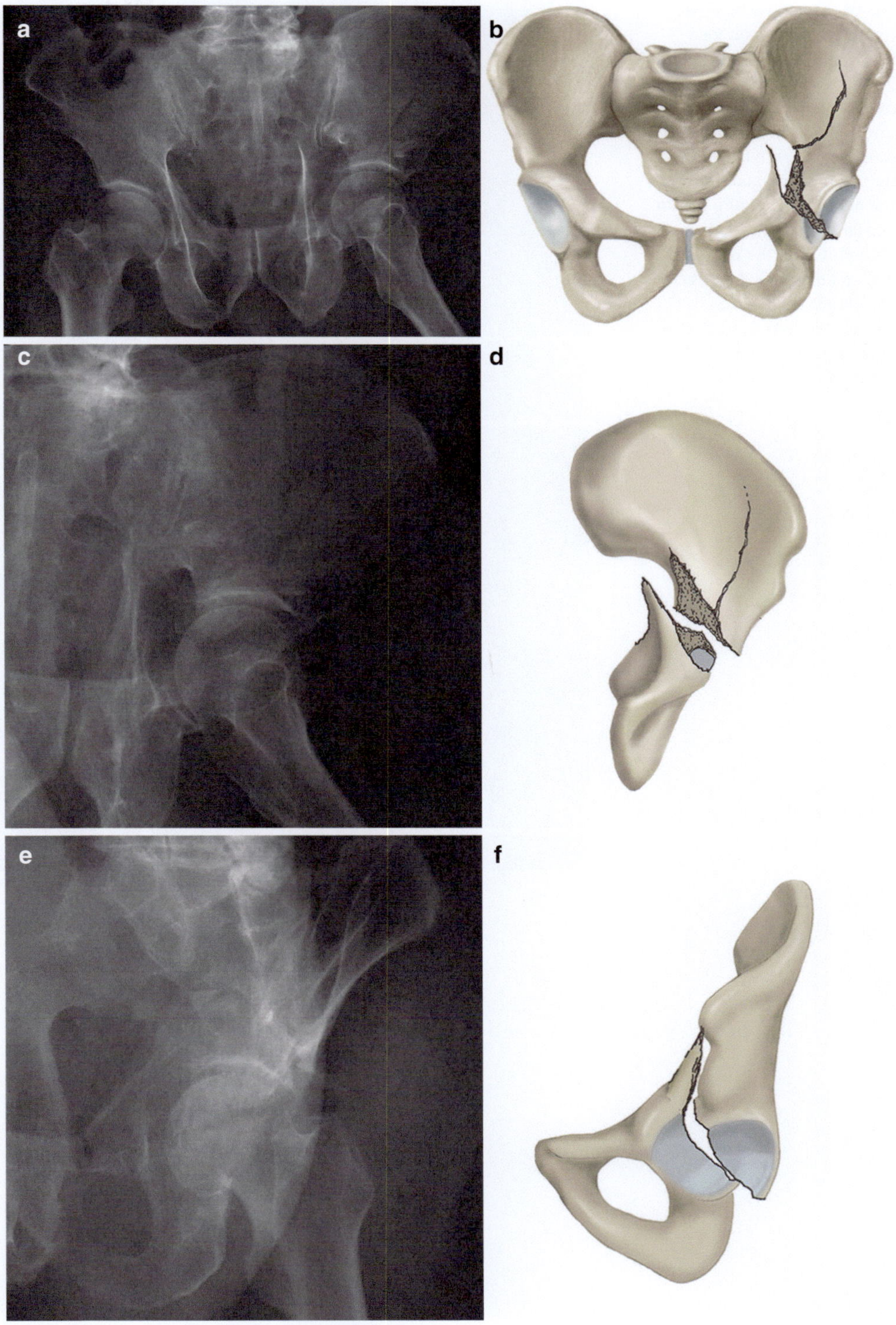

Fig. 8.14 (**a**) (anteroposterior views), (**b**, **c**) (obturator oblique views), (**d**, **e**) (iliac oblique views) and (**f**) show the discontinuity of iliopubic line and ilioischial line. The fracture involves the obturator ring (which is not clearly shown on the X-ray film and can be easily ignored) and extends to the ilium

14.2 CT scan (Fig. 8.14g–j)

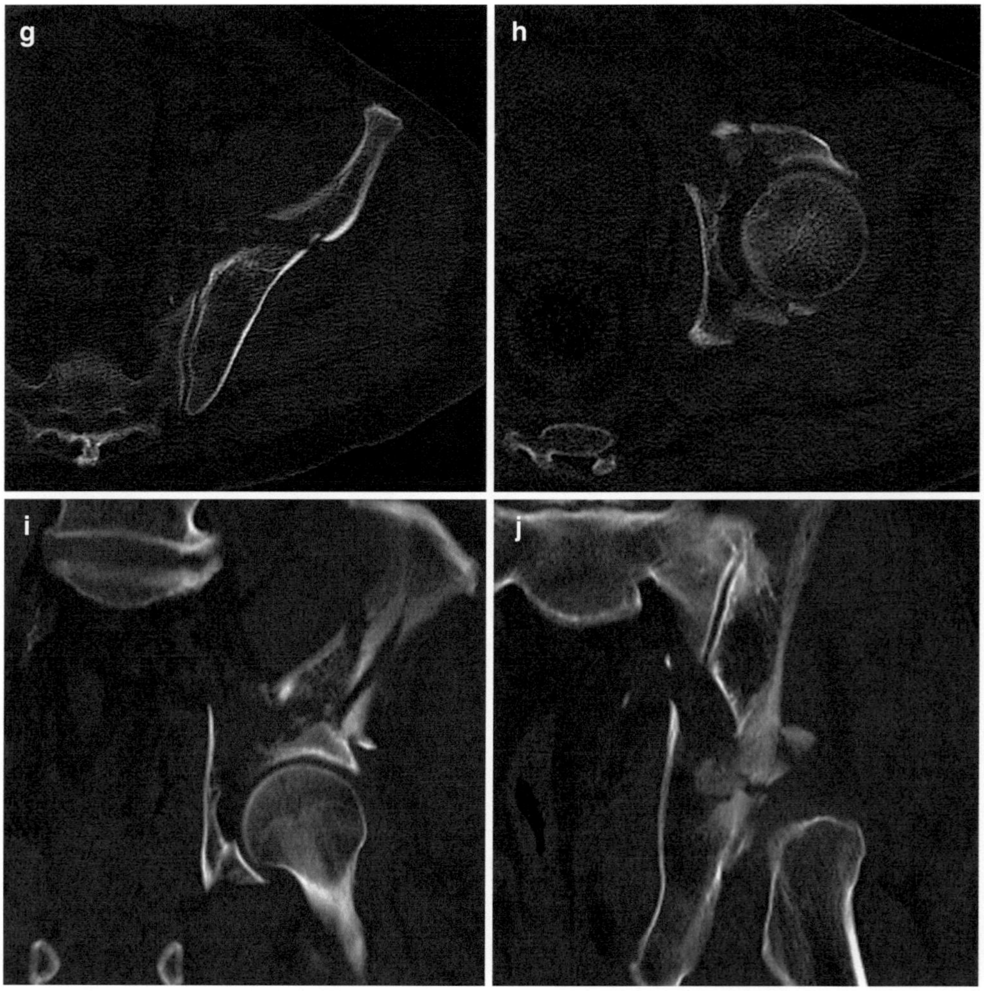

Fig. 8.14 (**g**, **h**) The fracture line of iliac and acetabular fracture is shown on the horizontal axis CT of different layers, respectively. (**i**, **j**) CT reconstruction of coronal revealed anterior column and posterior column fractures of the acetabulum, and iliac fractures. The fracture line in this case involves the obturator ring, the iliopubic line and the ilioischial line are discontinuous, and the fracture extends to ilium, this fracture belonging to a both- column fracture

8.2 Proximal Femur Fractures

Proximal femur fractures refer to femoral head fracture and fracture within 5 cm of the subtrochanteric femur. It can be divided into femoral head fracture, femoral neck fracture, intertrochanteric fracture, and subtrochanteric fracture. Femoral head fractures refer to the fracture of the femoral head. Femoral neck fractures refer to the fracture between the distal femoral head and the proximal intertrochanteric line. Intertrochanteric fractures refer to the fracture between the distal intertrochanteric line and the level of the lesser trochanter. According to the anatomical location, proximal femur fractures can be divided into two groups: intra-articular and extracapsular fractures. Intra-capsular fractures include femoral head fractures and femoral neck fractures. Extracapsular fractures include intertrochanteric fractures and subtrochanteric fractures. Complications of intracapsular fractures are higher than extracapsular fractures, and the most common complication is ischemic necrosis of the femoral head.

8.2.1 Femoral Head Fractures

8.2.1.1 Classification

Pipkin divided femoral head fractures into four types

- Type I: fracture of the femoral head inferior to the fovea centralis and accompanied by dislocation of hip joint
- Type II: fracture of the femoral head superior to the fovea centralis and accompanied by dislocation of hip joint
- Type III: similar to a Type I or II injury but associated with fracture of the femoral neck
- Type IV: similar to a Type I injury or II but associated with fracture of the acetabular rim

8.2.1.2 Injury Mechanism

Femoral head fractures are caused by high-energy injuries, most of which are traffic accidents. This fracture usually results from a major force exerted onto a flexed knee and hip. The resulting force transmits to the hip joint through the axis of the femur and often leads to a femoral head fracture. Fracture of Pipkin Type I is caused by a major force when the femoral adduction, Type II occurs when the femur is abducted; when trauma continues, Type III and IV will occur.

8.2.1.3 Signs and Symptoms

Femoral head fractures are usually combined with a posterior dislocation of the hip joint. The clinical features of the affected limb are shortening of the limb, and limited rotation, adduction, and flexion. However, there are no characteristic symptoms of these patients if the dislocation is automatically restored or no dislocation occurs.

8.2.1.4 Radiographic Diagnosis

Large and displaced femoral head fractures are easy to diagnose using X-rays; however, small femoral head fractures or undisplaced fractures are difficult to diagnose. Therefore, CT examination should be carried out before reducing a posterior hip joint dislocation to eliminate the fracture of the femoral head. Otherwise, it is easy to cause the failure of hip joint reduction and the displacement of femoral head fracture and resulting in the necrosis of the femoral head and other serious complications.

1. Type I femoral head fractures
   1.1 X-ray film (Fig. 8.15a, b)

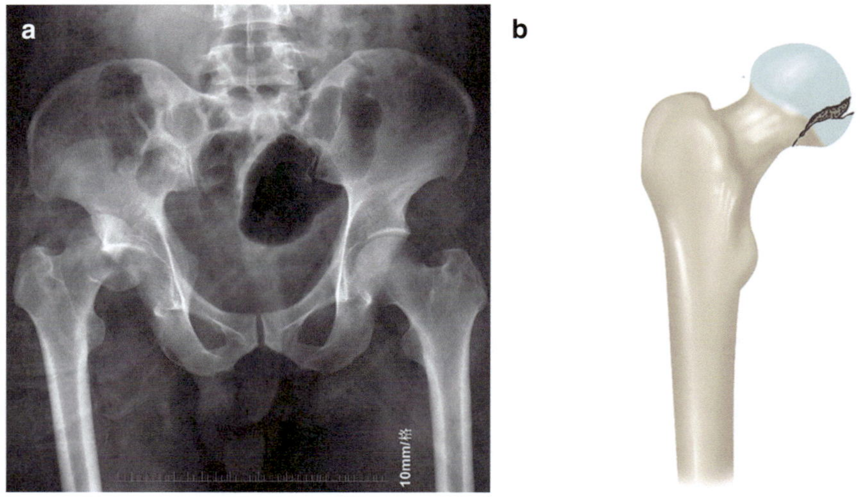

Fig. 8.15 X-ray film (**a**) shows fracture of the right hip joint with a fracture inferior to the fovea centralis. The fracture line is unclear, so the CT examination is performed (**b**)

   1.2 CT scan (Fig. 8.15c–f)

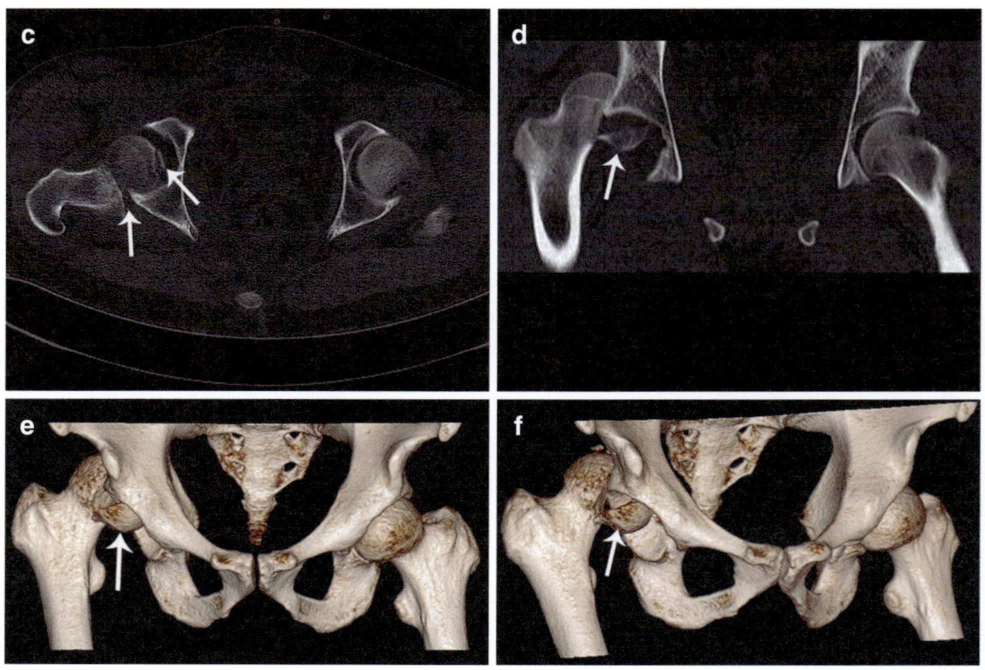

Fig. 8.15 Transverse axis of CT (**c**), coronal reconstruction of CT (**d**), anteroposterior views and anterolateral view of CT three-dimensional reconstruction (**e**, **f**) show posterior superior dislocation of the femoral head, femoral head fracture line inferior to the fovea centralis (white arrow)

2. Type I femoral head fractures
   2.1 X-ray film (Fig. 8.16a–d)

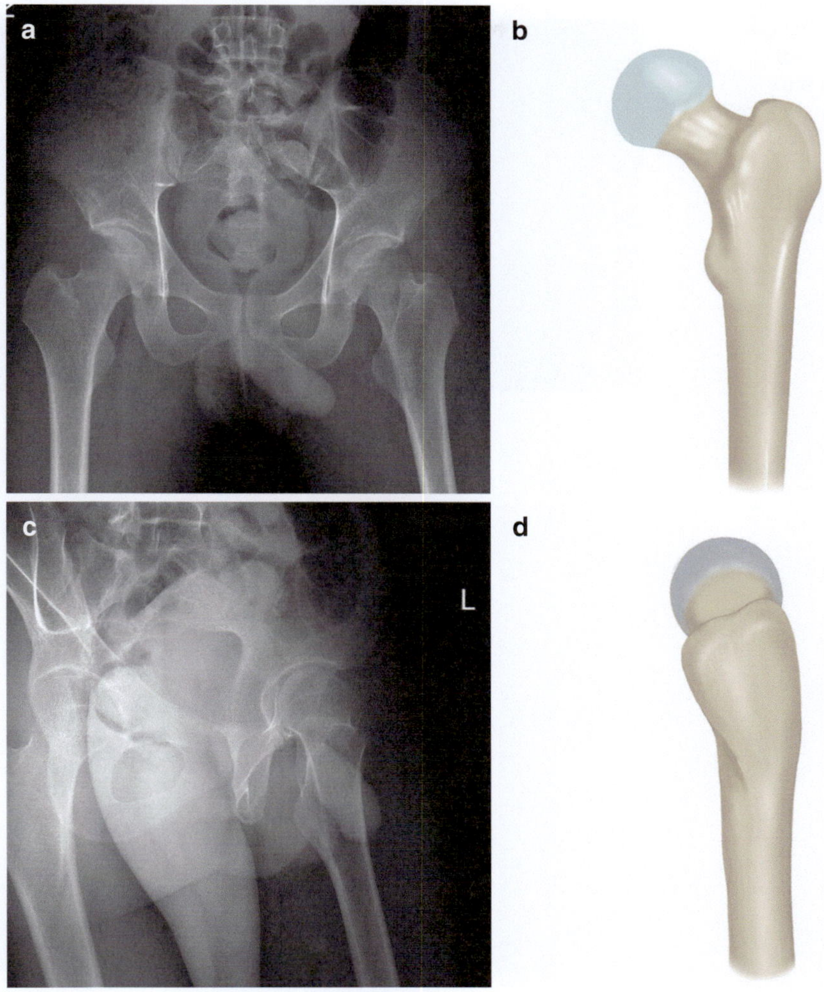

Fig. 8.16 X-ray anteroposterior views (**a**) and X-ray lateral view (**c**) show suspicious fracture of the left femoral head, the patient suffers from severe pain, so a CT examination is performed (**b**, **d**)

   2.2 CT scan (Fig. 8.16e, f)

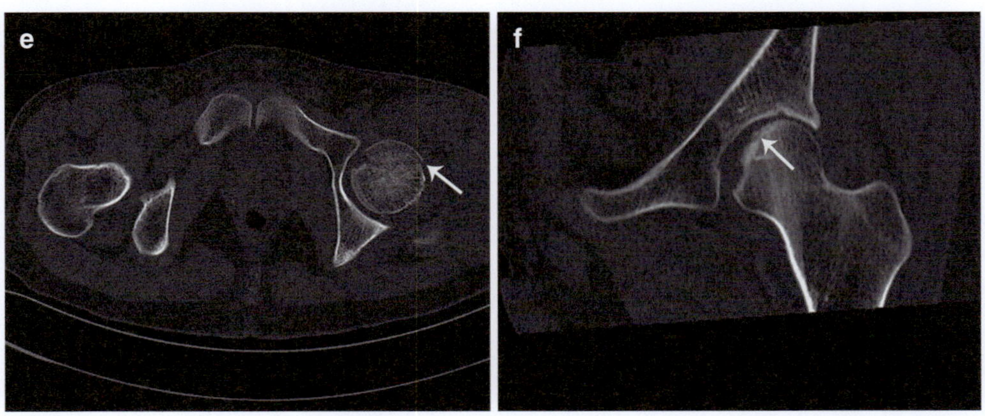

Fig. 8.16 Transverse axis of CT (**e**) and reconstruction of oblique coronal axis CT (**f**) show fractures superior to the fovea centralis (white arrow)

3. Comparison of Type III and Type I femoral head fractures
   3.1 CT scan (Fig. 8.17a, b)

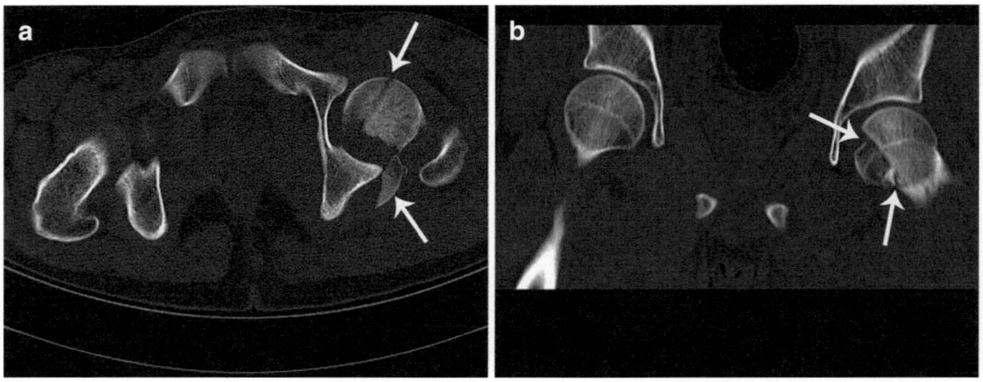

Fig. 8.17 Transverse axis of CT (**a**) and CT coronal reconstruction (**b**) show fracture inferior to the fovea centralis, and the fracture line involved the femoral neck (white arrow), it is a type III femoral head fracture

4. Comparison of Type III and Type II femoral head fractures
   4.1 CT scan (Fig. 8.18a–d)

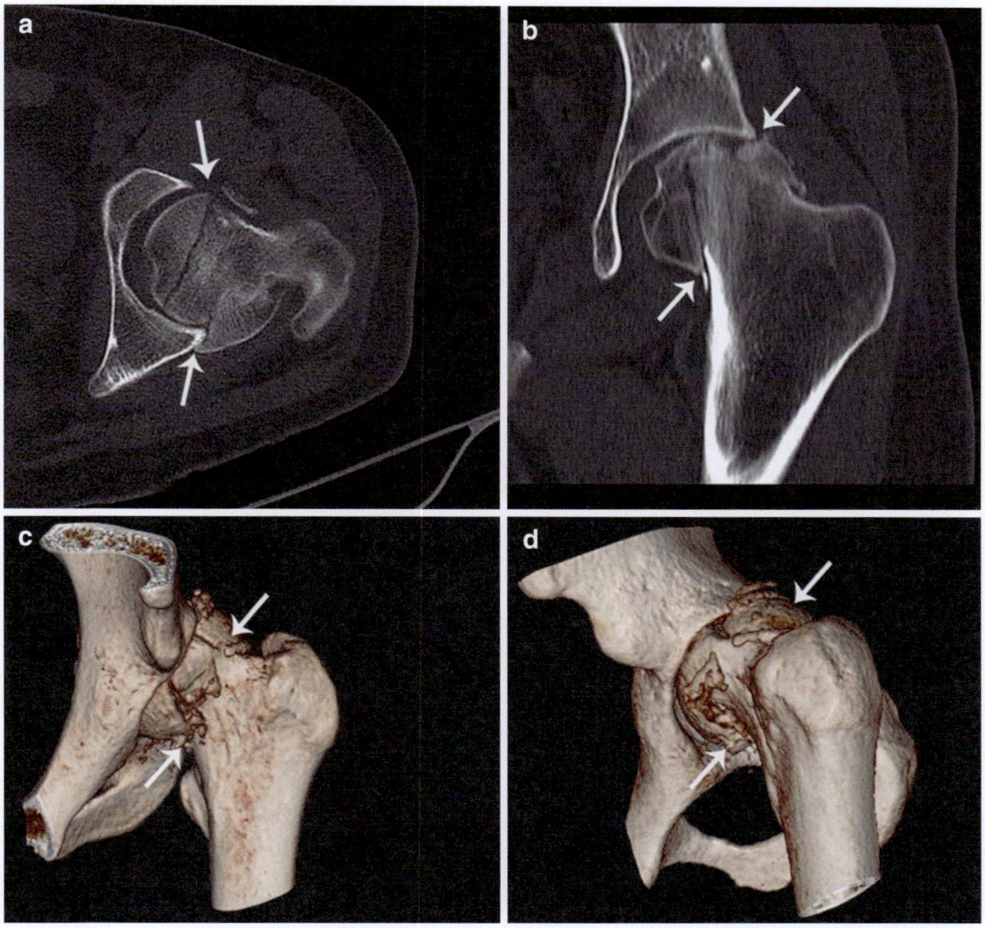

Fig. 8.18 Transverse axis of CT (**a**), CT coronal reconstruction (**b**), anteroposterior views and anterolateral view of CT three-dimensional reconstruction (**c**, **d**) show comminuted fracture superior to the fovea centralis. Comminuted fragments can be excised and dislocated, the fracture involving femoral neck (white arrow), it is a type III femoral head fracture (Fig. 8.19)

5. Type III femoral head fracture
   5.1 X-ray film (Fig. 8.19a, b)

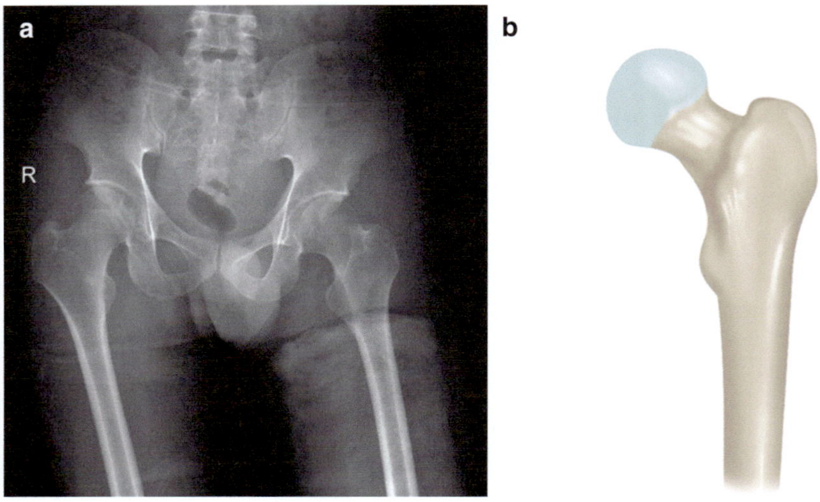

Fig. 8.19 X-ray film (**a**) shows the pelvis was tilted, no obvious fracture was observed, but the pain of the patient was serious, so a CT examination was performed (**b**)

5.2 CT scan (Fig. 8.19c–g)

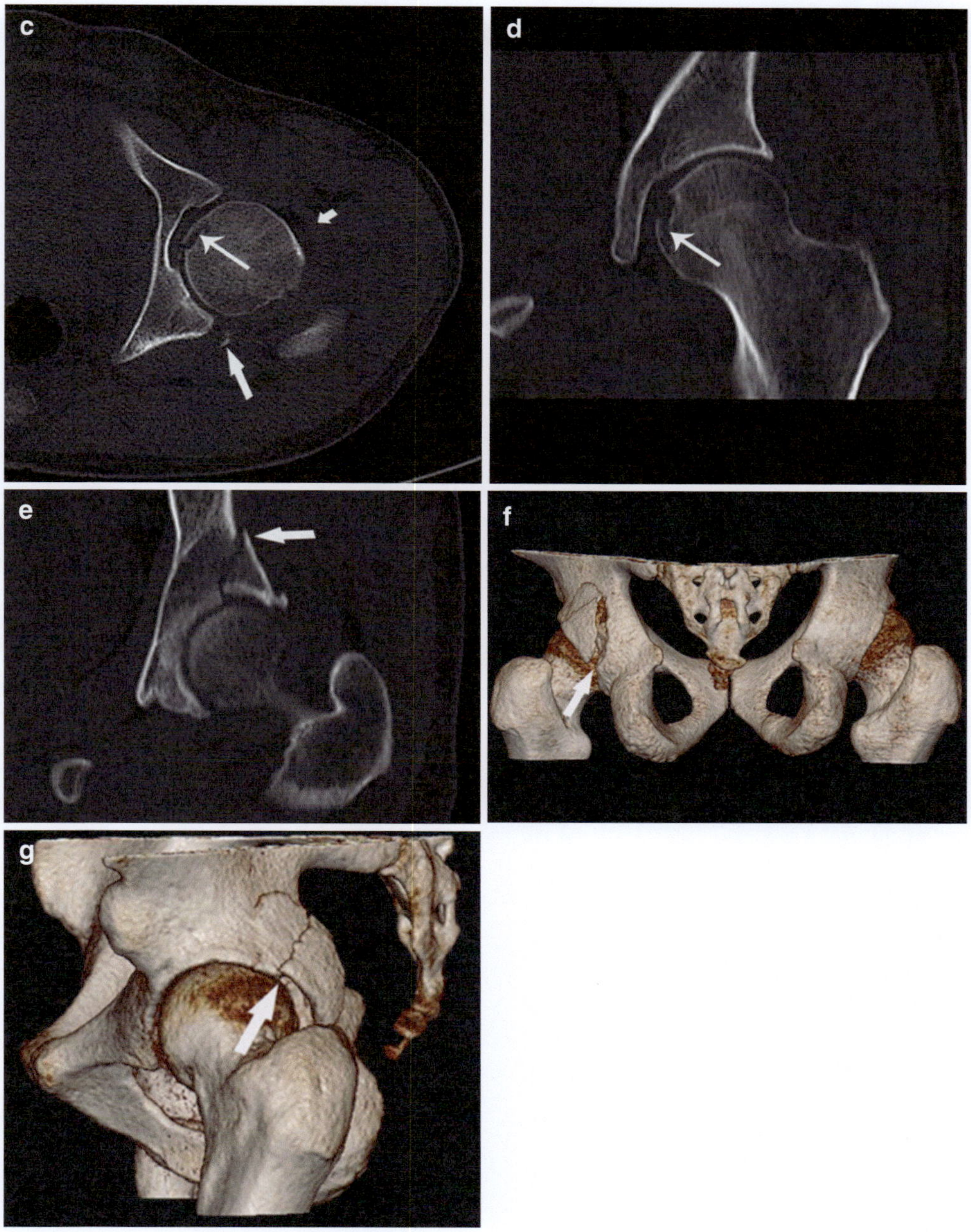

Fig. 8.19 Transverse axis of CT (**c**), CT coronal and sagittal reconstruction (**d**, **e**), shows the fracture of left femoral head. The fracture line inferior to the fovea centralis, involving the articular surface (thin white arrow), accompanied by the posterior margin fracture of the acetabulum (thick white arrow), and the intra-articular effusion was observed (white arrow). The posterior and lateral view of CT 3D reconstruction (**f**, **g**) shows the overall appearance of acetabular fracture (white arrow)

6. Comparison of Type IV and Type I femoral head fractures
   6.1 CT scan (Fig. 8.20a–d)

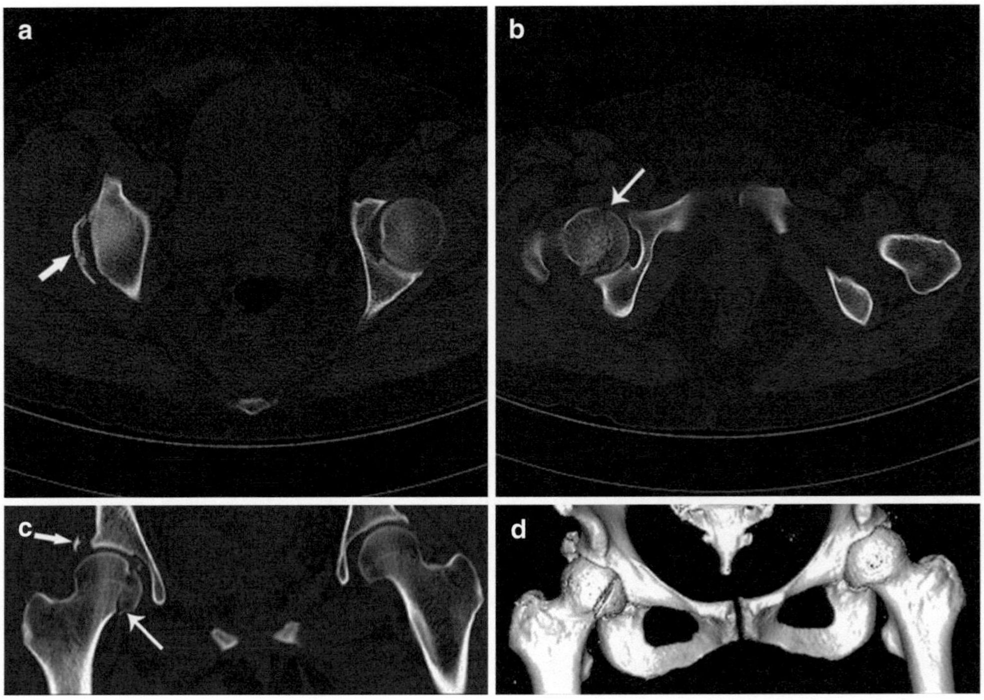

Fig. 8.20 Transverse axis of CT (**a**, **b**), coronal plane, and 3-dimensional reconstruction (**c**, **d**) show the fracture (fine white arrow) inferior to the fovea centralis, combined with the fracture of the right acetabulum (thick white arrow) and free bone fragments in the joint were observed

8.2.2 Femoral Neck Fractures

According to the anatomical site, the femoral neck fracture can be divided into sub fracture of the femoral head, fracture of pass-neck, and fracture of femoral neck base.

8.2.2.1 Injury Mechanism

Femoral neck fractures occur mostly in the elderly, with a higher incidence of women than men. Low-energy traumas are the common causes of this fracture in elderly patients. The cause of femoral neck fractures for young patients is high-energy trauma and often combined with other areas of injury.

8.2.2.2 Signs and Symptoms

Displaced femoral neck fractures are typically characterized by shortening of the limb and abnormal external rotation.

Un-displaced femoral neck fractures often have no obvious signs other than local pain. Some patients cannot walk to the hospital, which results in missed diagnosis, necrosis of femoral head, and various other serious complications. Meanwhile, femoral neck fractures must be excluded in patients with femoral shaft fractures.

8.2.2.3 Radiographic Diagnosis

Displaced femoral neck fractures are easy to diagnose by X-ray film, but difficult to diagnose if it is displaced. CT or MRI scans are needed to exclude fractures in these patients.

7. Diagnosis of femoral neck fracture with or without displacement
   7.1 X-ray film (Fig. 8.21a, b)

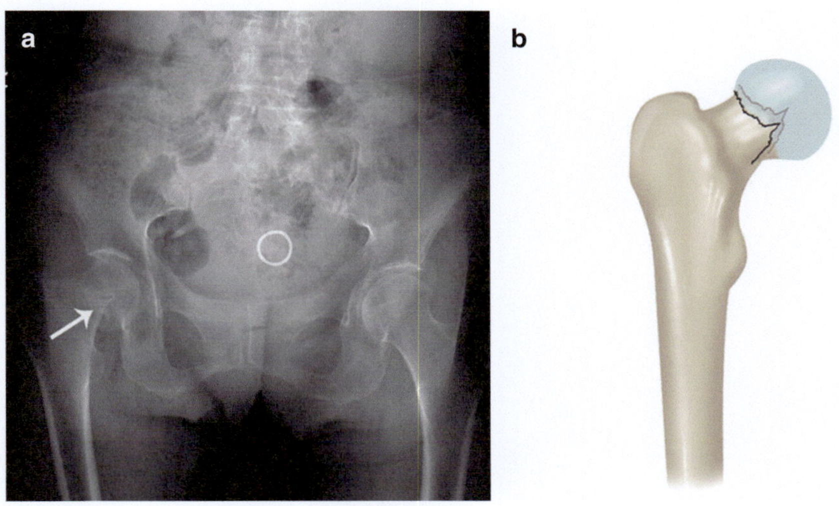

Fig. 8.21 X-ray films (**a**) show the right femoral neck shortened, small neck-shaft angle, the fracture line is unclear (white arrow). A CT examination is performed to ascertain displacement of this fracture (**b**)

7.2 CT scan (Fig. 8.21c–e)

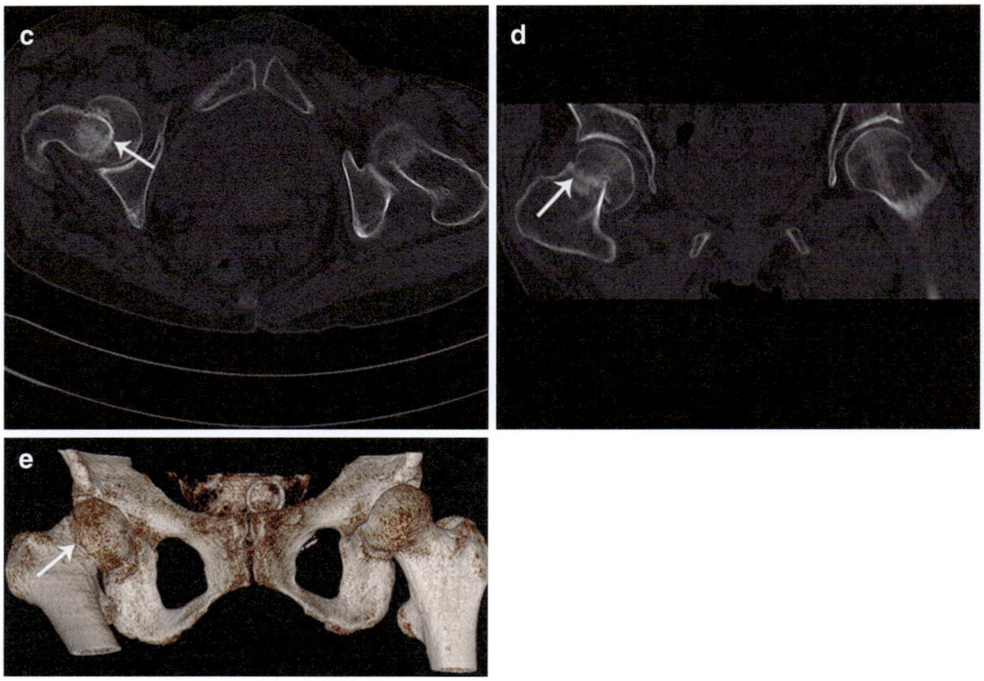

Fig. 8.21 Transverse axis of CT (**c**), coronal and three-dimensional reconstruction of CT (**d**, **e**), shows a right femoral neck fracture, the fracture site was inserted mutually, and the neck angle became smaller (white arrow)

8. Identification of femoral neck fracture
   8.1 X-ray film (Fig. 8.22a–d)

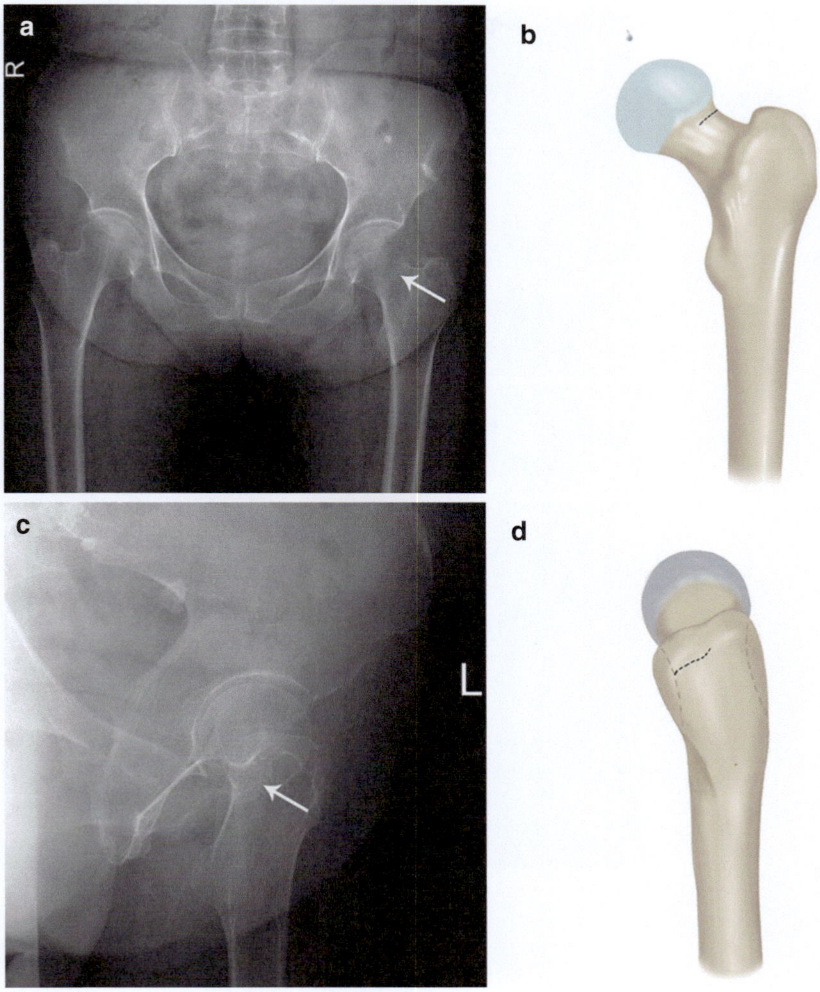

Fig. 8.22 The anteroposterior and oblique views of X-ray (**a**, **c**) show that the left femoral neck appears to have a slightly higher density shadow (white arrow). To determine whether there is a fracture or not, a CT examination is performed (**b**, **d**)

   8.2 CT scan (Fig. 8.22e, f)

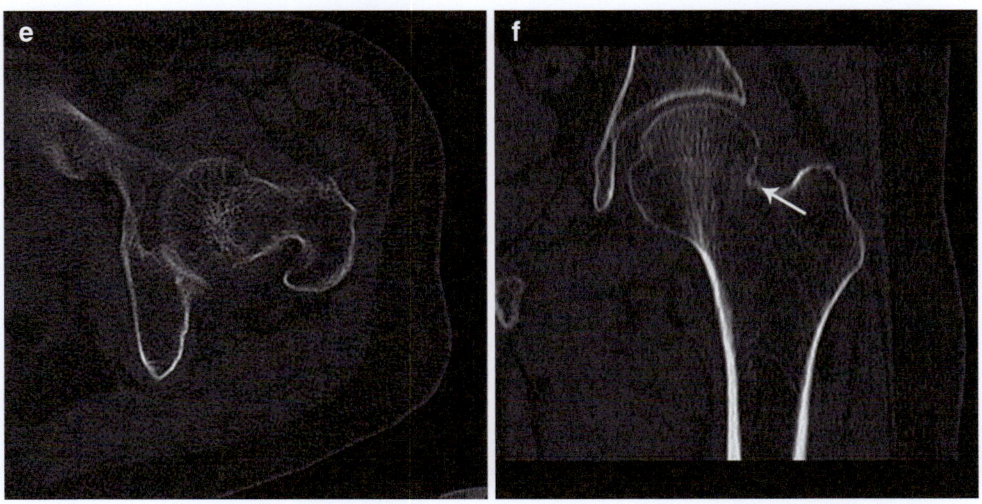

Fig. 8.22 Transverse axis of CT (**e**) shows unobvious fracture line, and coronal reconstruction of CT (**f**) shows discontinuity of cortex of femoral neck. For further diagnosis, MRI examination was performed

8.3 MRI examination (Fig. 8.22g–j)

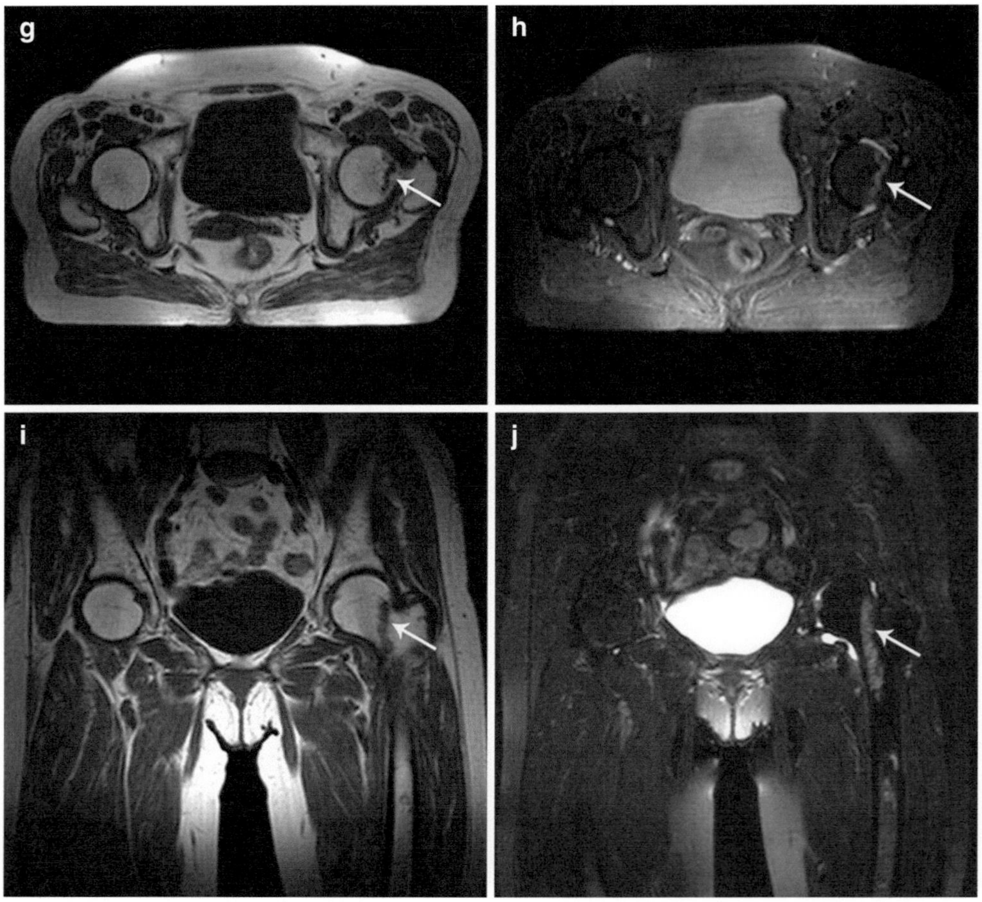

Fig. 8.22 T1WI on MRI horizontal axis (**g**), T2W on fat suppression (**h**), T1WI on coronal plane (**i**), and T2WI on fat suppression (**j**) show a fracture of the left femoral neck, T1WI shows low line-like signal (white arrow), T2WI shows high line-like signal (white arrow), and there was no dislocation in this fracture

9. Identification of femoral neck fracture
   9.1 X-ray film (Fig. 8.23a–f)

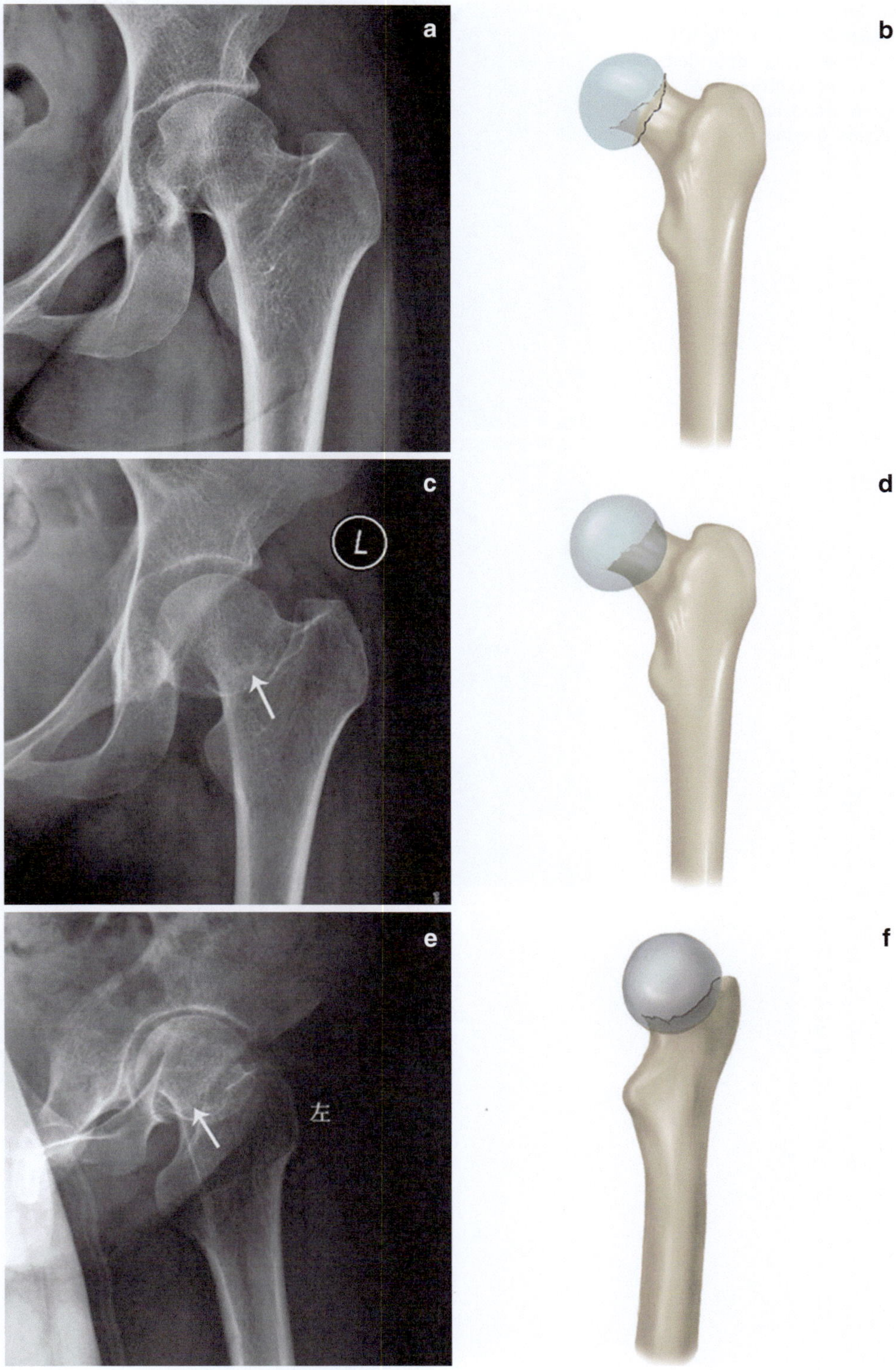

Fig. 8.23 No obvious fracture line was observed in the left femoral neck on the day of injury (**a**), no CT examination was performed and the patient suffered from pain in left hip joint (**b**). One month later, anteroposterior and lateral views of X-ray films (**c**, **e**) show high-density line-like shadows of femoral neck (white arrow) and the femoral neck became shorter (**d**, **f**)

9.2 CT scan (Fig. 8.23g–i)

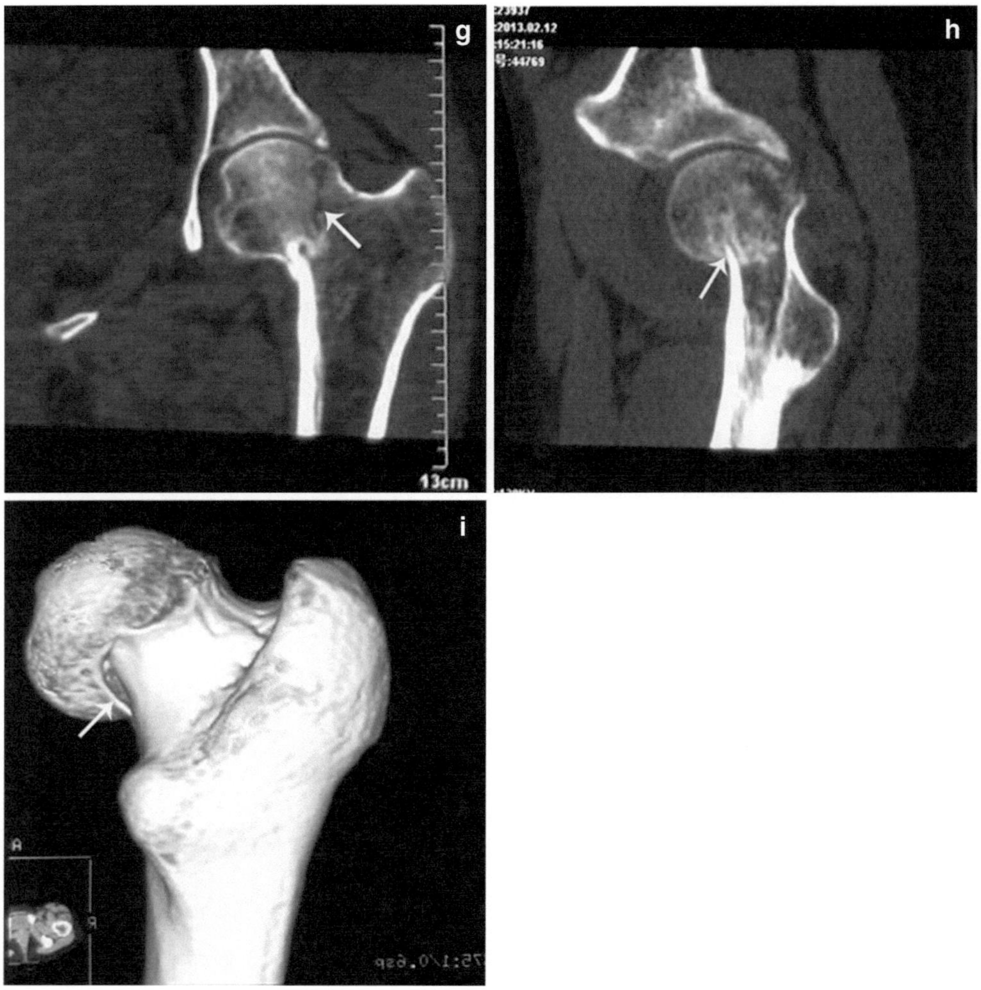

Fig. 8.23 Coronal, sagittal, and three-dimensional reconstruction of CT (**g**, **h**, **i**) shows the fracture of the left femoral neck, dislocation (white arrow), and joint effusion, one month after injury

10. Identification of complete and incomplete fractures of the femoral neck
    10.1 X-ray film (Fig. 8.24a–d)

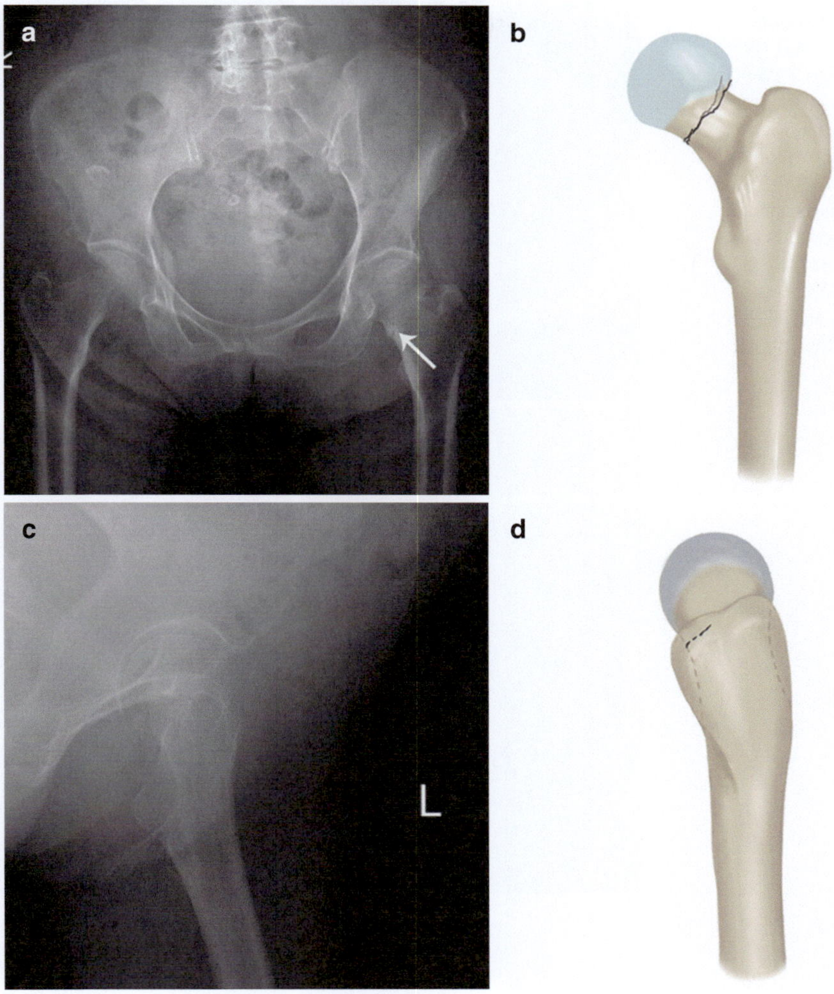

Fig. 8.24 Anteroposterior view of X-ray (**a**) shows a short strip of low-density shadow (white arrow) on the medial femoral neck of the left femur, and no fracture line was observed in the lateral view (**c**). To make a definitive diagnosis, CT and MRI are performed. (**b**, **d**)

    10.2 CT scan (Fig. 8.24e, f)

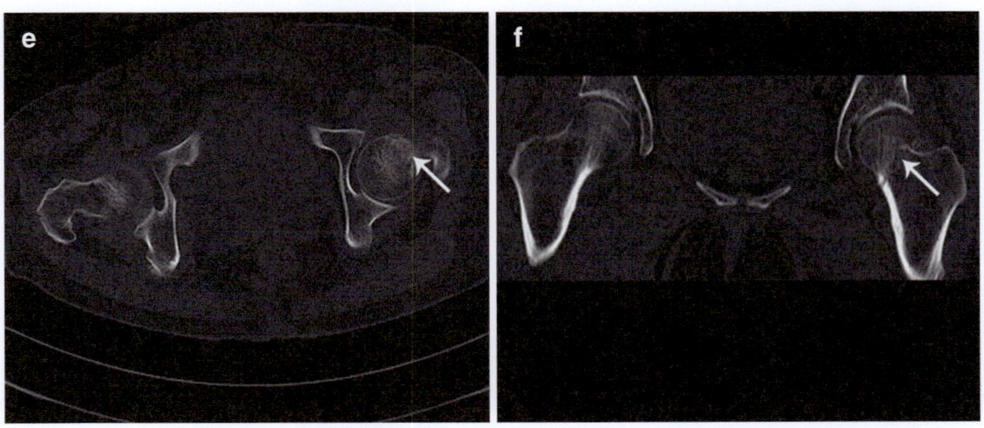

Fig. 8.24 Left femoral neck fracture (white arrow) can be seen in the transverse axis (**e**) and coronal reconstruction (**f**) of CT. Fracture fragment lightly inserted, and neck-shaft angle become larger

10.3 MRI examination (Fig. 8.24g–j)

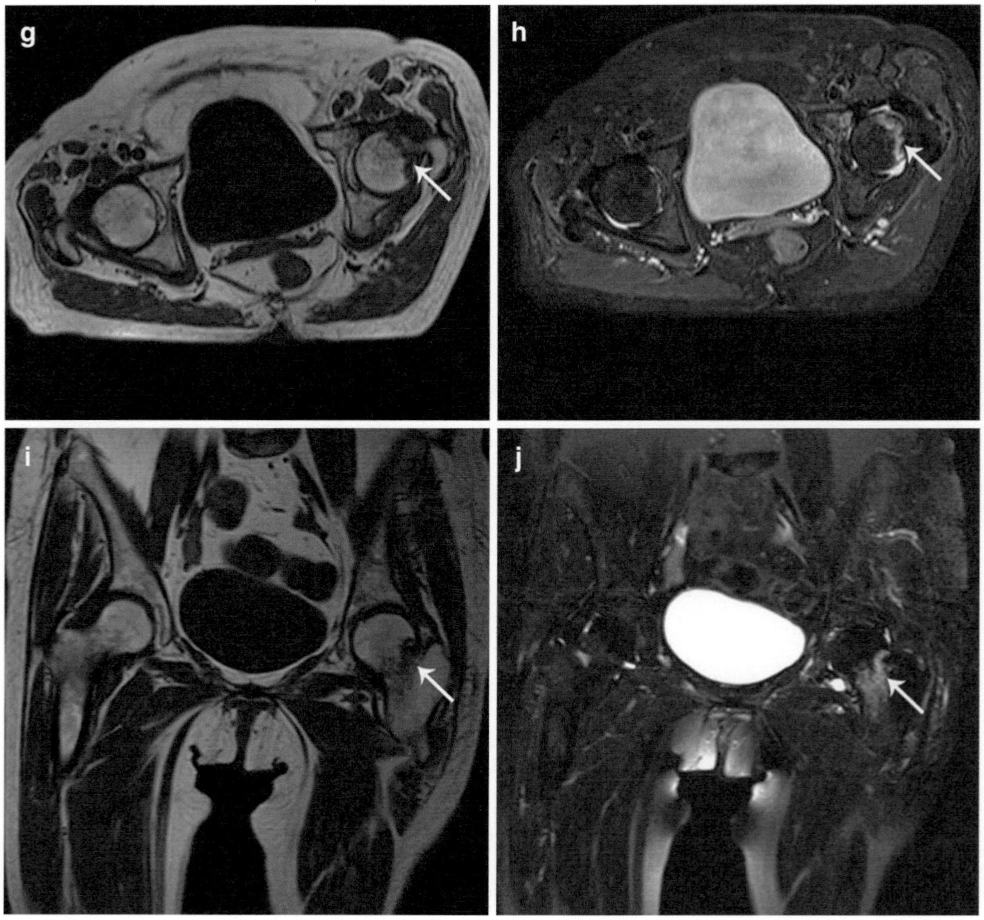

Fig. 8.24 T1WI of transverse axis MRI (**g**), T2WI of fat suppression (**h**), T1WI (**i**), and fat suppression T2WI (**j**) of coronal plane show fracture of left femoral neck, line-like low signal was shown on T1WI (white arrow), T2WI presents a line-like high signal (white arrow). There was edema around the fracture site, T1WI show a flaky low signal, and T2WI presents a flaky high signal

11. Identification of complete and incomplete fractures of the femoral neck

 11.1 X-ray film (Fig. 8.25a–d)

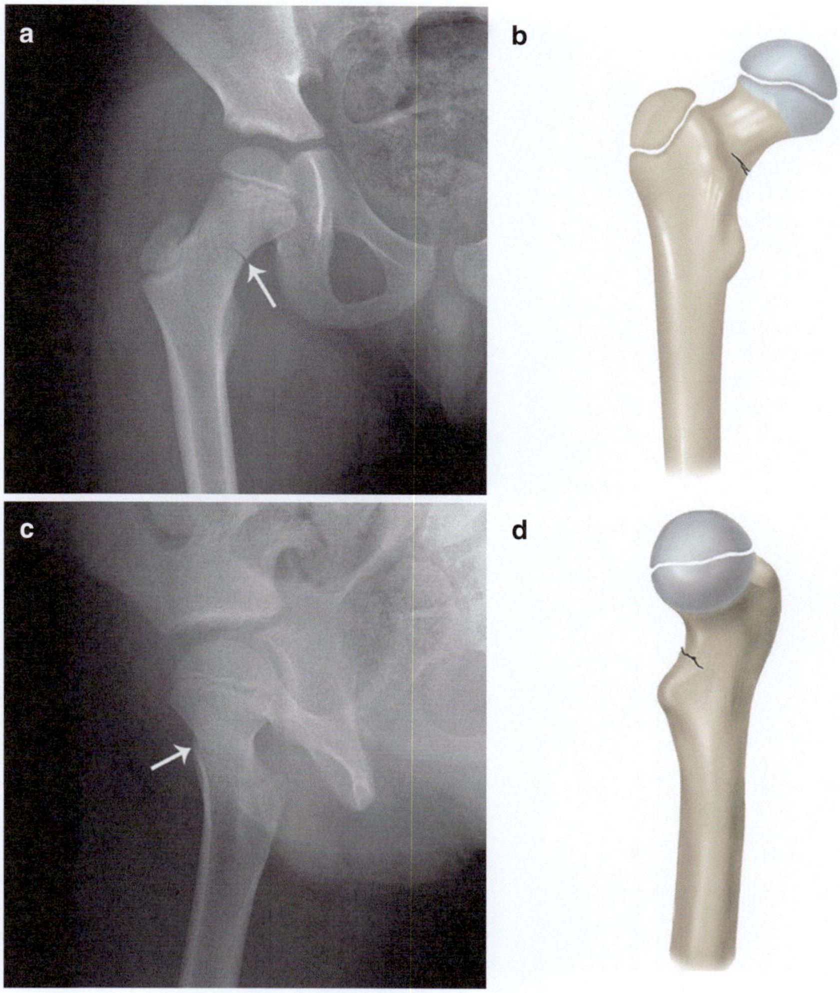

Fig. 8.25 Anteroposterior (**a**) and lateral view (**c**) of X-ray films shows a line-like low-density shadows (white arrows) of the right femoral neck, which seem to be an incomplete fracture. CT scan is preformed to verify the fracture complete or not (**b**, **d**)

 11.2 CT scan (Fig. 8.25e, f)

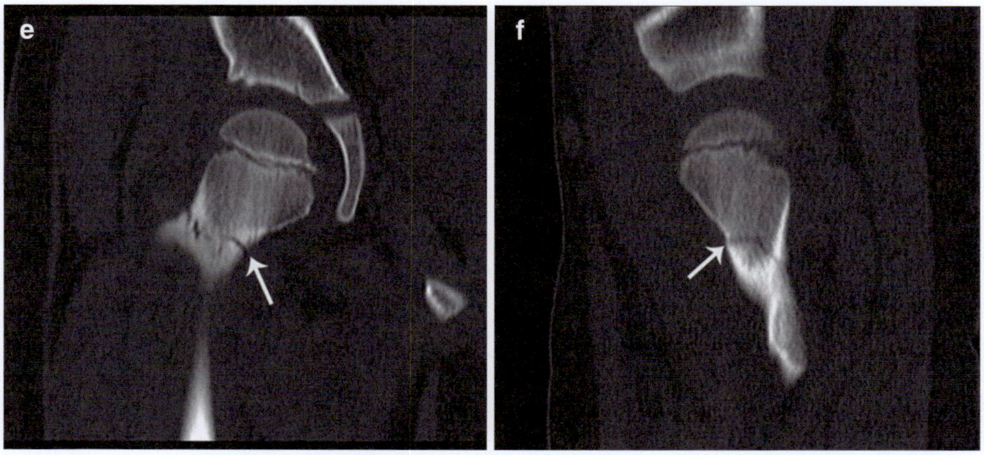

Fig. 8.25 Coronal and sagittal plane reconstruction of CT (**e**, **f**) shows complete fracture of the right femoral neck (white arrow)

12. Identification of basal femoral neck fracture and lesser trochanter fracture
    12.1 X-ray film (Fig. 8.26a–d)

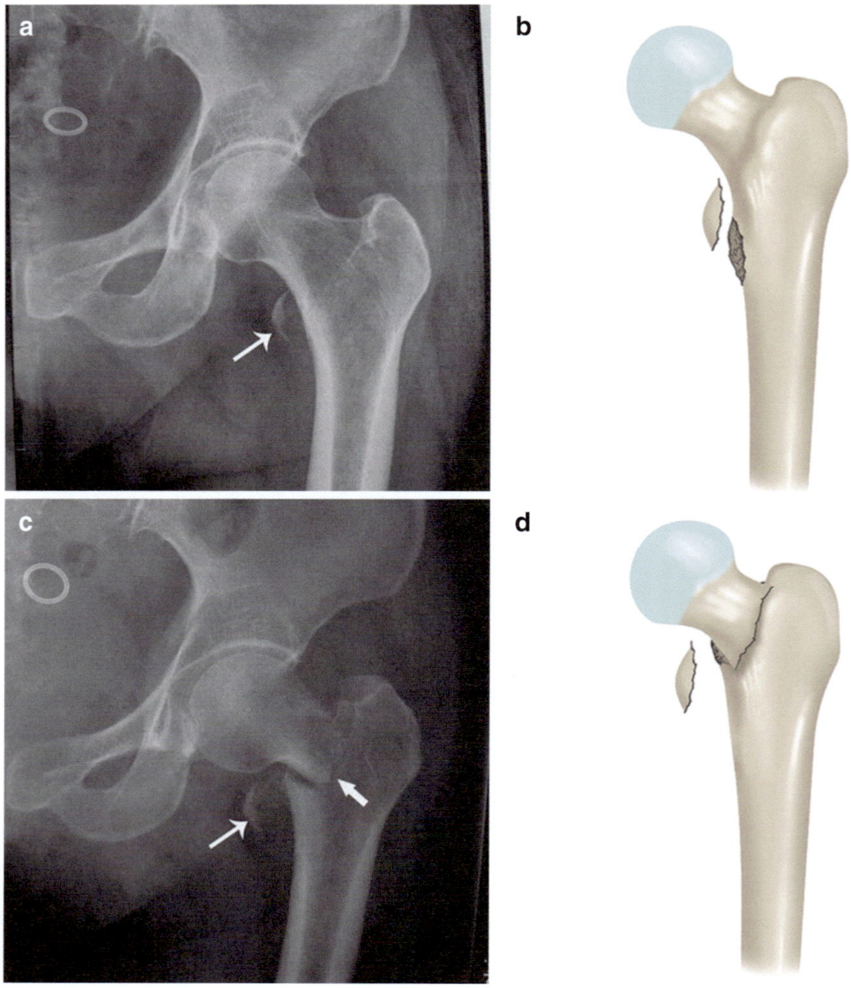

Fig. 8.26 On the day of the injury, the anteroposterior view of X-ray film (**a**) shows a displaced left femoral trochanter fracture (white arrow), no fracture line was seen at the base of the femoral neck, conservative treatment was performed for this patient, (**b**) 1 month later, the X-ray films (**c**) showing displaced left basal femoral neck fracture (rough white arrow), and lesser trochanter fracture (white arrow) (**d**)

    12.2 CT scan (Fig. 8.26e, f)

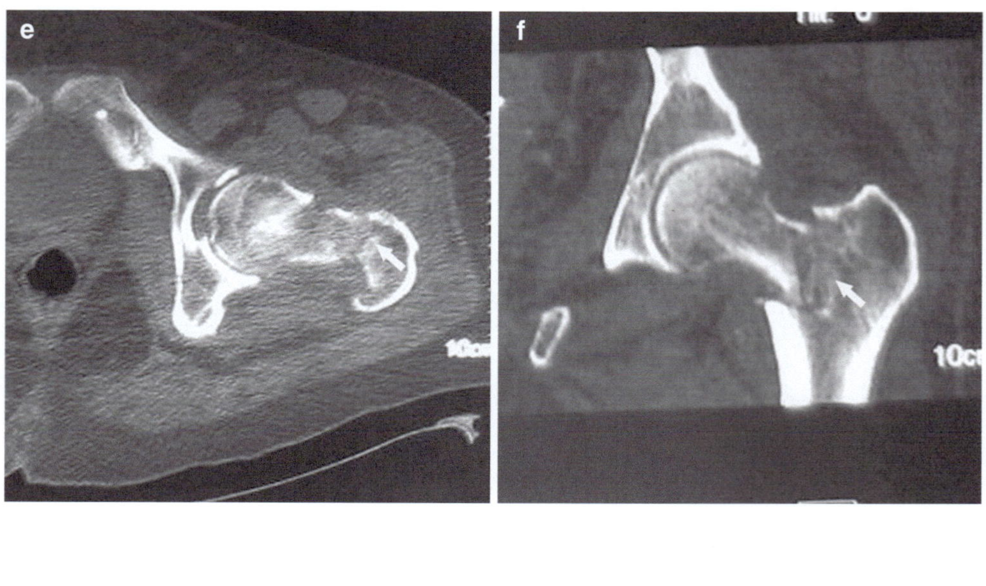

Fig. 8.26 Transverse axis CT (**e**) and coronal plane reconstruction (**f**) after 1 month of injury showed displaced left basal femoral neck fracture (rough white arrow), and lesser trochanter fracture (white arrow)

13. Identification of femoral neck giant osteophyte in osteoarthritis of hip and femoral neck fracture
    13.1 X-ray film (Fig. 8.27a, b)

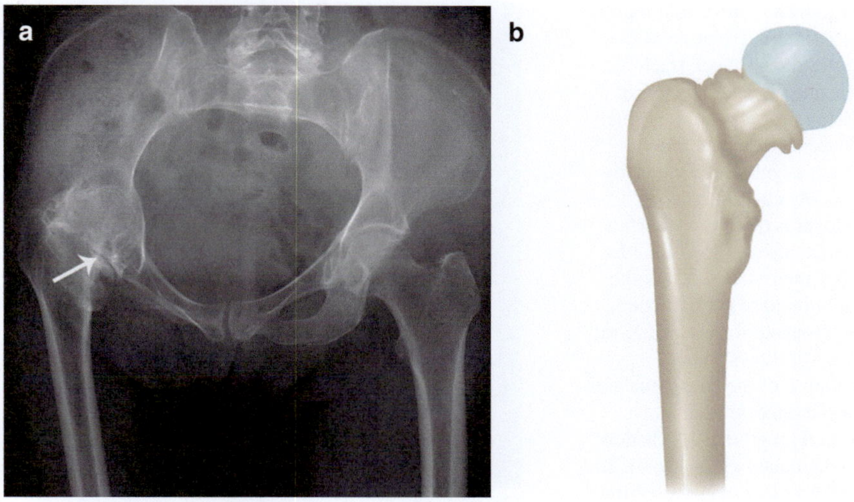

Fig. 8.27 Anteroposterior view of X-ray film (**a**) shows osteoarthritis of right hip, the linear low-density shadow between osteophyte of femoral head and lesser trochanteric is like the fracture line (white arrow). To make a clear diagnosis, a CT scan was conducted (**b**)

13.2 CT scan (Fig. 8.27c)

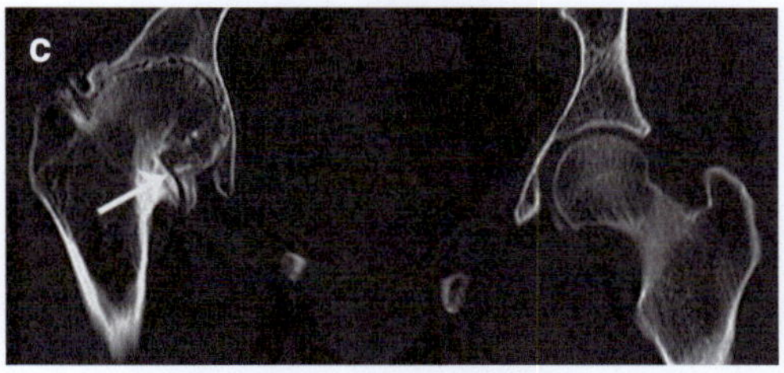

Fig. 8.27 CT coronal reconstruction (**c**) shows that the line-like low-density shadow is the space of osteophytes (white arrow), and the femoral neck has no fracture

14. Diagnosis of a femoral neck fracture combined with avascular necrosis of the femoral head (Male, 77 years old)
    14.1 X-ray film (Fig. 8.28a–d)

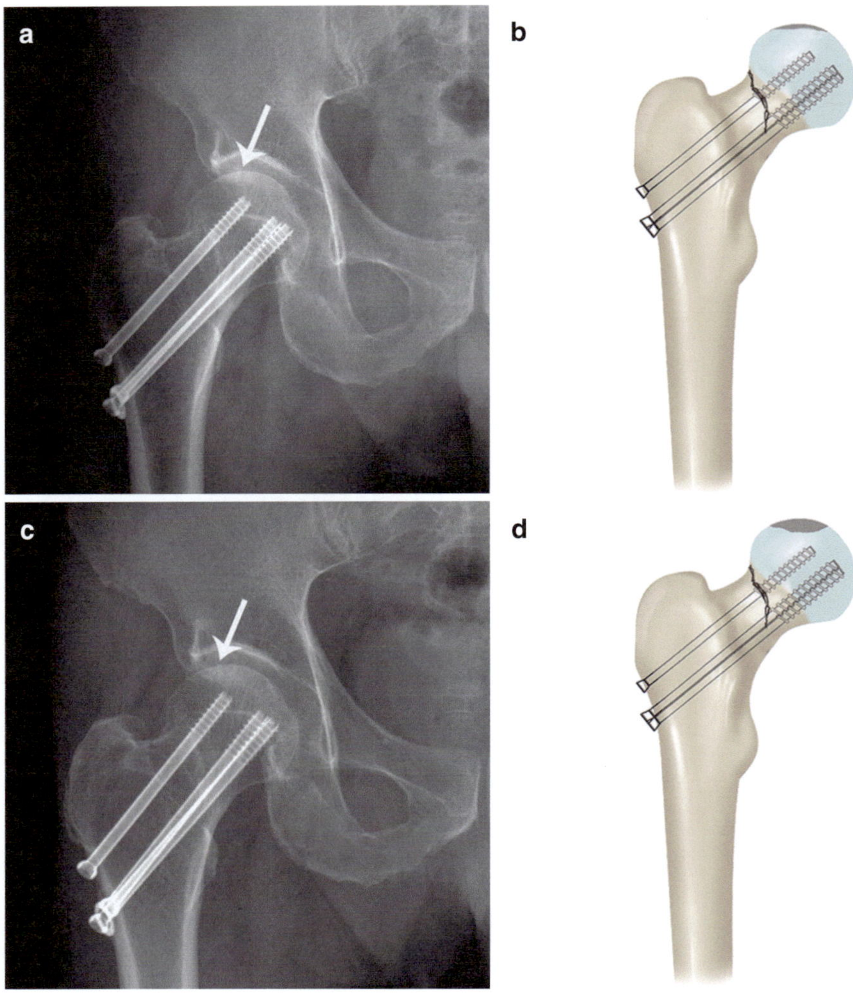

Fig. 8.28 Thirty-four months after internal fixation of the right femoral neck fracture, the anteroposterior view of X-ray film (**a**) shows normal shape of the right femoral head, slightly higher density shadow under the upper outwards of articular surface (white arrow, **b**); 37 months after internal fixation of the right femoral neck fracture, anteroposterior view of X-ray film (**c**) shows a slight collapse of the lateral surface of the femoral head and a slightly high-density shadow in the bone (white arrow). To make a clear diagnosis, MRI was performed (**d**)

14.2 MRI examination (Fig. 8.28e–l)

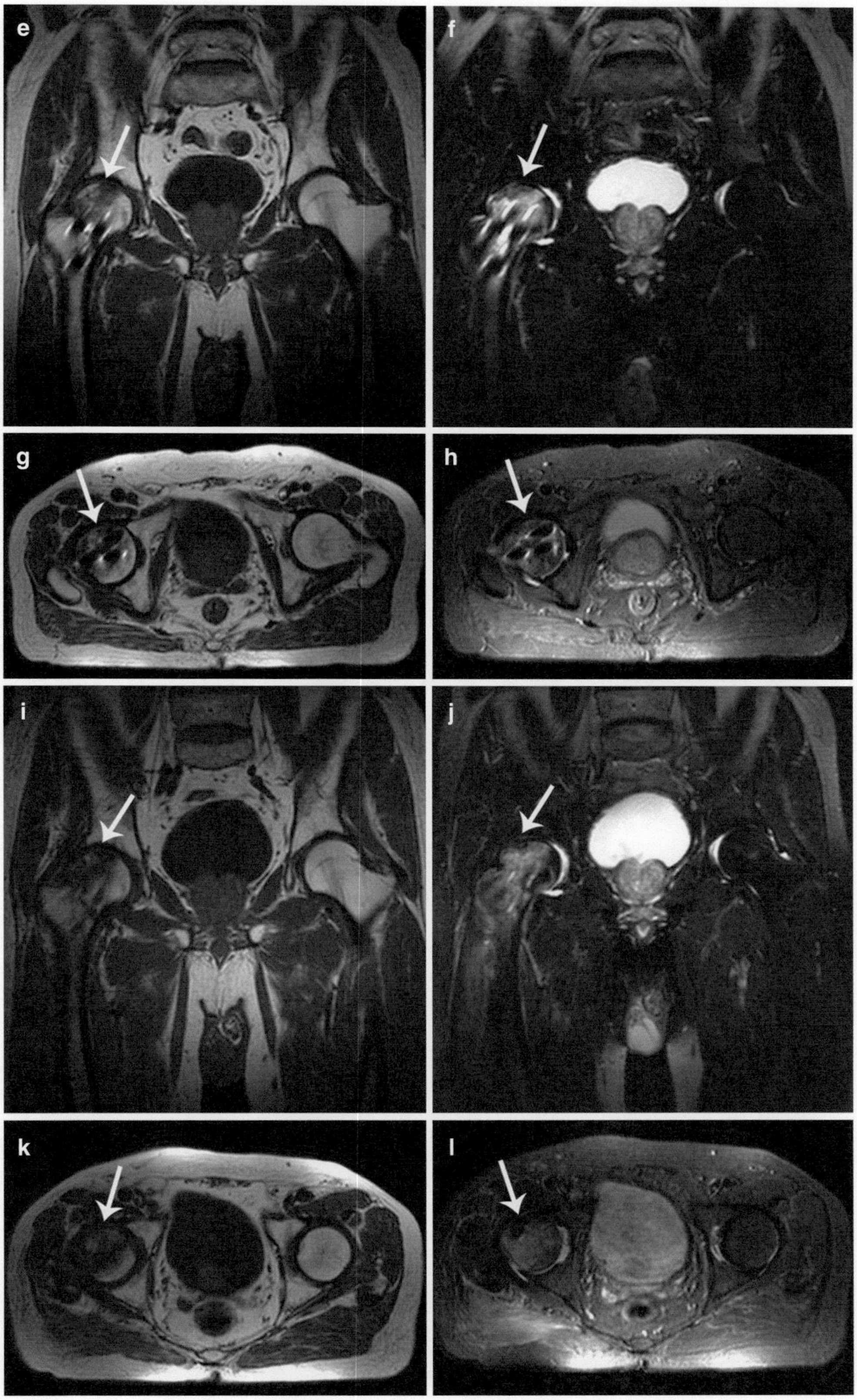

Fig. 8.28 Thirty-seven months after internal fixation of femoral neck fracture, coronal MRI of T1WI (**e**) and fat suppression T2WI (**f**), transverse axis T1WI (**g**), and fat suppression T2WI (**h**) show a slight collapse of the lateral surface of the femoral head and fracture of subarticular bone, line-like low and high signal shadow in T1WI, and fat suppression T2WI, respectively (white arrow), and metal artifacts caused by internal fixation. Internal fixation was removed 39 months after surgery. T1WI (**i**) and fat suppression T2WI (**j**) of coronal MRI; T1WI (**k**) and fat suppression T2WI of transverse MRI (**l**) show increased ischemic necrosis of the right femoral head, fragmentation in the subarticular, articular surface collapse (white arrow), edema in the surrounding bone, patchy low signal in T1WI and high signal in T2WI

15. Diagnosis of femoral neck fracture combined with avascular necrosis of the femoral head
    15.1 X-ray film (Fig. 8.29a–d)

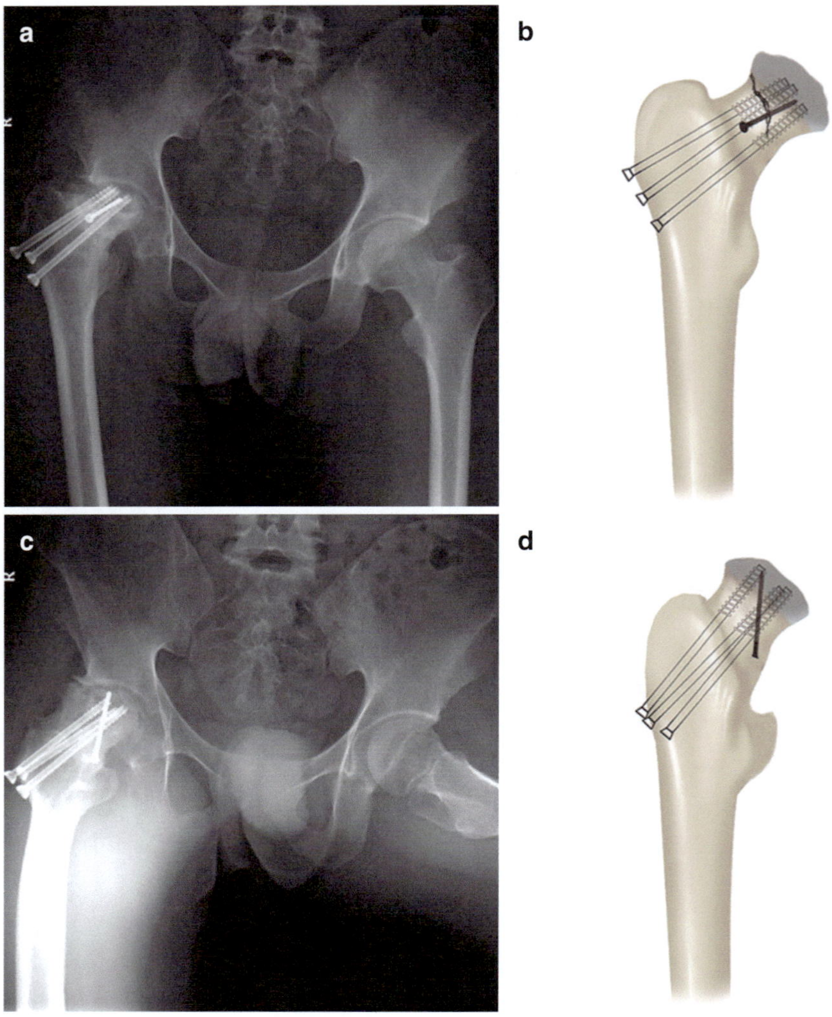

Fig. 8.29 Pain occurred 3.5 years after internal fixation of right femoral neck fracture. The anteroposterior view of X-ray film (**a**) and the frog position (**c**) shows the internal fixation of the right femoral neck fracture and the necrosis of the femoral head (**b**, **d**)

15.2 CT scan (Fig. 8.29e, f)

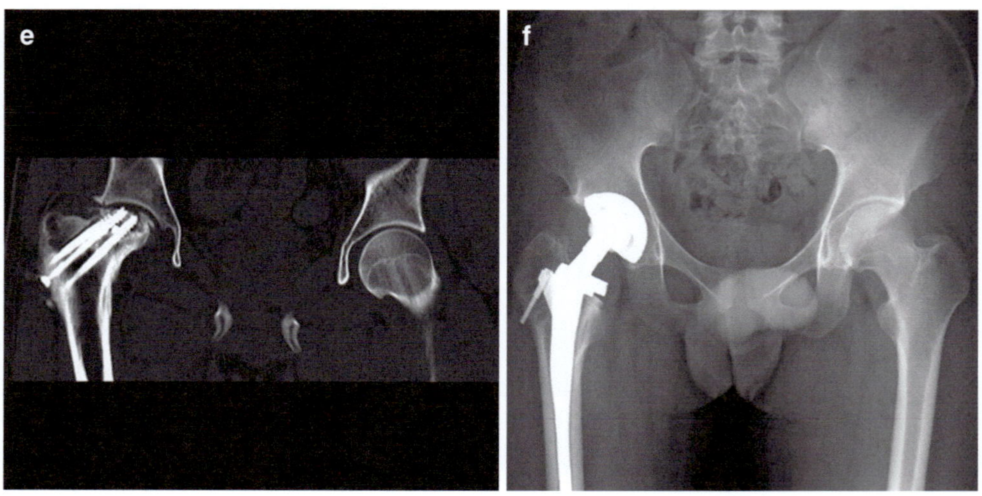

Fig. 8.29 CT coronal reconstruction (**e**) shows disappearance of the fracture line, avascular necrosis of the femoral head, and obvious collapse of the articular surface. Anteroposterior view of X-ray film after right hip arthroplasty (**f**)

8.2.3 Intertrochanteric Fracture

According to the AO/OTA classification, intertrochanteric fractures can be divided into simple fracture, comminuted fracture, and intertrochanteric fracture.

8.2.3.1 Injury Mechanism

Intertrochanteric fractures mostly occur in elderly patients, and its incidence in women is three times higher than that of men. Most common causes of this fracture in elderly patients are low-energy injuries. The most common causes of this injury in young patients are high-energy trauma, such as traffic accident or falling from a height. Attention should be paid to the head, chest, and abdominal injuries in these patients.

8.2.3.2 Signs and Symptoms

The typical clinical features of intertrochanteric fractures are shortening and external rotation deformity of the affected limb. However, if the fracture is not displaced, there is no characteristic symptoms, which needs to be identified by the clinician.

8.2.3.3 Radiographic Diagnosis

Displaced femoral intertrochanteric fractures are easy to diagnose by X-ray film, but it is difficult to diagnose by ordinary X-ray films if the fracture is not displaced. This requires CT or MRI scans to corroborate the fracture, otherwise, this fracture will be displaced after missed diagnosis.

16. Diagnosis of intertrochanteric fracture
    16.1 X-ray film (Fig. 8.30a, b)

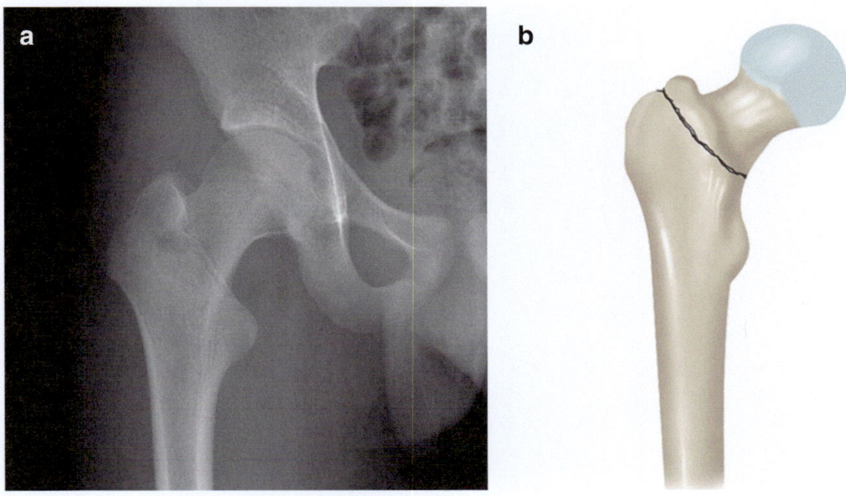

Fig. 8.30 Anteroposterior view of X-ray film (**a**) shows the irregular low-density shadow in the right femoral trochanter. To make a clear diagnosis, CT scan is performed (**b**)

    16.2 CT scan (Fig. 8.30c, d)

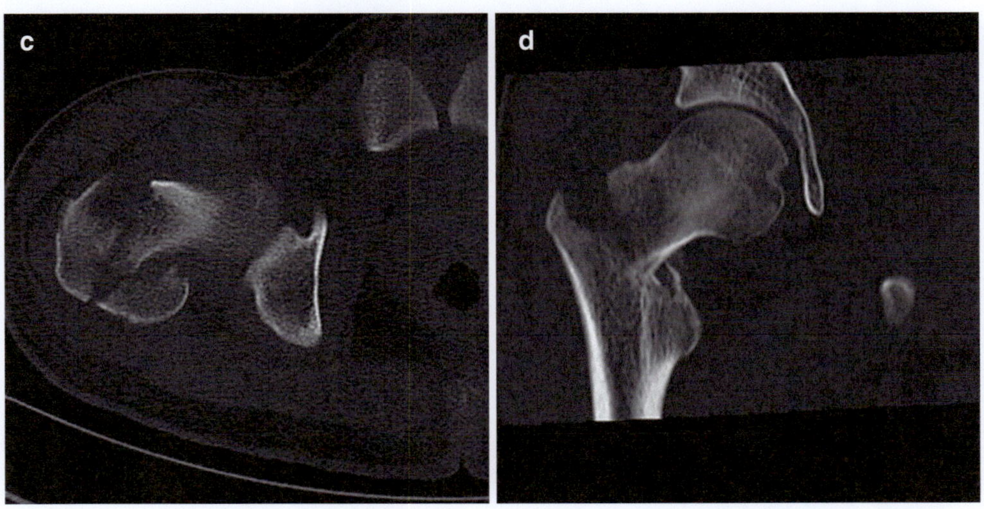

Fig. 8.30 Transverse axis of CT (**c**), CT coronal reconstruction (**d**) show comminuted intertrochanteric fracture

17. Identification of intertrochanteric fracture
    17.1 X-ray film (Fig. 8.31a, b)

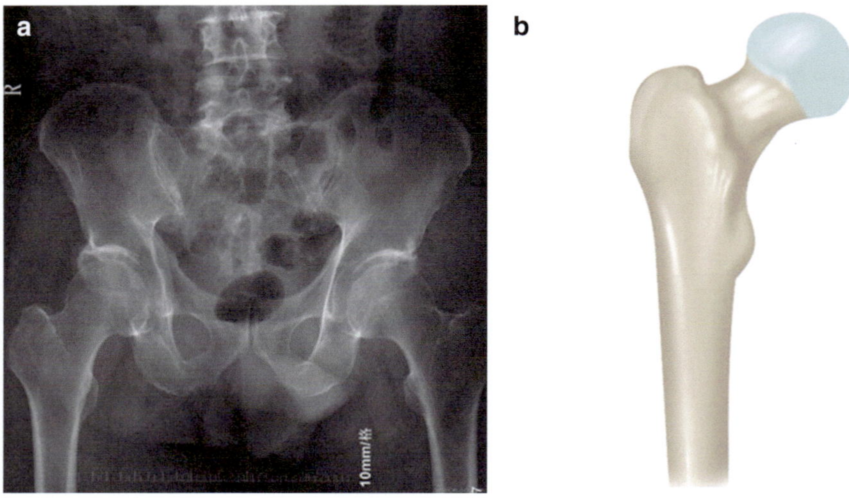

Fig. 8.31 Anteroposterior view of X-ray film (**a**) shows no obvious fractures, however, pain of this patient was serious, so an MRI examination is performed (**b**)

    17.2 MRI examination (Fig. 8.31c)

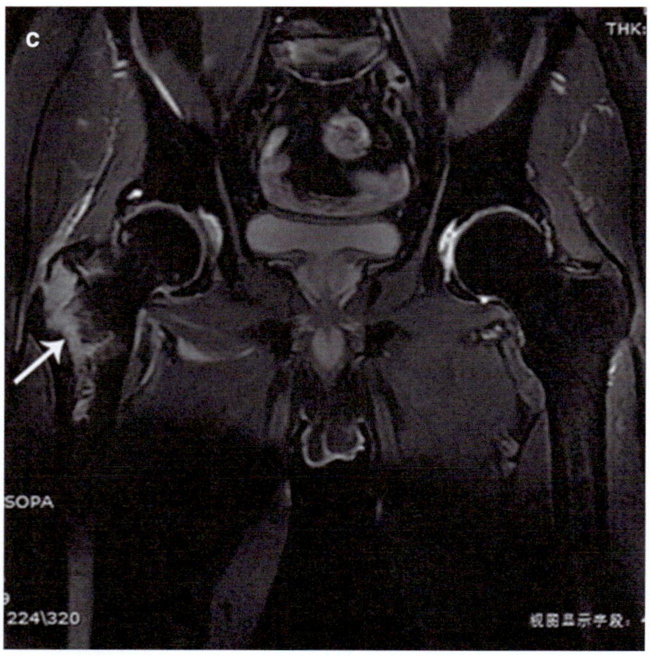

Fig. 8.31 T2WI of MRI coronal fat suppression (**c**) shows a right intertrochanteric fracture with a linear high signal shadow (white arrow), peripheral edema, there is no obvious dislocation

17.3 CT scan (Fig. 8.31d, e)

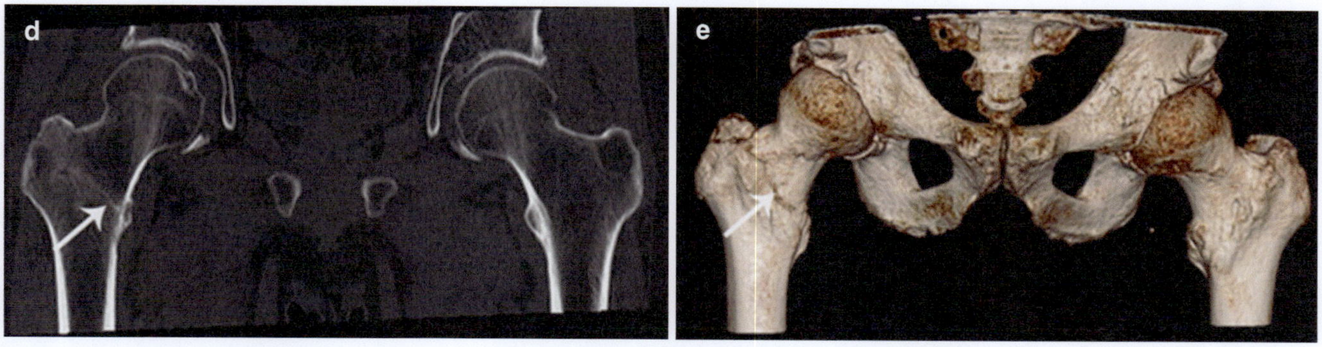

Fig. 8.31 Coronal and three-dimensional of CT reconstruction (**d**, **e**) after 1 month shows a clear intertrochanteric fracture line of the right femur and slight sclerosis of fracture site (white arrow)

18. Identification of comminuted and simple intertrochanteric fractures
    18.1 X-ray film (Fig. 8.32a, b)

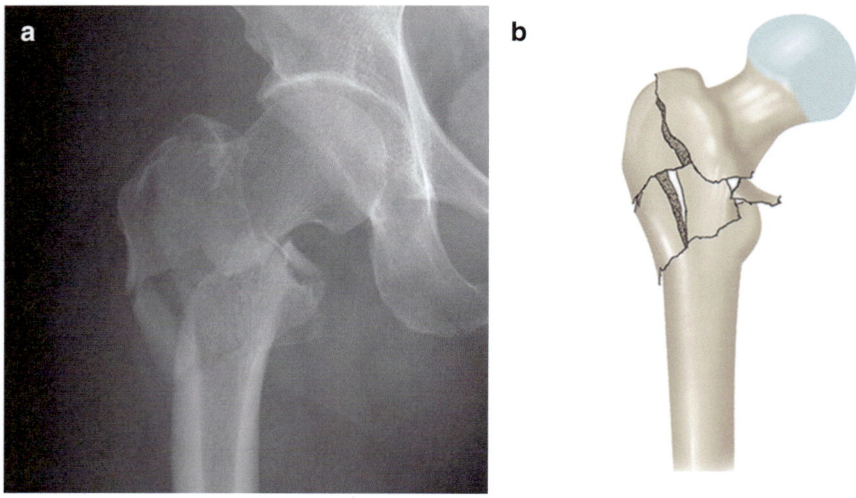

Fig. 8.32 Anteroposterior view of X-ray film (**a**) shows comminuted and displaced intertrochanteric fracture of the right femur (**a**, **b**)

    18.2 CT scan (Fig. 8.32c–e)

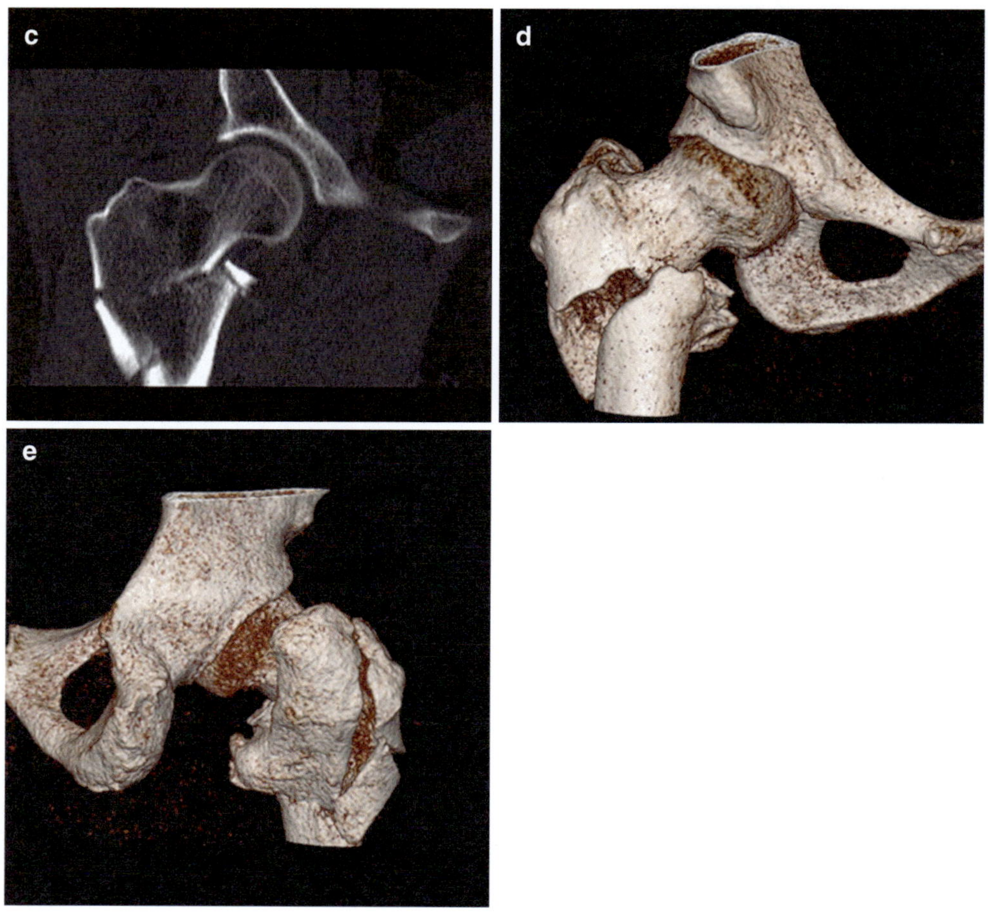

Fig. 8.32 Anteroposterior view of X-ray film (**a**) shows comminuted and displaced intertrochanteric fracture of the right femur (**a**, **b**). Coronal and three-dimensional reconstruction of CT (**c**, **d**, **e**) shows comminuted and displaced intertrochanteric fracture

8.3 Conclusion

1. Acetabular fractures are mostly caused by high-energy violence, which is transmitted from the femoral neck to the acetabulum. Acetabular fractures are complex type of fracture and are often accompanied by dislocation.
2. Anteroposterior and double oblique view are needed in the diagnosis of acetabular fractures.
3. The anatomical structure of a hip joint is complex, thus a CT scan and a three-dimensional reconstruction are necessary (besides X-ray film). These imagological examination can display types and involvement of fracture, micro fracture, information of the displacement of the fracture, and intra-articular fracture fragments.
4. Attention should be paid to pelvic vascular, urethral, and nerve injury in acetabular fractures.

Reference

1. Yingze Z, et al. Clinical epidemiology of orthopaedic trauma. Stuttgart: Thieme; 2016.

9 Knee Fracture

Xiaodong Lian and Yingze Zhang

9.1 Distal Femur Fractures

The distal femur refers to the position below 2–4 cm above the condyle of the femur. According to the location of fracture and the extension of the fracture line, it can be divided into supracondylar fracture of femur, condylar fracture of femur and intercondylar fracture of femur.

9.1.1 Injury Mechanism

At present, it is generally believed that axial load is the result of internal and external turning or rotating stress. In young people, most of them are injured by motorbikes.

9.1.2 Symptoms and Signs

The main symptoms are pain, swelling and restricted movement in the injured area, usually accompanied by obvious deformities. But it is difficult to make a definite diagnosis. Therefore, when a fracture is suspected, X-ray or CT scans should be conducted to prevent missed diagnosis.

9.1.3 Imaging Differential Diagnosis

In general, an X-ray can diagnose supracondylar fracture. CT scans can observe the internal collapse and defect of fracture, accurately locate the position of the bone fragments, whilst 3D reconstruction images are especially useful for intraoperative fracture reduction. MRI scans can simultaneously evaluate the degree of knee ligament and meniscus injury.

X. Lian · Y. Zhang (✉)
Department of Orthopaedics, The Third Hospital of Hebei Medical University, Shijiazhuang, Hebei, China

Y. Zhang (ed.), *Differential Diagnosis of Fracture*, https://doi.org/10.1007/978-981-13-8339-7_9

(1) Supracondylar fracture of the femur: These fracture types can be subdivided into non-displaced fracture, embedded fracture, displaced fracture and comminuted fracture

1. Differential displacement and non-displacement of femoral supracondylar fracture
   1.1 X-ray (Fig. 9.1a–d)

Fig. 9.1 (**a**, **c**) The positive and lateral position of the X-ray, respectively, indicating the fracture of the femoral condyle, dislocation and overlap, and angular deformity (**b**, **d**)

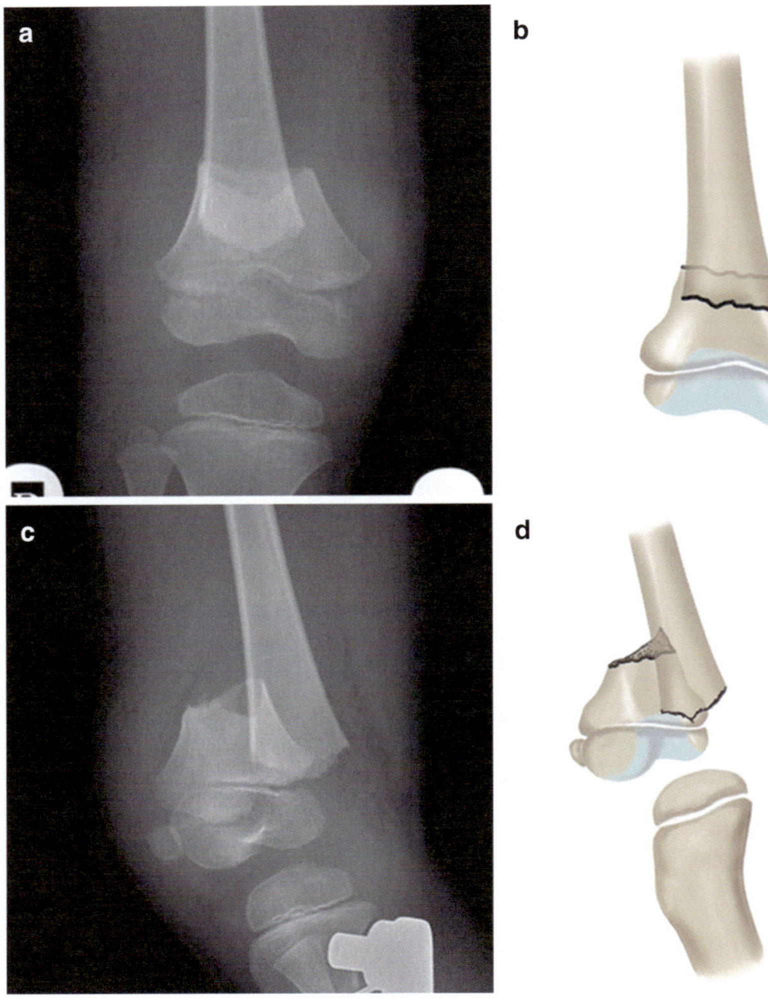

   1.2 CT (Fig. 9.1e, f)

Fig. 9.1 (**e**, **f**) are the sagittal plane of CT and the lateral view of 3D reconstruction, respectively, showing the fracture of the femoral condyle, dislocation, overlap and angular deformity, swelling of soft tissue and joint effusion. It is recommended to perform a tibial tuberosity traction

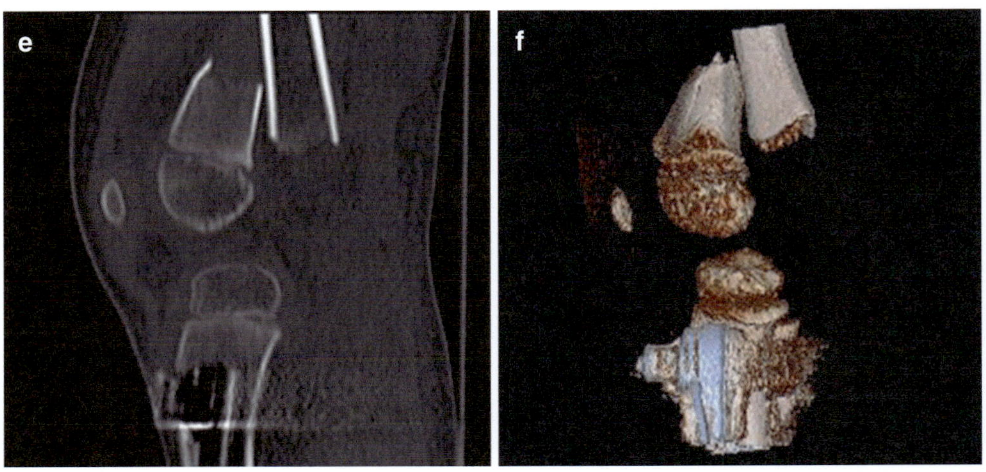

(2) Femoral condyle fracture

2. Differentiation between avulsion fracture and non-fracture of internal condyle of the femur
   2.1 X-ray (Fig. 9.2a–d)

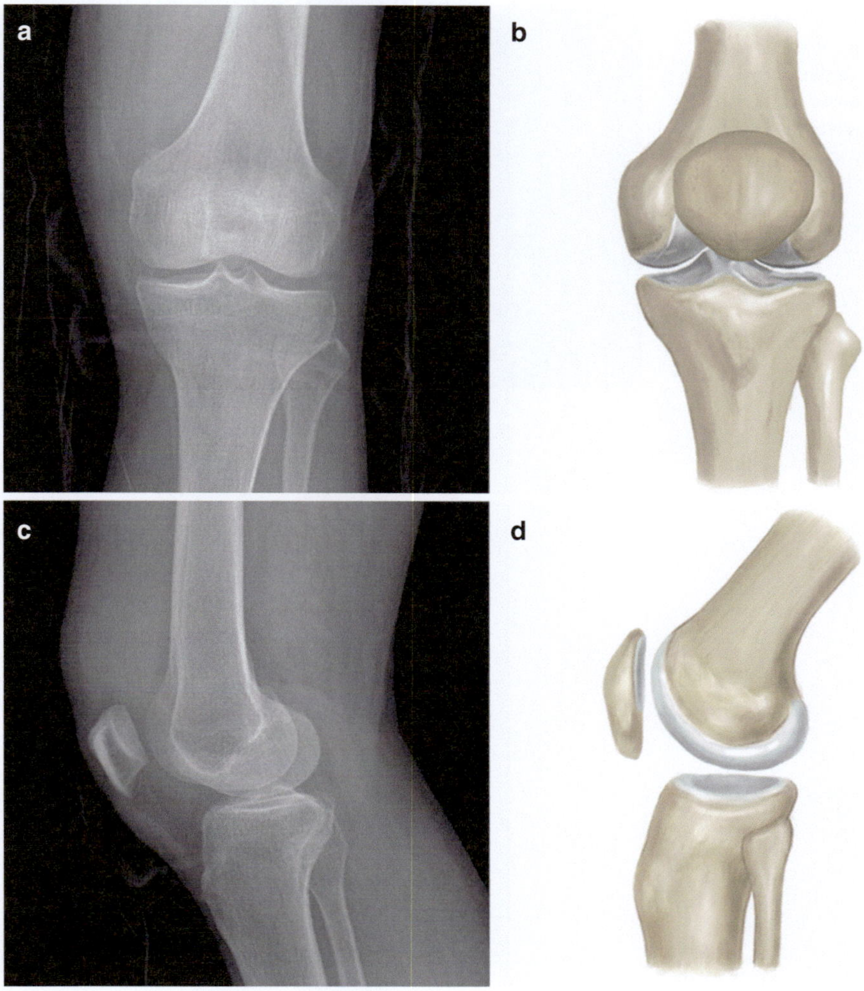

Fig. 9.2 (**a**, **c**) are in the positive and lateral positions of the X-ray, respectively, and no obvious signs of fracture have been observed (**b**, **d**). The superior patellar bursa is obviously swollen, and the texture of the condyle inside the femur is swollen

   2.2 CT (Fig. 9.2e, f)

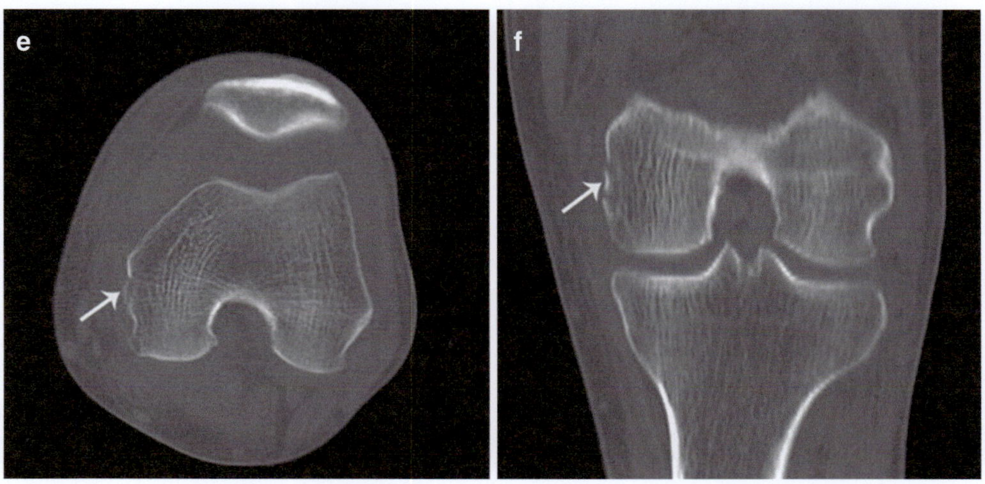

Fig. 9.2 (**e**, **f**) are, respectively, CT transverse plane and coronal plane reconstruction, showing avulsion fracture of left femoral condyle, no obvious dislocation (fine white arrow) and intra-articular effusion. In order to observe the ligament condition, a further MRI scan was performed

2.3 MRI (Fig. 9.2g, h)

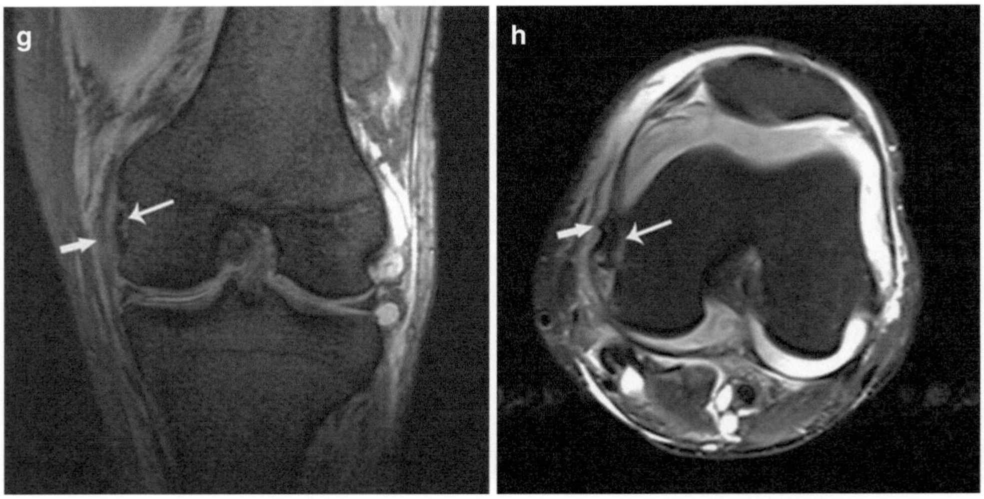

Fig. 9.2 (**g**, **h**) T2WI of MRI in the coronal and horizontal planes, respectively, showing the femoral internal condyle fracture tablet, without dislocation (fine white arrow), partial injury of the medial collateral ligament (thick white arrow), swelling of the soft tissue and massive fluid accumulation in the joints

3. Differentiation of femoral internal condyle fracture from non-fracture
   3.1 X-ray (Fig. 9.3a–d)

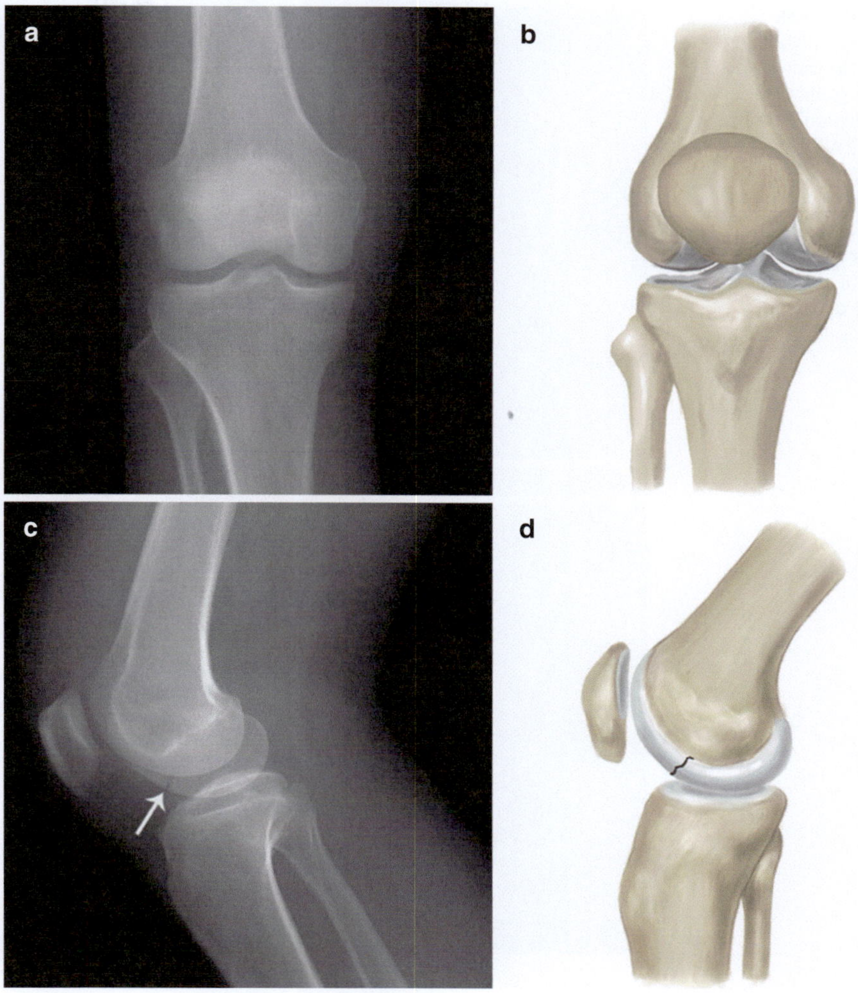

Fig. 9.3 (**a**) is the positive position of the X-ray, and no obvious fracture line is seen (**b**). (**c**) shows the lateral position of the X-ray showing the femoral internal condylar wire fracture (white arrow), and the schematic diagram (**d**)

3.2 MRI (Fig. 9.3e–h)

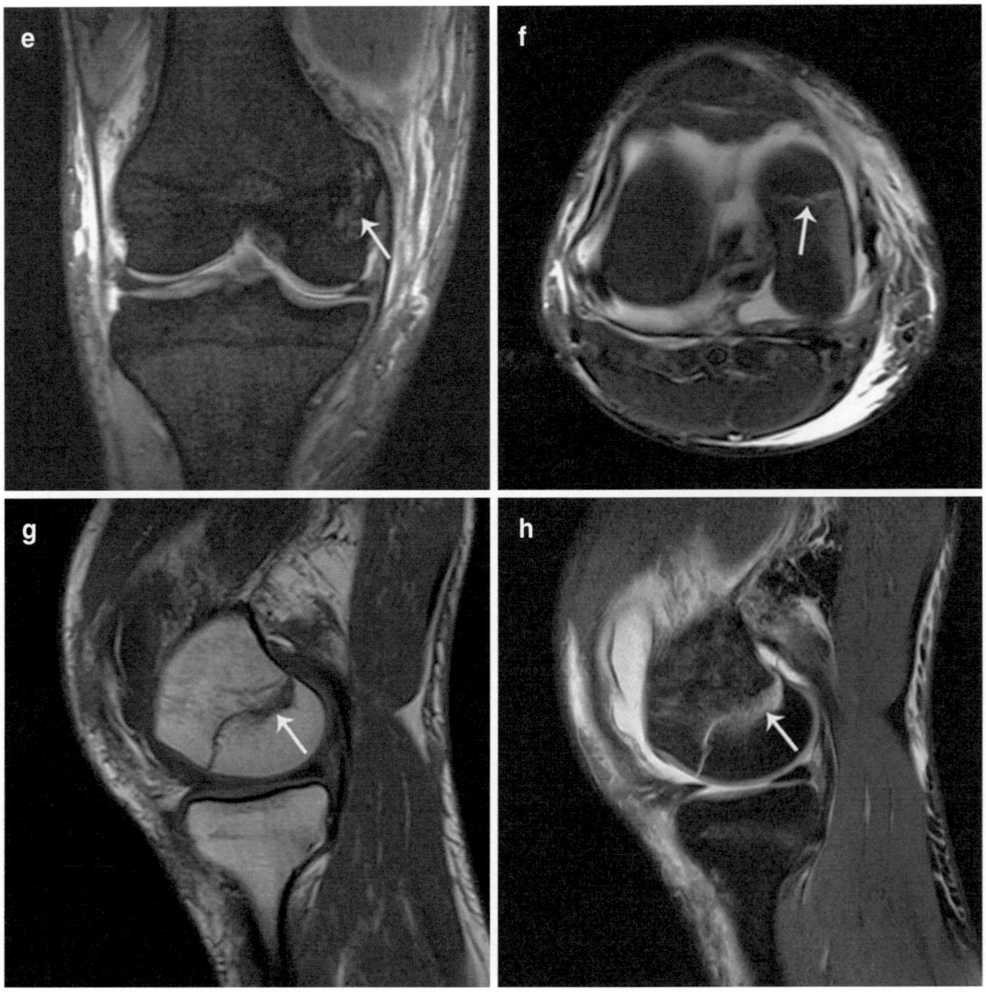

Fig. 9.3 In order to observe the ligament condition, further MRI examination was performed. (**e**–**h**) shows MRI coronal T2WI, transverse axial T2WI, sagittal T1WI and adipose T2WI, respectively, indicating femoral internal condyle fracture (white arrow), swelling of the surrounding soft tissue, joint effusion and normal medial collateral ligament

4. Differentiation of femoral condyle fracture from non-fracture
   4.1 X-ray (Fig. 9.4a–d)

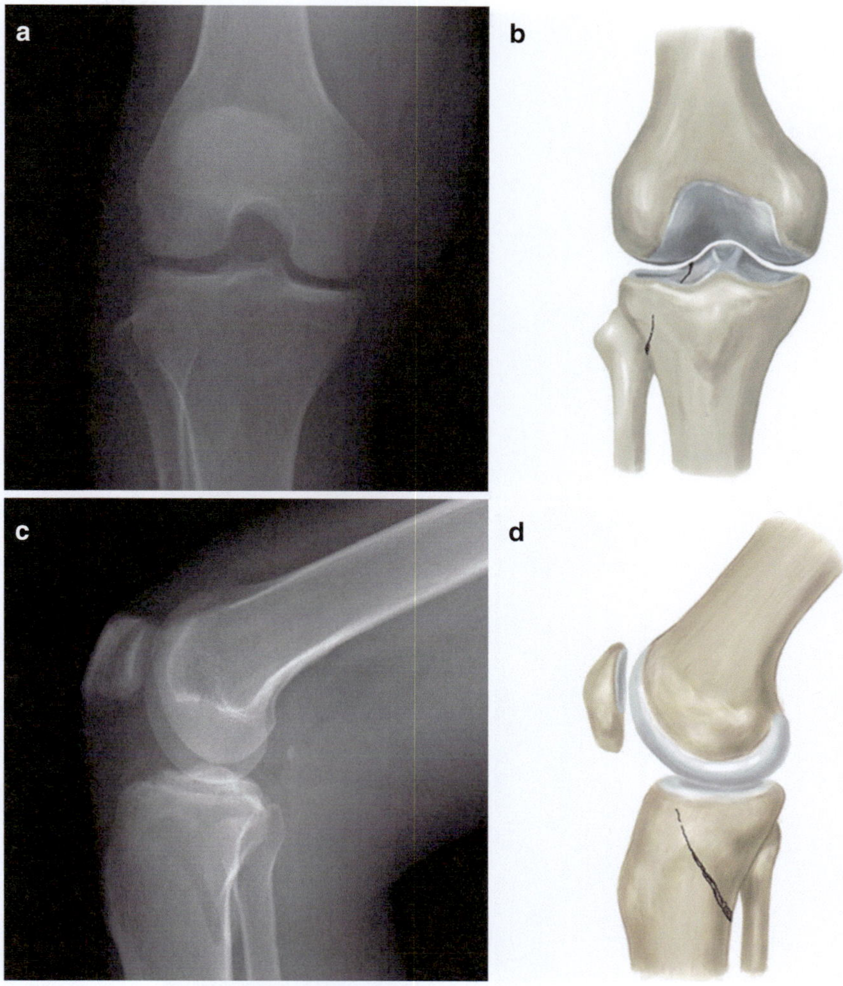

Fig. 9.4 (**a**, **c**) are X-ray positive and lateral position, respectively, showing tibial plateau fracture, no obvious femoral condyle fracture and schematic diagram (**b**, **d**)

   4.2 CT (Fig. 9.4e, f)

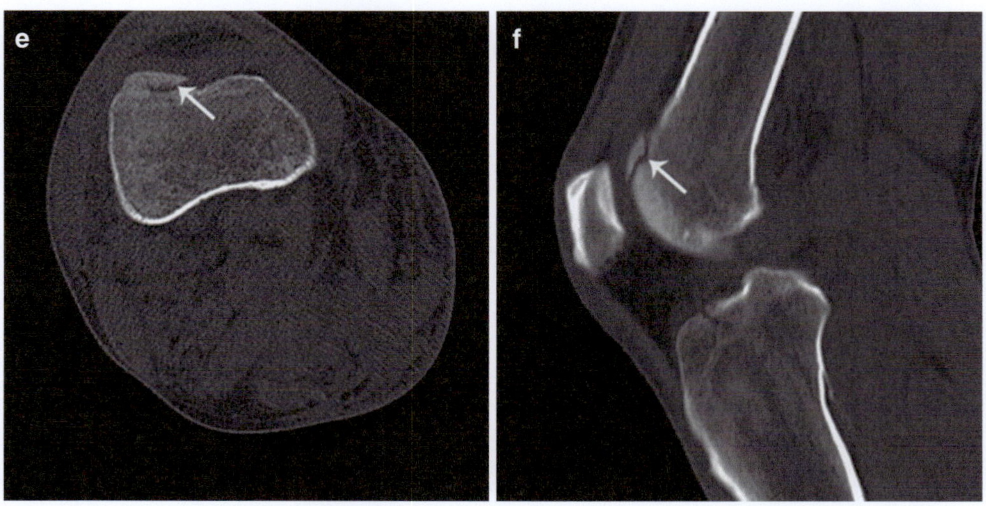

Fig. 9.4 (**e**, **f**) are CT transverse and sagittal reconstruction, showing avulsion fracture of external femoral condyle, no obvious dislocation (white arrow), tibial plateau fracture

5. Differential diagnosis between collapse and non-fracture of external condyle fracture of femur
   5.1 X-ray (Fig. 9.5a–d)

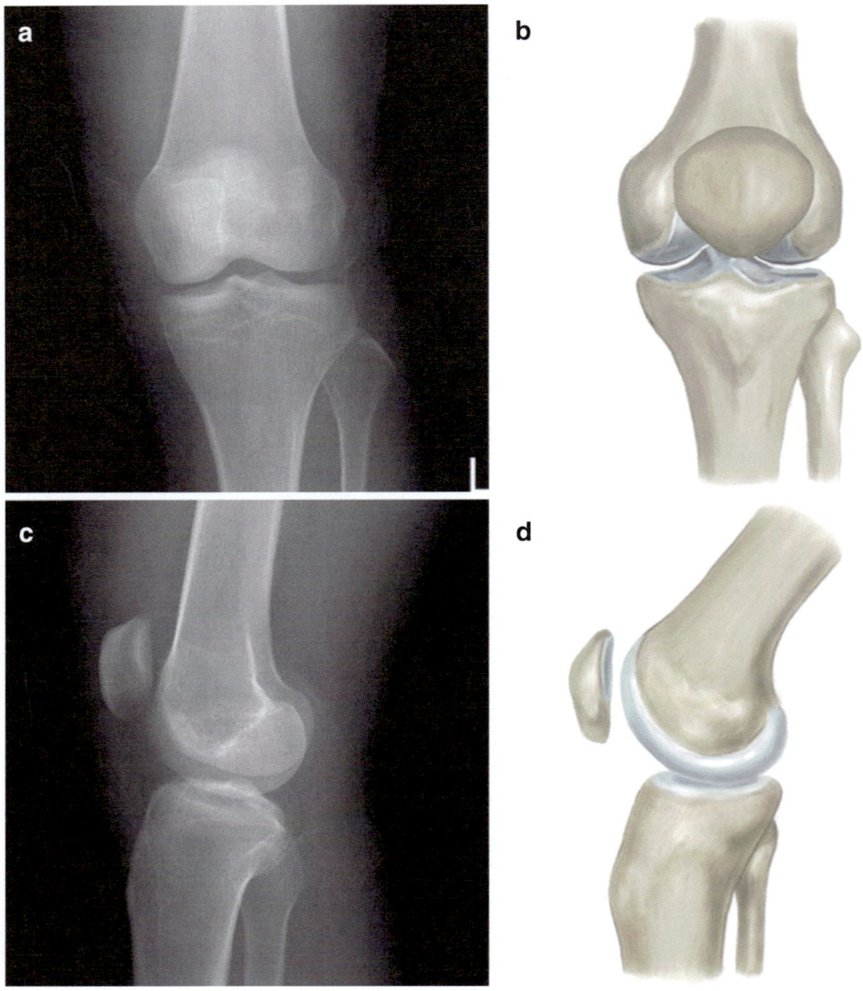

Fig. 9.5 (**a**, **c**) are the positive and lateral positions of X-ray, respectively, and the fracture line is not obvious, and the diagram (**b**, **d**) is shown, so further MRI scan is performed

5.2 MRI (Fig. 9.5e–h)

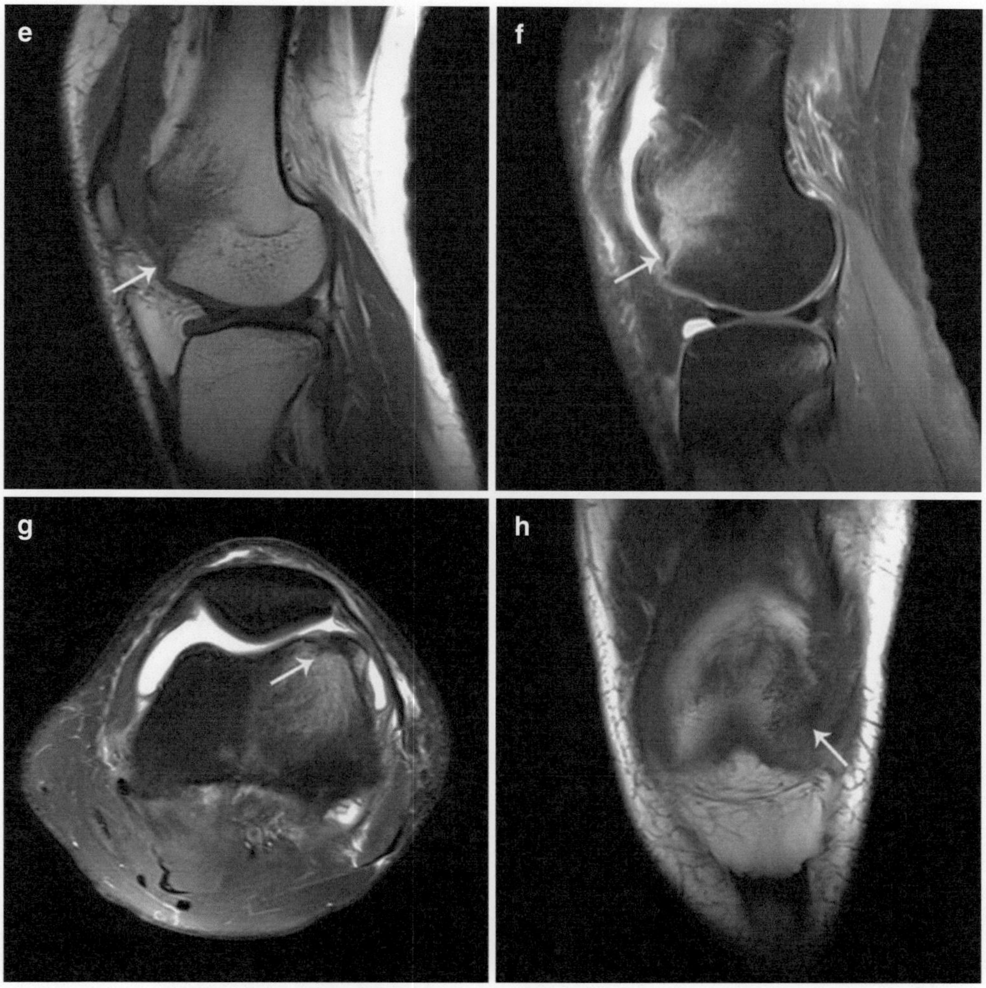

Fig. 9.5 (**e–h**) shows MRI sagittal plane T1WI, adipose inhibition T2WI, horizontal axis plane T2WI and coronal plane T1WI, respectively, showing femoral anterior condyle fracture, collapse (white arrow), peripheral bone marrow edema, soft tissue swelling and joint effusion

6. Differentiation of femoral external condyle fracture from non-fracture
   6.1 X-ray (Fig. 9.6a–d)

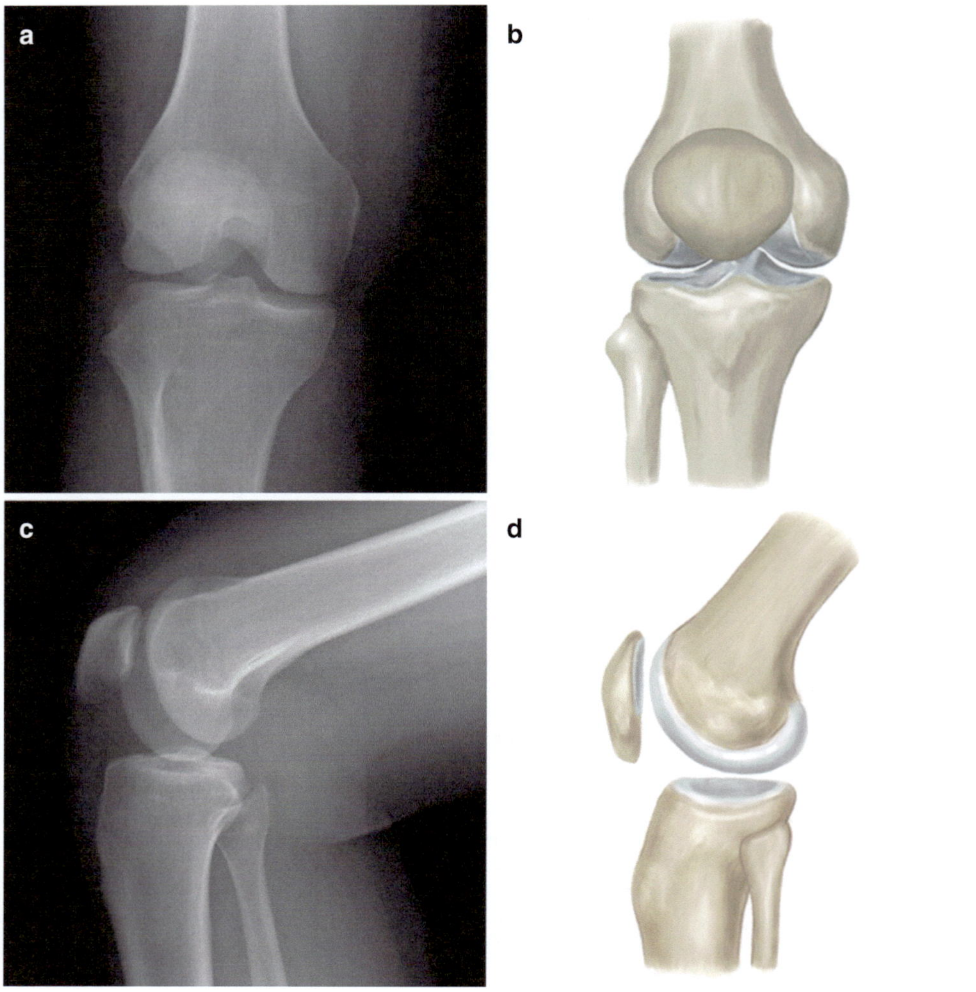

Fig. 9.6 (**a**, **c**) are X-ray positive and lateral position, respectively. No obvious fractures have been observed (**b**, **d**)

   6.2 CT (Fig. 9.6e, f)

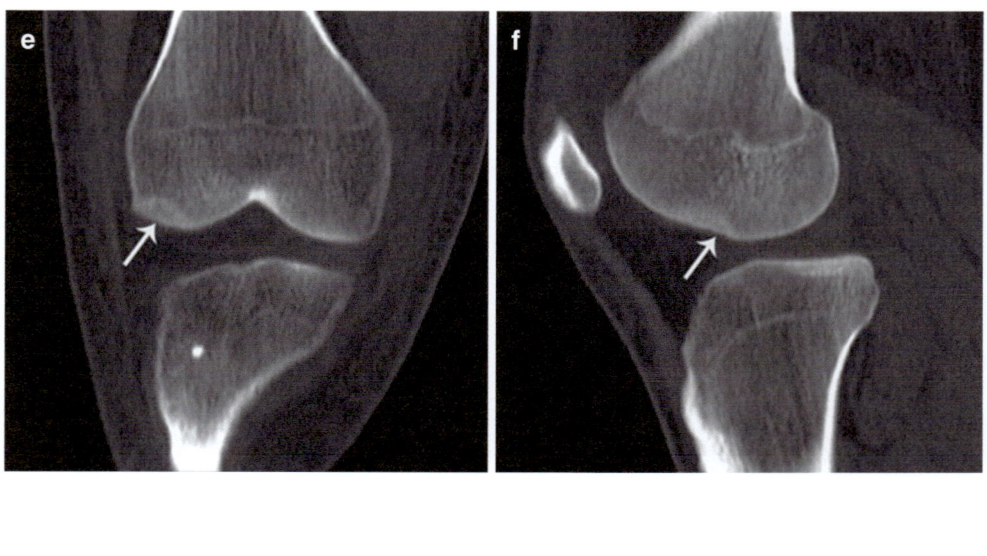

Fig. 9.6 (**e**, **f**) are, respectively, the coronal plane and sagittal plane reconstruction of CT, showing the local depression of the external condyle articular surface of femur, and the increase of bone density (white arrow)

6.3 MRI (Fig. 9.6g, h)

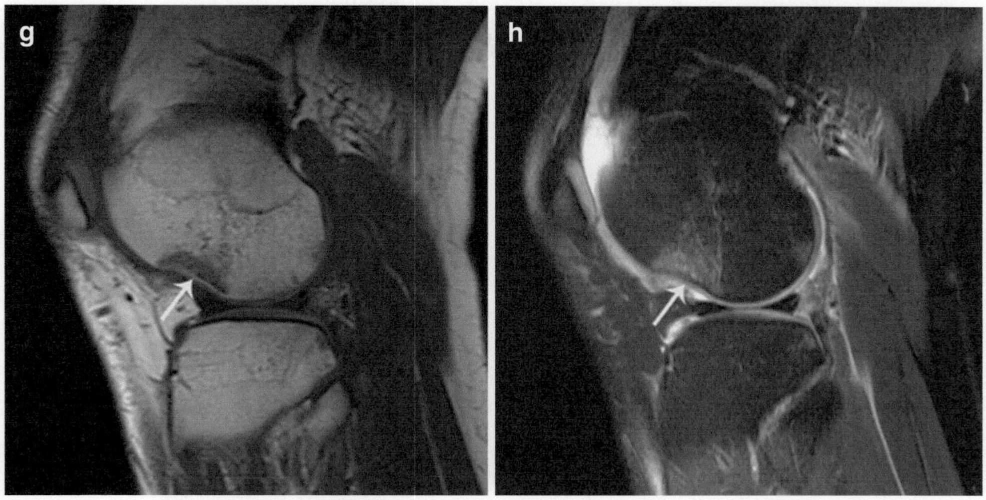

Fig. 9.6 (**g**, **h**) are MRI sagittal plane T1WI and fat suppression T2WI, respectively, showing the fractures and depressions (white arrow) of the femoral epicondyle cartilage, the surrounding bone marrow edema and the joint effusion

(3) Intercondylar fracture of the femur

7. Differentiation between intercondylar fracture and non-fracture of femur
   7.1 X-ray (Fig. 9.7a–d)

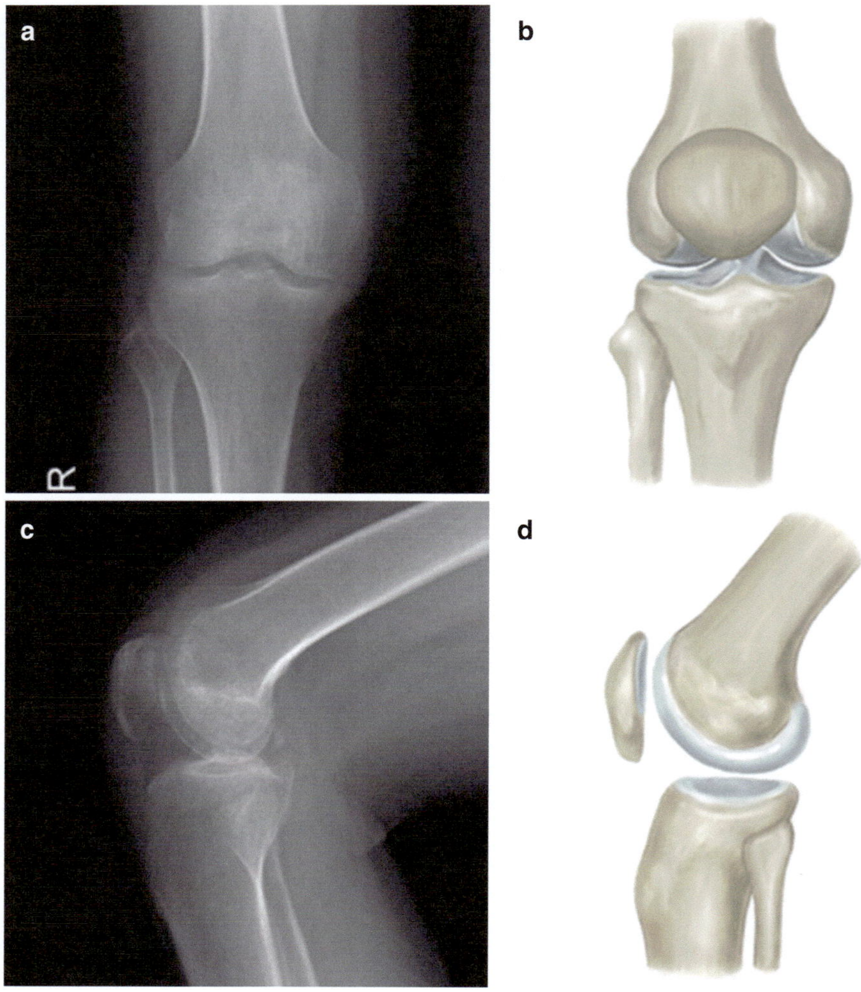

Fig. 9.7 (**a**, **c**) are X-ray positive and lateral position, respectively, showing osteoporosis of the right knee joint, no obvious fracture signs, and schematic diagram (**b**, **d**)

   7.2 CT (Fig. 9.7e, f)

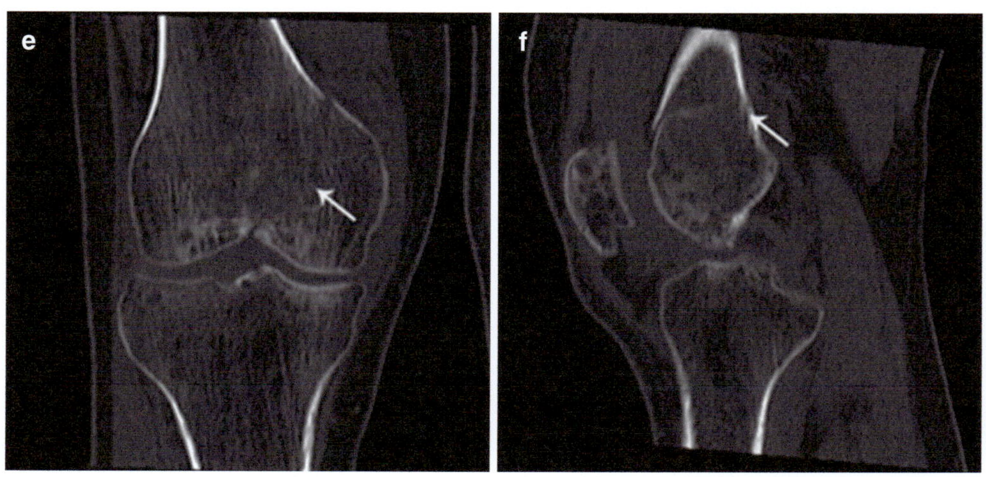

Fig. 9.7 (**e**, **f**) are, respectively, CT coronal reconstruction and sagittal reconstruction, showing intercondylar fracture of the femur (white arrow)

7.3 MRI (Fig. 9.7g–j)

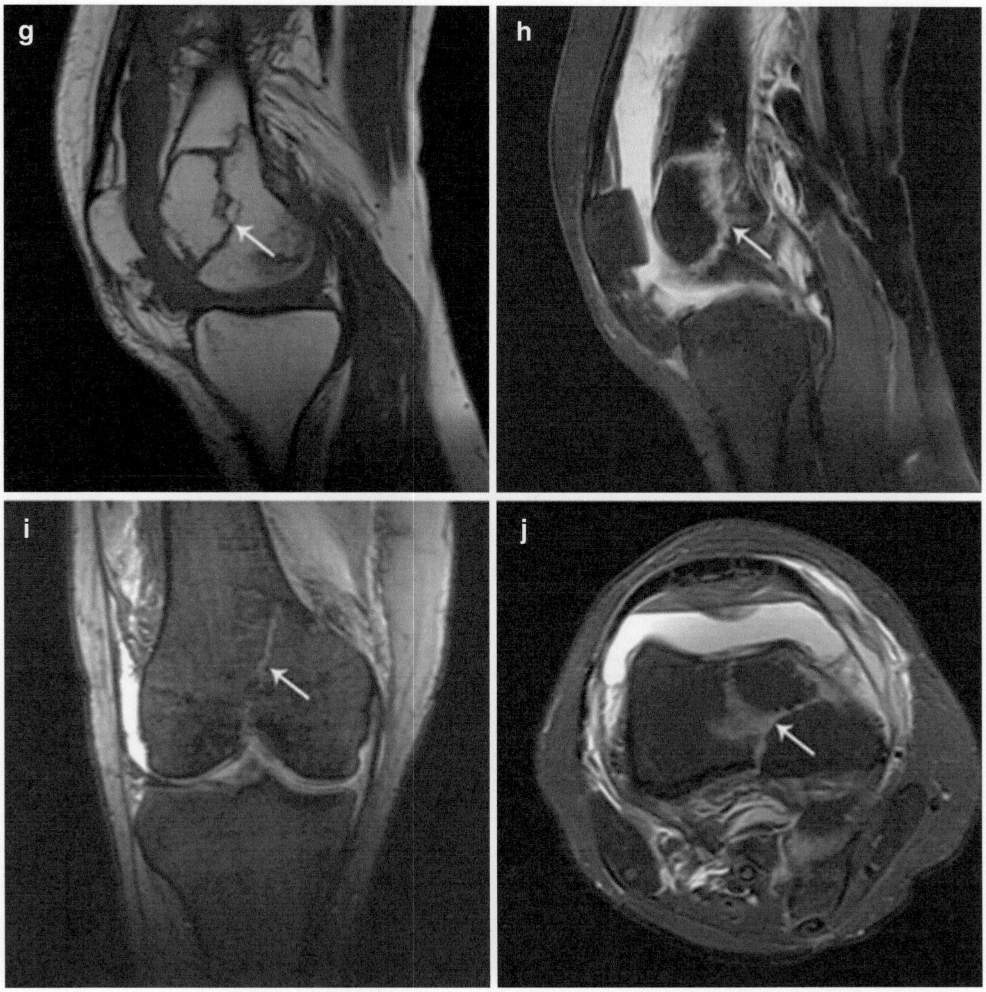

Fig. 9.7 (**g–j**) shows MRI sagittal plane T1WI, fat inhibition T2WI, coronal plane T2WI and horizontal axis plane fat inhibition T2WI, respectively, showing comminuted intercondylar fractures (white arrow), fluid accumulation in the joints and liquid-fluid plane

9.2 Tibiofibular Proximal Fracture

The medial and lateral platforms fractures of the tibia are the most common proximal tibial fractures. According to Schatzker type, the proximal tibial fracture is divided into six types: type I lateral platform pure cleavage fracture, there is no joint surface subsidence; type II lateral platform cleavage fracture with depression; type III lateral or centre platform simply collapse fractures; IV medial platform fractures, often combined ridge between tibial condyle fracture; V type bicondylar cleavage fracture; VI type tibial plateau fractures with epiphyseal end and backbone isolated. Avulsion fracture of tibial intercondylar ridge and posterior margin of tibial plateau is easy to occur.

9.2.1 Injury Mechanism

It is the result of strong axial stress combined with internal and external stress.

9.2.2 Symptoms and Signs

After a fracture, pain, swelling and limited activity in the injured area are present, but this lack of specificity for the symptoms makes it difficult to use as a definite diagnosis. Therefore, when a fracture is suspected, further X-ray or CT scans should be conducted to prevent missed diagnosis.

9.2.3 Imaging Differential Diagnosis

In general, X-rays can be used to diagnose tibial plateau fractures. A CT scan can observe the collapse, defect and bone fragment of a tibial plateau fracture and accurately show the scope of comminuted fracture. MRI can be multi-planar, multi-directional and multi-parameter imaging, showing more sensitive fractures.

1. Type I—Identification of simple cleft palate fractures and non-fractures on the lateral tibia.
   1.1 X-ray (Fig. 9.8a–d)

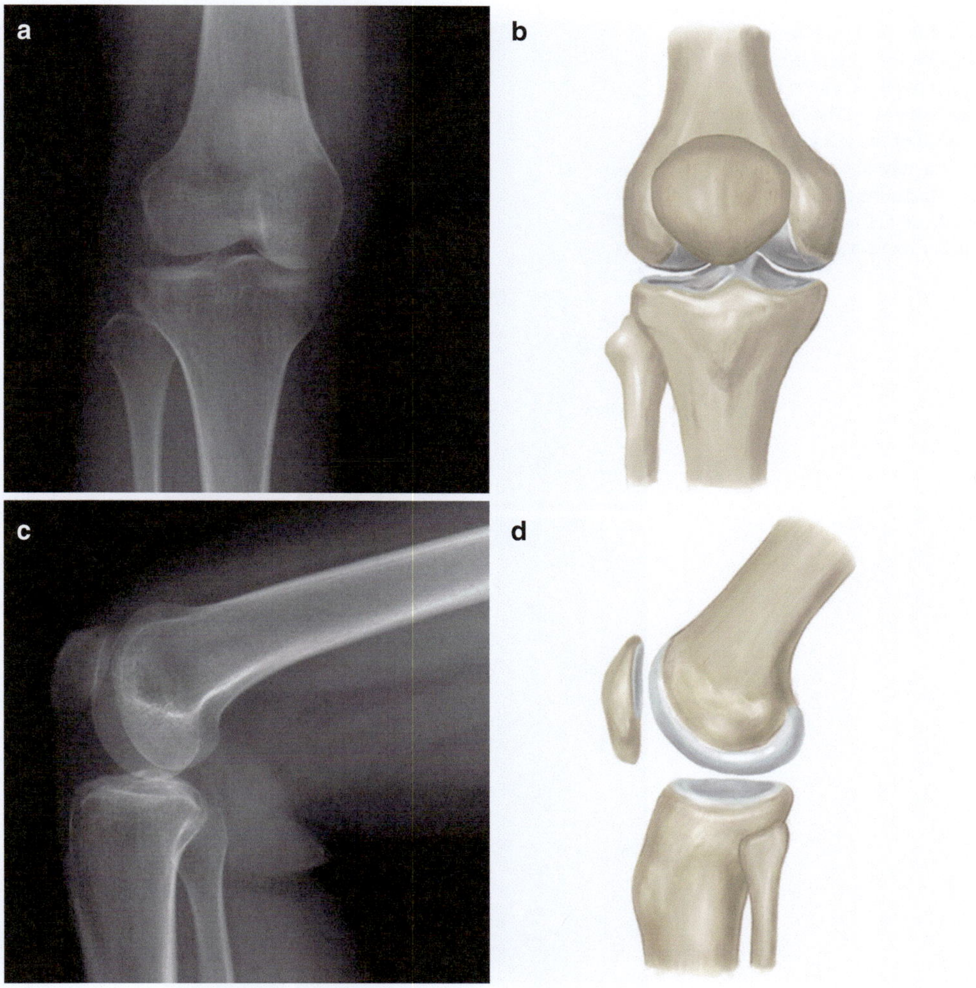

Fig. 9.8 (**a**, **c**) are X-ray positive and lateral positions, respectively, without obvious fractures, and the schematic diagrams are (**b**, **d**)

   1.2 CT (Fig. 9.8e, f)

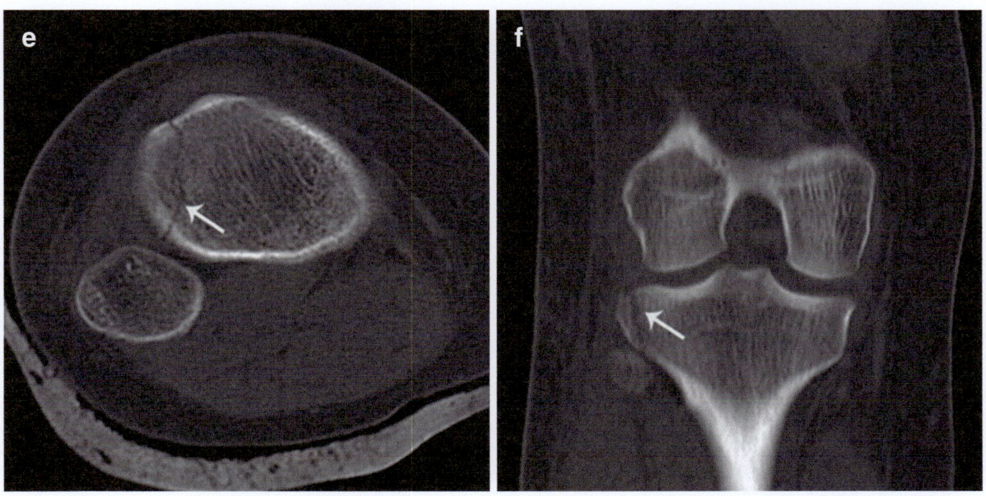

Fig. 9.8 (**e**, **f**) are CT transverse and coronal reconstructions. It shows the longitudinal fracture line (white arrow) of the lateral tibia of the right knee, without dislocation

2. Type II—Identification of collapse and fracture of the lateral tibial platform.
   2.1 X-ray (Fig. 9.9a–d)

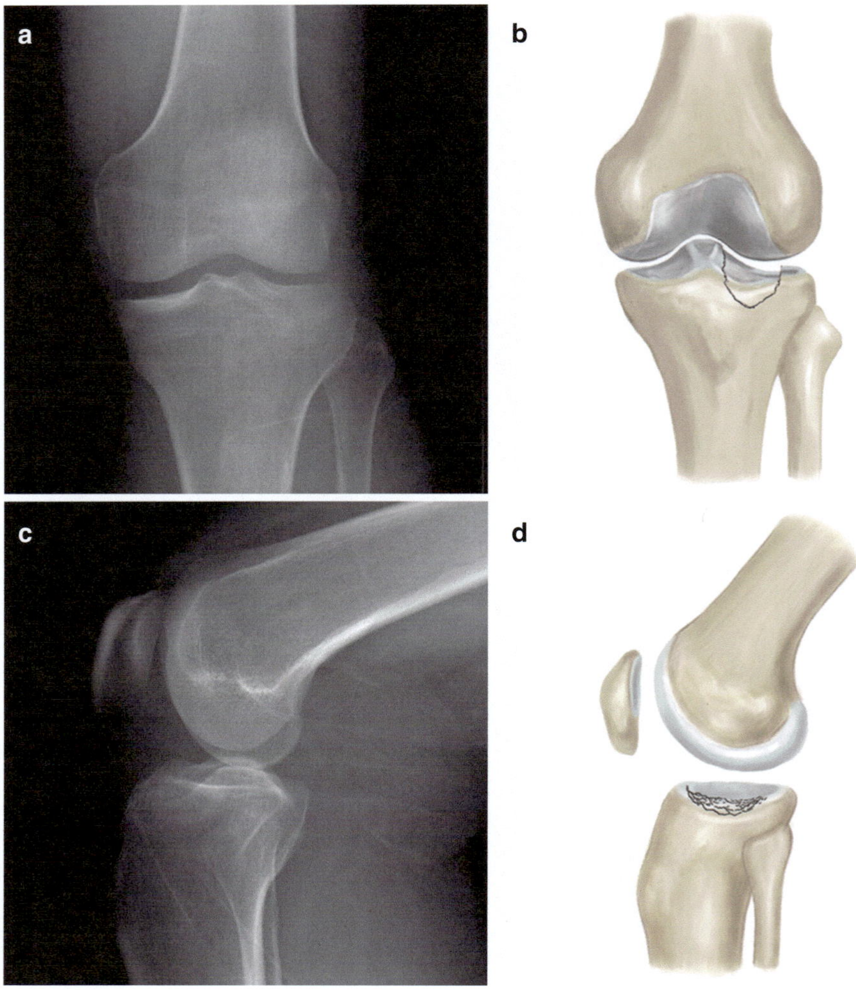

Fig. 9.9 (**a**, **c**) are X-ray positive and lateral position, respectively. It shows fracture and collapse of the lateral plateau of the left knee, and the fracture line was unclear. The diagrams are shown in (**b**, **d**), so CT and MRI were further requested

2.2 CT (Fig. 9.9e–g)

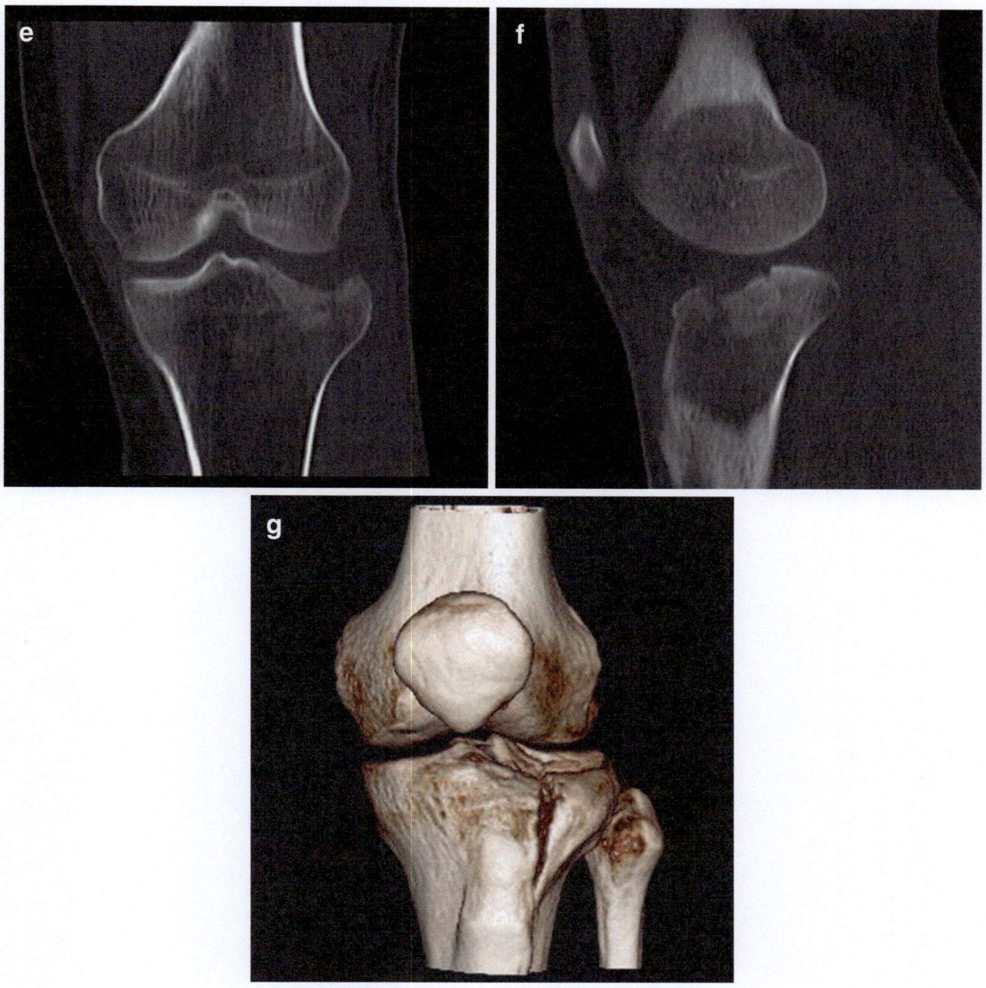

Fig. 9.9 (**e**, **f**, **g**) are CT coronal, sagittal and 3D reconstructions, respectively. It shows a fracture of the lateral tibia, collapse and a fracture of the anterior cleft

2.3 MRI (Fig. 9.9h–j)

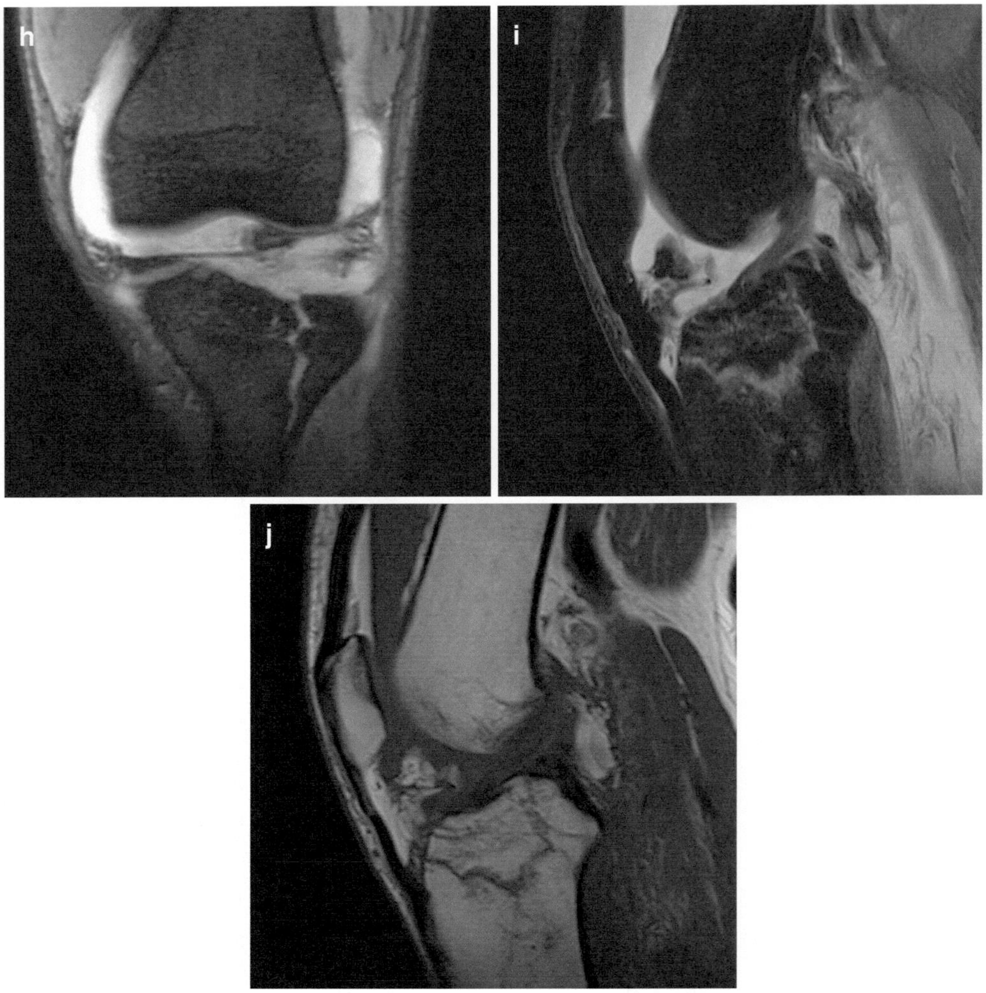

Fig. 9.9 (**h**, **i**, **j**) are MRI coronal T2WI, sagittal fat suppression T2WI and T1WI, respectively. It shows comminuted fracture of the tibial plateau, collapse, anterior cleft palate fracture and intra-articular effusion

3. Type III—lateral collapse of the tibial plateau with simple fracture and no fracture identification.
   3.1 X-ray (Fig. 9.10a–d)

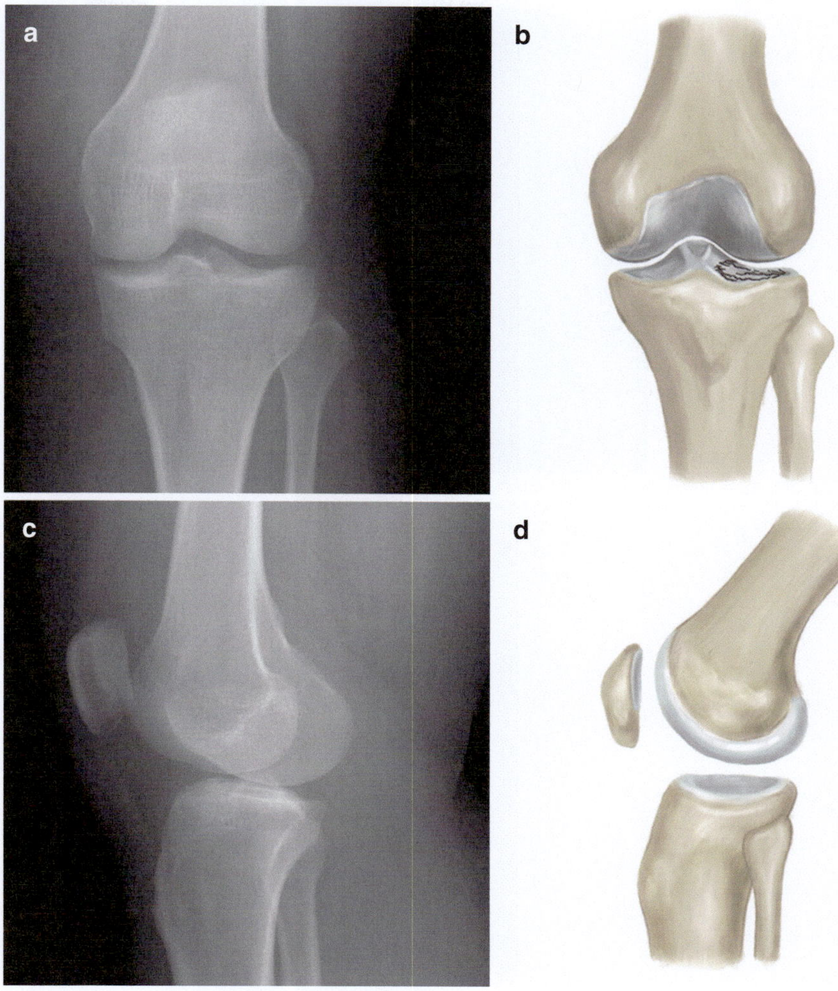

Fig. 9.10 (**a**, **c**) show the X-ray positive and lateral positions, respectively, and the left lateral tibial platform collapses. The fracture line is unclear, so CT is performed, and the diagrams are shown in (**b**, **d**)

   3.2 CT (Fig. 9.10e, f)

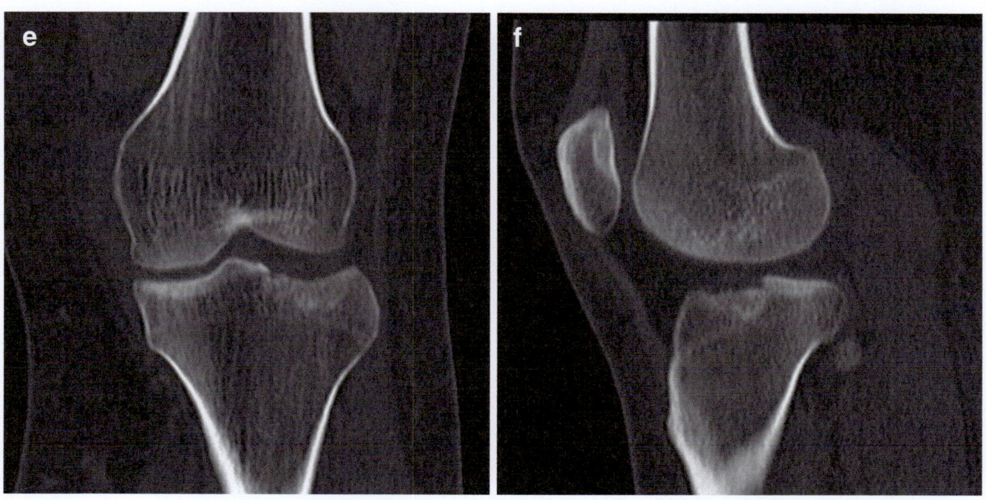

Fig. 9.10 (**e**, **f**) are CT coronal and sagittal reconstructions showing collapse of the lateral tibial plateau

3.3 MRI (Fig. 9.10g, h)

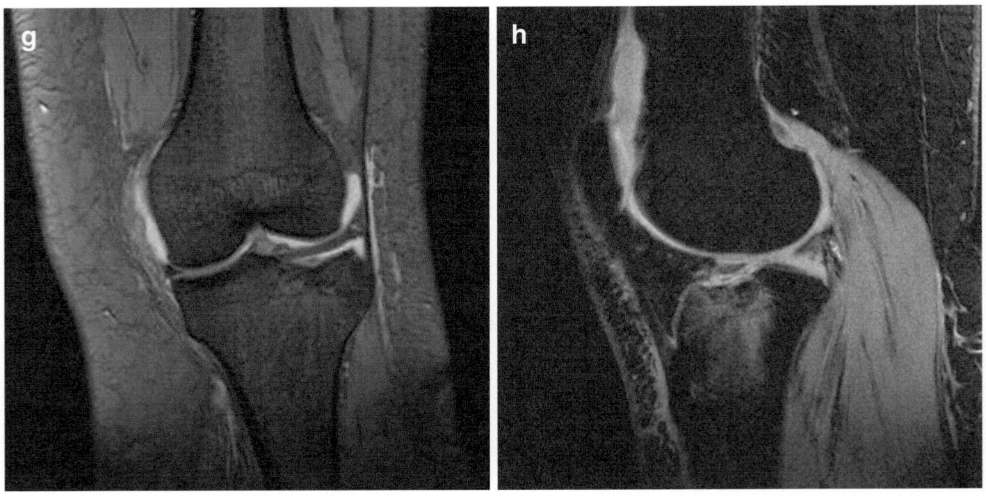

Fig. 9.10 (**g**, **h**) show MRI coronal and sagittal fat suppression T2WI, showing a lateral tibial plateau fracture and an articular surface collapse

4. Type IV—medial platform fracture combined with intercondyle fracture and no fracture identification.
   4.1 X-ray (Fig. 9.11a–d)

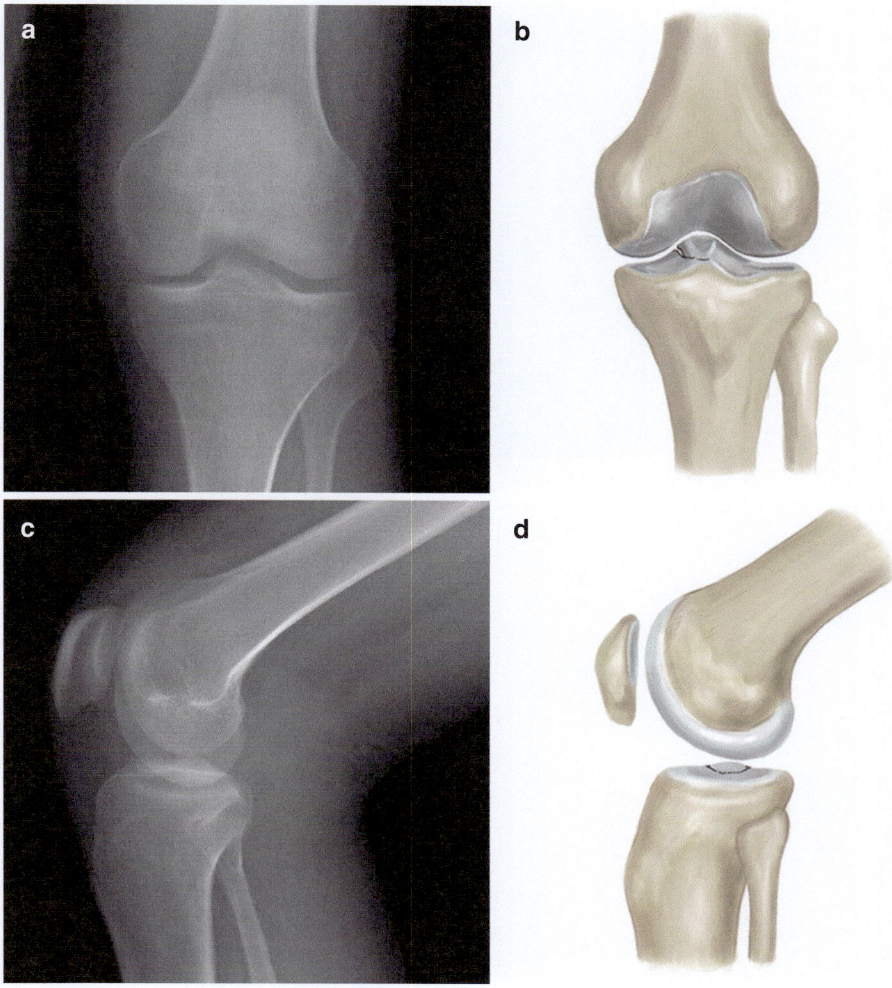

Fig. 9.11 (**a**, **c**) are the X-ray positive and lateral positions, respectively, showing the tibial intercondylar fracture, mild dislocation, and the diagrams are shown in (**b**, **d**)

   4.2 CT (Fig. 9.11e, f)

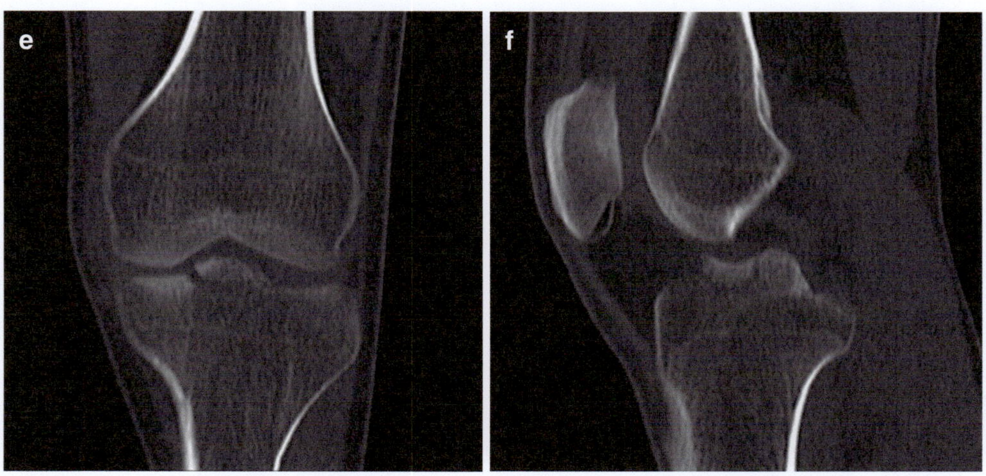

Fig. 9.11 (**e**, **f**) are CT coronal and sagittal reconstructions showing medial tibial plateau fractures with intercondylar fractures

4.3 MRI (Fig. 9.11g, h)

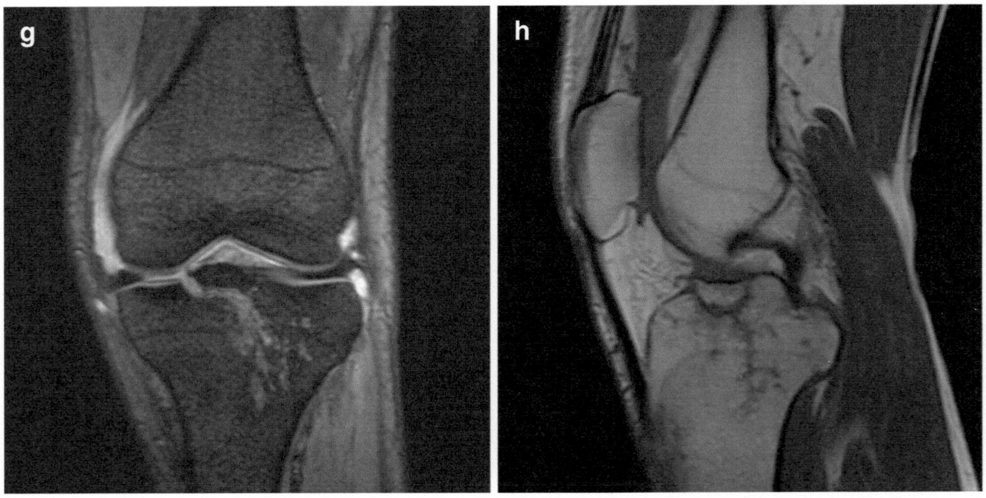

Fig. 9.11 (**g**, **h**) show the MRI coronal plane T2WI and the sagittal plane T1WI, showing the medial tibial plateau and intercondylar fractures

5. Double tibial condyle cleavage fracture
   5.1 X-ray (Fig. 9.12a, b)

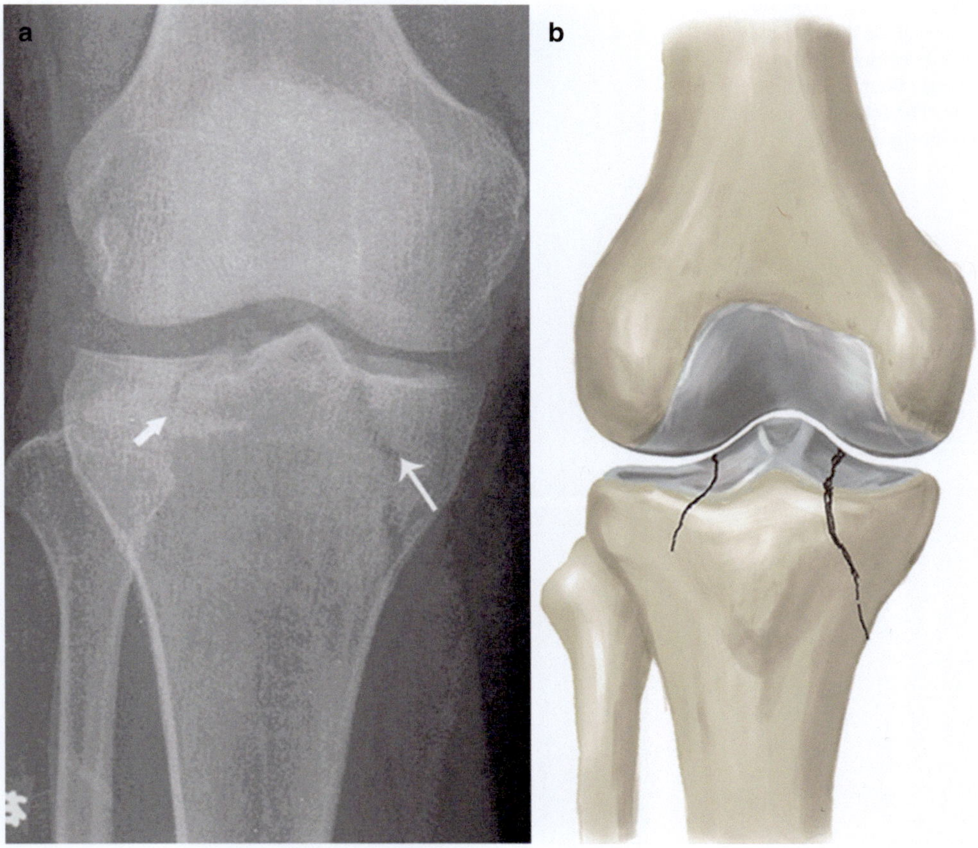

Fig. 9.12 (**a**) X-ray positive position shows the right medial condyle fracture (white arrow) and lateral cleft palate (rough white arrow). The schematic diagram is (**b**)

6. Double tibial condyle cleavage fracture
   6.1 X-ray (Fig. 9.13a–d)

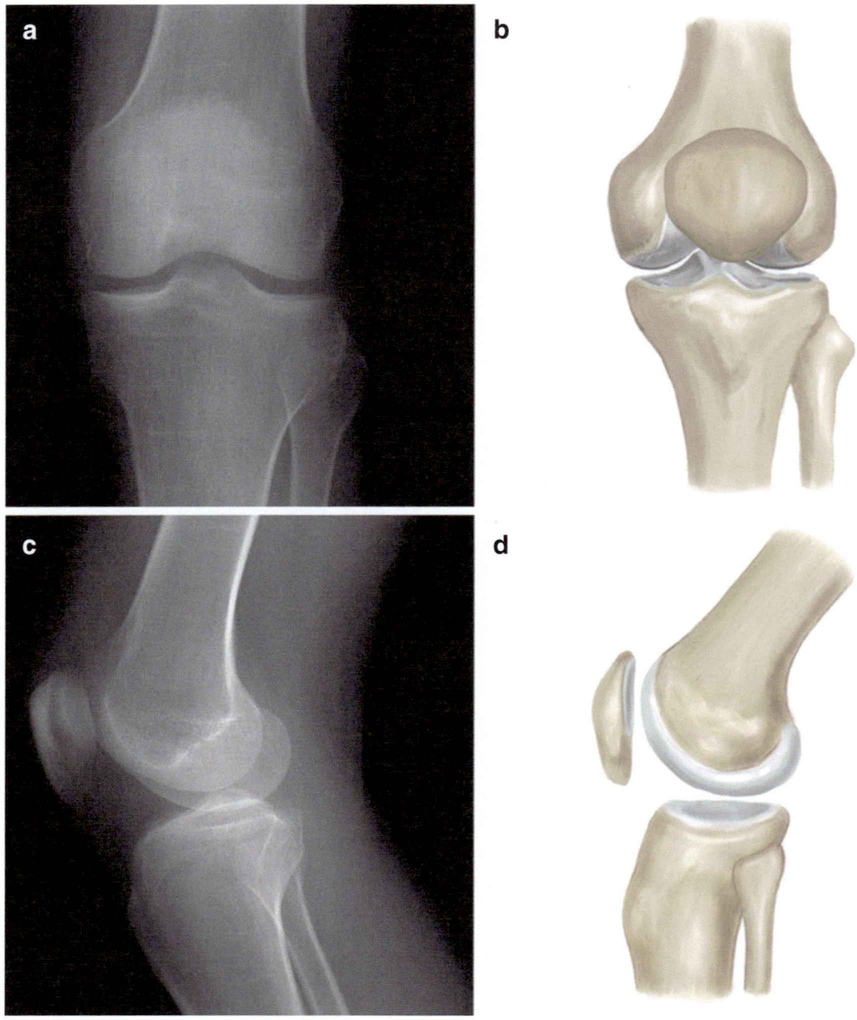

Fig. 9.13 (**a**, **c**) show the X-rays in the positive and lateral positions, and no obvious fracture lines are seen. The schematic diagrams are shown in (**b**, **d**)

6.2 CT (Fig. 9.13e)

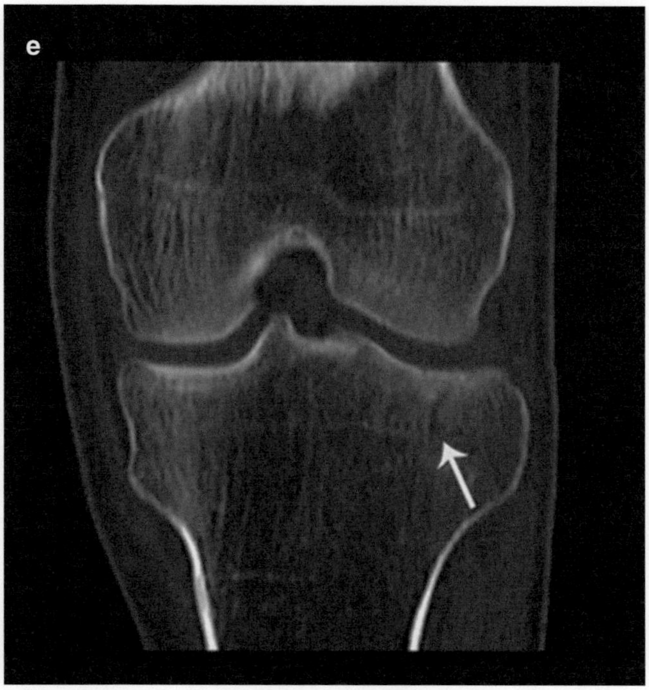

Fig. 9.13 (**e**) is a CT scan of the coronal plane, showing a tibial lateral condyle fracture (white arrow)

6.3 MRI (Fig. 9.13f–h)

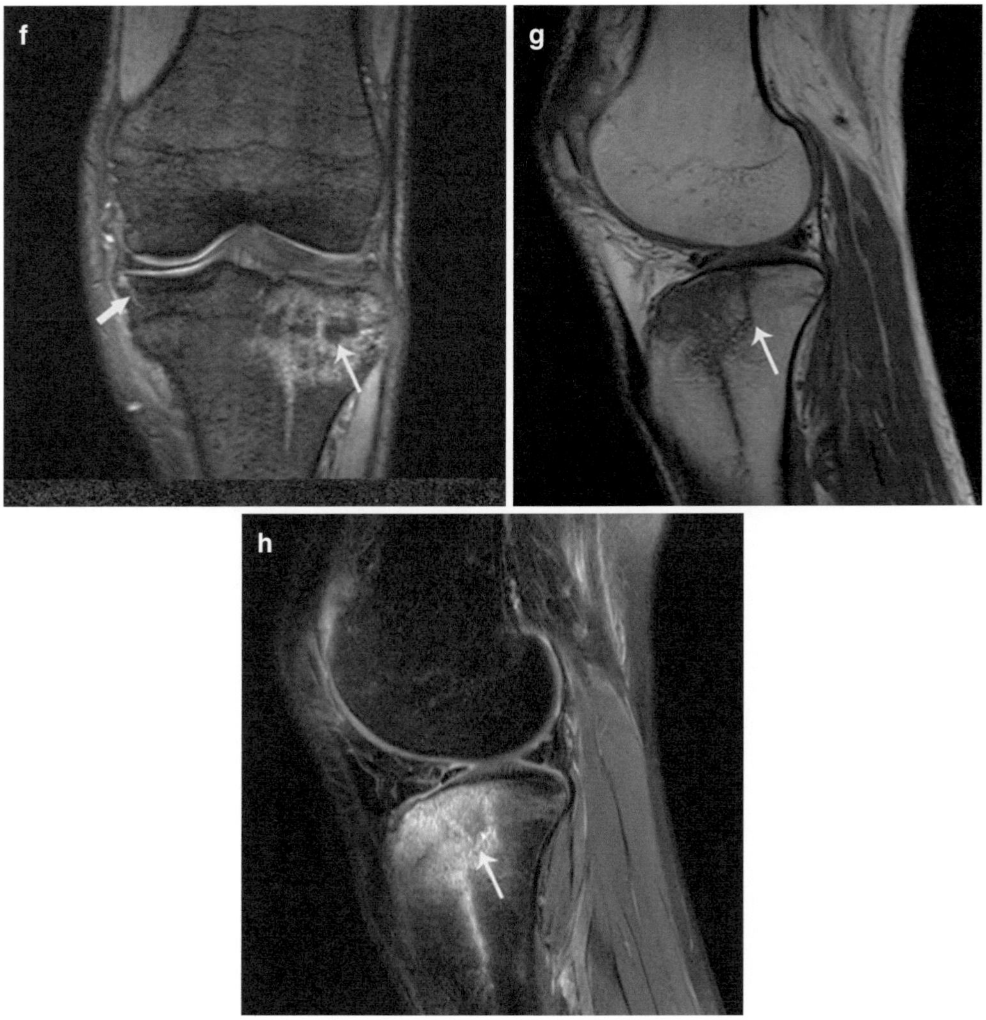

Fig. 9.13 (**f**) T2WI of MRI in coronal plane shows a tibial lateral condyle fracture (white arrow), peripheral edema and a tibial condyle fracture (rough white arrow). (**g**, **h**) are the MRI sagittal planes T1WI and T2WI, respectively, which show tibial lateral condyle fractures (white arrows) and peripheral edema

7. Proximal tibia fracture and obvious fracture identification
   7.1 X-ray (Fig. 9.14a–d)

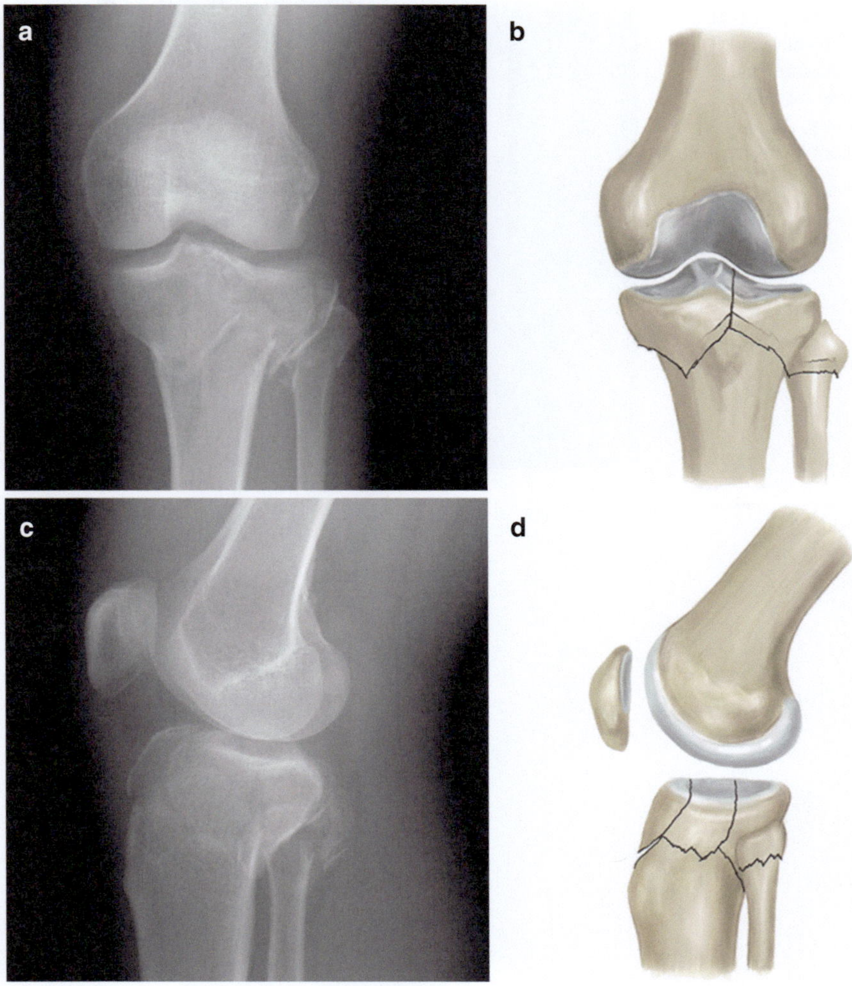

Fig. 9.14 (**a**, **c**) show the X-ray positive and lateral position, respectively, showing the comminuted fracture of the upper end of the tibia. The schematic diagrams are shown in (**b**, **d**)

   7.2 CT (Fig. 9.14e, f)

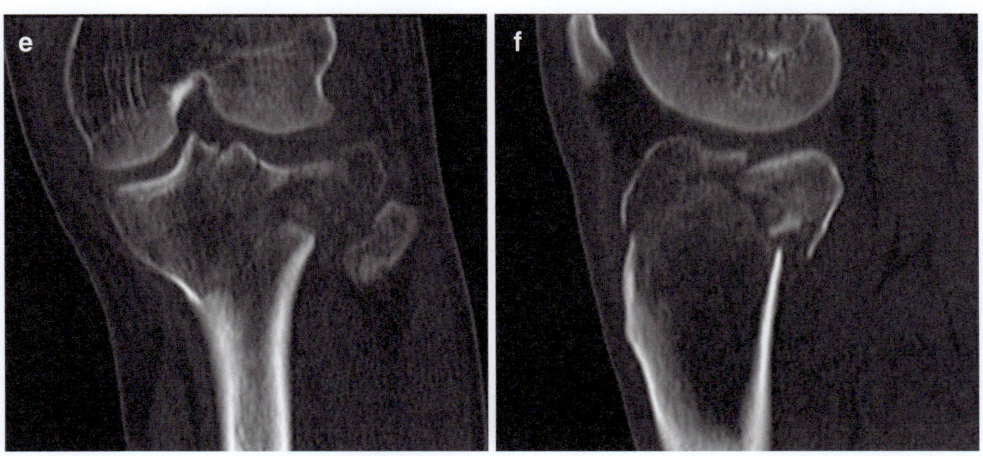

Fig. 9.14 (**e**, **f**) are CT coronal and sagittal reconstructions showing comminuted fractures of the upper tibia and collapse of the lateral tibia

7.3 MRI (Fig. 9.14g, h)

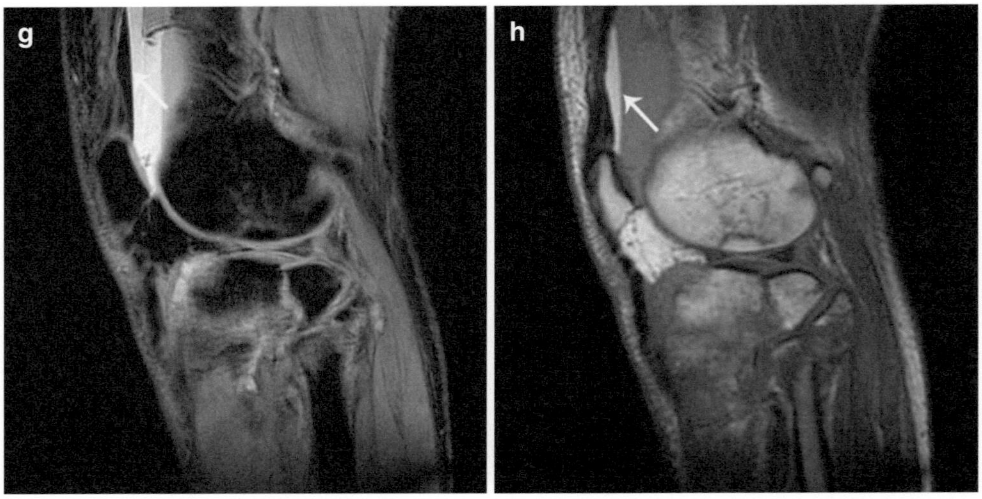

Fig. 9.14 (**e**, **h**) show MRI sagittal fat suppression T2WI and T1WI, which show intra-articular effusion, and can be seen in the fat fluid plane (white arrow), as well as the distal femoral fracture

8. Intercondylar spine tibial fractures
   8.1 X-ray (Fig. 9.15a–d)

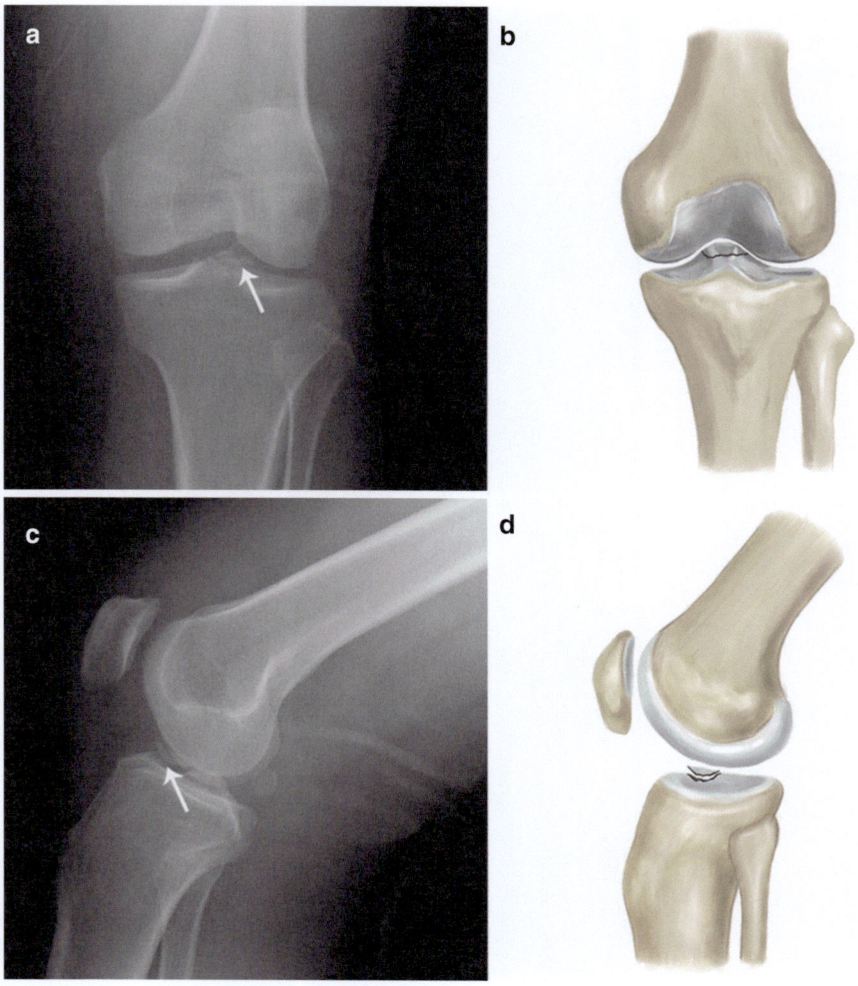

Fig. 9.15 (**a**, **c**) are X-ray positive lateral slices showing an intercondylar spine tibial fracture (white arrow), a schematic of which is shown in (**b**, **d**)

   8.2 CT (Fig. 9.15e, f)

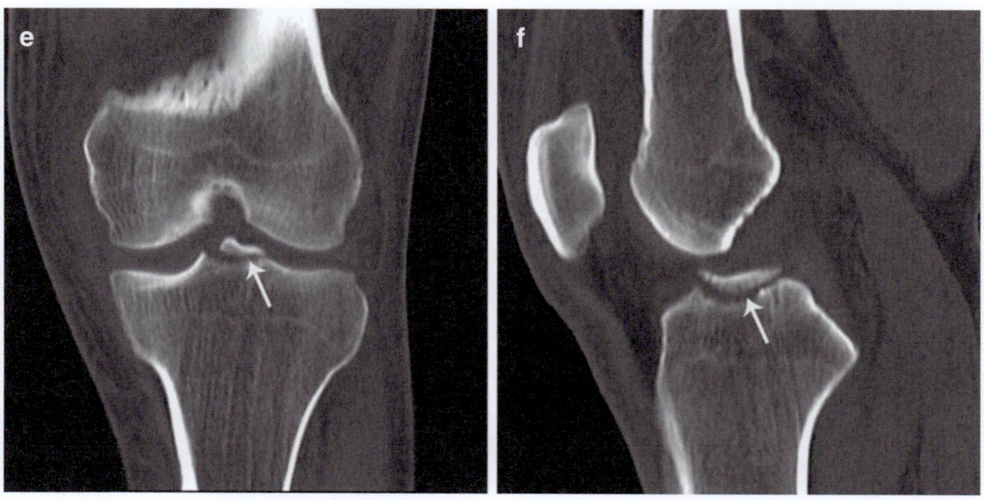

Fig. 9.15 (**e**, **f**) are CT coronal and sagittal reconstructions showing an intercondylar spine tibial fracture and a dislocation (white arrow)

9. The avulsion fracture of the posterior margin of the tibial plateau was identified.
   9.1 X-ray (Fig. 9.16a–d)

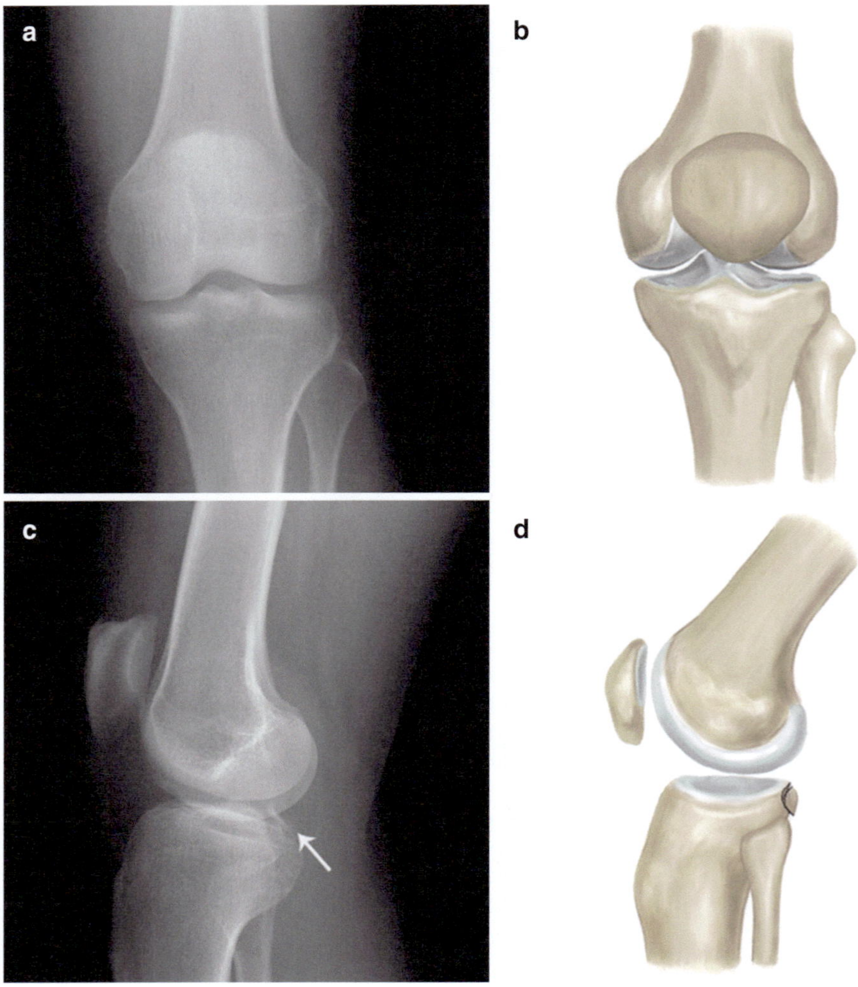

Fig. 9.16 (**a**) is an X-ray positive position, no obvious fracture line is seen, and its schematic view is (**b**). (**c**) is an X-ray lateral slice showing the posterior margin fracture of the tibial plateau (white arrow), the schematic of which is (**d**)

   9.2 CT (Fig. 9.16e, f)

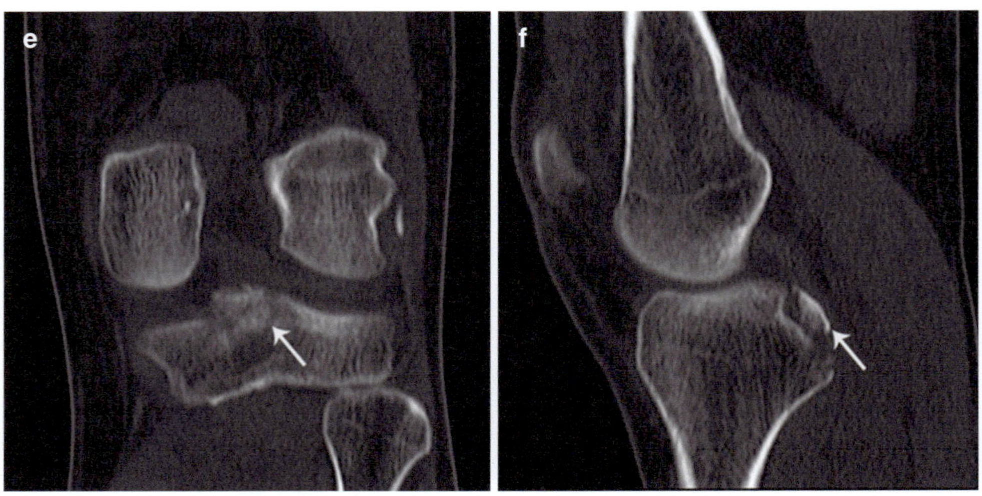

Fig. 9.16 (**e**, **f**) are CT coronal and sagittal reconstructions that clearly show avulsion fractures (white arrows) at the posterior border of the tibial plateau

9.3 MRI (Fig. 9.16g, h)

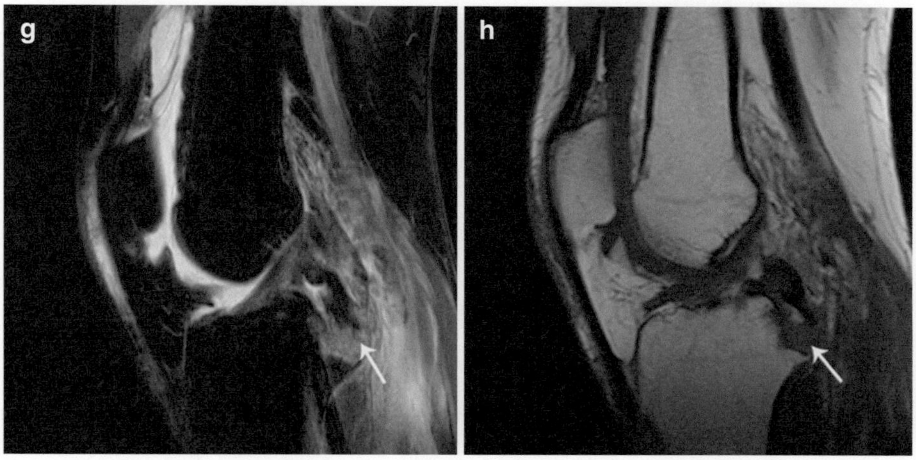

Fig. 9.16 (**g**, **h**) show MRI sagittal fat suppression T2WI and T1WI, which shows avulsion fractures of the posterior cruciate ligament attachment of the posterior tibial plateau and posterior cruciate ligament rupture (white arrow)

9.3 Patellar Fractures

9.3.1 Injury Mechanism

It is caused by direct trauma to the front of the knee or indirect force on the quadriceps tendon.

9.3.2 Symptoms and Signs

After the fracture, it appears pain in the injured area, and the knee is weak and cannot be stretched. If the fracture with a large displacement can touch the fracture gap, a diagnosis can be confirmed. If there is a suspected fracture, a further X-ray or CT scan should be taken to prevent missed diagnosis.

9.3.3 Imaging Differential Diagnosis

Simple longitudinal and transverse patellar fractures cannot be found on the X-ray posteroanterior or lateral position, whilst a CT scan can show the fracture line. CT 3D reconstruction images can clearly show multiple fracture lines and identify comminuted fractures. Avulsion fractures can also be seen clearly on CT. It should be differentiated from the bipartite patella and multi-division patella. The bipartite patella or multi-division patella is a normal variation. The distal part of the fibular fissure can be seen in the cortical bone. MRI shows no edema.

1. The longitudinal comminuted fracture of the patella was identified by displacement and no displacement.
   1.1 X-ray (Fig. 9.17a–d)

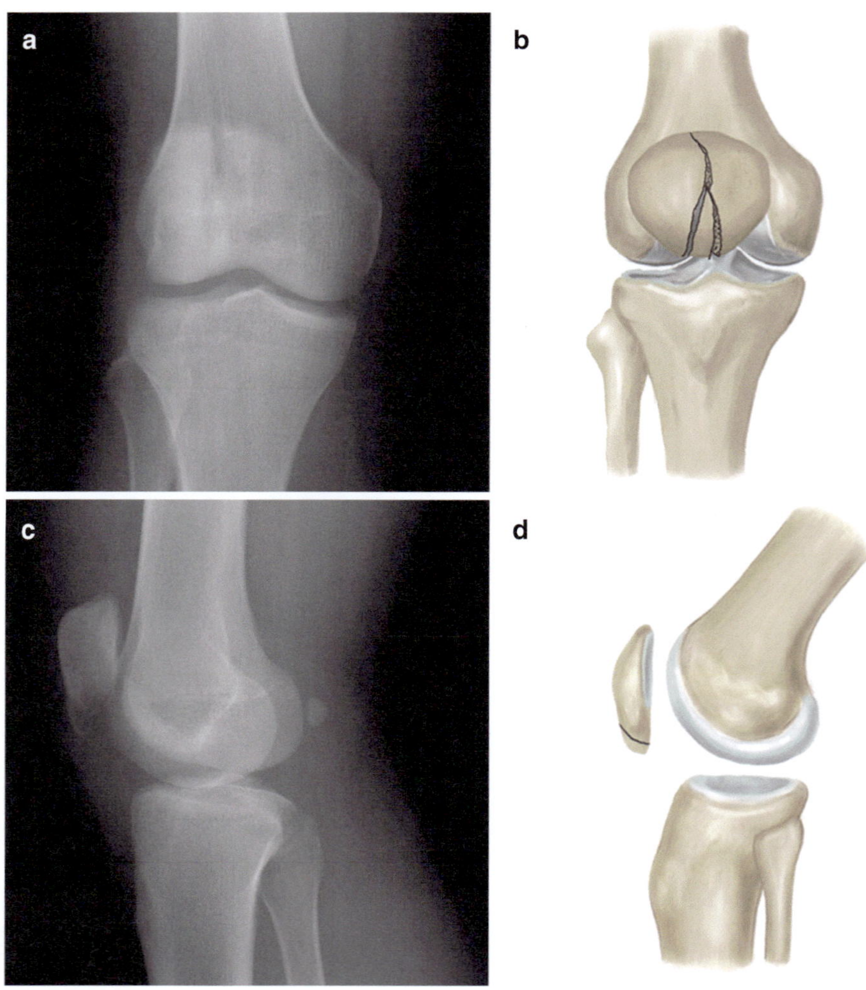

Fig. 9.17 (**a**) is an X-ray anterior piece, which can be seen as a longitudinal fracture line of the patella (**b**). (**c**) shows the X-ray lateral position, and the fracture line is not obvious. Therefore, CT is performed, and the schematic diagram is (**d**)

1.2 CT (Fig. 9.17e–h)

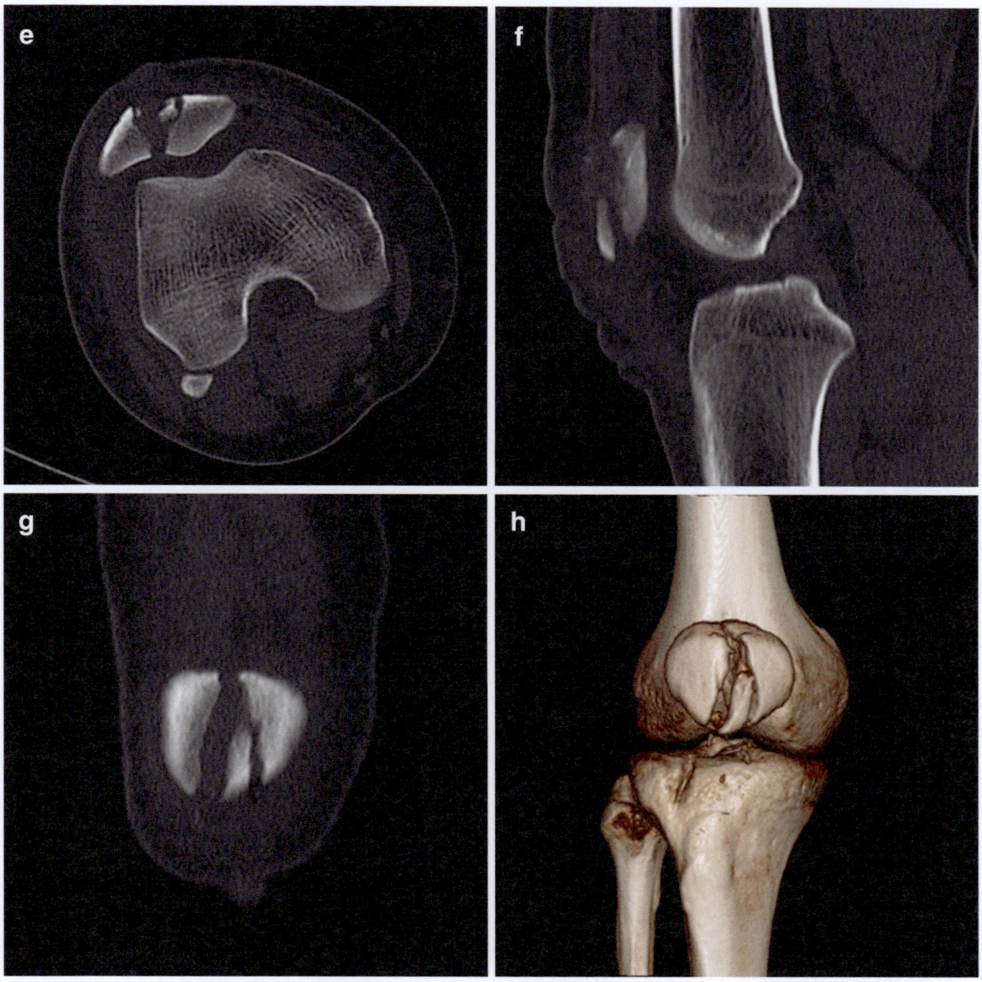

Fig. 9.17 (**e**–**h**) are CT transverse axis, sagittal reconstruction, coronal reconstruction and three-dimensional reconstruction. It shows a longitudinal comminuted fracture of the patella of the right knee, displacement, joint effusion and swelling of surrounding soft tissue

2. The patella transverse fracture was identified without displacement and displacement.
   2.1 X-ray (Fig. 9.18a–d)

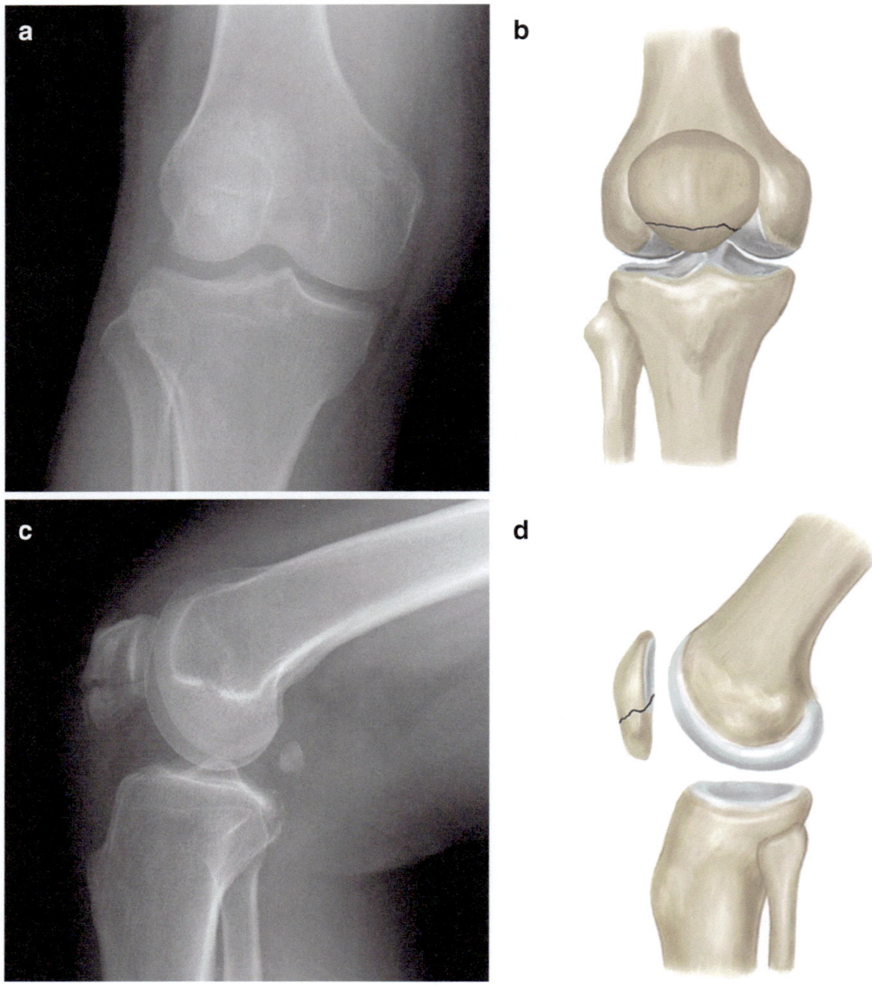

Fig. 9.18 (**a**) is an X-ray positive position, the fracture line is not obvious, and its schematic view is (**b**). (**c**) is a X lateral position showing a transverse patella fracture, the schematic of which is (**d**)

2.2 CT (Fig. 9.18e–h)

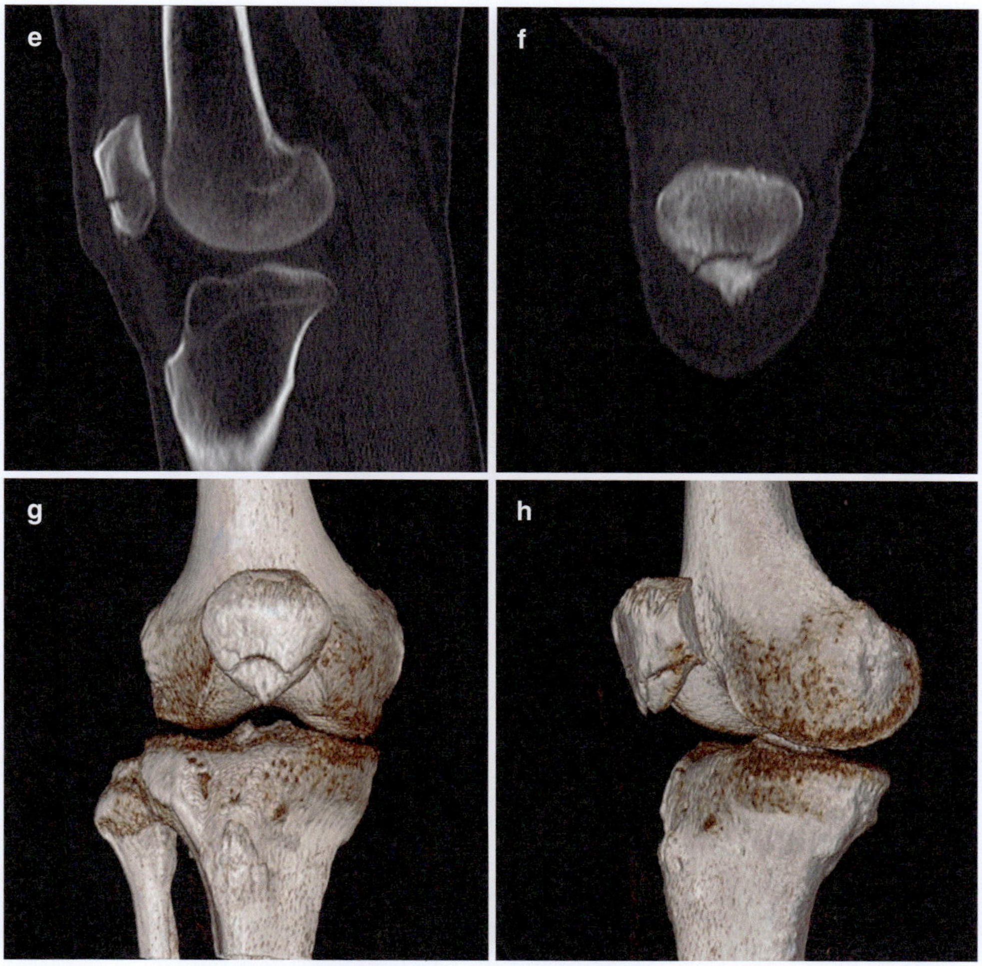

Fig. 9.18 (**e**–**h**) are CT sagittal reconstruction, coronal reconstruction, three-dimensional reconstruction of the anterior and lateral view, which show transverse fractures of the right patella and no displacement

3. Distal patella fracture displacement and no displacement identification.
   3.1 X-ray (Fig. 9.19a–d)

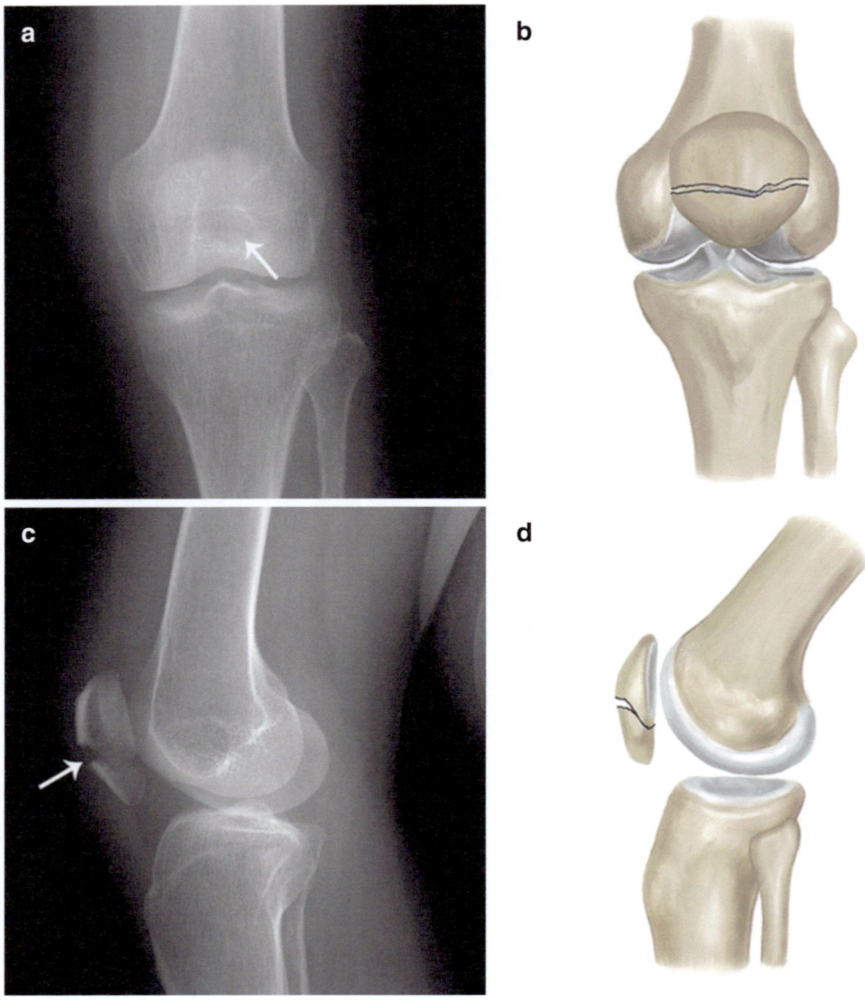

Fig. 9.19 (**a**) is an X-ray anteroposterior, the patella fracture line is faintly visible, and its schematic view is (**b**). (**c**) is an X-ray lateral slice, a transverse patella fracture line (white arrow), and its schematic view is (**d**)

3.2 CT (Fig. 9.19e–h)

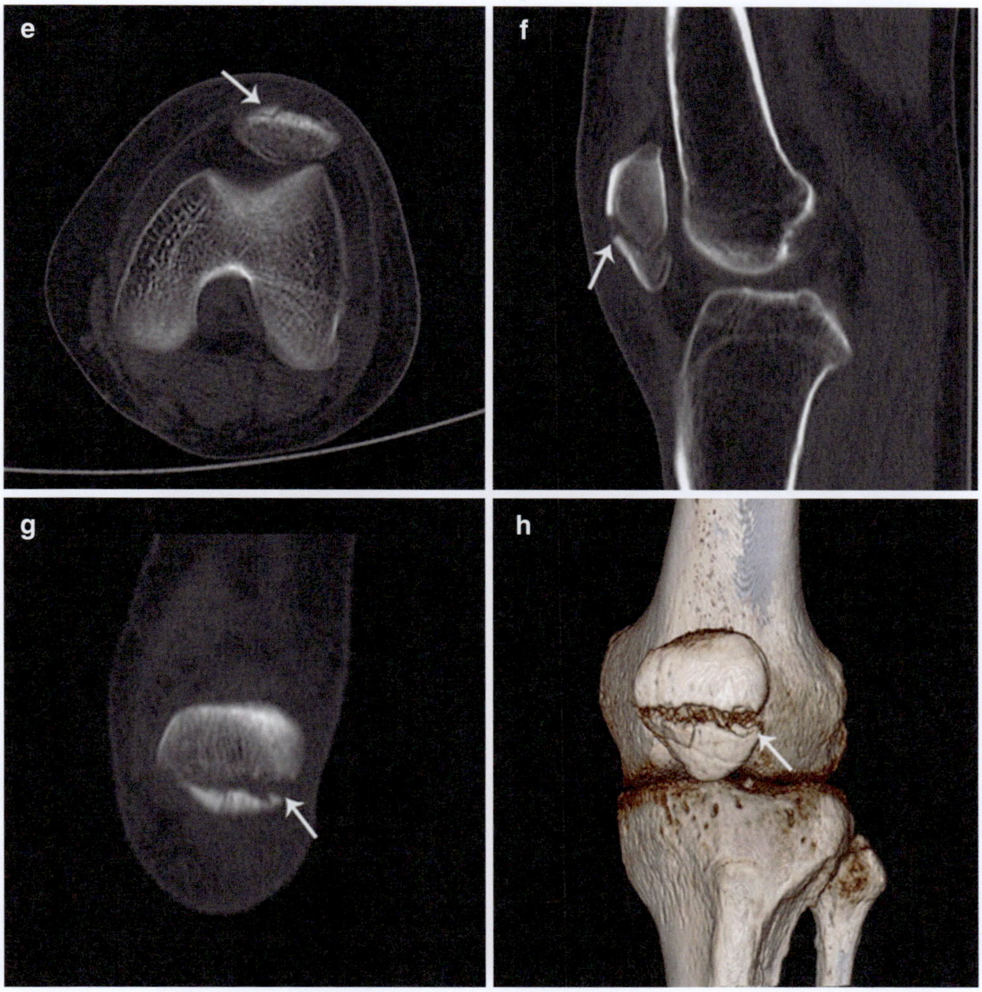

Fig. 9.19 (**e–h**) are CT transverse axis, sagittal reconstruction, coronal reconstruction and 3D reconstruction. They show transverse bone fracture and displacement (white arrow) in the middle of the left patella

4. Identification of comminuted fractures of the patella and without fractures.
   4.1 X-ray (Fig. 9.20a–d)

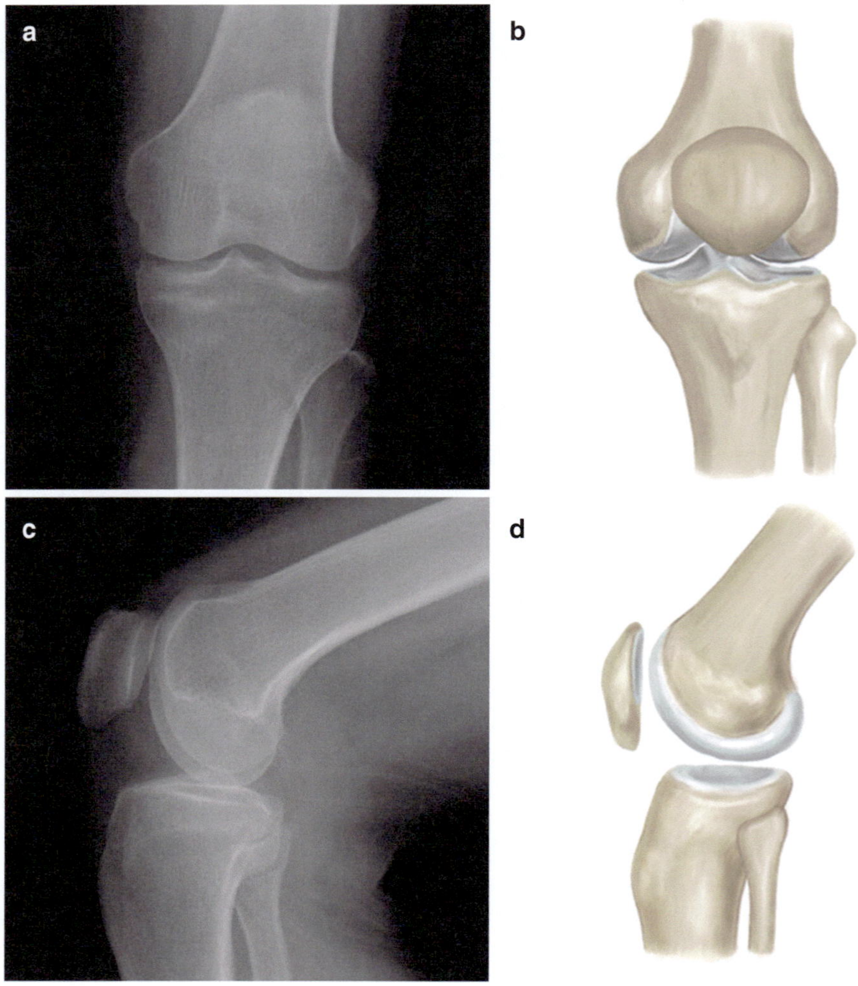

Fig. 9.20 (**a**, **c**) are X-ray positive and lateral positions, respectively, and the patellar fracture line is not obvious. In order to confirm the diagnosis, CT examination is performed, and the schematic diagrams are shown in (**b**, **d**)

4.2 CT (Fig. 9.20e–h)

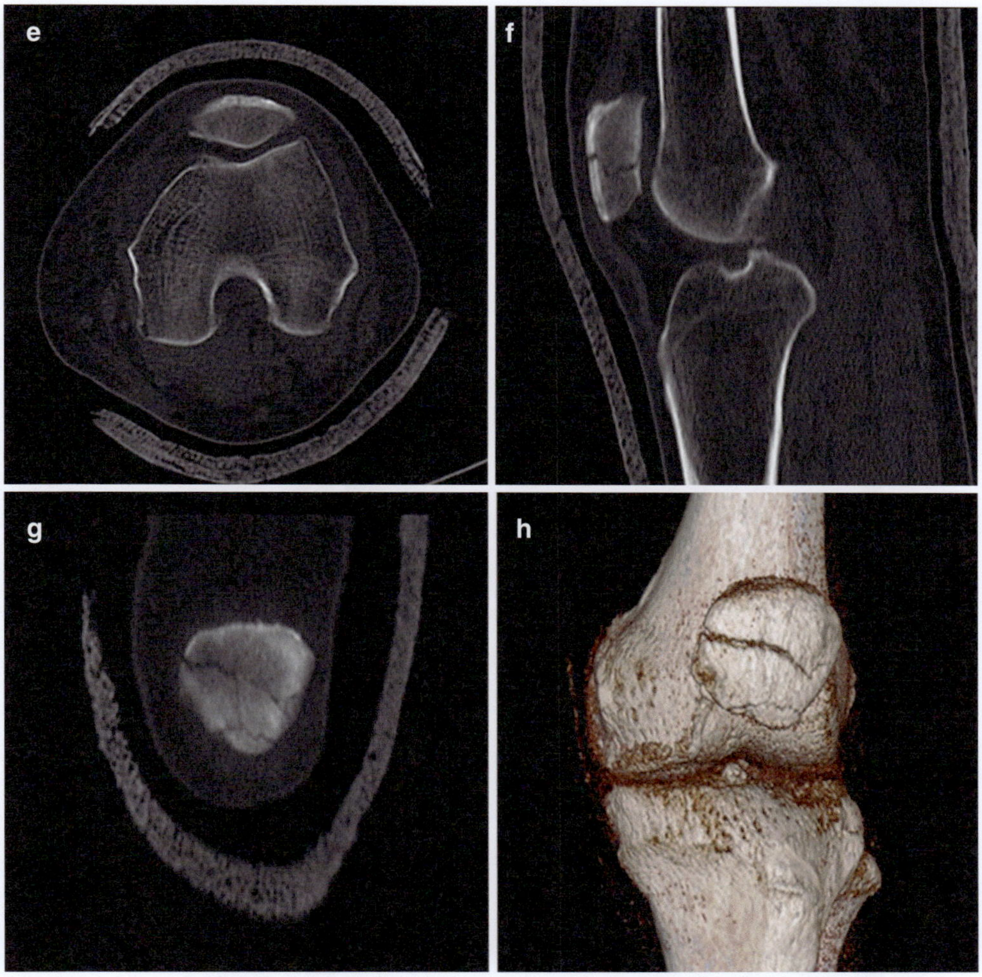

Fig. 9.20 (**e**–**h**) are CT transverse axis, sagittal reconstruction, coronal reconstruction and three-dimensional reconstruction. It shows comminuted fracture of the middle and lower end of the left patella without displacement. It can be seen that the plaster is fixed externally

5. Distal patellar fracture displacement and no displacement identification.
   5.1 CT (Fig. 9.21a–d)

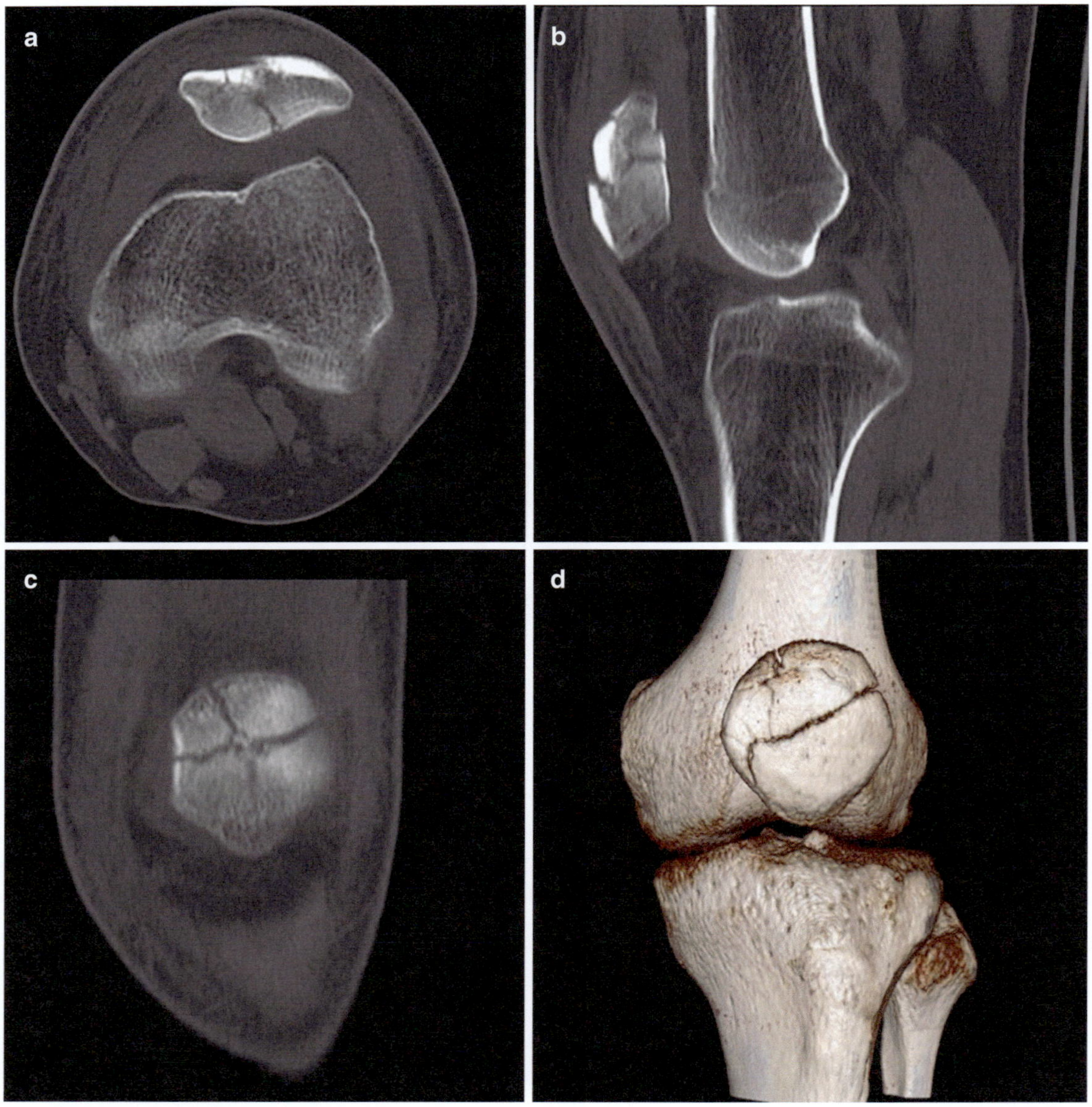

Fig. 9.21 (**a**–**d**) are CT transverse axis, sagittal reconstruction, coronal reconstruction and three-dimensional reconstruction. It shows a comminuted fracture of the middle and upper bones of the left patella, with displacement, and associated with effusion

6. Distal displacement and mild displacement of comminuted fractures of the patella.
   6.1 CT (Fig. 9.22a–d)

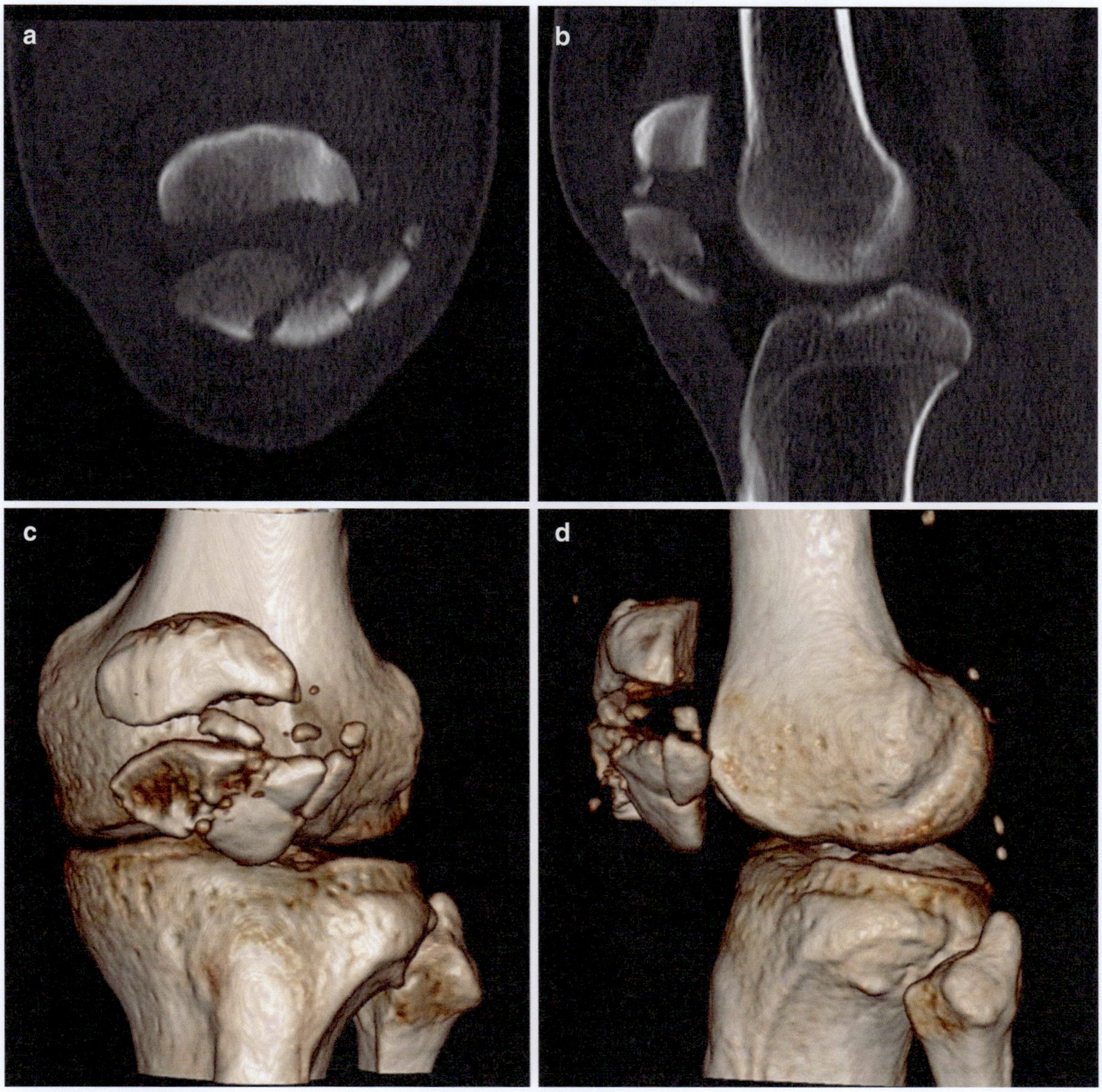

Fig. 9.22 (**a**–**d**) are CT coronal reconstruction, sagittal reconstruction and 3D reconstruction of anterior and lateral view, respectively. It shows a comminuted fracture of the left patella with a significant displacement

7. Identification of avulsion fractures of the patella and no fractures.
   7.1 X-ray (Fig. 9.23a–d)

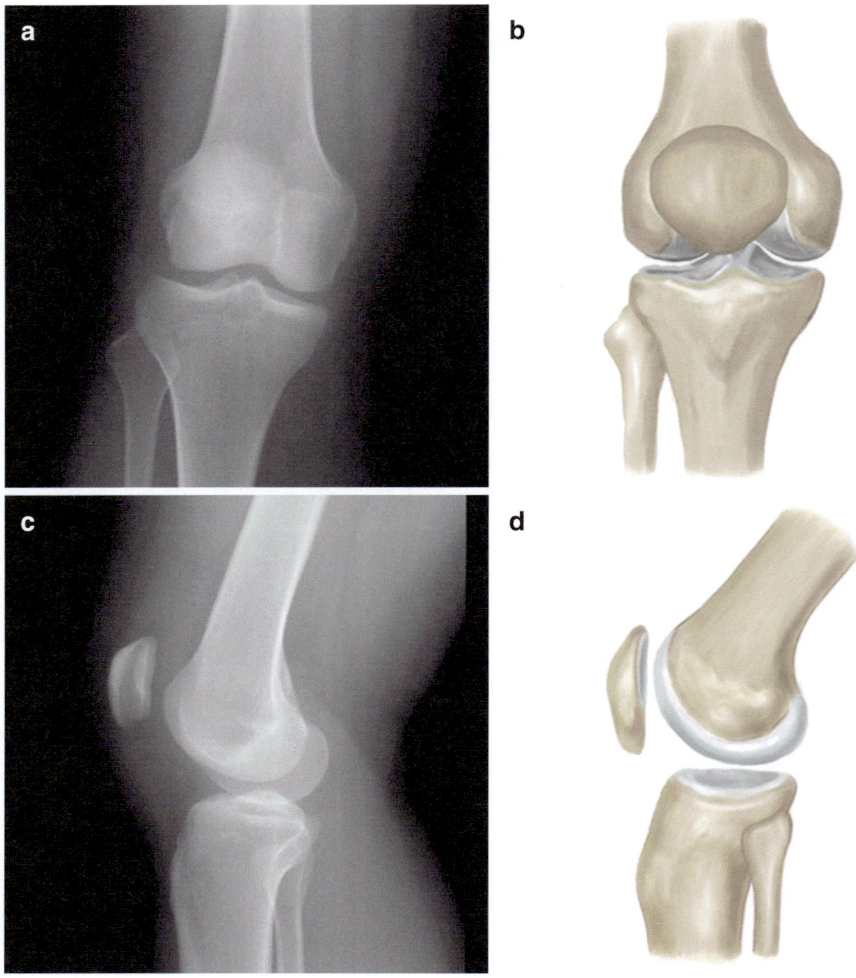

Fig. 9.23 (**a**, **c**) are X-ray positive and lateral position, respectively. The fracture line is not obvious, and a large amount of effusion is visible in the joint. In order to confirm the diagnosis, CT examination is performed, and the diagrams are shown in (**b**, **d**)

7.2 CT (Fig. 9.23e–h)

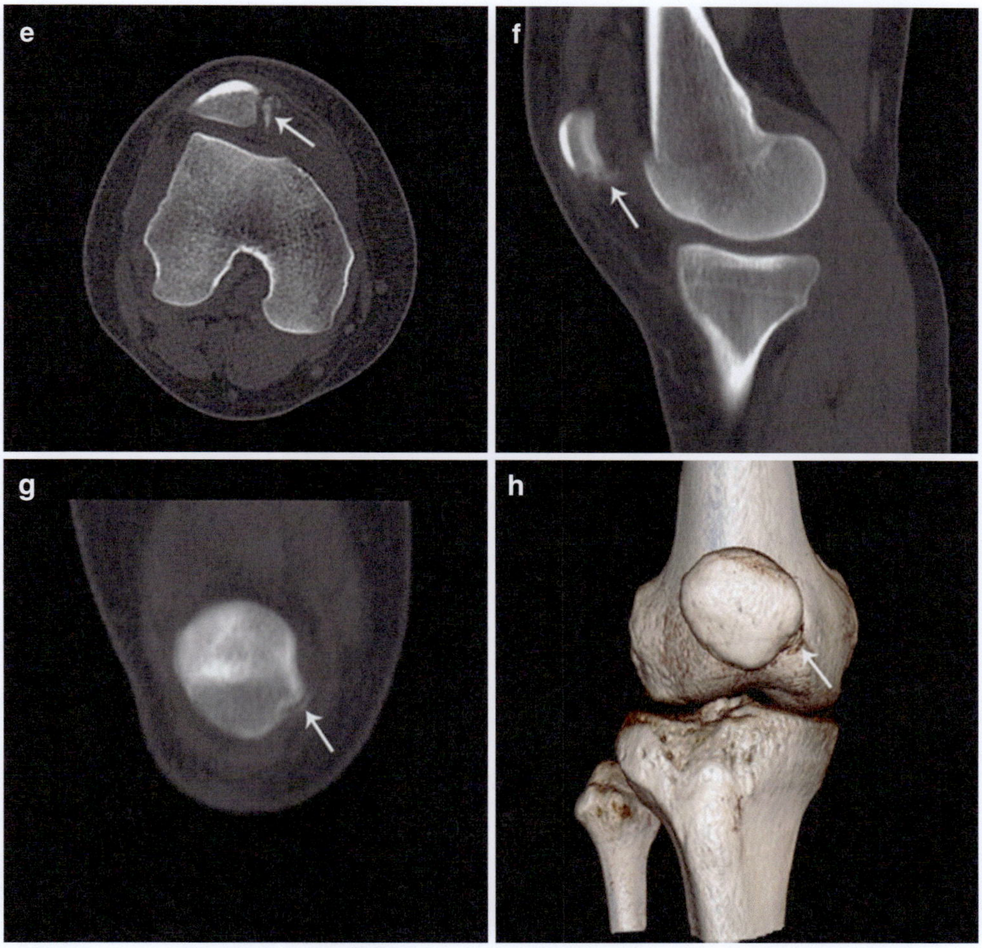

Fig. 9.23 (**e–h**) are CT transverse axis, sagittal reconstruction, coronal reconstruction and three-dimensional reconstruction. It shows avulsion fracture of the lower edge of the patella, mild displacement (white arrow) and joint effusion

8. The patellar comminuted avulsion fracture displacement and non-displacement identification.
   8.1 CT (Fig. 9.24a–d)

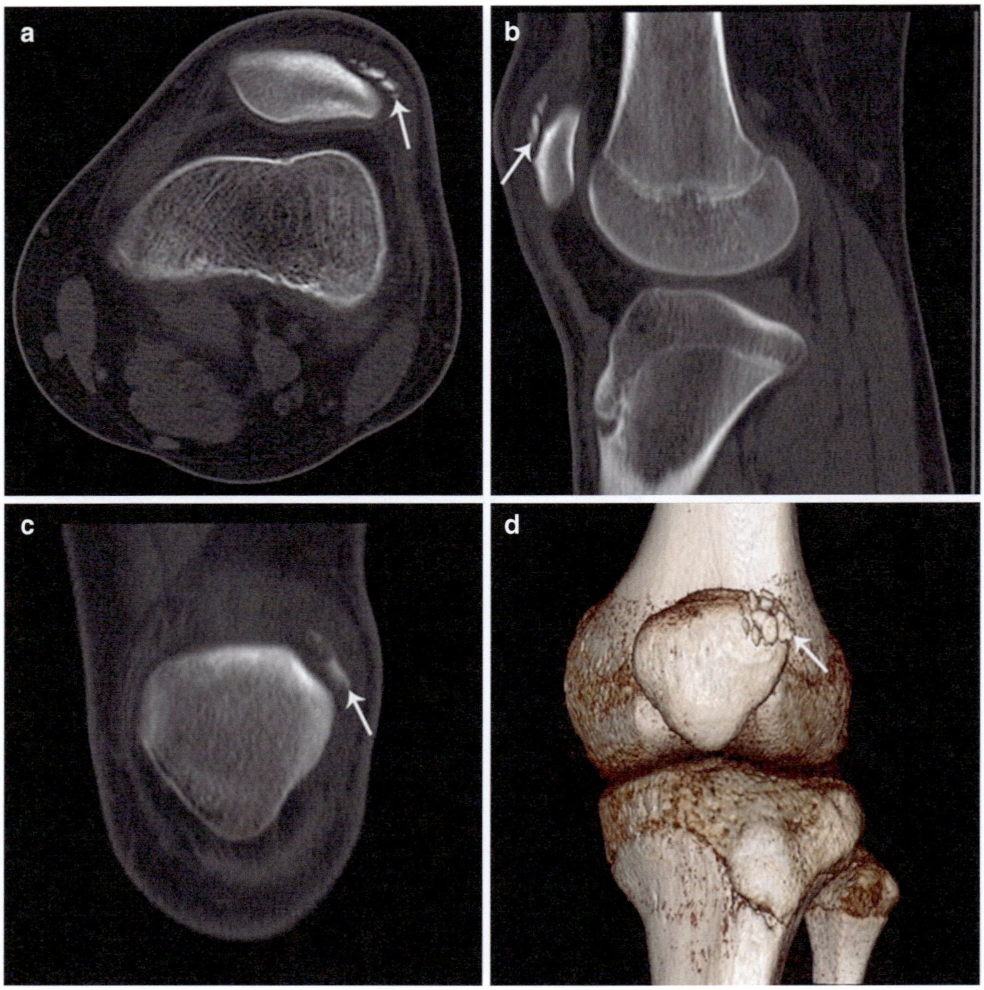

Fig. 9.24 (**a**–**d**) are CT transverse axis, sagittal reconstruction, coronal reconstruction and 3D reconstruction. It shows avulsion fracture of the superior patella, multiple fractures and displacement (fine white arrow)

   8.2 MRI (Fig. 9.24e, f)

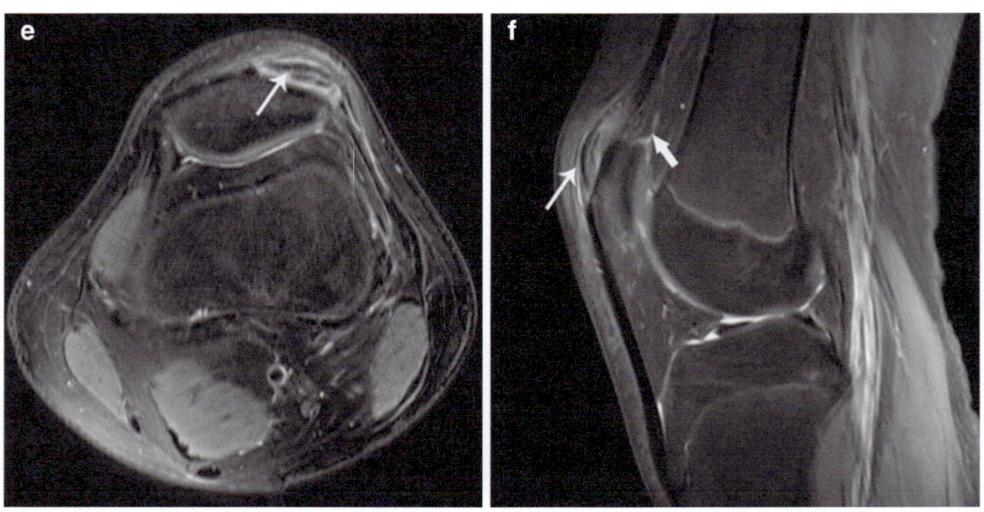

Fig. 9.24 (**e**, **f**) are MRI transverse axis and sagittal fat suppression T2WI, respectively. It shows avulsion fracture of the superior patella (white arrow), quadriceps injury (rough white arrow)

9. Identification of the bipartite and multiple fracture.
   9.1 X-ray (Fig. 9.25a–d)

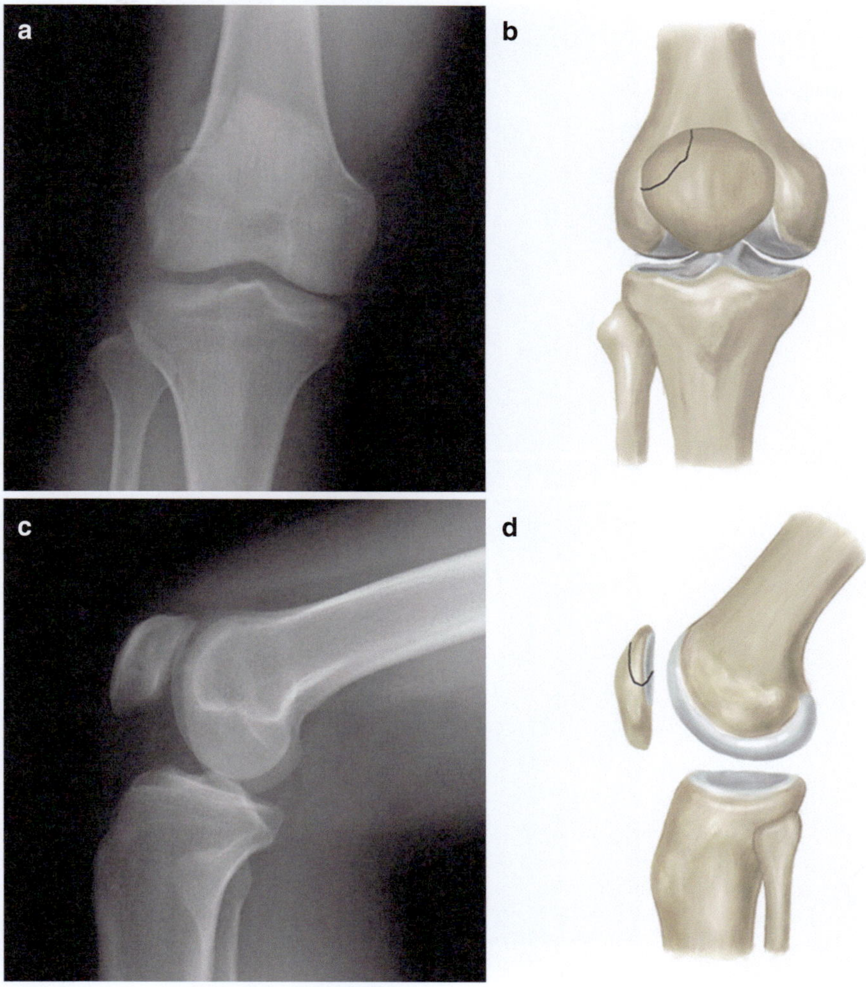

Fig. 9.25 (**a**) is an X-ray anterior piece. The outer edge of the patella is visible like a linear or radiolucent shadow. The schematic view is (**b**). (**c**) is the X-ray lateral position. No obvious linear or radiolucent is seen. Therefore, CT is further examined. The schematic diagram is (**d**)

9.2 CT (Fig. 9.25e–h)

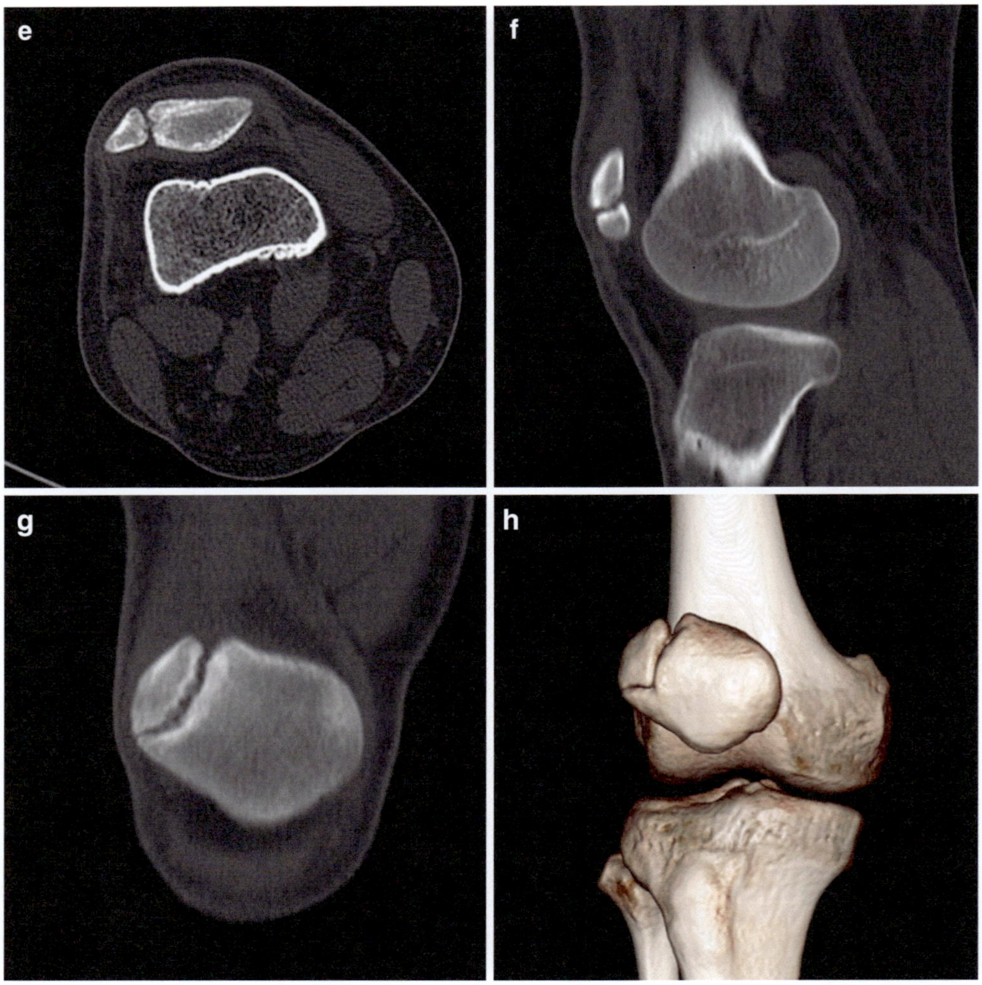

Fig. 9.25 (**e**–**h**) are CT transverse axis, sagittal reconstruction, coronal reconstruction and 3D reconstruction images. It shows that the right patella is divided into two parts, the edges are smooth, and the cortical bone is visible

9.4 Summary of Key Points

1. Fractures and dislocations around the knee can be conventionally diagnosed by a plain film. A CT can clearly show subtle fractures and non-displaced fractures. It can also evaluate the collapse and defect of the articular surface and accurately locate the location and extent of bone fragments. MRI is mainly used to show the degree of damage to soft tissues, tendons, ligaments and meniscus around the knee joint.
2. Non-displaced patellar fractures should be differentiated from bipartite patella and multi-division patella. The bipartite patella or multi-division patella is a normal variation. Identification points: the latter sacral fissure is blunt, visible cortical bone, MRI showed no edema.

Malleolar Fractures

10

Bo Wang and Yingze Zhang

10.1 Malleolar Fractures

The ankle joint consists of the tibia, the distal fibula and the talus. The medial malleolus is the medial of the distal tibia, the lateral malleolus is the distal fibula, whereas the posterior malleolus is the posterior border of the distal tibia which is labial. The lateral malleolus is longer than the medial malleolus, and the posterior malleolus is smaller than both of them. The lateral and medial malleolus form the ankle mortise together, and the ankle joint space presents an inverted U shape. The joint of the tibiofibular syndesmosis is formed by the fibular notch on the lateral side of the distal tibia, and the distal part of the fibula. Malleolar fractures can be divided into single malleolar fracture, bi-malleolar fractures, tri-malleolar fractures, compound fractures and special type fracture determined by its location. The incidence of single ankle fracture is the highest, which is common in the lateral malleolus. The bi-malleolar fracture is the simultaneous fracture of both medial and lateral ankles. The tri-malleolar fracture is the simultaneous fracture of the medial, lateral and posterior malleolus. Compound fracture is comminuted fractures of the distal tibia and distal fibula. Common special types of fractures are: Dupuytren fracture, which refers to the simultaneous avulsion fracture of the medial malleolus, the rupture of the distal tibiofibular ligament, the separation of the distal tibiofibular syndesmosis, the fracture of the distal fibula, lower 1/3 spiral fracture of the tibia which often combines with a posterior malleolus fracture and finally a Tillaux fracture which is the avulsion fracture of the anterior tubercle of distal tibia caused by traction of distal tibiofibular syndesmosis, etc.

10.1.1 Identification of Injury Mechanism

Ankle fractures are usually caused by indirect violence. The isolated fractures of the lateral malleolus are caused by indirect violence when the ankle is sprained. The isolated fractures of the medial malleolus are mostly caused by valgus injury, and a few cases are varus injury. Posterior malleolar fractures, often seen with the lower 1/3 spiral fractures of the tibia, are often caused by external rotation. The bi-malleolar fractures are mainly caused by indirect violence such as external rotation, varus and valgus. The tri-malleolar fractures are usually caused by severe rotation forces.

10.1.2 Identification of Symptoms and Signs

The most obvious manifestations are pain, swelling, limited ankle activity; however, these clinical features lack specificity, and therefore cannot be used for diagnosis. If the fracture displacement is obvious, the malleolus can have obvious deformity which is helpful to diagnosis, but the fracture cannot be ruled out when there are no specific manifestations such as malformation. Therefore, the patients with a history of ankle sprain often need to take X-ray to exclude fracture.

B. Wang · Y. Zhang (✉)
Department of Orthopaedics, The Third Hospital of Hebei Medical University, Shijiazhuang, Hebei, China

Y. Zhang (ed.), *Differential Diagnosis of Fracture*, https://doi.org/10.1007/978-981-13-8339-7_10

10.1.3 Imaging Differential Diagnosis

For malleolar fractures, a routine X-ray of the ankle joint contributes to an accurate diagnosis. A CT scan is mainly used for patients with obvious clinical symptoms, whilst X-ray shows no fracture. An MRI scan can effectively diagnose the tendon and soft tissue injury around the ankle joint, especially an epiphyseal injury and ligament injury in children. The accessory bone of the ankle should be carefully identified on the X-ray film. The common accessory bones include the sub-tibial bone, sub-fibular bone and the triangular accessory bone. The shape is mostly round, with a smooth edge and complete bone cortex, all characteristics that should be identified with the fracture. Posterior malleolar fractures caused by the spiral tibial fractures are often unclear on the X-ray film due to an overlap of the radiographic position in the anteroposterior lateral view. The CT reconstruction image or an MRI can detect posterior malleolar fractures that cannot be revealed by an X-ray.

10.1.3.1 The Single Malleolar Fractures

1. Identification of lateral malleolar fractures without displacement and non-fracture
   1.1. The X-ray (Fig. 10.1a–d)

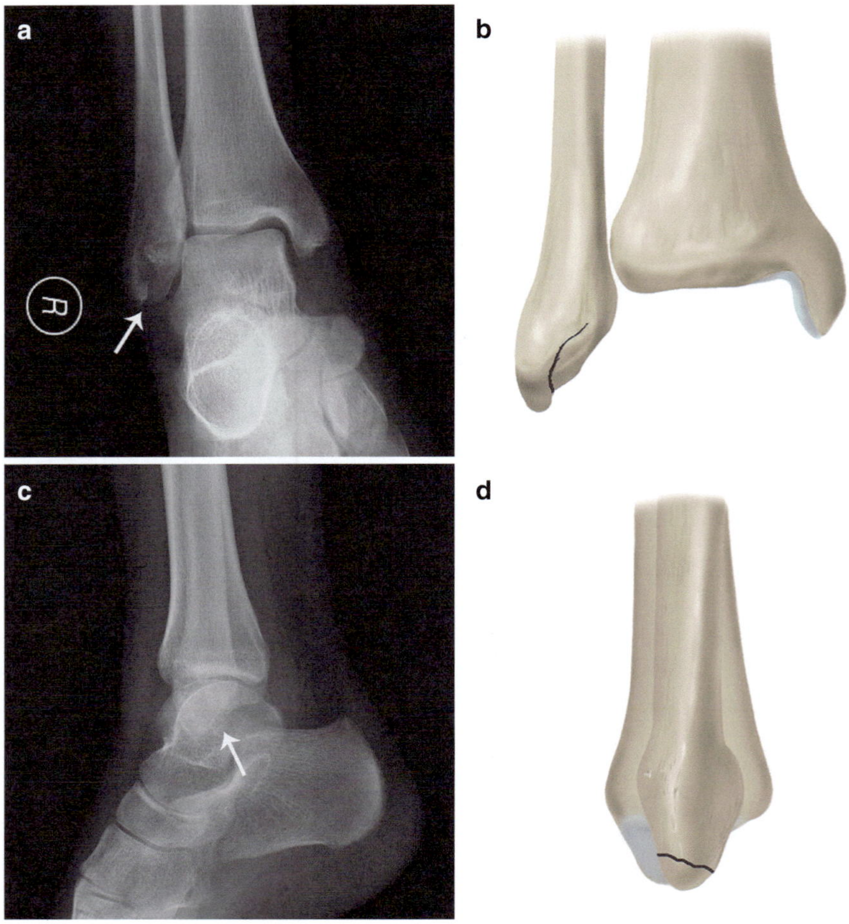

Fig. 10.1 (**a**) and (**c**) are the anteroposterior and lateral view of X-ray, showing suspicious fracture of the right lateral malleolus (white arrow). (**b**, **d**)

1.2. CT scan (Fig. 10.1e–h)

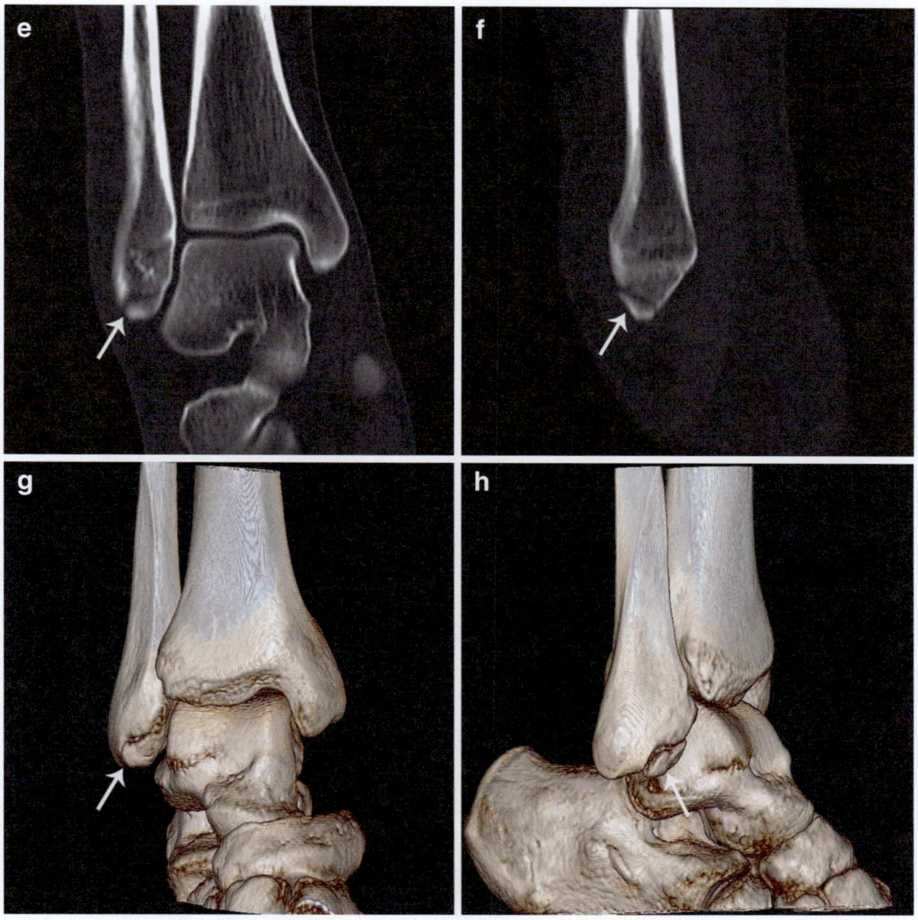

Fig. 10.1 (**e–h**) are CT reconstruction in coronal and sagittal plane, CT three-dimensional reconstruction of the positive and external view, respectively, showing the right lateral malleolus fracture, without displacement (white arrow)

2. Identification of avulsion fracture of the lateral malleolus with ligament injury and non-fracture
   2.1. CT scan (Fig. 10.2a–d)

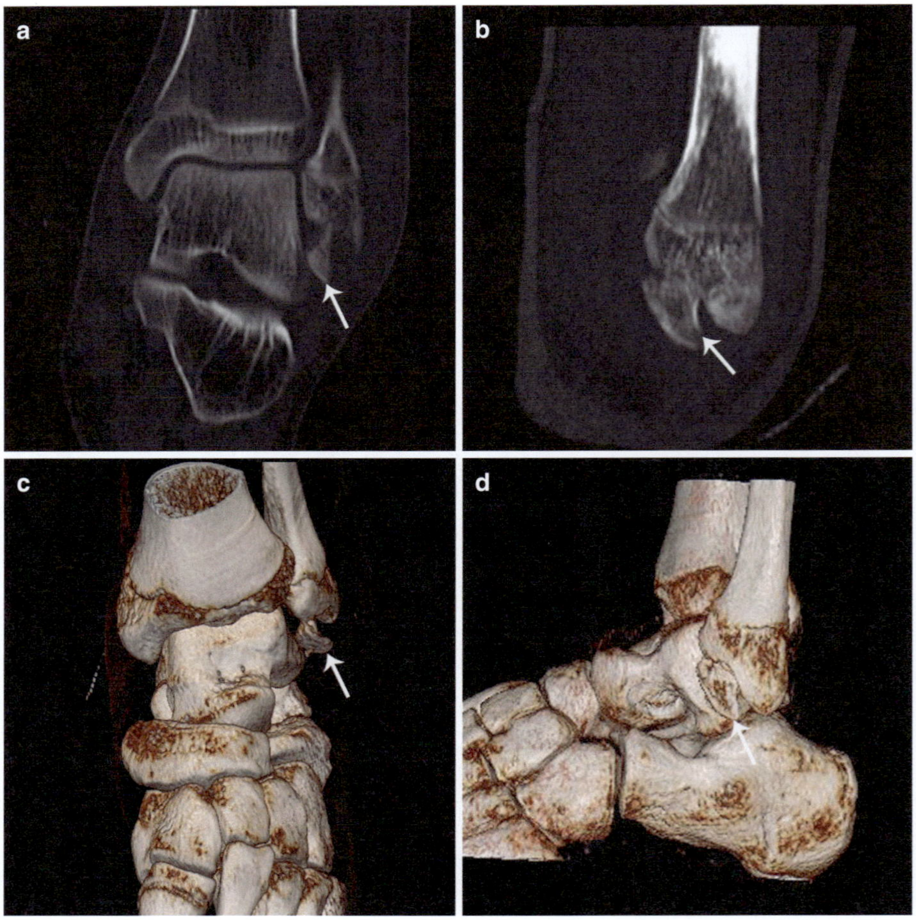

Fig. 10.2 (**a**–**d**) are CT reconstruction in coronal and sagittal plane, CT three-dimensional reconstruction of the positive and external view, respectively, showing the left lateral malleolus fracture and displacement (coarse white arrow). To observe the ligament condition, the MRI examination is performed

2.2. MRI scan (Fig. 10.2e–h)

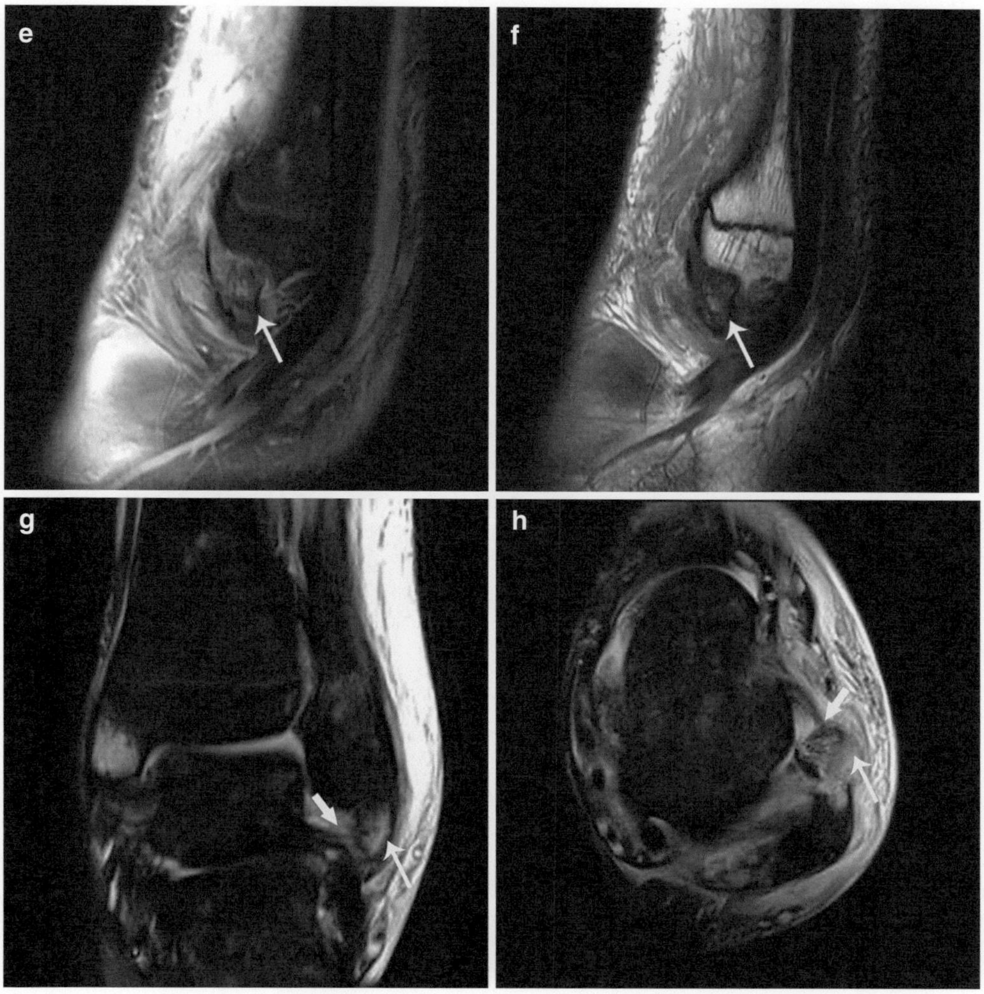

Fig. 10.2 (**e**–**h**) are MRI sagittal T2WI, sagittal T1WI, coronal T2WI and transverse axis T2WI, respectively, showing the left lateral malleolus fracture, displacement (coarse white arrow) and the ligament injury (fine white arrow)

3. Identification of the medial malleolus fractures with slight displacement and non-displacement
   3.1. The X-ray (Fig. 10.3a–d)

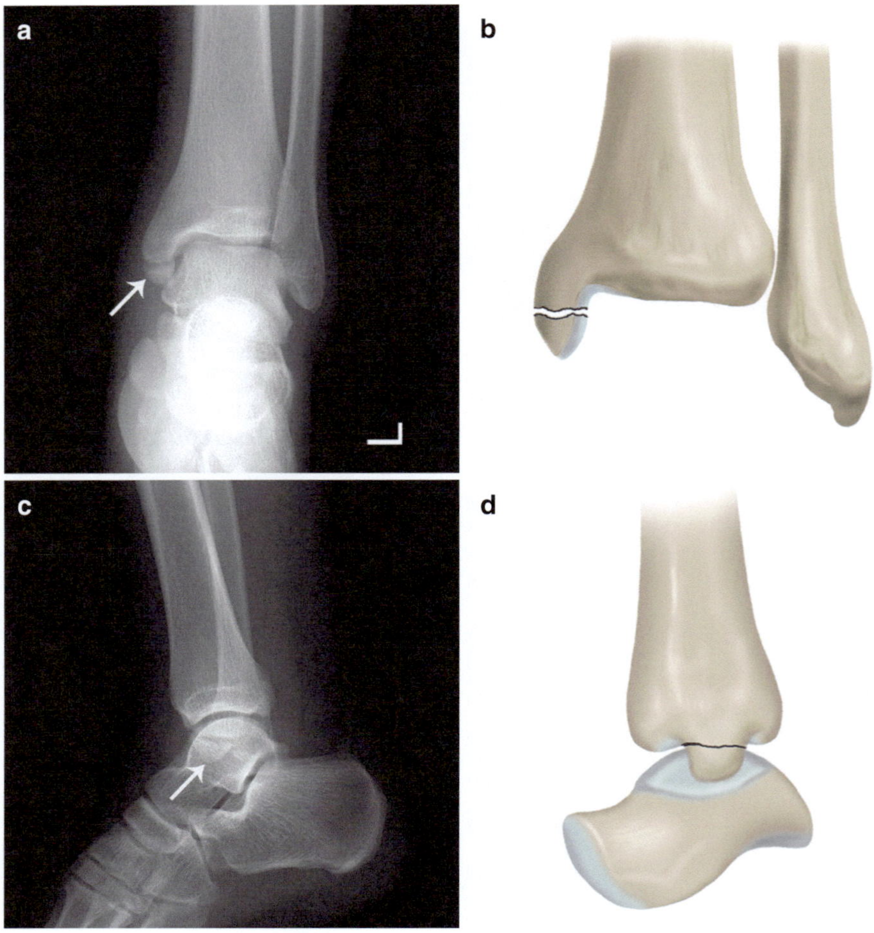

Fig. 10.3 (**a**, **c**) are the anteroposterior and lateral view of X-ray, respectively, showing a left medial malleolus fracture and slight dislocation (white arrow), (**b**, **d**)

3.2. CT scan (Fig. 10.3e–h)

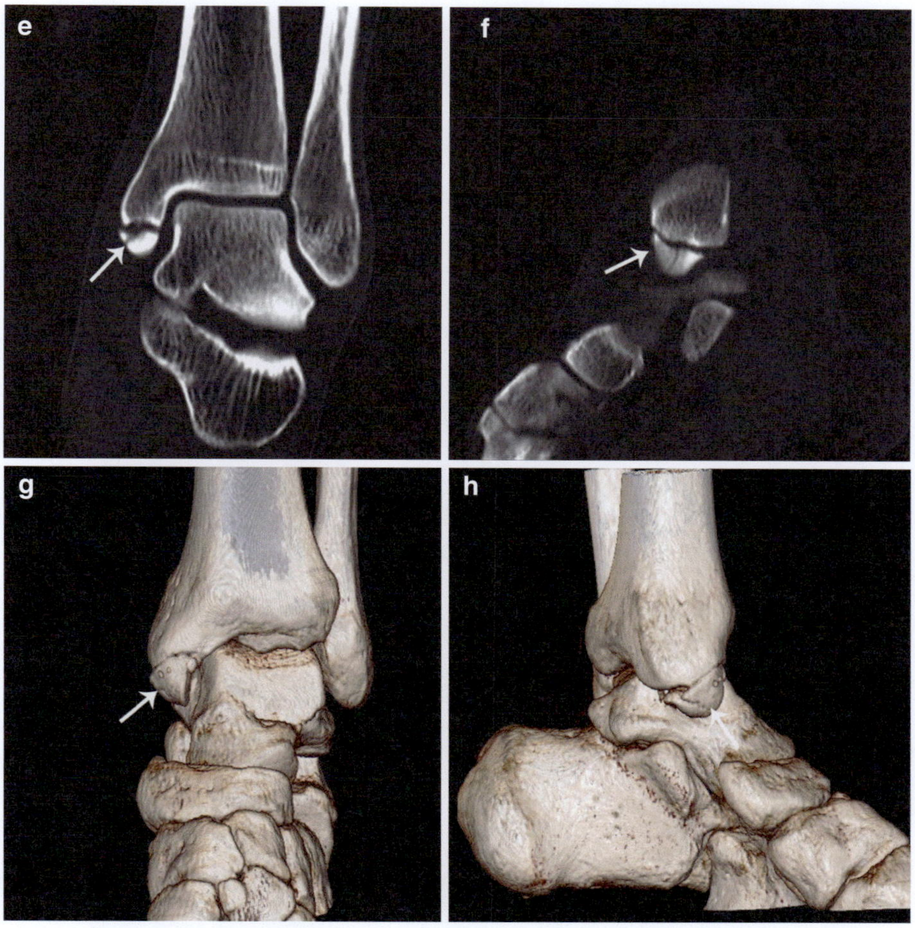

Fig. 10.3 (e–h) are CT reconstruction in coronal and sagittal plane, CT three-dimensional reconstruction of the positive and internal view, respectively, showing the left medial malleolus fracture, slight displacement (white arrow)

4. Identification of the medial malleolus fracture without displacement and non-fracture
   4.1. The X-ray (Fig. 10.4a–d)

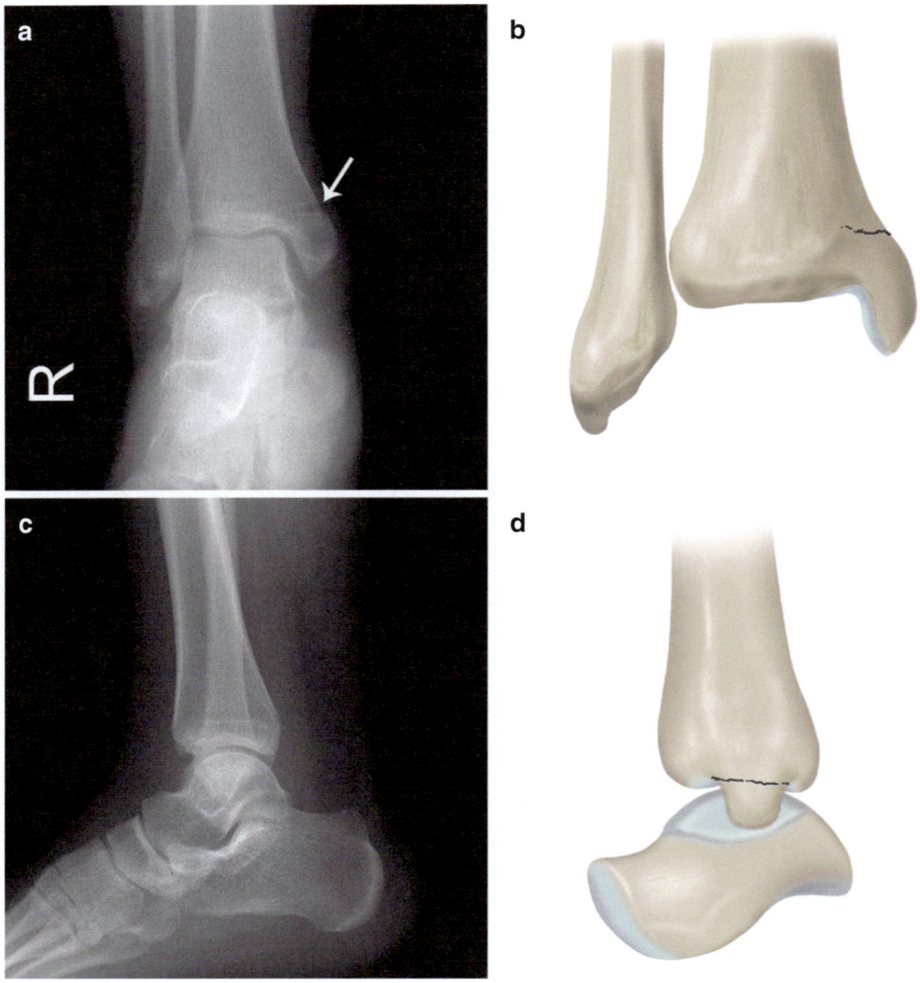

Fig. 10.4 (**a**, **c**) are the anteroposterior and lateral position of X-ray, respectively, showing suspicious fracture of the right medial malleolus (white arrow). (**b**, **d**) take the CT scan to make a definite diagnosis

4.2. CT scan (Fig. 10.4e–h)

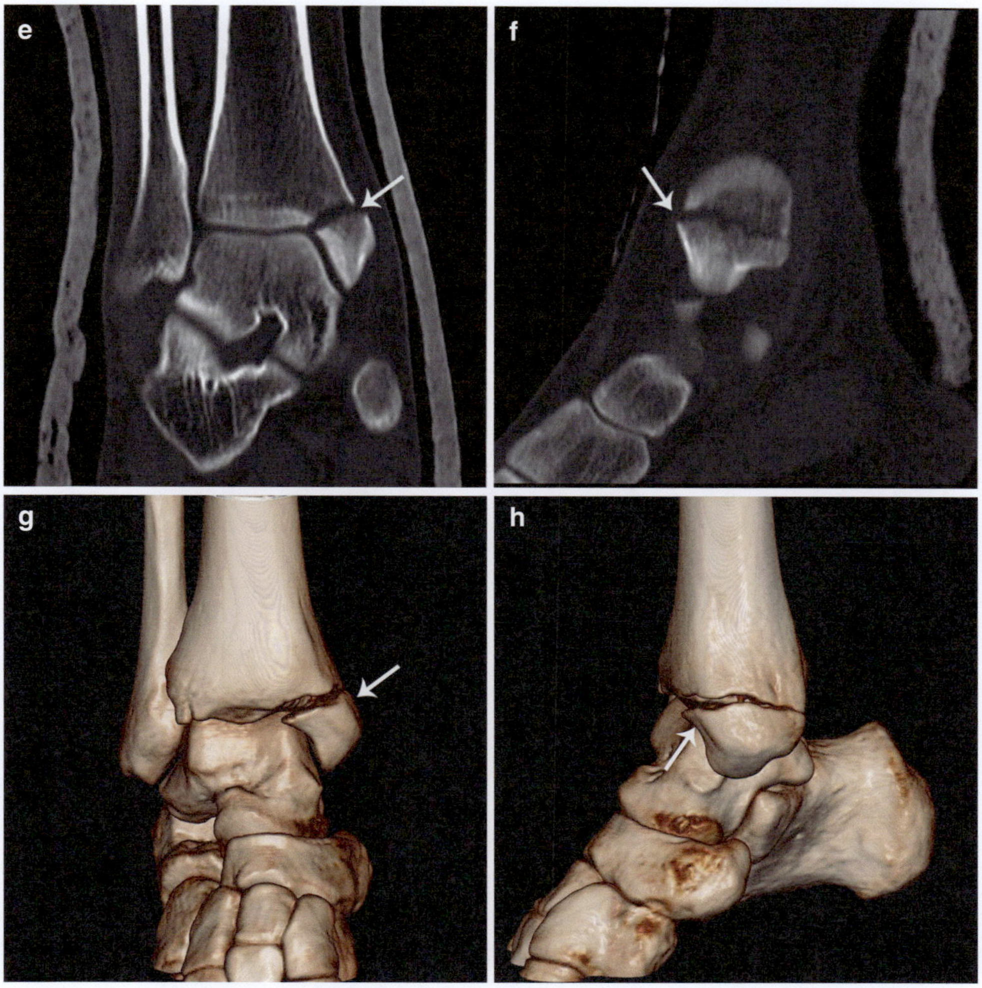

Fig. 10.4 (**e**–**h**) are CT reconstructions in the coronal and sagittal plane, CT three-dimensional reconstruction of the positive and internal view, respectively, showing the right medial malleolus fracture, without displacement (white arrow)

5. Identification of the posterior malleolus fracture and non-fracture
   5.1. The X-ray (Fig. 10.5a–d)

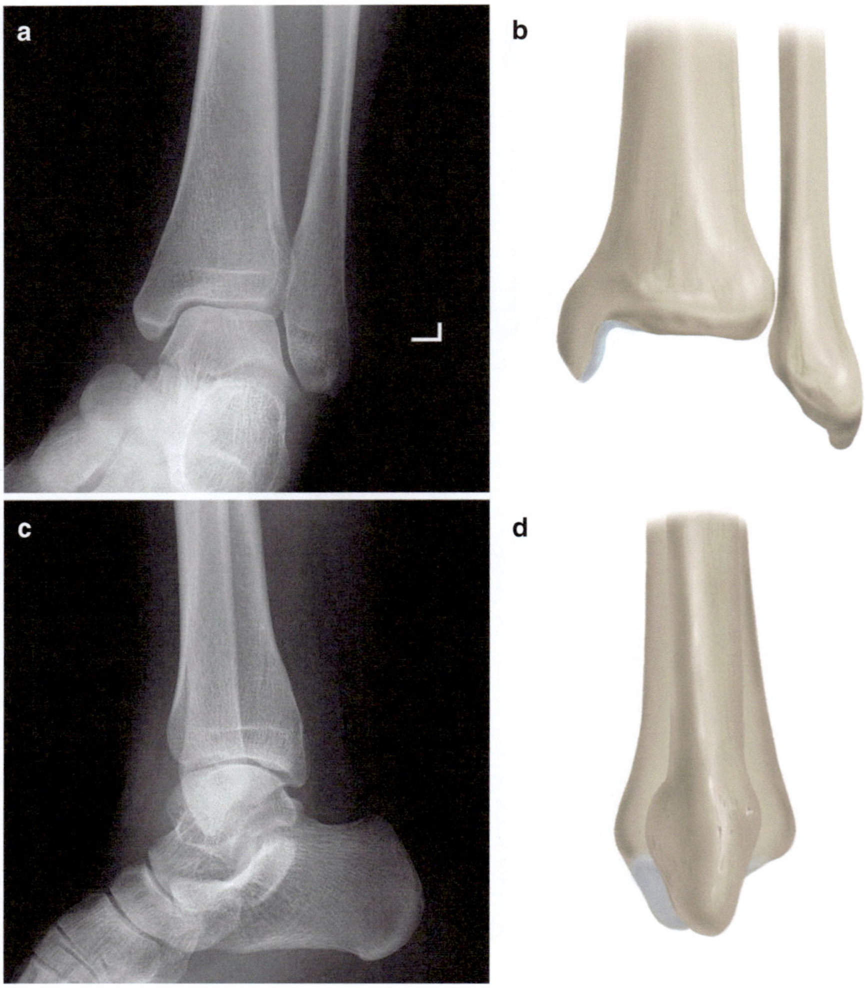

Fig. 10.5 (**a**, **c**) are the anteroposterior and lateral view of X-ray, respectively, showing the fracture line is not obvious, and the articular capsule is swelling. (**b**, **d**) therefore take the CT scan to make a definite diagnosis

5.2. CT scan (Fig. 10.5e–h)

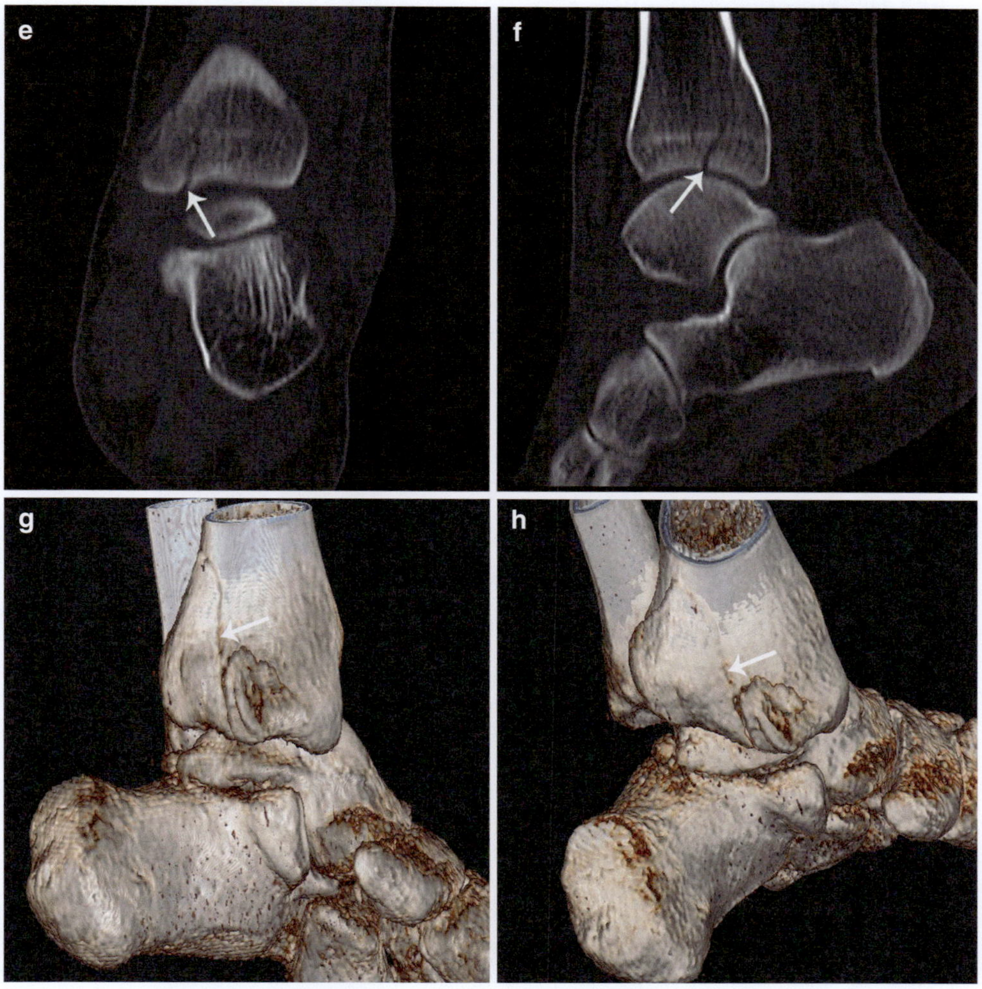

Fig. 10.5 (**e–h**) are CT reconstruction in coronal and sagittal plane, CT three-dimensional reconstruction of the positive and internal view, respectively, showing the left posterior malleolus fracture, without displacement (white arrow)

10.1.3.2 The Bi-malleolar Fracture

6. Identification of the bi-malleolar fracture and non-fracture
   6.1. The X-ray (Fig. 10.6a–d)

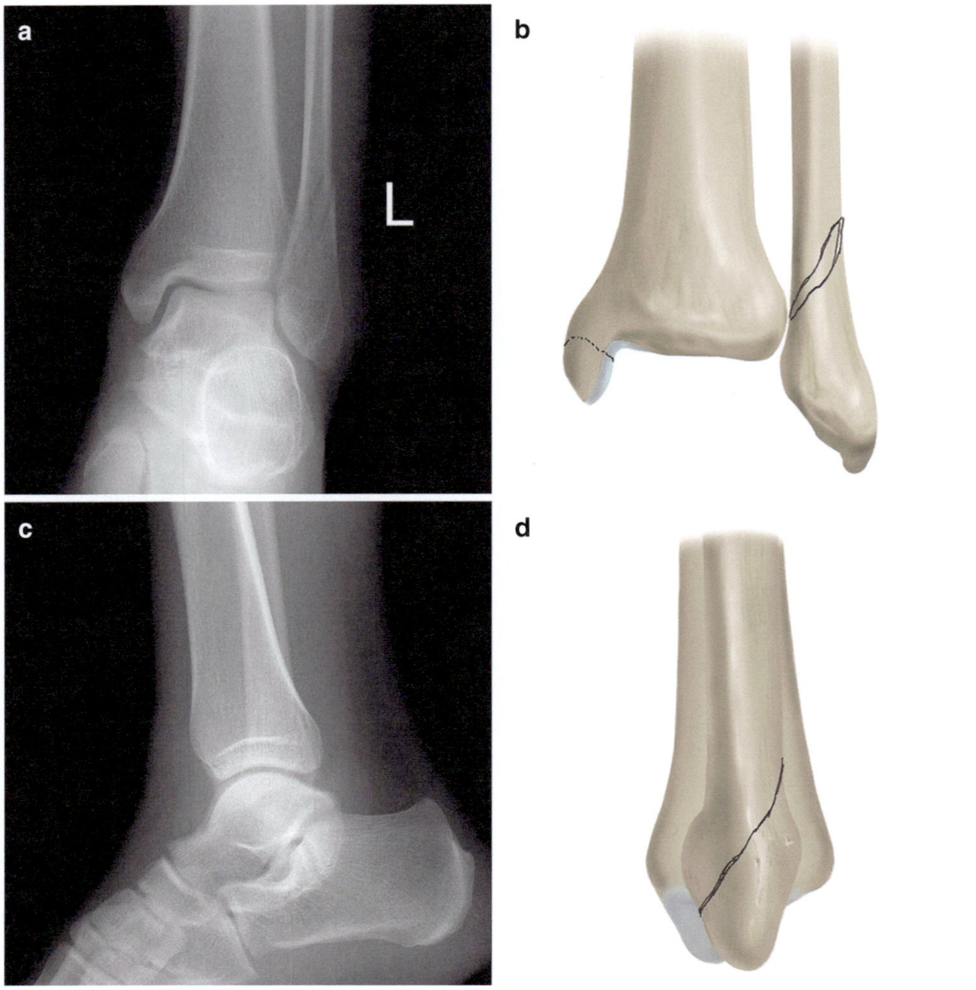

Fig. 10.6 (**a**, **c**) are the anteroposterior and lateral view of X-ray, respectively, showing the lateral malleolus fracture without displacement, and no obvious fracture line in the medial malleolus. (**b**, **d**) Therefore, CT examination was performed

   6.2. CT scan (Fig. 10.6e, f)

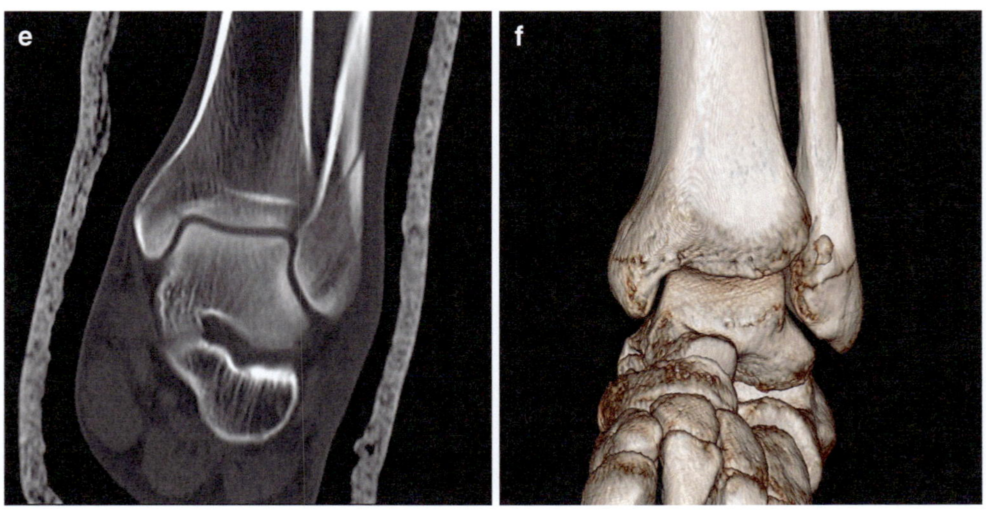

Fig. 10.6 (**e**, **f**) are CT reconstruction in coronal plane, CT three-dimensional reconstruction of the anterior view, respectively, showing the fracture of the medial and lateral malleolus, without displacement

7. Identification of the bi-malleolar fracture and non-fracture
   7.1. The X-ray (Fig. 10.7a–d)

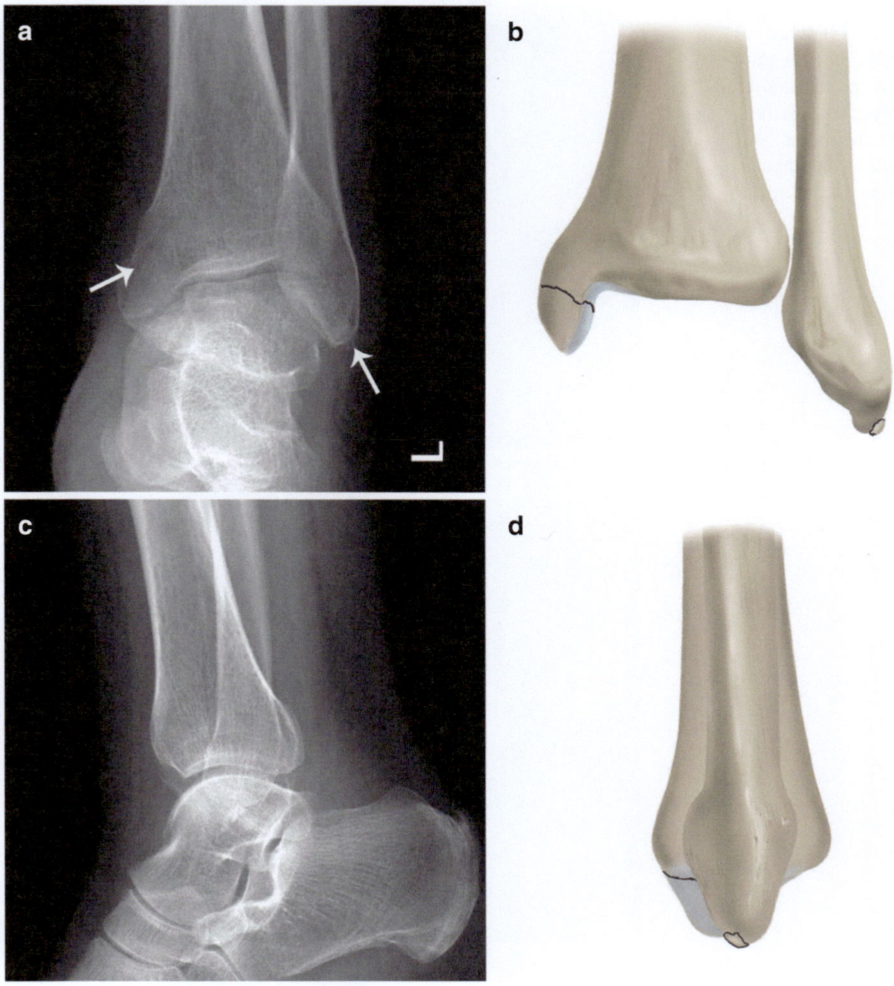

Fig. 10.7 (**a**, **c**) are the anteroposterior and lateral view of X-ray, respectively, showing the medial malleolus fracture without displacement (white arrow) and the suspicious lateral malleolus fracture (white arrow) (**b**, **d**)

7.2. CT (Fig. 10.7e–h)

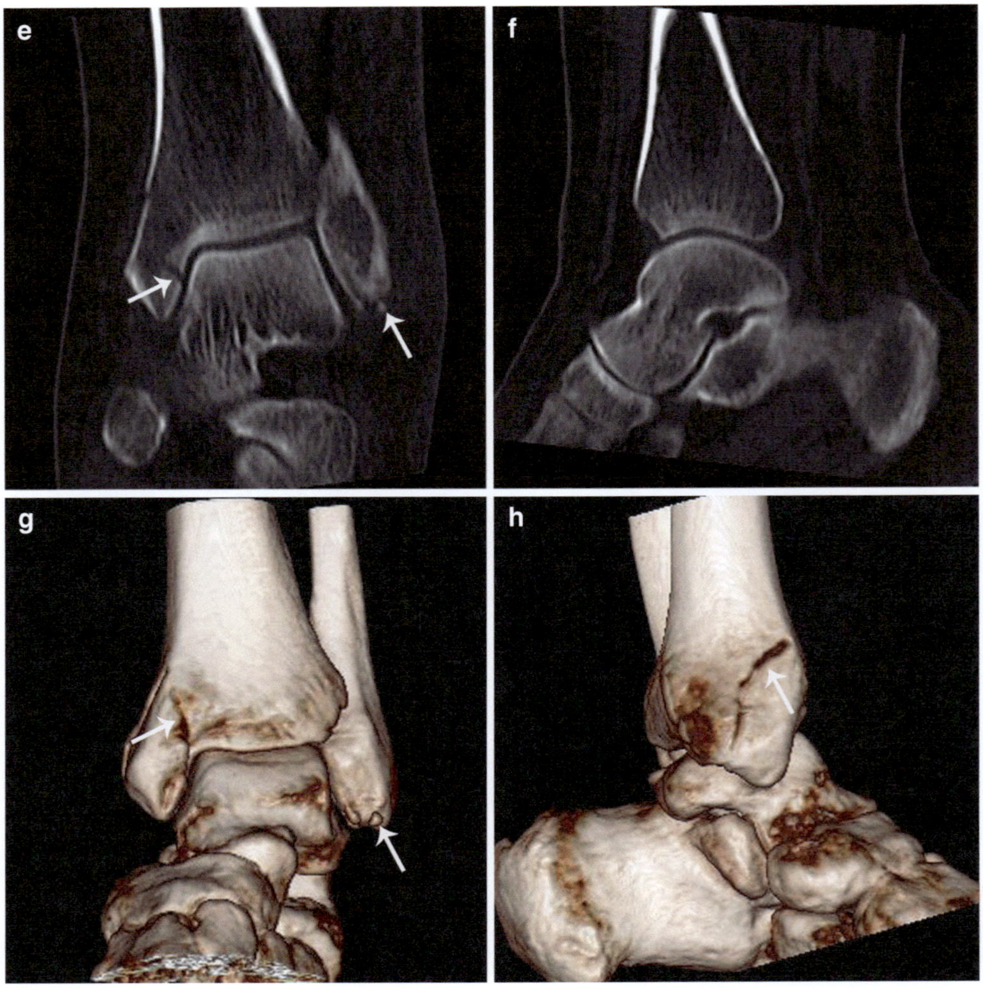

Fig. 10.7 (**e**–**h**) are CT reconstruction in coronal and sagittal plane, CT three-dimensional reconstruction of the positive and internal view respectively, showing the fractures of the medial and lateral malleolus without displacement (white arrow)

8. Identification of the posterior malleolus, lateral malleolus fractures and isolated lateral malleolus fracture
   8.1. The X-ray (Fig. 10.8a–d)

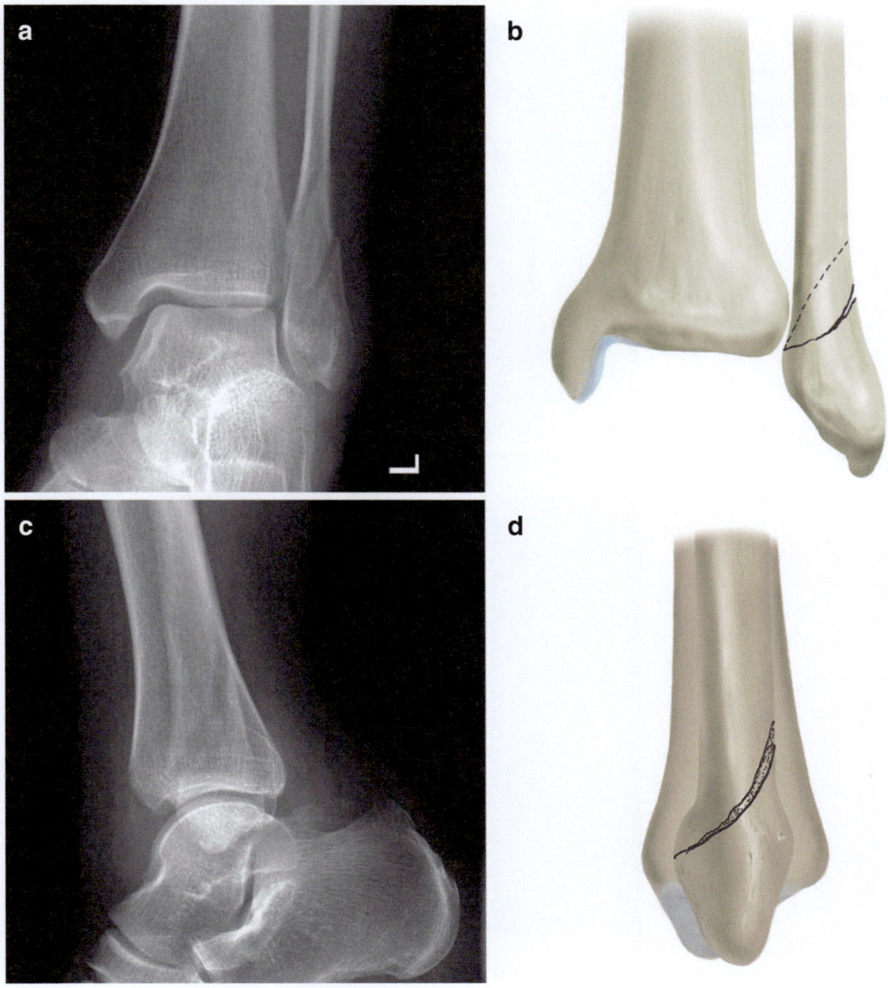

Fig. 10.8 (**a**, **c**) are the anteroposterior and lateral view of X-ray, respectively, showing the lateral malleolus fracture, and the posterior malleolus without obvious fracture line (**b**, **d**)

8.2. MRI scan (Fig. 10.8e–h)

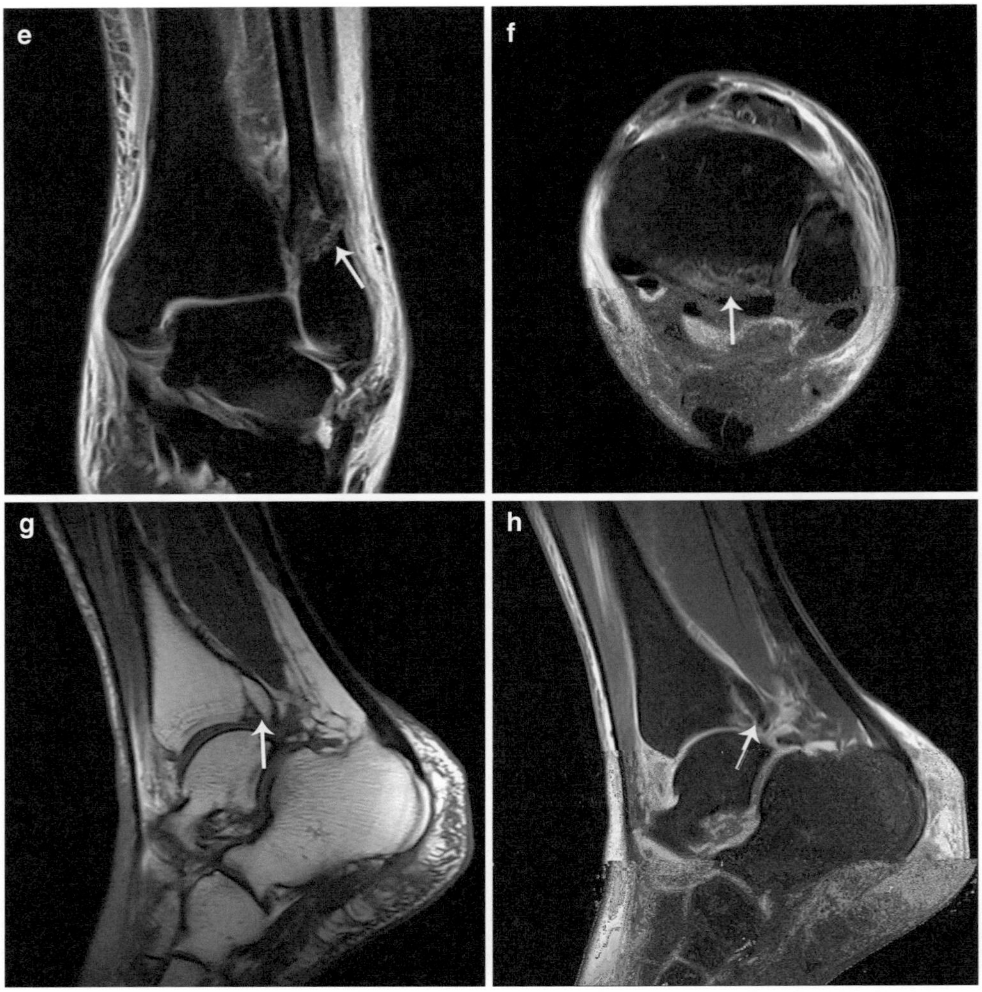

Fig. 10.8 (**e**–**h**) are MRI: coronal T2WI, transverse axial fat suppression T2WI, sagittal T1WI and fat suppression T2WI, showing lateral malleolus and posterior malleolus fractures (white arrow)

9. Identification of the posterior malleolus medial malleolus fractures and isolated medial malleolus fracture
    9.1. The X-ray (Fig. 10.9a–d)

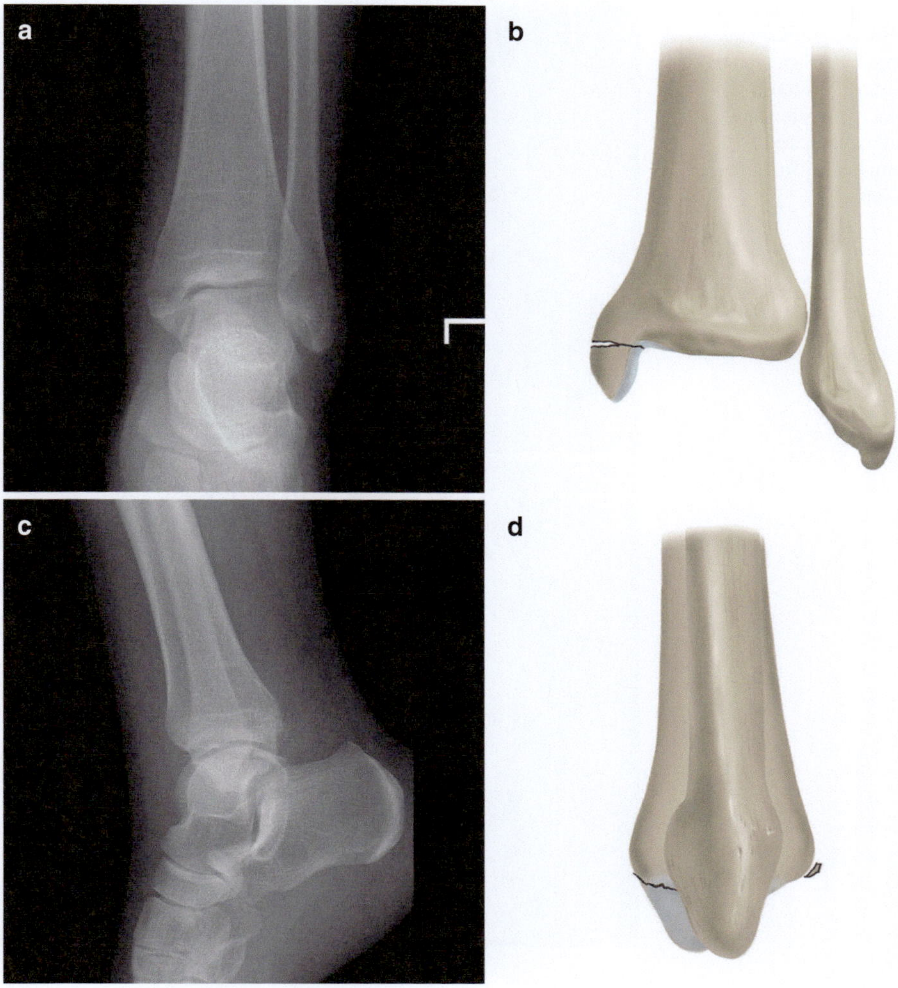

Fig. 10.9 (**a**, **c**) are the anteroposterior and lateral view of X-ray, respectively, showing the medial malleolus fracture and the posterior malleolus without obvious fracture line (**b**, **d**)

9.2. CT examination (Fig. 10.9e–h)

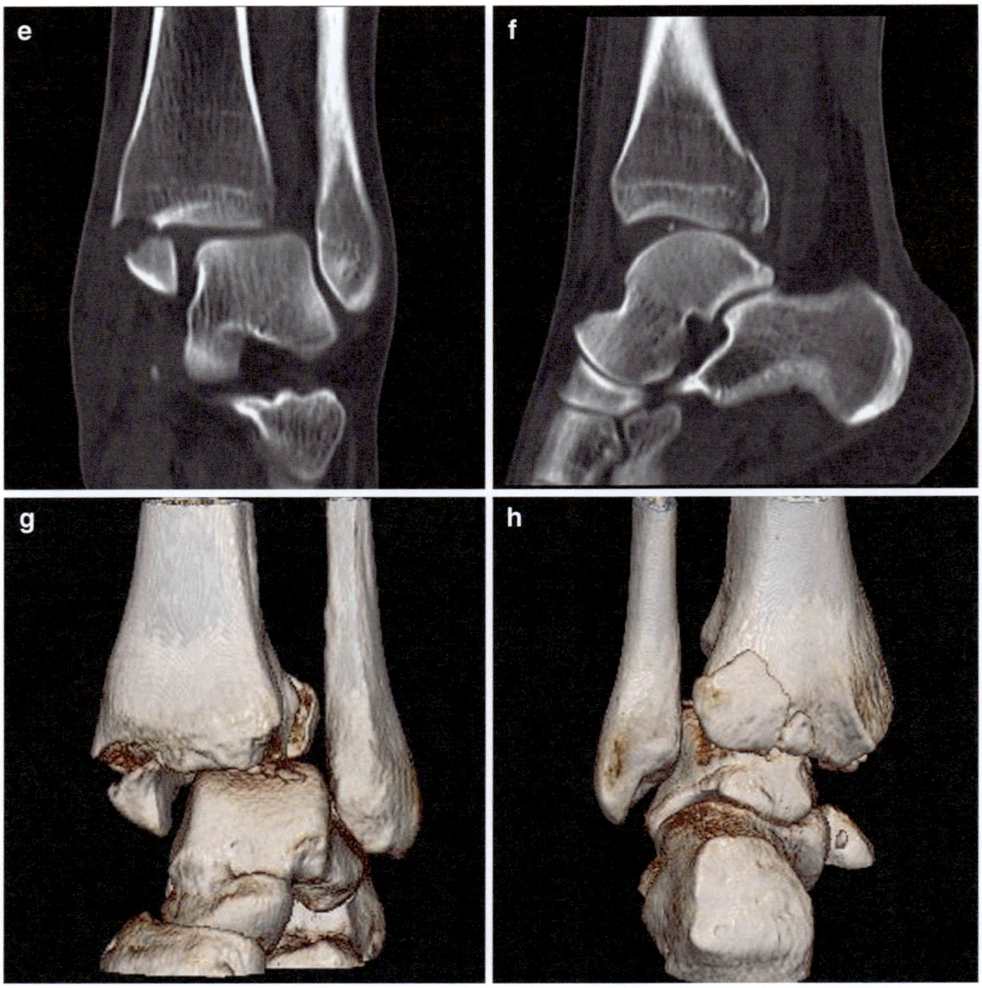

Fig. 10.9 (**e**–**h**) are CT reconstruction in coronal and sagittal plane, CT three-dimensional reconstruction of the anterior and posterior view, respectively, showing the medial malleolus and posterior malleolus fractures, displacement

10.1.3.3 The Tri-malleolar Fracture

10. Identification of a tri-malleolar fracture with displacement and the bi-malleolar fracture
    10.1. The X-ray (Fig. 10.10a–d)

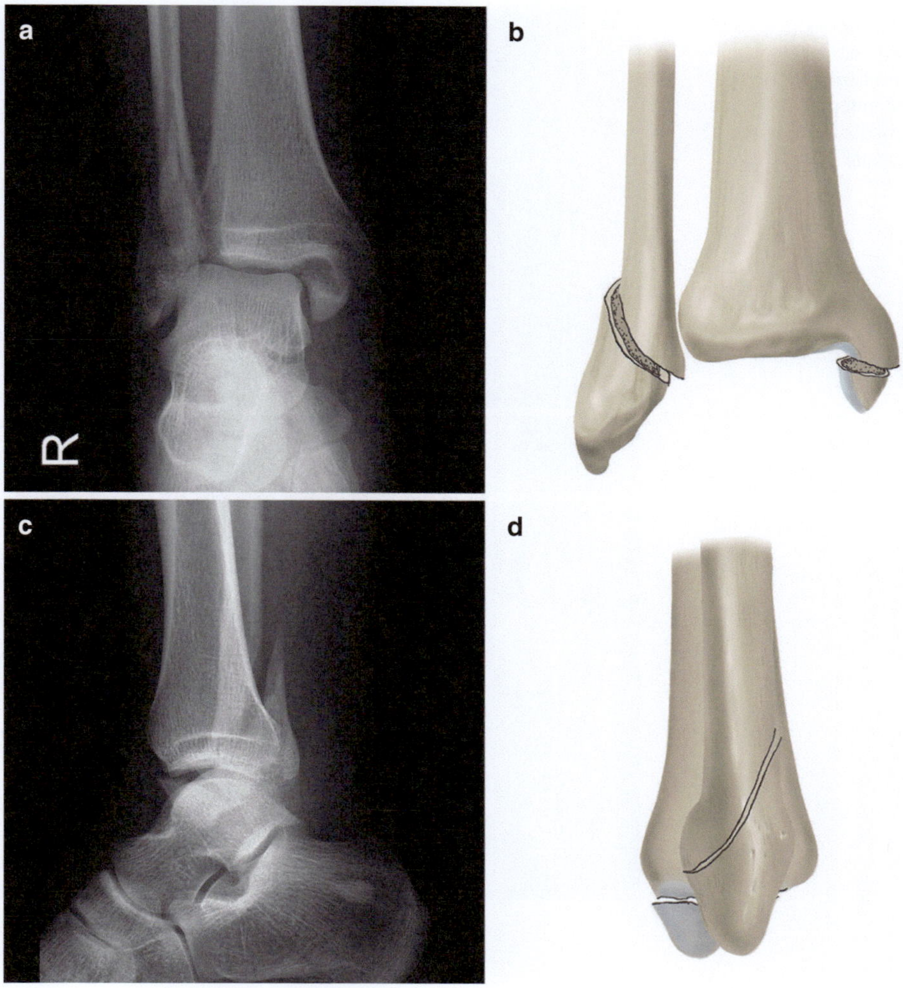

Fig. 10.10 (**a**, **c**) are the anteroposterior and lateral view of X-ray, respectively, showing medial malleolus and lateral malleolus fractures, displacement and the posterior malleolus unclear (**b**, **d**)

10.2. CT scan (Fig. 10.10e–h)

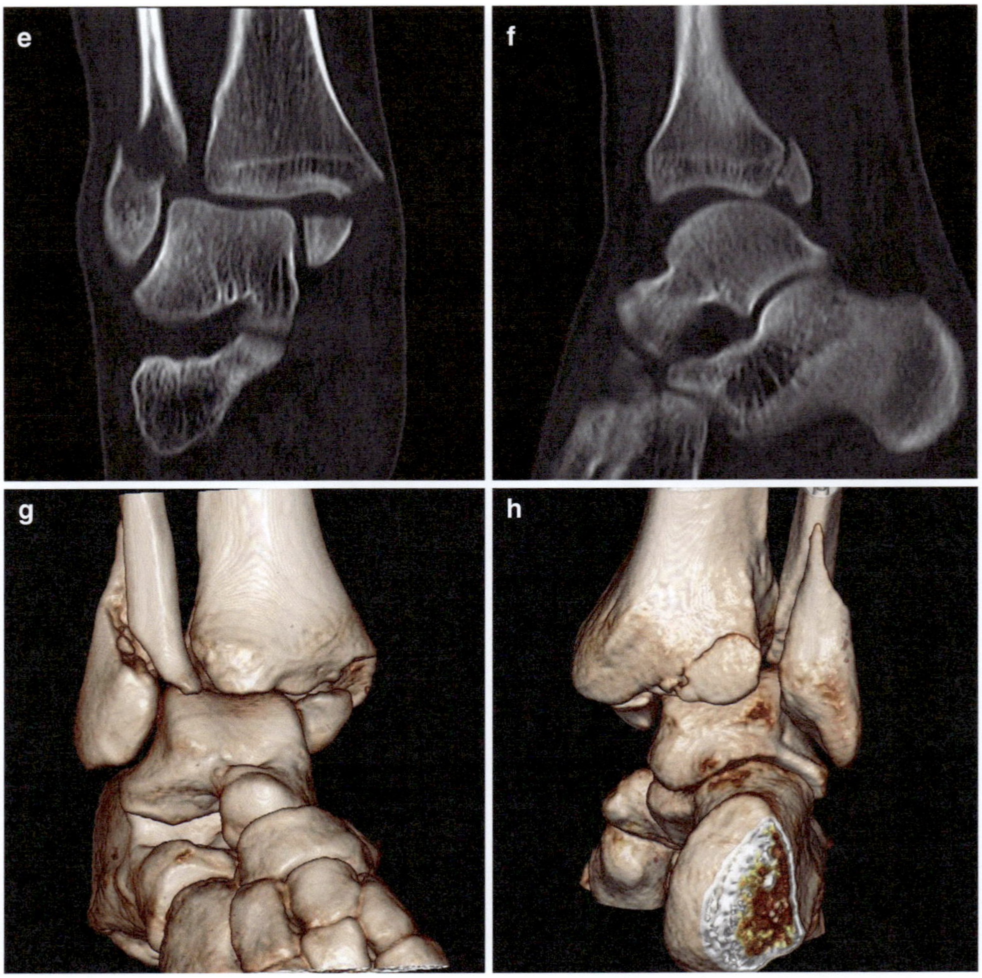

Fig. 10.10 (**e**–**h**) are CT reconstruction in coronal and sagittal plane, CT three-dimensional reconstruction of the anterior and posterior view, respectively, showing the medial, internal and posterior malleolus fractures, and displacement

10.1.3.4 The Compound Fracture

11. Identification of comminuted fractures of distal tibia and fibula with dislocation of ankle joint and that without dislocation
    11.1. The X-ray (Fig. 10.11a–d)

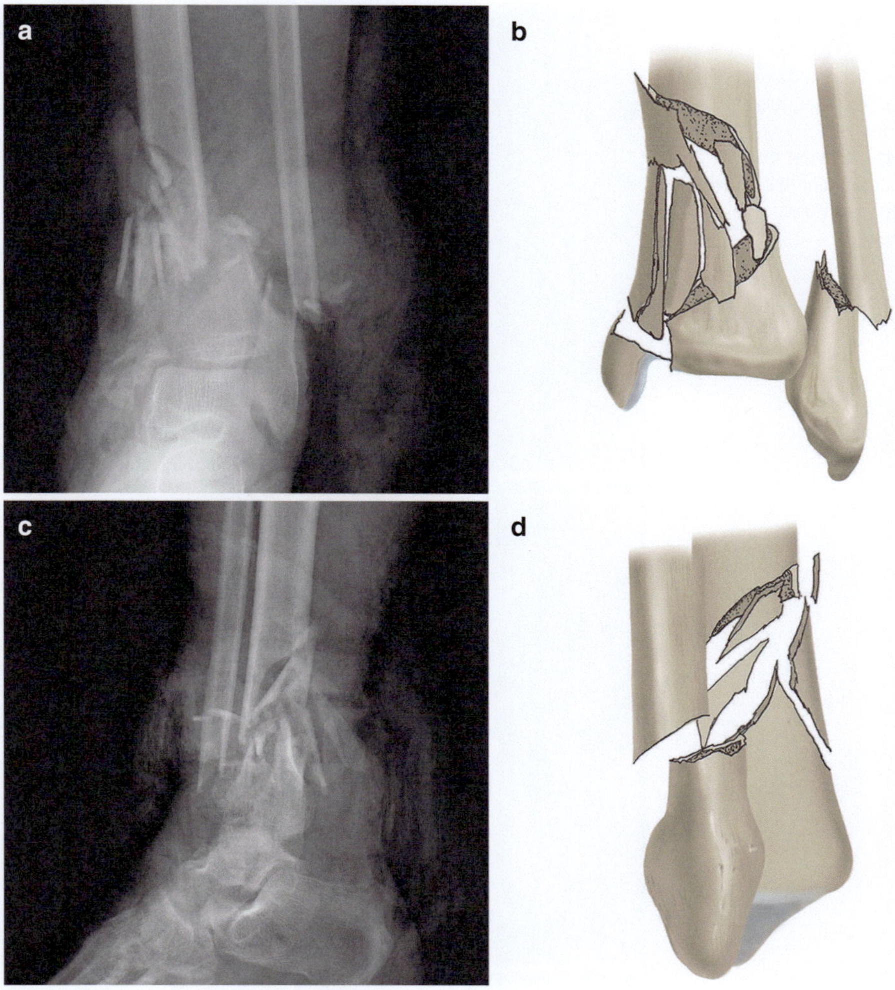

Fig. 10.11 (**a**, **c**) are the anteroposterior and lateral view of X-ray, respectively, showing the left distal tibiofibula comminuted fractures, displacement, with a good correspondence of the ankle joint. (**b**, **d**) in order to observe the correspondence of the ankle joint, the CT scan is performed

    11.2. CT scan (Fig. 10.11e, f)

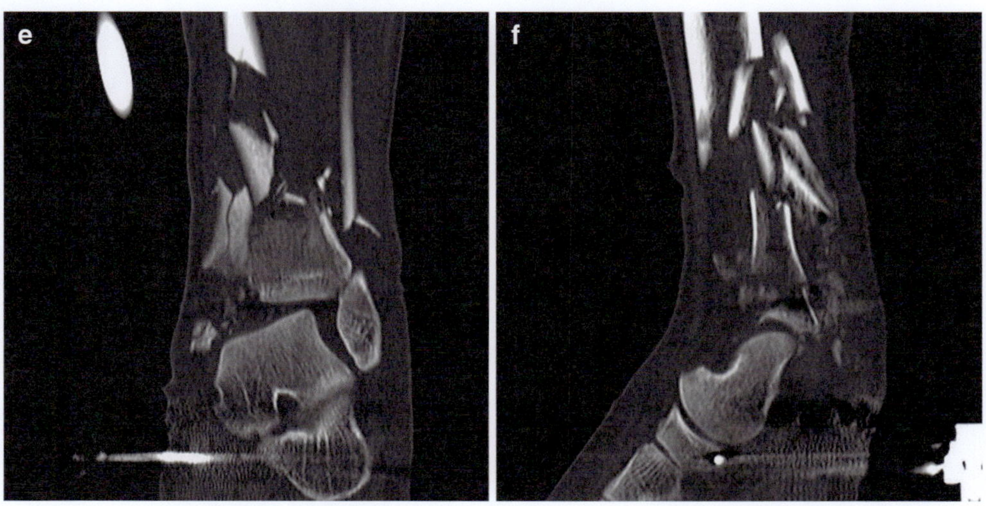

Fig. 10.11 (**e**, **f**) are CT reconstruction in coronal and sagittal plane, respectively, showing the distal tibiofibula comminuted fractures, displacement, with the dislocation of the ankle joint

12. Identification of comminuted fractures of distal tibia and fibula with dislocation of ankle joint and that without dislocation
    12.1. CT scan (Fig. 10.12a–f)

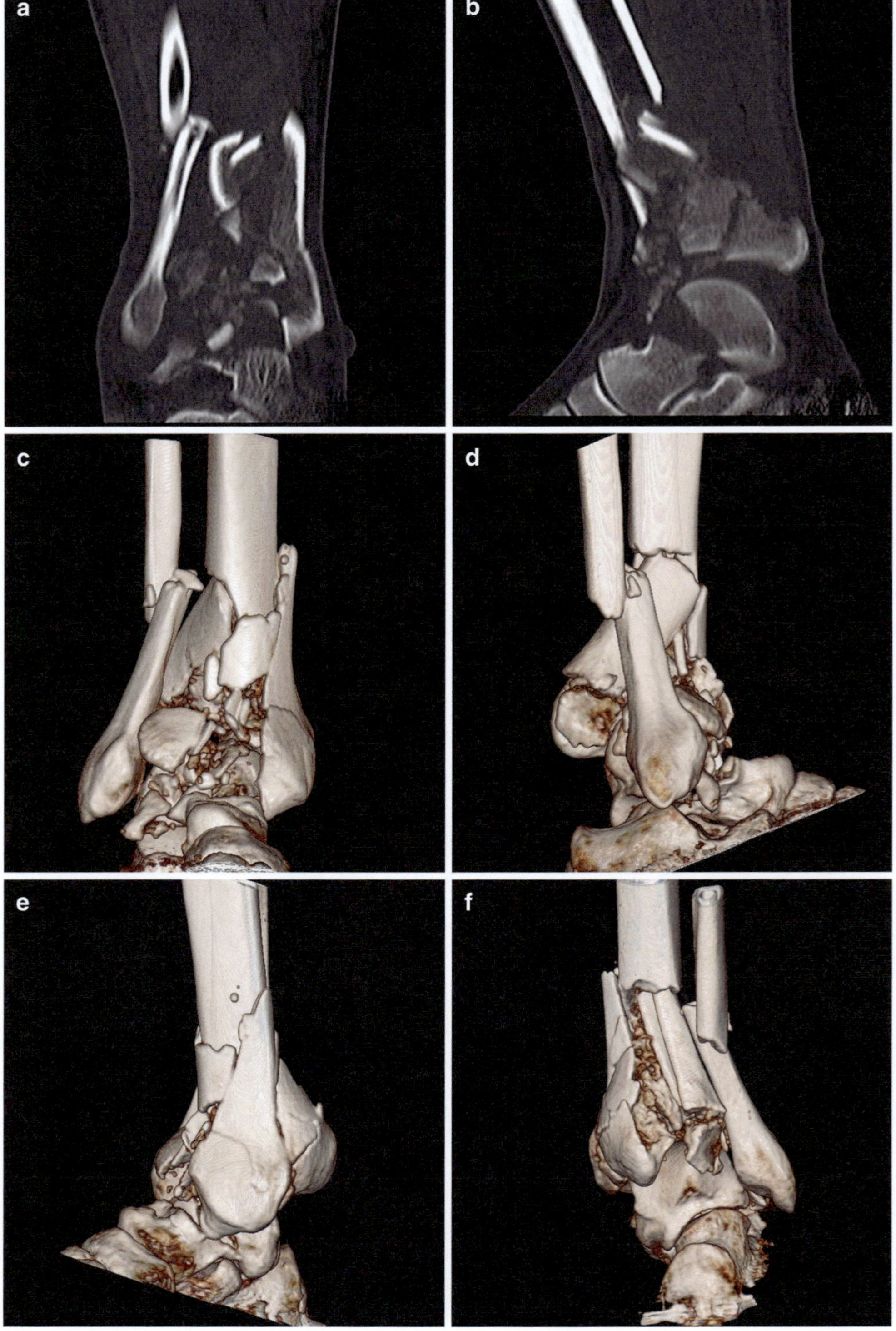

Fig. 10.12 (**a**–**f**) are CT reconstruction in coronal and sagittal plane, CT three-dimensional reconstruction of the anterior, internal, medial and posterior view, respectively, showing the distal tibiofibula and the talus comminuted fractures, displacement

10.1.3.5 The Special Type Fracture

Common special types of fractures are: Dupuytren fracture, which refers to the simultaneous avulsion fracture of the medial malleolus, the rupture of the distal tibiofibular ligament, the separation of the distal tibiofibular syndesmosis and the fracture of the distal fibula. And the distal spiral fracture of the tibia combining with posterior malleolus fracture.

13. Dupuytren identification of the Dupuytren fracture and the bi-malleolar fracture
    13.1. The X-ray (Fig. 10.13a–d)

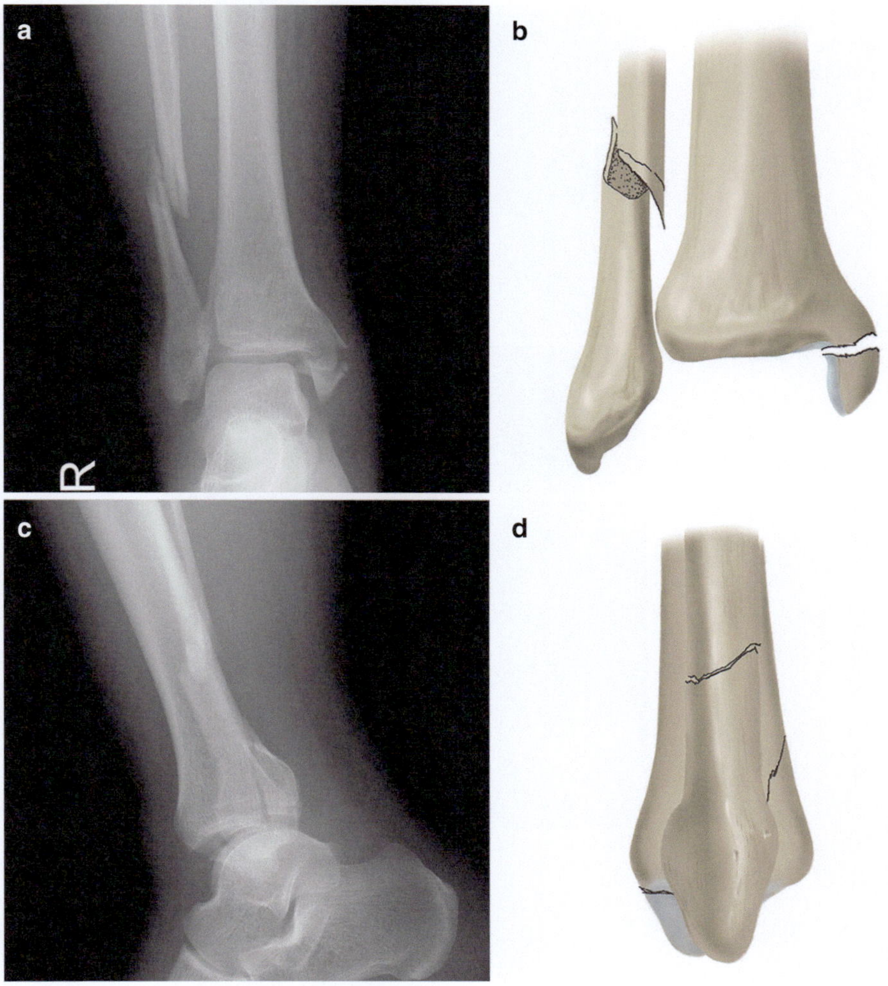

Fig. 10.13 (**a**, **c**) are the anteroposterior and lateral view of X-ray, respectively, showing the fractures of the right distal fibula and medial malleolus, and a good correspondence between ankle joint and the distal tibiofibular joint (**b**, **d**)

    13.2. CT scan (Fig. 10.13e, f)

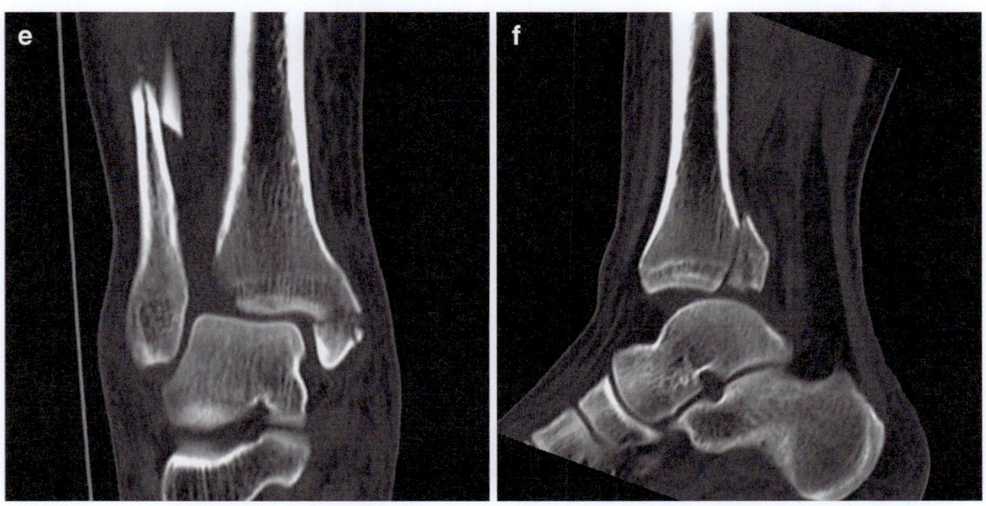

Fig. 10.13 (**e**, **f**) are CT reconstruction in coronal and sagittal plane, respectively, showing the avulsion fracture of medial malleolus, the fracture of distal fibula, combining the separation of distal tibiofibular syndesmosis

14. Identification of the Dupuytren fracture and the bi-malleolar fracture
    14.1. The X-ray (Fig. 10.14a–d)

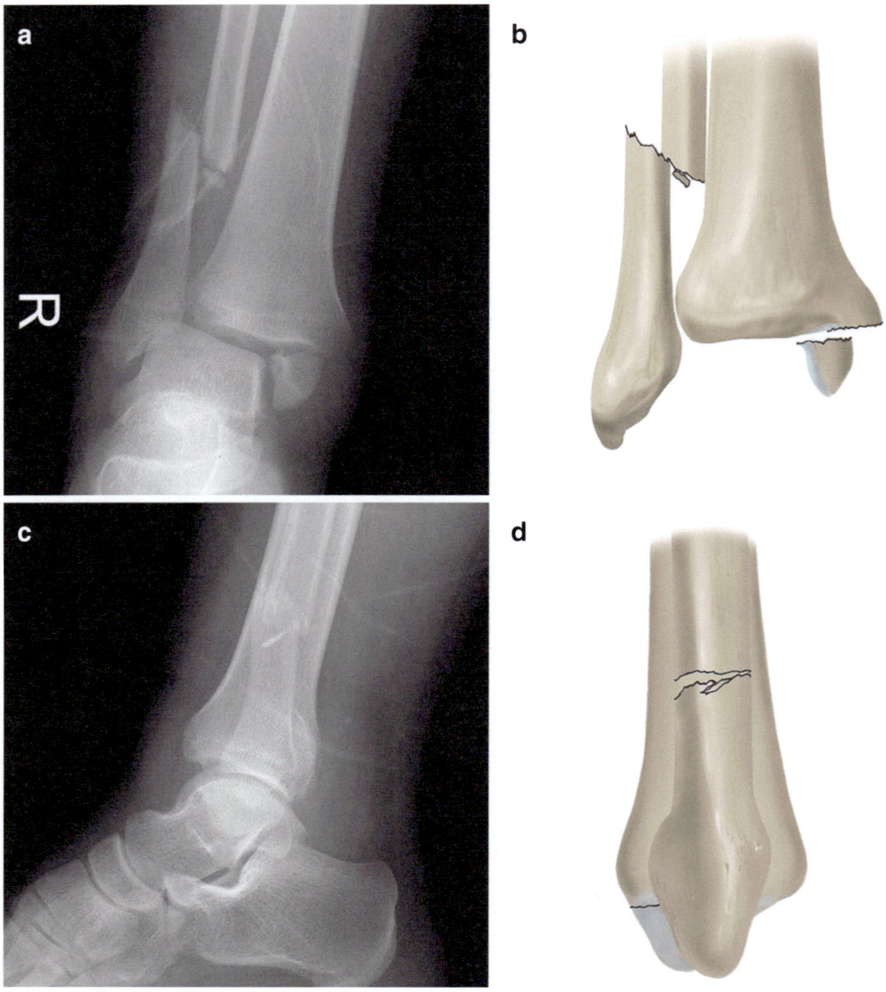

Fig. 10.14 (**a**, **c**) are the anteroposterior and lateral view of X-ray, respectively, showing the fractures of the right distal fibula and medial malleolus, and a good correspondence between ankle joint and the distal tibiofibular joint (**b**, **d**)

    14.2. CT scan (Fig. 10.14e, f)

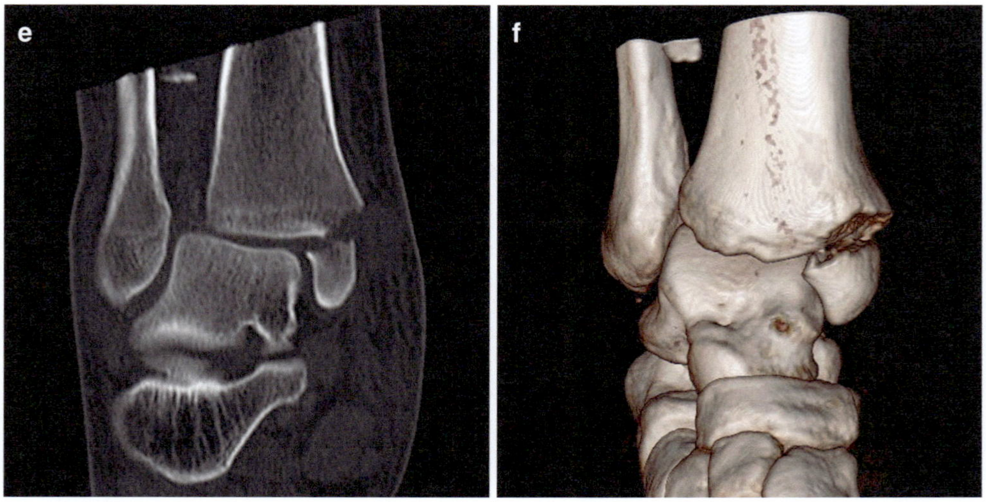

Fig. 10.14 (**e**, **f**) are CT reconstruction in coronal plane and CT three-dimensional reconstruction of the anterior view, respectively, showing the avulsion fracture of medial malleolus, the fracture of distal fibula, combining the separation of distal tibiofibular syndesmosis

15. Identification of the spiral fracture of distal tibia and fibula combining posterior malleolus fracture and that without posterior malleolus fracture
    15.1. The X-ray (Fig. 10.15a–d)

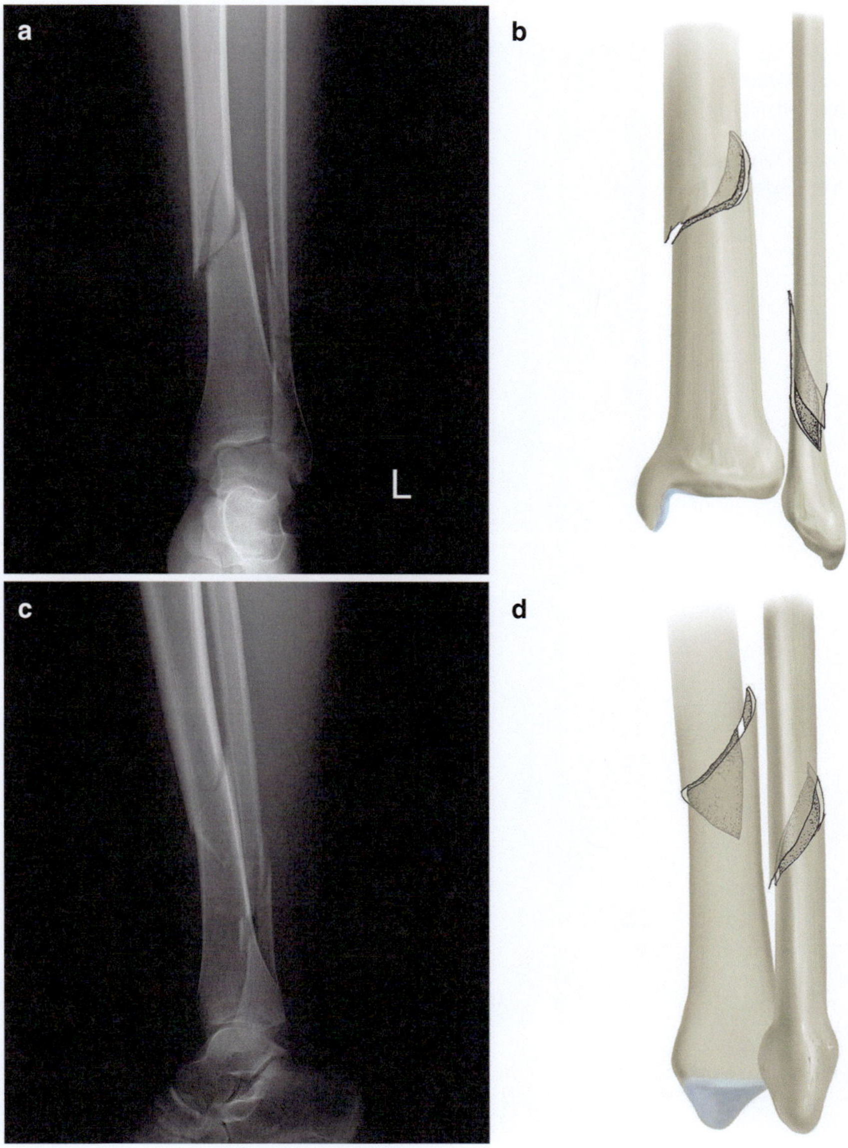

Fig. 10.15 (**a**, **b**) are the anteroposterior and lateral view of X-ray, respectively, showing the spiral fractures of the left distal tibiofibular, and the posterior malleolus without obvious fracture line (**b**, **d**)

    15.2. CT scan (Fig. 10.15e, f)

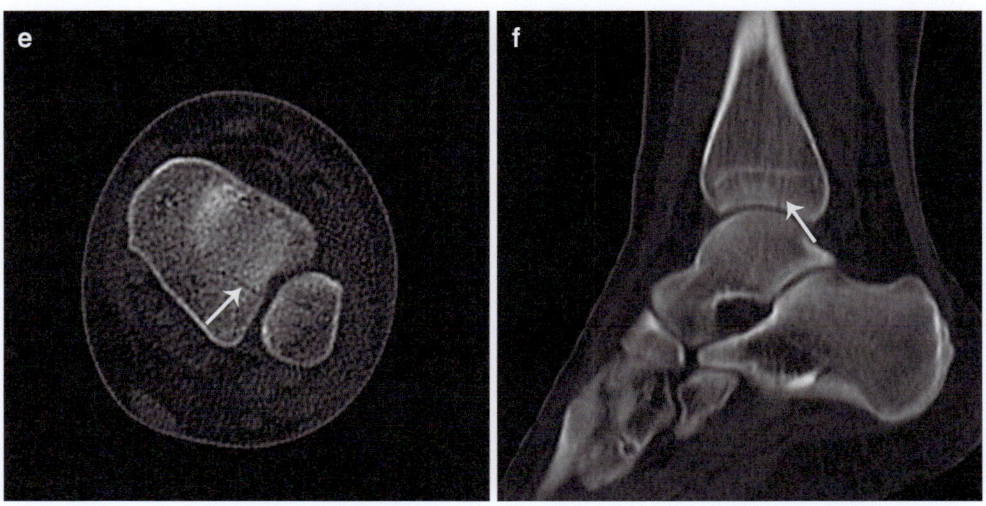

Fig. 10.15 (**e**, **f**) are CT reconstruction in the transverse axial plane and sagittal plane, respectively, showing the fracture of posterior malleolus

10.1.3.6 Accessory Bone of Ankle Joint

16. Identification of the fracture of sub-fibular bone and avulsion fracture of the distal fibula
    16.1. The X-ray (Fig. 10.16a–d)

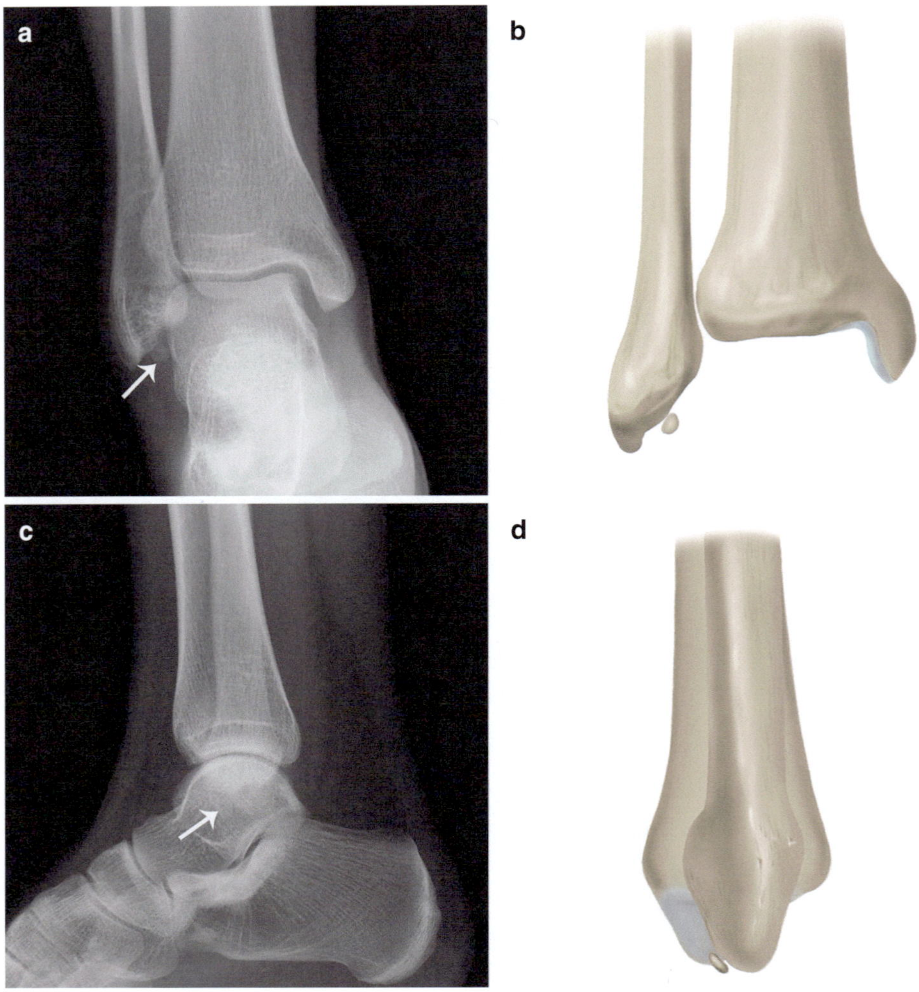

Fig. 10.16 (**a**, **c**) are the anteroposterior and lateral view of X-ray, respectively, showing a round-like bone mass below the fibula with smooth edges (white arrow) (**b**, **d**)

16.2. CT scan (Fig. 10.16e–h)

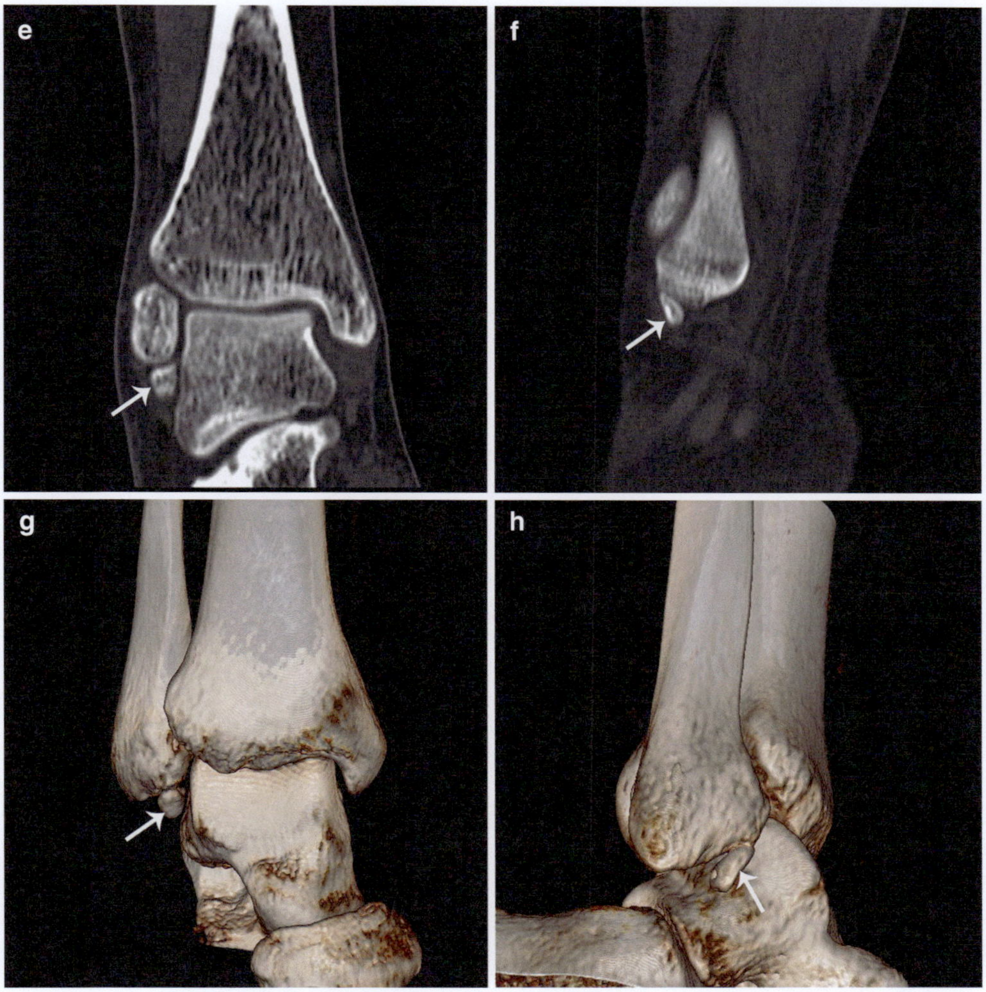

Fig. 10.16 (**e–h**) are CT reconstruction in coronal and sagittal plane, CT three-dimensional reconstruction of the anterior and internal view, respectively, showing the accessory bone below the fibula with smooth edges and intact cortical bones (white arrow)

17. The sub-fibular bone and the avulsion fracture of the distal fibula
    17.1. The X-ray (Fig. 10.17a–d)

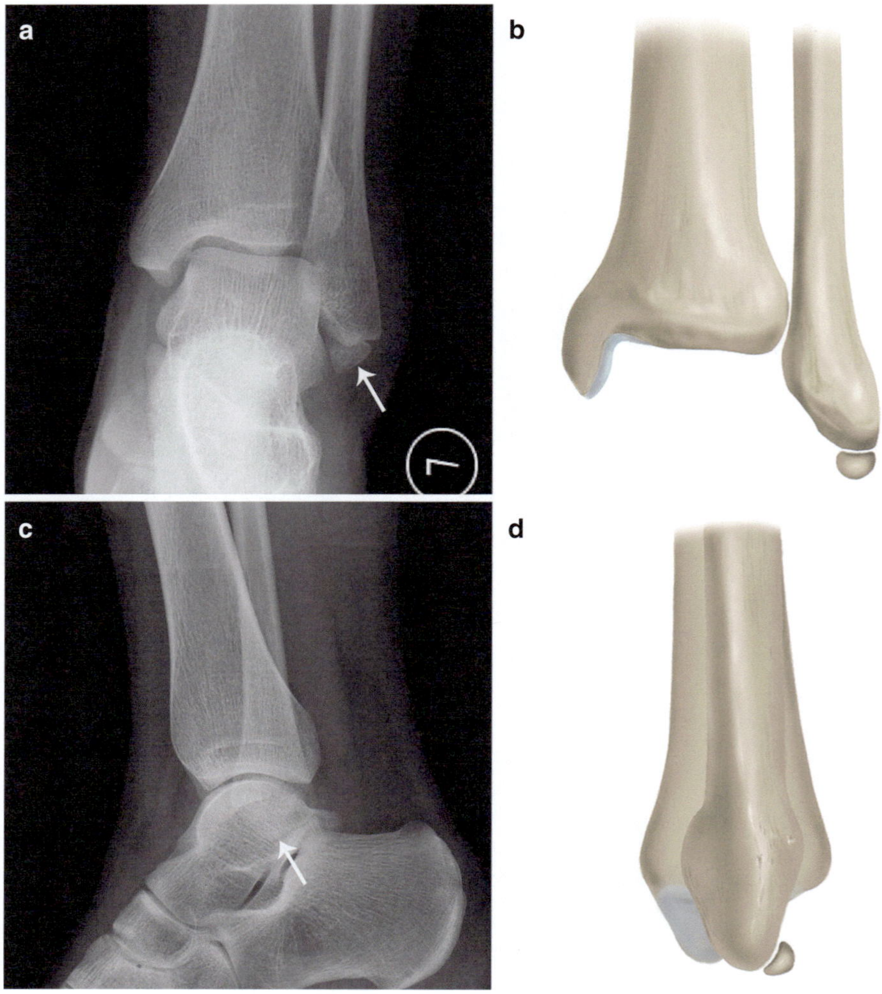

Fig. 10.17 (**a**, **c**) are the anteroposterior and lateral view of X-ray, respectively, showing an accessory bone below the fibula with smooth edges and intact cortical bones (white arrow) (**b**, **d**)

18. Identification of the sub-tibial bone and the avulsion fracture of the distal tibia
    18.1. The X-ray (Fig. 10.18a–d)

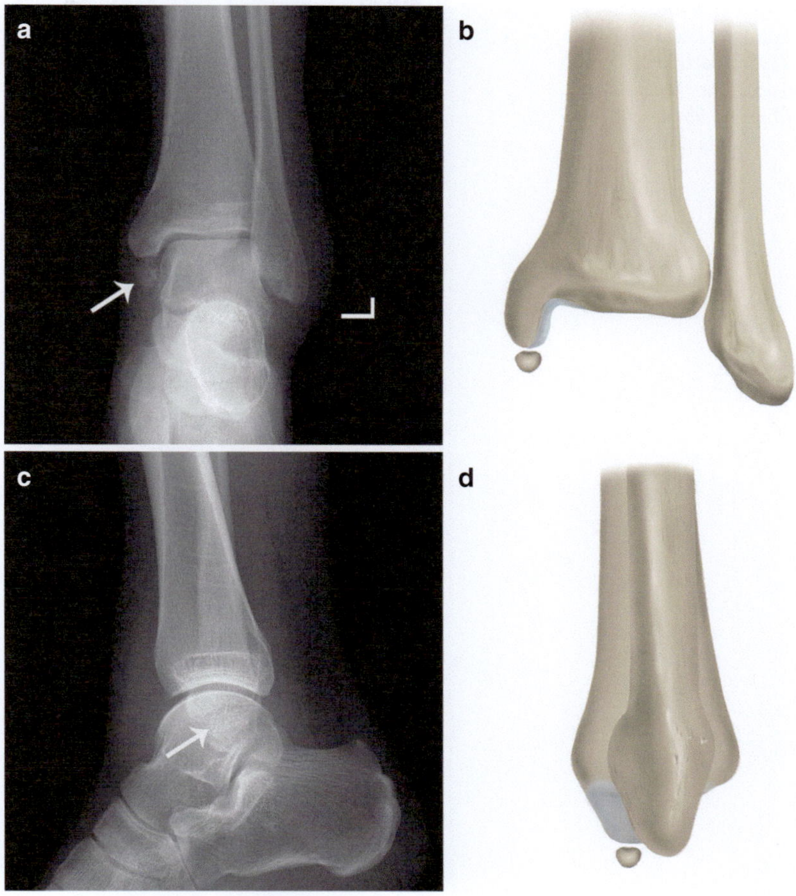

Fig. 10.18 (**a**, **c**) are the anteroposterior and lateral view of X-ray, respectively, showing an accessory bone below the tibia with smooth edges and intact cortical bones (white arrow) (**b**, **d**)

19. Identification of the sub-tibial bone, sub-fibular bone and the avulsion fracture of the distal tibiofibula
    19.1. The X-ray (Fig. 10.19a–d)

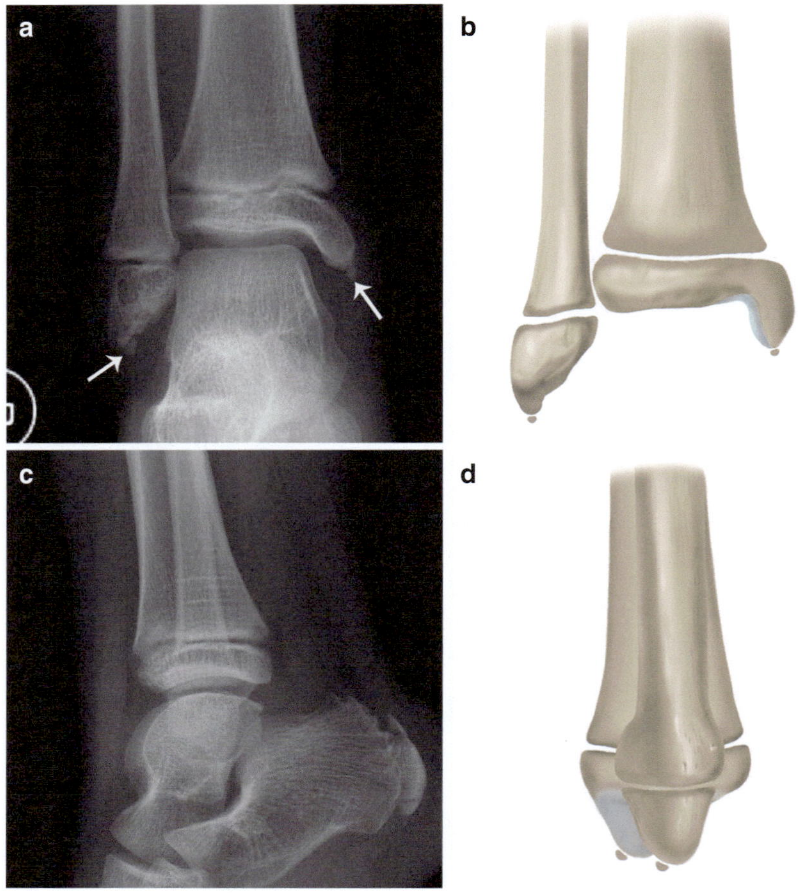

Fig. 10.19 (**a**, **c**) are the anteroposterior and lateral view of X-ray, respectively, showing an accessory bone below the tibia and fibula with smooth edges (white arrow) (**b**, **d**)

20. Identification of triangulated accessory bone and talus tail fracture
    20.1. The X-ray (Fig. 10.20a–d)

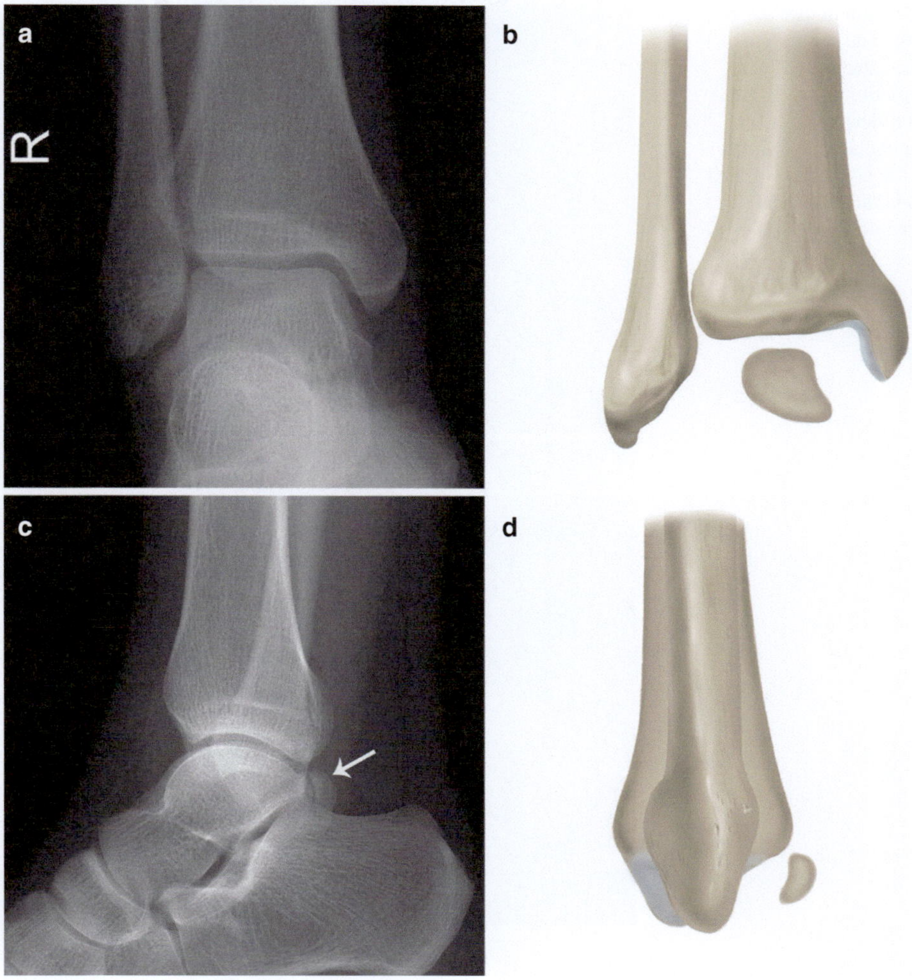

Fig. 10.20 (**a**, **c**) are the anteroposterior and lateral view of X-ray, respectively, showing an accessory bone below the tibia and fibula with smooth edges (white arrow) (**b**, **d**)

20.2. CT scan (Fig. 10.20e–h)

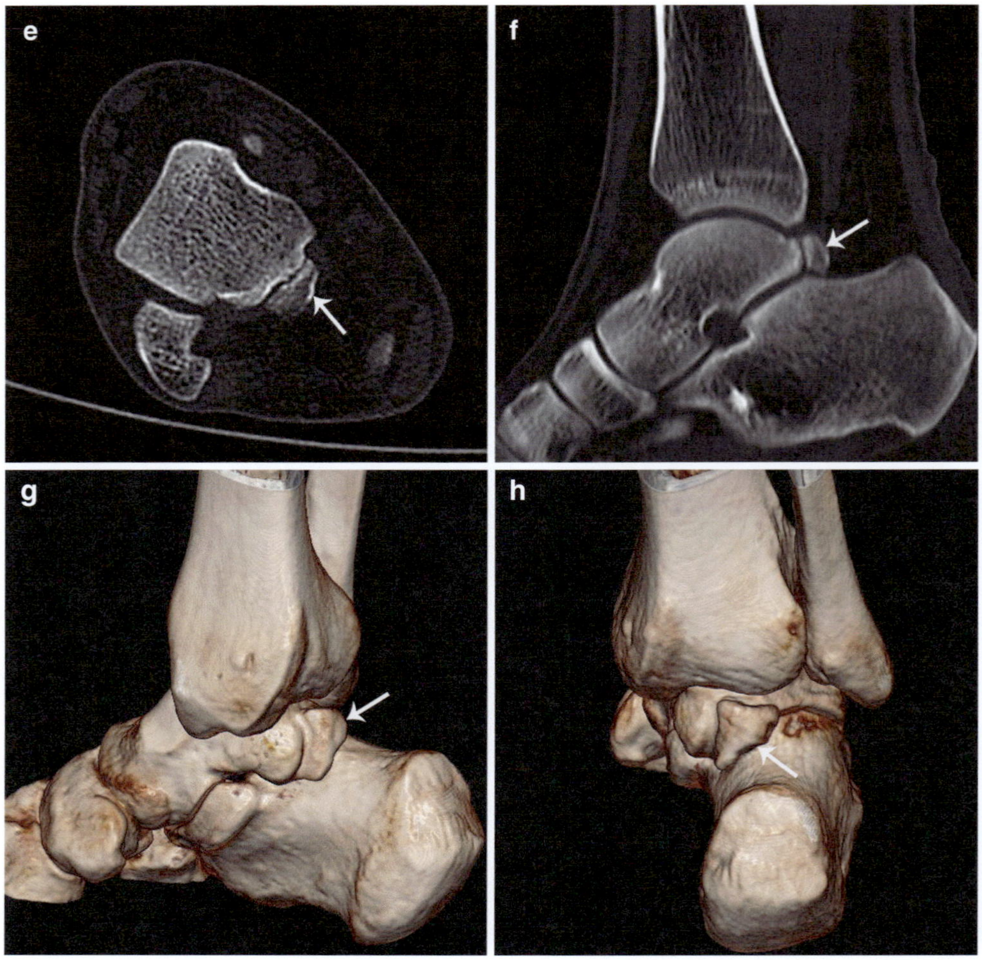

Fig. 10.20 (**e**–**h**) are CT reconstruction in the horizontal and sagittal plane, CT three-dimensional reconstruction of the internal posterior view, respectively, showing the accessory bone behind the talus, with smooth edges and intact cortical bones (white arrow)

10.2 Talus Fractures

According to the anatomical location, talus fractures can be divided into: fractures of the lateral talar process, fractures of the posterior talar process, fractures of the talar head, fractures of the talar body and fracture of the talar neck. The talar neck is the most vulnerable part and is most easy to fracture.

10.2.1 Identification of Injury Mechanism

Given the strength of talus is high, most talar fractures are caused by serious injuries, such as the traffic accidents or high falling injuries. The usual mechanism is associated with hyper-dorsiflexion of the ankle, as the talar neck impacts the anterior margin of the tibia, resulting in non-displaced fractures of the talus. If the force of dorsiflexion continues to increase, it will result in the displaced fracture of talus and dislocation of the sub-talar joint.

10.2.2 Identification of Symptoms and Signs

The most obvious manifestations are pain, swelling, limited ankle activity, yet these lack specificity, and therefore cannot be used for diagnosis. When a talar fracture cannot be ruled out, the patients need to take X-ray to exclude the possibility of a fracture.

10.2.3 Imaging Differential Diagnosis

For displaced talar fractures, conventional X-ray films can basically make accurate diagnosis. The CT scan is mainly used for patients with obvious clinical symptoms, whilst an X-ray shows no obvious fracture. At the same time, it can help to assess the degree of talus comminution. An MR scan helps to diagnose the injury of tendon and soft tissue around the talus. The triangular accessory bone is easily misdiagnosed as fractures of the posterior talar process, and CT horizontal and sagittal reconstruction can be used to differentiate it.

1. Identification of the fractures of lateral talar process and non-fractures
   1.1. The CT scan (Fig. 10.21a–d)

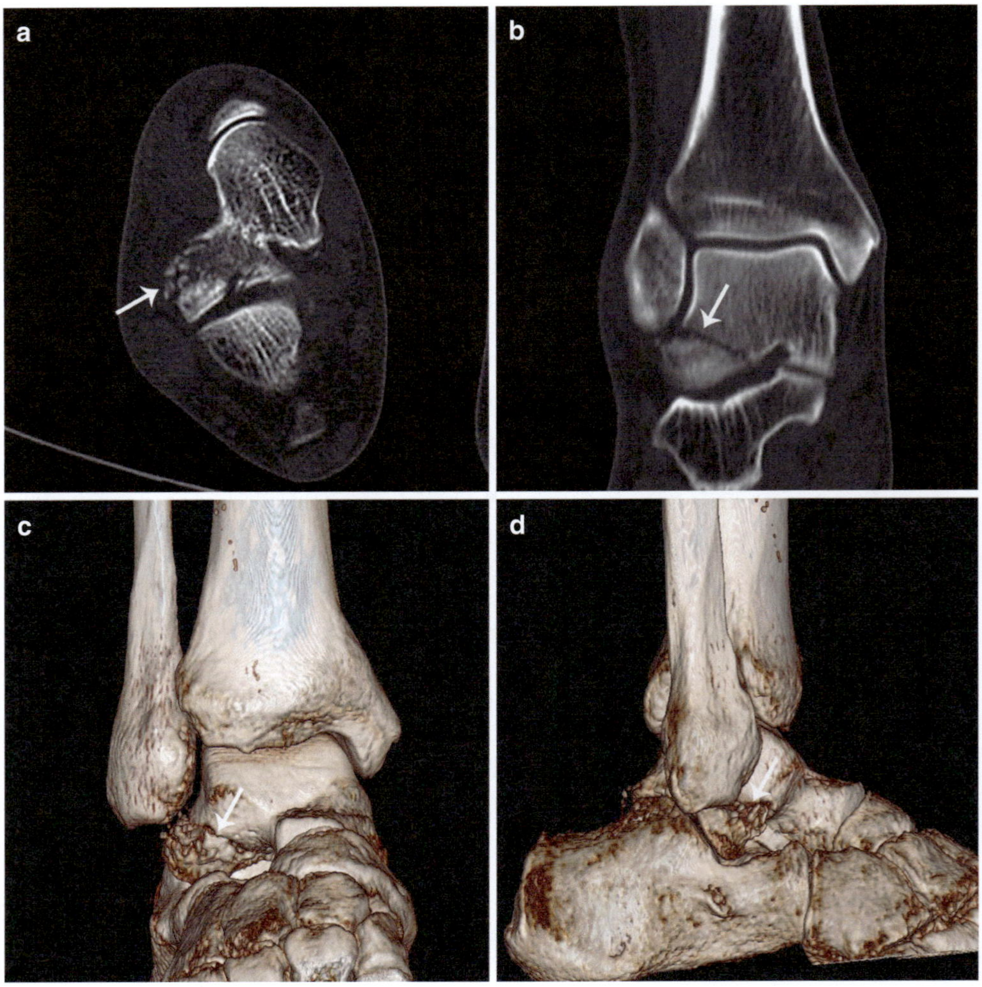

Fig. 10.21 (**a**–**d**) are CT reconstruction in horizontal and sagittal plane, CT three-dimensional reconstruction of the anterior and lateral view, respectively, showing the fractures of lateral talar process (white arrow)

2. Identification of the fractures of the posterior talar process and non-fractures
   2.1. The X-ray (Fig. 10.22a–d)

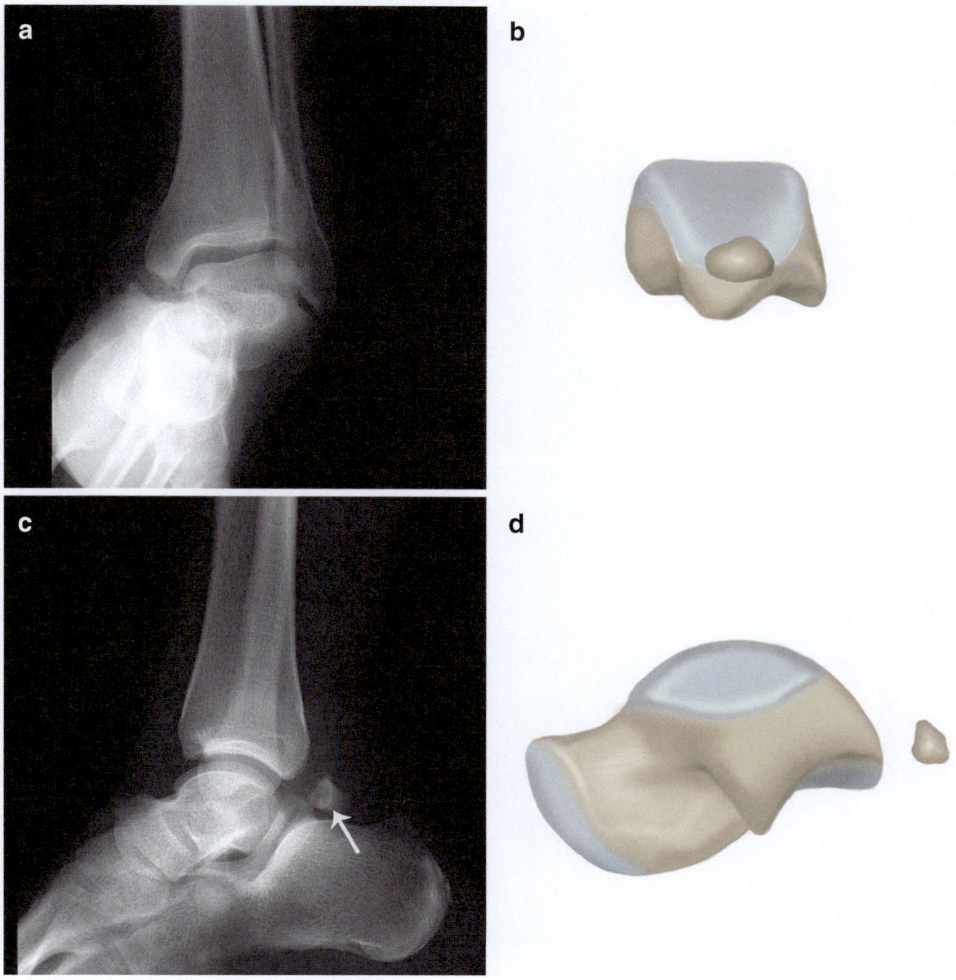

Fig. 10.22 (**a**, **c**) are the anteroposterior and lateral view of X–ray, respectively, showing the fractures of posterior talar process (**b**, **d**)

2.2. CT scan (Fig. 10.22e–h)

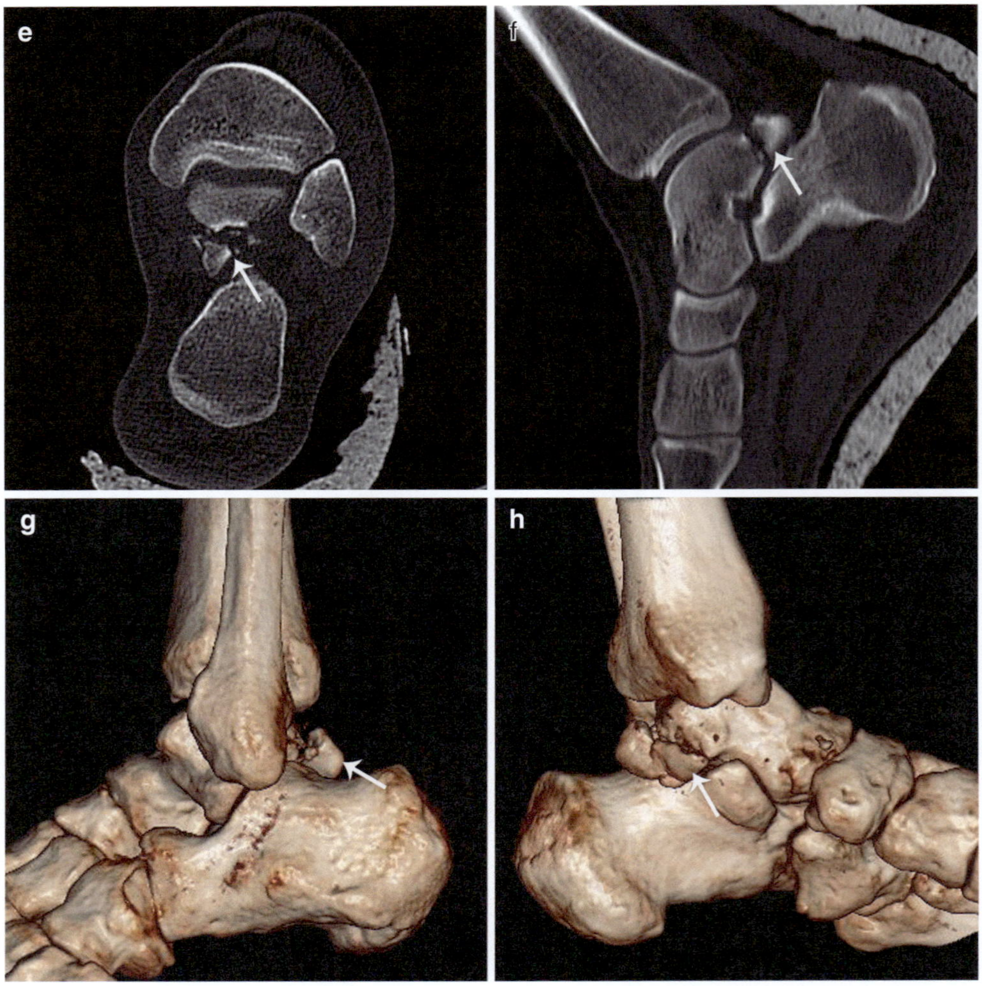

Fig. 10.22 (**e**–**h**) are CT reconstruction in horizontal and sagittal plane, CT three-dimensional reconstruction of the lateral and posterior view, respectively, showing the fractures of posterior talar process (white arrow)

3. The fractures of the talar body and the talar neck
   3.1. The X-ray (Fig. 10.23a–d)

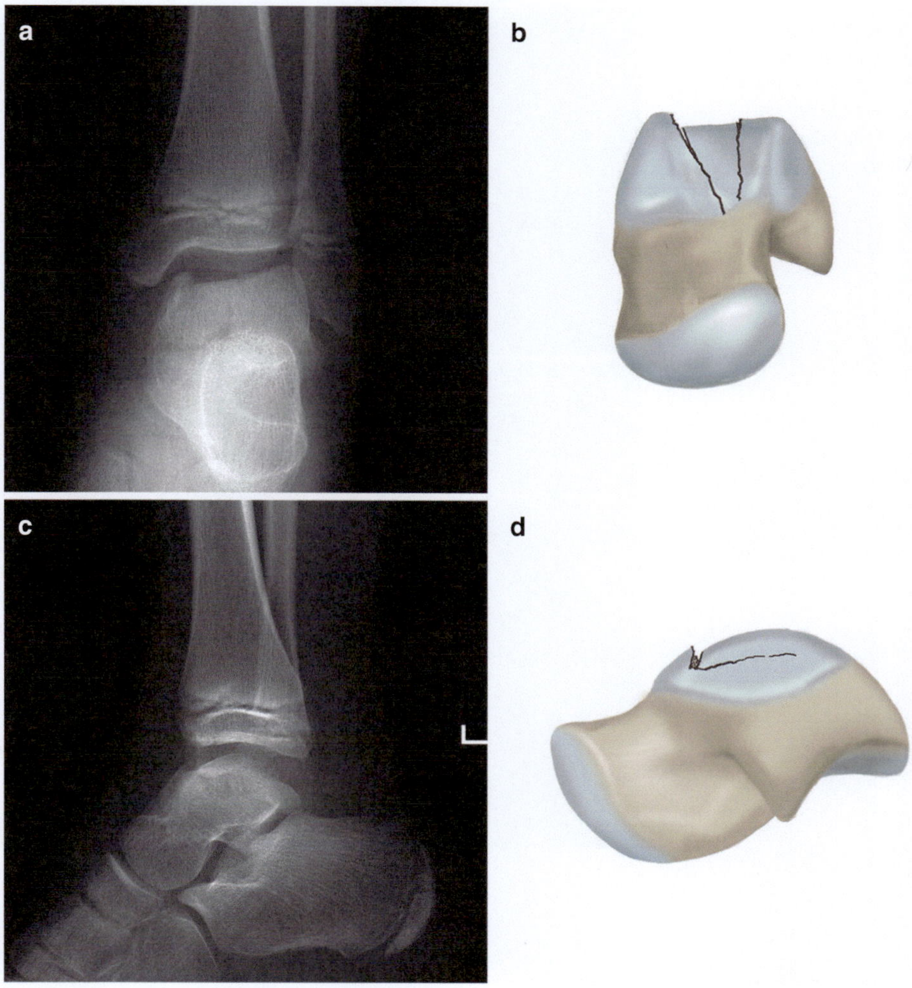

Fig. 10.23 (**a**, **c**) are the anteroposterior and lateral view of X-ray, respectively, showing the fractures of the talar body and the talar neck (**b**, **d**)

3.2. CT scan (Fig. 10.23e–h)

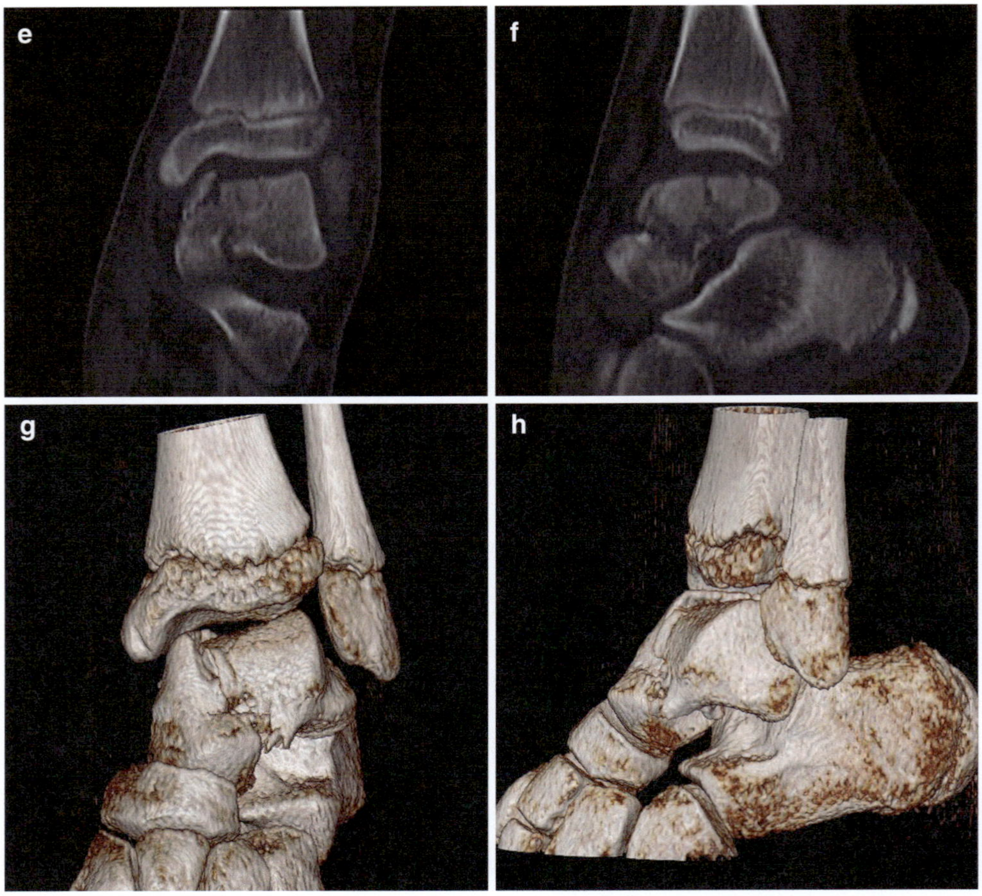

Fig. 10.23 (**e**–**h**) are CT reconstruction in coronal and sagittal plane, CT three-dimensional reconstruction of the anterior and lateral view, respectively, showing the fractures of the talar body and the talar neck

4. The fractures of talar head
   4.1. CT scan (Fig. 10.24a–d)

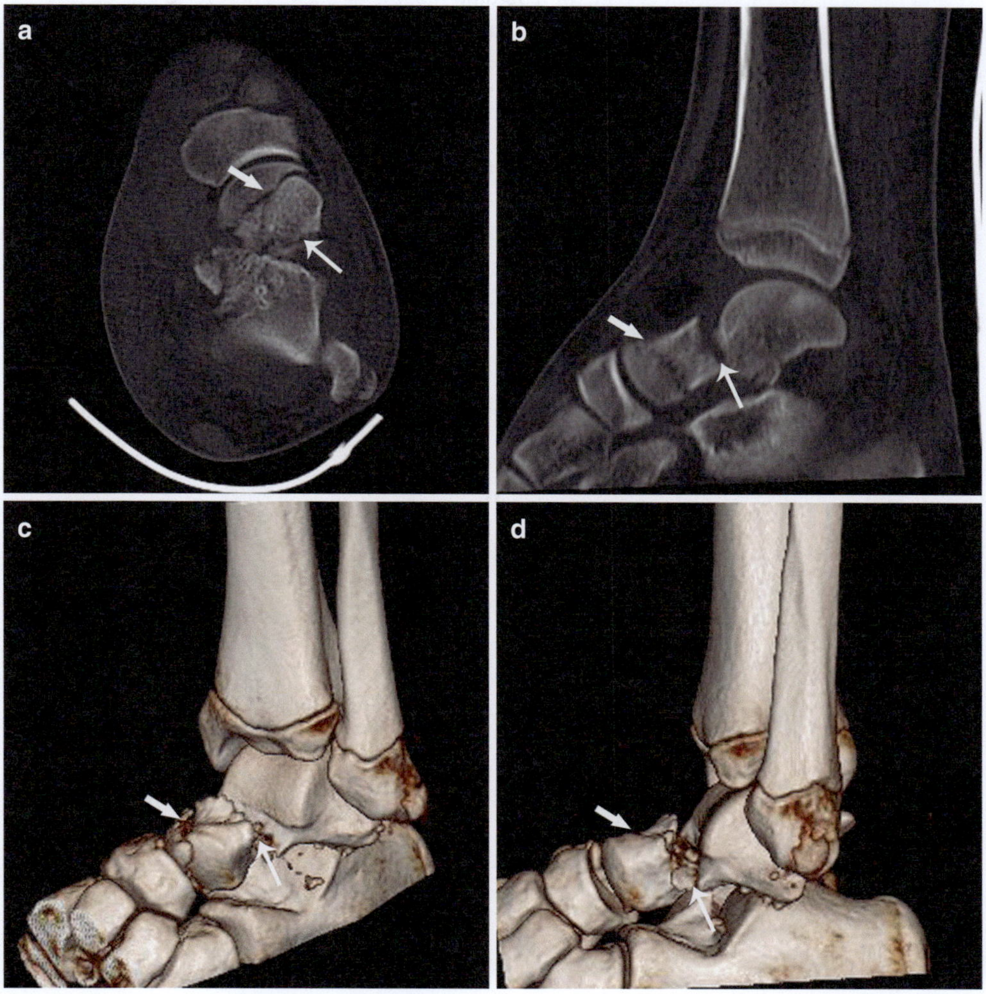

Fig. 10.24 (**a–d**) are CT reconstruction images in horizontal and sagittal plane, CT three-dimensional reconstruction of the anterior and lateral view, respectively, showing the fractures of the talar neck and the talar head

10.3 Summary

1. Anatomical features of the ankle joint: the lateral malleolus is 1–1.5 cm longer than the medial malleolus and is lower, and the talar trochlear joint is wide in front and narrow in back. Therefore, it is easy to cause the plantar flexion and varus injury of the ankle joint.
2. The ligaments are strengthened around the ankle joint; therefore, ankle injuries often cause fracture and/or ligament damage. Fractures of the anterior, inferior and lateral edge of the tibia at the attachment of the inferior tibiofibular ligament and the posterior malleolus fracture are easy to misdiagnosis on plain film; therefore, a CT scan is necessary. When combined ligament damage occurs, it requires an MRI scan to assess. The outline of the MRI is parallel to the inspected ligament to scan.
3. Attention should be paid to the concomitant high fibular fractures in valgus and external rotation ankle injuries.
4. Epiphyseal injuries and ligament injuries in children are also good indications for MR examination.
5. The accessory bone of the ankle should be carefully identified on the X-ray film. Common accessory bones include the sub-tibial bone, the sub-fibular bone and the triangular accessory bone. The shape is mostly round, the edge is smooth, the bone cortex is complete, all of which should be identified with the fracture.

Foot Fractures

11

Qi Zhang and Yingze Zhang

11.1 Calcaneal Fracture

The calcaneus is the largest tarsal bone, resembling a rectangular-like structure, with 3 talus joints and 1 cuboid joint. The heel joint is divided into three groups, which is located above the calcaneus. The posterior articular surface is oval, located in the middle of the calcaneus, whilst the middle articular surface is the flat protuberance of the medial calcaneus. The front of the articular surface is situated in front of the calcaneus and the joint from the bone. The calcaneal joint is located in front of the calcaneus. A fracture of the calcaneus accounts for 29.77% of the foot fracture. Calcaneal fractures are commonly categorized using the Sanders classification: The Sanders classification of calcaneal fractures is divided into four types: non-displaced intra-articular fracture; two parts fractures of the posterior articular surface, displacement greater than 2 mm, three parts fractures of the posterior articular surface, and more than four parts of the posterior articular surface. Furthermore, the two parts fracture of the posterior articular surface fracture, whereby its displacement is greater than or equal to 2 mm, is divided into three parts: IIA, lateral fracture line, IIB, medial fracture line, and IIC, fracture line adjacent to the loading process. Overall, the three parts of the posterior articular surface were divided into three parts: IIIAB, IIIAC, IIIBC.

11.1.1 Identification of Injury Mechanism

The most common injury mechanism of calcaneal fractures are landing with force exerted onto the high heel. Identifying this mechanism of injury is easy.

11.1.2 Symptoms and Signs

Symptoms of the fracture are pain, swelling, and limited activity of the heel. Thus, the patient experiences difficulty in walking. Due to the symptoms lacking specificity, it is difficult to make a definite diagnosis. Therefore, an X-ray or CT scan should be carried out when a fracture is suspected. We should pay attention to calcaneal fractures given it is combined with spinal fractures to prevent a missed diagnosis.

11.1.3 Imaging Differential Diagnosis

Conventional X-ray films can be used to diagnose calcaneal fractures, but CT 3D reconstruction can show the position of the fracture line more clearly. Thus, calcaneus CT scan is vital in the clinic.

Q. Zhang · Y. Zhang (✉)
Department of Orthopaedics, The Third Hospital of Hebei Medical University, Shijiazhuang, Hebei, China

Y. Zhang (ed.), *Differential Diagnosis of Fracture*, https://doi.org/10.1007/978-981-13-8339-7_11

1. X-ray film versus CT for intra-articular fractures of the calcaneus without displacement
   1.1 X-ray film (Fig. 11.1a, b)

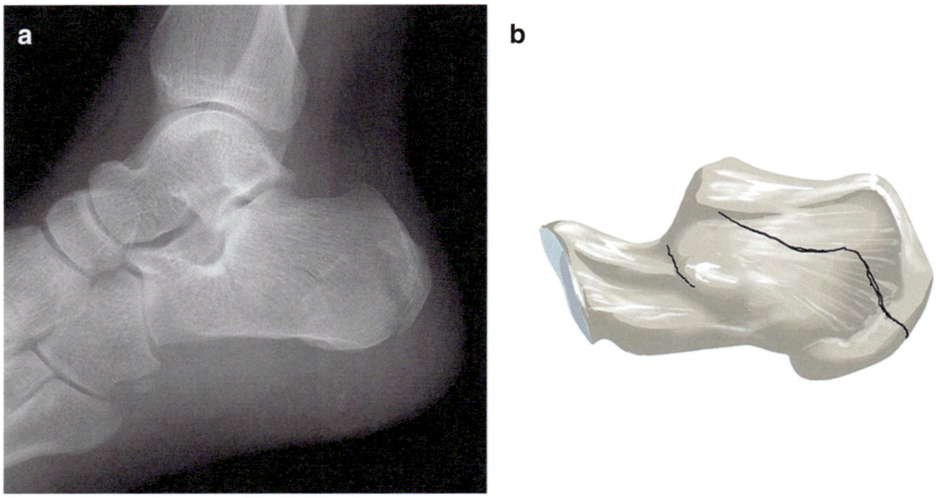

Fig. 11.1 X-ray film (**a**) shows a fracture of the calcaneal body. The fracture line involved the heel to the articular surface. There was no obvious dislocation at the end of the calcaneus (**b**)

   1.2 CT scan (Fig. 11.1c–e)

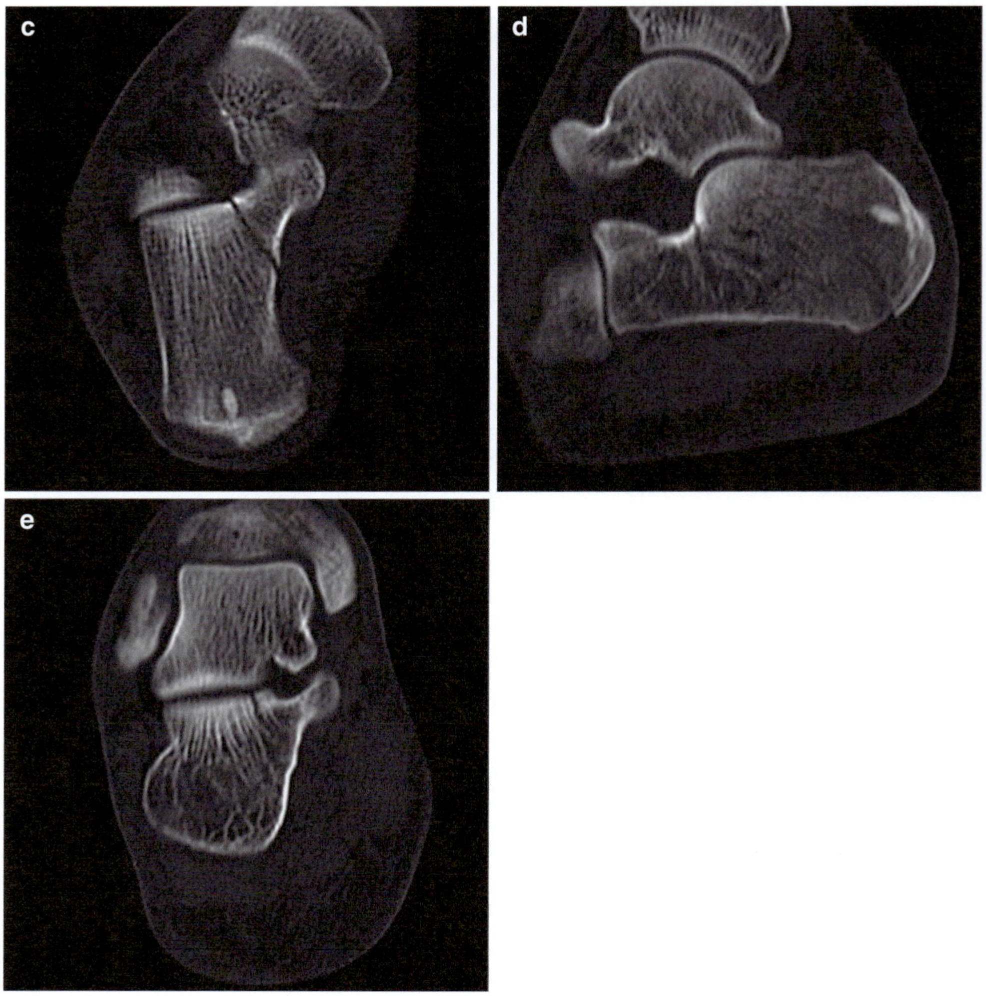

Fig. 11.1 CT cross section (**c**), sagittal plane (**d**), and oblique coronal surface (**e**) show an oblique bone fracture of the calcaneus body. Fracture line involves the inner block of the heel and the medial part of the articular surface, and there is no obvious dislocation in the broken end

2. X-ray film versus CT for intra-articular fractures of the calcaneus without displacement
   2.1 X-ray film (Fig. 11.2a–d)

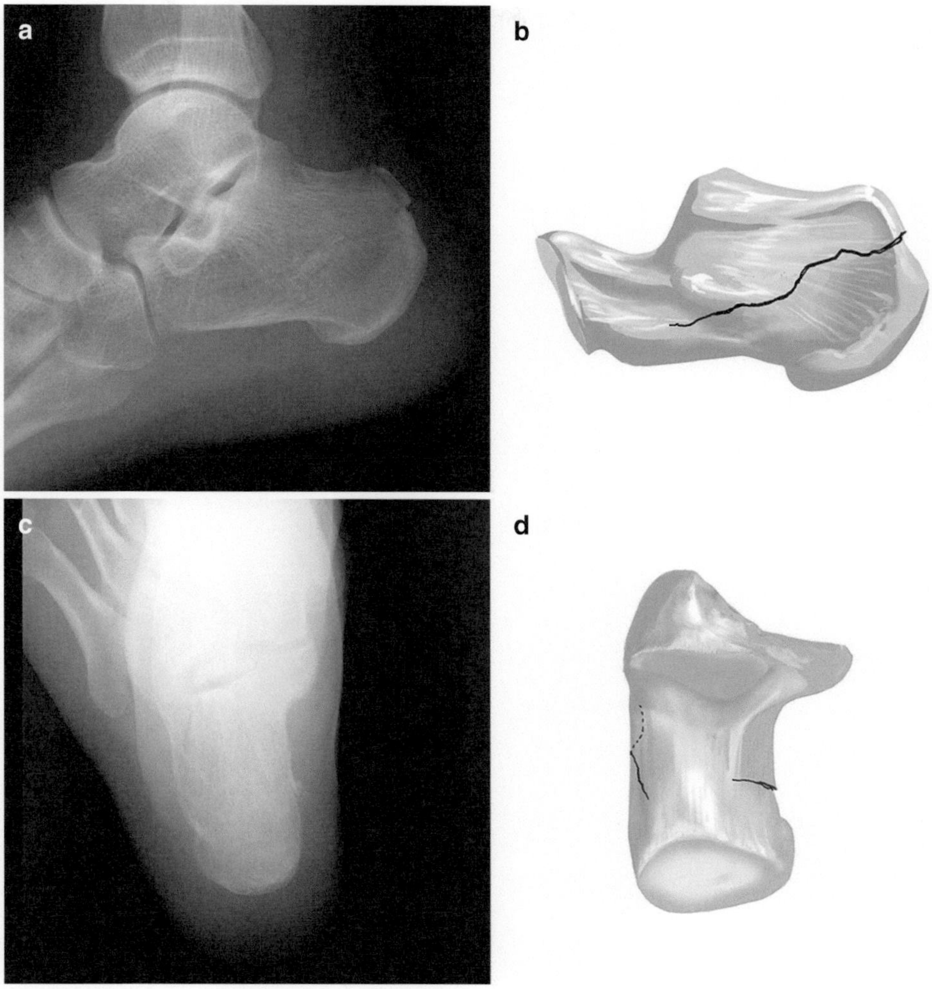

Fig. 11.2 X-ray plain film (**a**, **c**) shows the fracture of the calcaneal body, and the dislocation of the ends was not obvious. The schematic diagram (**b**, **d**)

   2.2 CT scan (Fig. 11.2e, f)

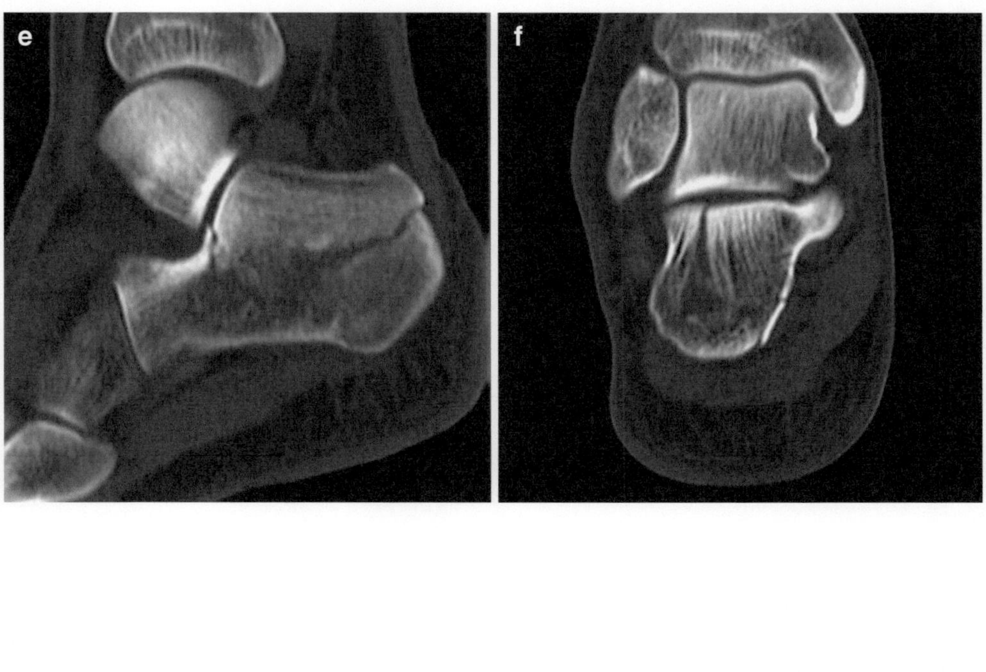

Fig. 11.2 CT sagittal plane (**e**) and oblique coronal surface (**f**) show an oblique bone fracture of the calcaneal body. The fracture line involves the lateral mass of the heel and the lateral part of the articular surface. There is no obvious dislocation in the broken end

3. X-ray film with simple intra-articular fracture of calcaneus compared with CT
   3.1 X-ray film (Fig. 11.3a–d)

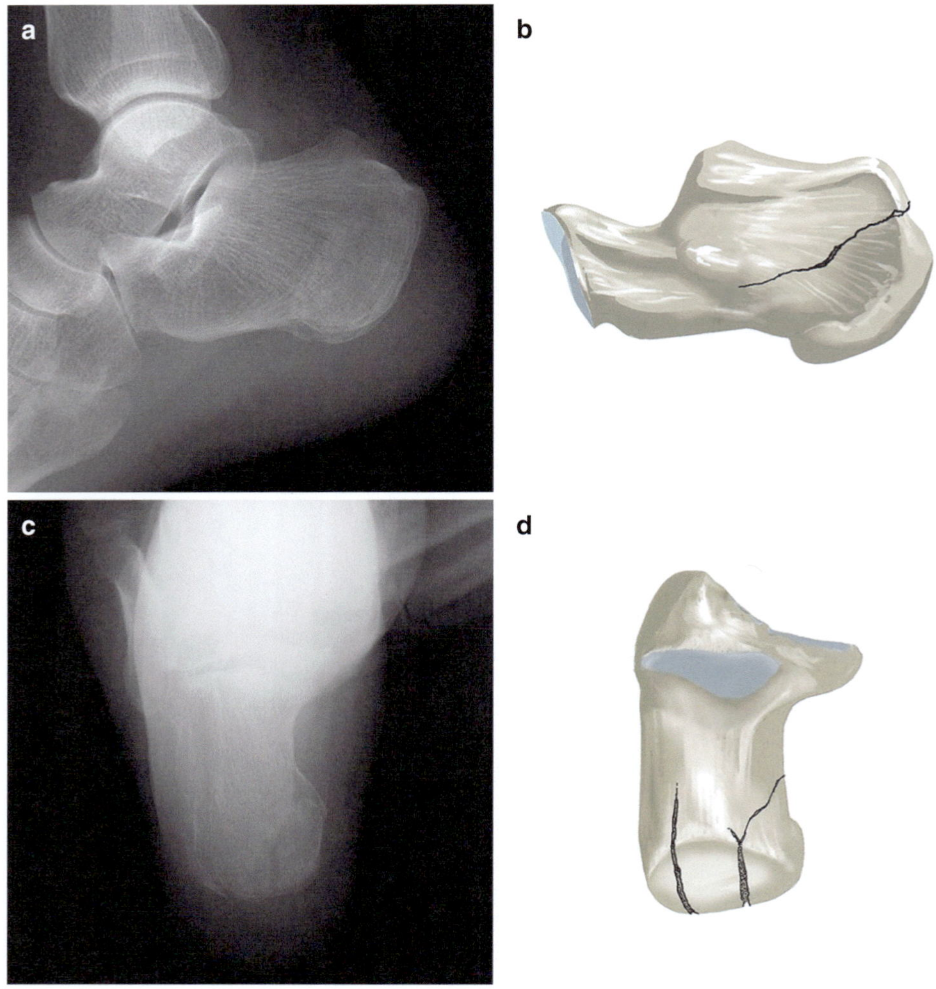

Fig. 11.3 X-ray film (**a**, **c**) shows a fracture of the calcaneal body, with a slightly inserted end and a misplaced position. The schematic diagram (**b**, **d**)

   3.2 CT scan (Fig. 11.3e, f)

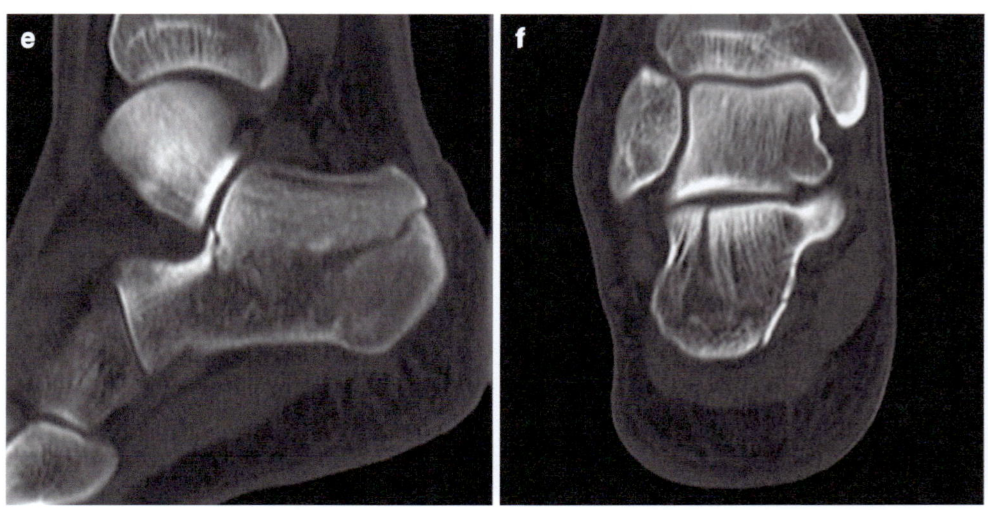

Fig. 11.3 CT sagittal plane (**e**) and oblique coronal plane (**f**) show a bone fracture of the calcaneus. The fracture line involved the posterior heel from the central part of the articular surface and there was no obvious dislocation at the end of the fracture

4. Comparison between plain film and CT of calcaneal type II A fracture
   4.1 X-ray film (Fig. 11.4a–d)

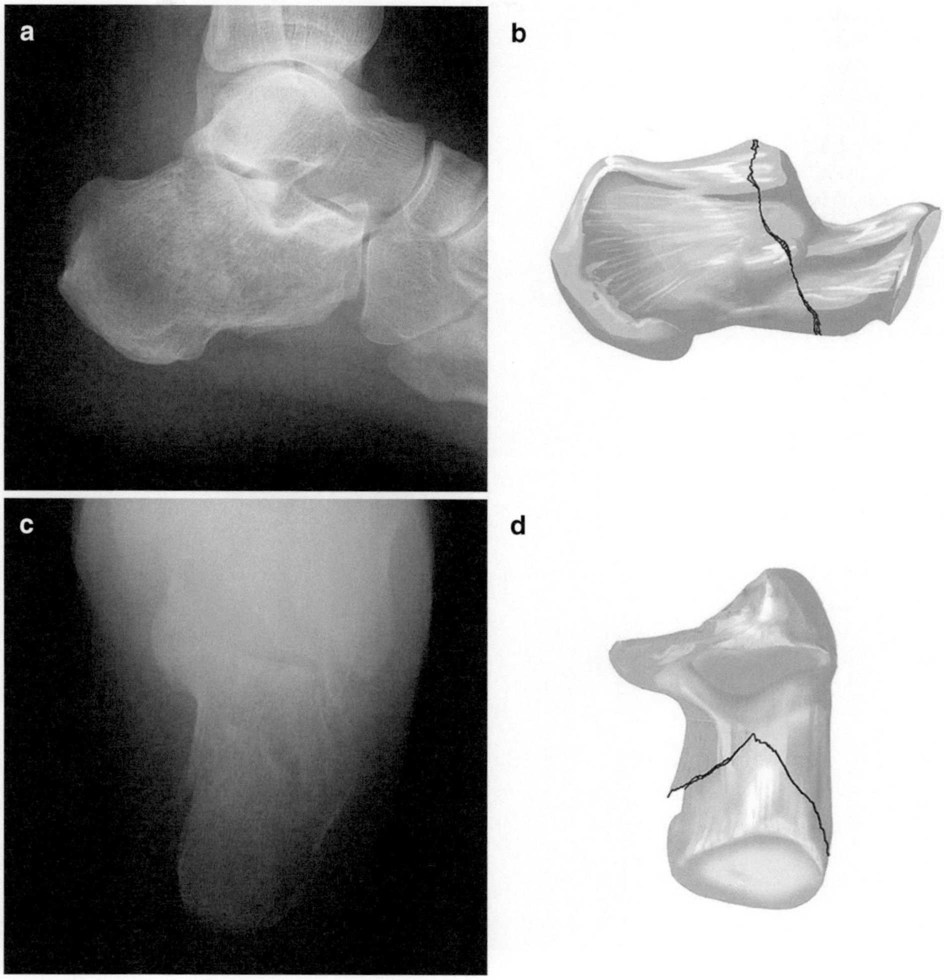

Fig. 11.4 X-ray film (**a**, **c**) shows the fracture of the calcaneal body, the dislocation was not obvious, and the lateral side of the calcaneus was raised outward (**b**, **d**)

4.2 CT scan (Fig. 11.4e–h)

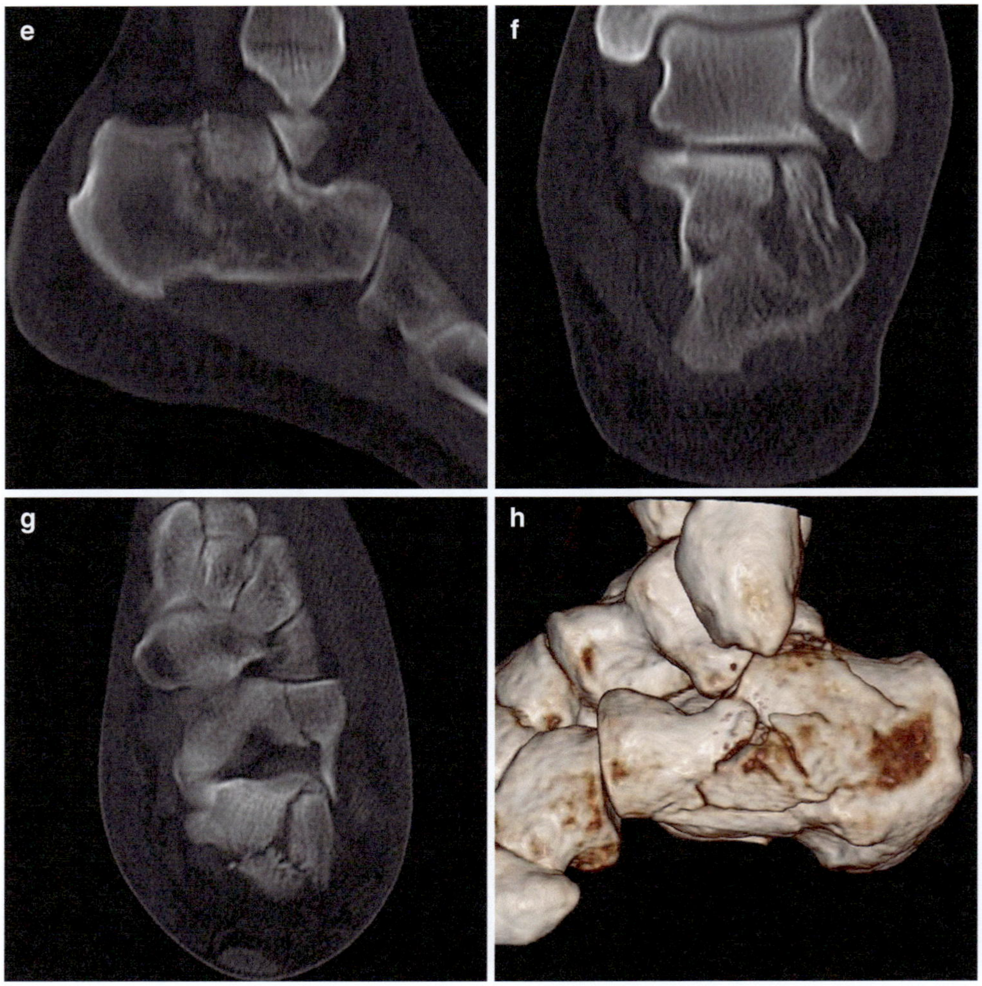

Fig. 11.4 CT sagittal plane (**e**), oblique coronal surface (**f**), cross section (**g**), and three-dimensional reconstruction (**h**) show the fracture of the calcaneal body and bone. The fracture line involves the lateral mass of the heel to the articular surface, the fracture line widened, and the calcaneus to the lateral bulge

5. Comparison between plain film and CT of calcaneal type II A fracture
   5.1 X-ray plain film (Fig. 11.5a–d)

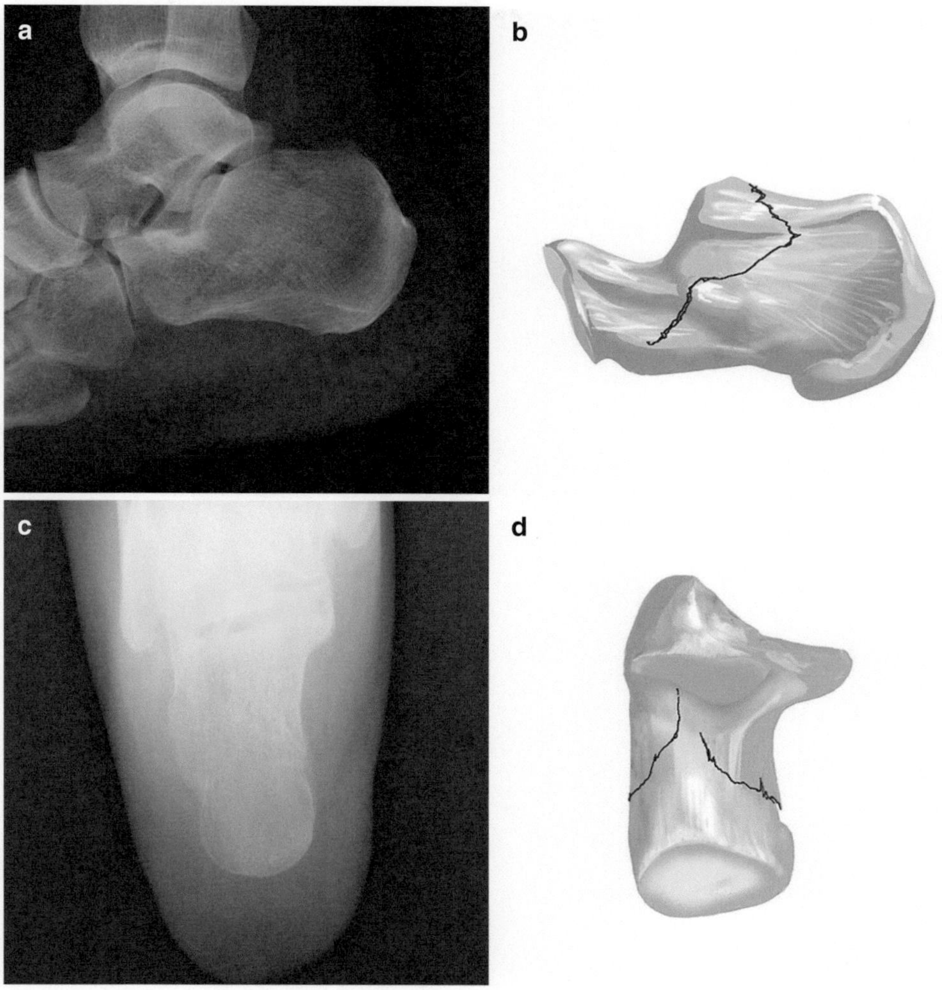

Fig. 11.5 X-ray film (**a**, **c**) shows a fracture of the calcaneal body, with a slightly inserted end and a misplaced position. The schematic diagram (**b**, **d**)

   5.2 CT scan (Fig. 11.5e, f)

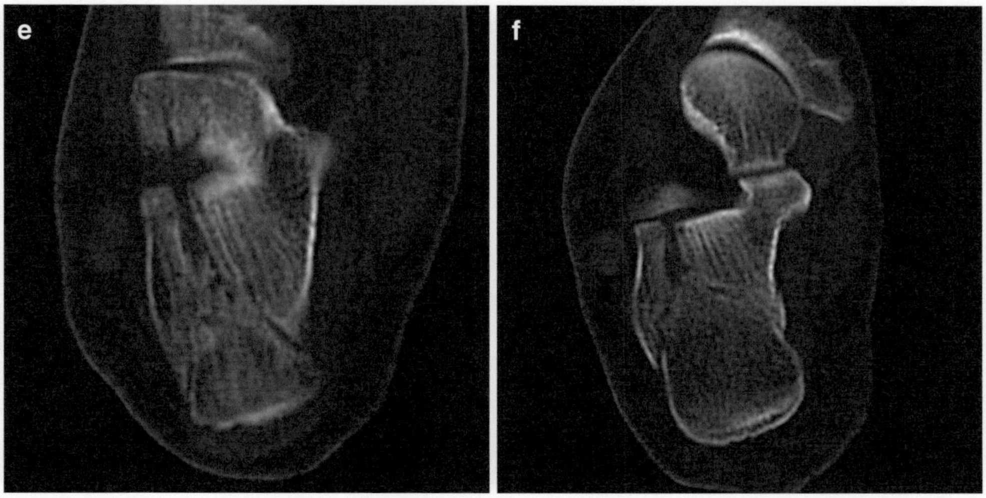

Fig. 11.5 CT sagittal plane (**e**) and oblique coronal surface (**f**) show the fracture of the calcaneal body and bone. The fracture line involves the lateral mass of the heel and the lateral part of the articular surface. The joint surface is slightly dislocation and the fracture line is wide

6. Comparison between plain film and CT of calcaneal type II A fracture
   6.1 X-ray film (Fig. 11.6a–d)

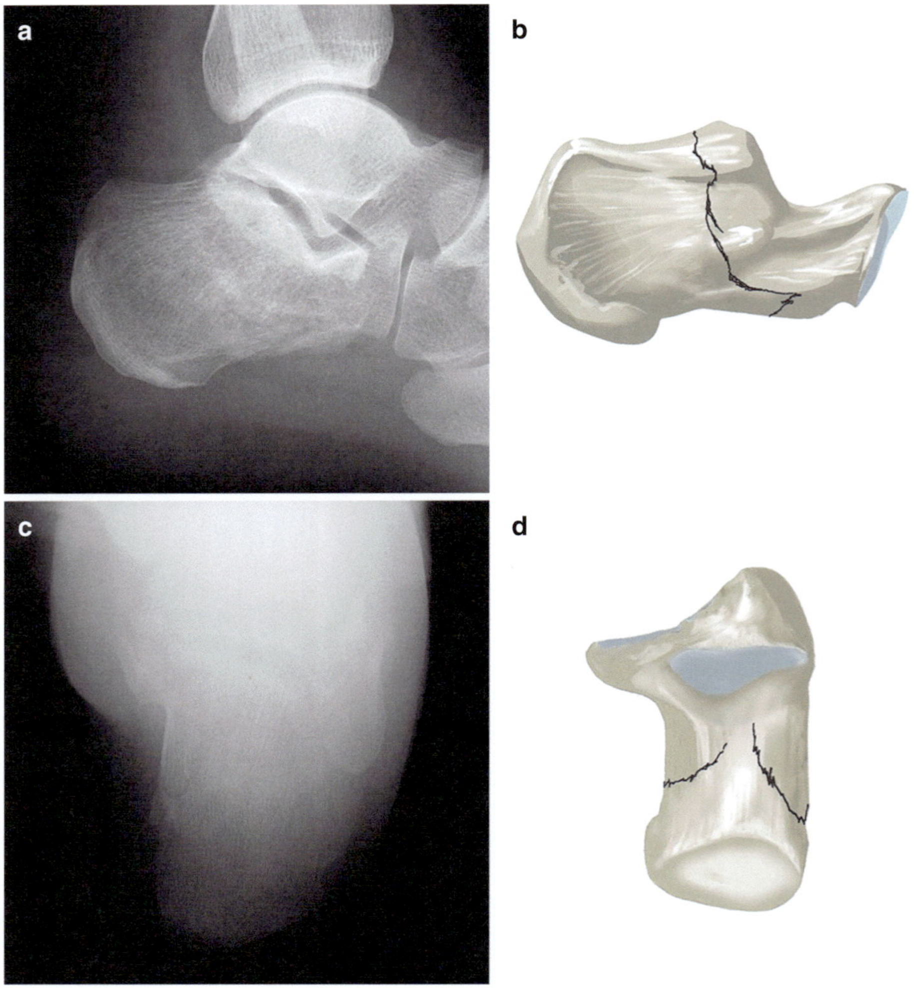

Fig. 11.6 X-ray film (**a**, **c**) shows a fracture of the calcaneal body, with a slightly inserted end of the calcaneus and a lateral uplift of the calcaneus (**b**, **d**)

   6.2 CT scan (Fig. 11.6e, f)

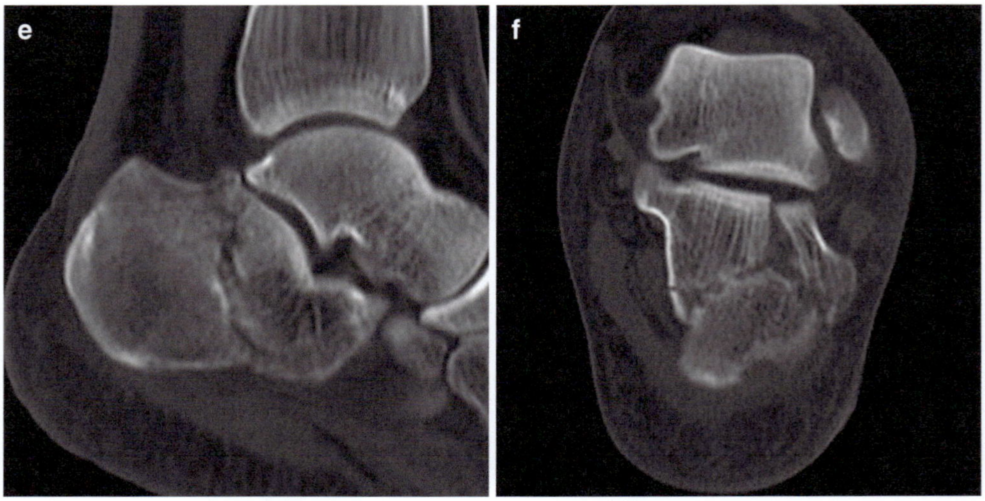

Fig. 11.6 CT sagittal plane (**e**) and oblique coronal surface (**f**) show the fracture of the calcaneal body and bone. The fracture line involves the lateral mass of the heel and the lateral part of the articular surface. The joint surface is slightly dislocation, the fracture line is wide, and the lateral calcaneus is outward

7. Comparison between plain film and CT of calcaneal type II A fracture
   7.1 X-ray film (Fig. 11.7a, b)

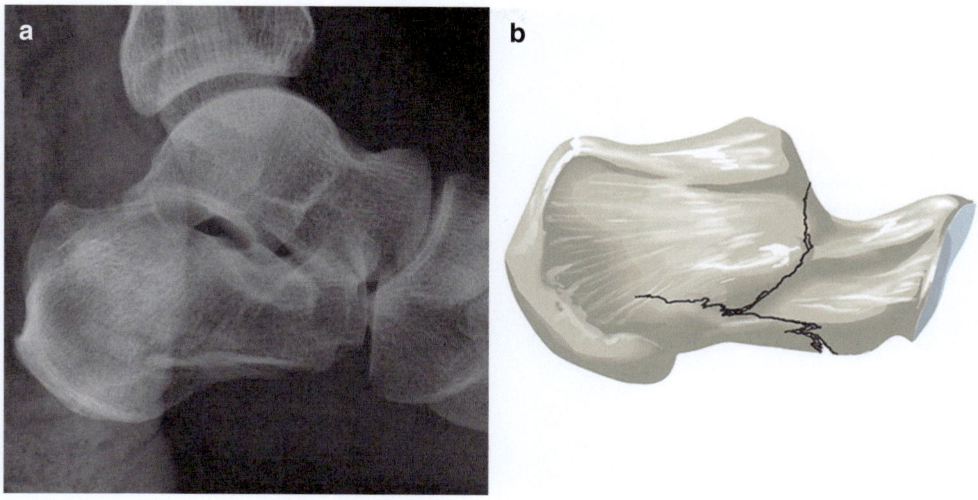

Fig. 11.7 X-ray plain film (**a**) shows the calcaneal heel was collapsed from the articular surface, the end of the calcaneus was embedded, and the angle of the talus was smaller. The schematic diagram (**b**)

   7.2 CT scan (Fig. 11.7c–e)

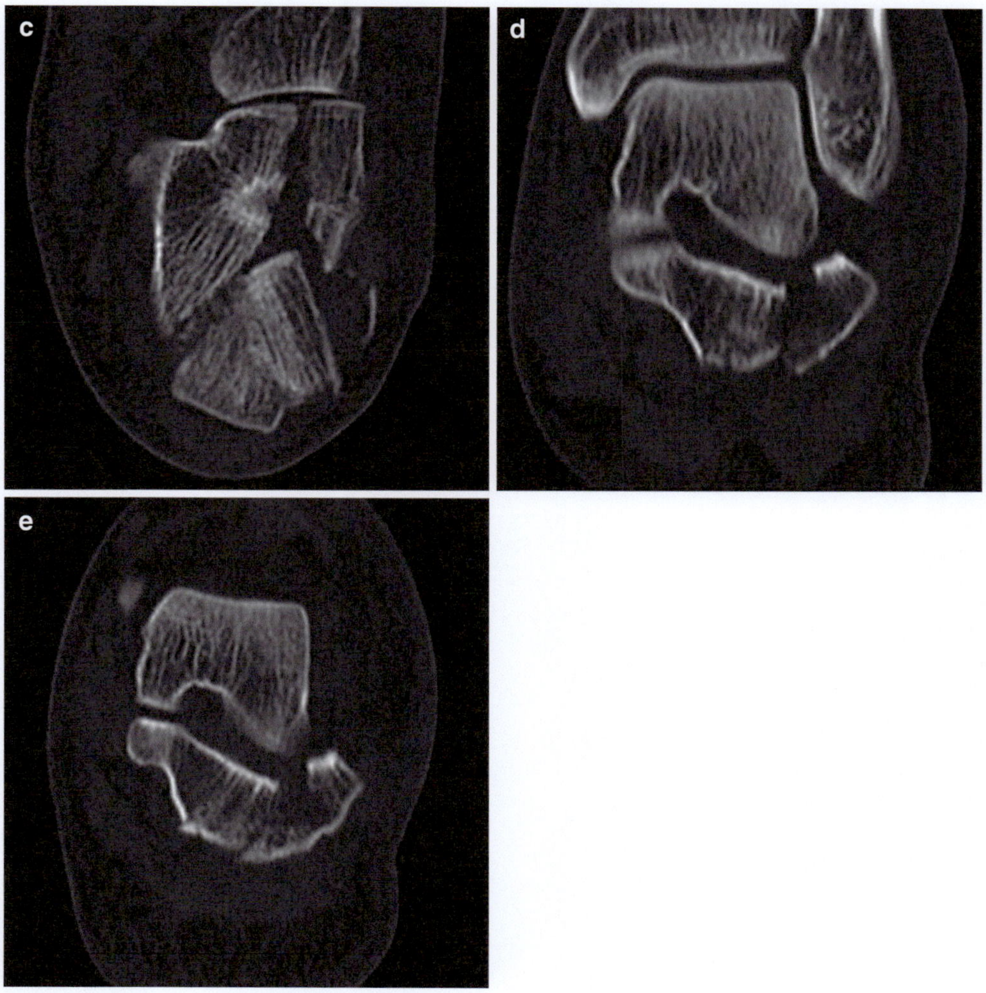

Fig. 11.7 CT transverse section (**c**) and oblique coronal plane (**d**, **e**) show the fracture of the calcaneus, and the fracture line involved the lateral heel from the lateral surface of the joint

8. Comparison between X-ray film and CT of calcaneal type IIB fracture
   8.1 X-ray film (Fig. 11.8a–d)

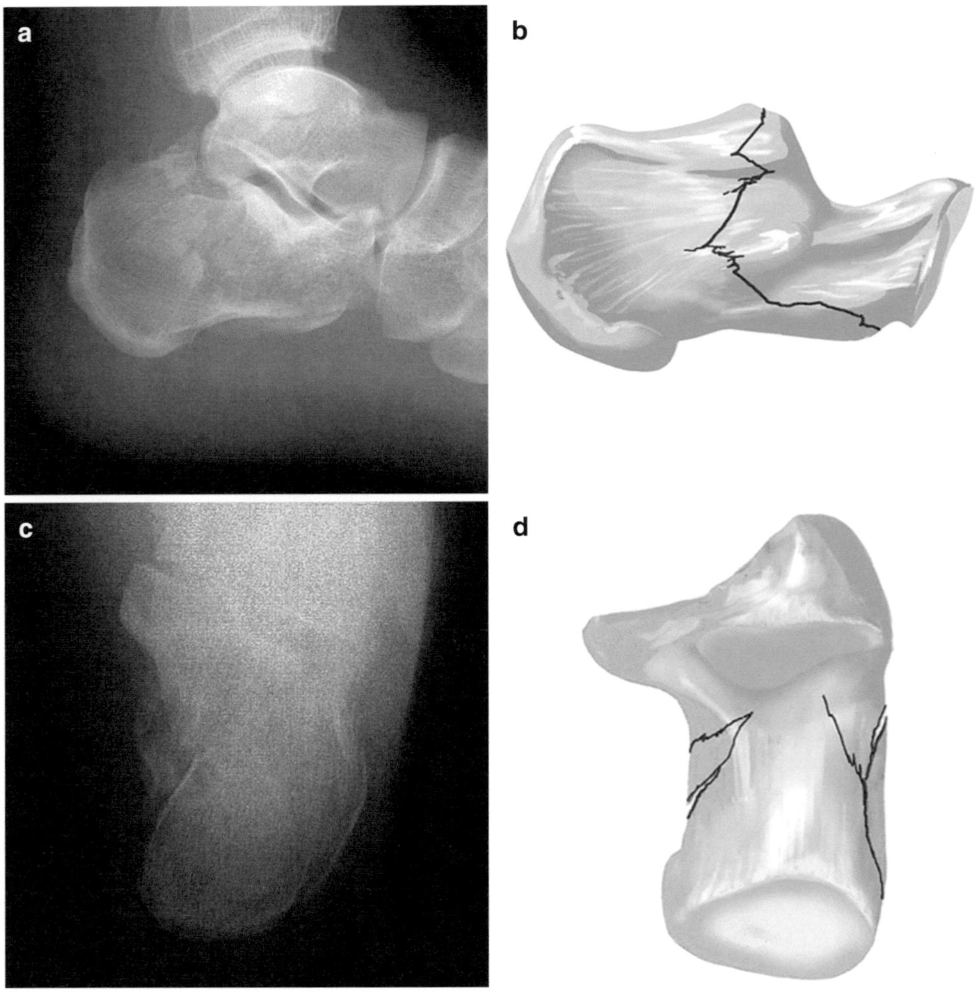

Fig. 11.8 X-ray film (**a**, **c**) shows that the calcaneal heel was collapsed from the articular surface, the end of the calcaneus was embedded and misplaced, and the calcaneus widened outward to show its elevation (**b**, **d**)

   8.2 CT scan (Fig. 11.8e, f)

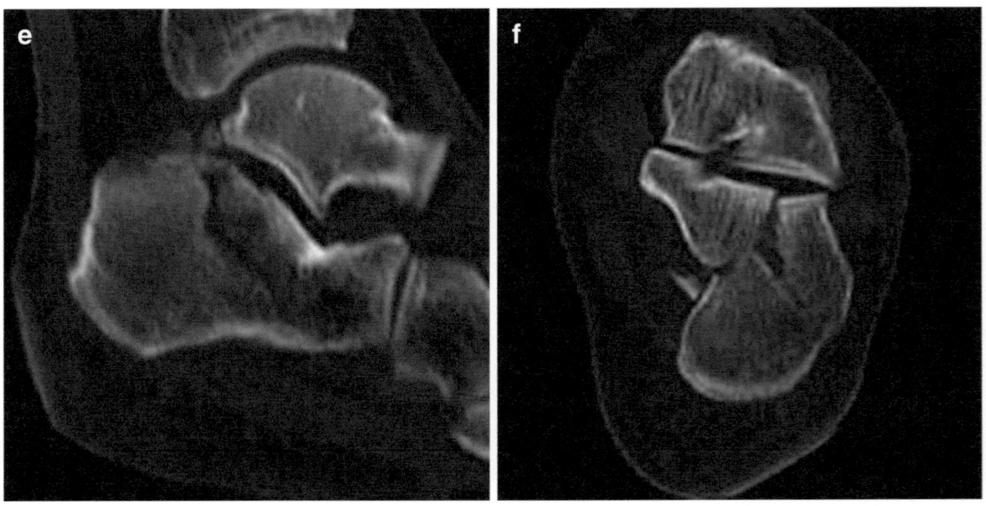

Fig. 11.8 CT sagittal plane (**e**) and oblique coronal surface (**f**) show the collapse of the heel of the calcaneus. The fracture line involves the central block of the heel, the dislocation of the articular surface, the width of the fracture line, the widening of the calcaneus, and the outward eminence

9. Comparison between X-ray film and CT of calcaneal type II B fracture
   9.1 X-ray film (Fig. 11.9a–d)

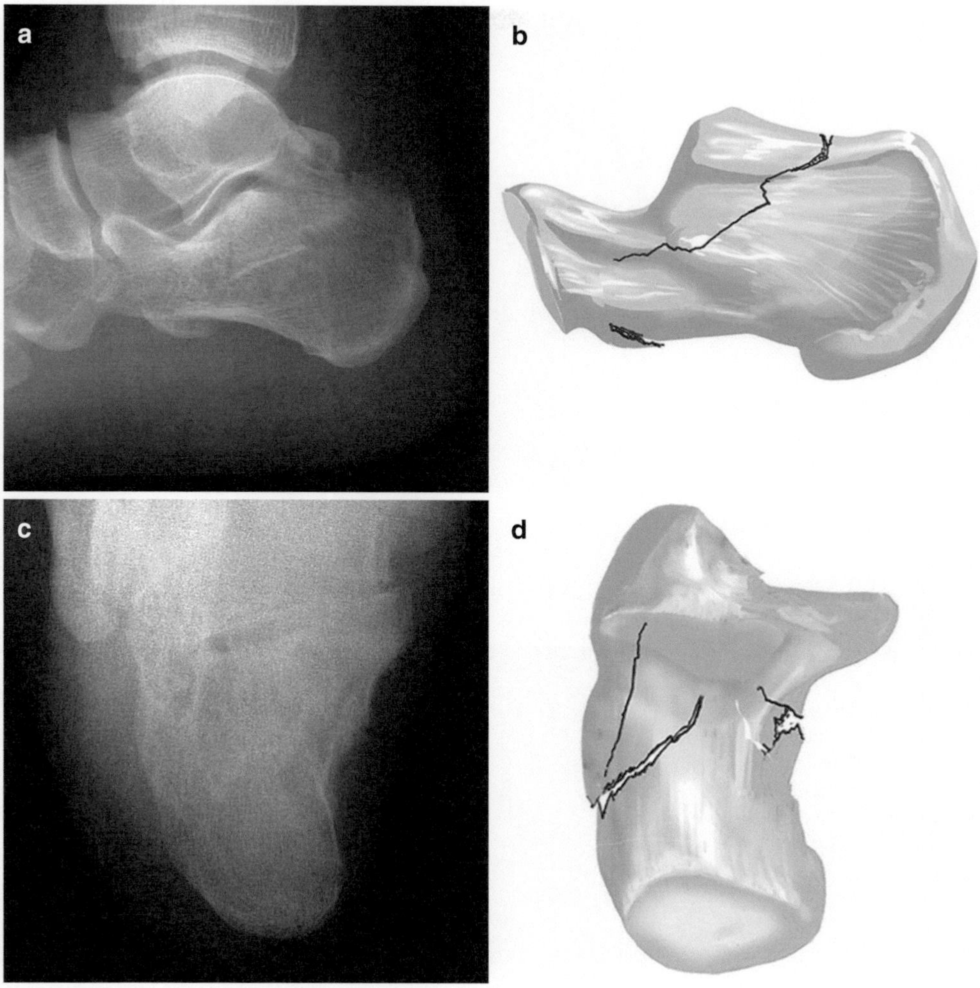

Fig. 11.9 X-ray film (**a**, **c**) shows the posterior calcaneal talar articular surface collapse, insertion of the broken end, slightly dislocation, calcaneal widening, schematic diagram (**b**, **d**)

   9.2 CT scan (Fig. 11.9e, f)

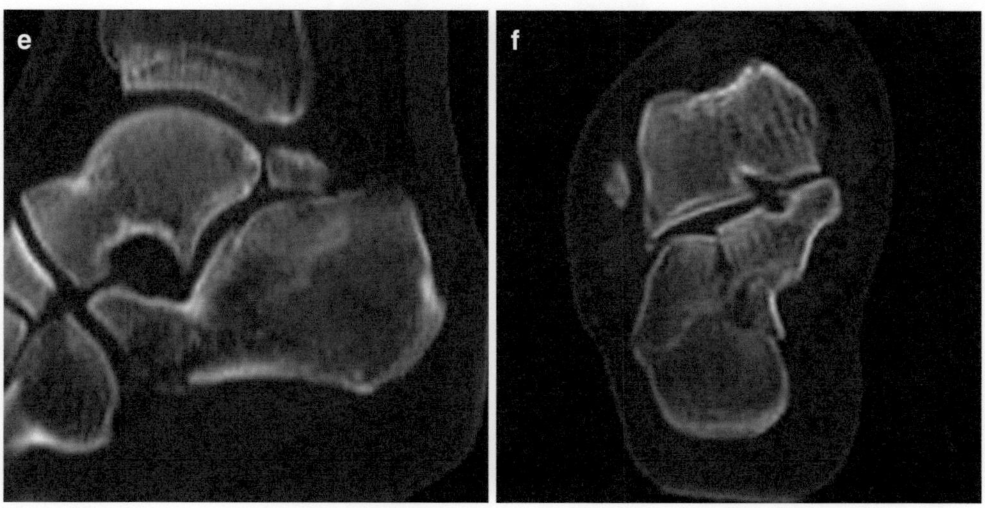

Fig. 11.9 CT sagittal plane (**e**) and oblique coronal surface (**f**) show the collapse of the heel of the calcaneus. The fracture line involves the central block of the heel, the dislocation of the articular surface, and the widening of the calcaneus

10. Comparison between X-ray film and CT of calcaneal type II B fracture
    10.1 X-ray film (Fig. 11.10a, b)

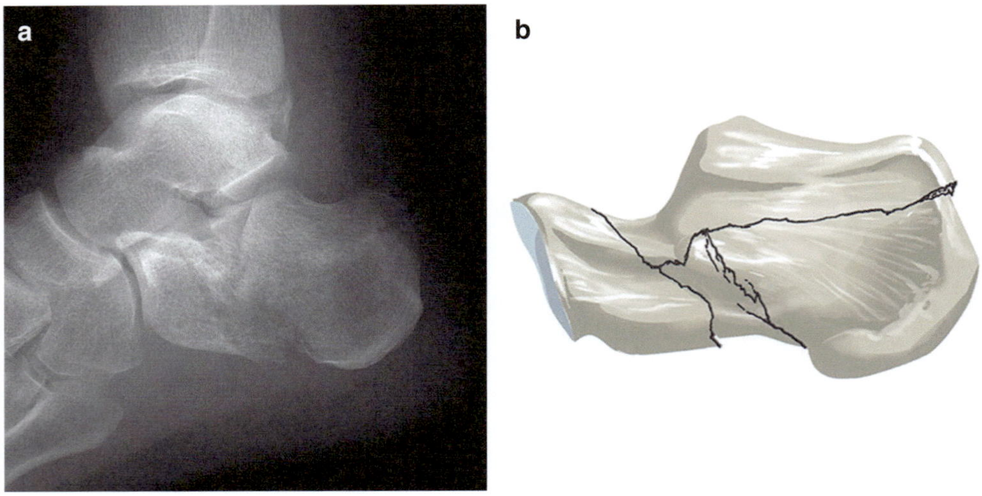

Fig. 11.10 X-ray film (**a**) showed bone fracture of calcaneus, broken ends embedded, and smaller angles (**b**)

10.2 CT scan (Fig. 11.10c–e)

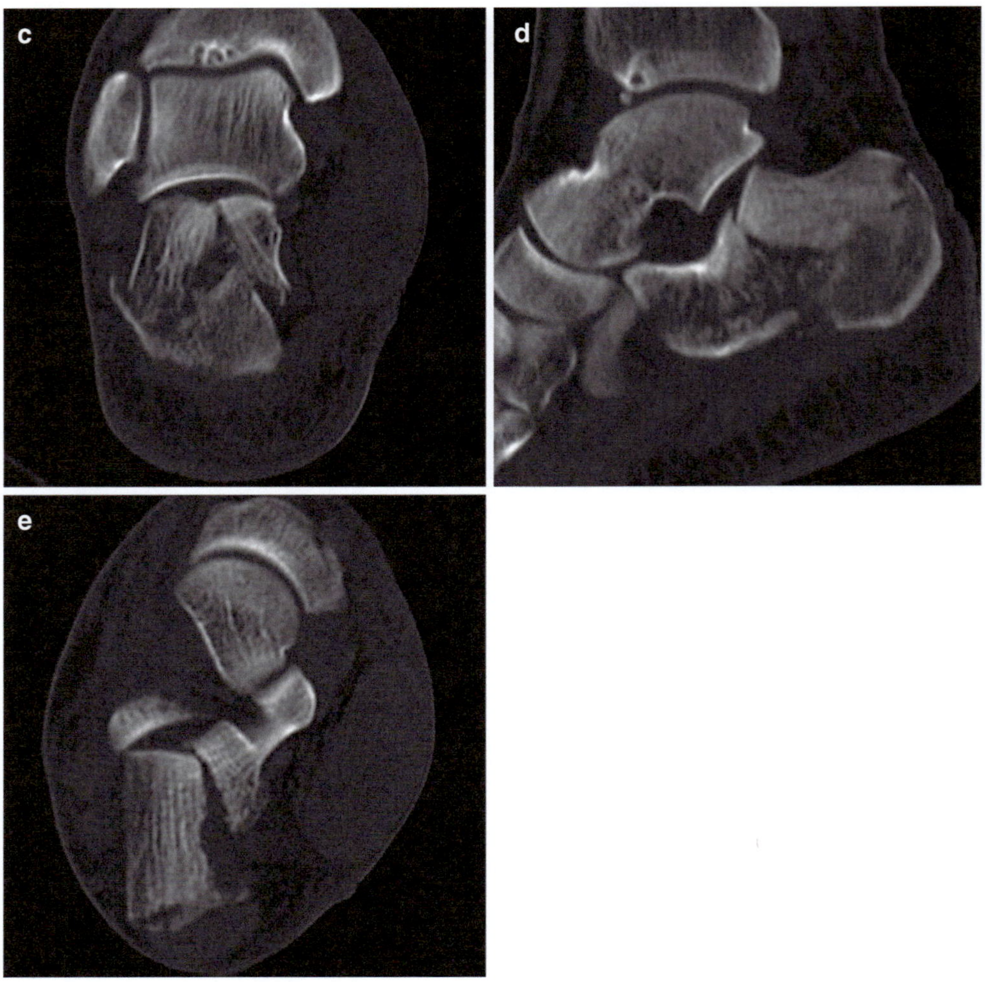

Fig. 11.10 CT oblique coronal surface (**c**), sagittal plane (**d**), and cross section (**e**) display the fracture of the calcaneus, and the fracture line involves the central block of the heel and the dislocation of the articular surface

11. Comparison between X-ray film and CT of calcaneal type II C fracture
  11.1 X-ray film (Fig. 11.11a–d)

Fig. 11.11 X-ray film (**a** and **c**) shows an oblique fracture of calcaneal bone, slight insertion of the broken end, smaller heel distance angle, schematic diagram (**b** and **d**)

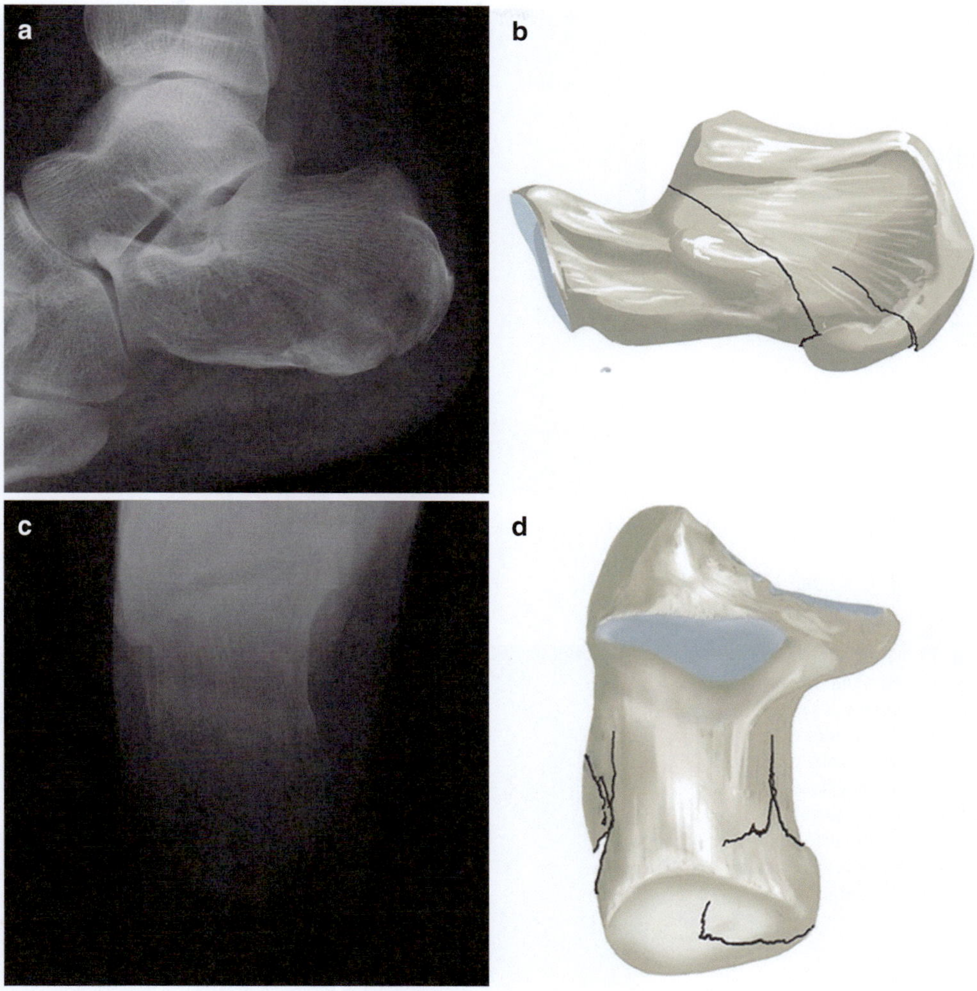

  11.2 CT scan (Fig. 11.11e, f)

Fig. 11.11 CT sagittal plane (**e**) and oblique coronal surface (**f**) show the fracture of the calcaneal bone. The fracture line involved the heel of the articular surface, adjacent to the distance, dislocation of the articular surface, and the widening of the fracture line

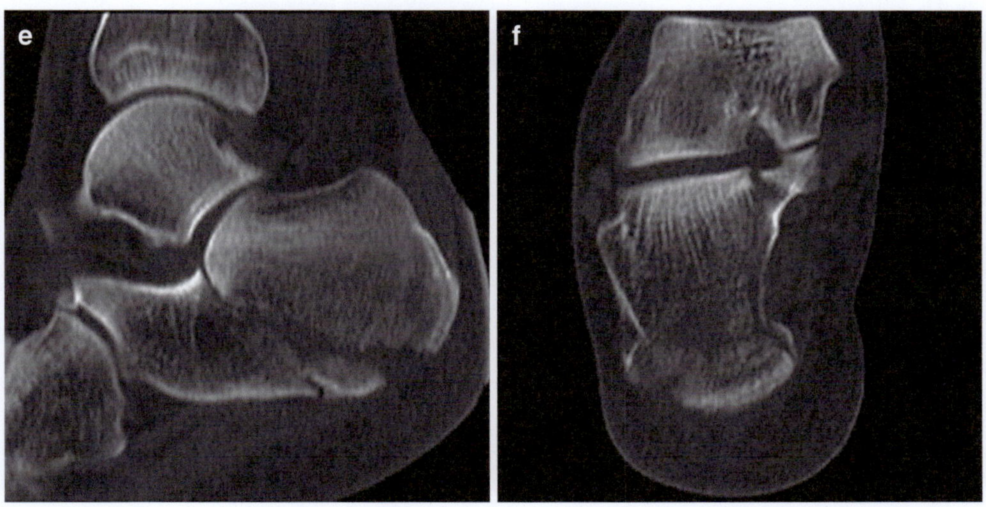

12. Comparison between X-ray film and CT of calcaneal type II C fracture
    12.1 X-ray film (Fig. 11.12a, b)

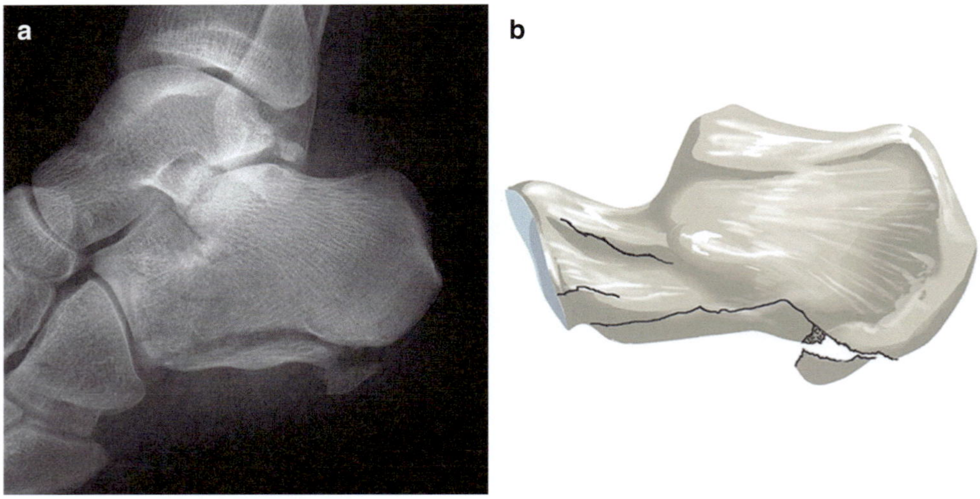

Fig. 11.12 X-ray plain film (**a**) shows a fracture of the calcaneal body and a displacement of the bone in the lower edge of the calcaneus (**b**)

    12.2 CT scan (Fig. 11.12c–e)

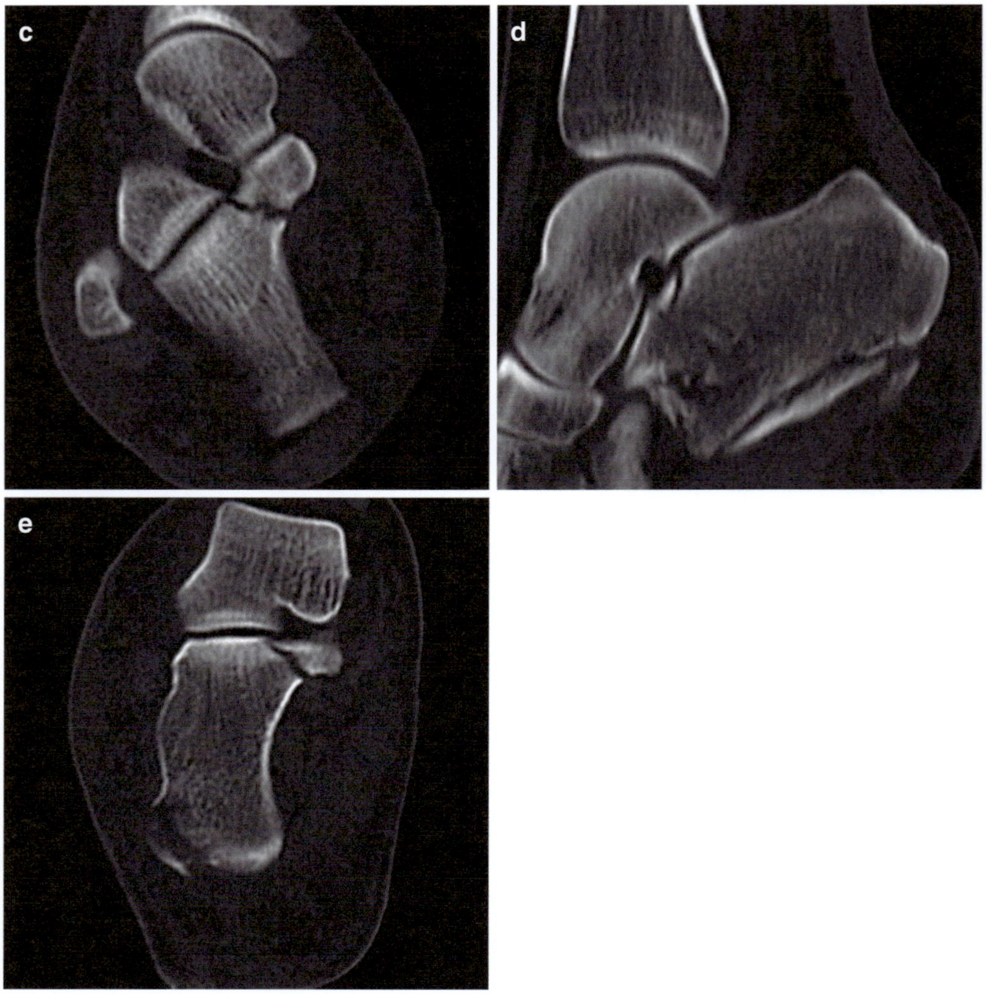

Fig. 11.12 CT cross section (**c**), sagittal plane (**d**), oblique coronal surface (**e**) show fracture of calcaneus bone, fracture line involved the heel distance joint surface, adjacent to the carrier distance, joint surface slightly dislocation, and the fracture line widened slightly

13. Comparison between X-ray film and CT of calcaneus type III A B fracture
    13.1 X-ray film (Fig. 11.13a–d)

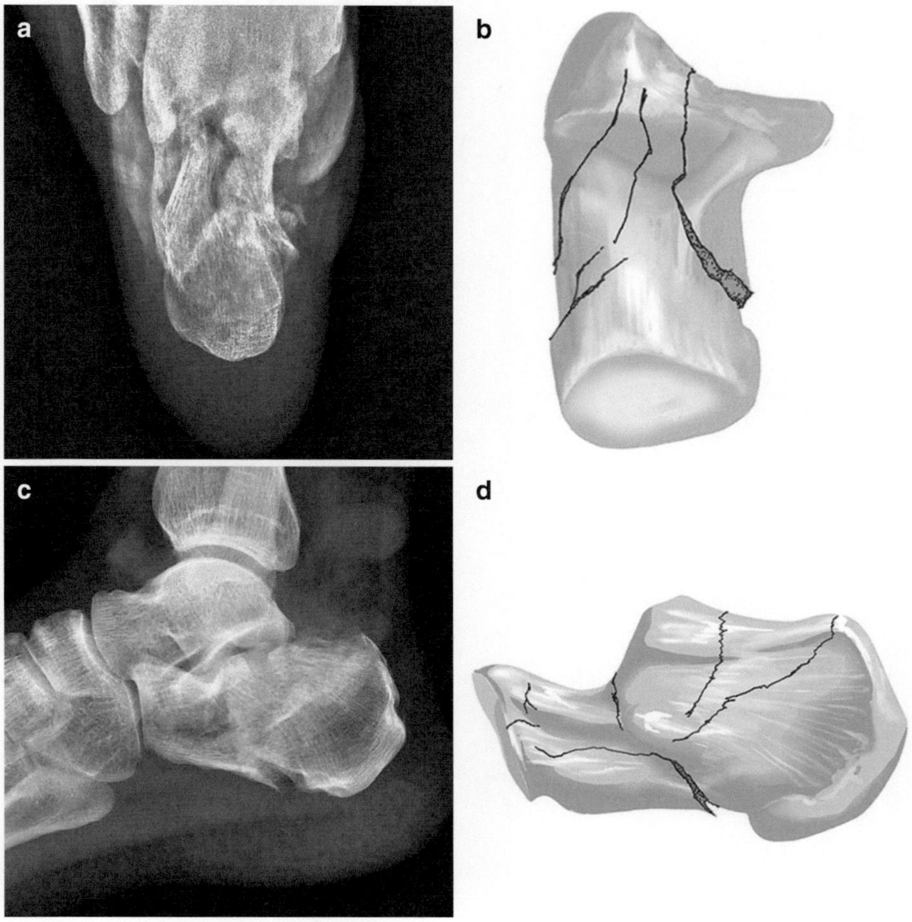

Fig. 11.13 X-ray film (**a**, **c**) shows bone fracture of calcaneus, broken ends embedded, and smaller angles (**b**, **d**)

13.2 CT scan (Fig. 11.13e–h)

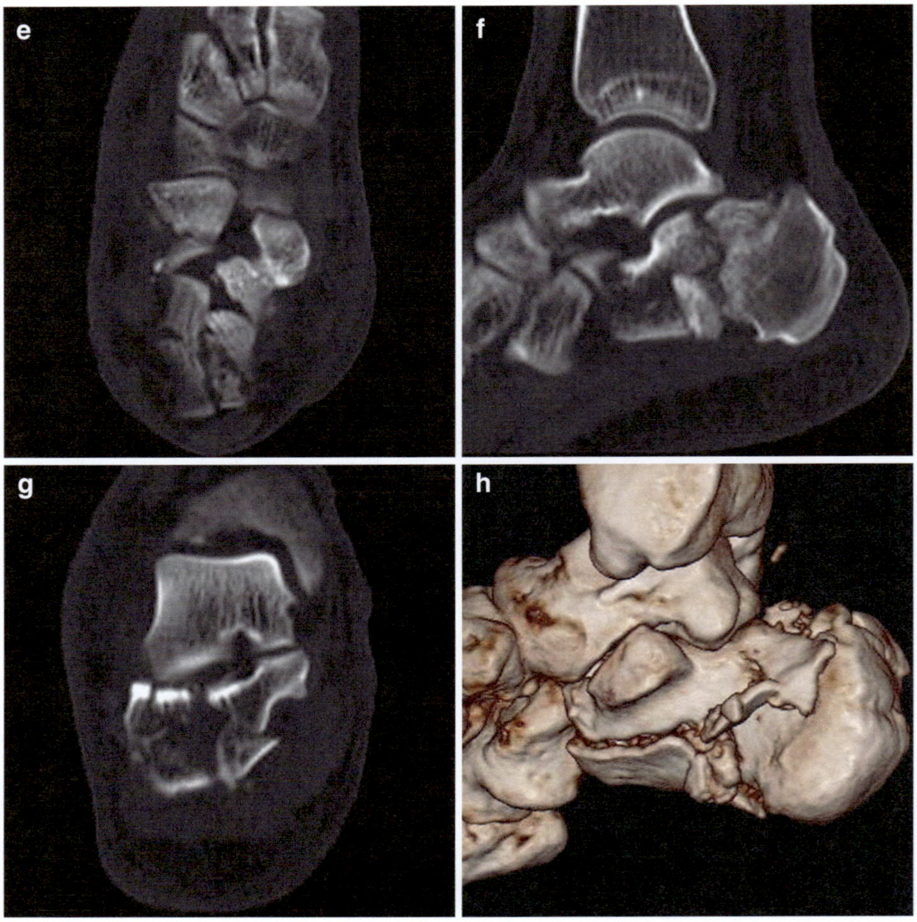

Fig. 11.13 CT cross section (**e**), sagittal plane (**f**), oblique coronal surface (**g**), and three-dimensional reconstruction (**h**) display the fracture of the calcaneus. The fracture line involves the lateral mass of the heel and the central block, the joint surface is slightly dislocation, and the fracture line is widened

14. Comparison between X-ray film and CT of calcaneus type III A B fracture
    14.1 X-ray film (Fig. 11.14a–d)

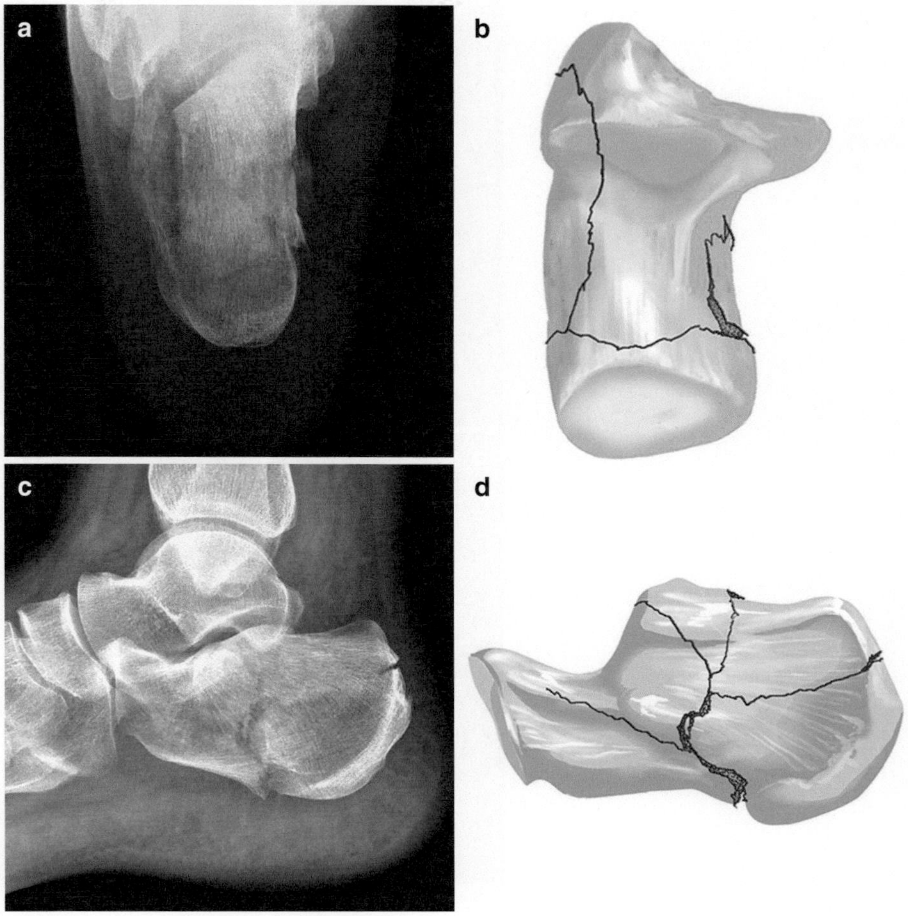

Fig. 11.14 X-ray film (**a**, **c**) shows bone fracture of calcaneus, broken ends embedded, and smaller angles (**b**, **d**)

14.2 CT scan (Fig. 11.14e–h)

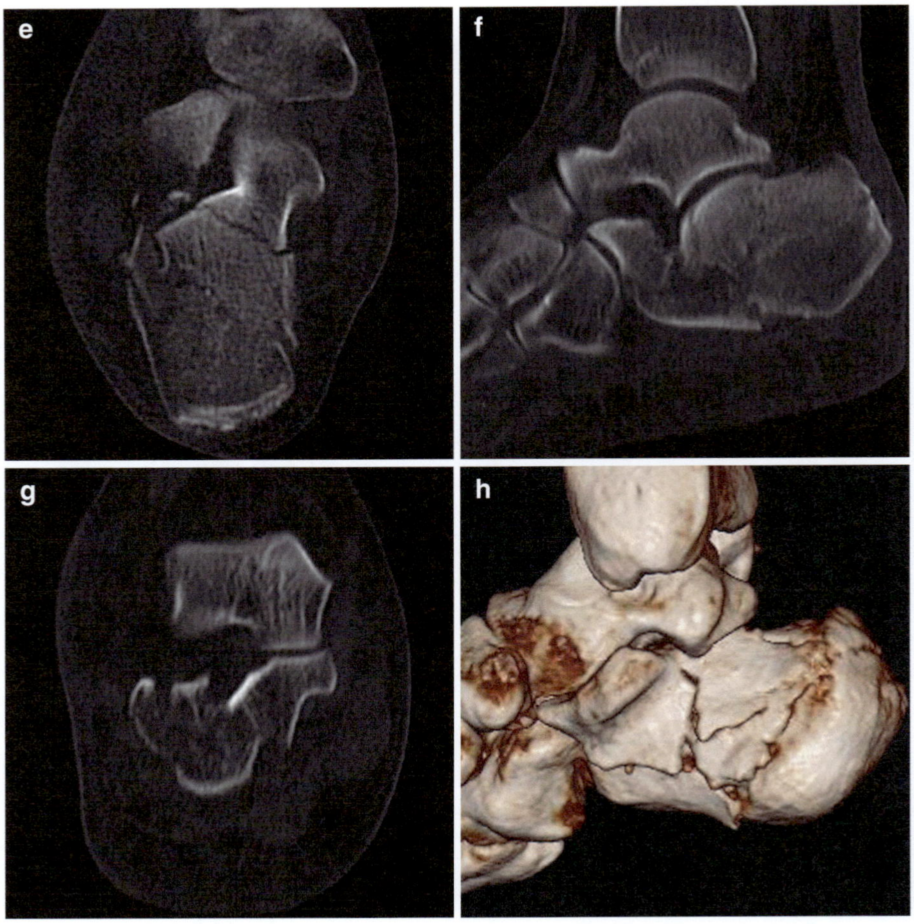

Fig. 11.14 CT cross section (**e**), sagittal plane (**f**), oblique coronal surface (**g**), and three-dimensional reconstruction (**h**) display the fracture of the calcaneus. The fracture line involves the lateral and medial blocks of the heel, the dislocation of the articular surface, and the widening of the fracture line

15. Comparison between X-ray film and CT of calcaneus type III A B fracture
15.1 X-ray film (Fig. 11.15a–d)

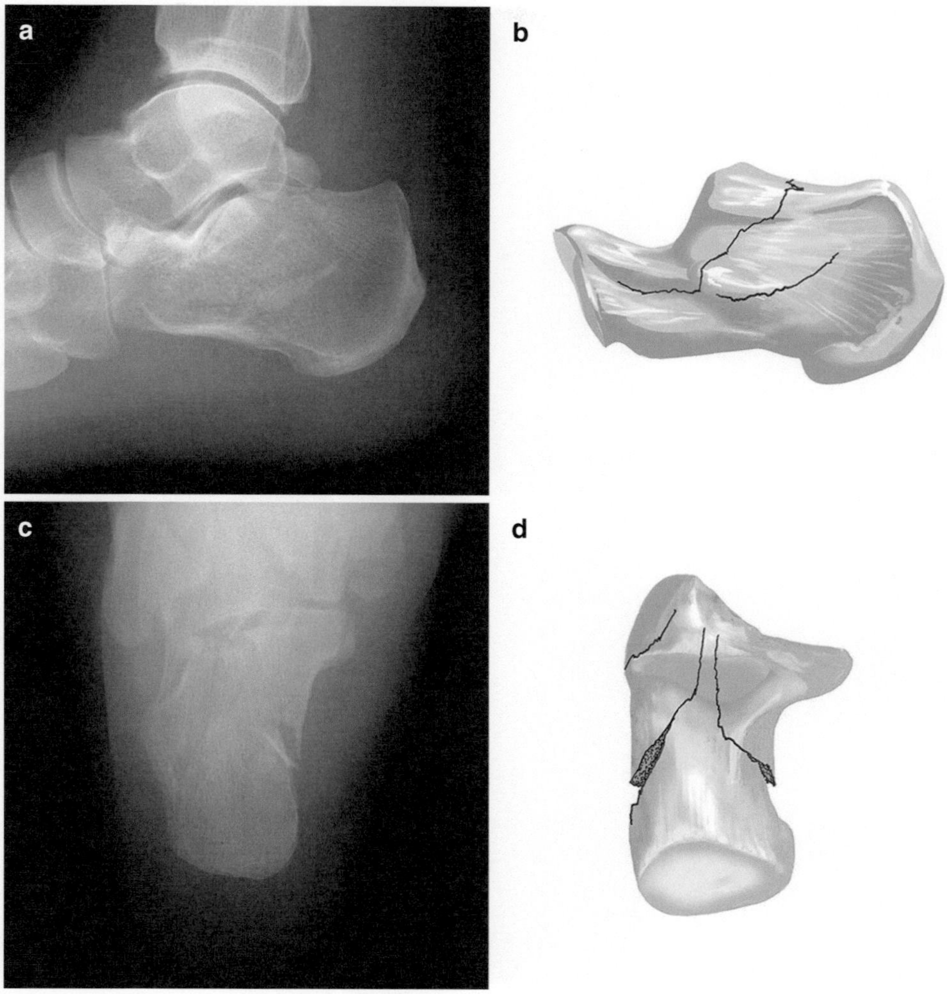

Fig. 11.15 X-ray film (**a**, **c**) shows that the calcaneal heel was collapsed from the articular surface, the end of the calcaneus was embedded, and the talus was smaller. The schematic diagram (**b**, **d**)

15.2 CT scan (Fig. 11.15e, f)

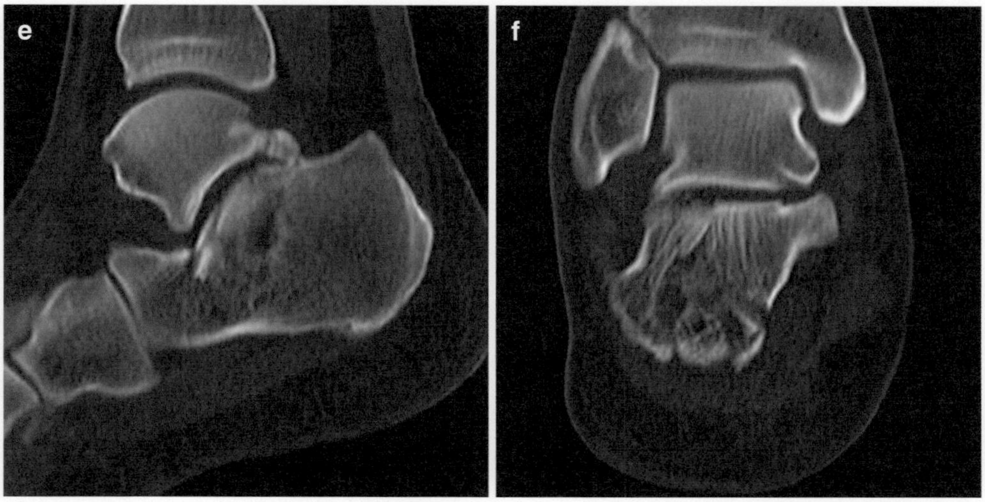

Fig. 11.15 CT sagittal plane (**e**) and oblique coronal surface (**f**) show the fracture and collapse of the heel distance of the calcaneus, and the fracture line involves the lateral mass of the heel and the central part of the articular surface. Dislocation is present in the broken end

16. Comparison between X-ray film and CT of calcaneus type III A B fracture
    16.1 X-ray film (Fig. 11.16a–d)

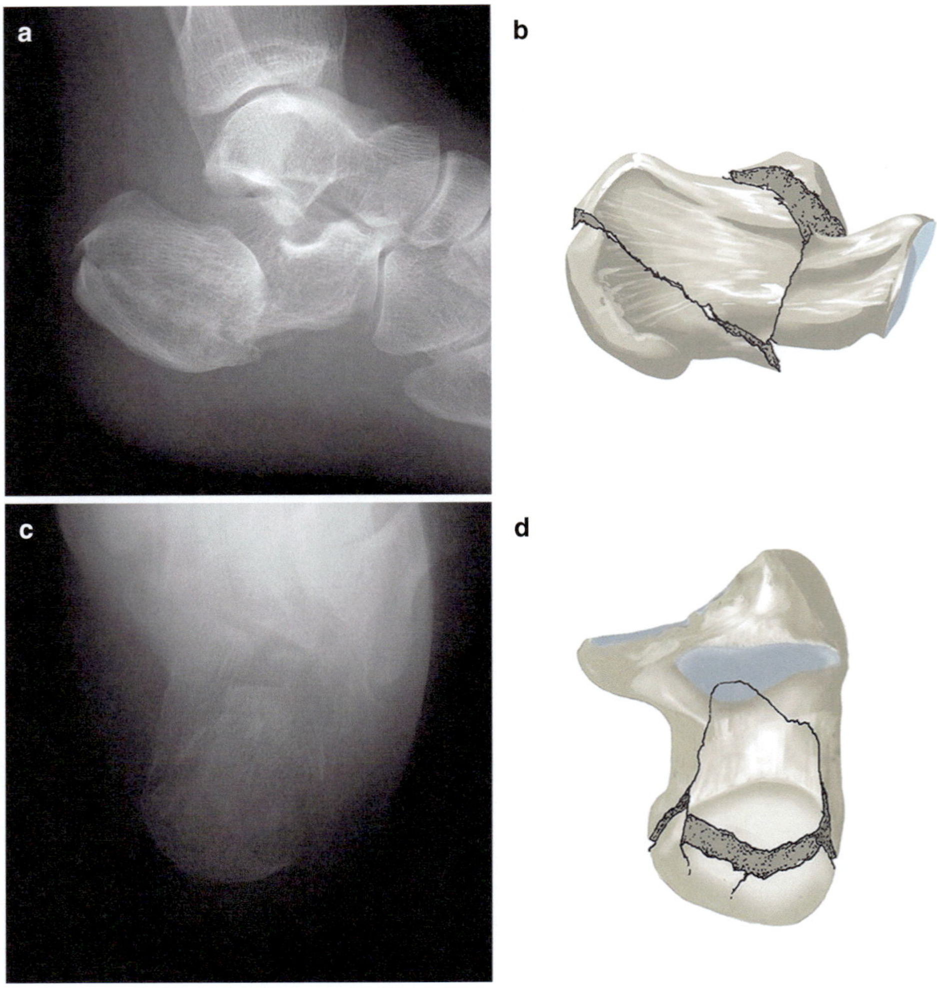

Fig. 11.16 X-ray film (**a** and **c**) shows bone fragmentation of calcaneus, slightly inserted ends of the calcaneus, dislocation of the articular surface, and smaller angle of the calcaneus (**b**, **d**)

16.2 CT scan (Fig. 11.16e, f)

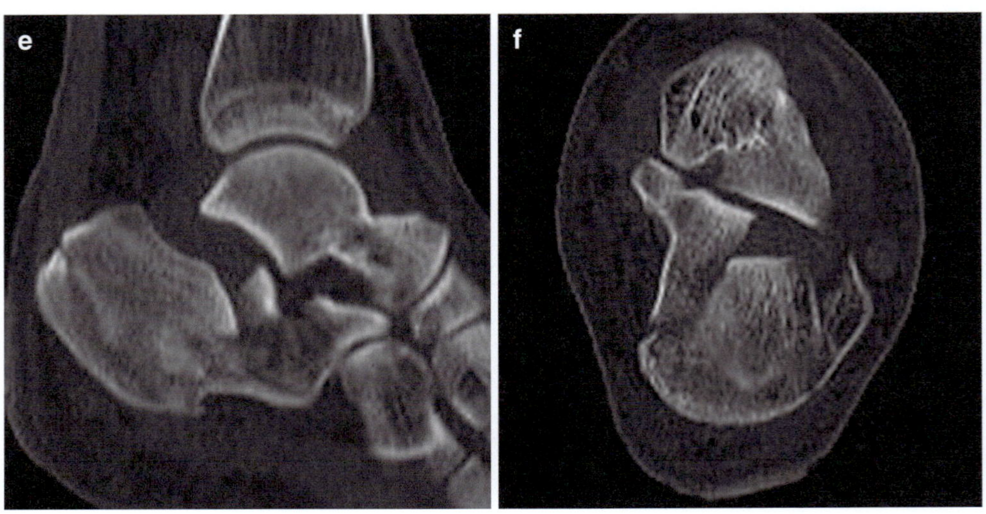

Fig. 11.16 CT sagittal plane (**e**) and oblique coronal surface (**f**) show fracture of the calcaneus bone, the broken end was inserted, the fracture line involved the lateral mass of the heel and the central block. The dislocation of the articular surface was obvious, and the fracture line was widened

17. Comparison between X-ray film and CT of calcaneus type III A C fracture
    17.1 X-ray film (Fig. 11.17a–d)

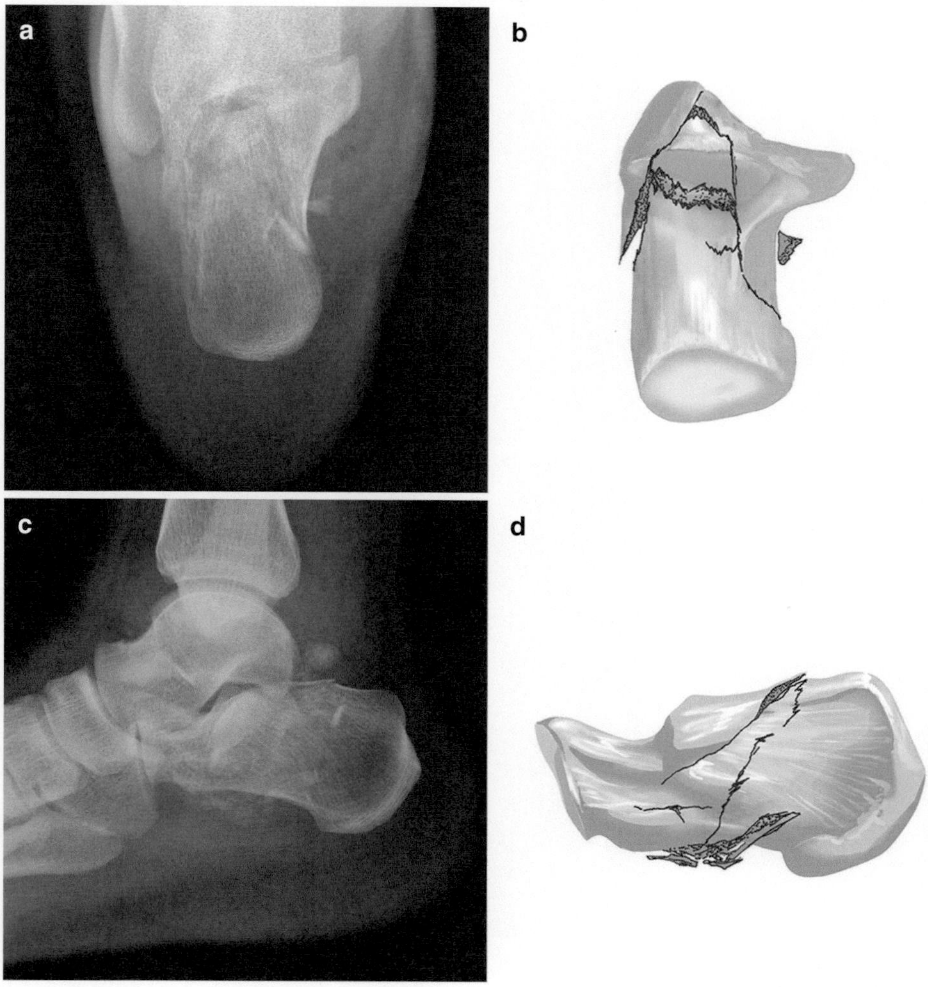

Fig. 11.17 X-ray film (**a**, **c**) shows that the calcaneal heel was collapsed from the articular surface, the end of the calcaneus was embedded, and the talus was smaller. The schematic diagram (**b**, **d**)

17.2 CT scan (Fig. 11.17e–h)

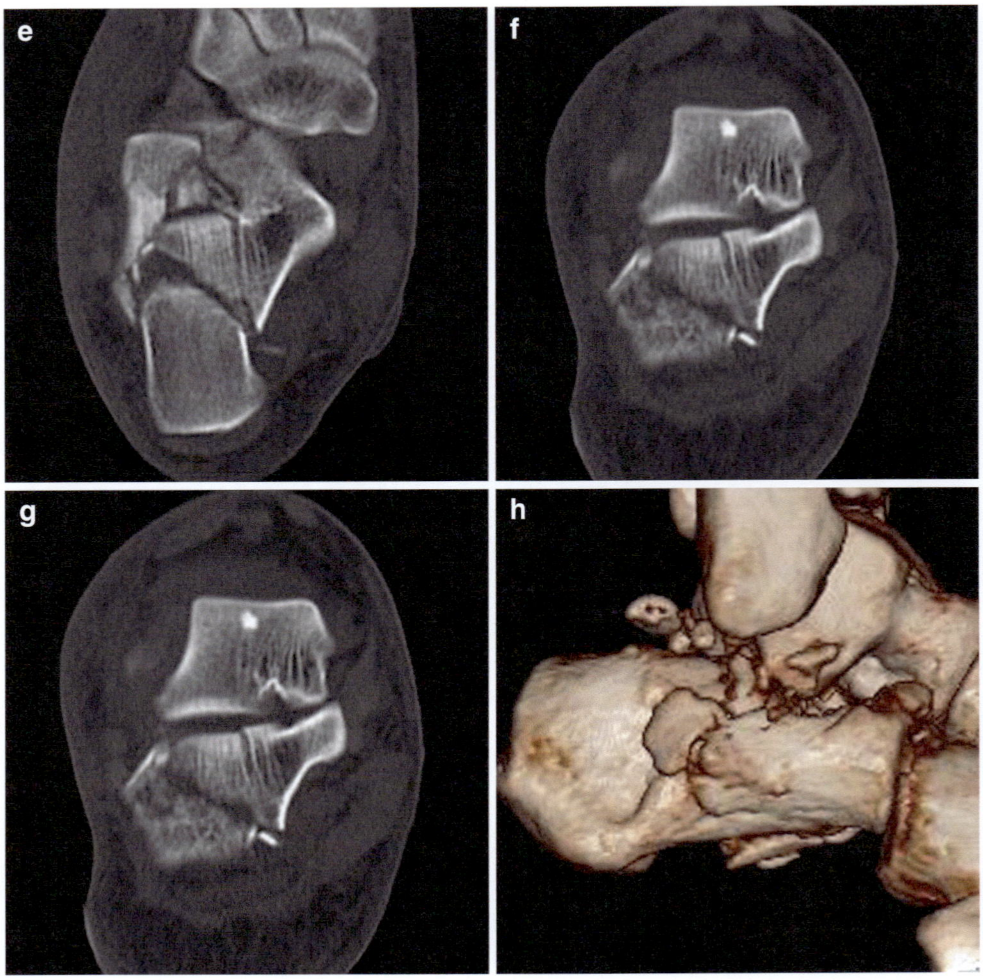

Fig. 11.17 CT cross section (**e**), oblique coronal surface (**f**, **g**), and three-dimensional reconstruction (**h**) show the fracture of the calcaneus. The fracture line involved the lateral mass of the heel and the medial block. The joint surface was slightly dislocation, and the fracture line was widened

18. Comparison between X-ray film and CT of calcaneus type III A C fracture
    18.1 X-ray film (Fig. 11.18a, b)

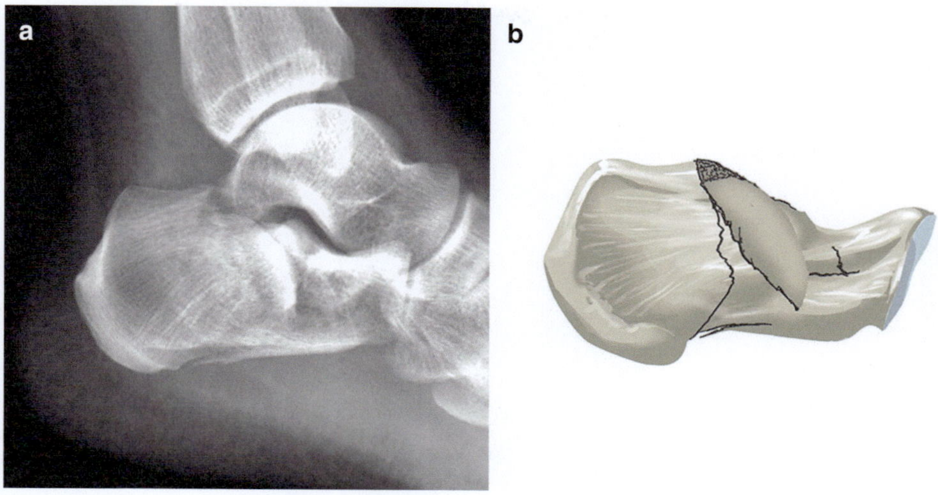

Fig. 11.18 X-ray film (**a**) shows the calcaneal heel from the articular surface collapse, the broken ends are inserted, and the schematic diagram (**b**)

    18.2 CT scan (Fig. 11.18c–e)

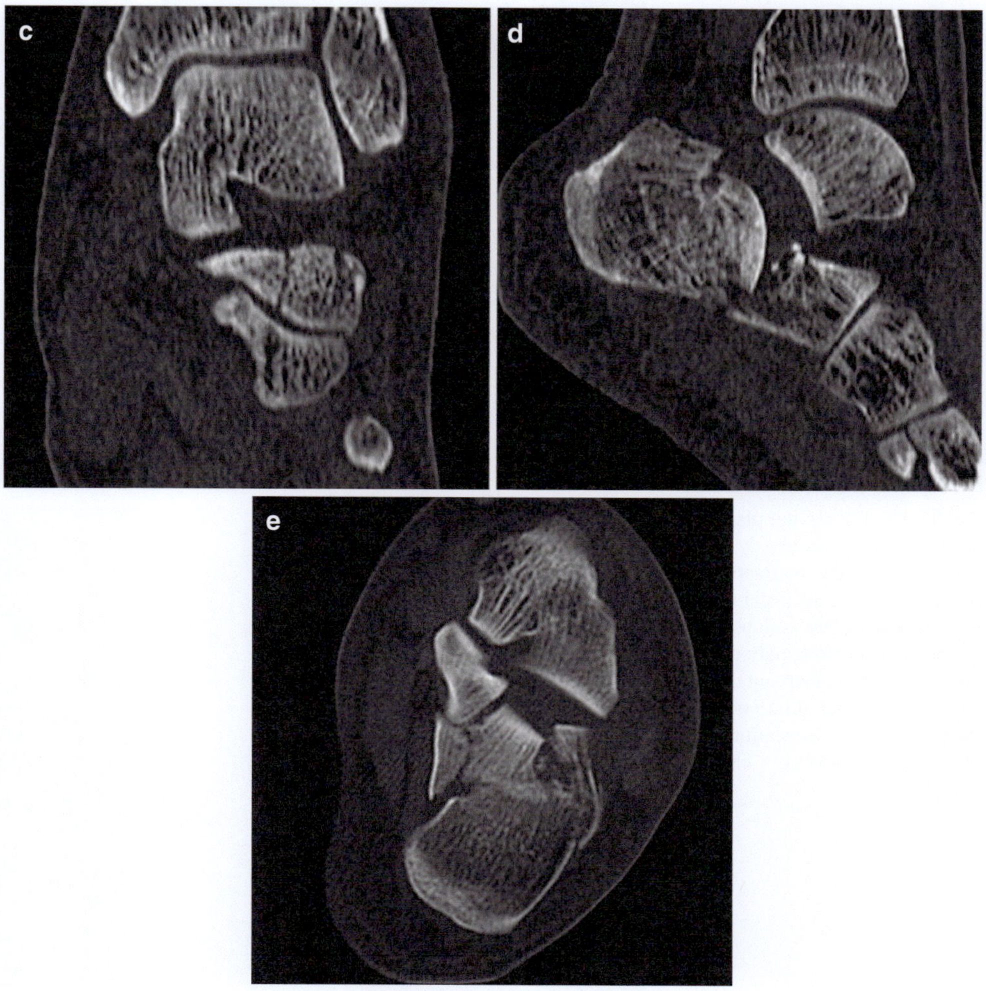

Fig. 11.18 CT oblique coronal plane (**c**), sagittal plane (**d**), cross section (**e**) show the collapse of the heel of the calcaneus, intercalation of the broken end, the fracture line involving the lateral and medial blocks of the heel, the dislocation of the articular surface, and the fracture line Shao Zengkuan

19. Comparison between X-ray film and CT of calcaneus type III A C fracture
    19.1 X-ray film (Fig. 11.19a–d)

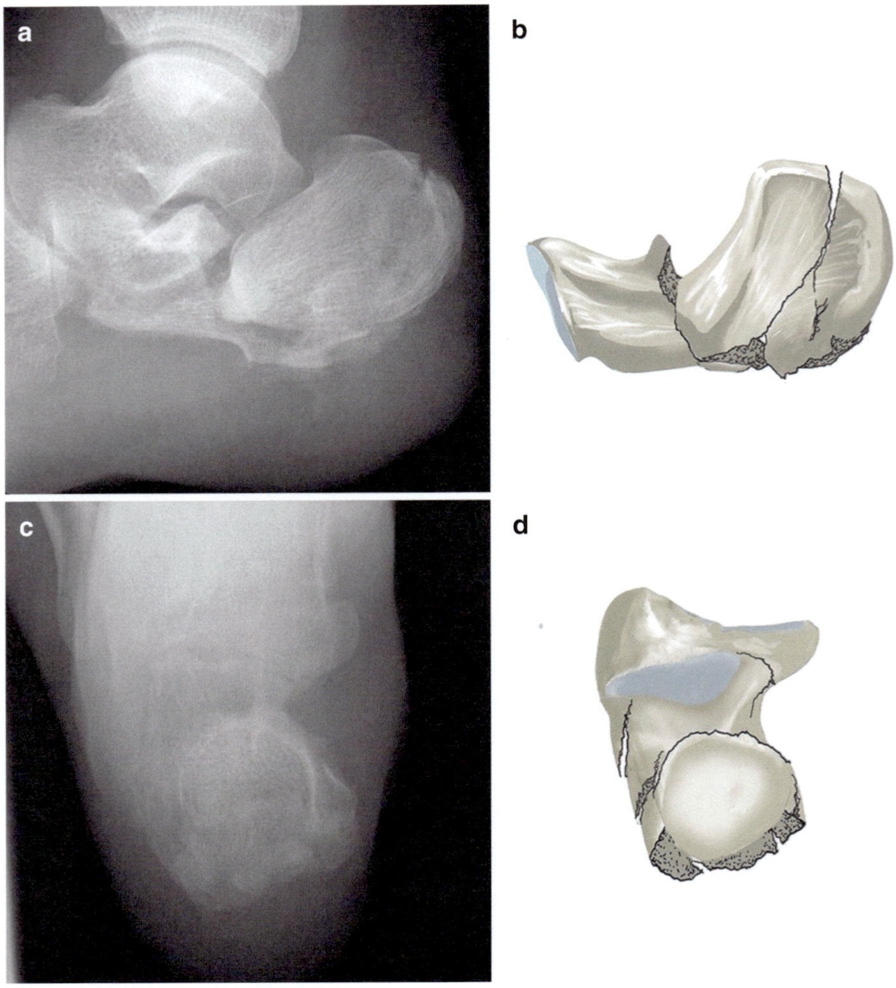

Fig. 11.19 X-ray film (**a**, **c**) shows calcaneal collapse, broken ends embedded, smaller with the angle of the calcaneus, widening the lateral calcaneus, schematic diagram (**b**, **d**)

19.2 CT scan (Fig. 11.19e, f)

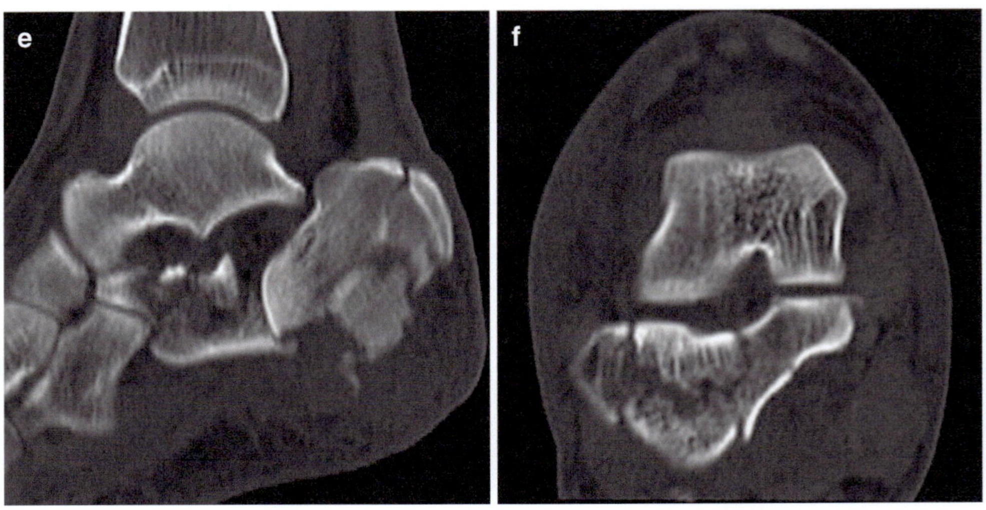

Fig. 11.19 CT sagittal plane (**e**) and oblique coronal surface (**f**) display the fracture of the calcaneus, the heel of the articular surface collapse, the broken end intercalation, the fracture line involving the lateral and medial blocks of the heel, and the dislocation of the articular surface

20. Comparison between X-ray film and CT of calcaneus type III A C fracture
    20.1 X-ray film (Fig. 11.20a–d)

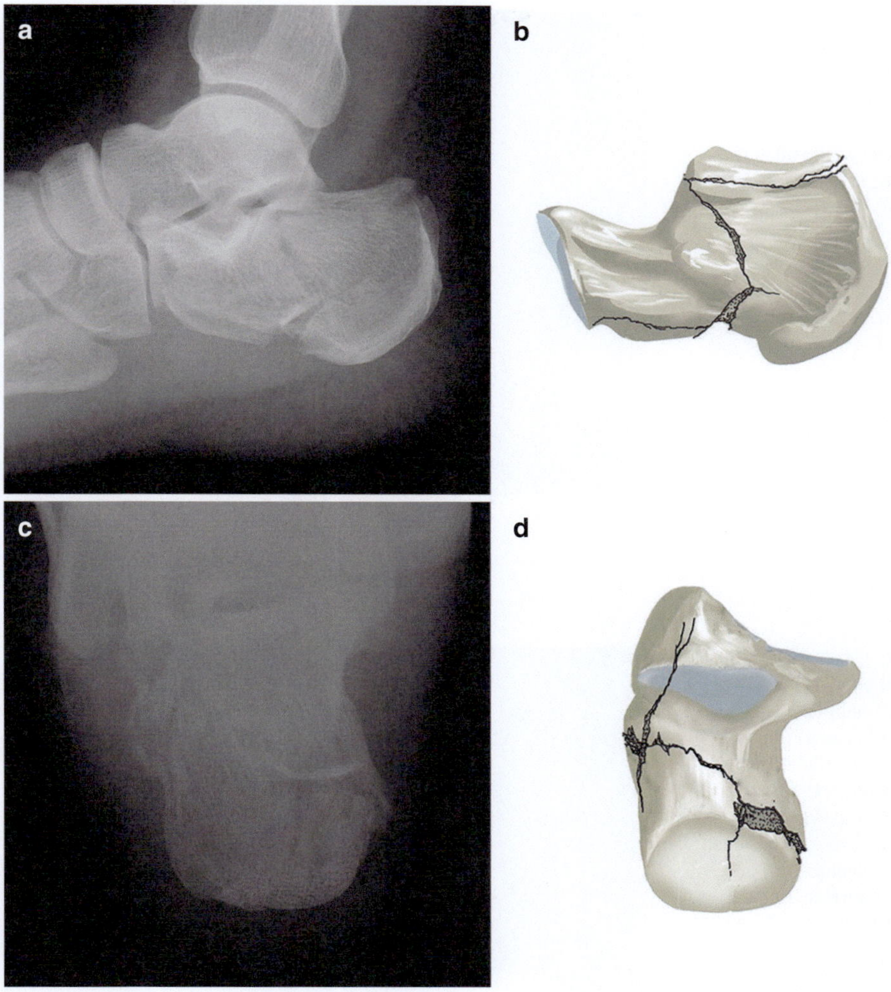

Fig. 11.20 X-ray plain film (**a**, **c**) shows calcaneal collapse, broken ends embedded, smaller with the angle of the calcaneus, widening the lateral calcaneus, and schematic diagram (**b**, **d**)

20.2 CT scan (Fig. 11.20e, f)

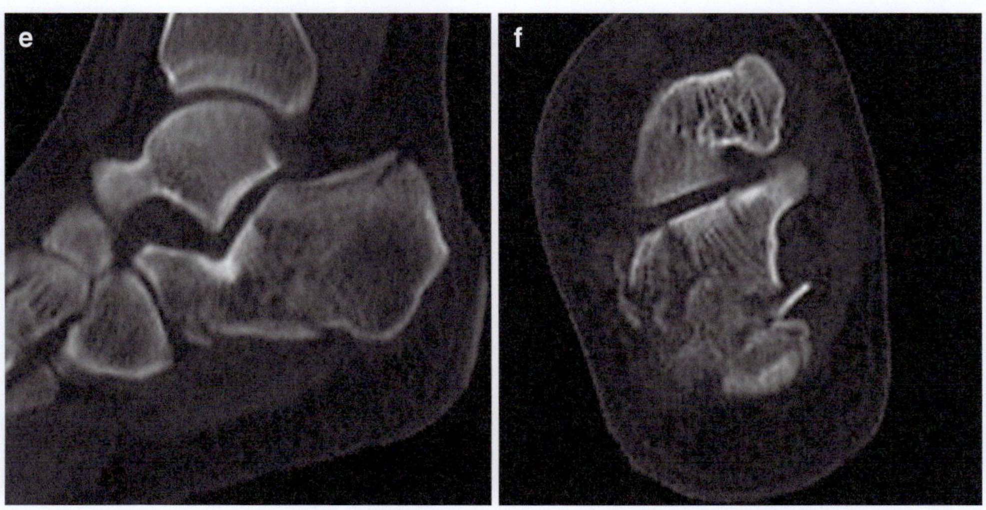

Fig. 11.20 CT sagittal plane (**e**) and oblique coronal surface (**f**) show fracture of calcaneus bone, intercalation end, and fracture line involving the lateral and medial blocks of the heel and dislocation of the articular surface

21. Comparison between X-ray film and CT of calcaneus type III B C fracture
    21.1 X-ray film (Fig. 11.21a, b)

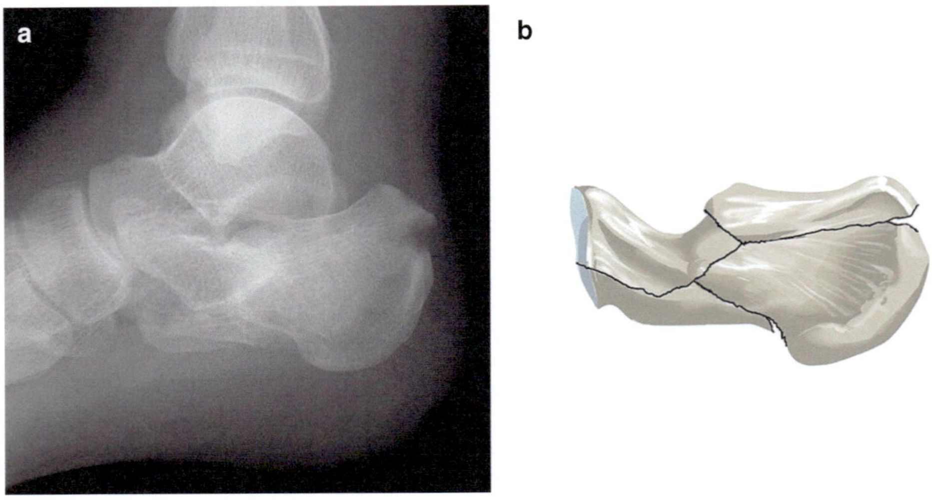

Fig. 11.21 X-ray film (**a**) shows that the calcaneal heel was collapsed from the articular surface, the end of the calcaneus was embedded, and the angle of the talus was smaller. The schematic diagram (**b**)

21.2 CT scan (Fig. 11.21c–e)

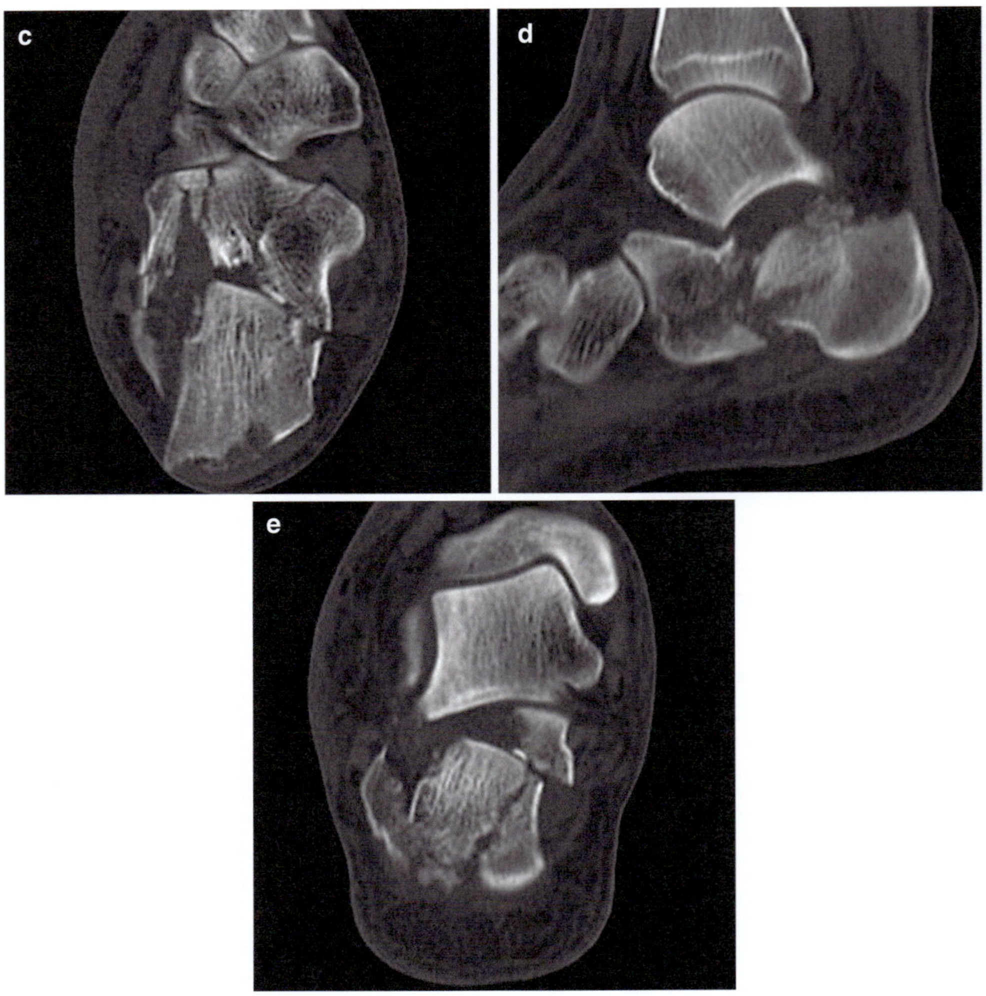

Fig. 11.21 CT cross section (**c**), sagittal plane (**d**), and oblique coronal plane (**e**) show the collapse of the heel of the calcaneus, the broken end is embedded, the fracture line involves the central block and the inner block of the heel distance, the dislocation of the articular surface, and the fracture line Shao Zengkuan

22. Comparison between X-ray film and CT of calcaneus type IV fracture
    22.1 X-ray film (Fig. 11.22a–d)

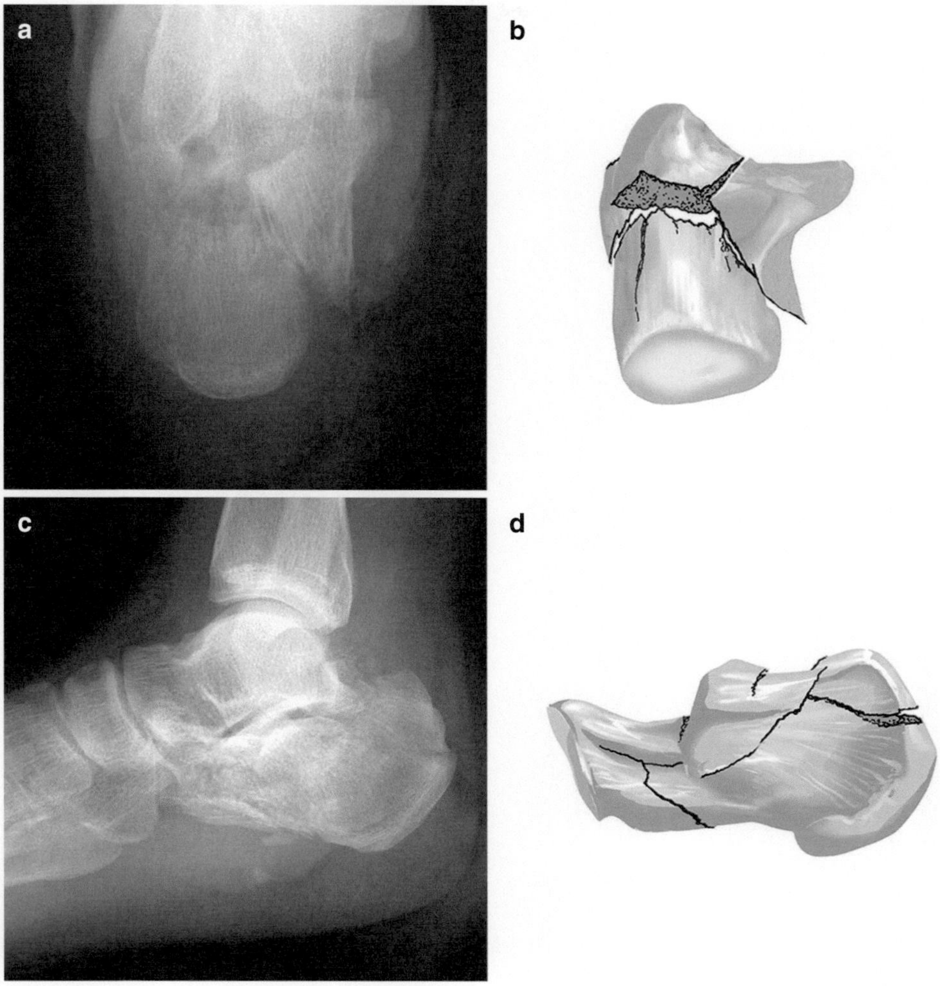

Fig. 11.22 X-ray plain film (**a**, **c**) shows that the calcaneal heel was collapsed from the articular surface, the end of the calcaneus was embedded, the talus was smaller, and the calcaneus was widened (**b**, **d**)

22.2 CT scan (Fig. 11.22e–h)

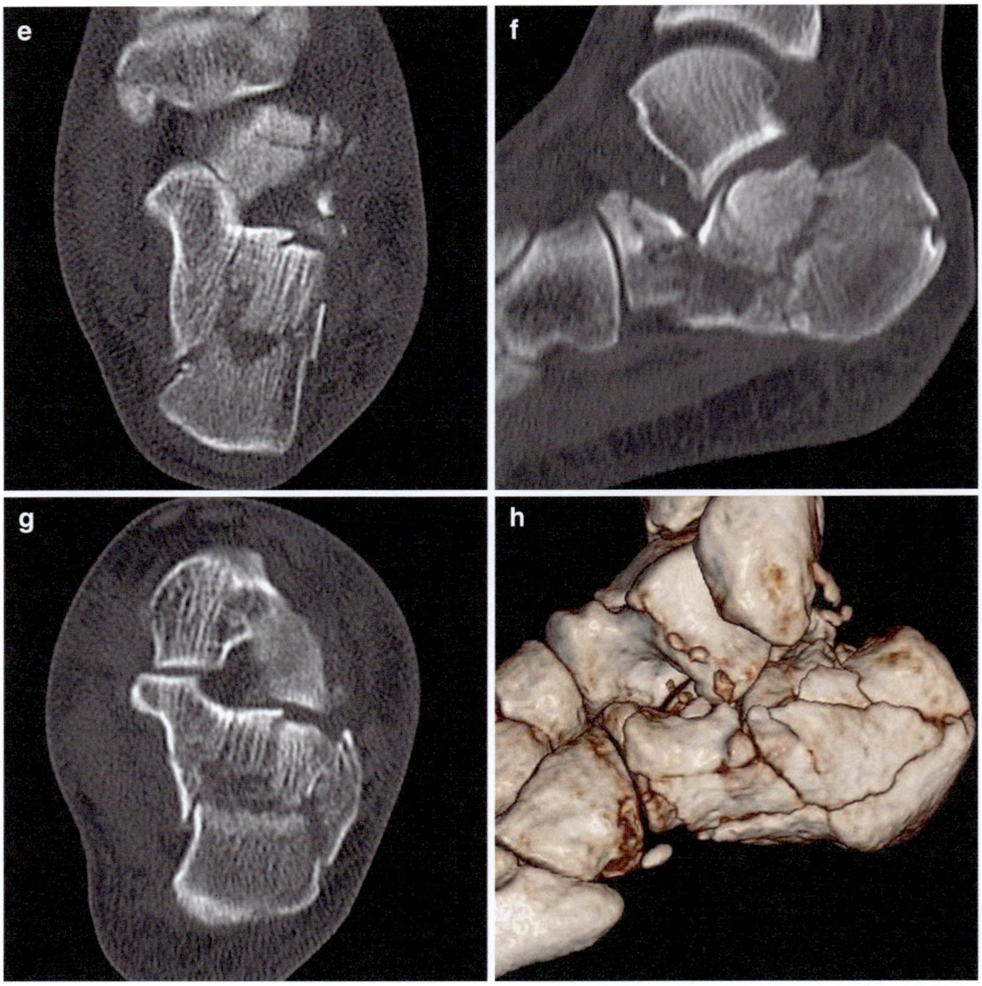

Fig. 11.22 CT cross section (**e**), sagittal plane (**f**), oblique coronal surface (**g**), and three-dimensional reconstruction (**h**) display calcaneal bone fragmentation, broken end intercalation, heel distance joint surface fracture, joint surface slightly dislocation, fracture line widening

23. Comparison between X-ray film and CT of a calcaneus type IV fracture
    23.1 X-ray film (Fig. 11.23a–d)

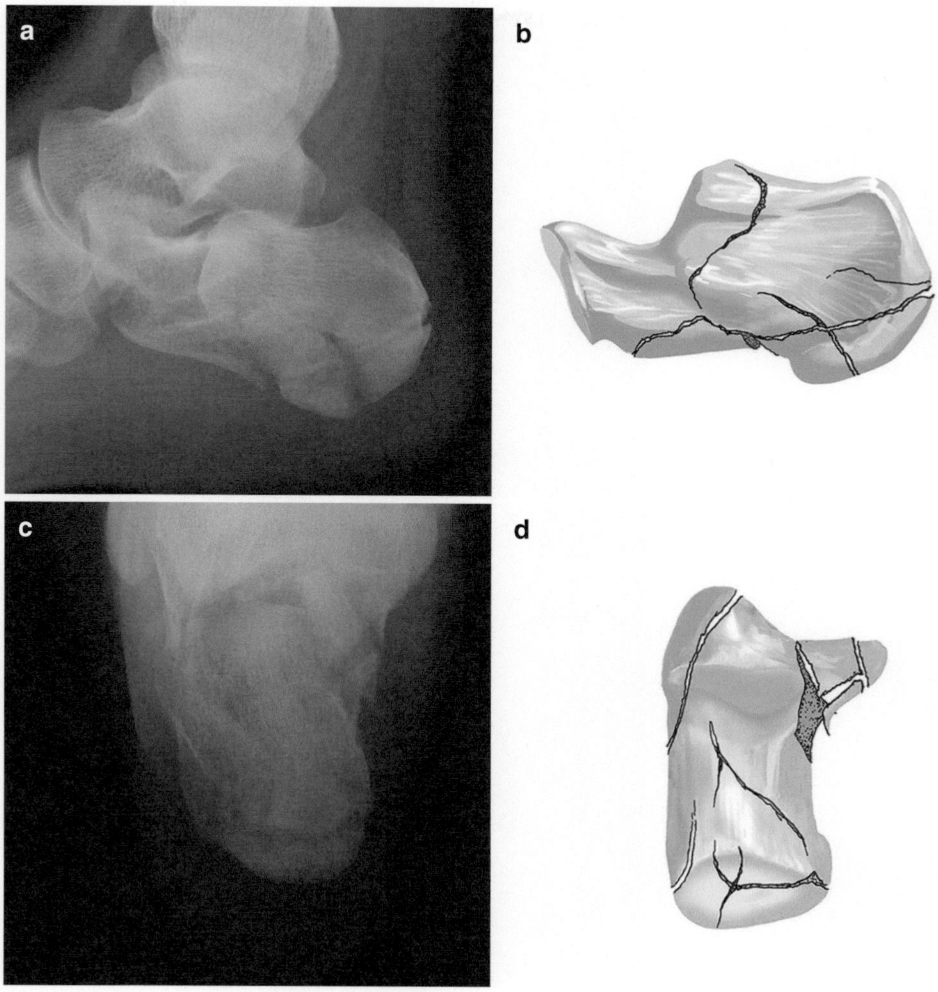

Fig. 11.23 X-ray film (**a**, **c**) shows calcaneal collapse, broken ends embedded, smaller with the angle of the calcaneus, widening the lateral calcaneus, and schematic diagram (**b**, **d**)

23.2 CT scan (Fig. 11.23e, f)

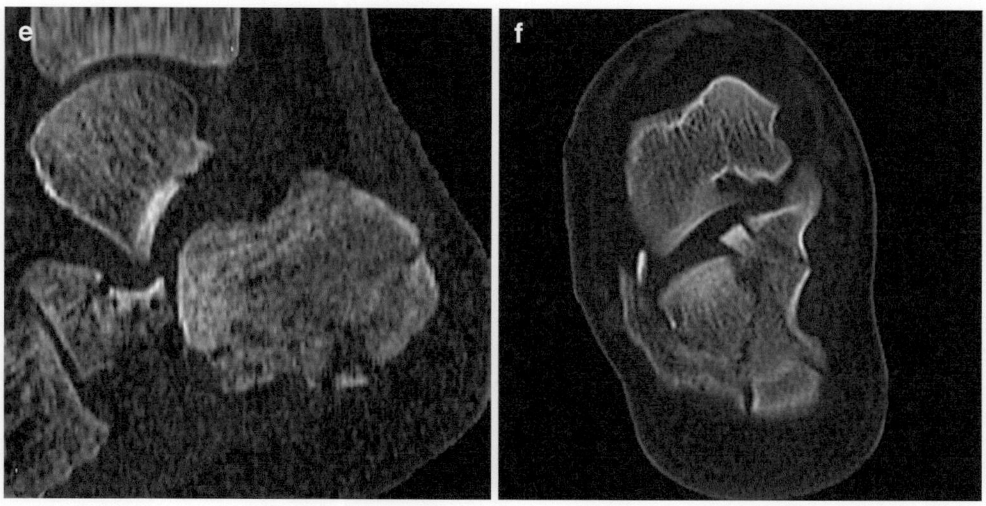

Fig. 11.23 CT sagittal plane (**e**) and oblique coronal plane (**f**) show bone fragmentation of calcaneus, broken ends embedded, posterior heel fracture, articular surface dislocation

24. Comparison between X-ray film and CT of calcaneus type IV fracture
    24.1 X-ray film (Fig. 11.24a–d)

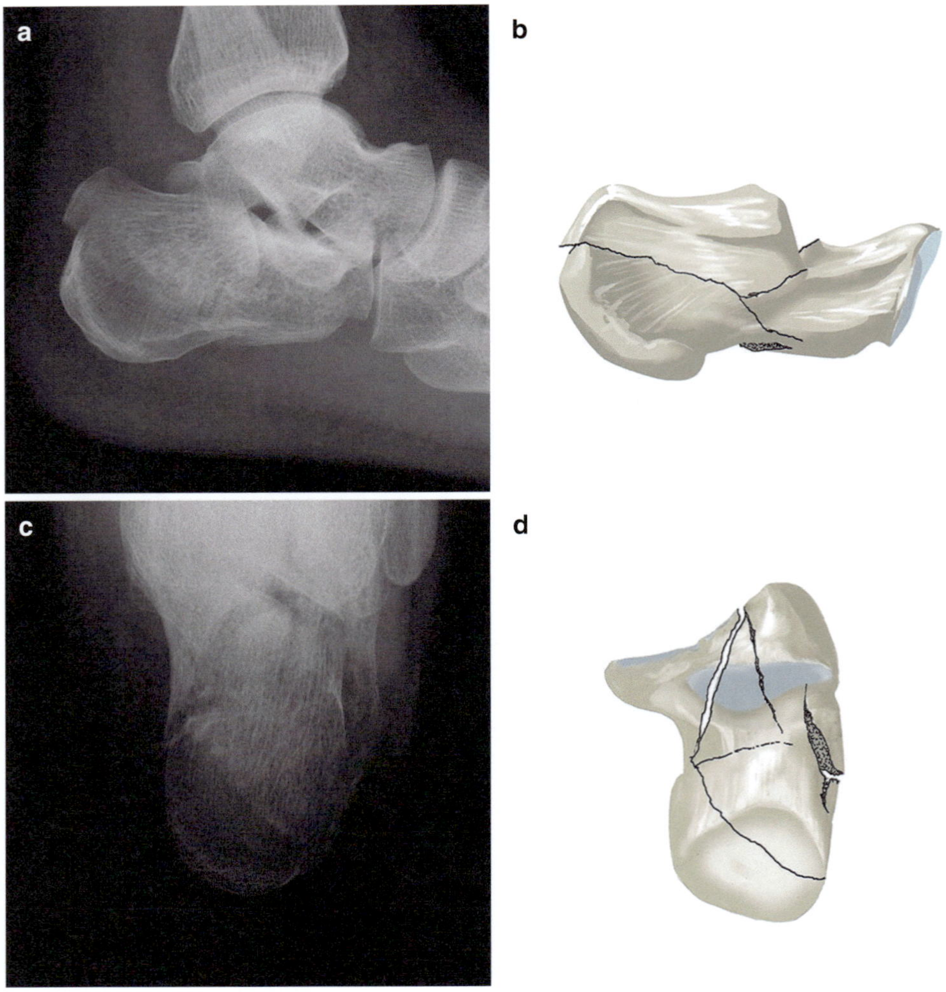

Fig. 11.24 X-ray film (**a**, **c**) shows a calcaneal collapse, broken ends embedded, smaller with the angle of the calcaneus, widening the lateral calcaneus, and schematic diagram (**b**, **d**)

24.2 CT scan (Fig. 11.24e, f)

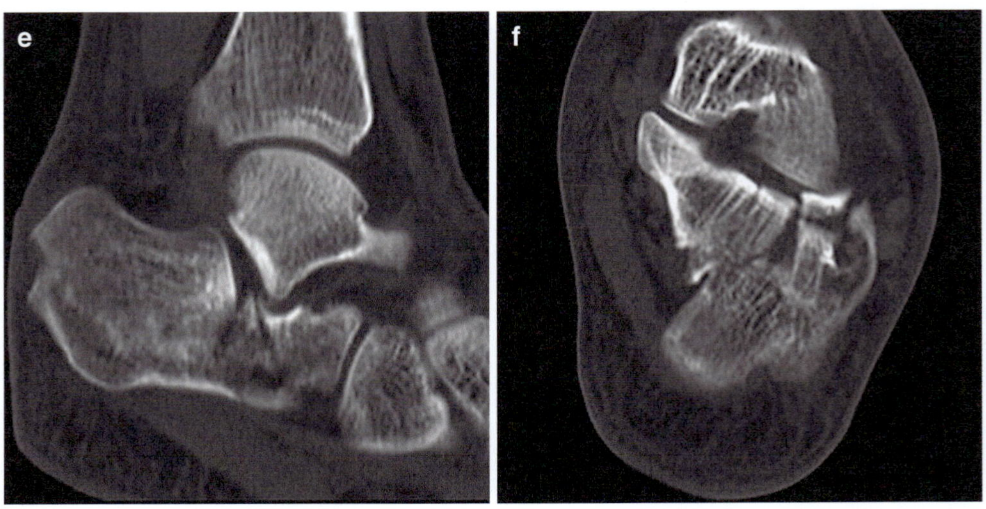

Fig. 11.24 CT sagittal plane (**e**) and oblique coronal plane (**f**) show bone fragmentation of calcaneus, broken ends embedded, posterior heel fracture, articular surface dislocation

25. Comparison between X-ray film and CT of calcaneus type IV fracture
    25.1 X-ray film (Fig. 11.25a–d)

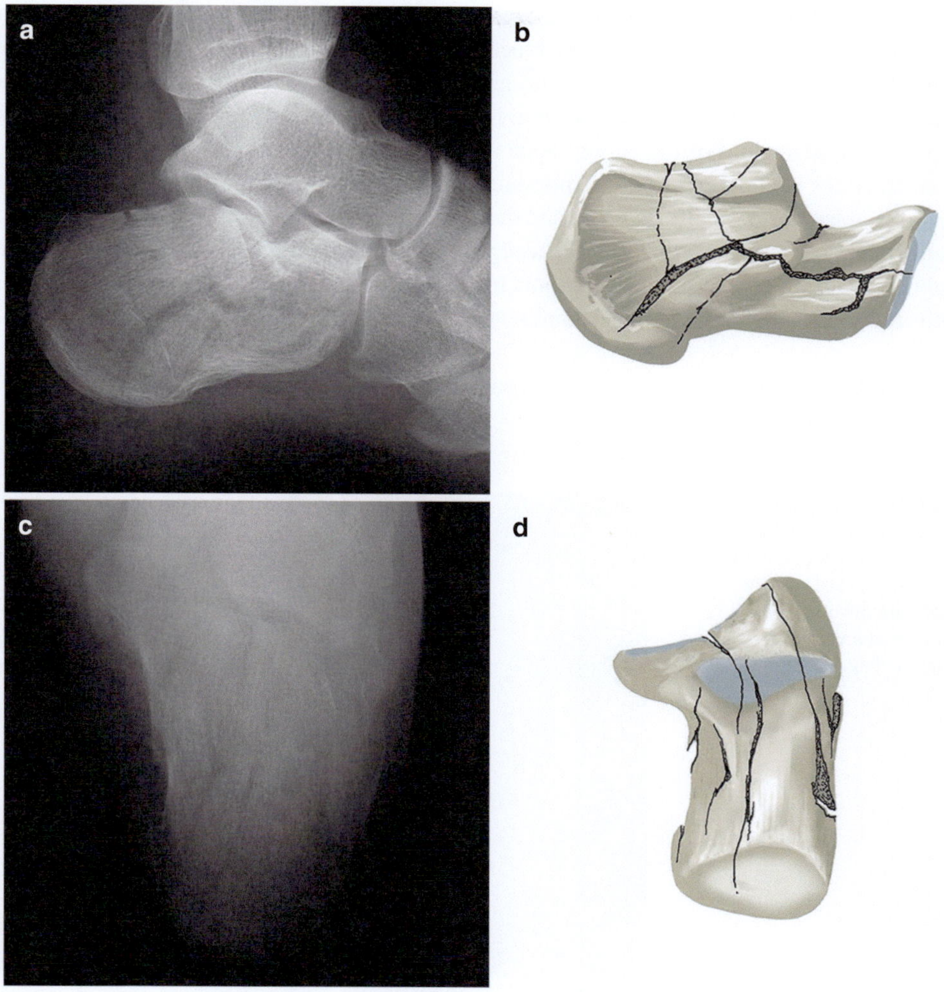

Fig. 11.25 X-ray film (**a**, **c**) shows calcaneal collapse, broken ends inserted, and calcaneus widened laterally (**b**, **d**)

25.2 CT scan (Fig. 11.25e, f)

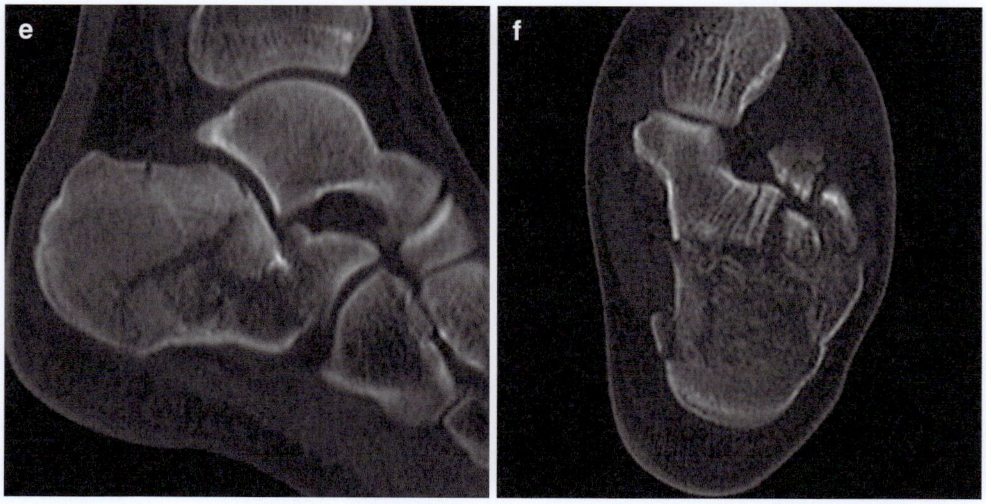

Fig. 11.25 CT sagittal plane (**e**) and oblique coronal plane (**f**) show bone fragmentation of calcaneus, broken ends embedded, posterior heel fracture, articular surface dislocation

11.2 Other Tarsal Fractures

Besides the talus and calcaneus, other tarsal bones include scaphoid bone, 3 cuneiform bone, and the cuboid bone. The medial aspect of the scaphoid bone is wider and the outer side is narrower. The posterior part of the scaphoid is concave to the articular surface of the canthus, with 3 facet joints and 3 articulatory joints of the cuneiform bone. The AO/OTA classification of scaphoid fractures is divided into non-comminuted fractures and comminuted fractures. The cuboid is irregular, located on the lateral side of the middle foot, forming a joint behind the calcaneus and joint with the base of the 4/5 metatarsal in front. The fracture of the cuboid bone accounts for 1.17% of the fracture of the foot. The AO/OTA classification of cuboid fractures is classified as non-comminuted fracture and comminuted fracture. There are 3 cuneus, the medial cuneiform bone, the middle cuneiform bone, and the lateral cuneiform bone. The medial cuneiform bone is the longest, the middle cuneiform bone is the shortest, and the 3-wedge bone forms the mortise and mortise structure, with the corresponding metatarsal base. The cuneiform fracture accounts for 2.01% of the foot fracture. The AO/OTA classification of the fracture of the cuneiform bone is divided into non-comminuted fracture and comminuted fracture.

1. Comparison of X-ray film and CT between scaphoid non-comminuted fractures
   1.1 X-ray film (Fig. 11.26a–d)

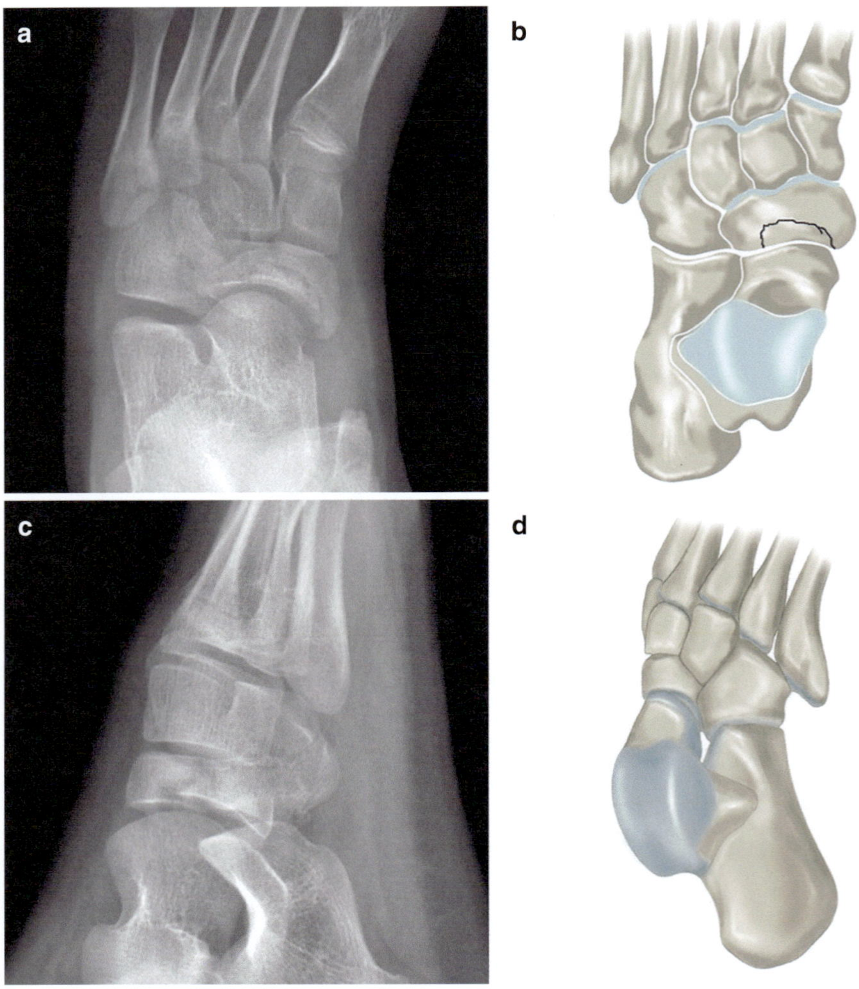

Fig. 11.26 X-ray film (**a**, **c**) shows scaphoid bone fracture, no obvious dislocation at the end of the fracture, and the fracture line involved the articular surface. The schematic diagram (**b**, **d**)

1.2 CT scan (Fig. 11.26e, f)

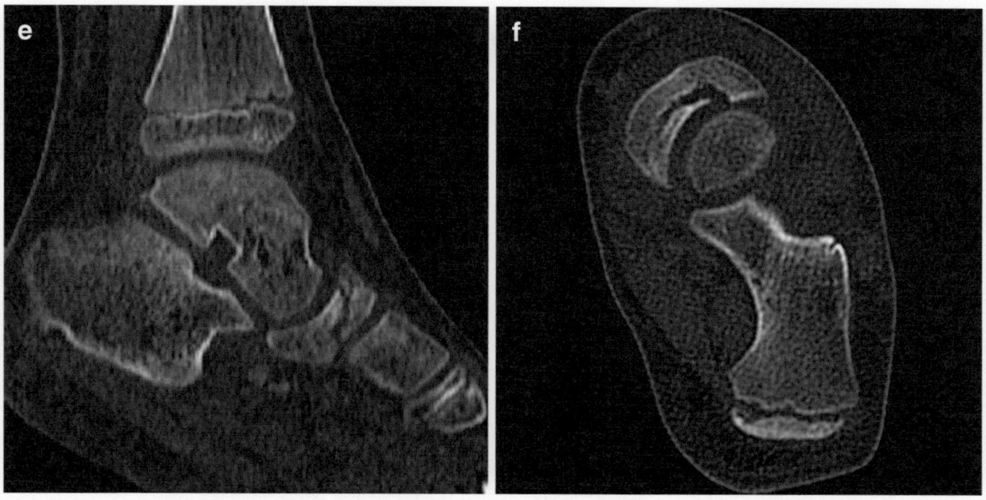

Fig. 11.26 CT sagittal plane (**e**) and cross section (**f**) show scaphoid bone fracture, slightly dislocated ends, and uneven joints

2. Comparison of X-ray film and CT between scaphoid non-comminuted fractures
   2.1 X-ray film (Fig. 11.27a–d)

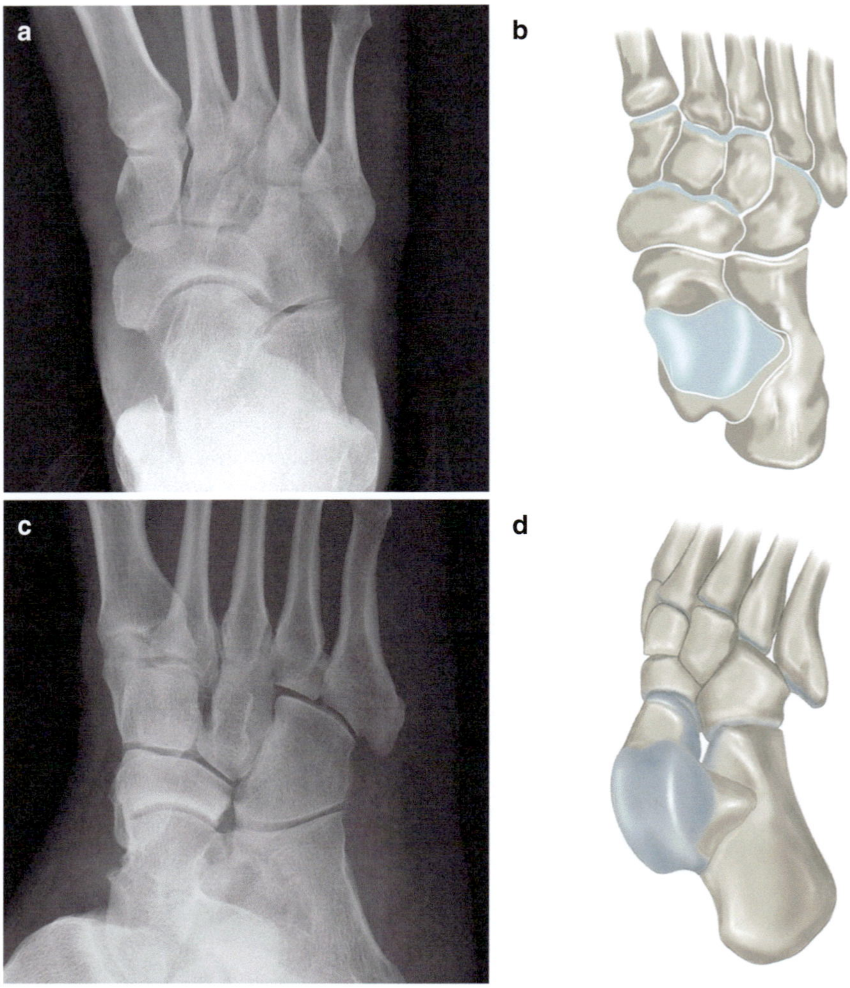

Fig. 11.27 X-ray film (**a**, **c**) scaphoid shows no definite signs of fracture, schematic diagram (**b**, **d**)

   2.2 CT scan (Fig. 11.27e, f)

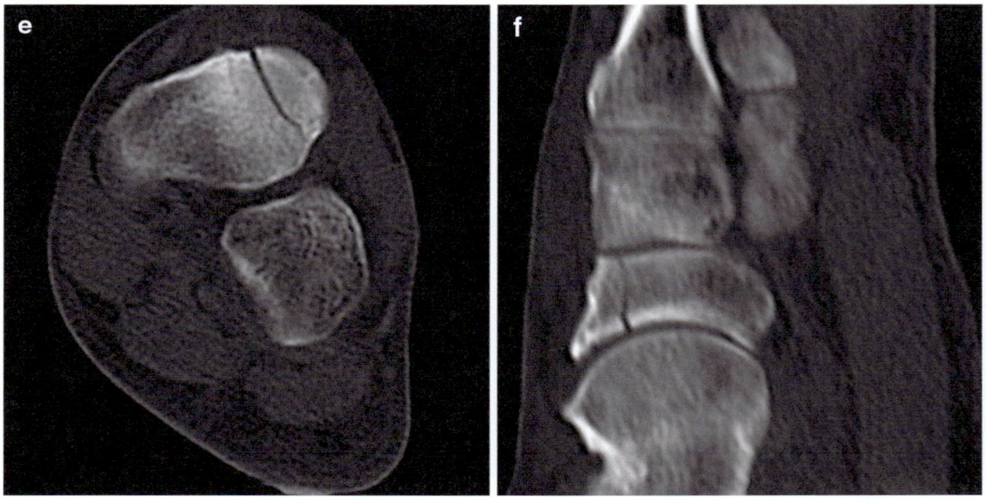

Fig. 11.27 CT coronal plane (**e**) and sagittal plane (**f**) show a fracture of the anterior margin of the scaphoid, with no obvious dislocation at the end of the fracture, and the fracture line involved the articular surface

3. Comparison of X-ray film and CT between scaphoid comminuted fractures
 3.1 X-ray film (Fig. 11.28a–d)

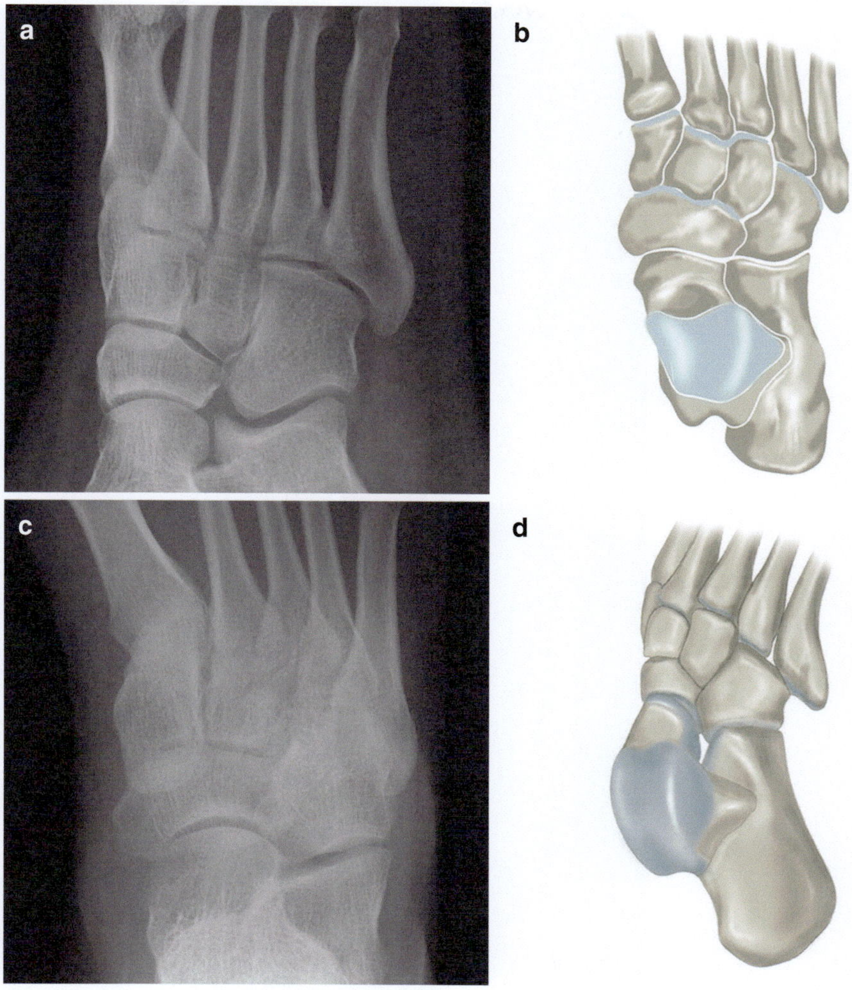

Fig. 11.28 X-ray film (**a**, **c**) shows that the structure of the scaphoid joint near the talus was slightly disturbed, and no definite fracture line was found. The schematic diagram (**b**, **d**)

 3.2 CT scan (Fig. 11.28e, f)

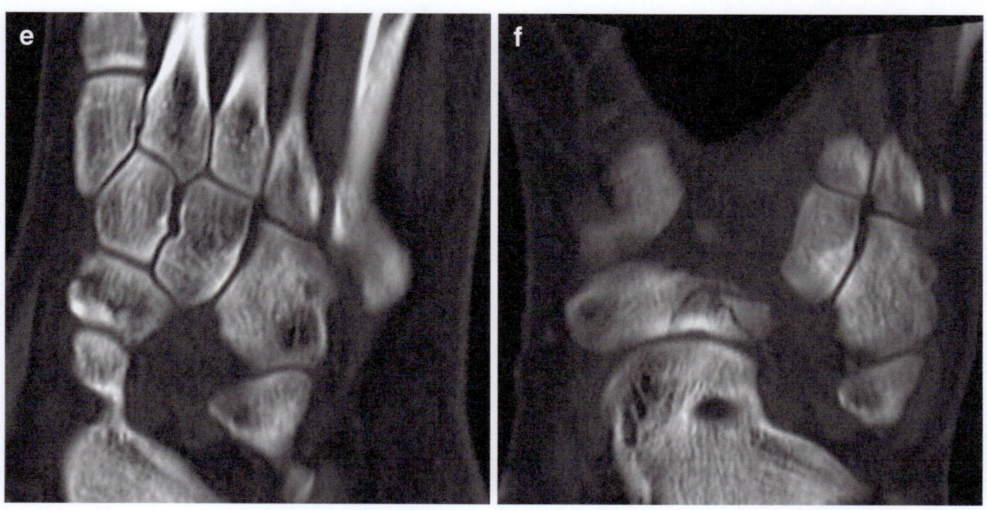

Fig. 11.28 CT sagittal plane (**e**) and transect (**f**) show bone fragmentation on the lateral part of scaphoid, showing multiple bones. The fracture line involved the articular surface, and the dislocation was not obvious

4. Comparison of X-ray film and CT between scaphoid comminuted fractures
   4.1 X-ray film (Fig. 11.29a–d)

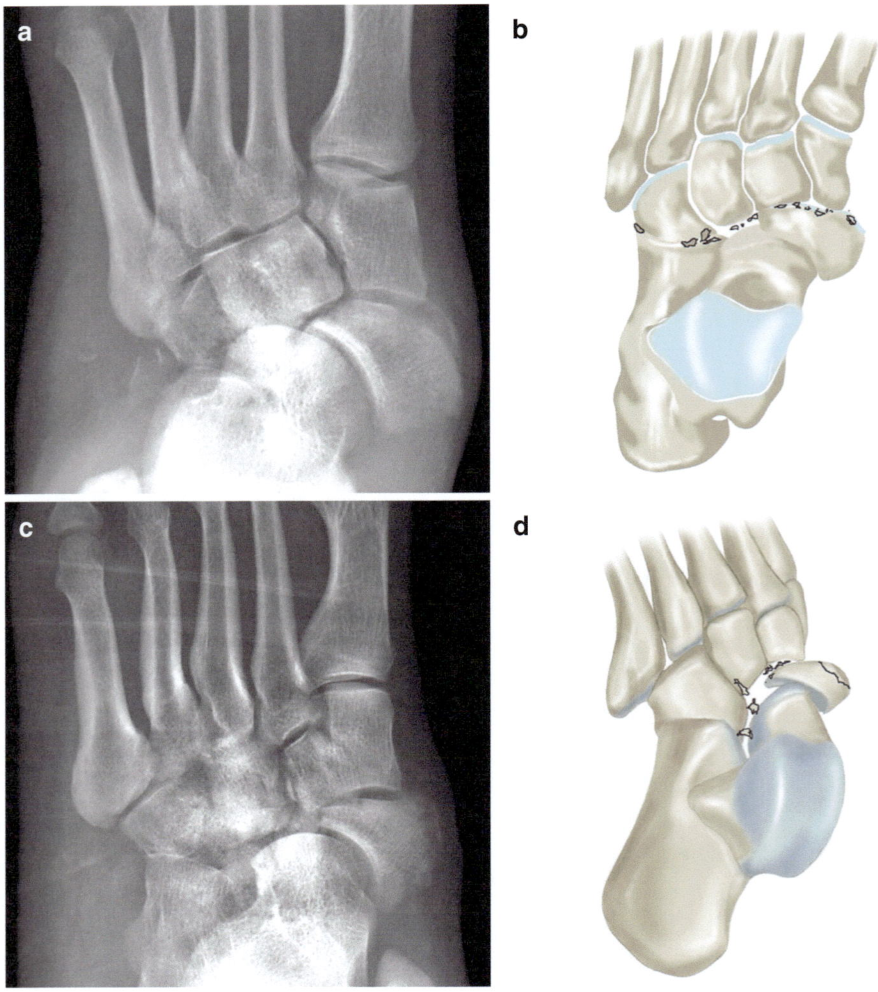

Fig. 11.29 The X-ray plain film (**a**, **c**) shows the dislocation of the canoe joint, the displacement of the cuneiform to the outside, the fracture of the outer margin of the scaphoid, and the shadow of the bone in the outer edge of the cuboid bone, and the schematic (**b**, **d**)

   4.2 CT scan (Fig. 11.29e, f)

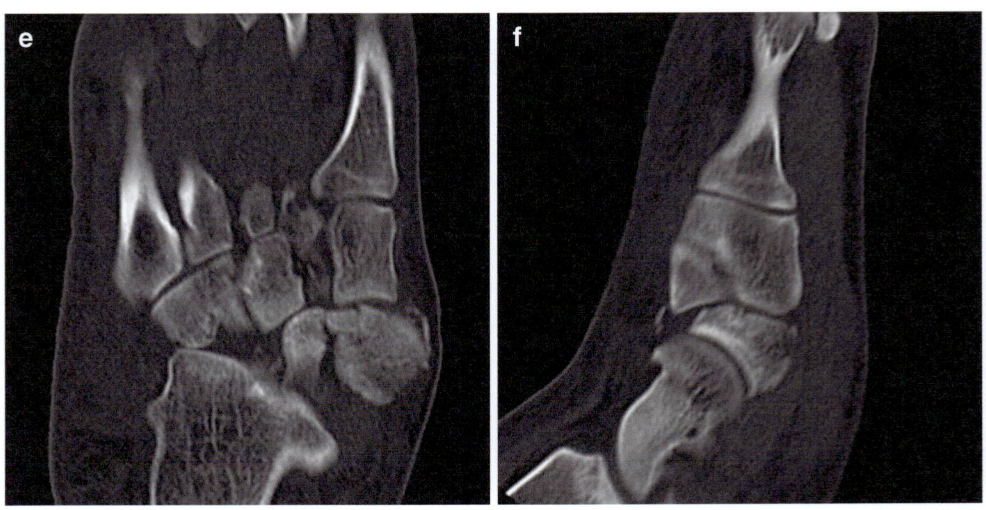

Fig. 11.29 CT cross section (**e**) and sagittal plane (**f**) show the dislocation of the canoe joint, the cuneiform bone moved to the lateral and dorsal side, the scaphoid bone fragmentation, multiple bone mass, the fracture line involving the articular surface, and the dislocation of the articular surface

5. Comparison between X-ray film and CT for comminuted fracture of cuboid bone
   5.1 X-ray film (Fig. 11.30a–d)

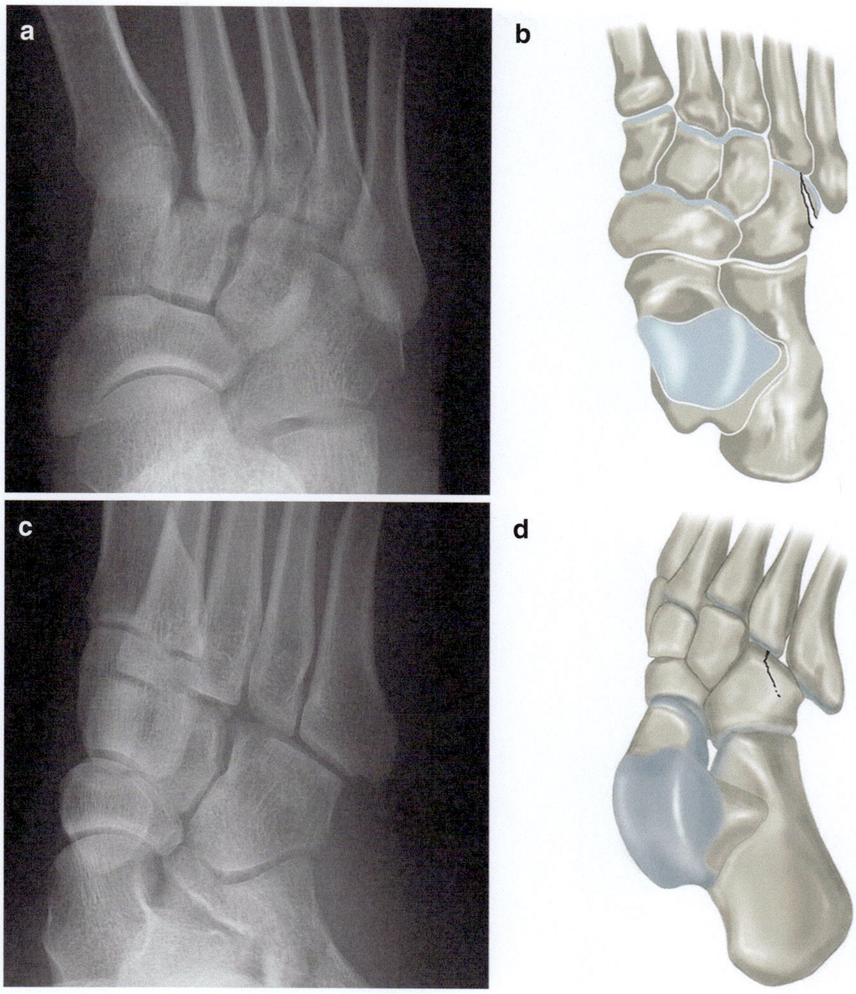

Fig. 11.30 X-ray film (**a** and **c**) shows bone fracture outside the cuboid bone, and the fragment moved outward, and the fracture line involved the articular surface. The schematic diagram (**b**, **d**)

   5.2 CT scan (Fig. 11.30e, f)

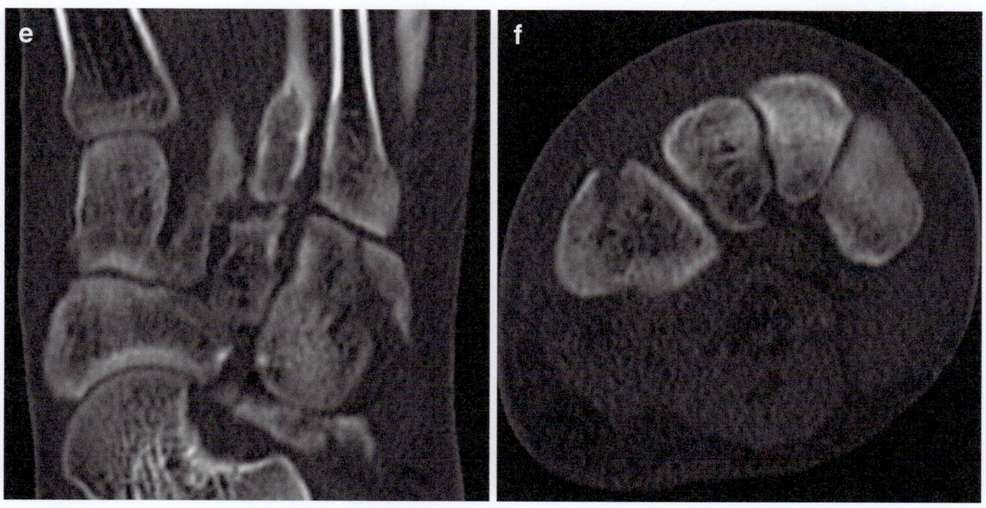

Fig. 11.30 CT transect (**e**) and coronal plane (**f**) show bony fracture of the lateral border of the cuboid bone, dislocation of the end of the fracture, and the fracture line involving the articular surface

6. Comparison between X-ray film and CT for comminuted fracture of cuboid bone
   6.1 X-ray film (Fig. 11.31a–d)

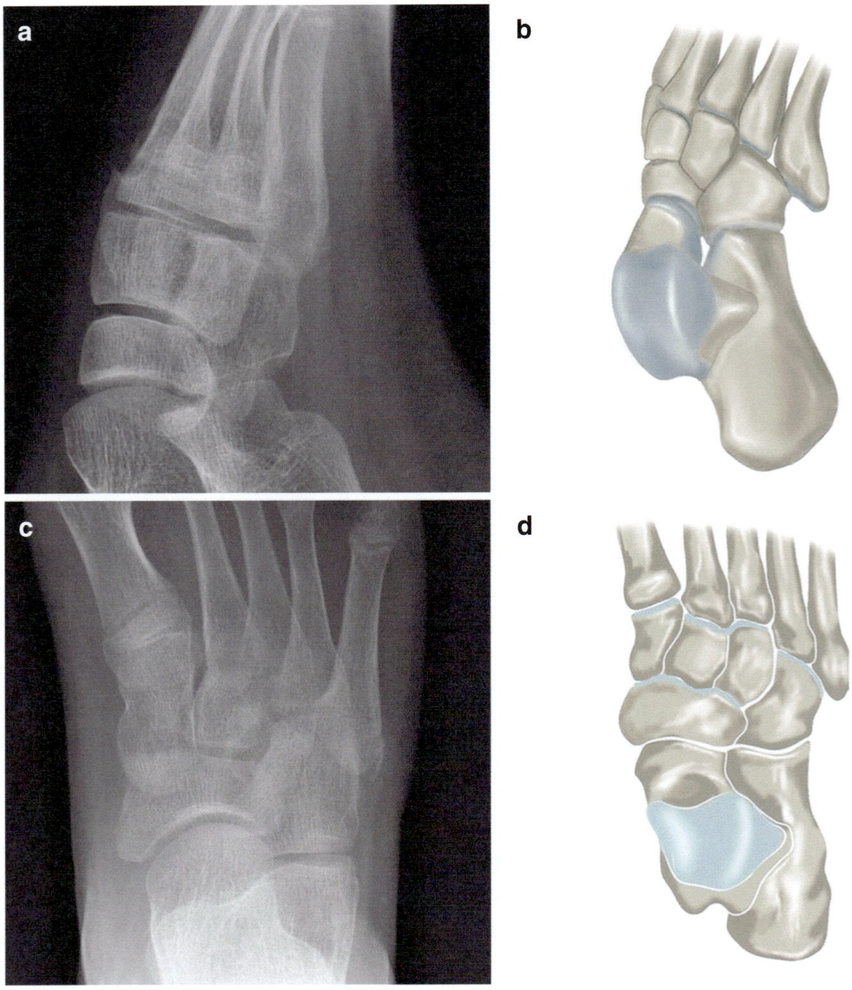

Fig. 11.31 X-ray film (**a**, **c**) shows no definite fracture signs of the cuboid bone, and the schematic diagram (**b**, **d**)

   6.2 CT scan (Fig. 11.31e, f)

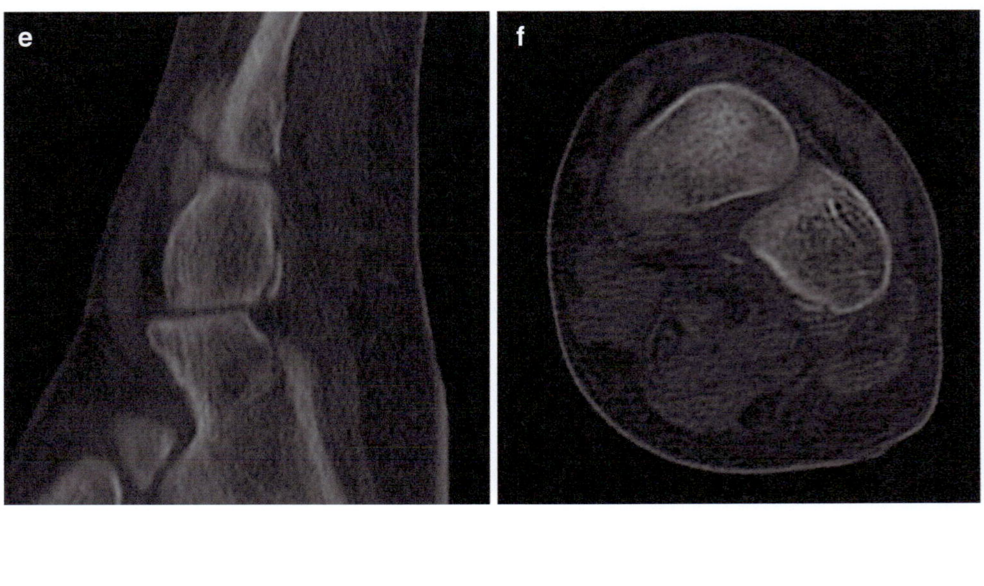

Fig. 11.31 CT sagittal plane (**e**) and coronal plane (**f**) show bone fracture of the lateral border of the cuboid bone, showing an arc bone shadow

7. Comparison between X-ray film and CT in comminuted fracture of the cuboid bone
   7.1 X-ray film (Fig. 11.32a–d)

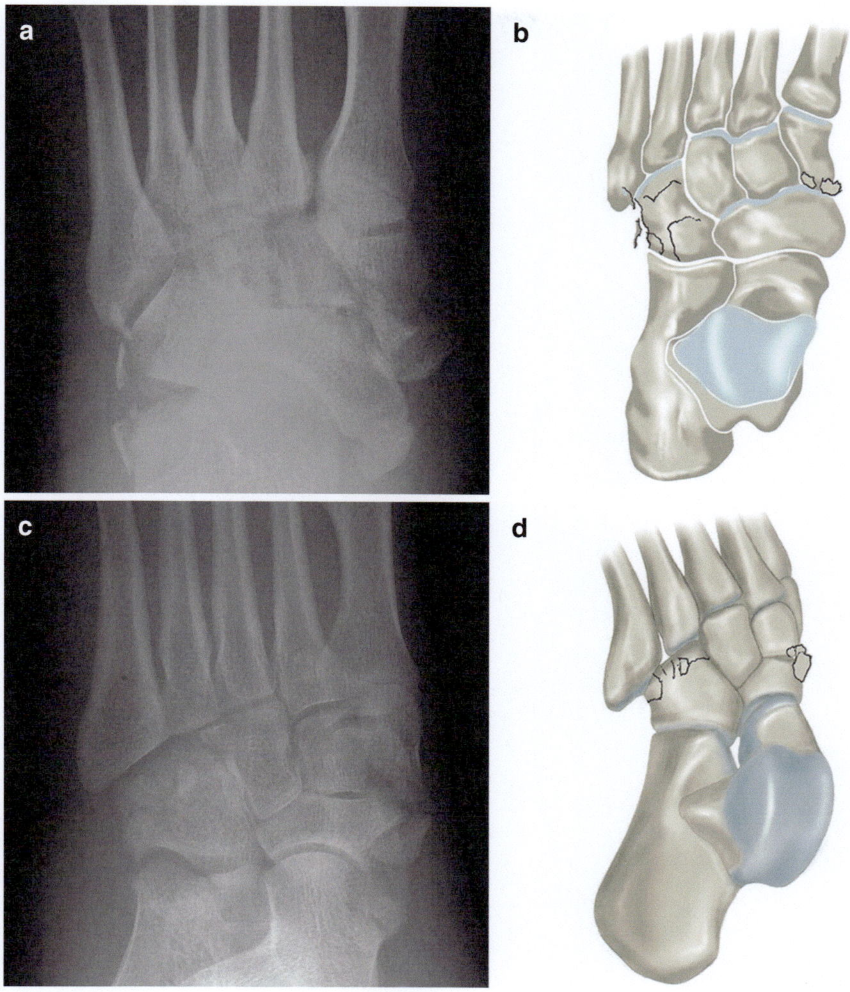

Fig. 11.32 X-ray film (**a**, **c**) shows bone fracture of cuboid bone, broken bone of medial cuneiform, dislocation, and bone fracture of anterior edge of calcaneus (**b**, **d**)

   7.2 CT scan (Fig. 11.32e, f)

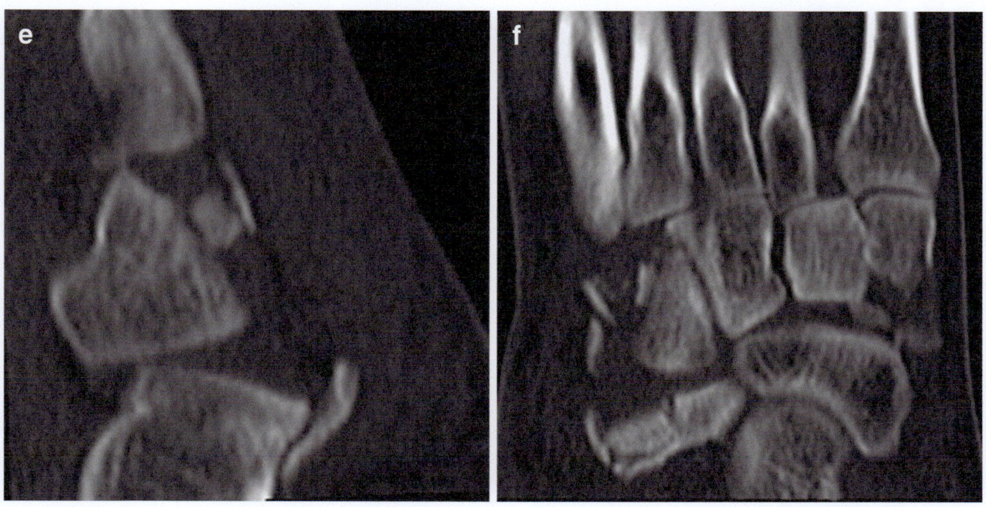

Fig. 11.32 CT sagittal plane (**e**) and cross section (**f**) show bone fragmentation of the dice bone, dislocation of the dice and dice metatarsal joints, the collapse of the calcaneus anterior margin, and the fracture of the medial cuneiform bone

8. Comparison between X-ray film and CT in comminuted fracture of the cuboid bone
   8.1 X-ray film (Fig. 11.33a–d)

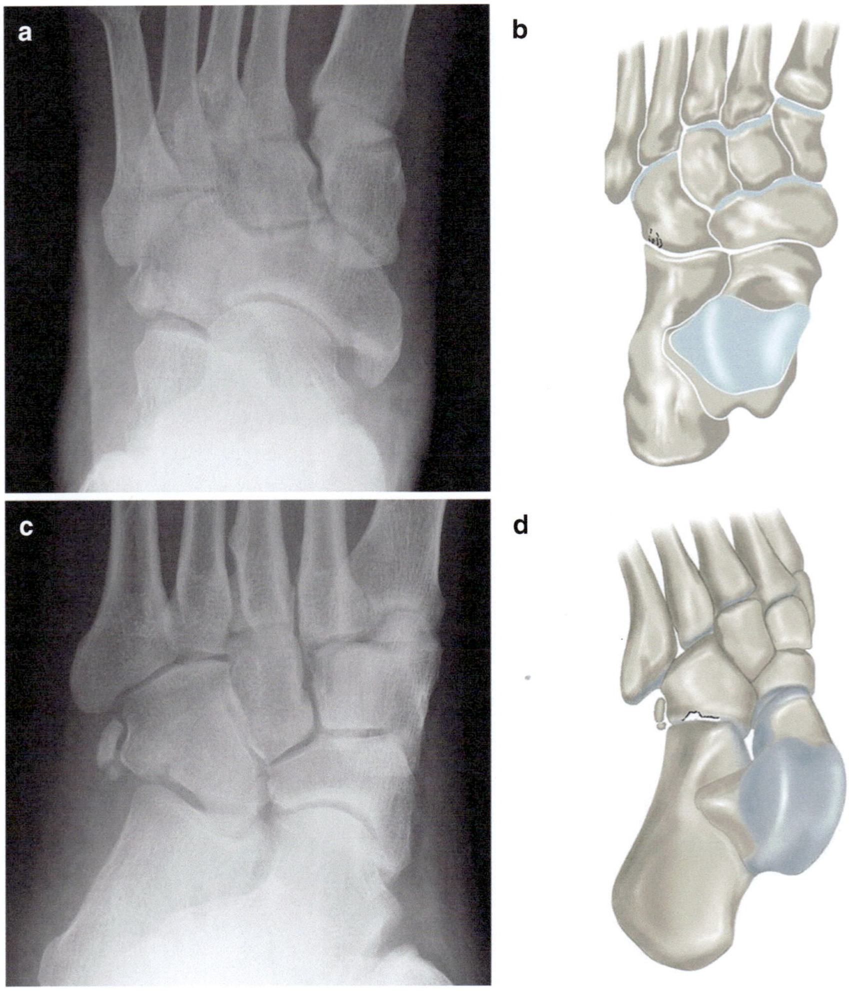

Fig. 11.33 X-ray film (**a**, **c**) shows the collapse of the articular surface of the proximal part of the cuboid bone, trabecular bone fracture, and the widening of the base space of the first, second metatarsus (**b**, **d**)

   8.2 CT scan (Fig. 11.33e, f)

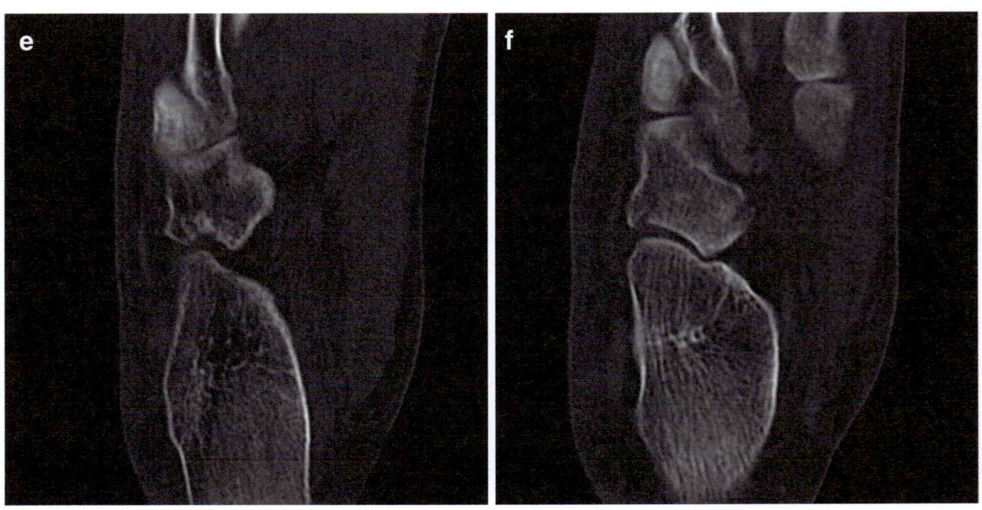

Fig. 11.33 The CT cross section (**e**, **f**) shows the collapse of the articular surface of the cuboid proximal part and the fracture of bone

9. Comparison between X-ray film and CT for comminuted fracture of cuneiform bone
   9.1 X-ray film (Fig. 11.34a–d)

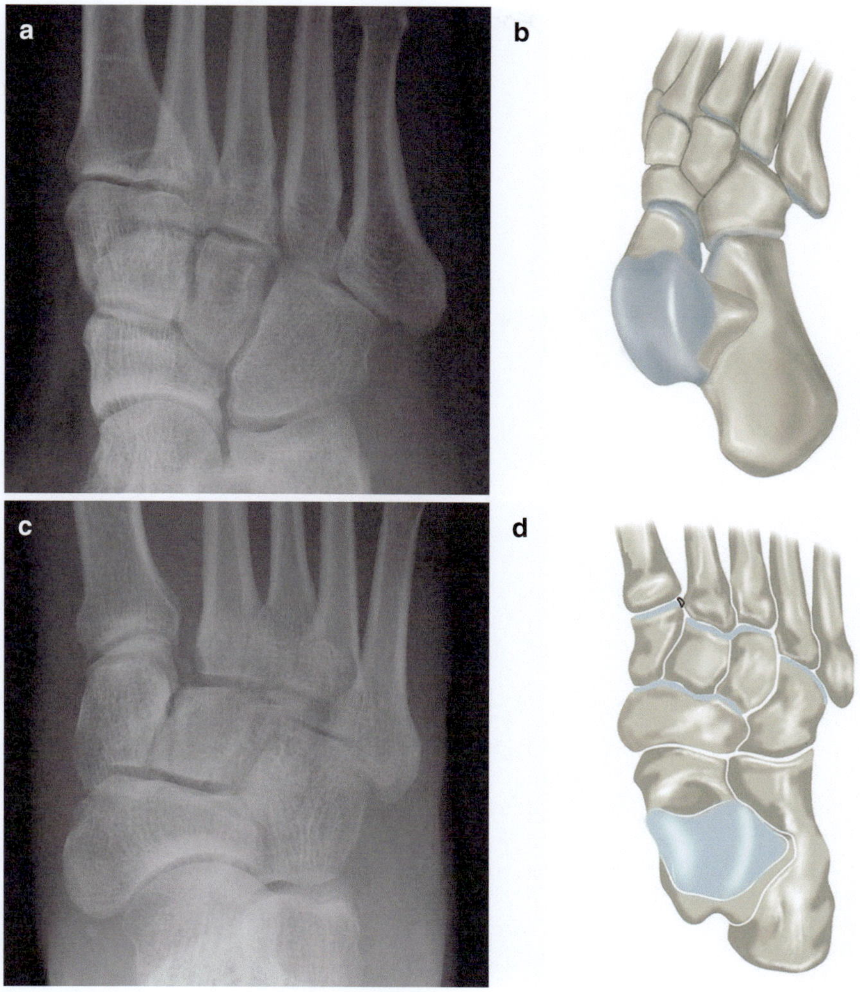

Fig. 11.34 X-ray film (**a**, **c**) shows widening of the base space of the first, second metatarsus. Small bone fragments were seen. Wedge bone showed no definite signs of fracture. The schematic diagram (**b**, **d**)

   9.2 CT scan (Fig. 11.34e, f)

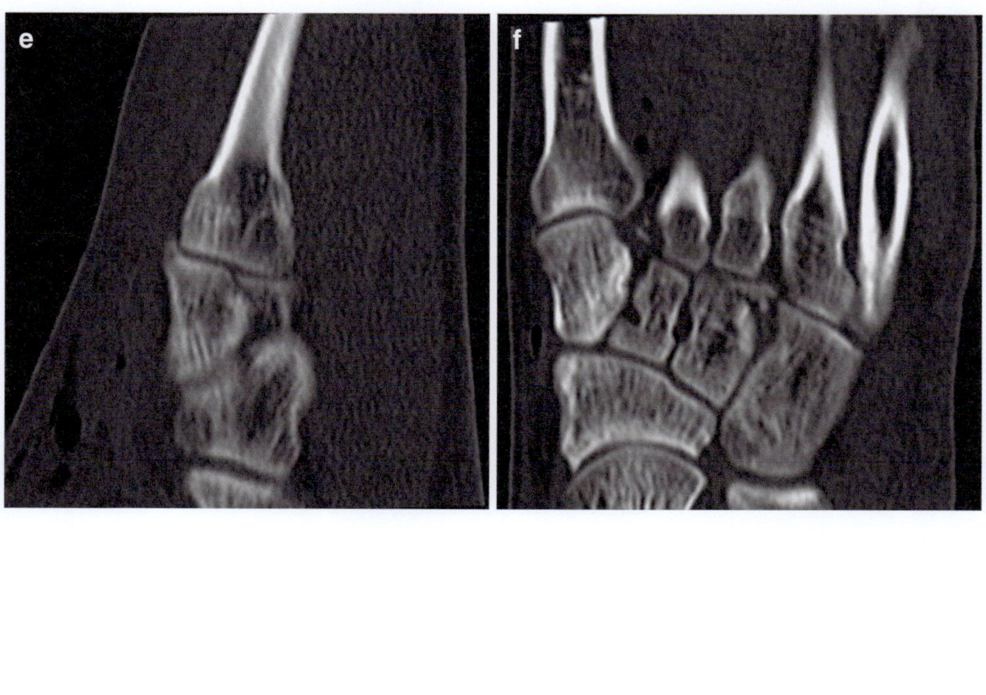

Fig. 11.34 CT sagittal plane (**e**) and cross section (**f**) show the fracture of the lateral wedge bone. The dislocation of the broken end was not obvious. The fracture line involved the articular surface. The second metatarsal basement was seen in the small bone slices

10. Comparison between X-ray film and CT for comminuted fracture of cuneiform bone
    10.1 X-ray film (Fig. 11.35a–d)

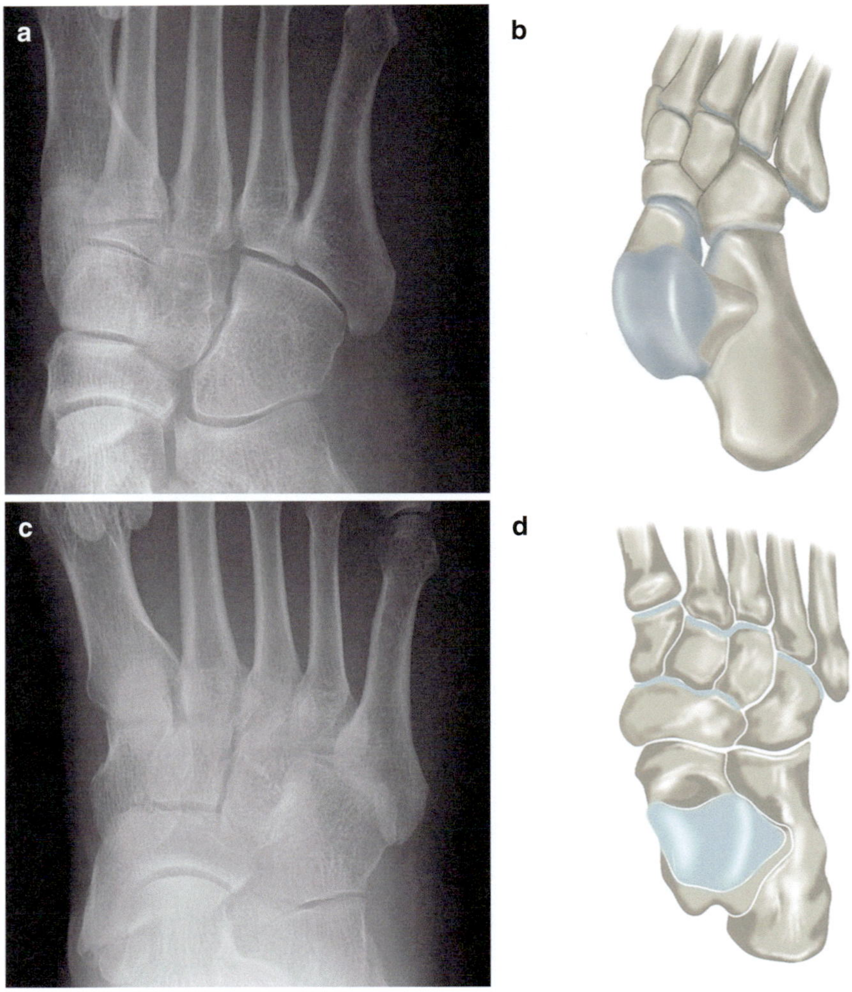

Fig. 11.35 X-ray films (**a**, **c**) shows no definite signs of fracture in the tarsal metatarsal joint, and the schematic diagram (**b**, **d**)

10.2 CT scan (Fig. 11.35e, f)

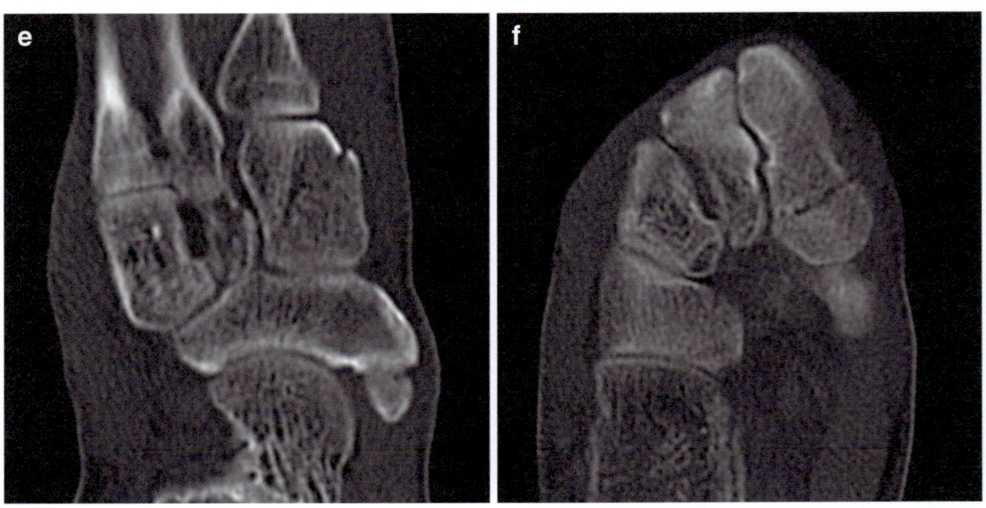

Fig. 11.35 CT cross section (**e**) and coronal plane (**f**) show bone fracture of medial wedge bone and dislocation of the ends

11. Comparison of X-ray film and CT for comminuted fracture of the cuneiform bone
    11.1 X-ray film (Fig. 11.36a–d)

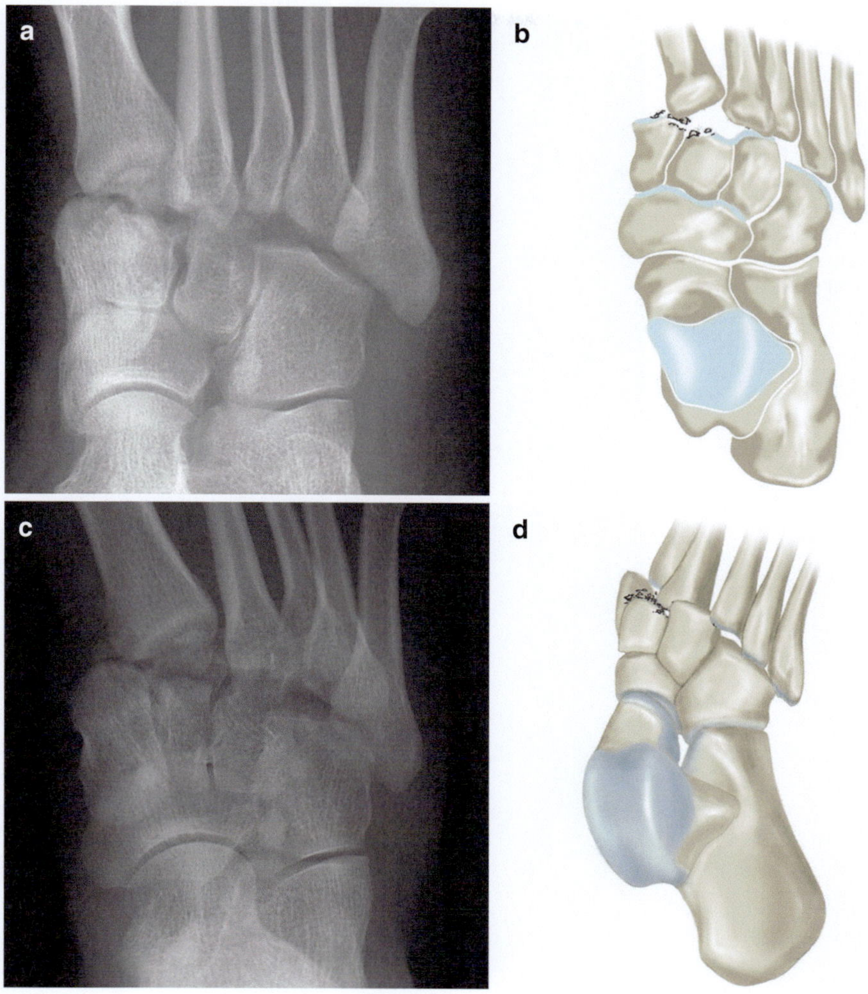

Fig. 11.36 X-ray film (**a** and **c**) shows the lateral displacement of the base of the first to 5 metatarsal base, with irregular base and small bone fragments. The schematic diagram (**b**, **d**)

    11.2 CT scan (Fig. 11.36e, f)

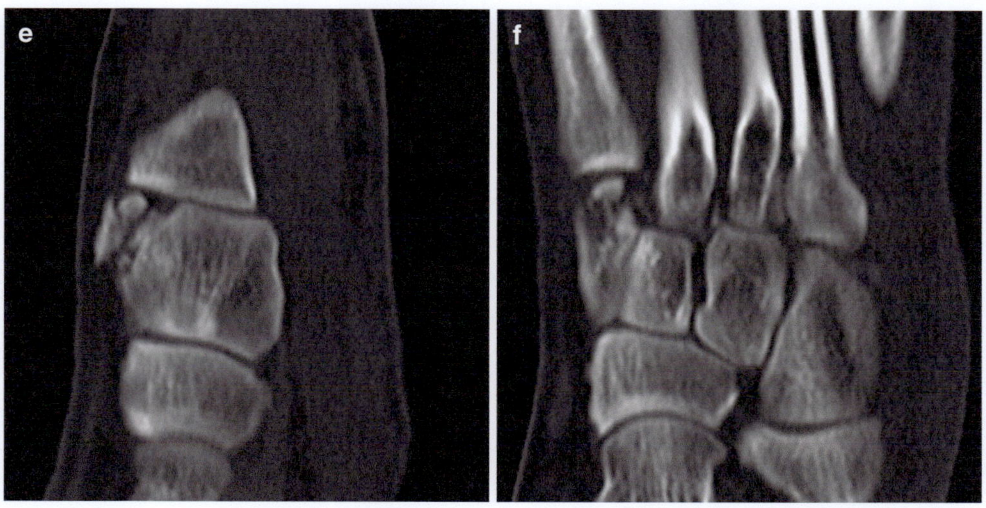

Fig. 11.36 CT sagittal plane (**e**) and cross section (**f**) show bone fragmentation of the medial cuneiform bone, dislocation of the broken end, fracture line involving the articular surface, and small slices of bone in the base of the second, third metatarsal

12. Comparison of X-ray film and CT for comminuted fracture of the cuneiform bone
    12.1 X-ray film (Fig. 11.37a–d)

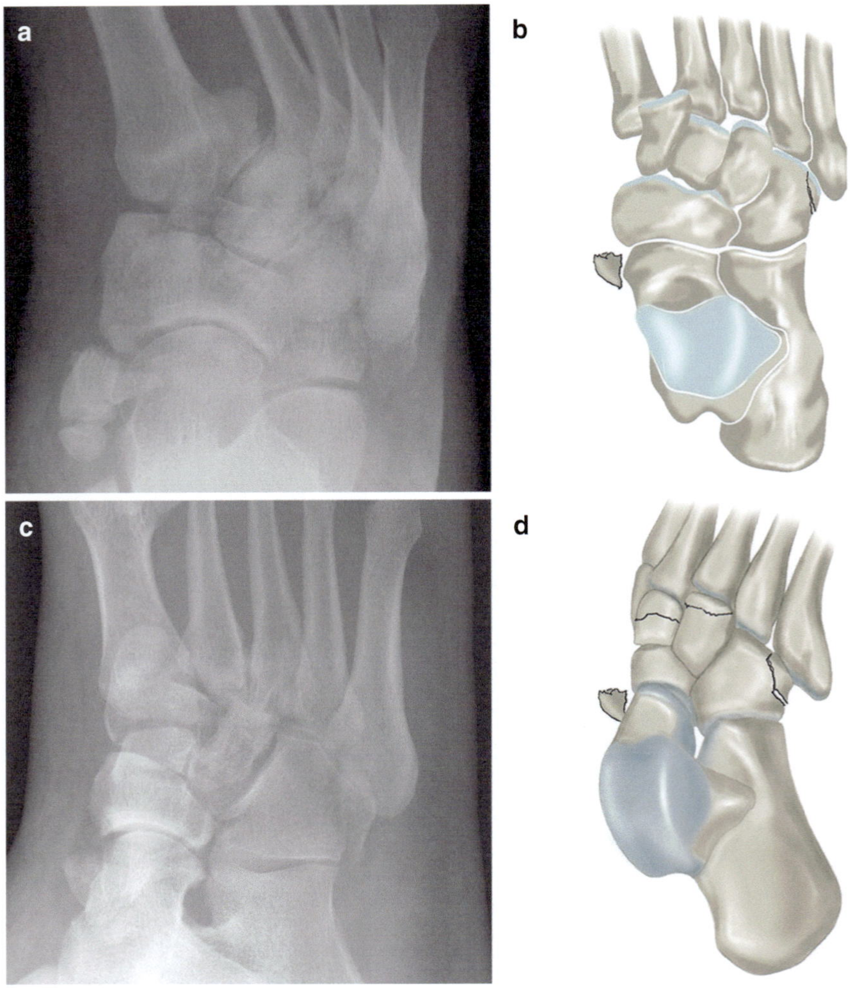

Fig. 11.37 X-ray film (**a**, **c**) shows the displacement of the first metatarsal basement to the medial side, the second metatarsal basement translocation, the medial wedge bone, the middle wedge bone fracture, the medial scaphoid bone fracture, the outer bone fracture of the cuboid bone, and the schematic diagram (**b**, **d**)

    12.2 CT scan (Fig. 11.37e, f)

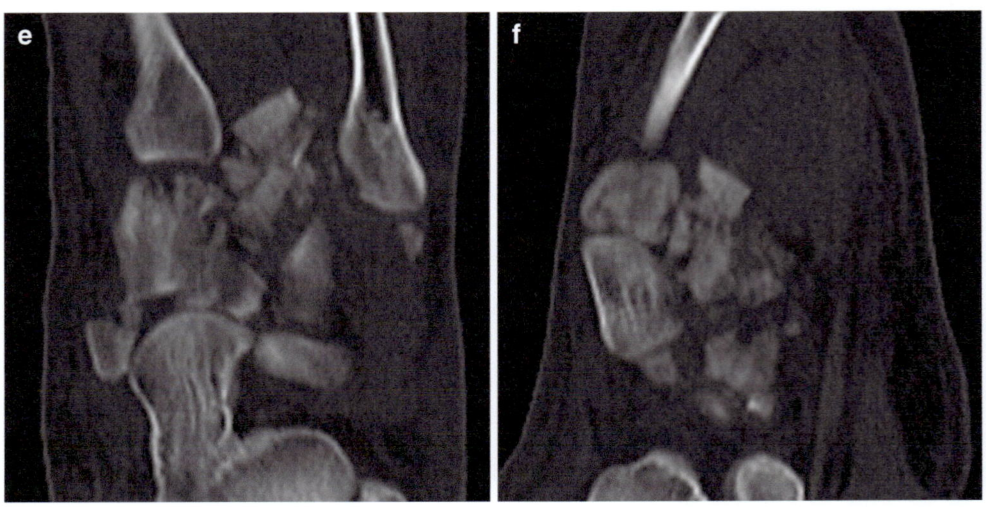

Fig. 11.37 CT cross section (**e**) and sagittal plane (**f**) show scaphoid, medial wedge-shaped bone, and middle wedge-shaped bone fracture

13. Comparison of X-ray film and CT for comminuted fracture of the cuneiform bone
    13.1 X-ray film (Fig. 11.38a–d)

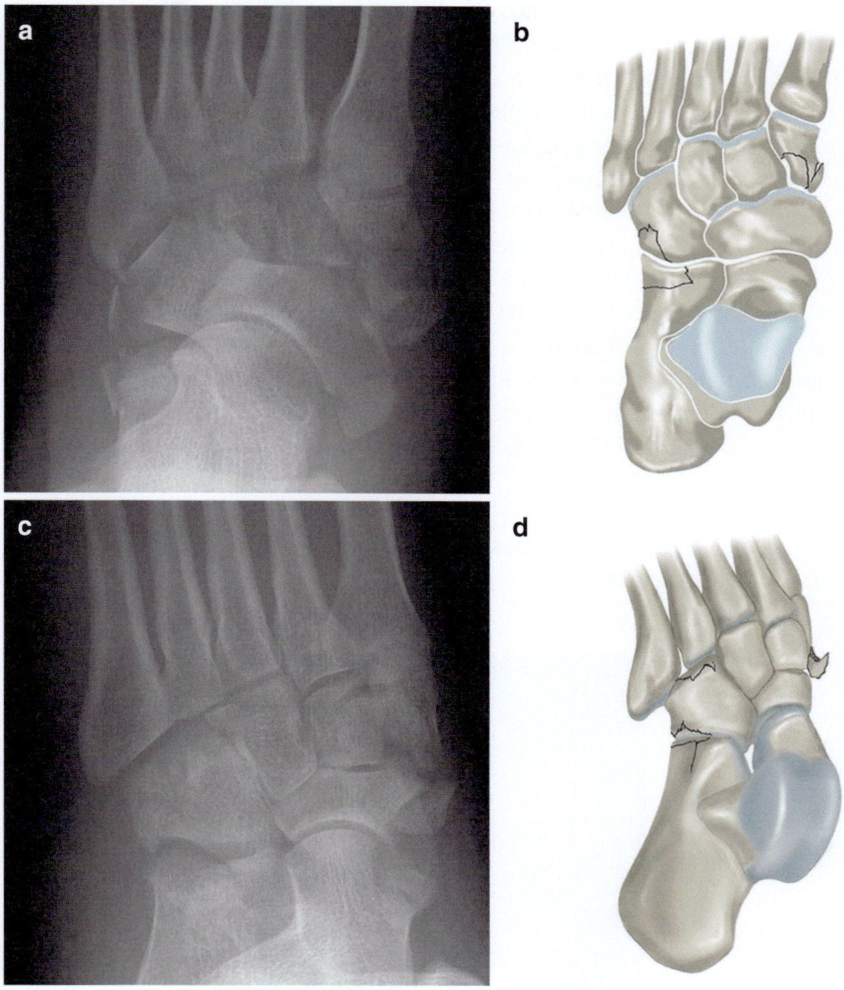

Fig. 11.38 X-ray film (**a**, **c**) shows bone fracture of medial wedge bone, dislocation, fracture of cuboid and anterior calcaneal bone, and schematic diagram (**b**, **d**)

13.2 CT scan (Fig. 11.38e, f)

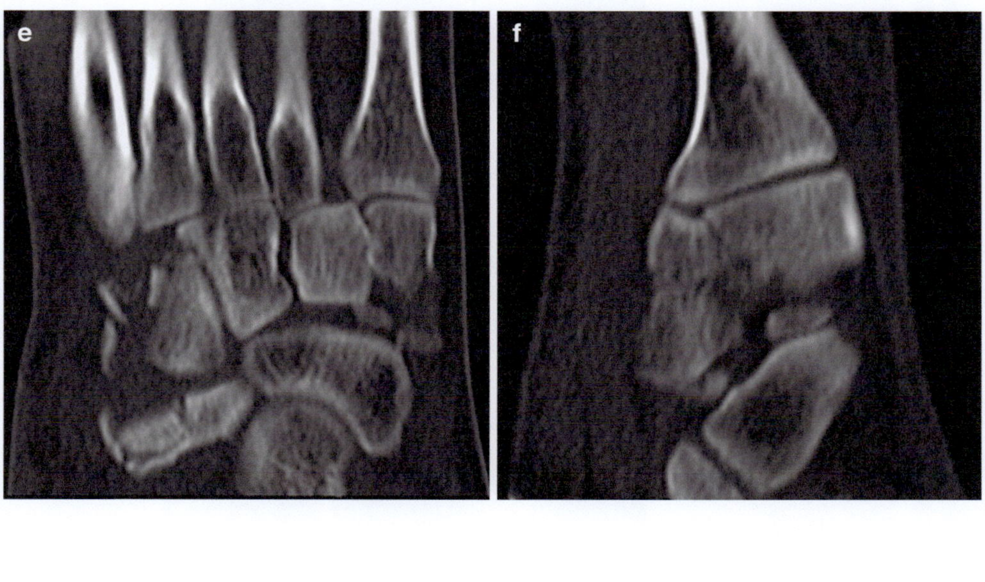

Fig. 11.38 CT cross section (**e**) and sagittal plane (**f**) show the bone fracture of the medial wedge bone, dislocation of the broken end, the fracture line involving the articular surface, the cataclastic bone, the calcaneus bone, the dislocation, and the irregular joint surface

11.3 Metatarsal Fracture

The metatarsus is a long tubular bone with five pieces, divided into three parts: the bottom, the body, and the head. The metatarsus is slightly expanded near the end of the metatarsal, which is cuneiform, called the bottom. The bottom is articulated with the long tarsus. The distal end of the metatarsus is a head with a protruding joint surface, which is articulated with the proximal phalanges. The body is between the head and the bottom. The metatarsal fracture accounts for 37.54% of the foot fracture. The AO/OTA classification of metatarsal fractures is divided into extra-articular fractures of the proximal metatarsal, simple metatarsal shaft fractures, extra-articular fractures of the distal metatarsal, intra-articular fractures of the proximal metatarsal, wedge-shaped fractures of the metatarsal, intra-articular fractures of the distal metatarsal, complete intra-articular fractures of the proximal metatarsal, comminuted fracture of the metatarsal shaft, and complete intra-articular fracture of the distal metatarsal. The extra-articular fractures of the proximal metatarsal accounted for 13.30% of the foot fracture, the simple metatarsal shaft fractures accounted for 6.78% of the foot fracture, and extra-articular fractures of the distal metatarsal accounted for 5.52% of the foot fracture. The incomplete intra-articular fracture of proximal metatarsal accounted for 6.20% of the foot fractures, the wedge-shaped fractures of the metatarsal accounted for 1.62% of the foot fractures, and intra-articular fractures of the distal metatarsal accounted for 0.43% of the foot fractures. The complete intra-articular fractures of the proximal metatarsal accounted for 2.41% of the foot fractures. The comminuted fracture of the metatarsal shaft accounted for 0.84% of the foot fracture, and the complete intra-articular fracture of the distal metatarsal accounted for 0.44% of the foot fracture.

1. Multiple metatarsal proximal fractures were identified with suspected fractures
   1.1 X-ray plain film (Fig. 11.39a–d)

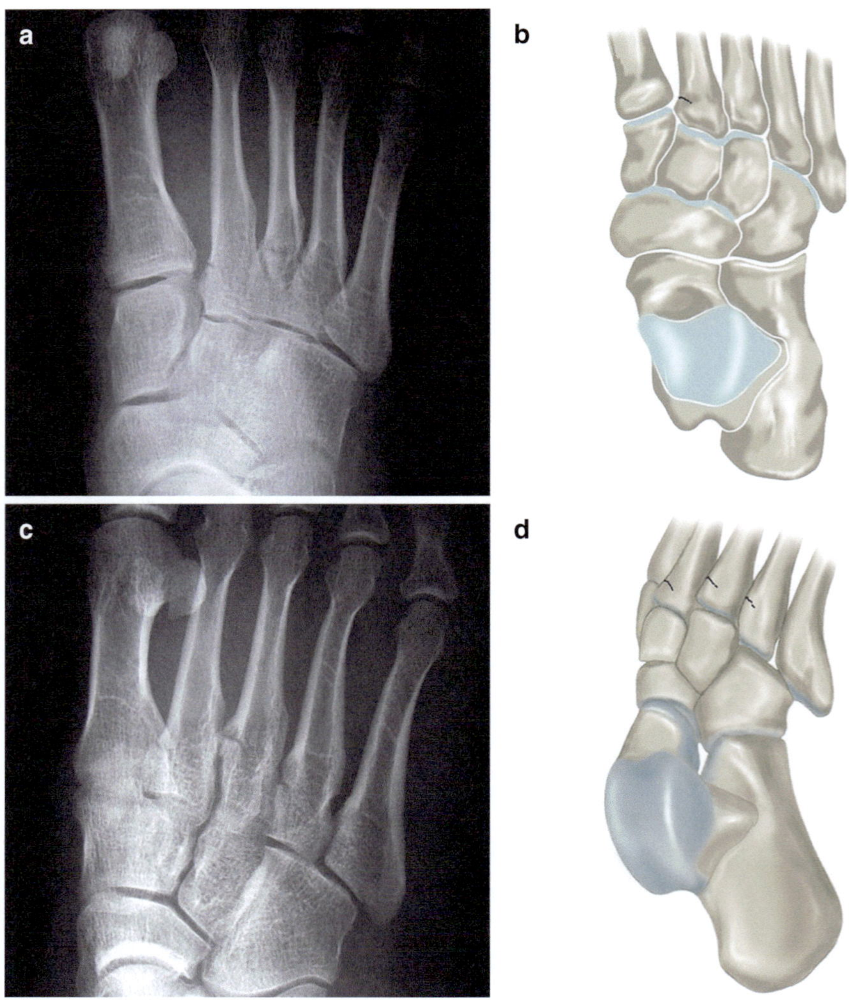

Fig. 11.39 X-ray plain film (**a**, **c**) shows the bone cortex of the base of the 2–4 metatarsal interrupted continuously without obvious dislocation. The schematic diagram (**b**, **d**)

1.2 CT scan (Fig. 11.39e, f)

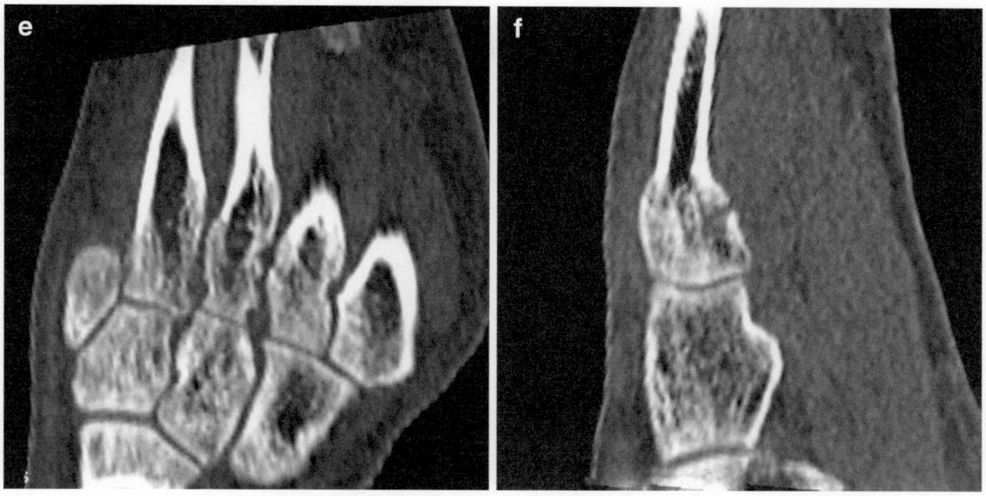

Fig. 11.39 CT transect (**e**) and sagittal plane (**f**) show bone fracture in the medial border of metatarsal base and metatarsal border, and no obvious malposition at the end of the metatarsus

2. Comminuted fracture of proximal metatarsal bone and fracture
   2.1 X-ray plain film (Fig. 11.40a–d)

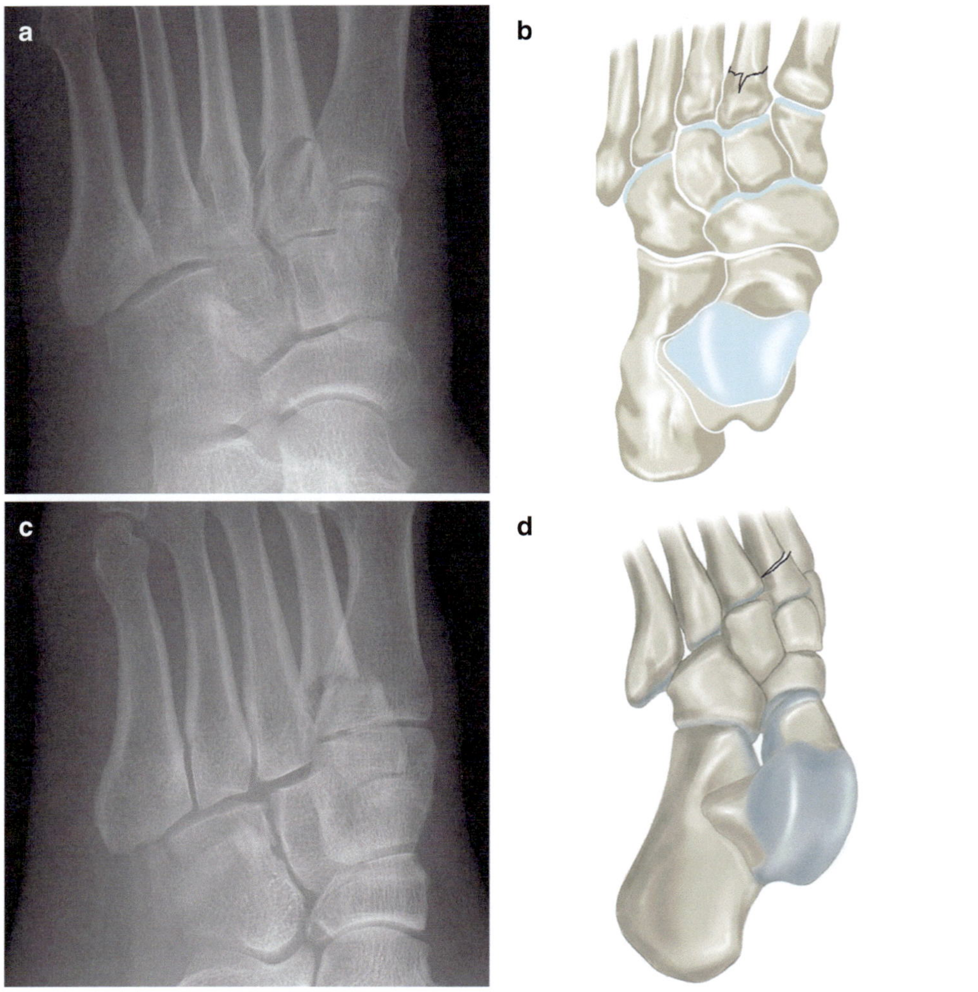

Fig. 11.40 X-ray plain film (**a**, **c**) shows a transverse fracture of the base of the second metatarsal bone, with a slightly dislocated end, and a schematic diagram (**b**, **d**)

   2.2 CT scan (Fig. 11.40e, f)

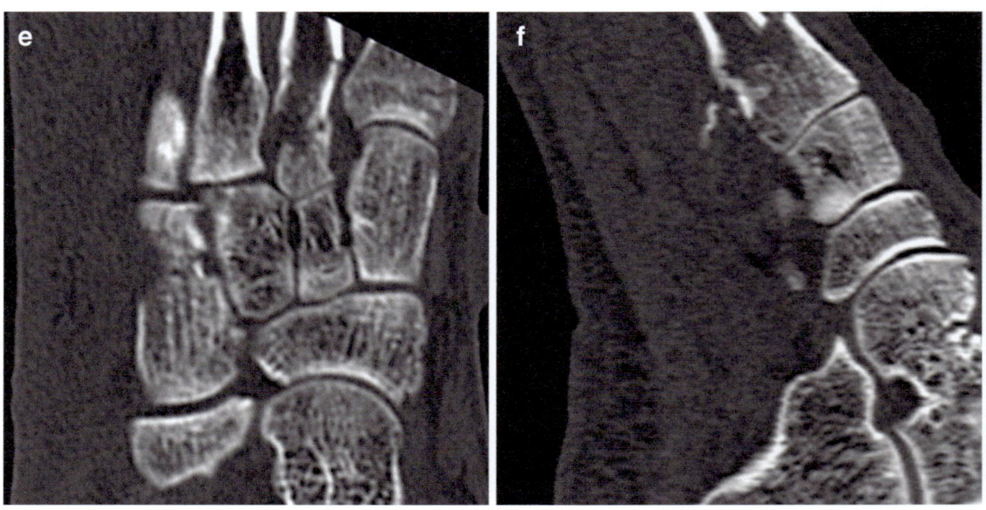

Fig. 11.40 The CT transect (**e**) and sagittal plane (**f**) show that the base of the second metatarsal bone was fragmented, and the ends of the metacarps were slightly mal-positioned

3. Identification of proximal metatarsal fractures and suspicious fractures
   3.1 X-ray plain film (Fig. 11.41a–d)

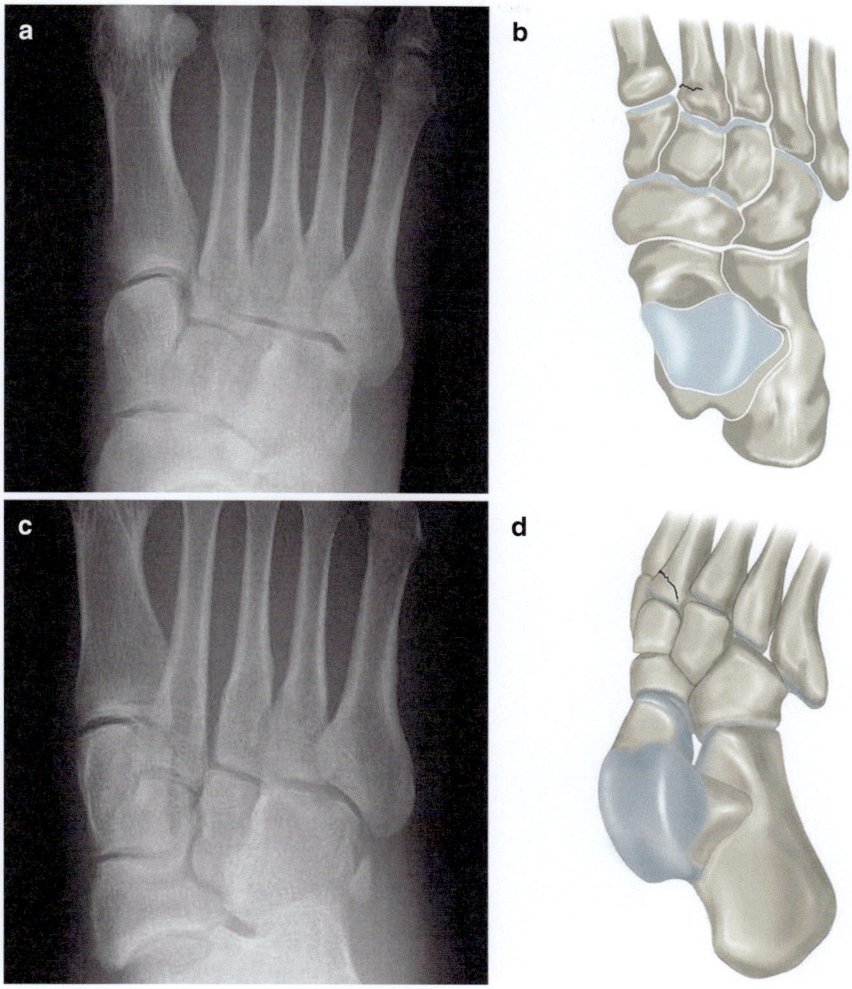

Fig. 11.41 X-ray plain film (**a** and **c**) shows a translucent shadow between the medial border of the base of the second metatarsal bone (**b**, **d**)

   3.2 CT scan (Fig. 11.41e, f)

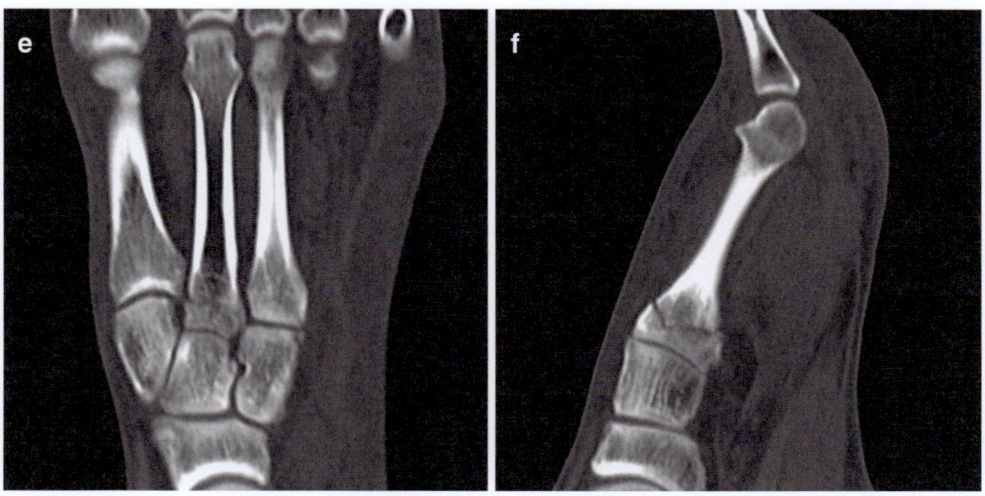

Fig. 11.41 CT transverse section (**e**) and sagittal plane (**f**) show a transverse fracture of the base of the second metatarsal bone with no obvious dislocation at the end of the fracture

4. Comparison between plain film and CT for spiral fracture of metatarsal stem
   4.1 X-ray plain film (Fig. 11.42a–d)

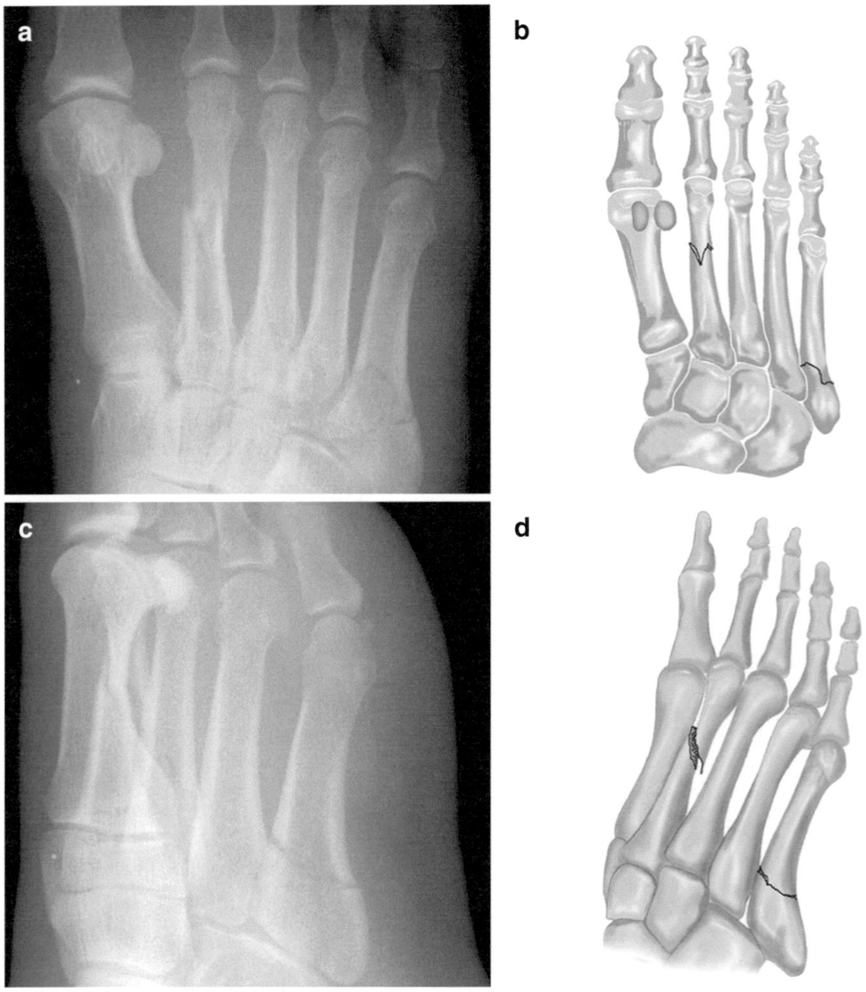

Fig. 11.42 X-ray plain film (**a**, **c**) shows the fracture of the middle bone of the second metatarsal bone, a slight dislocation of the broken end, the fracture of the proximal bone of the fifth metatarsal, and no obvious dislocation in the broken end, and the schematic (**b**, **d**)

   4.2 CT scan (Fig. 11.42e, f)

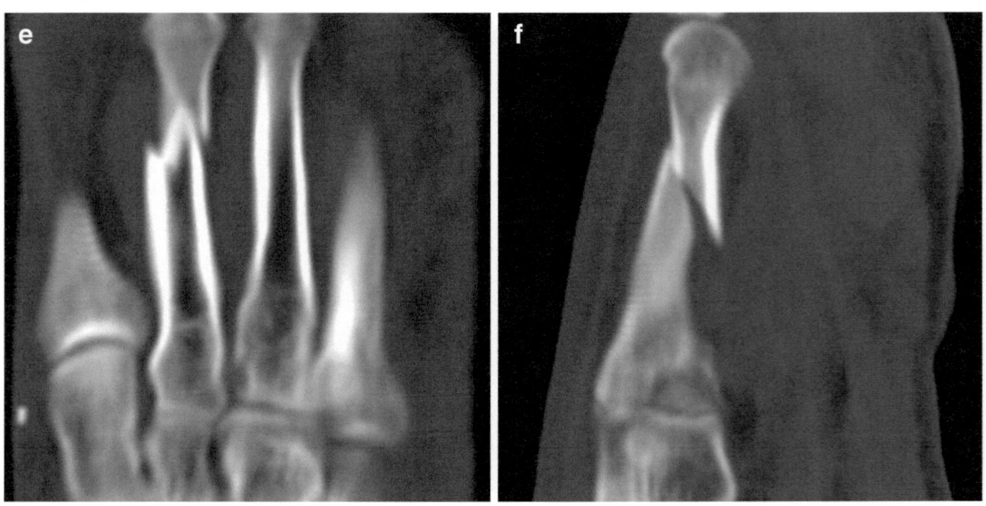

Fig. 11.42 CT transect (**e**) and sagittal plane (**f**) show spiral bone fracture in the middle part of the second metatarsal shaft, and the dislocation was slightly angled

5. Comparison of plain films with CT for multiple distal metatarsal fractures
   5.1 X-ray plain film (Fig. 11.43a–d)

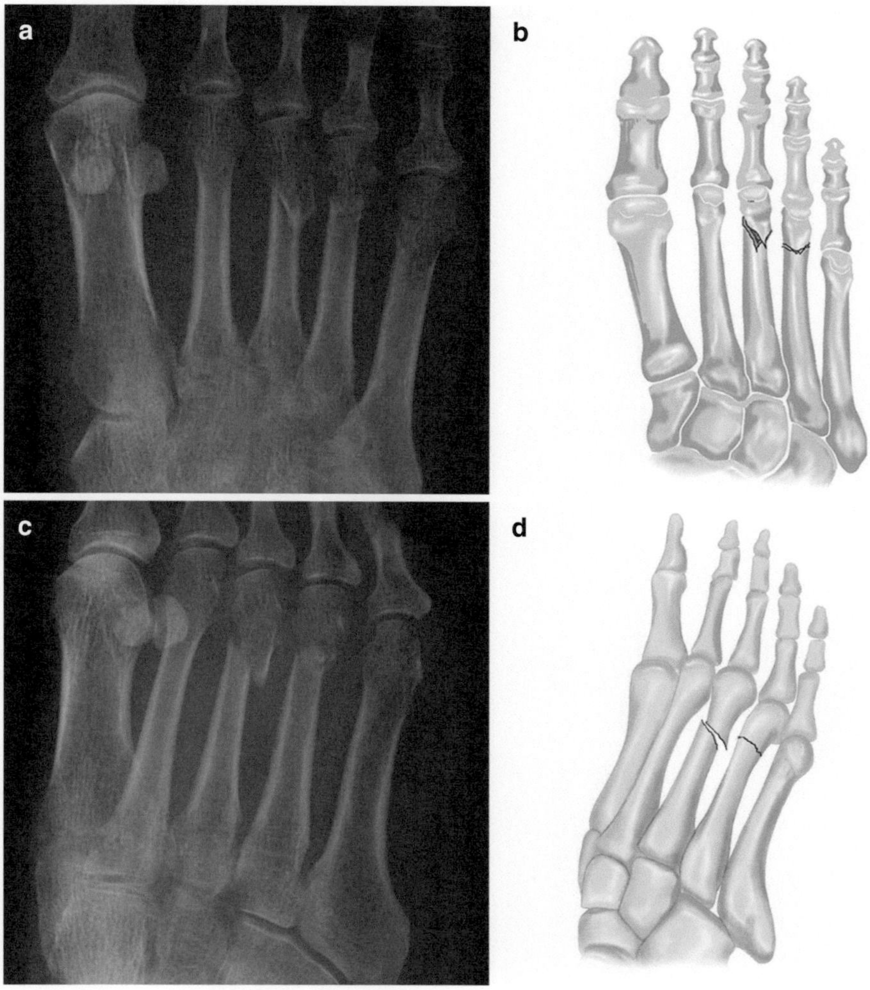

Fig. 11.43 X-ray plain film (**a**, **c**) shows a fracture of the distal part of the third, fourth metatarsal shaft, with a slightly dislocated end, and a schematic diagram (**b**, **d**)

   5.2 CT scan (Fig. 11.43e, f)

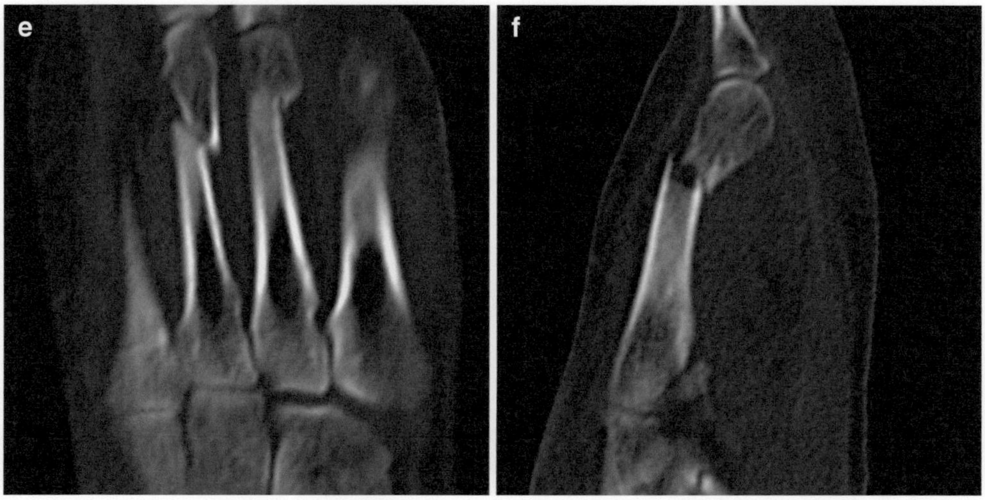

Fig. 11.43 CT transect (**e**) and sagittal plane (**f**) show fracture of distal bone of the third, fourth metatarsal shaft, dislocation of the ends, slightly angled

6. Comparison between plain film and CT for distal metatarsal fractures
   6.1 X-ray plain film (Fig. 11.44a–d)

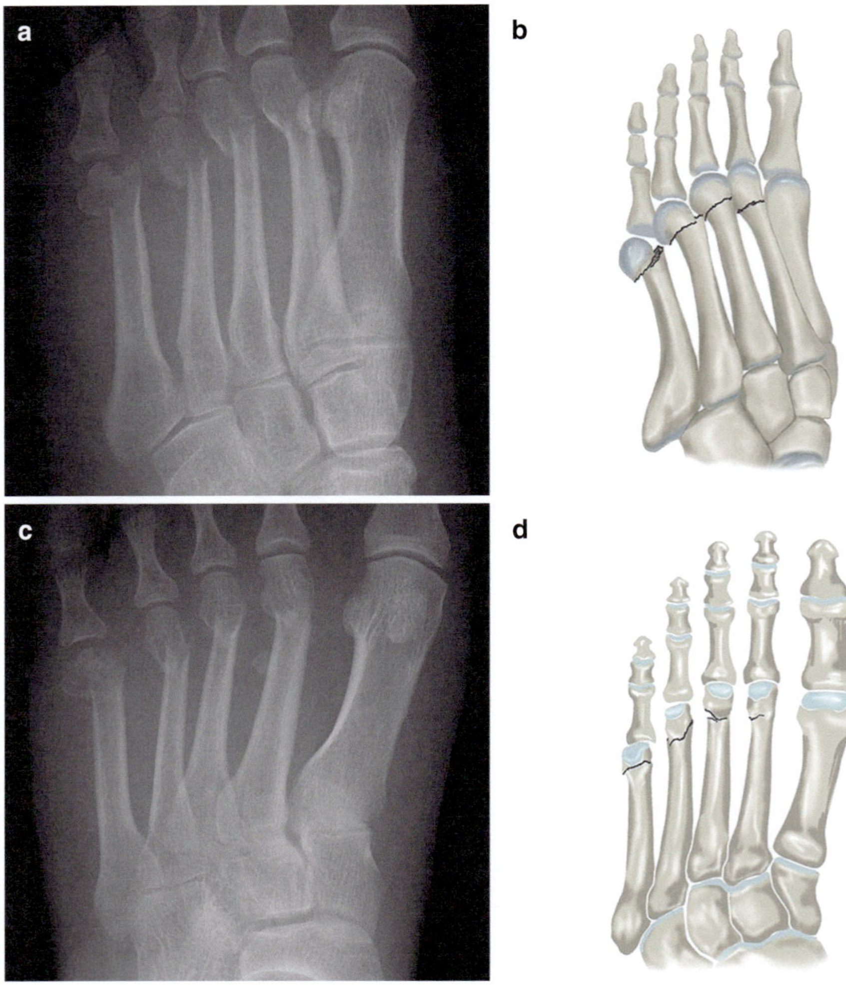

Fig. 11.44 X-ray plain film (**a**, **c**) shows a fracture of the distal part of the 3–5 metatarsal bone, with a slightly broken end and second irregular shape of the distal metatarsus (**b**, **d**)

   6.2 CT scan (Fig. 11.44e, f)

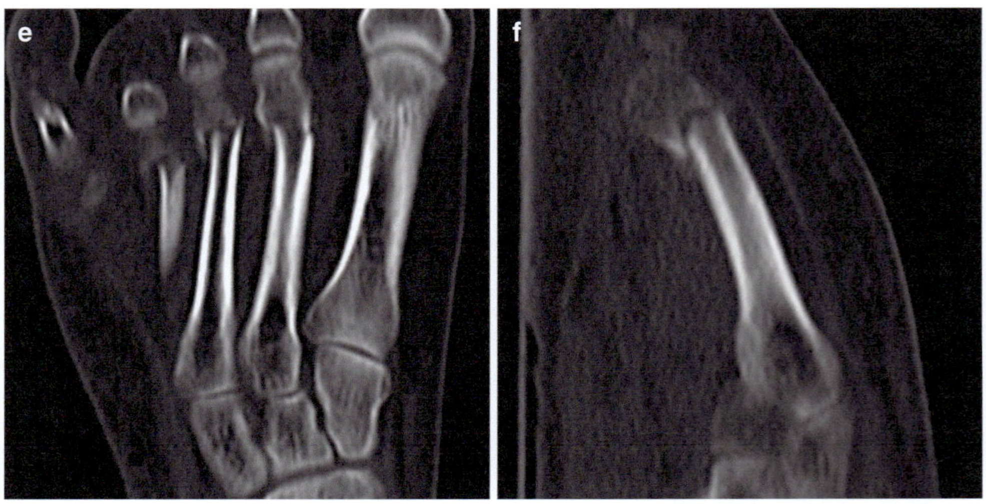

Fig. 11.44 CT transect (**e**) and sagittal plane (**f**) show a fracture of the distal 2–5 metatarsal bone with a slightly inserted dislocation at the end of the fracture

7. Comparison of plain films with CT for multiple distal metatarsal fractures
    7.1 X-ray plain film (Fig. 11.45a–d)

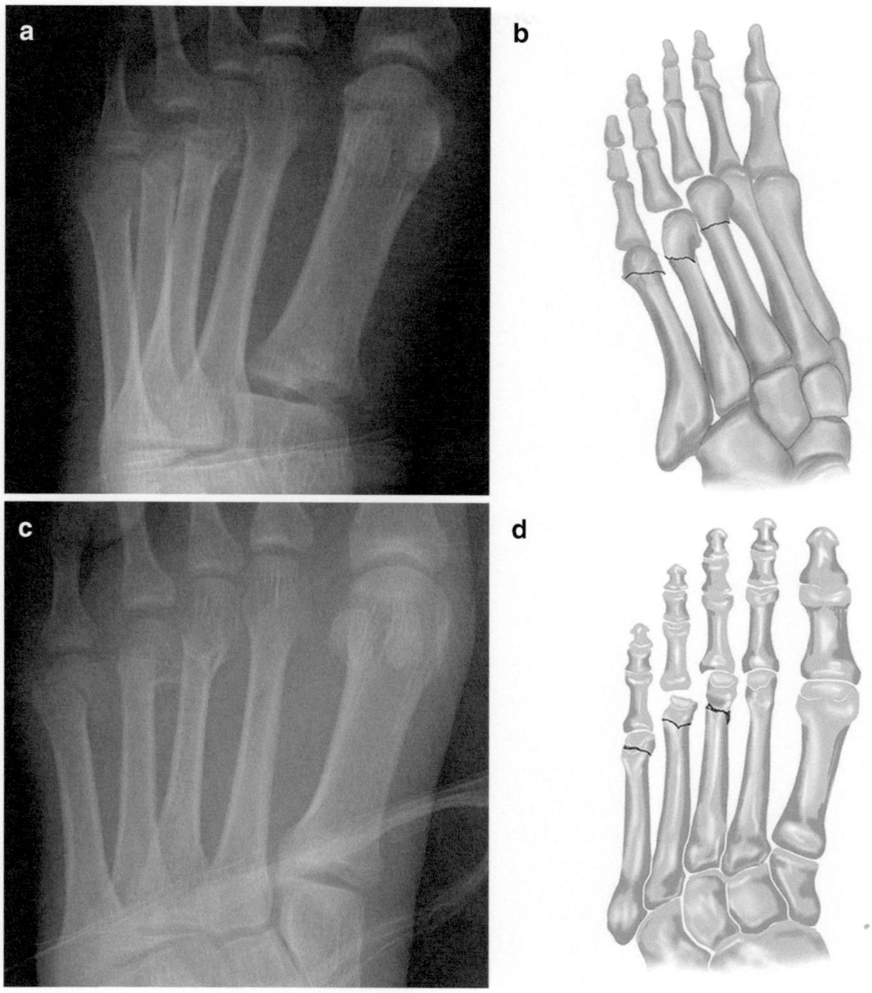

Fig. 11.45 X-ray plain film (**a**, **c**) shows a fracture of the distal 3–5 metatarsal bone with a slightly inserted end, and a schematic diagram (**b**, **d**)

7.2 CT scan (Fig. 11.45e, f)

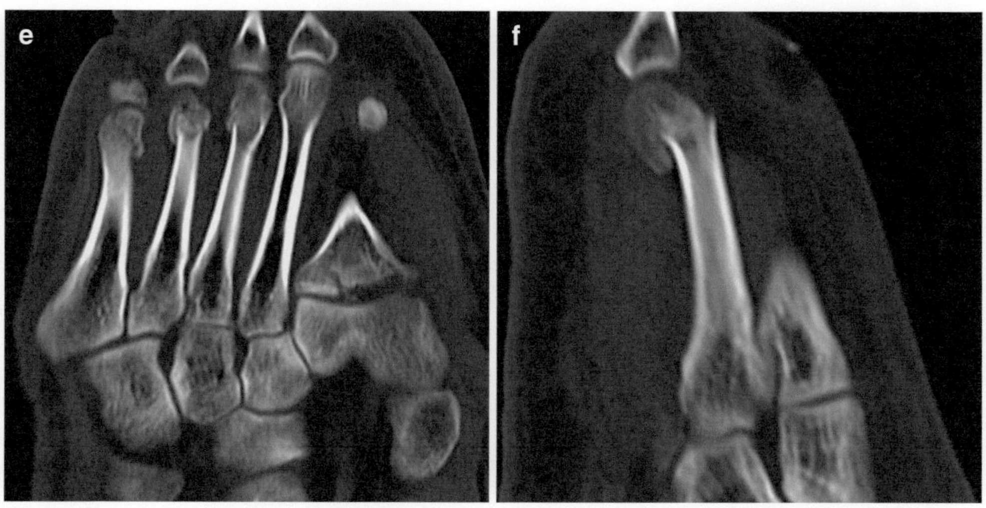

Fig. 11.45 CT transect (**e**) and sagittal plane (**f**) show the fracture of the distal bone of the 3–5 metatarsal, a slight dislocation of the broken end, the fifth metatarsal fracture line involving the distal articular surface, and the collapse of the proximal articular surface of the first metatarsal

8. Comparison between plain film and CT for proximal intra-articular fracture of metatarsus
   8.1 X-ray plain film (Fig. 11.46a–d)

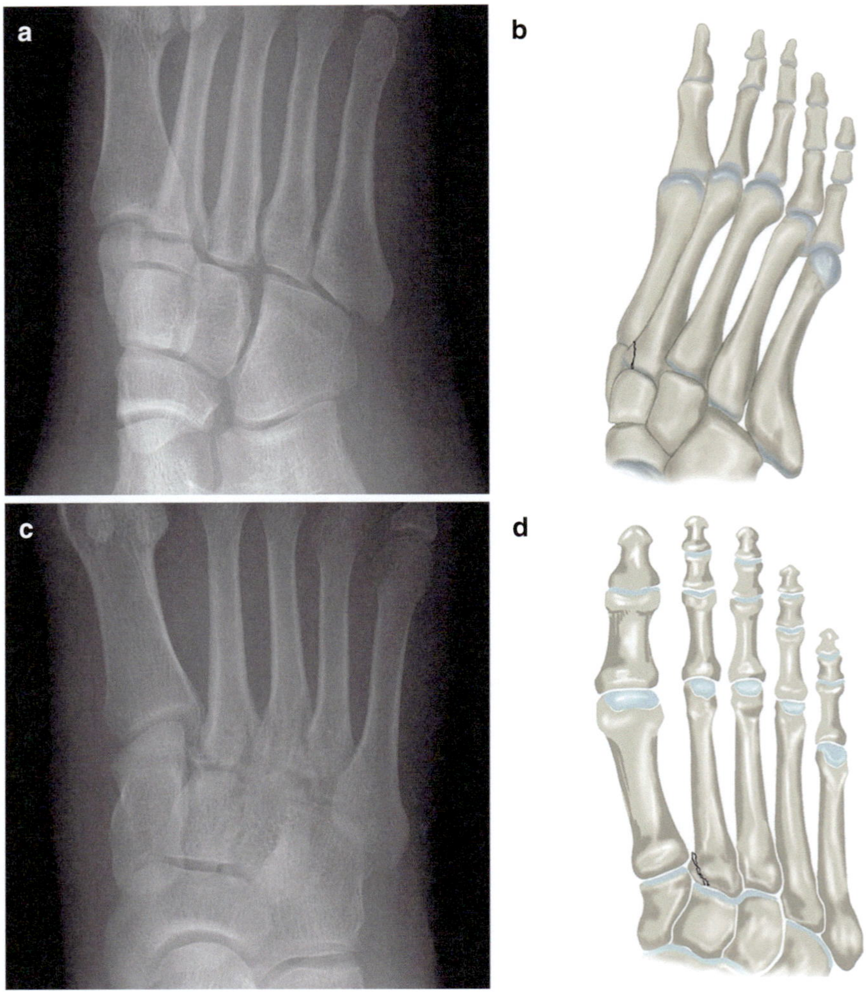

Fig. 11.46 X-ray plain film (**a**, **c**) shows the split of the base of the second metatarsal base, and bone fragments were seen. The fracture line involved the articular surface. The schematic diagram (**b**, **d**)

   8.2 CT scan (Fig. 11.46e, f)

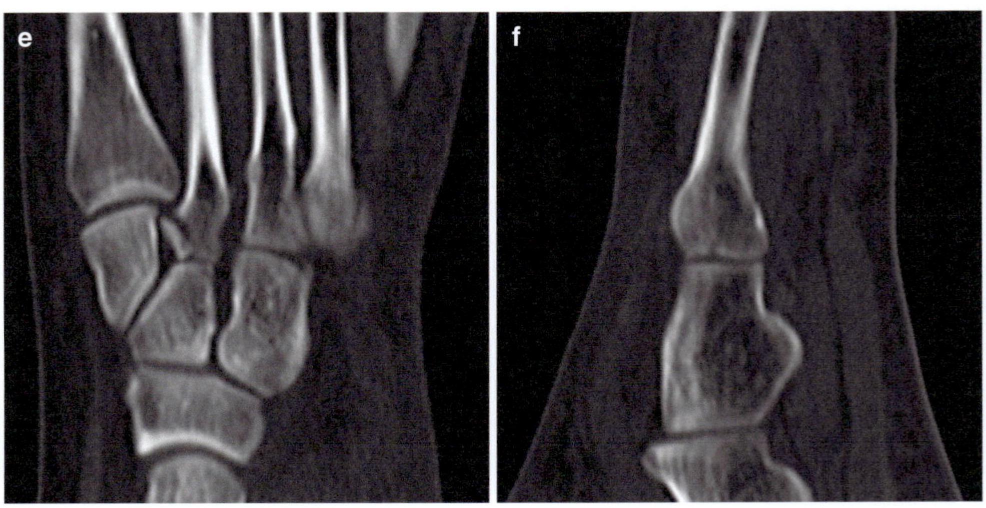

Fig. 11.46 CT transect (**e**) and sagittal plane (**f**) show bone fracture of the base of the second metatarsus, and the fracture line involved the articular surface

9. Comparison between plain film and CT for proximal intra-articular fracture of metatarsus
   9.1 X-ray plain film (Fig. 11.47a–d)

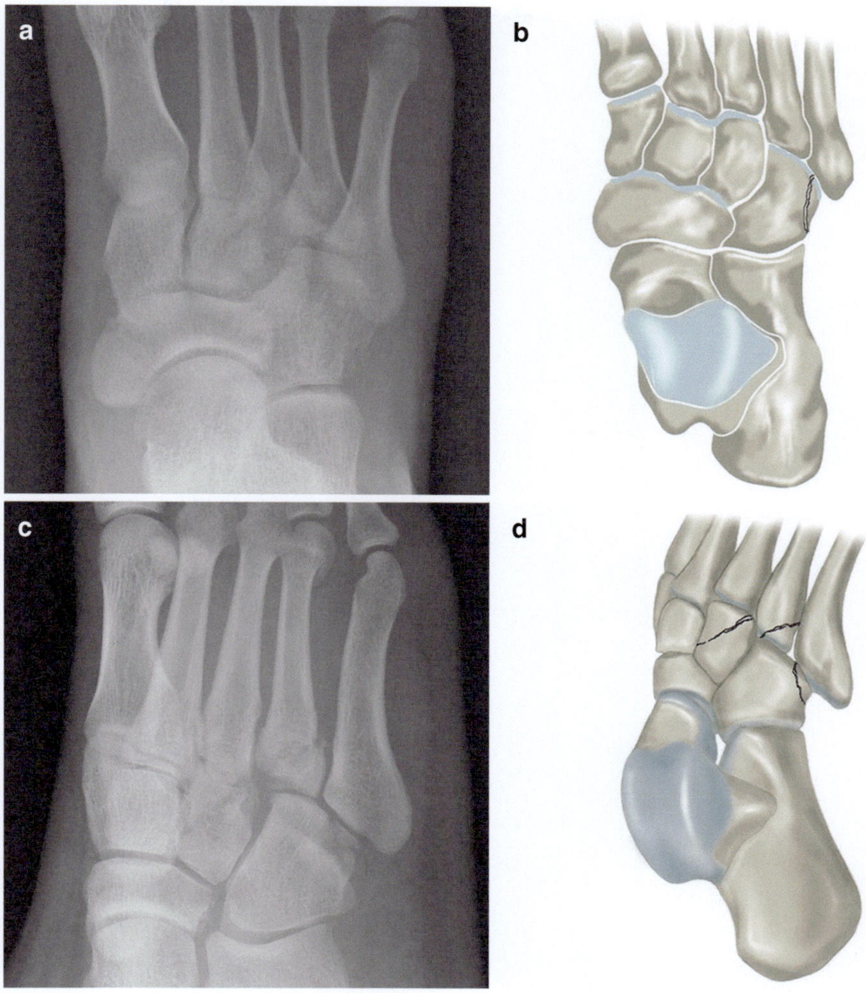

Fig. 11.47 X-ray plain film (**a**, **c**) shows the cleavage of the outer edge of the fourth metatarsal, the shadow of the bone, the fracture line involving the articular surface, and the shadow of the bone in the outer edge of the cuboid bone, and the schematic (**b**, **d**)

   9.2 CT scan (Fig. 11.47e, f)

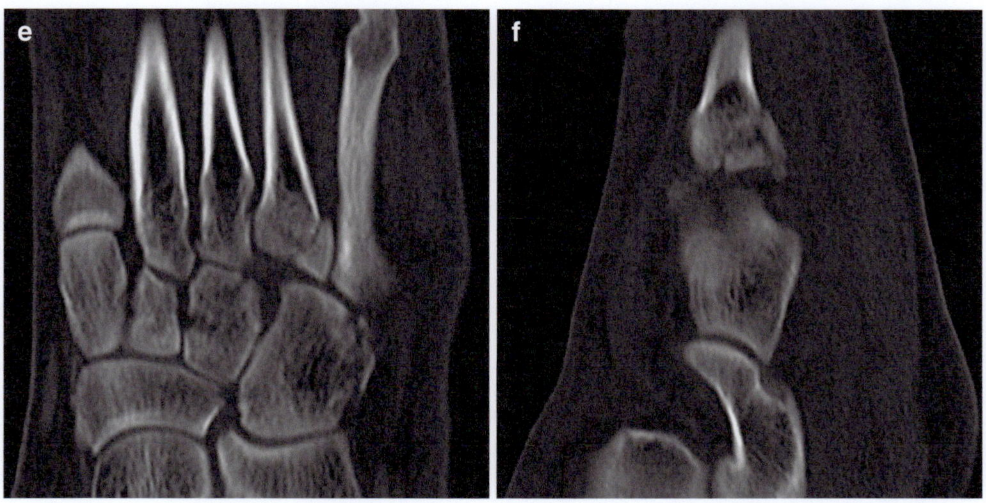

Fig. 11.47 CT transverse section (**e**) and sagittal plane (**f**) show bone fracture of the base of the fourth metatarsal bone, involving the articular surface of the fracture line and the fracture of the external border of the cuboid bone

10. Comparison between plain film and CT for proximal intra-articular fracture of metatarsus
    10.1 X-ray plain film (Fig. 11.48a–d)

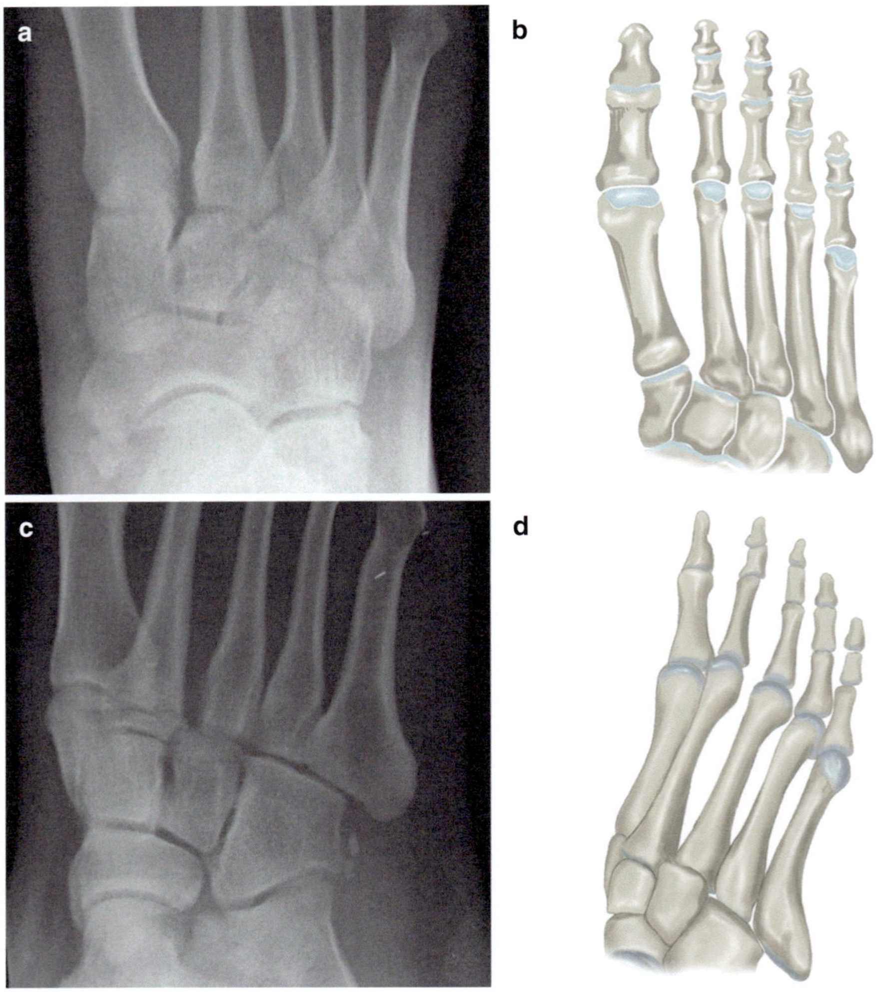

Fig. 11.48 Plain films (**a**, **c**) show no definite signs of fracture of the tarsal joint bones, and the base of the 2–5 metatarsal slightly shifted laterally (**b**, **d**)

    10.2 CT scan (Fig. 11.48e, f)

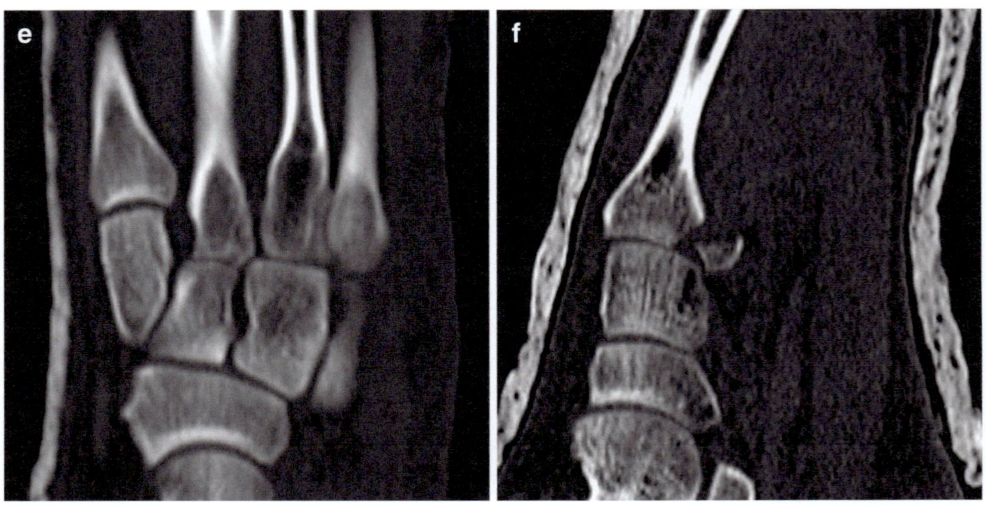

Fig. 11.48 CT transect (**e**) and sagittal plane (**f**) show bone fracture of the basal metatarsal border of the second metatarsal, the fracture line involved the articular surface, and the second, third metatarsal basement shifted outward

11. Comparison between plain film and CT for proximal intra-articular fracture of metatarsus
    11.1 X-ray plain film (Fig. 11.49a–d)

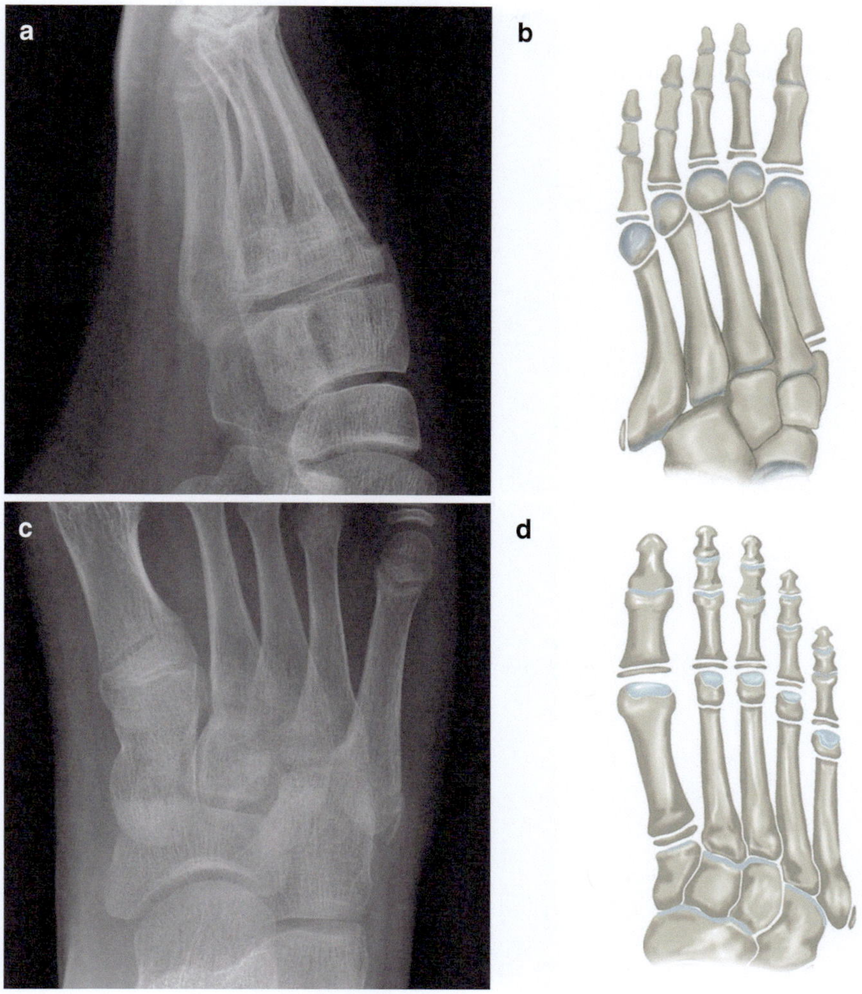

Fig. 11.49 X-ray plain films (**a**, **c**) show no definite fracture signs of the tarsal joint bones, schematic diagram (**b**, **d**)

11.2 CT scan (Fig. 11.49e, f)

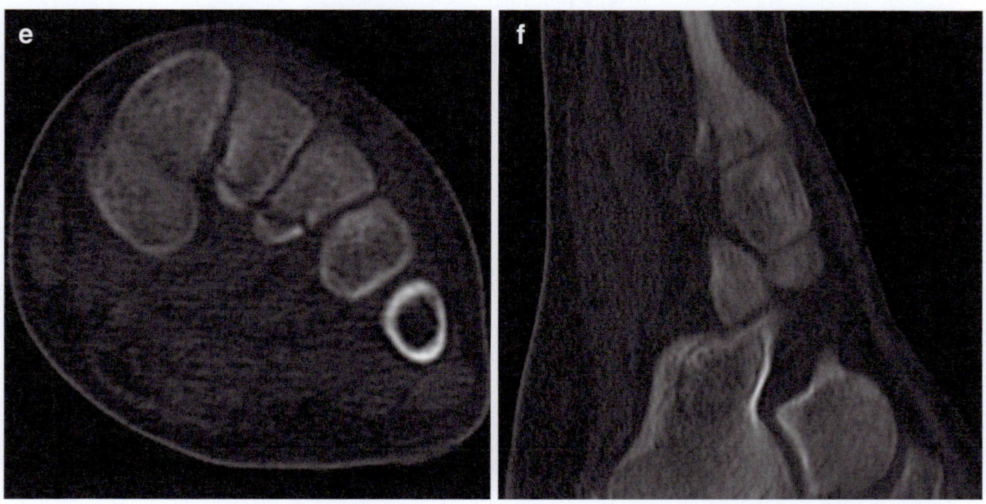

Fig. 11.49 CT coronal plane (**e**) and sagittal plane (**f**) show bone fracture of the base of the second, third metatarsal base, and the fracture line involved the articular surface

12. Comparison between plain film and CT for wedge fracture of metatarsal stem
    12.1 X-ray plain film (Fig. 11.50a–d)

Fig. 11.50 X-ray plain films (**a**, **c**) show no definite fracture signs of the tarsal joint bones, schematic diagram (**b**, **d**)

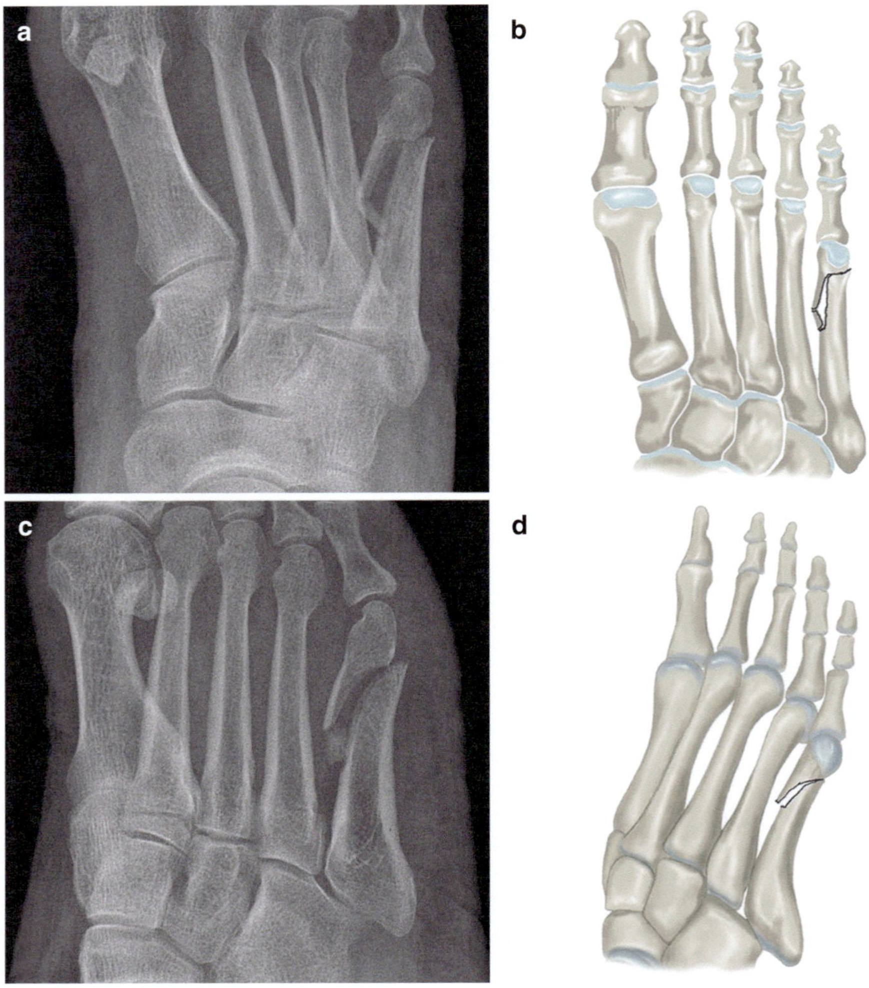

12.2 CT scan (Fig. 11.50e, f)

Fig. 11.50 CT coronal plane (**e**) and sagittal plane (**f**) show bone fracture of the base of the second, third metatarsal base, and the fracture line involved the articular surface

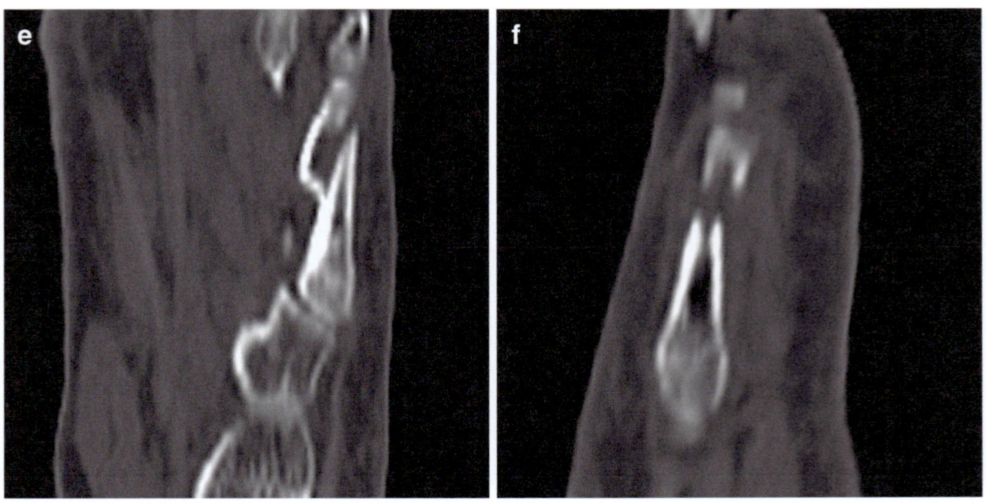

13. Comparison between plain film and CT for wedge fracture of metatarsal stem
    13.1 X-ray plain film (Fig. 11.51a, b)

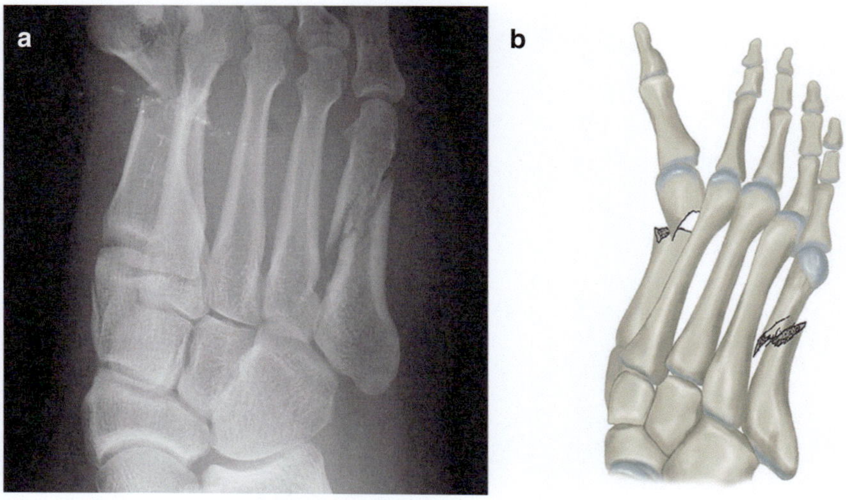

Fig. 11.51 X-ray plain film (**a**) shows a fracture of fifth metatarsal diaphysis wedge-shaped bone, partial visible wedge bone shadow, first metatarsal distal bone fracture, and dislocation of the broken end into angle, and a schematic diagram (**b**)

    13.2 CT scan (Fig. 11.51c–e)

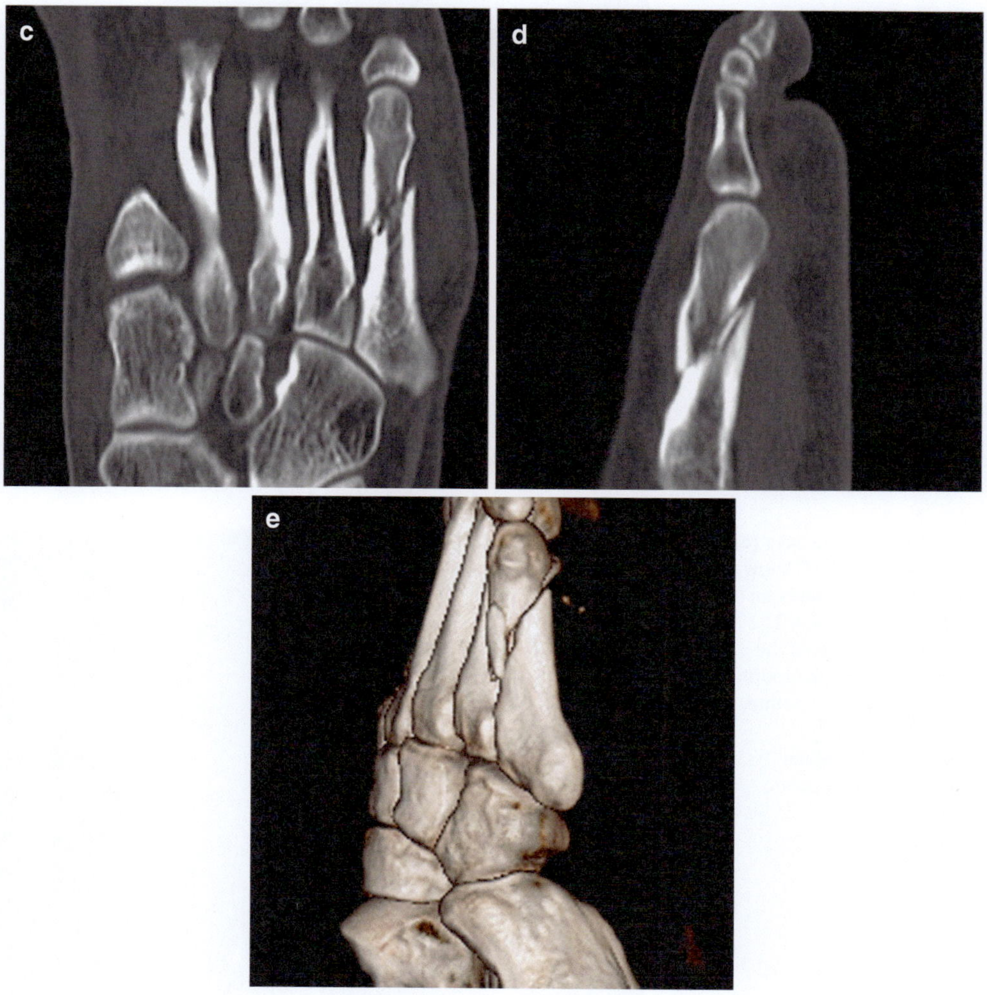

Fig. 11.51 CT cross section (**c**), sagittal plane (**d**), and three-dimensional reconstruction (**e**) show wedge bone fracture of the fifth metatarsal shaft, and wedge-shaped bone on dorsal side

14. Comparison of plain intra-articular fractures of the distal metatarsal bone with CT
    14.1 X-ray plain film (Fig. 11.52a–d)

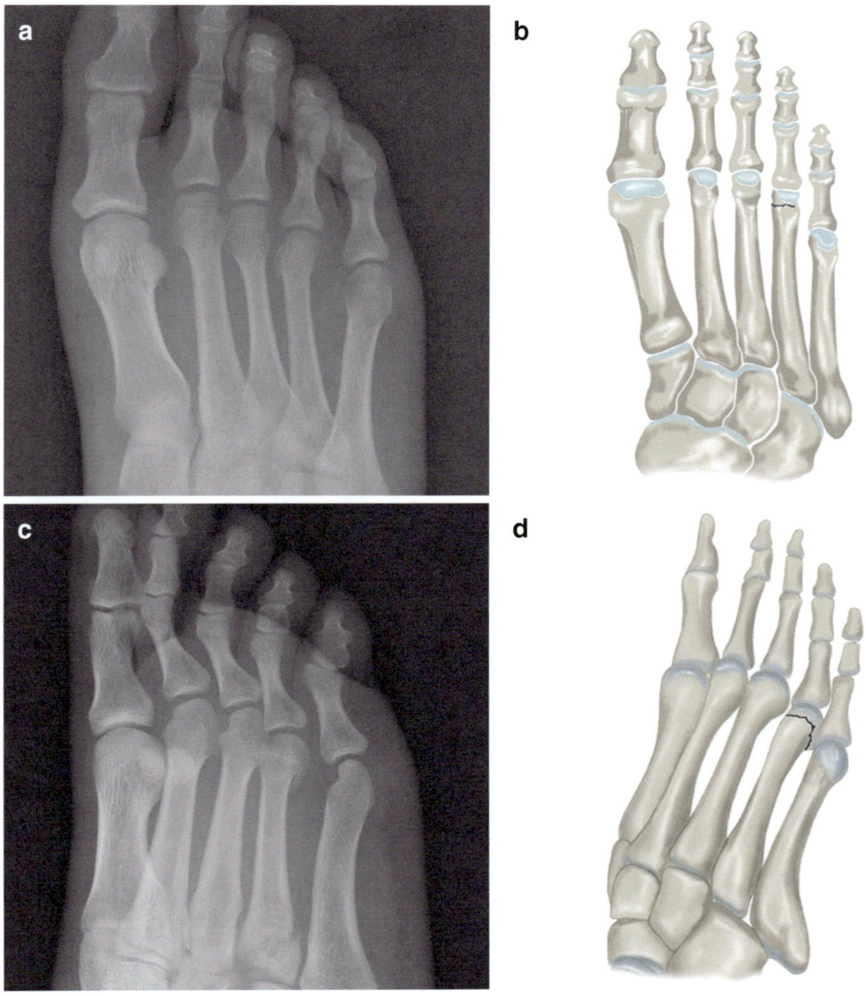

Fig. 11.52 X-ray plain film (**a**, **c**) shows a fracture of the distal fourth metatarsal bone, slightly dislocated ends, and irregular base of the fourth metatarsal bone (**b**, **d**)

14.2 CT scan (Fig. 11.52e, f)

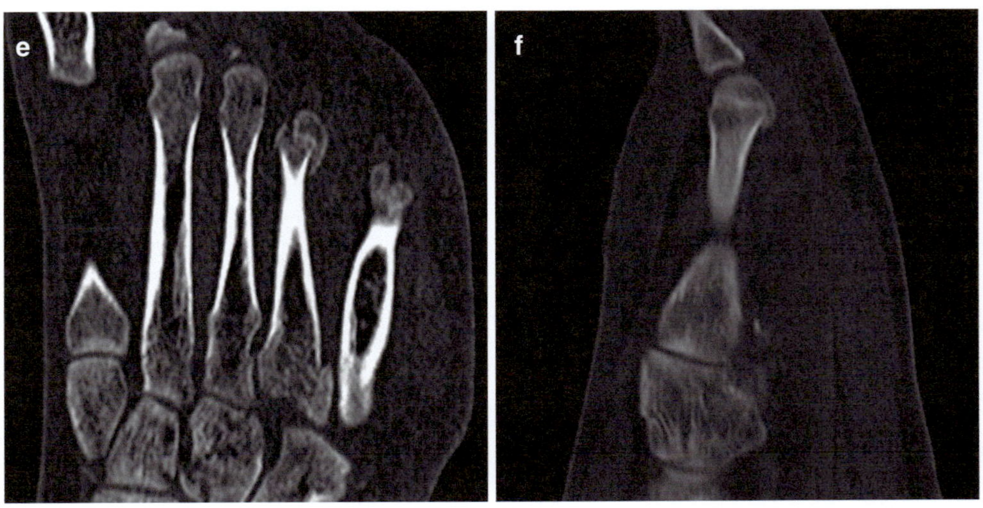

Fig. 11.52 CT transect (**e**) and sagittal plane (**f**) show the fracture of the distal bone of the fourth metatarsal. The fracture line involved the articular surface, the fourth metatarsal basilar fracture, the broken end slightly dislocation, the lateral cuneiform bone fracture

15. Comparison of plain film with CT in distal metatarsal fractures
    15.1 X-ray plain film (Fig. 11.53a–d)

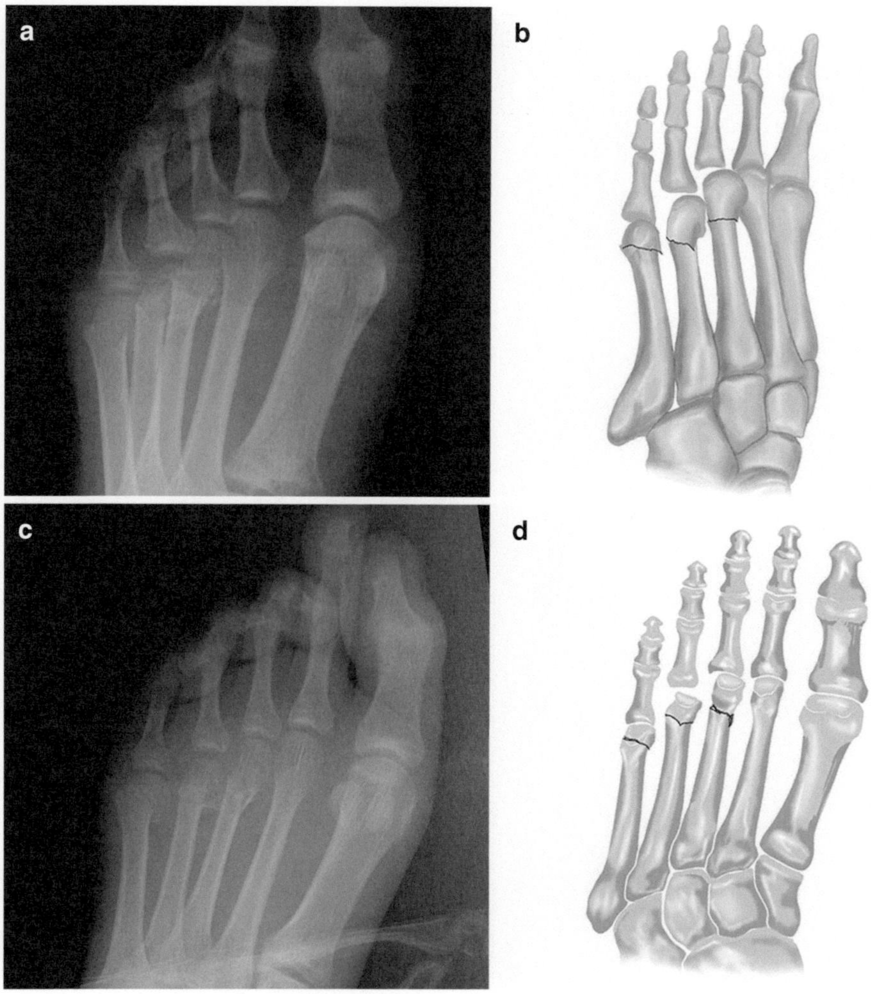

Fig. 11.53 X-ray plain film (**a**, **c**) shows a fracture of the distal part of the fourth, fifth metatarsal bone, a slightly dislocated end, and a fracture of the distal third metatarsal bone (**b**, **d**)

15.2 CT scan (Fig. 11.53e, f)

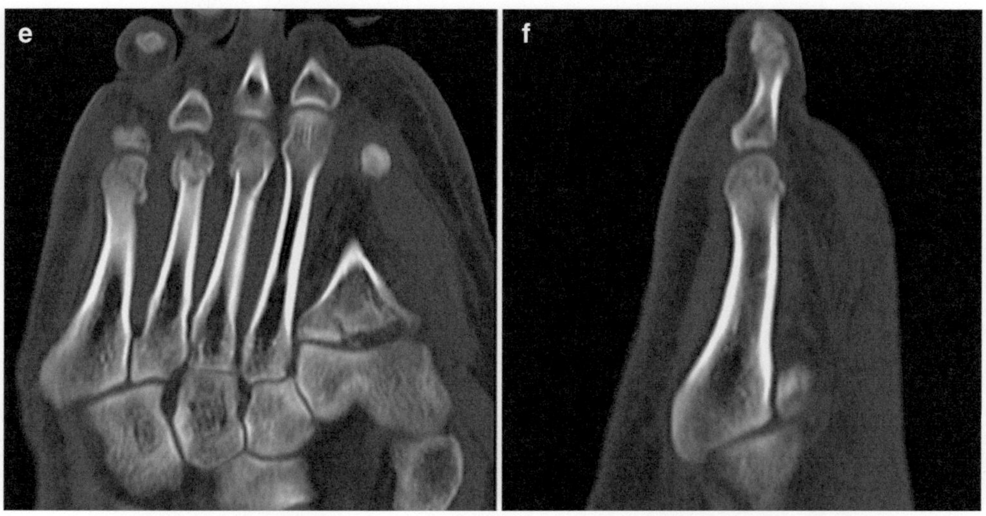

Fig. 11.53 CT transect (**e**) and sagittal plane (**f**) show the fracture of the distal bone of the fifth metatarsal. The fracture line involved the articular surface, the third, fourth metatarsus distal bone fracture, the broken end a little insert, and the first metatarsal fracture

16. Comparison of plain intra-articular fractures with CT in proximal metatarsal fractures
    16.1 X-ray plain film (Fig. 11.54a–d)

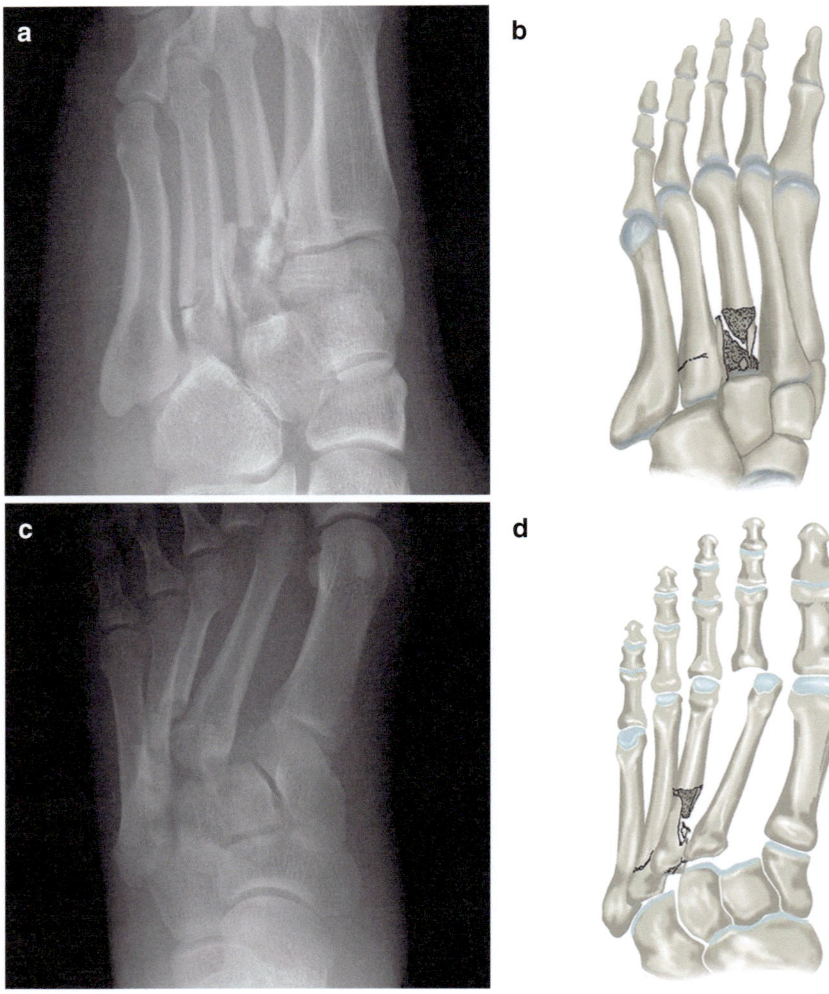

Fig. 11.54 X-ray plain film (**a**, **c**) shows the fracture of third, fourth metatarsal basilar bone, a slight dislocation of the broken end, second tarsus and metatarsal joint dislocation, and metatarsal displacement to the lateral (**b**, **d**)

16.2 CT scan (Fig. 11.54e, f)

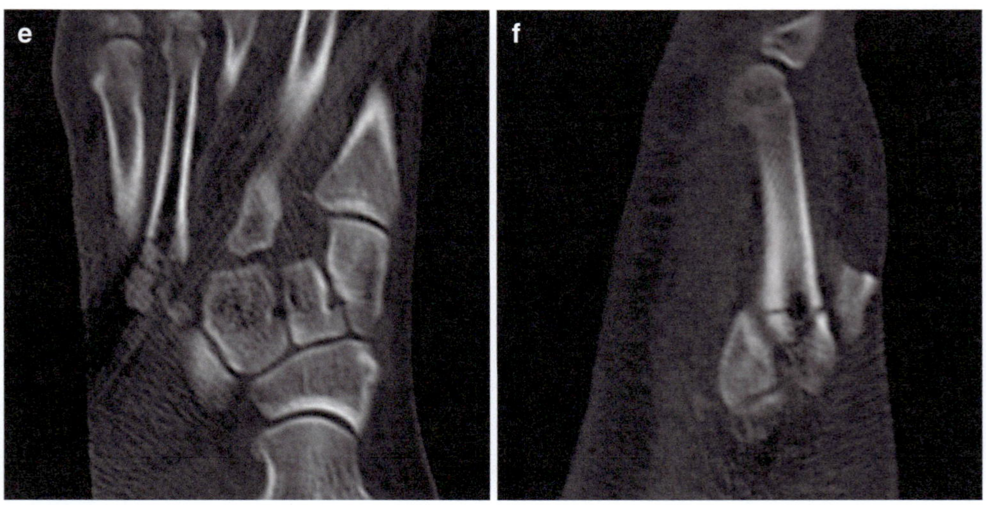

Fig. 11.54 CT cross section (**e**) and sagittal plane (**f**) show the proximal bone fragmentation of the fourth metatarsal, the fracture line is involved in the articular surface, the second, third metatarsal basement is shifted outward, and the bone mass is visible locally

17. Comparison of plain intra-articular fractures with CT in proximal metatarsal fractures
    17.1 X-ray plain film (Fig. 11.55a–d)

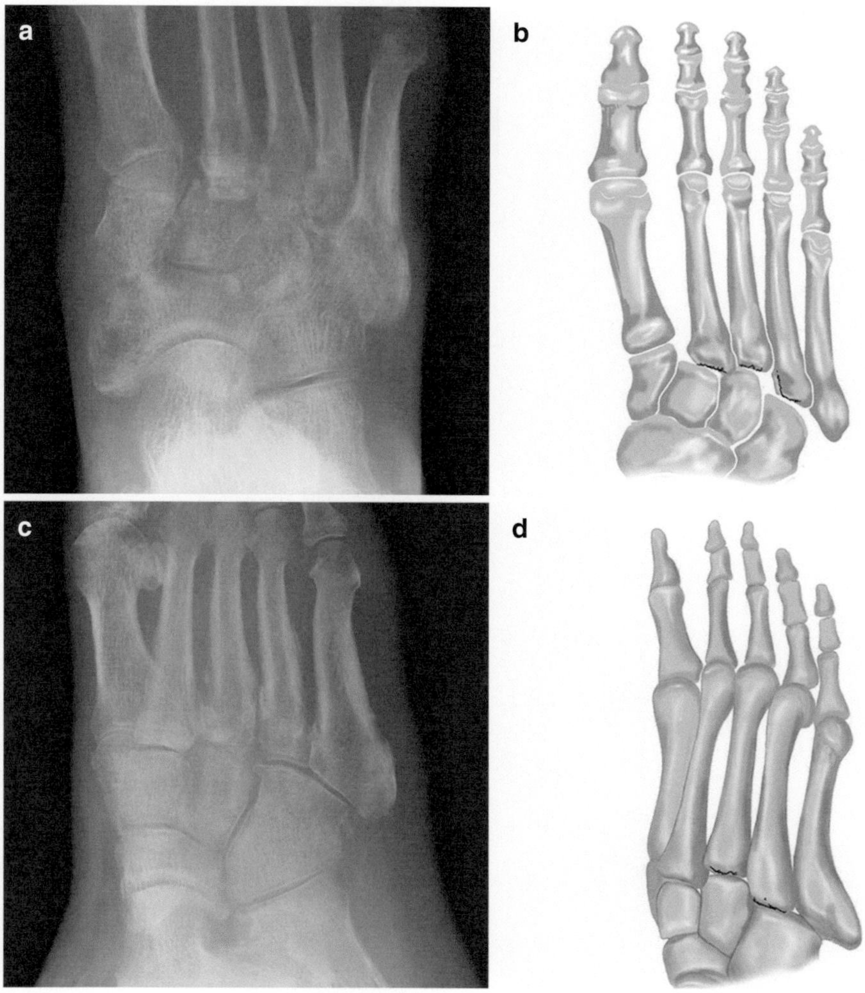

Fig. 11.55 X-ray plain film (**a**, **c**) shows the lateral displacement of the 2–4 metatarsal bone, the disorder of bone structure, the small bone fragments are seen, and the osteoporosis of bones (**b**, **d**)

    17.2 CT scan (Fig. 11.55e, f)

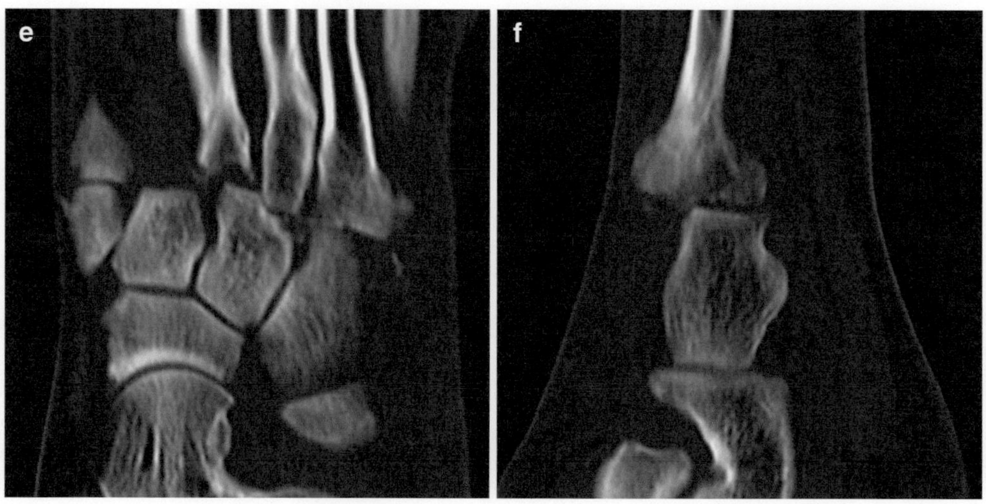

Fig. 11.55 CT transect (**e**) and sagittal plane (**f**) show the displacement of the 2–4 metatarsal to the lateral. The bone structure is disorderly, the small bone fragments are seen, the fourth metatarsus is fragmented near the end of the metatarsal, and the fracture line involves the articular surface

18. Comparison of plain intra-articular fractures with CT in proximal metatarsal fractures
    18.1 X-ray plain film (Fig. 11.56a–d)

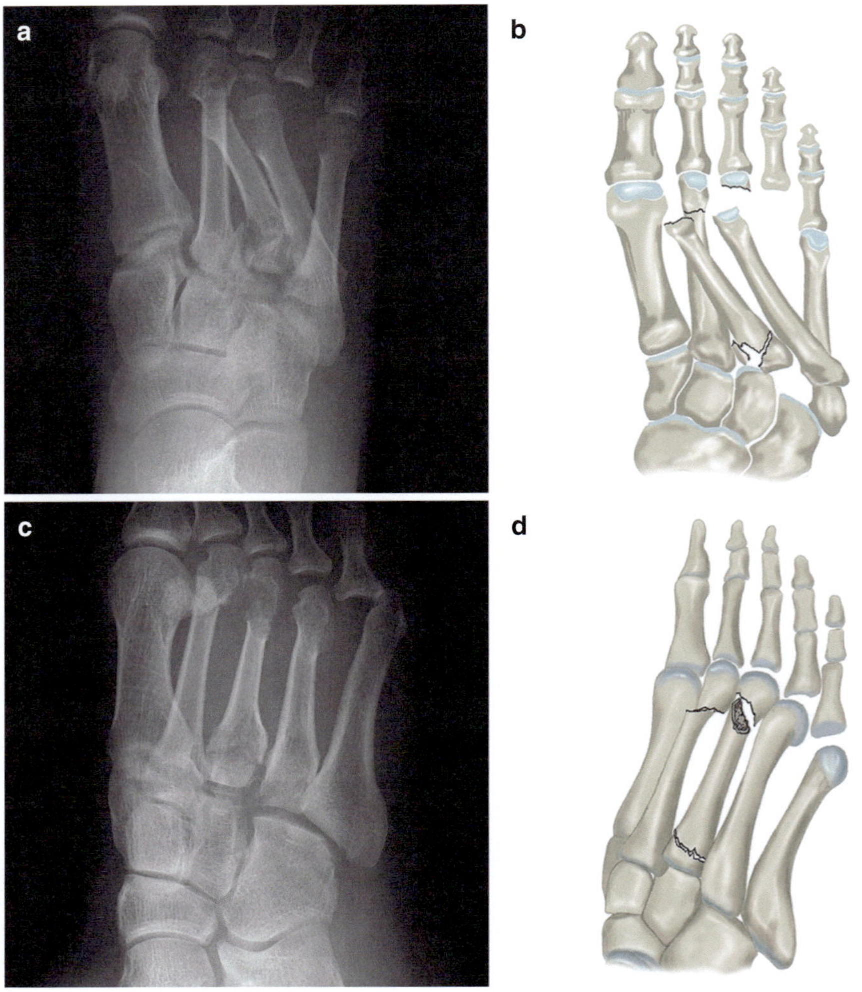

Fig. 11.56 X-ray film (**a**, **c**) shows the lateral displacement of the third, fourth metatarsal basement, the fracture of the metatarsal basilar bone, the fracture of the third metatarsal bone, the dislocation of the broken end, the dislocation of the fourth, fifth metatarsophalangeal joint, and the schematic (**b**, **d**)

18.2 CT scan (Fig. 11.56e, f)

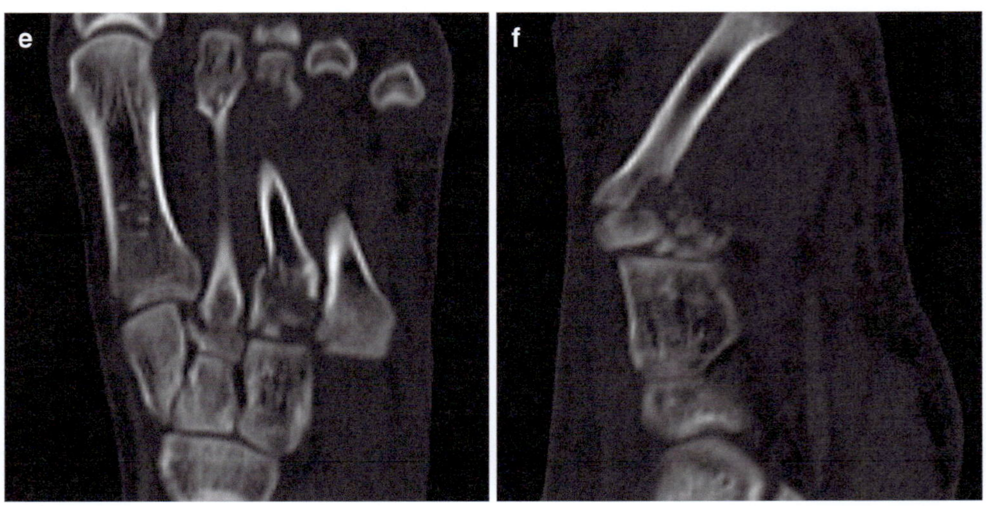

Fig. 11.56 CT transect (**e**) and sagittal plane (**f**) show basal bone fracture of the 2–4 metatarsal bone, and third metatarsal base bone fragmented, involving the articular surface

19. Comparison of comminuted fracture of metatarsal bone with CT
    19.1 X-ray film (Fig. 11.57a, b)

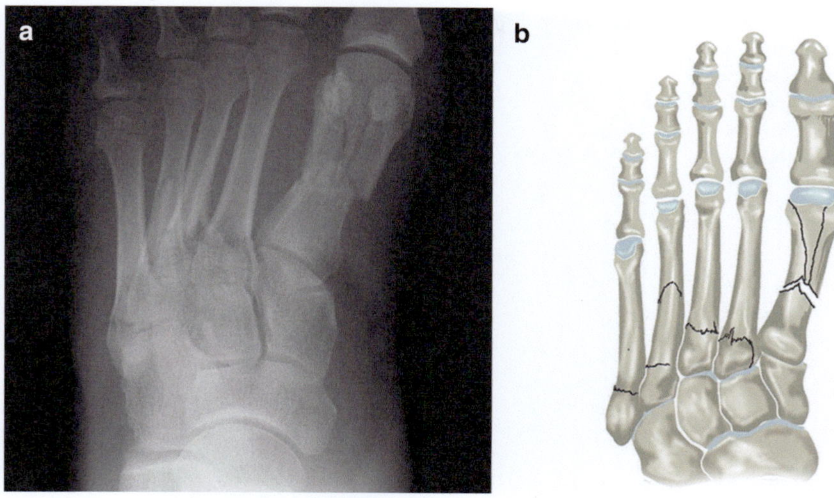

Fig. 11.57 X-ray plain film (**a**) shows bone fracture of the first metatarsal shaft, slightly dislocated ends, and 2–5 metatarsal base fractures (**b**)

19.2 CT scan (Fig. 11.57c–e)

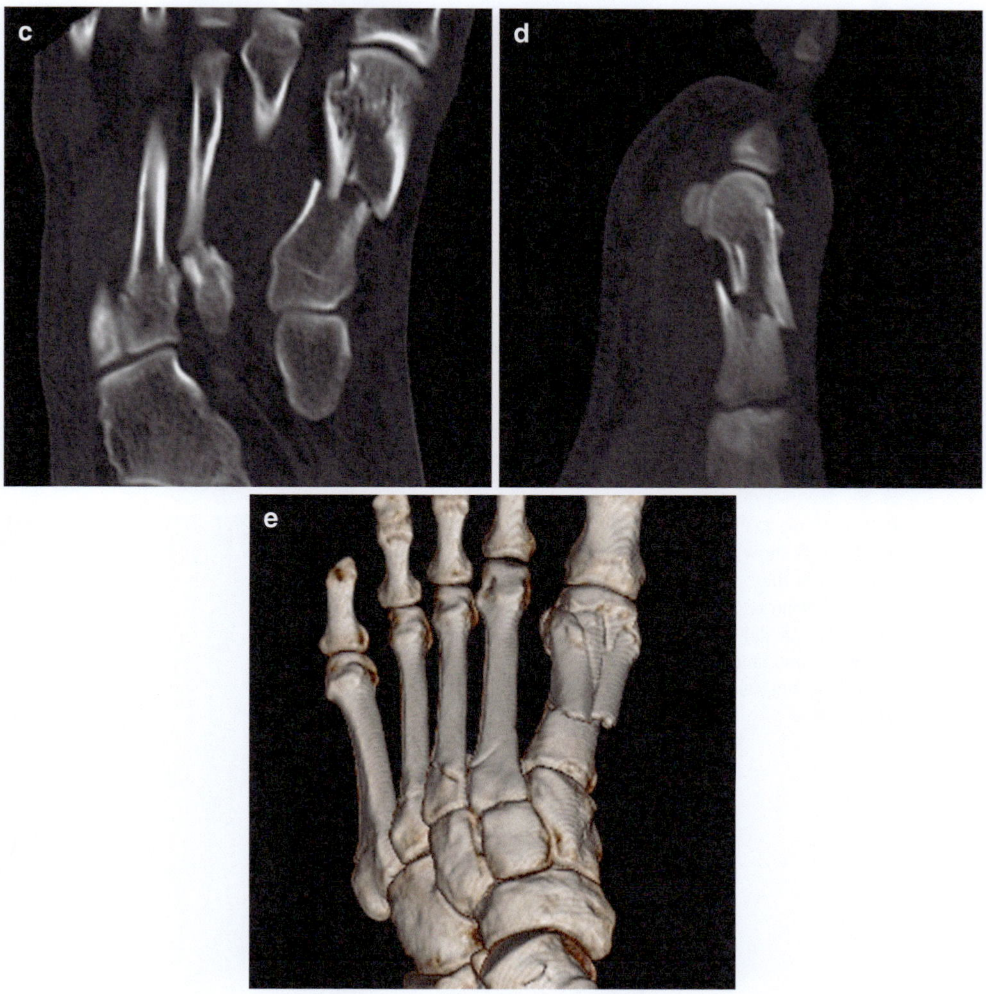

Fig. 11.57 CT transect (**c**), sagittal plane (**d**), and three-dimensional reconstruction (**e**) show bone fragmentation of the 1 metatarsal shaft, slightly dislocated ends, and basal bone fracture of the 2–5 metatarsal bone

20. Comparison between plain film and CT for comminuted distal metatarsal fractures
    20.1 X-ray film (Fig. 11.58a–d)

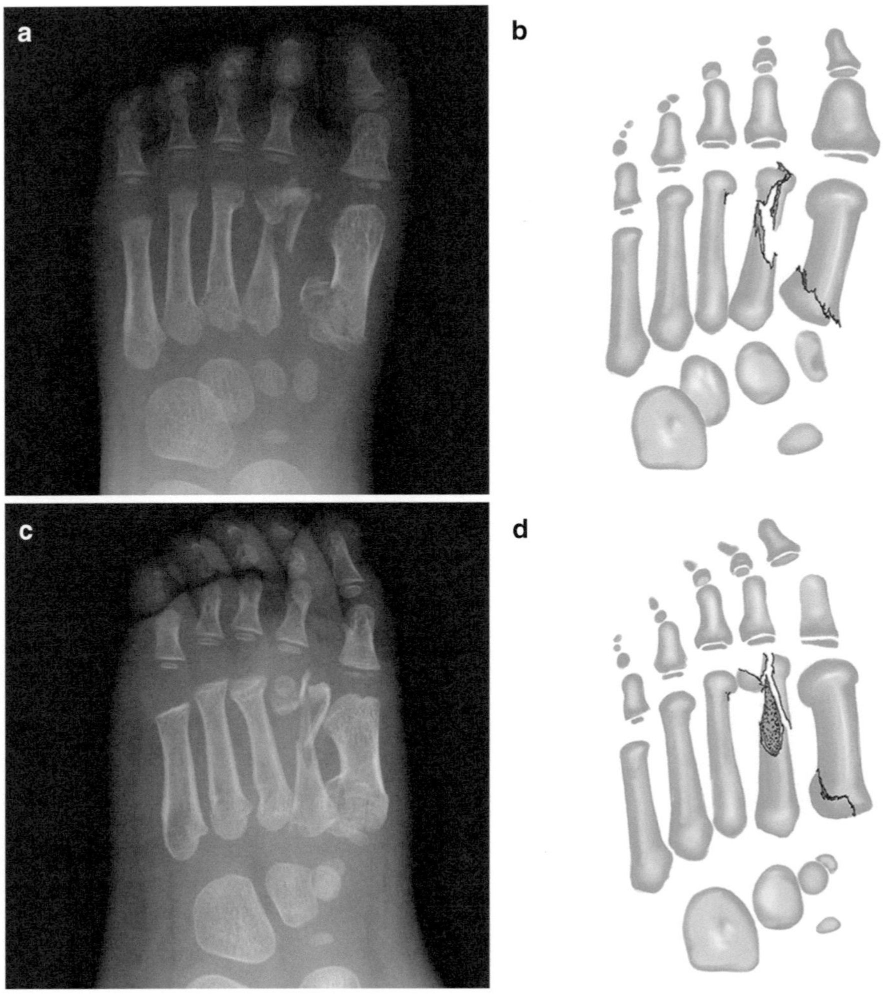

Fig. 11.58 X-ray plain film (**a**, **c**) shows bone fracture of distal second metatarsal bone, dislocation of broken ends, and fracture of basal bone of first metatarsal bone (**b**, **d**)

20.2 CT scan (Fig. 11.58e, f)

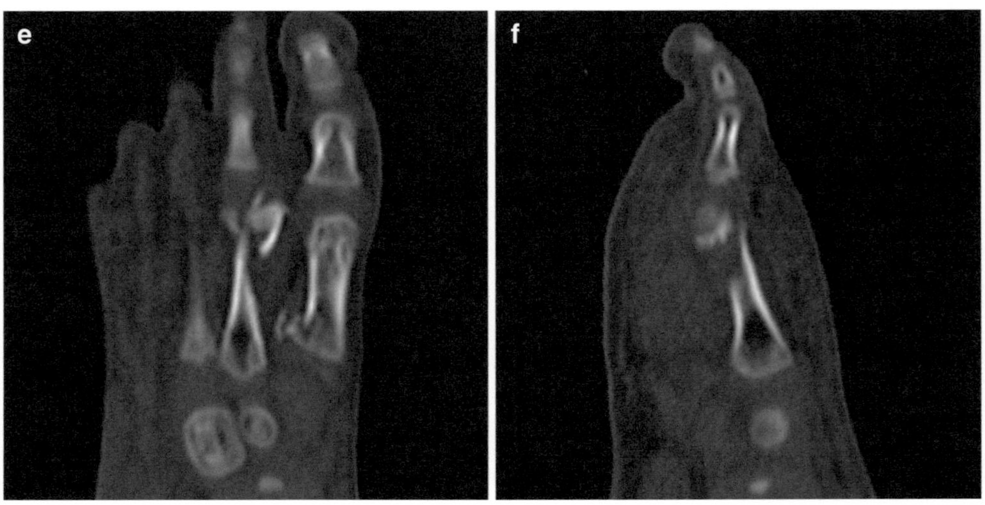

Fig. 11.58 CT transect (**e**) and sagittal plane (**f**) show that the distal part of the second metatarsal bone is fragmented, the end of the fracture was dislocated, and the base of the first metatarsal bone was fragmented

11.4 Phalangeal Fracture

The phalanges are divided into proximal, middle, and distal segments. The first toe has no middle segment, and the fifth toe often has only 2 phalanges. The fracture of the phalanges accounts for 23.48% of the fracture of the foot. The AO/OTA classification of phalangeal fractures is divided into the proximal articular fracture of the phalanges, simple fracture of the diaphysis of the toe, external fracture of the distal phalanges, the proximal part of the phalanges, the proximal part of the phalanges, the wedge-shaped fracture of the toe diaphysis, partial intra-articular fracture of distal phalanges, the complete intra-articular fracture of the proximal end of the phalanges, the comminuted fracture of the toe diaphysis, and the distal total articular fracture of the phalanges. The proximal fracture of the phalanx accounts for 4.53% of the foot fracture, 4.50% of the simple fracture of the toe diaphysis, 4.92% of the distal fracture of the phalanges, 1.57% of the proximal part of the phalanges, 1.15% of the toe bone fracture, and the distal part of the phalanx of the phalanges. 1.58% of the partial intra-articular fracture of distal phalanges, 1.01% of the total articular fracture of the proximal end of the phalanges, 1.47% of the broken toe bone fracture, and 2.76% of the distal total articular fracture of the phalanges.

11.4.1 Identification of Injury Mechanism

The injury mechanism is due to direct violence, most of which are heavy objects, thus the fracture is induced due to a crush. The indirect violence is subjected to the internal and external stress in the presence of axial pressure, whereby the deformity is more obvious.

11.4.2 Symptoms and Signs

After a fracture, there is pain, swelling, and limited activity of the toe. The patient cannot walk normally, however, these symptoms lack of specificity; thus, it is difficult to make a definite diagnosis. Therefore, an X-ray scan should be carried out when the fracture is suspected.

11.4.3 Imaging Differential Diagnosis

Though conventional X-ray films usually diagnose fractures, a CT three- dimensional reconstruction should be performed if the fracture is difficult to diagnose.

1. Distal articular fracture of the proximal phalanx
   1.1 X-ray plain film (Fig. 11.59a–d)

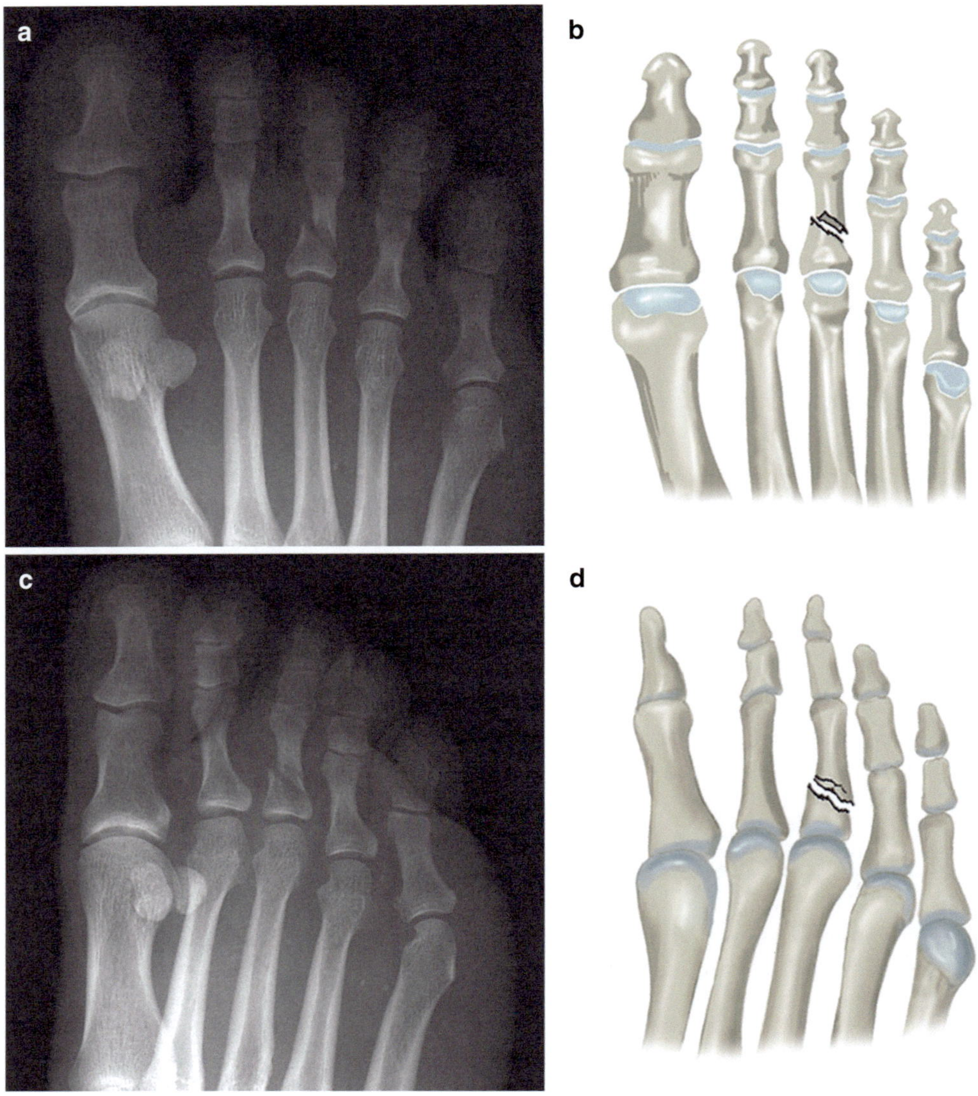

Fig. 11.59 X-ray plain film (**a**, **c**) shows that the proximal phalangeal base of the third toe was fractured. The broken ends were slightly misplaced. The fracture line did not involve the articular surface. The schematic diagram (**b**, **d**)

2. Distal articular fracture of the proximal phalanx
   2.1 X-ray plain film (Fig. 11.60a–d)

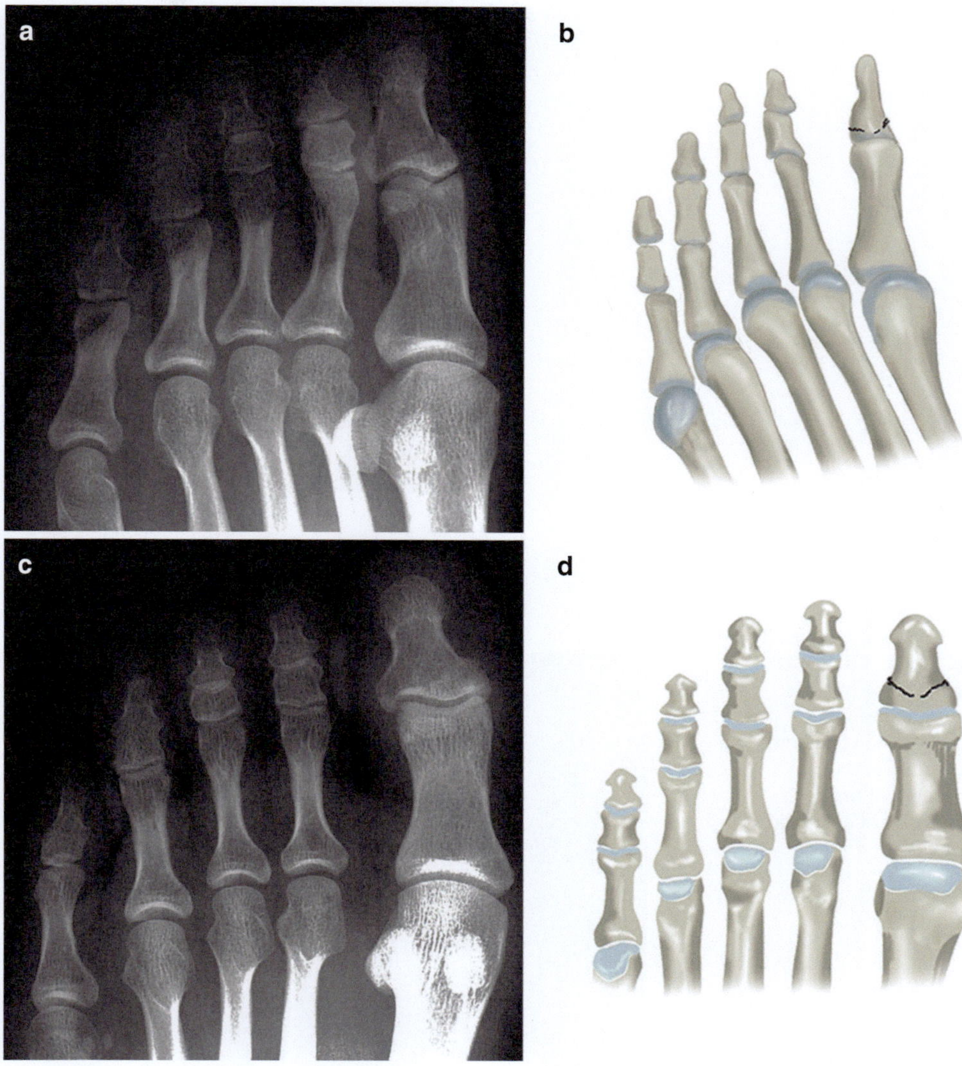

Fig. 11.60 X-ray plain film (**a**, **c**) shows basal bone fracture of distal phalanges of first toes, and no obvious dislocation at the ends of the phalanges (**b**, **d**)

3. Simple fracture of the toe backbone
   3.1 X-ray plain film (Fig. 11.61a, b)

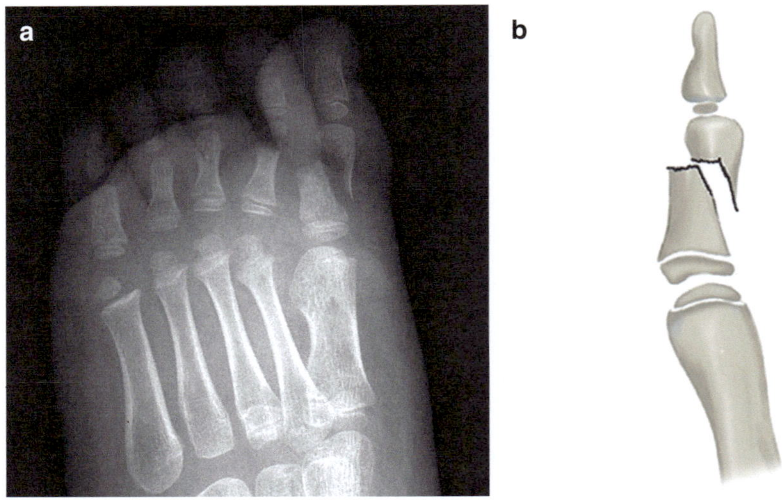

Fig. 11.61 X-ray plain film (**a**) shows a fracture of the proximal phalanx of the first toe and a slight dislocation of the ends of the phalanx (**b**)

   3.2 CT scan (Fig. 11.61c–e)

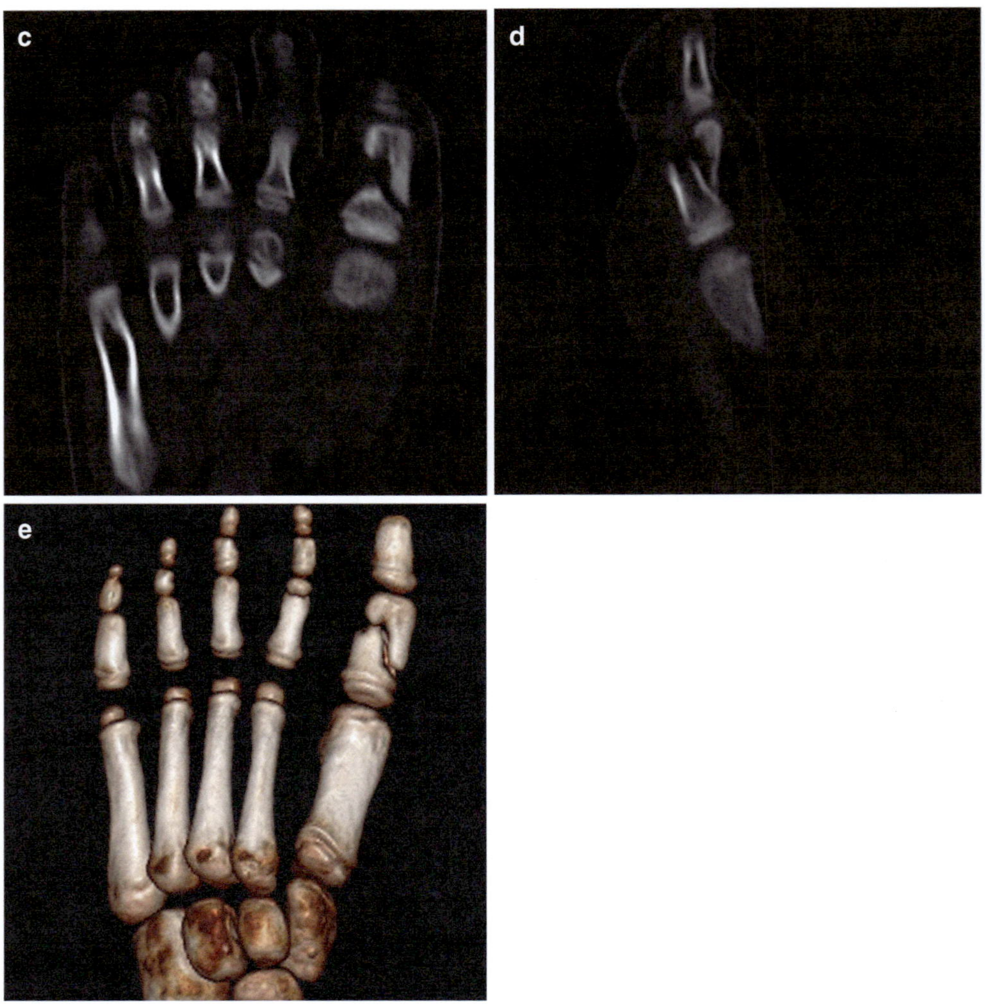

Fig. 11.61 CT transect (**c**), sagittal plane (**d**), and three-dimensional reconstruction (**e**) show bone fracture of proximal phalanges of first toe, dislocation of ends, and angulation

4. Distal articular fracture of the distal end of the phalanx
   4.1 X-ray plain film (Fig. 11.62a–d)

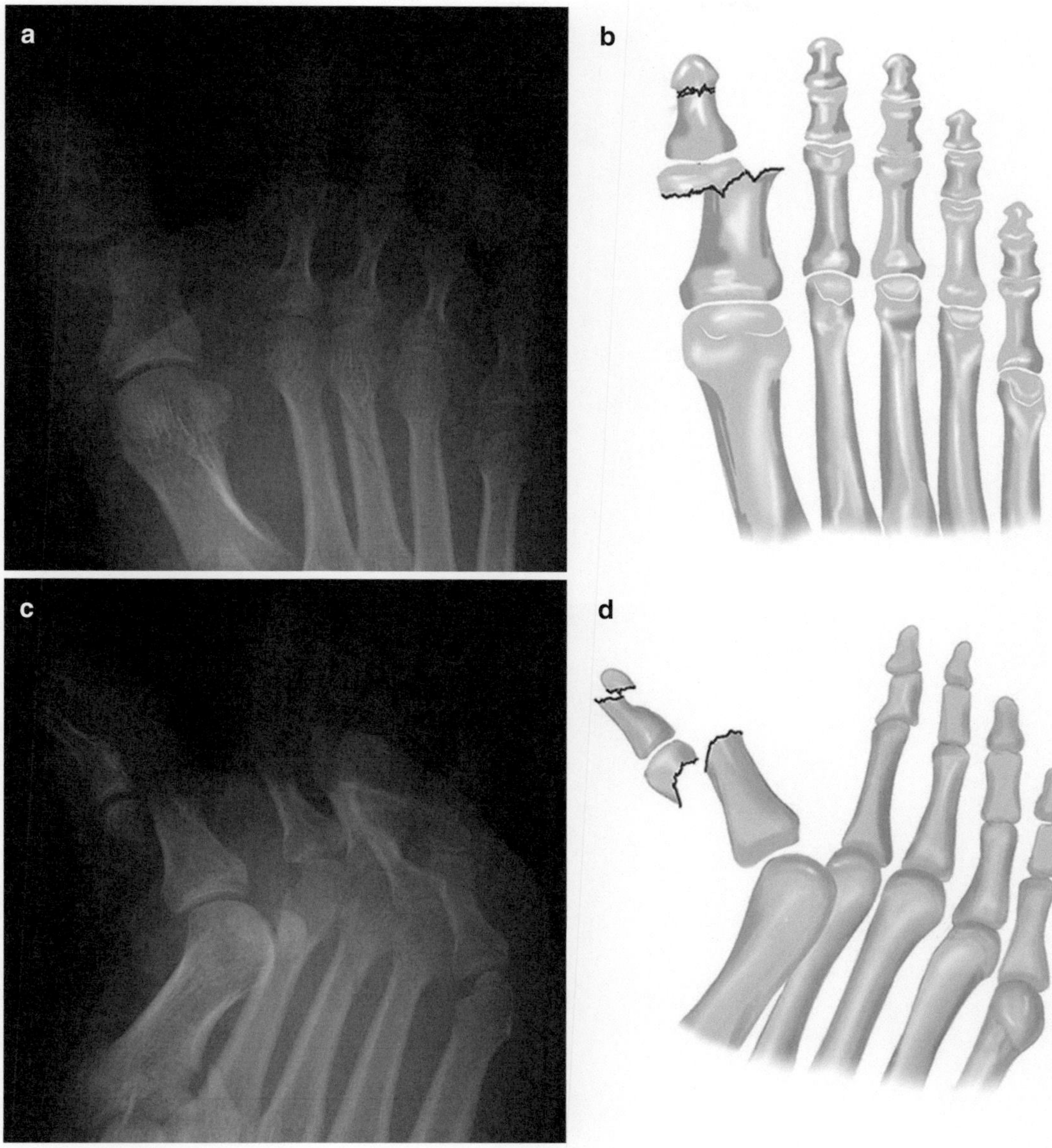

Fig. 11.62 The X-ray plain film (**a**, **c**) shows the fracture of the distal bone of the first toe near the phalanges, dislocation of the broken end, the distal bone fracture of the distal phalanges, and the irregular base of the first metatarsal (**b**, **d**)

5. Distal articular fracture of the distal end of the phalanx
   5.1 X-ray plain film (Fig. 11.63a–d)

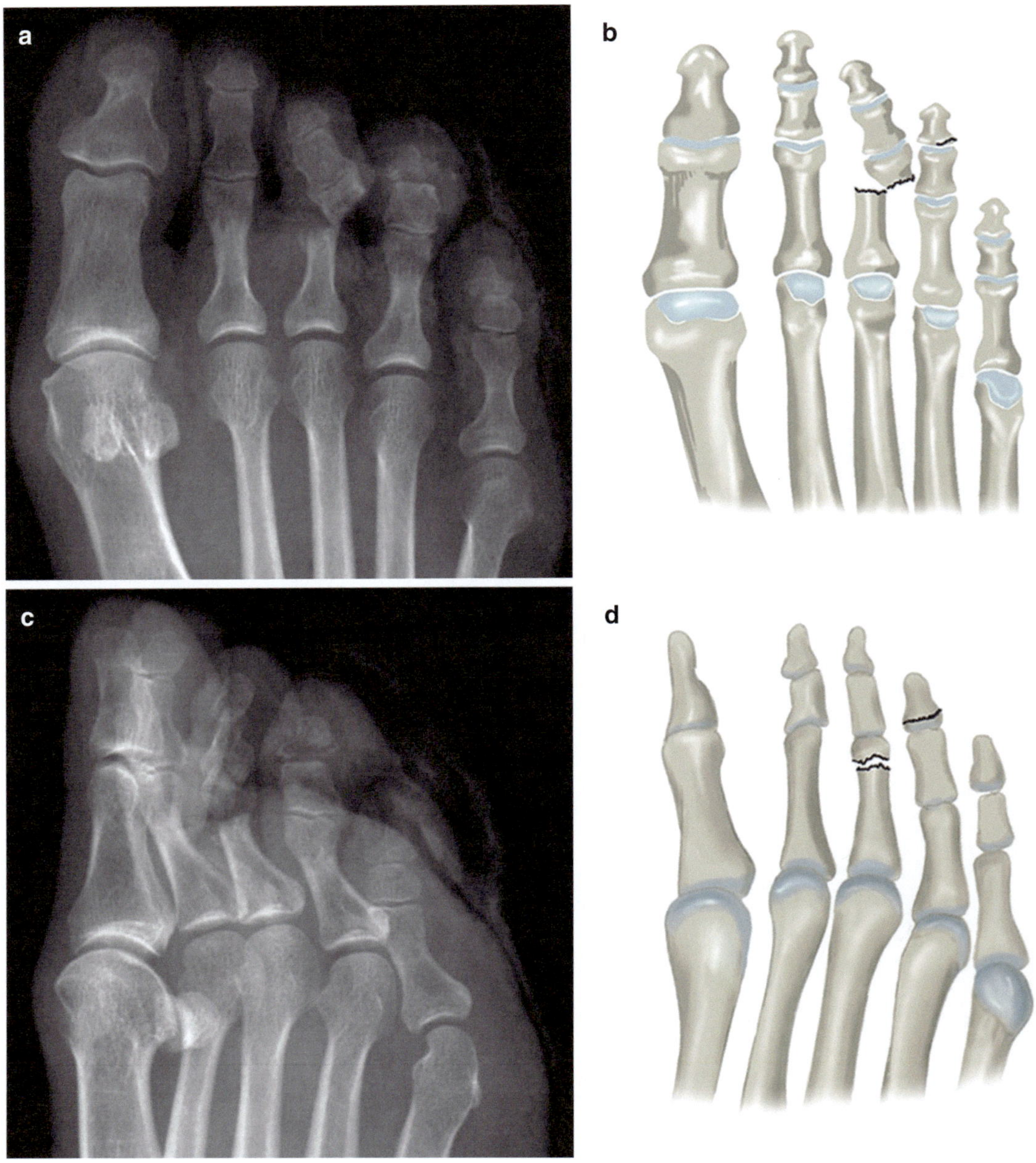

Fig. 11.63 The X-ray plain film (**a**, **c**) shows the fracture of the distal bone of the third toe near the phalanges, dislocation of the broken end, the angle, the fracture of the fourth toe bone of the distal phalangeal bone, and a schematic diagram (**b**, **d**)

6. Intra-articular fractures of the proximal part of the phalanx
   6.1 X-ray plain film (Fig. 11.64a–d)

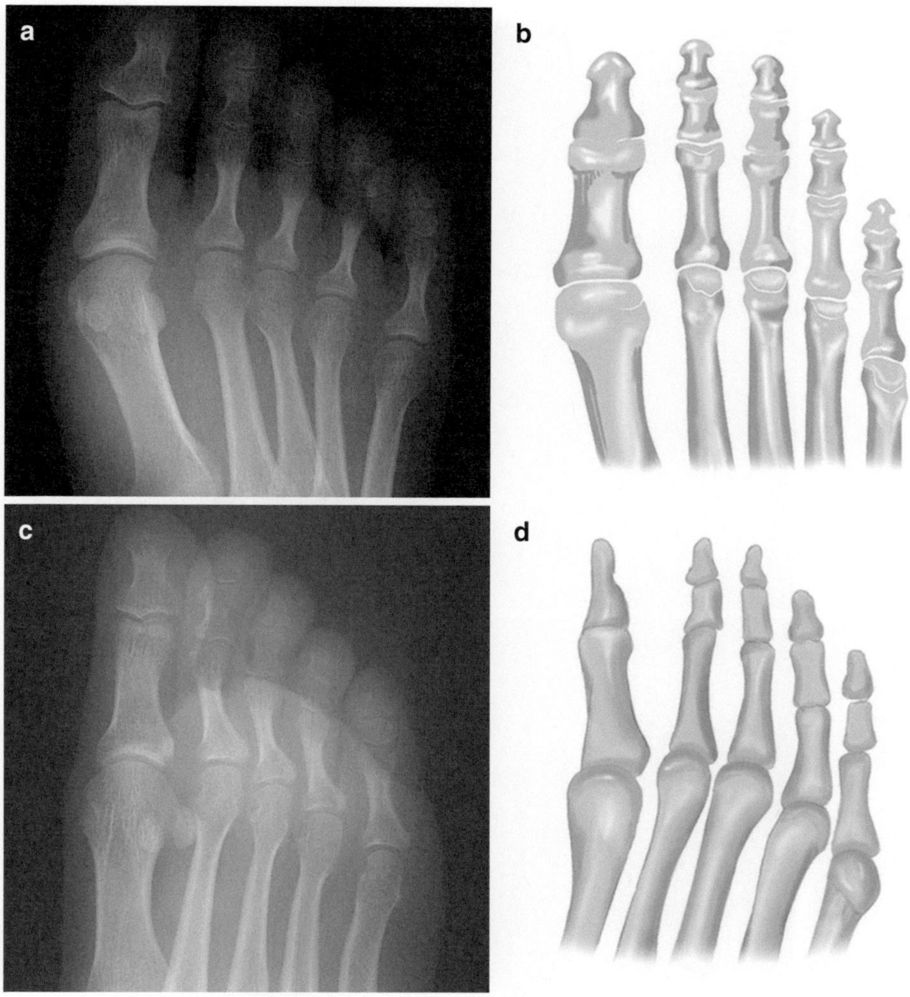

Fig. 11.64 X-ray plain film (**a**, **c**) shows no definite signs of fracture in the bones of the feet (**b**, **d**)

   6.2 CT scan (Fig. 11.64e, f)

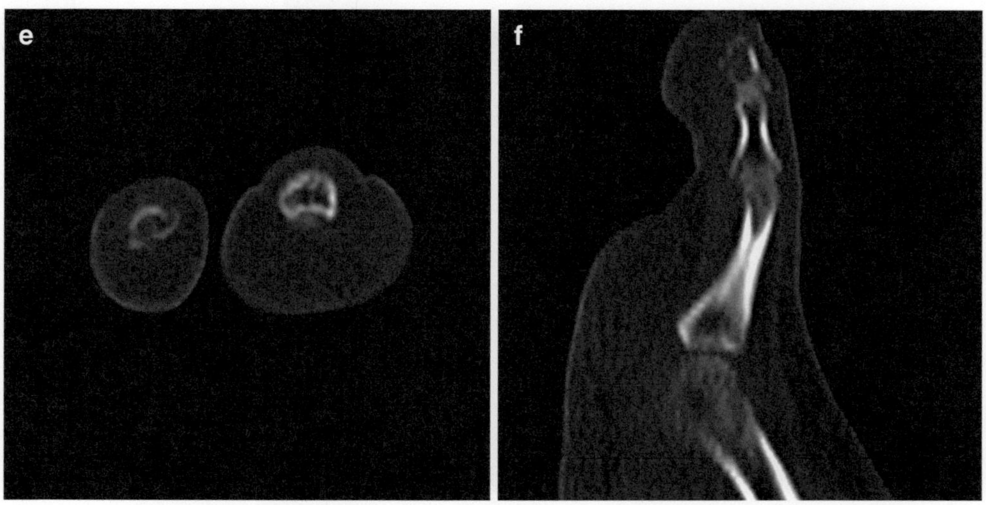

Fig. 11.64 CT coronal plane (**e**) and sagittal plane (**f**) show basal bone fracture of distal phalanges of second toes and slightly dislocated ends

7. Toe cuneiform fracture
   7.1 X-ray plain film (Fig. 11.65a–d)

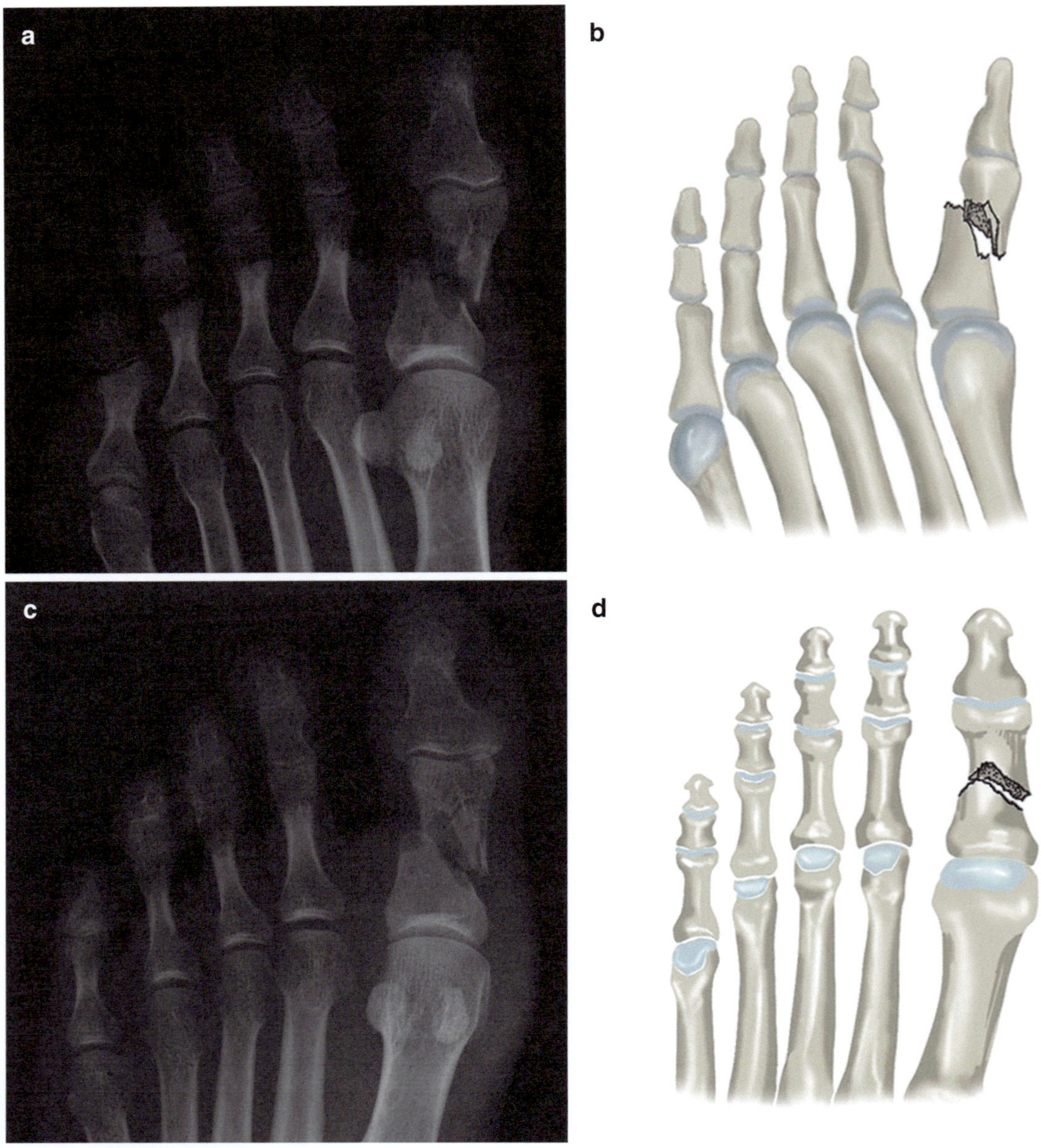

Fig. 11.65 X-ray plain film (**a**, **c**) shows bone fracture of the proximal phalanx of the first toes and visible wedge bone mass. The schematic diagram (**b**, **d**)

8. Distal part of the articular fracture of the phalanx
   8.1 X-ray plain film (Fig. 11.66a–d)

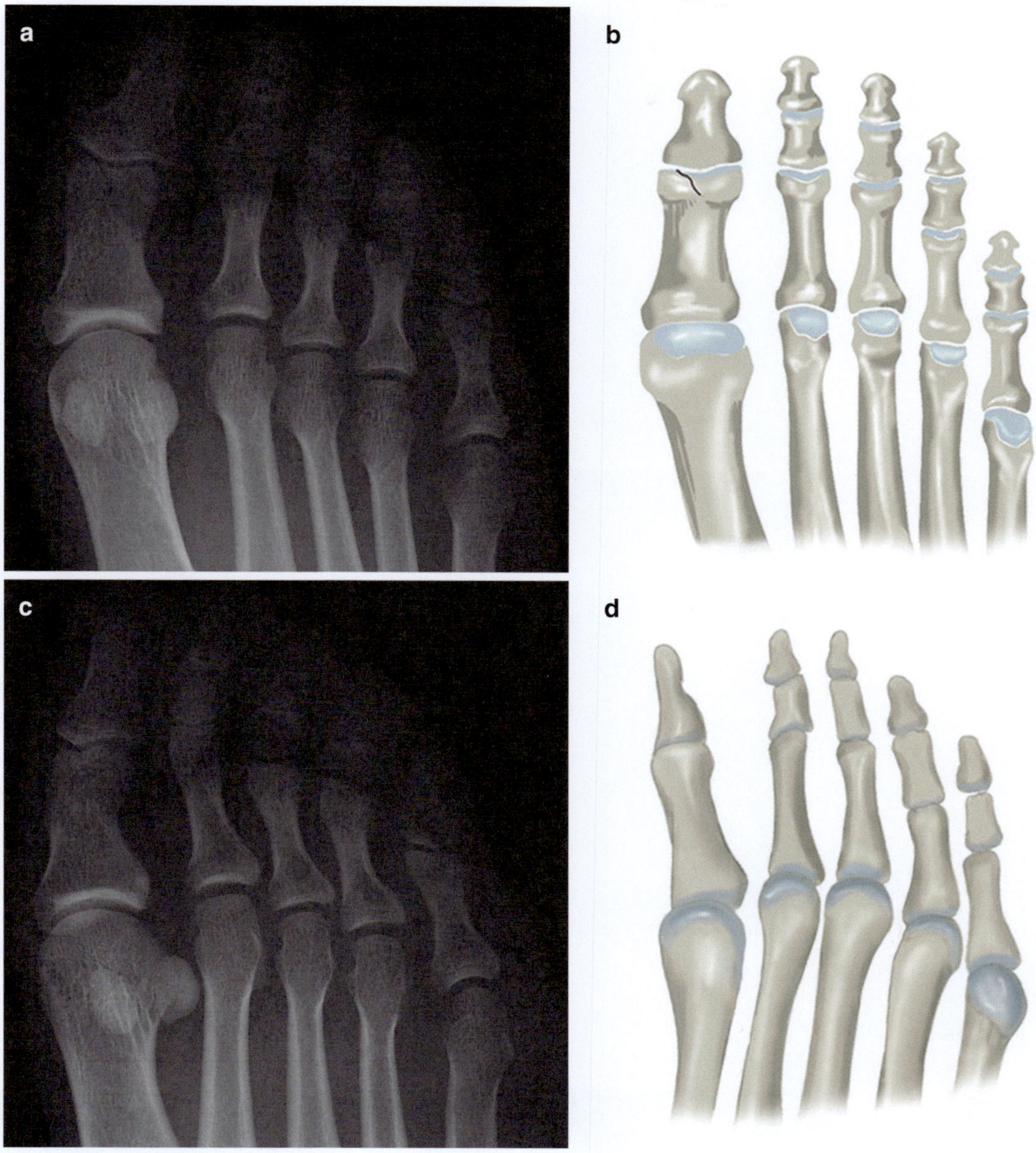

Fig. 11.66 X-ray plain film (**a**, **c**) shows the distal phalangeal fracture of the first phalanges near the phalanx of the distal phalanx, the fracture line reached the articular surface, and the dislocation was not obvious. The schematic diagram (**b**, **d**)

9. Complete intra-articular fracture of the proximal end of the phalanges
   9.1 X-ray plain film (Fig. 11.67a–d)

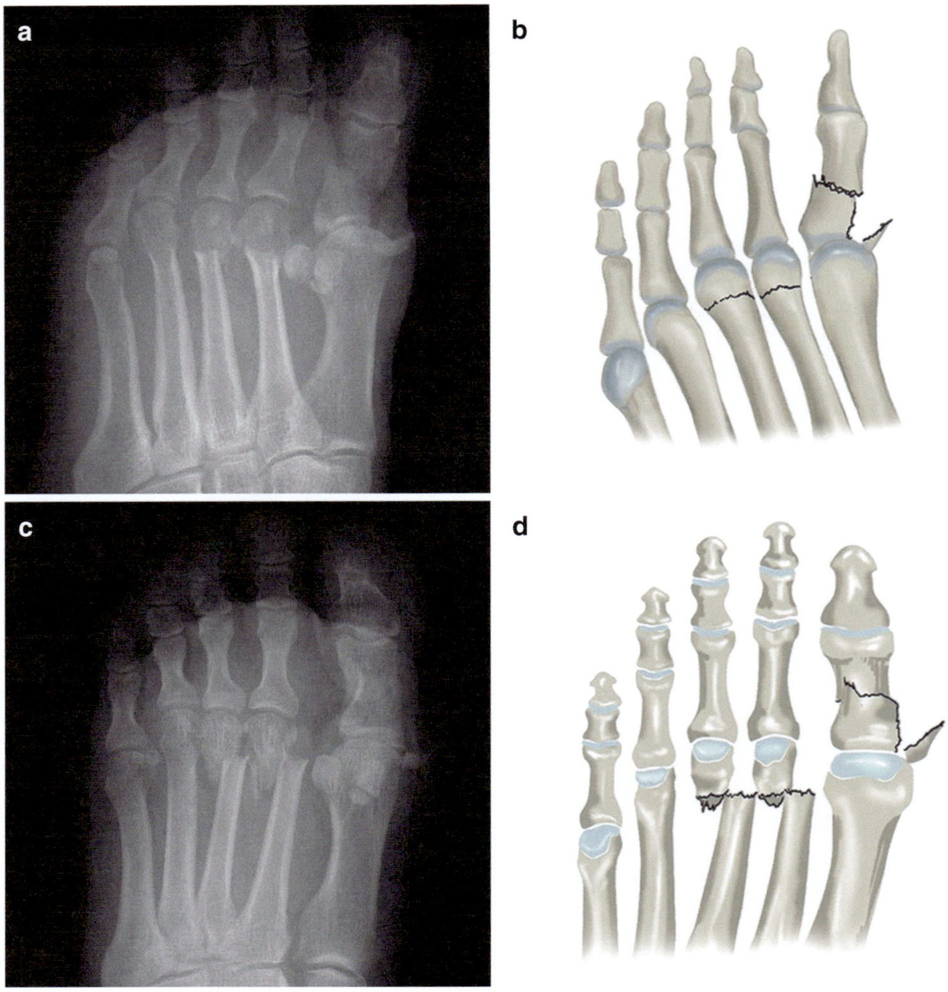

Fig. 11.67 X-ray plain film (**a**, **c**) shows the proximal bone fragmentation of the first toe near the phalanges, dislocation of the broken end, irregular articular surface, fracture of the second, third metatarsal neck bone, and a schematic diagram (**b**, **d**)

   9.2 CT scan (Fig. 11.67e, f)

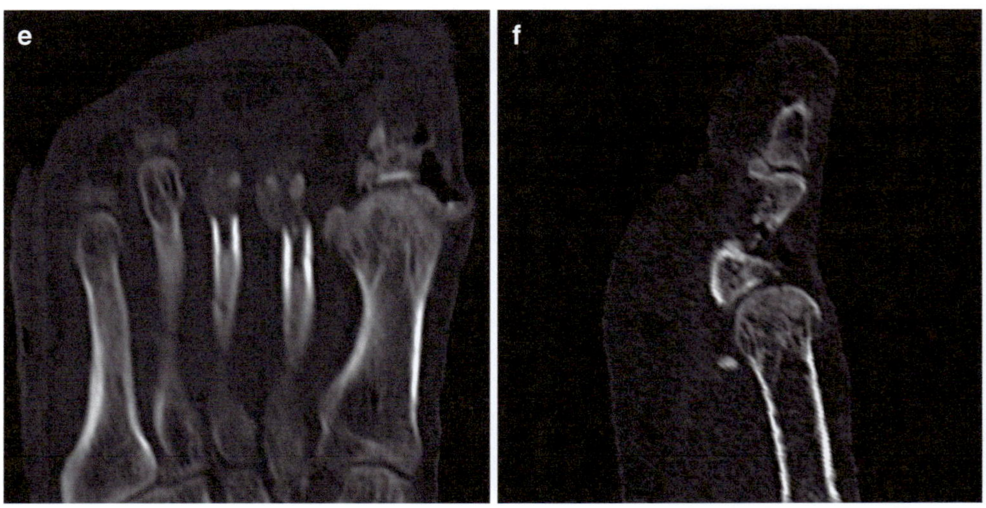

Fig. 11.67 CT cross section (**e**) and sagittal plane (**f**) show the bone fragmentation of the first toe near the phalanges, involving the joints, the visible gas shadow in the soft tissue, and the fracture of the second, third metatarsal bone

10. Complete intra-articular fracture of the proximal end of the phalanges
    10.1 X-ray plain film (Fig. 11.68a–d)

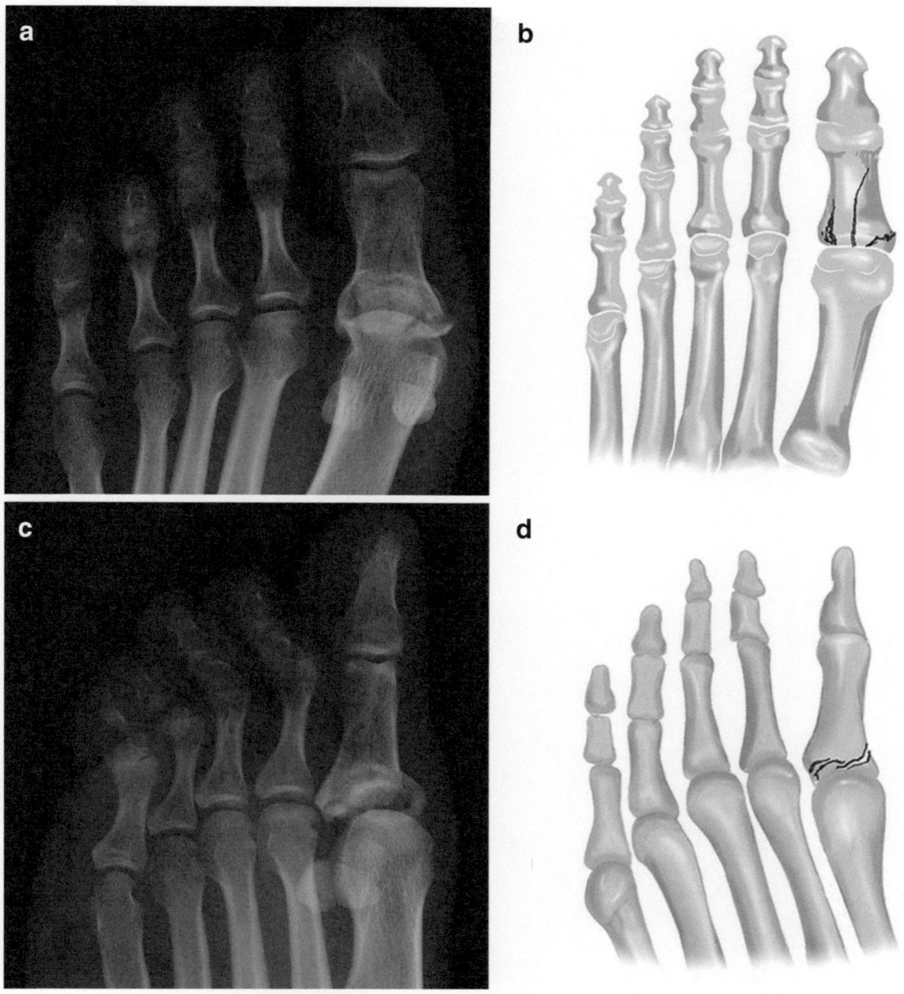

Fig. 11.68 X-ray plain film (**a**, **c**) shows bone fracture of proximal phalanges near the first phalanges, dislocation of the ends, irregular joints, and schematic diagram (**b**, **d**)

    10.2 CT scan (Fig. 11.68e, f)

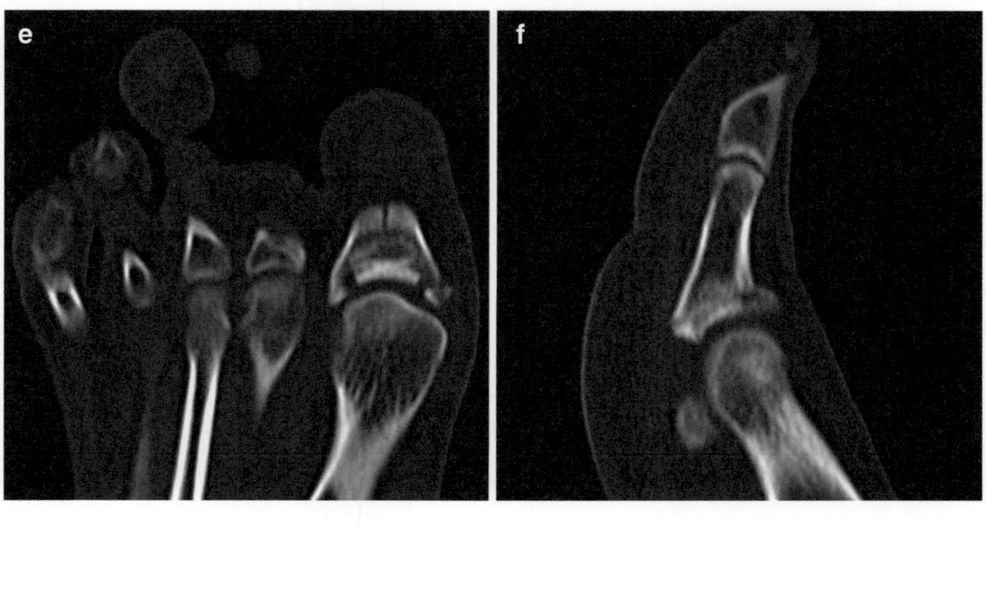

Fig. 11.68 CT transect (**e**) and sagittal plane (**f**) show bone fracture of the proximal phalanges of first toes involving the joints

11. Comminuted fracture of the diaphysis of the toes
    11.1 X-ray plain film (Fig. 11.69a–d)

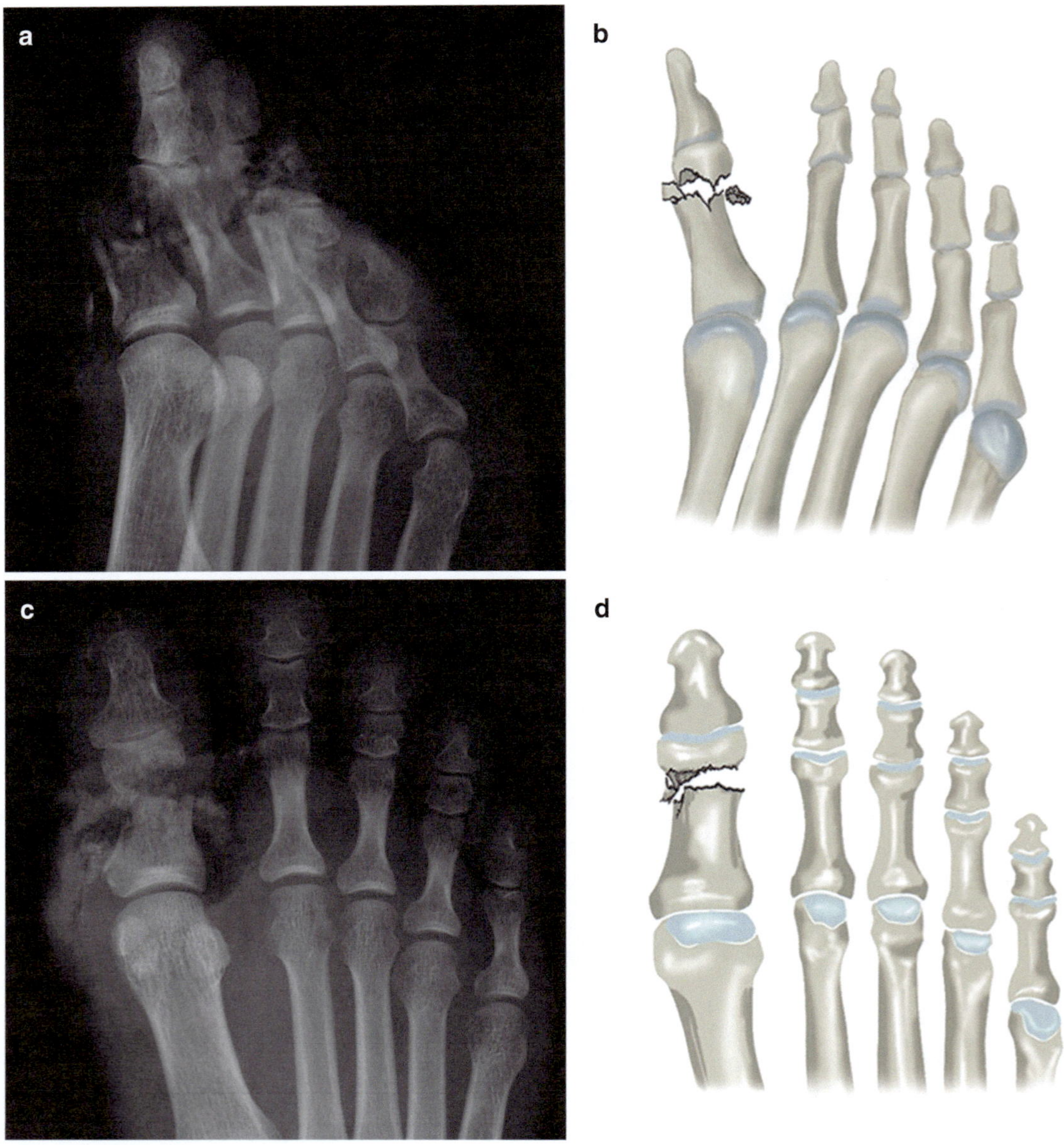

Fig. 11.69 X-ray plain film (**a**, **c**) shows bone fracture of proximal phalanx of the first toes, dislocation of the ends, irregular soft tissue, and schematic diagram (**b**, **d**)

12. Comminuted fracture of the diaphysis of the toes
    12.1 X-ray plain film (Fig. 11.70a–d)

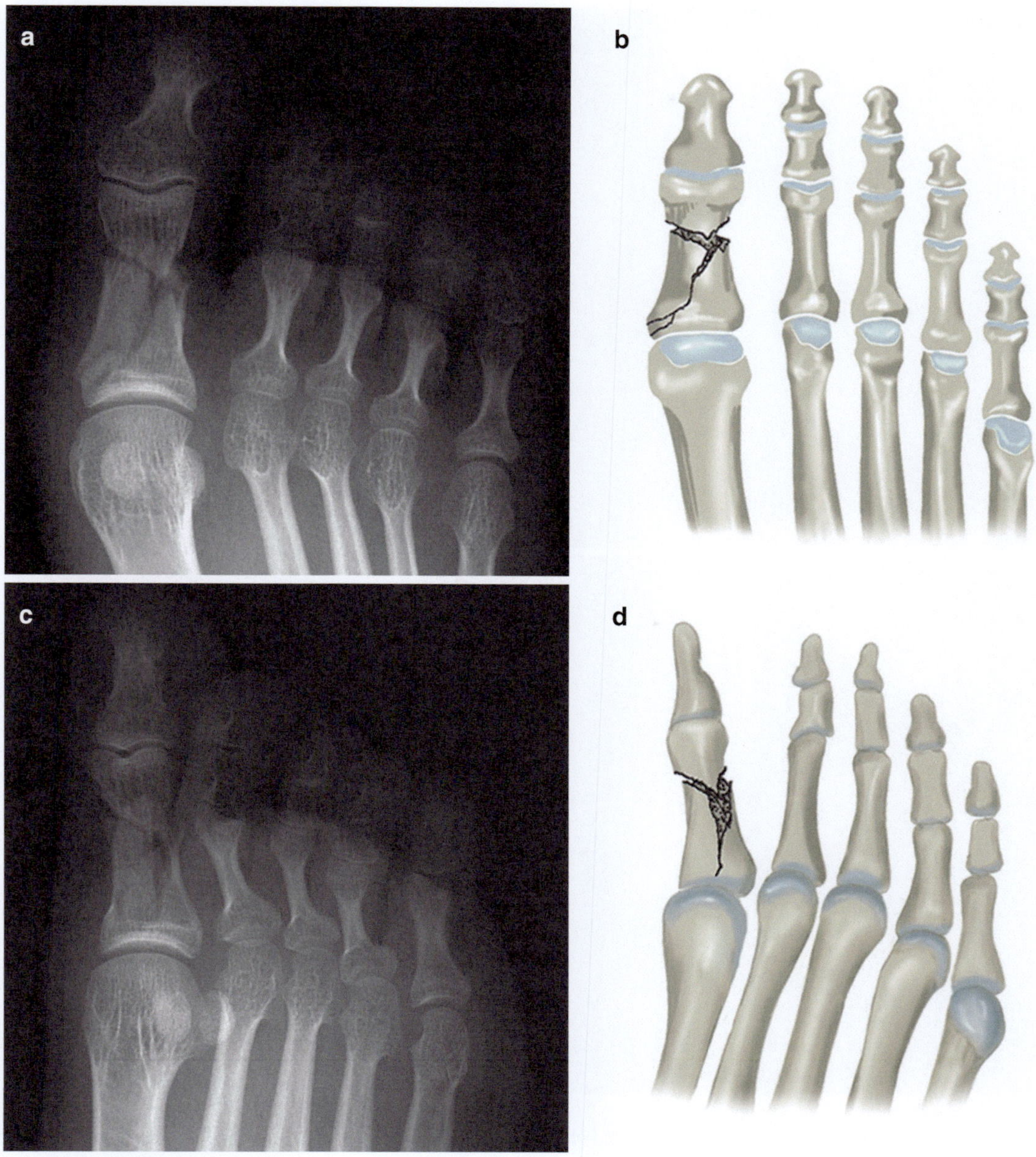

Fig. 11.70 X-ray plain film (**a**, **c**) shows bone fracture of the proximal phalanx of the first toes and slightly dislocation of the ends of the phalanx (**b**, **d**)

13. Complete intra-articular fracture of the distal phalanx
    13.1 X-ray plain film (Fig. 11.71a–d)

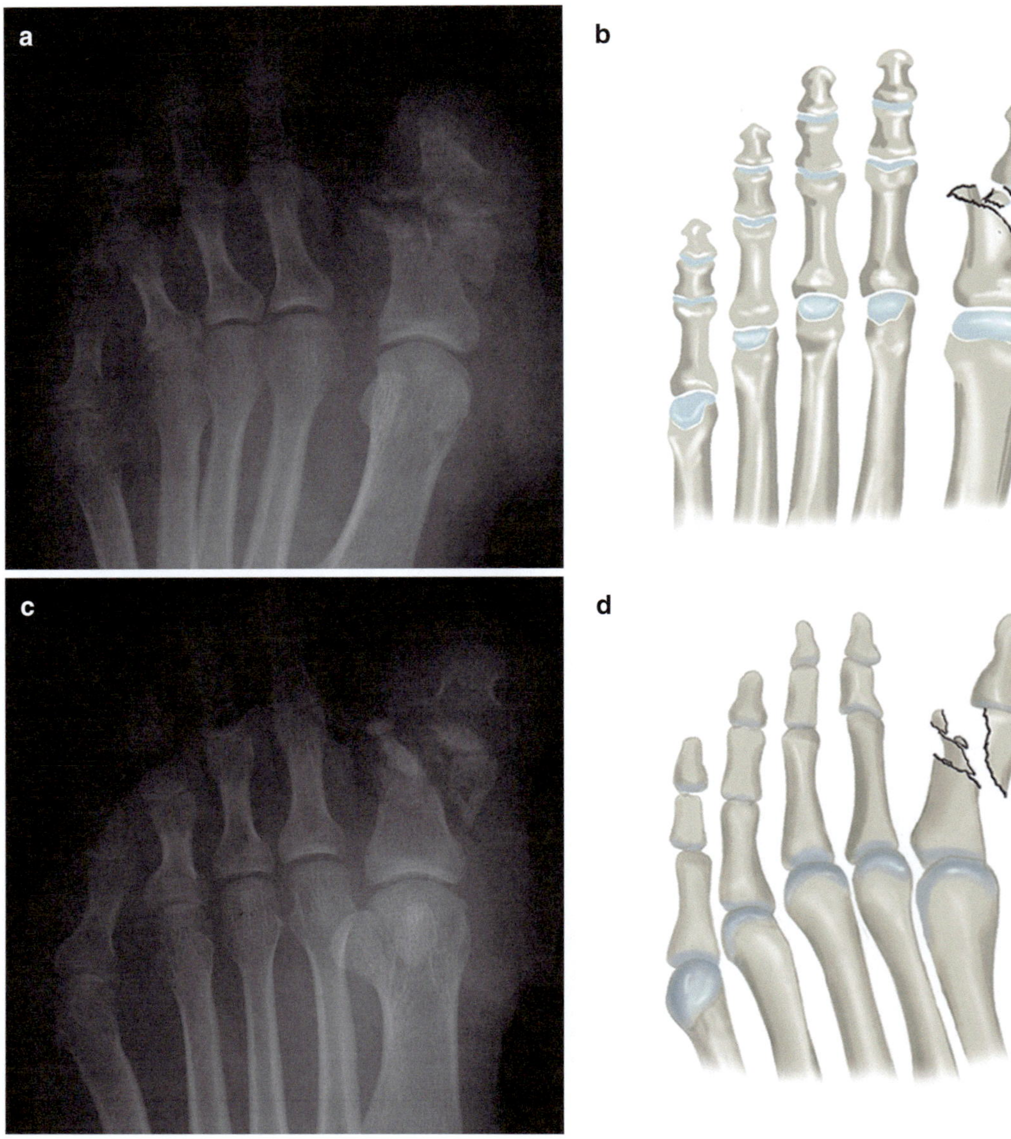

Fig. 11.71 X-ray plain film (**a**, **c**) shows bone fracture of distal phalanges of distal first phalanges, dislocation of ends, disorder of articular surface, irregular soft tissue, and schematic diagram (**b**, **d**)

14. Complete intra-articular fracture of the distal phalanx
    14.1 X-ray plain film (Fig. 11.72a–d)

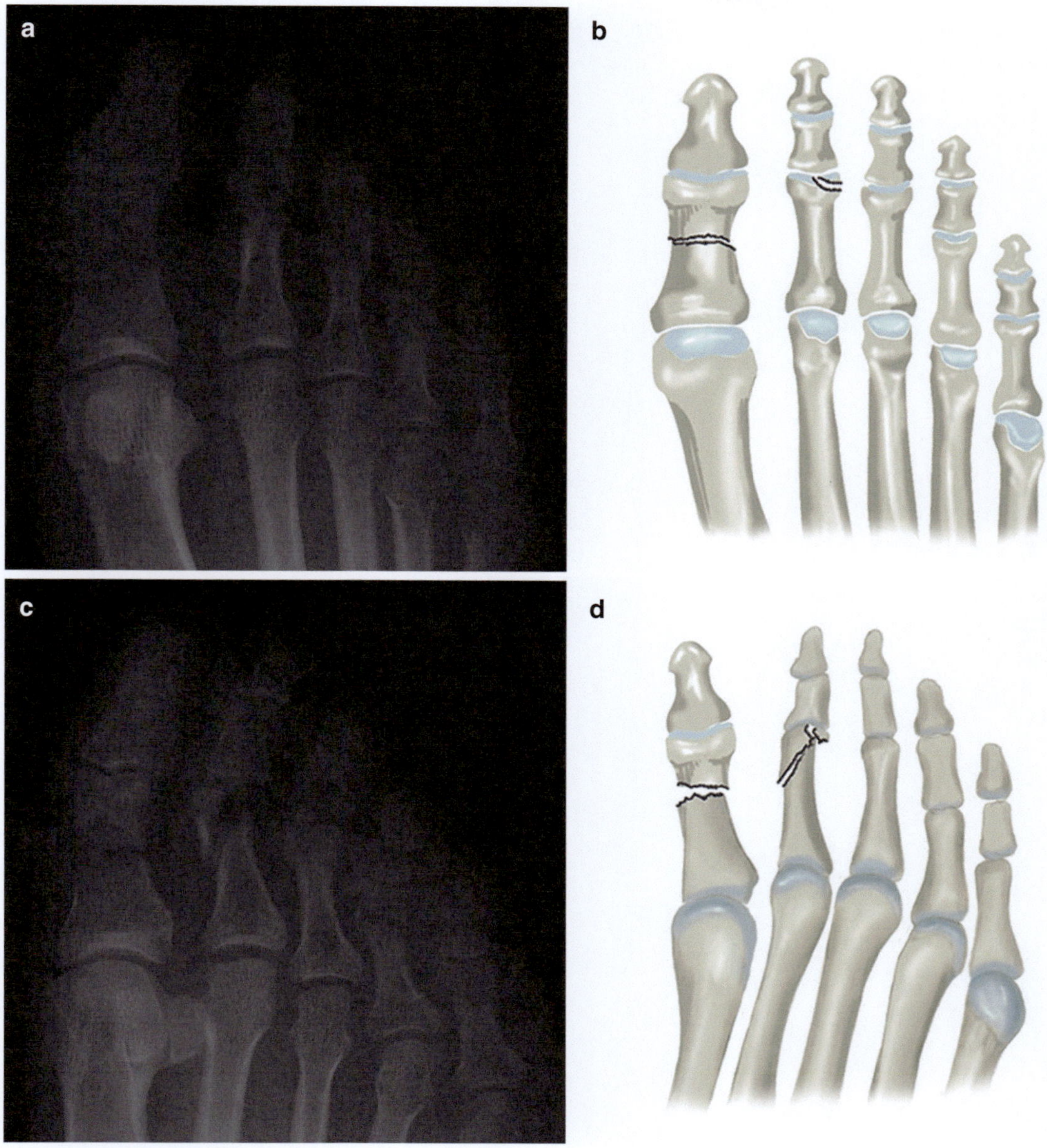

Fig. 11.72 The X-ray plain film (**a**, **c**) shows the distal bone fragmentation of the second toe near the phalanges, dislocation of the broken end, involvement of the joint, and the fracture of the first toe near the diaphysis of the diaphysis of the phalanx (**b**, **d**)

15. Complete intra-articular fracture of the distal phalanx
    15.1 X-ray plain film (Fig. 11.73a–d)

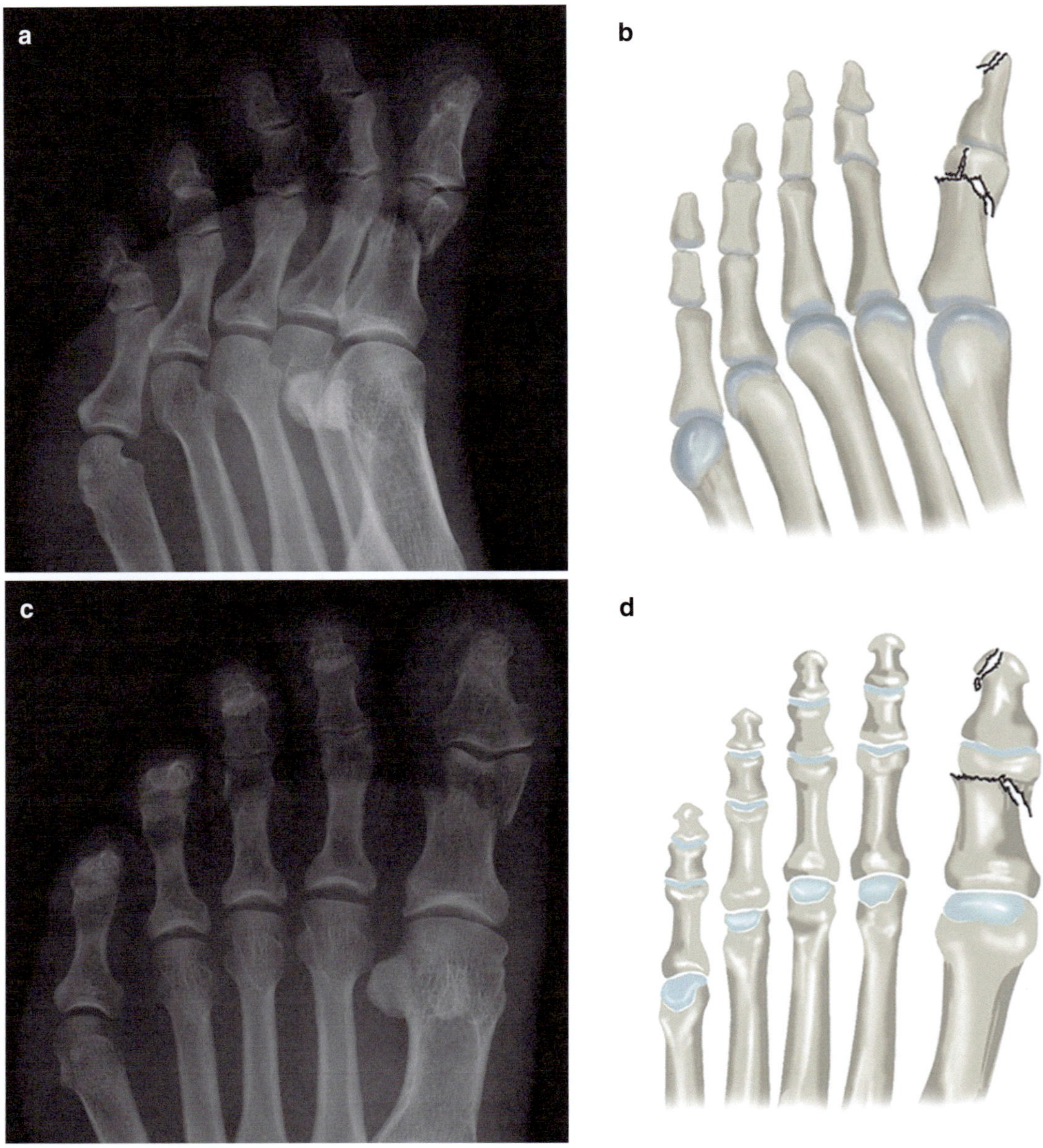

Fig. 11.73 X-ray plain film (**a**, **c**) shows bone fracture of distal phalanges of distal first phalanges, dislocation of the ends, and fracture line involving the articular surface. The schematic diagram (**b**, **d**)

11.5 Fracture of the Sesamoid Bone

The sesamoid bone is a round or oval small bone, commonly found in the tendons of the hip joints, hands, knees, and feet. They can protect the tendons and increase the muscle torque. There are large anatomical variation of the seed bone, which manifests in its total quantity, the incidence and morphology of various parts. According to the literature most people have 42 bones. In some locations, the incidence of a seed bone was as high as 100%, whilst it was less than 1% in other parts. The sesamoid bone of the patella and the first metatarsophalangeal joint are a relatively constant sesamoid bone which almost everyone has. The percentage prevalence of febella and os perineum is 31% and 14%, respectively, but the incidence of os talotibiale and os intercuneiforme is less than 1%.

Like other parts of the skeleton, fractures of the sesamoid bones and other pathological changes can also occur. The patella is the largest and the most constant sesamoid bone in the human body. Its fracture has been described in the former chapter. The first metatarsophalangeal joint is also a relatively constant sesamoid bone, but its incidence of fractures is unknown, the existing literature is only reported in a case report, whilst the fracture of the other sesamoid bones is also reported.

According to the morphology of the fracture of the sesamoid bone, it can be divided into the avulsion fracture (A type), the simple fracture (type B), the complex fracture (type C), and the special fracture (type B3). The avulsion fracture can be divided into the near pole (A1 type) or the distal (A2) avulsion fracture. The simple fracture is divided into the transverse fracture (B1 type), the oblique line, and the longitudinal fracture (B2 type) according to the fracture line, and the complex fracture is divided into 3 fracture blocks (C1 type) and the complete comminuted fracture of more than 3 fracture blocks (C2 type). Apart from a fracture, the dislocation of the first metatarsophalangeal joint occasionally occurs.

11.6 Identification of Injury Mechanism

The most common mechanism of injury is due to indirect trauma, usually a sprain.

11.7 Symptoms and Signs

Symptoms following a fracture present as pain, swelling, and limited activity in the region of the bone, yet these clinical features lack specify.

11.7.1 Imaging Differential Diagnosis

If the pain and swelling are obvious in the region of the sesamoid bone, an X-ray of the regular foot and oblique shows the abnormal shape of the sesamoid bone. The possibility of a sesamoid bone fracture should be considered, thus the axial position of the seed bone should be further added, and a CT scan should be performed when necessary. If there is a dislocation of the sesamoid bone it is usually between two points of the sesamoid bone, but the gap between the two poles of the sesamoid bone is not regular. MRI scan is feasible.

1. Avulsion fracture of the sesamoid bone
   1.1 X-ray plain film (Fig. 11.74a–d)

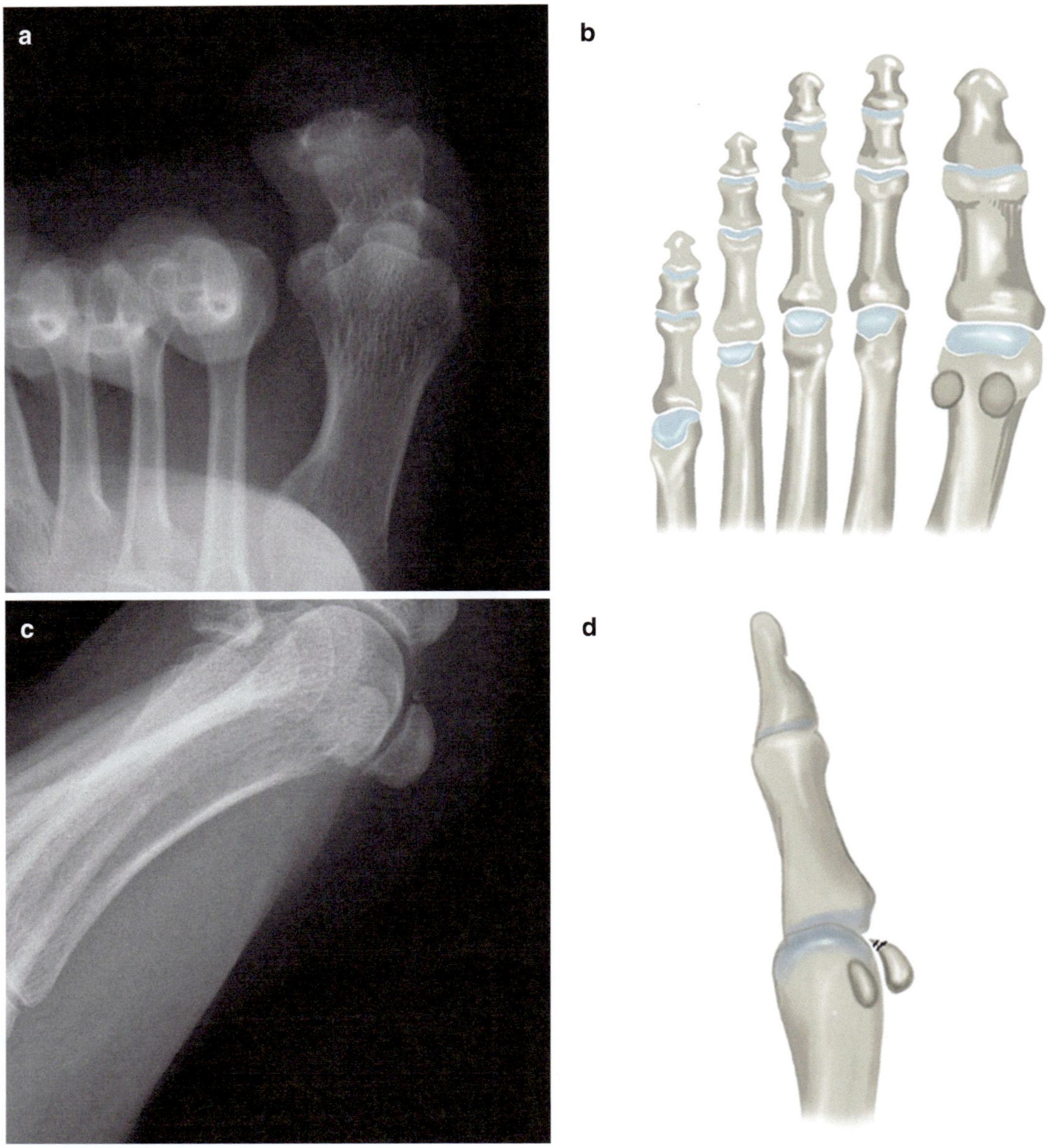

Fig. 11.74 X-ray plain film (**a**, **c**) shows the distal avulsion fracture of the first metatarsophalangeal joint and the fracture line is very clear in the lateral position of ankle joint, the schematic diagram (**b**, **d**)

2. Sesamoid bone
   2.1 X-ray (Fig. 11.75a–d)

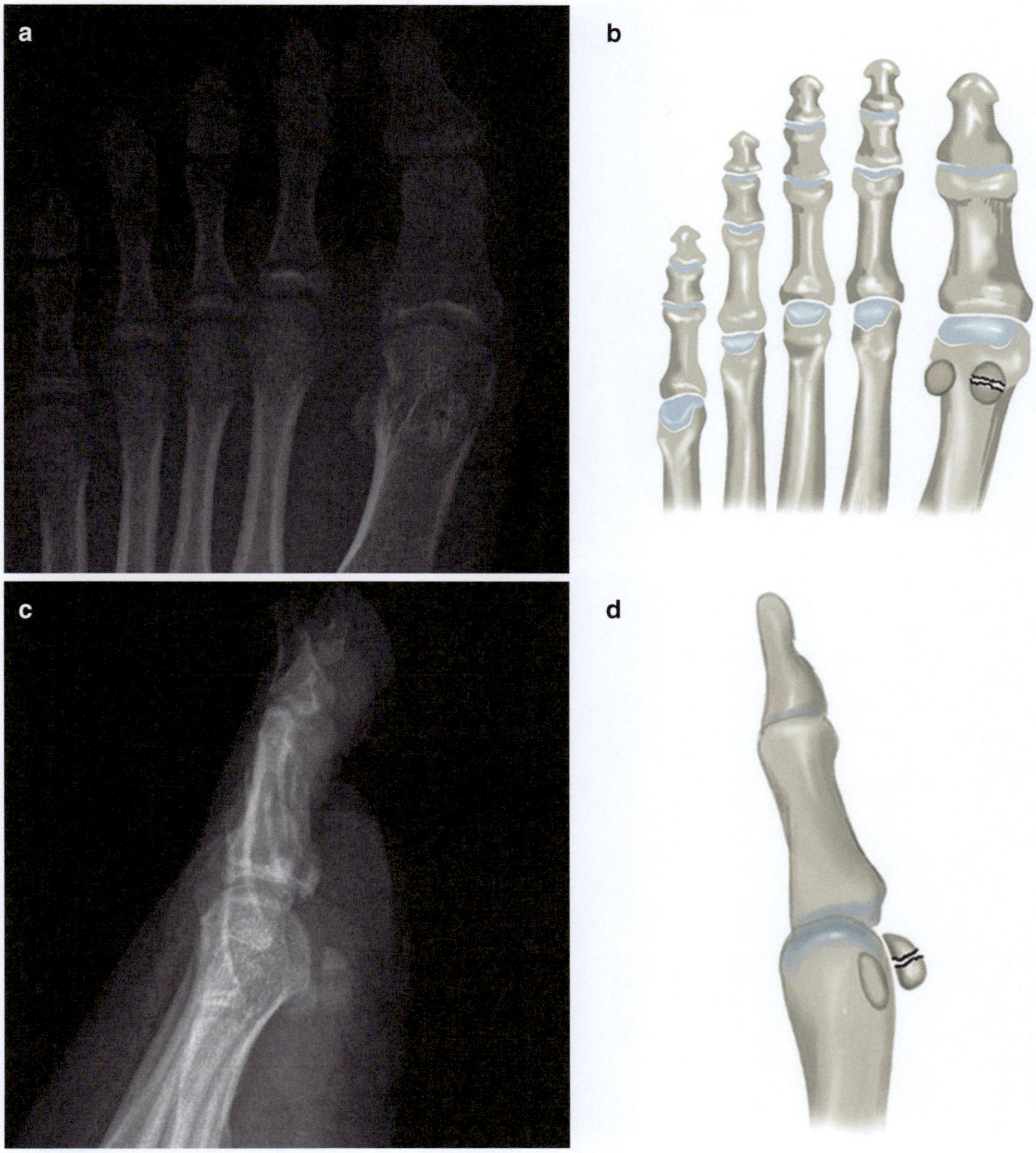

Fig. 11.75 X-ray plain film (**a**, **c**) shows transverse fracture of the medial side of the first metatarsophalangeal joint of the left foot, and the schematic diagram (**b**, **d**)

3. Sesamoid bone
   3.1 X-ray plain film (Fig. 11.76a–d)

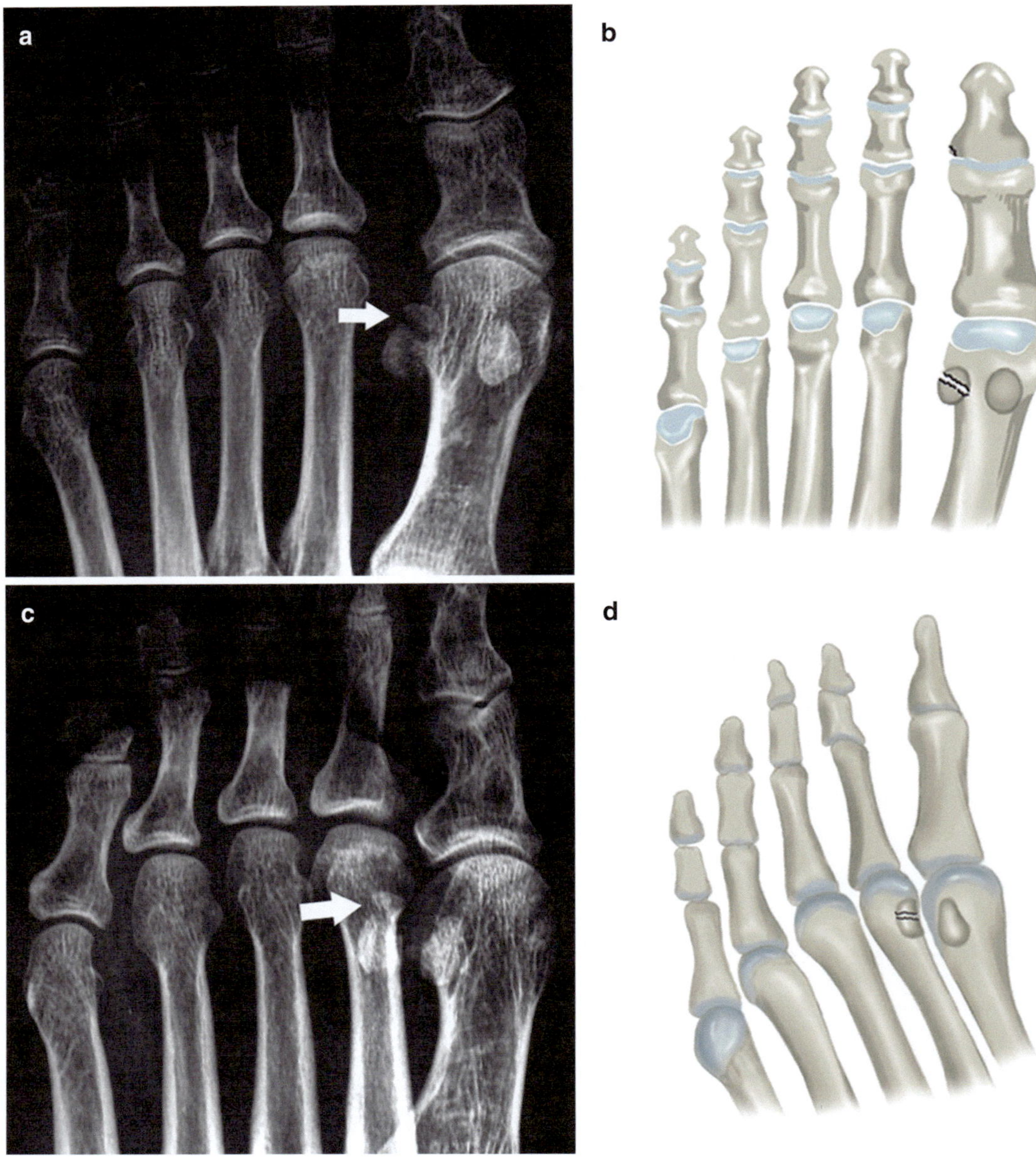

Fig. 11.76 X-ray plain film (**a**, **c**) shows a fracture of the first metatarsal bone (arrow), a slight dislocation, and a schematic diagram (**b**, **d**)

4. Sesamoid bone
   4.1 CT scan (Fig. 11.77a, b)

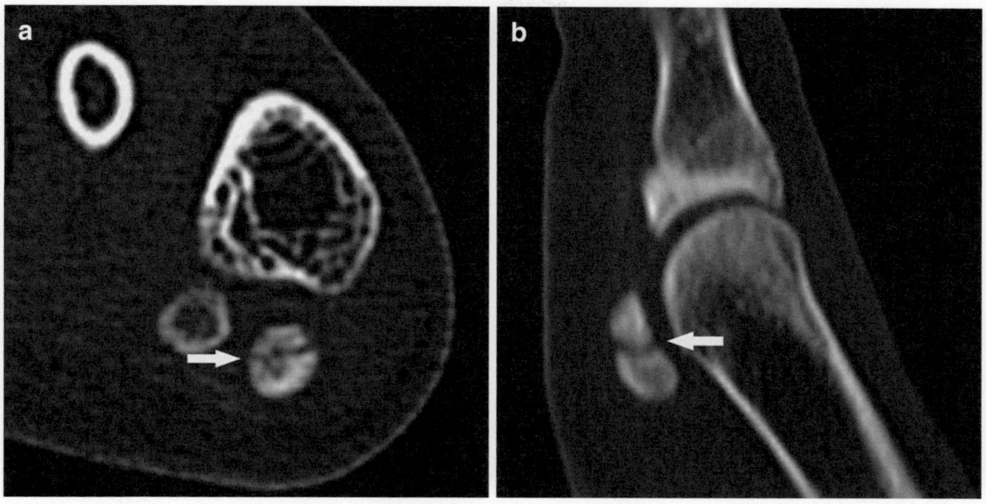

Fig. 11.77 CT coronal plane (**a**) and sagittal plane (**b**) show a fracture of the first metatarsal bone (arrow), and slightly separated dislocation

5. Dislocation of the sesamoid bone
   5.1 X-ray plain film (Fig. 11.78a–d)

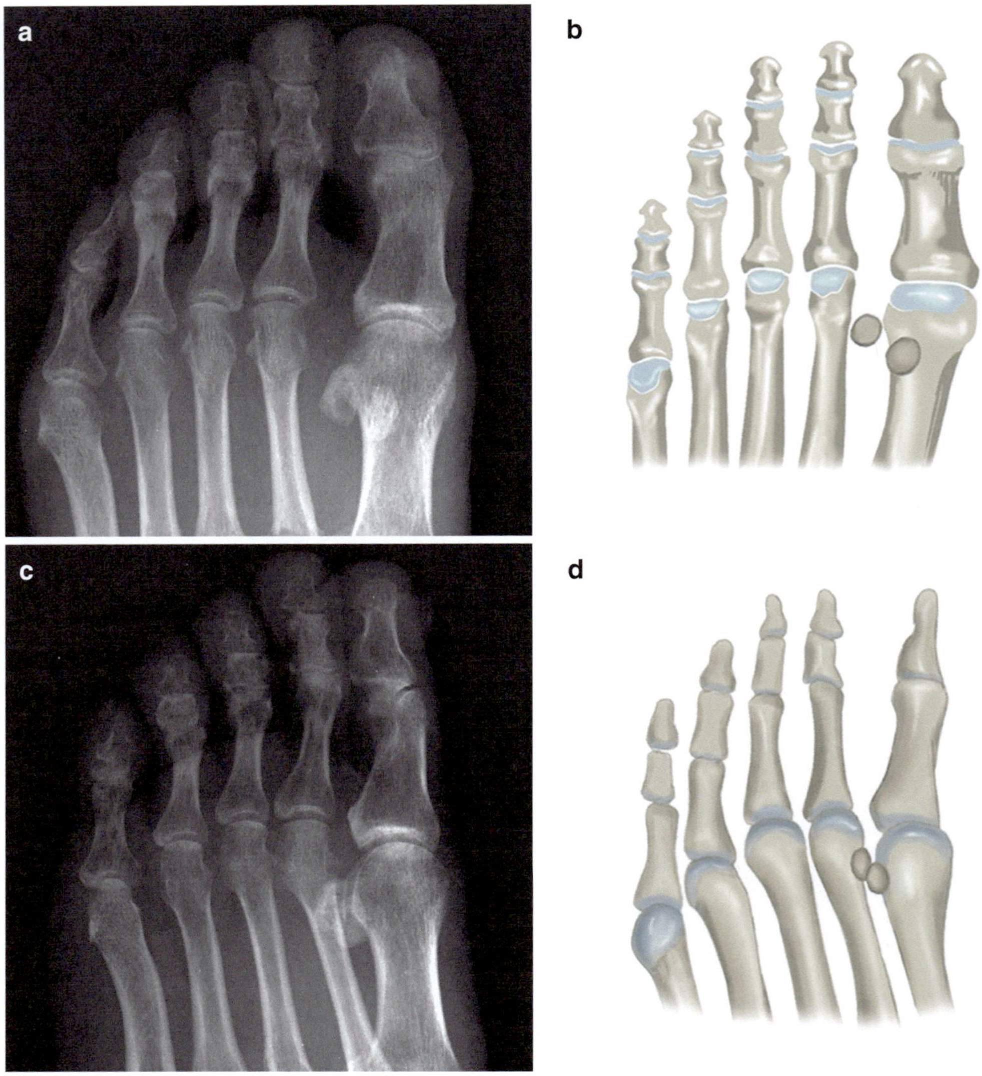

Fig. 11.78 X-ray plain film (**a**, **c**) shows multiple metatarsal fractures of the left foot, accompanied by dislocation of the first metatarsophalangeal joint. The schematic diagram (**b**, **d**)

Key Points

1. The most common fracture of tarsal bone is a calcaneal fracture, which is usually caused by the falling on heel of the foot, often accompanied with compression burst fracture of vertebral body.
2. Lateral and oblique radiographs are of great clinical significance given it shows avulsion fracture of tarsal bone.
3. CT plain scan and multiplane reconstruction can show the structure and anatomical relationship of the tarsus efficiently. It has important clinical value when judging the range of fracture, the condition of the joint surface, the fracture, and dislocation.
4. Intra-articular fracture is the main cause of calcaneal fracture. CT scan and reconstruction should be parallel or perpendicular to the talar joint surface.
5. Normal fractures of the metatarsal and phalangeal fractures can meet the clinical needs.

12 Lower Limb Shaft Fracture

Zhanle Zheng and Yingze Zhang

12.1 Femoral Shaft Fracture

Femoral shaft fractures refer to the fracture of the femur from 5 cm under the lesser trochanter to 2 cm above the femoral condyle. According to the 2007 AO/OTA classification, it can be divided into 3 types: type A simple fracture, type B wedge fracture, and type C comminuted fracture.

12.1.1 Identification of Injury Mechanism

Most fractures are caused by traffic accidents and falls, often combined with injuries of other parts of the body, such as head and chest trauma.

12.1.2 Identification of Symptoms and Signs

The clinical features are pain, swelling, restricted movement, and deformity, which are easy to diagnose.

12.1.3 Imaging Differential Diagnosis

X-ray is applied to diagnose femoral shaft fracture; meanwhile it is necessary to take an image of both femoral neck and knee joint to prevent missed diagnosis.

12.1.3.1 Type A Simple Fracture

Type A simple fracture can be divided into: simple spiral fracture, simple oblique fracture, and simple transverse fracture. In addition, incomplete fractures can occur in young children, where a part of the bone remains intact and unbroken, which are also called greenstick fracture.

Z. Zheng · Y. Zhang (✉)
Department of Orthopaedics, The Third Hospital of Hebei Medical University, Shijiazhuang, Hebei, China

Y. Zhang (ed.), *Differential Diagnosis of Fracture*, https://doi.org/10.1007/978-981-13-8339-7_12

1. Differential diagnosis between simple spiral fracture and oblique fracture of the femoral shaft
   1.1 X-ray (Fig. 12.1a–d)

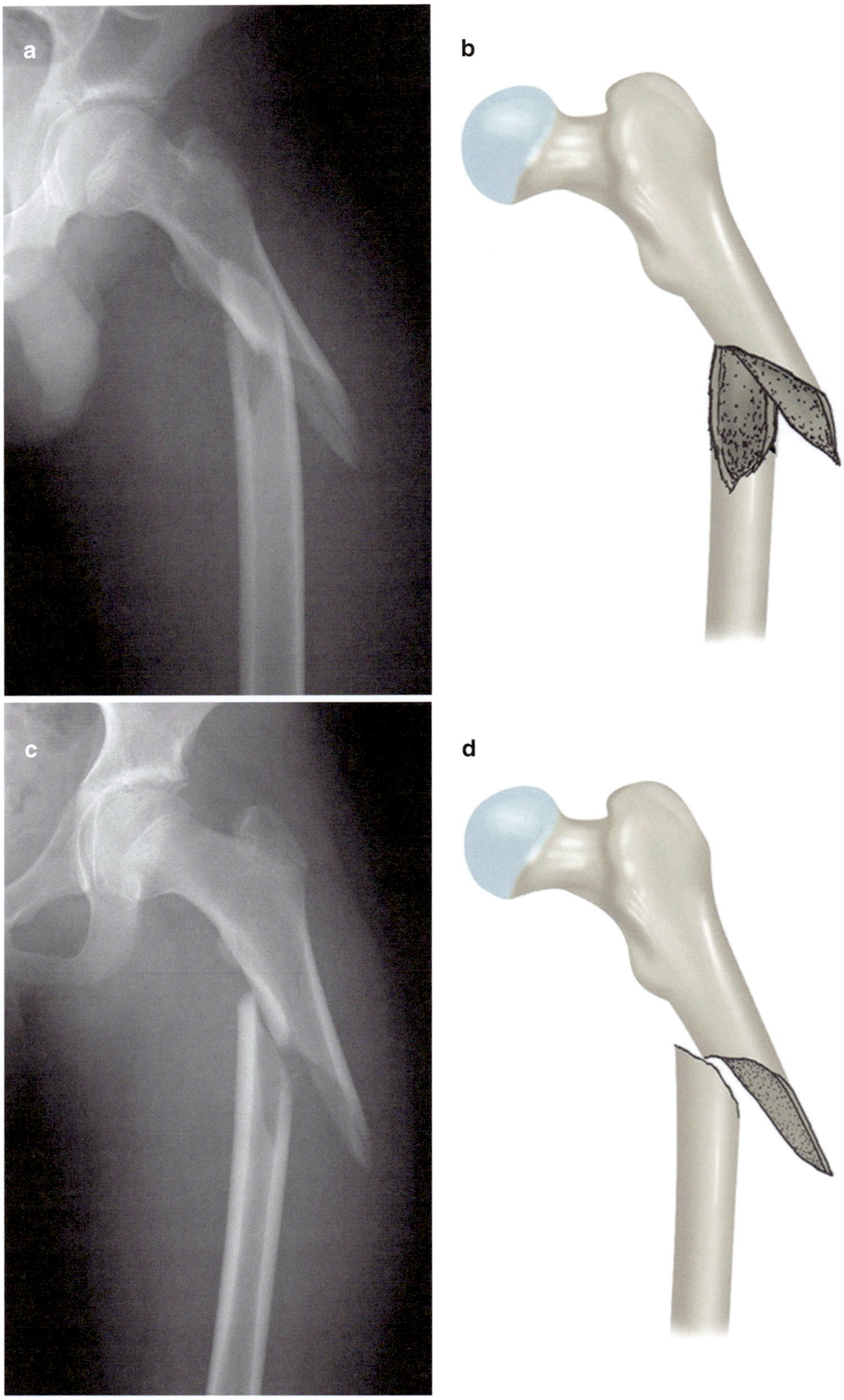

Fig. 12.1 (**a**, **c**) are respectively the lateral and anteroposterior (AP) views of the X-ray, showing the spiral fracture of the femoral shaft. Schematic diagram (**b**, **d**)

2. Differential diagnosis between simple oblique fracture and simple transverse fracture of the femoral shaft
   2.1 X-ray (Fig. 12.2a–d)

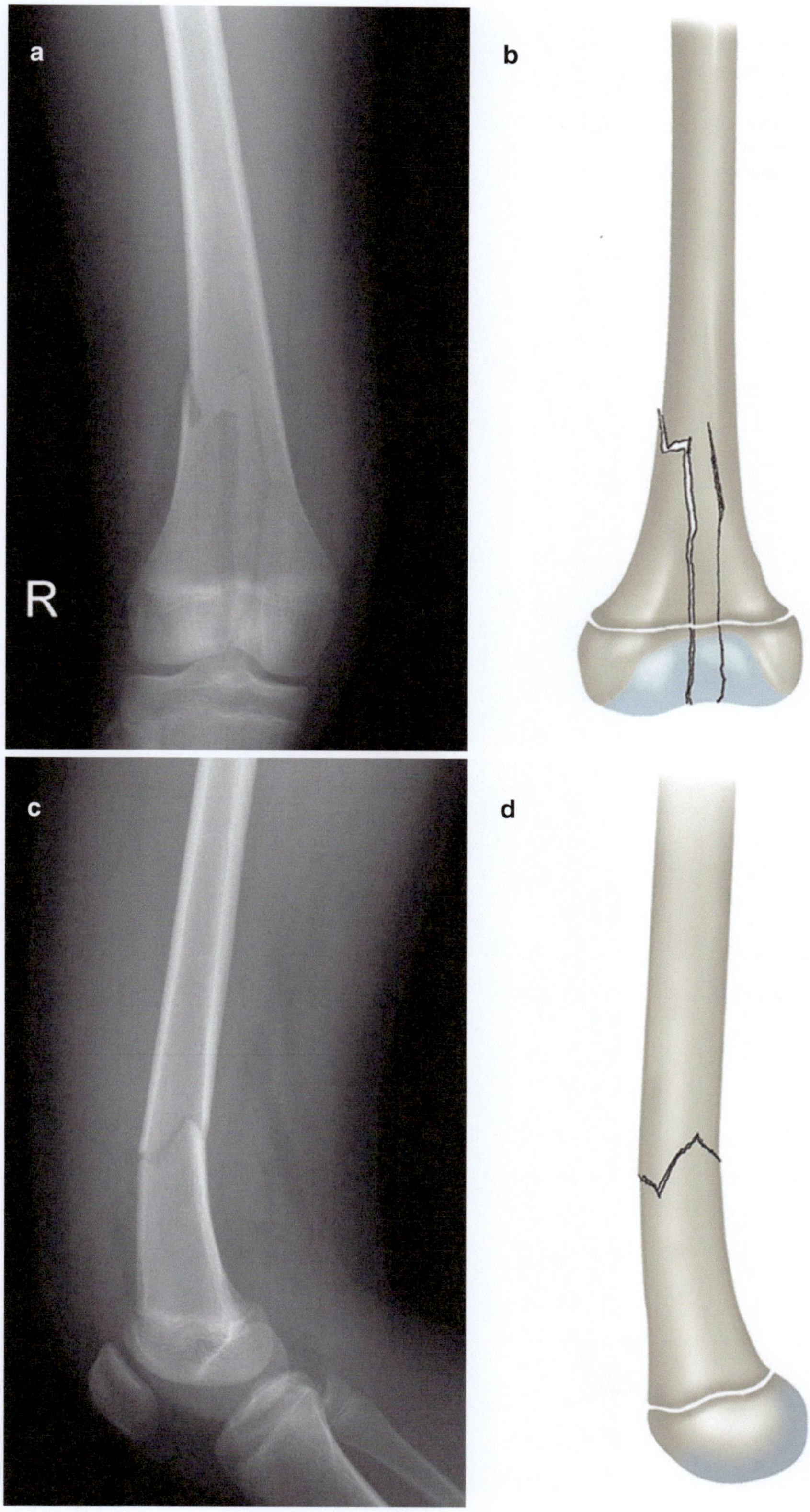

Fig. 12.2 (**a**, **c**) are respectively the lateral and anteroposterior (AP) views of the X-ray, showing the oblique fracture of the femoral shaft, without dislocation, and the schematic diagram (**b**, **d**)

3. Differential diagnosis between simple transverse femoral shaft fractures and simple oblique fractures
   3.1 X-ray (Fig. 12.3a–d)

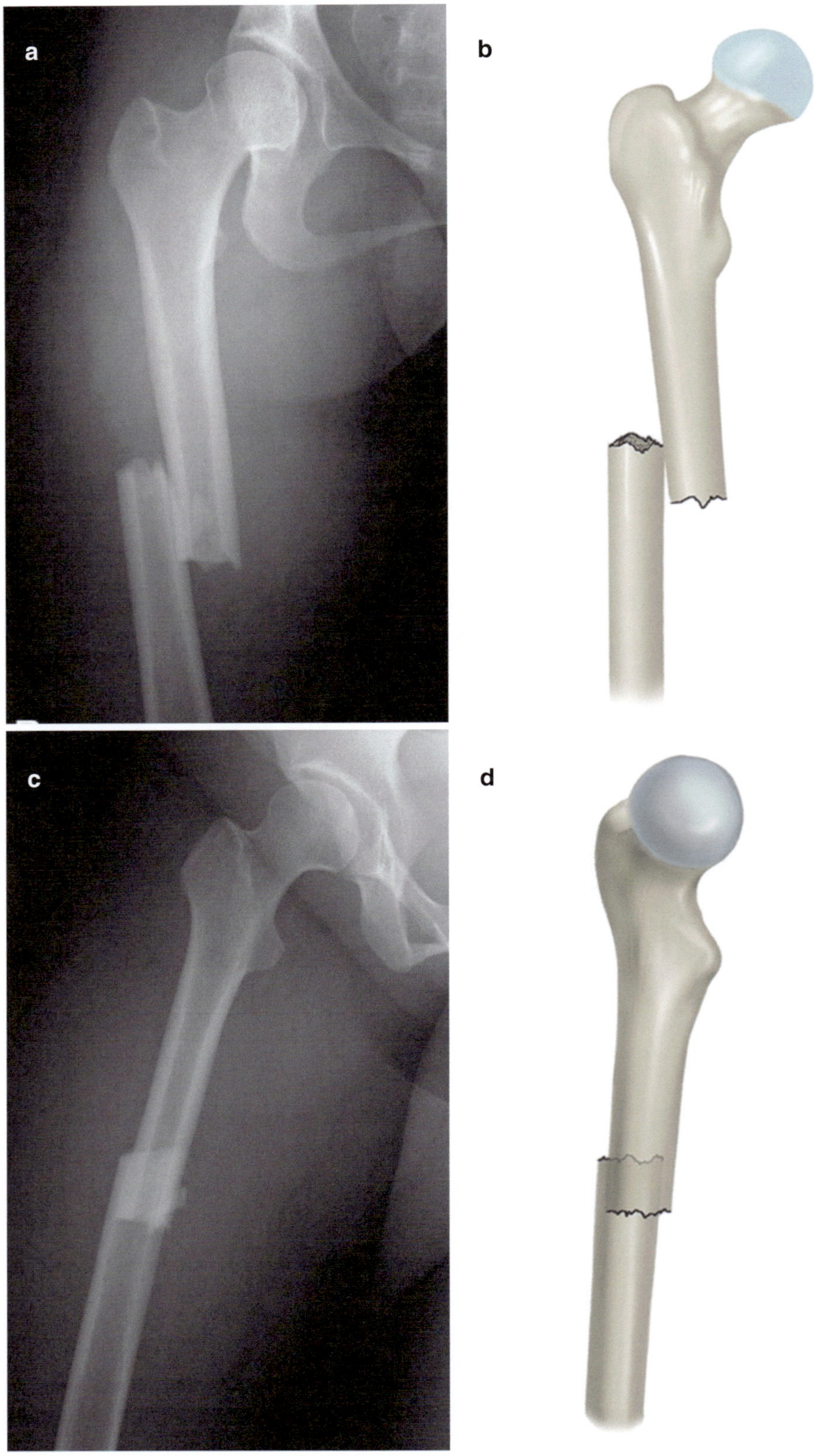

Fig. 12.3 (**a**, **c**) are respectively the lateral and anteroposterior (AP) views of the X-ray, showing the transverse fracture and overlapping dislocation of the femoral shaft. Schematic diagram (**b**, **d**)

4. Differential diagnosis between femoral shaft greenstick fracture and nonfracture
   4.1 X-ray (Fig. 12.4a–d)

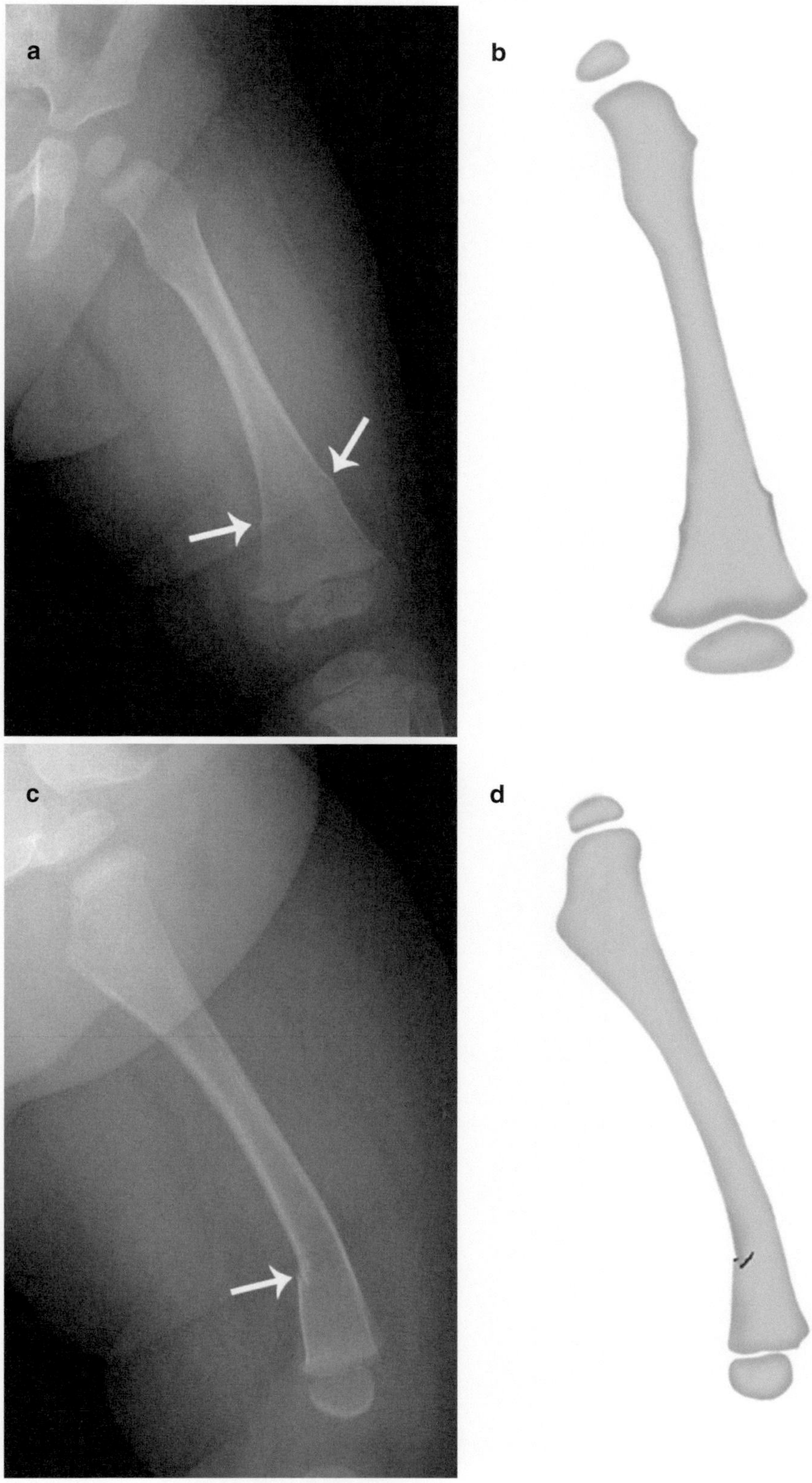

Fig. 12.4 (**a**, **c**) are respectively the lateral and anteroposterior (AP) views of the X-ray, showing the osteocortical fold (white arrow) of the lower femur, and the schematic diagram (**b**, **d**)

12.1.3.2 Type B Wedge Fracture

Wedge fractures are classified as spiral wedge fractures, curved wedge fractures, and comminuted wedge fractures.

5. Differential diagnosis between spiral wedge fracture and simple spiral fracture of the femoral shaft
   5.1 X-ray (Fig. 12.5a–d)

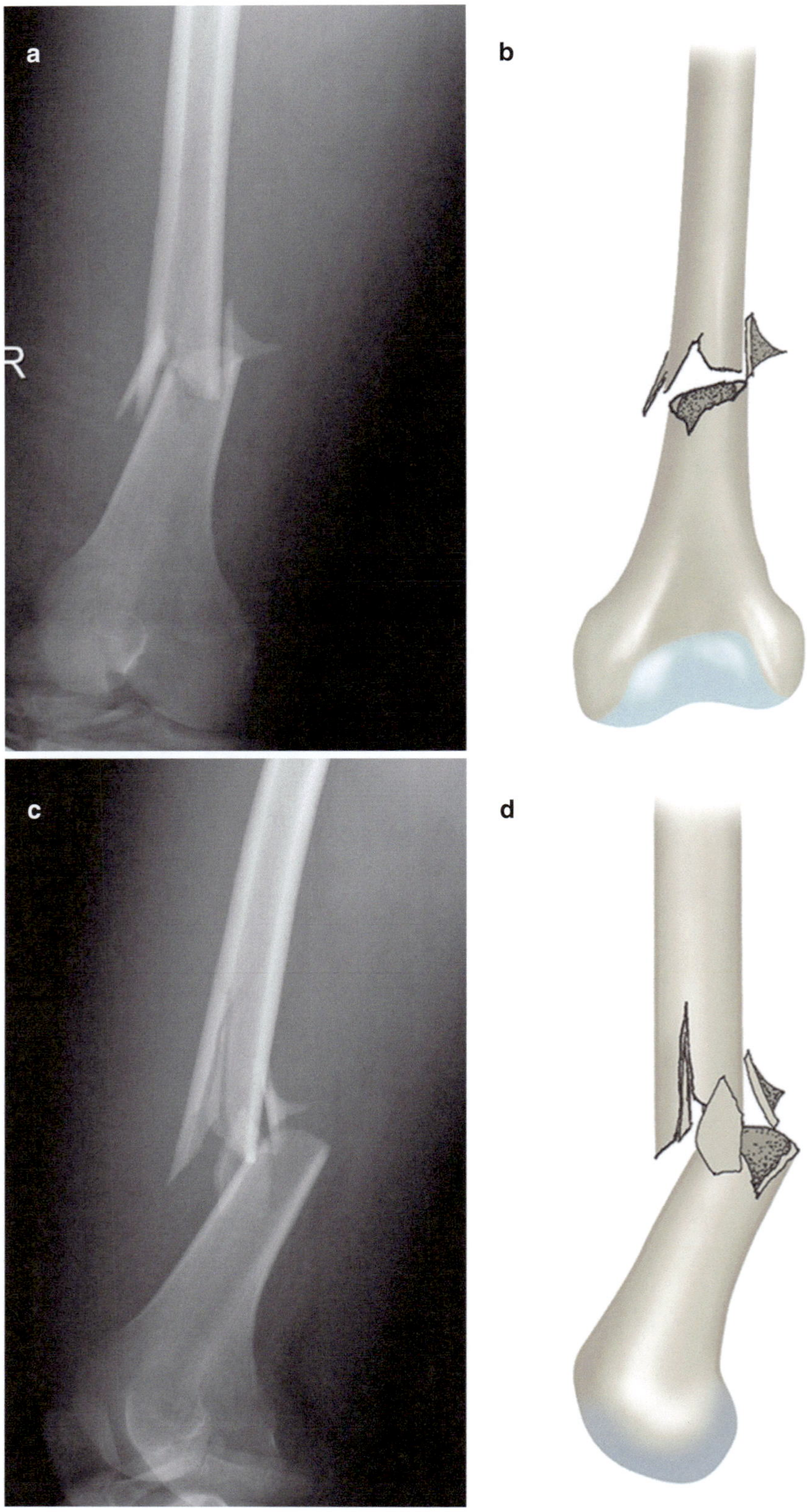

Fig. 12.5 (**a**, **c**) are respectively the lateral and anteroposterior (AP) views of the X-ray, showing the spiral fracture of the femoral shaft with wedge-shaped fragment, and the schematic diagram (**b**, **d**)

6. Differential diagnosis between curved wedge fracture and spiral wedge fracture of the femoral shaft
   6.1 X-ray (Fig. 12.6a–d)

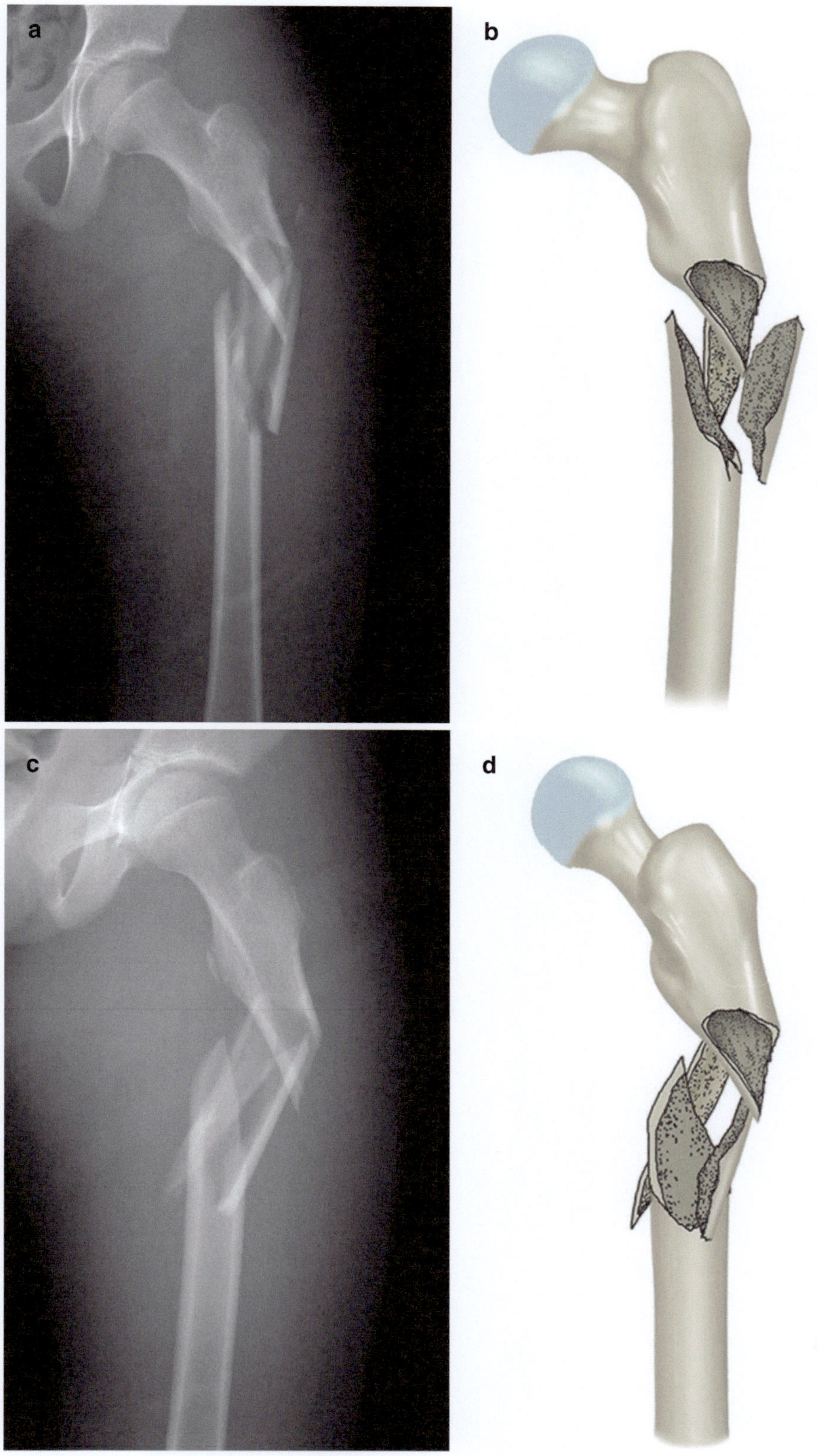

Fig. 12.6 (**a**, **c**) are respectively the lateral and anteroposterior (AP) views of the X-ray, showing curved fracture of the femoral shaft with wedge-shaped fragment, and the schematic diagram (**b**, **d**)

7. Differential diagnosis between comminuted wedge fracture and spiral wedge fracture of the femoral shaft
   7.1 X-ray (Fig. 12.7a–d)

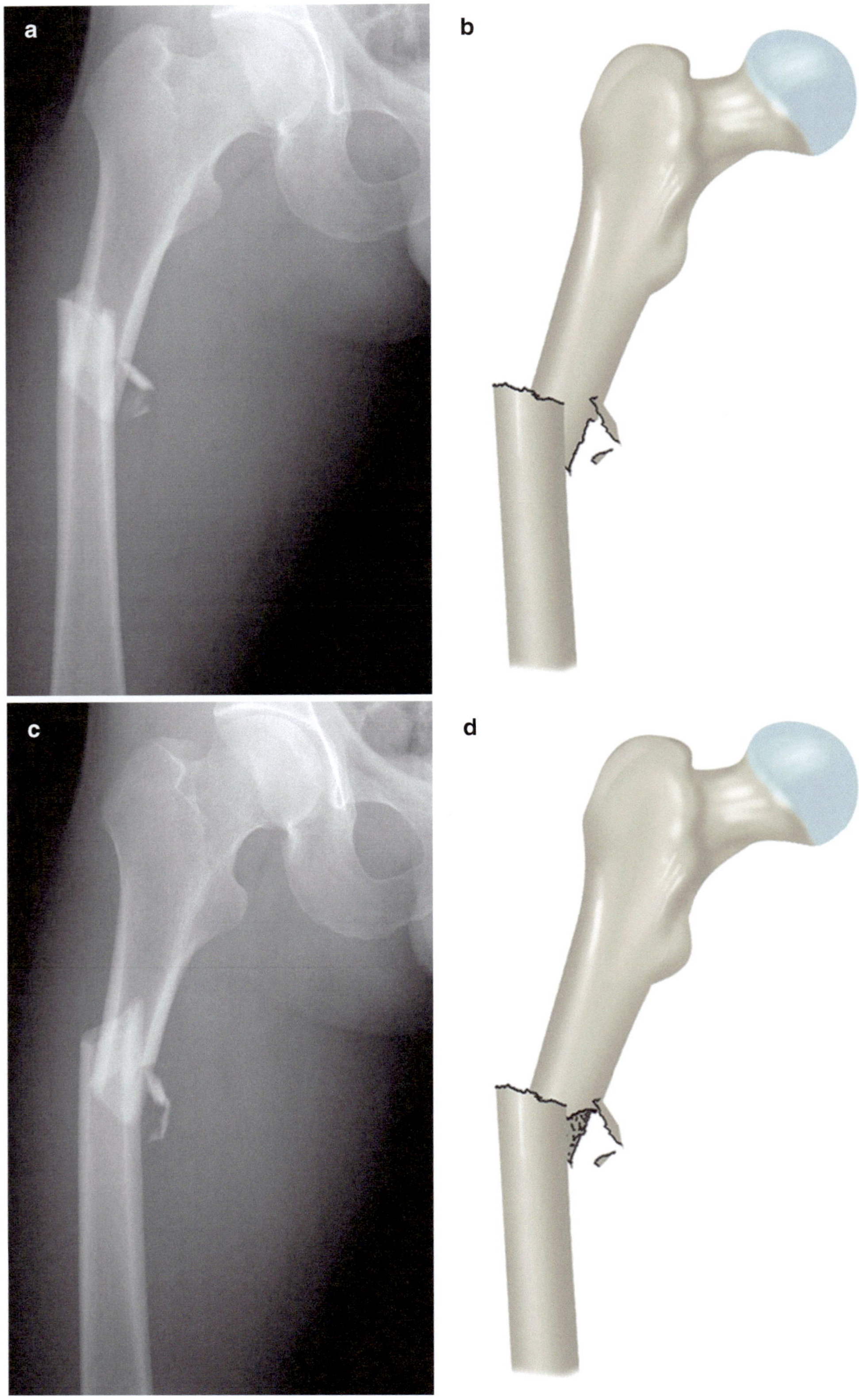

Fig. 12.7 (**a**, **c**) are respectively the lateral and anteroposterior (AP) views of the X-ray, showing a comminuted fracture of the femoral shaft with wedge-shaped fragment, and the schematic diagram (**b**, **d**)

12.1.3.3 Type C Comminuted Fracture

Comminuted fractures are divided into: comminuted spiral fractures, segmental comminuted fractures, and irregular comminuted fractures.

8. Differential diagnosis between comminuted spiral fracture and spiral fracture of the femoral shaft
   8.1 X-ray (Fig. 12.8a–d)

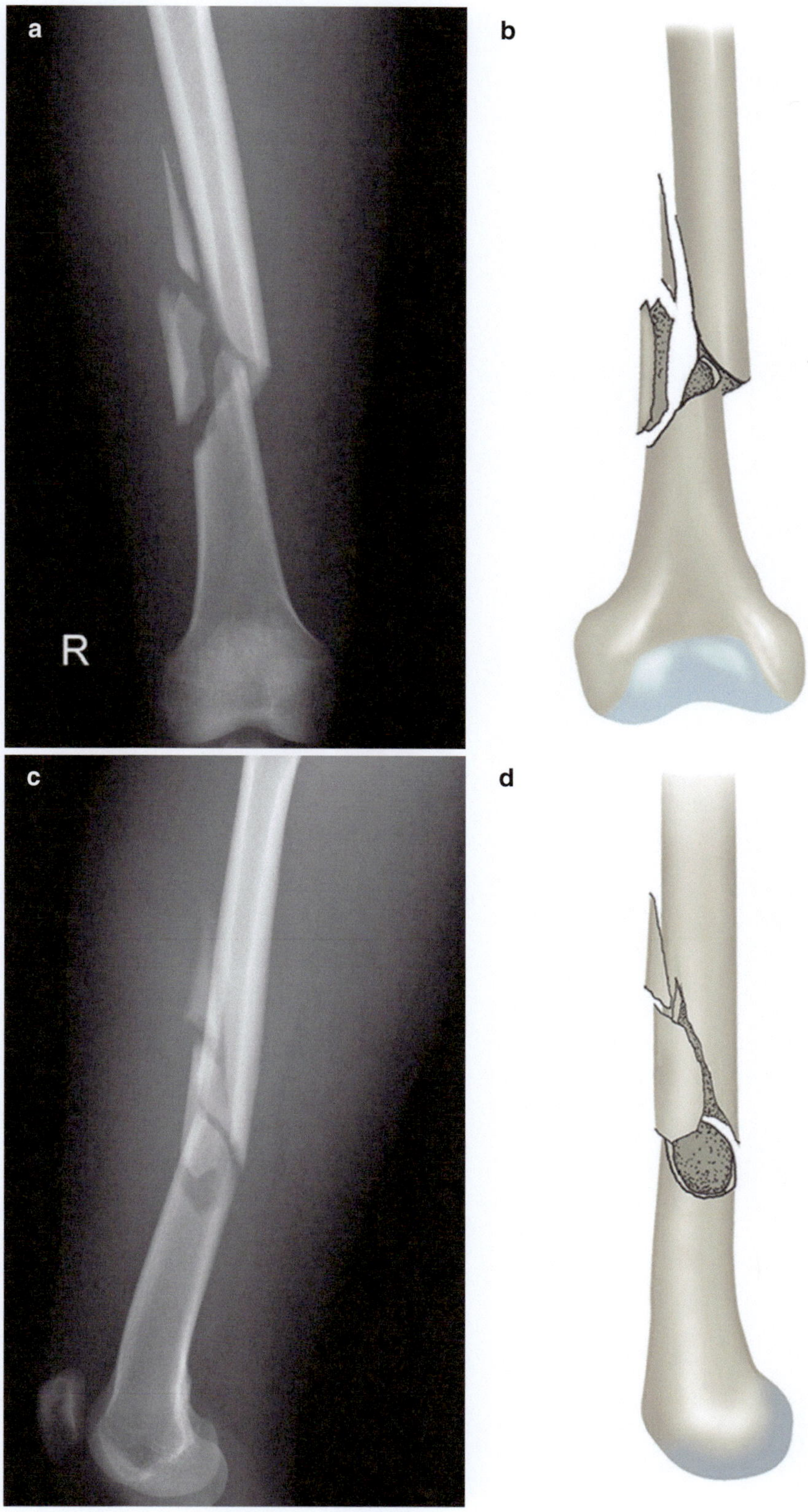

Fig. 12.8 (**a**, **c**) are respectively the lateral and anteroposterior (AP) views of the X-ray, showing a comminuted spiral fracture of the femoral shaft, and the schematic diagram (**b**, **d**)

9. Differential diagnosis between segmental comminuted fracture and single fracture of the femoral shaft
    9.1 X-ray (Fig. 12.9a–d)

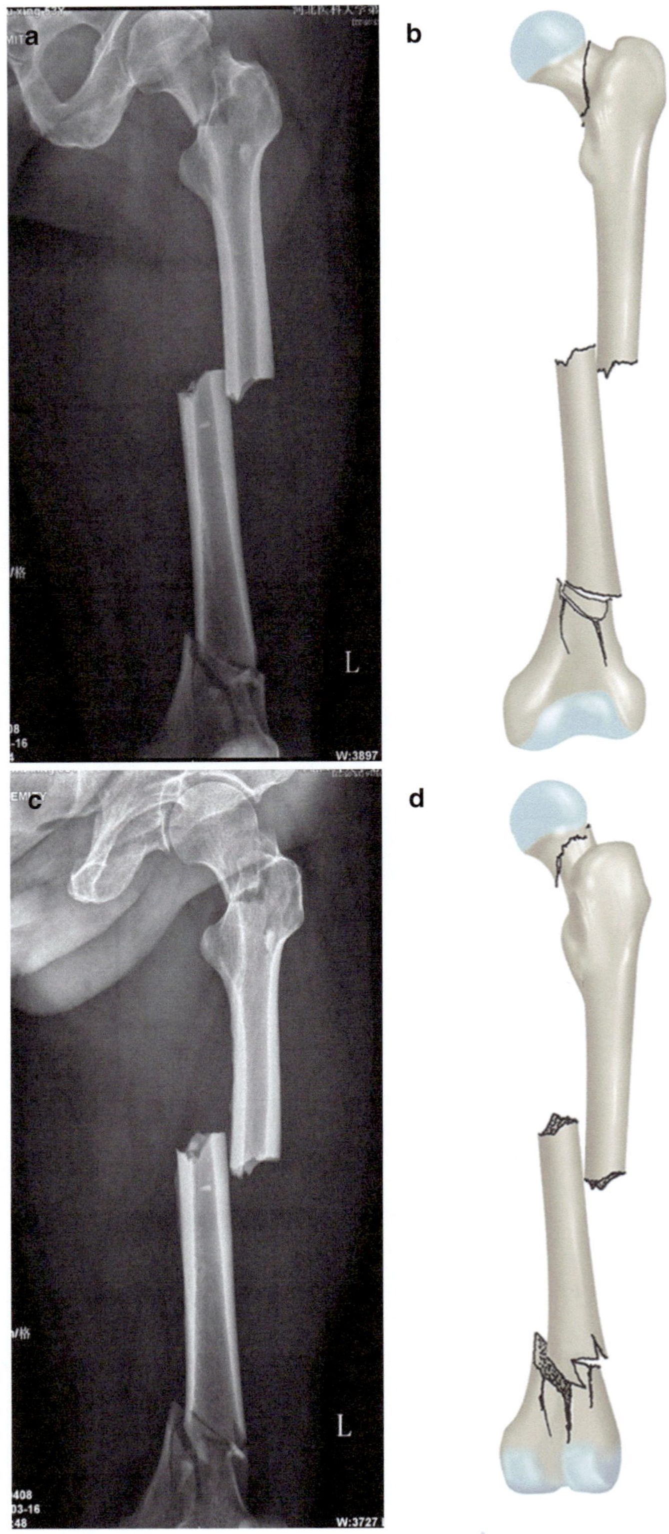

Fig. 12.9 (**a**, **c**) are respectively the lateral and anteroposterior (AP) views of the X-ray, showing multiple segment comminuted fracture of femoral neck, femoral shaft and distal femur. Schematic diagram (**b**, **d**)

10. Differential diagnosis between irregular comminuted fracture and transverse fracture of the femoral shaft
    10.1 X-ray (Fig. 12.10a–d)

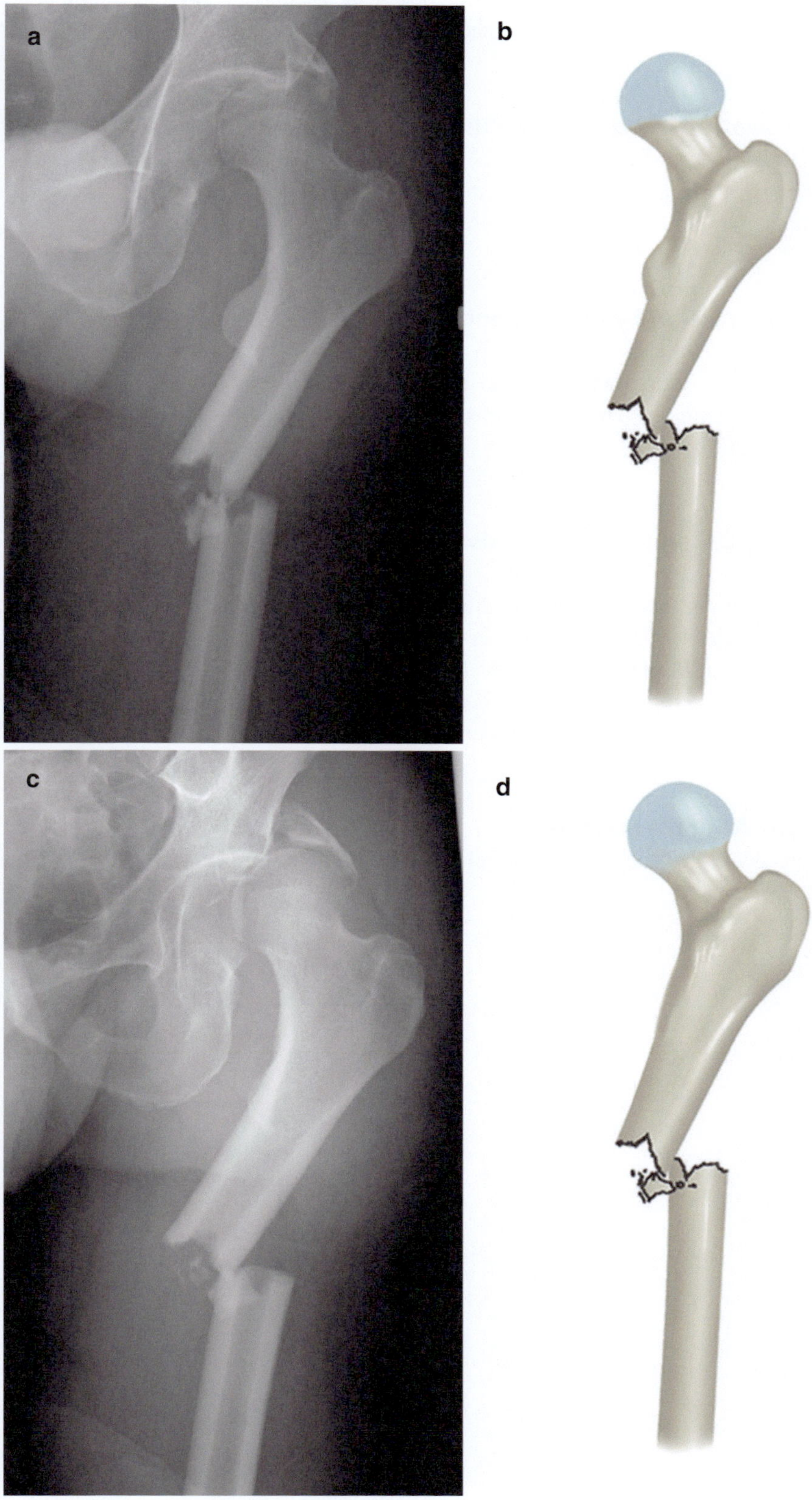

Fig. 12.10 (**a**, **c**) are respectively the lateral and anteroposterior (AP) views of the X-ray, showing an irregular comminuted fracture of the femoral shaft, and schematic diagram (**b**, **d**)

12.2 Tibiofibular Shaft Fracture

An interruption in bone continuity of the tibiofibular shaft is defined as tibiofibular shaft fracture, which is commonly seen in long tubular bone fractures. According to the 2007 AO/OTA classification, it can be divided into: type A simple fracture, type B wedge fracture, and type C comminuted fracture.

12.2.1 Identification of Injury Mechanism

Most of the fractures are caused by traffic accidents, falls, and athletic injuries, which is a result of strong axial stress combined with rotating stress.

12.2.2 Identification of Symptoms and Signs

The clinical features are pain in injured areas, swelling, and restricted movement but difficult to make a definitive diagnosis due to the lack of specificity. Therefore, when a fracture is suspected, further X-ray or CT scans should be conducted to prevent missed diagnosis.

12.2.3 Imaging Differential Diagnosis

In general, X-rays can be used to diagnose tibial fractures. When a distal 1/3 tibia spiral fracture occurs, CT or MRI scan on ankle joint is necessary to determine whether there is a posterior malleolus fracture. The fracture of the tibiofibular shaft should be distinguished from the diaphyseal vascular groove and growth retardation line. The fracture line is sharp while the vascular groove is smooth, with a certain direction pointing to the joint surface. Growth retardation line in X-ray and CT scans are shown as transversely linear high-density shadow, while in MRI, it was a low-signal line, perpendicular to the long axis of the shaft.

12.2.3.1 Type A Simple Fracture

Simple fracture is divided into: simple spiral fractures, simple oblique fractures ($\geq 30°$), and simple transverse fractures ($<30°$).

1. Differential diagnosis between simple spiral fracture and simple oblique fracture of the tibia
   1.1 X-ray (Fig. 12.11a–d)

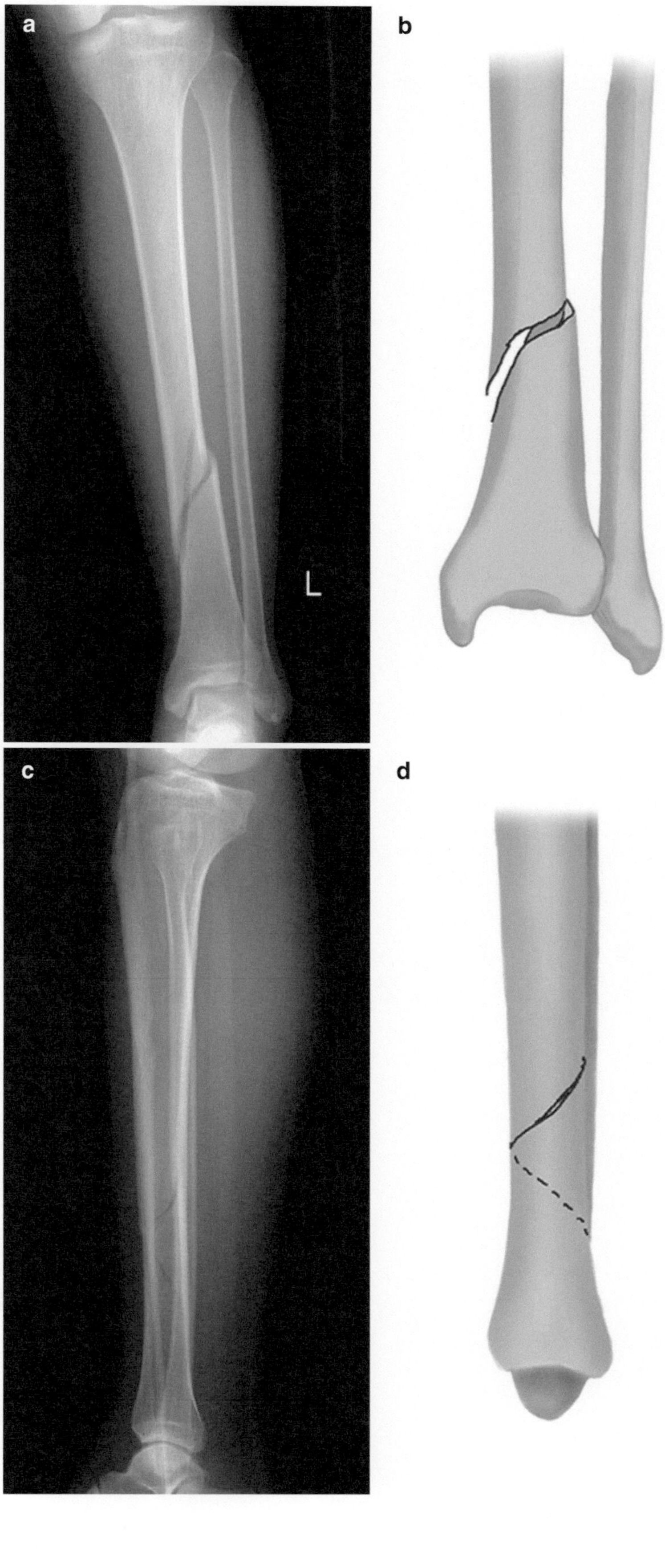

Fig. 12.11 (**a**, **c**) are respectively the lateral and anteroposterior (AP) views of the X-ray, showing a simple spiral fracture of the middle and lower tibial shaft, and schematic diagram (**b**, **d**)

2. Differential diagnosis between simple spiral fracture and simple oblique fracture of the fibula
   2.1 X-ray (Fig. 12.12a–d)

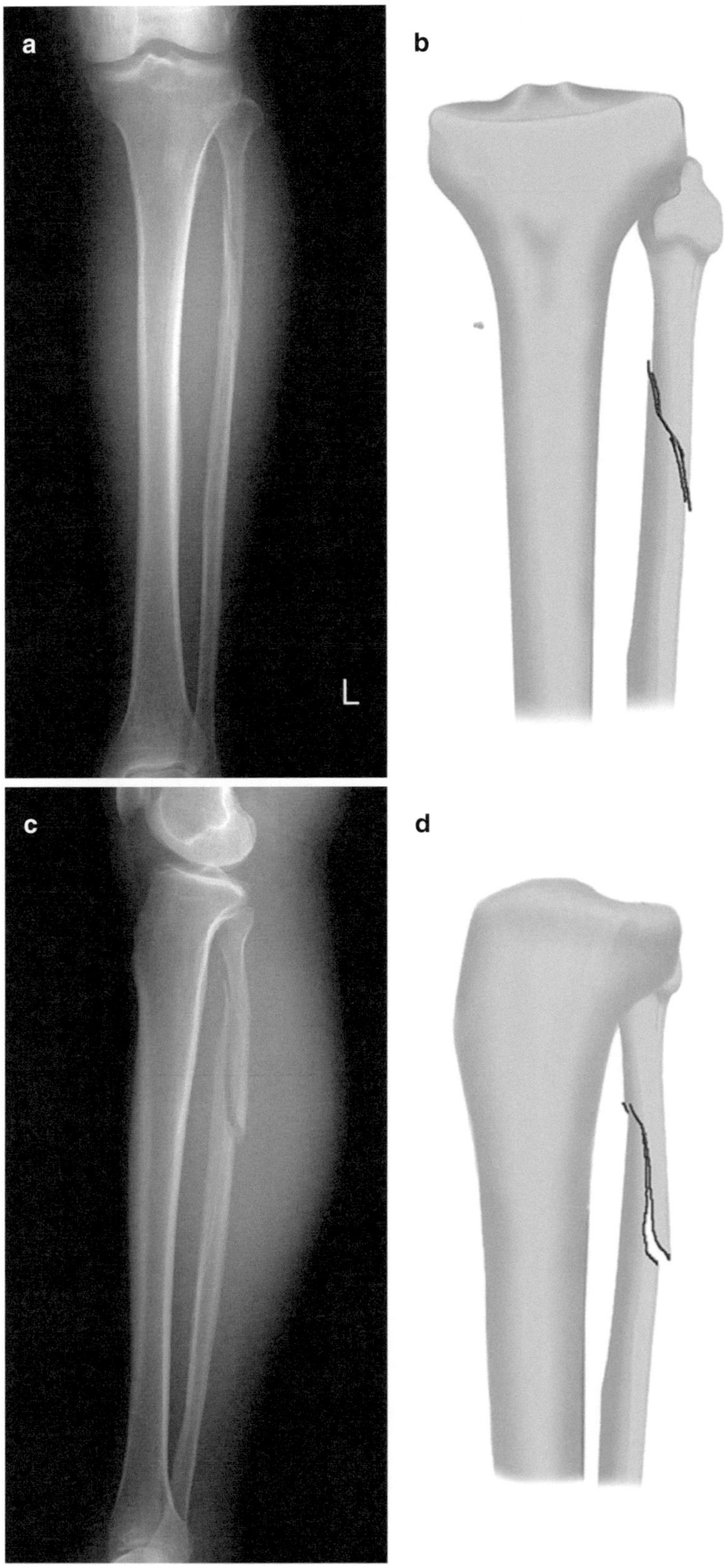

Fig. 12.12 (**a**, **c**) are respectively the lateral and anteroposterior (AP) views of the X-ray, showing a simple spiral fracture of the upper fibular shaft without tibial fracture, and schematic diagram (**b**, **d**)

3. Differential diagnosis between spiral fracture and oblique fracture of the tibiofibular fractures at the same level
   3.1 X-ray (Fig. 12.13a–d)

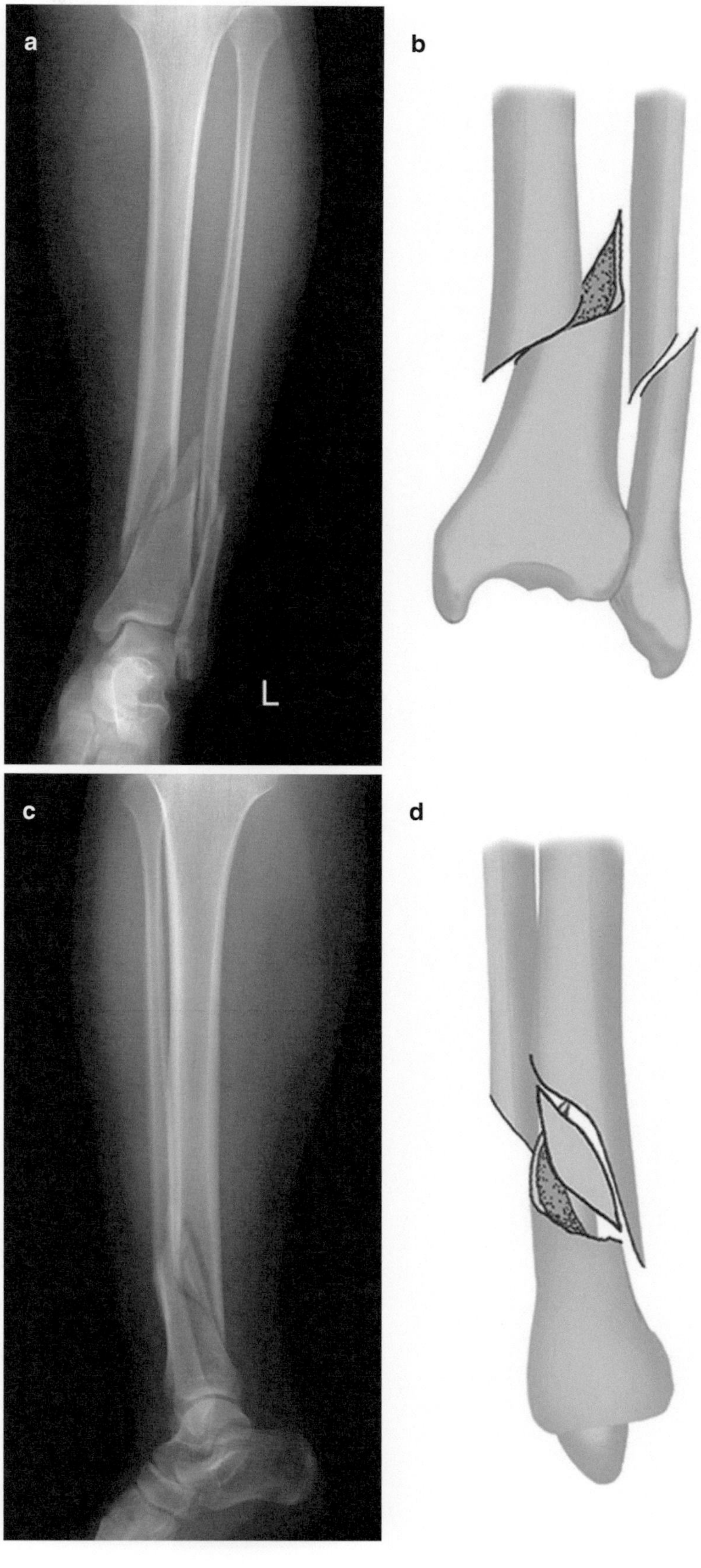

Fig. 12.13 (**a**, **c**) are respectively the lateral and anteroposterior (AP) views of the X-ray, showing a lower tibiofibular fracture at the same level, and schematic diagram (**b**, **d**)

4. Differential diagnosis between spiral fracture and oblique fracture of the tibiofibular fractures at different levels
   4.1 X-ray (Fig. 12.14a–d)

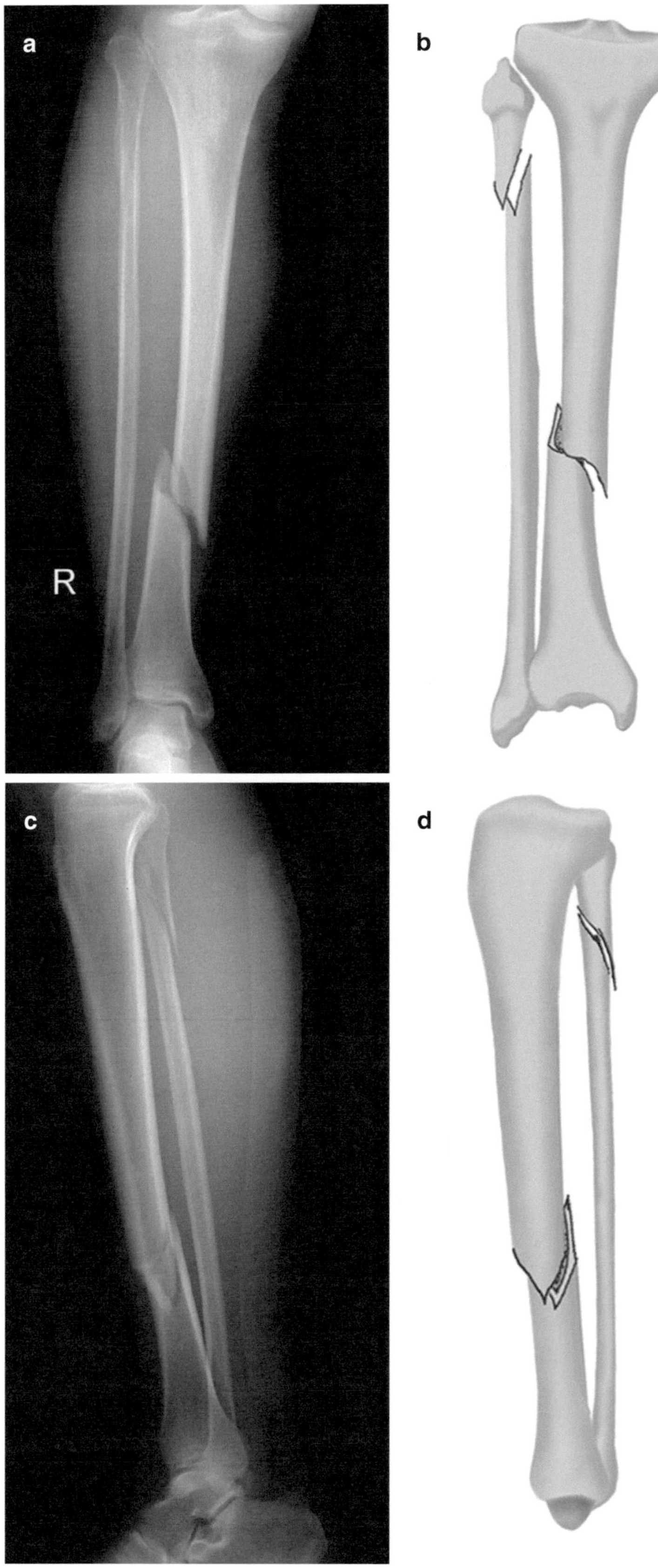

Fig. 12.14 (**a**, **c**) are respectively the lateral and anteroposterior (AP) views of the X-ray, showing an ipsilateral lower tibial and upper fibula fractures, and schematic diagram (**b**, **d**)

5. Differential diagnosis between tibial oblique with fibular transverse fractures and tibiofibular transverse fractures
   5.1 X-ray (Fig. 12.15a–d)

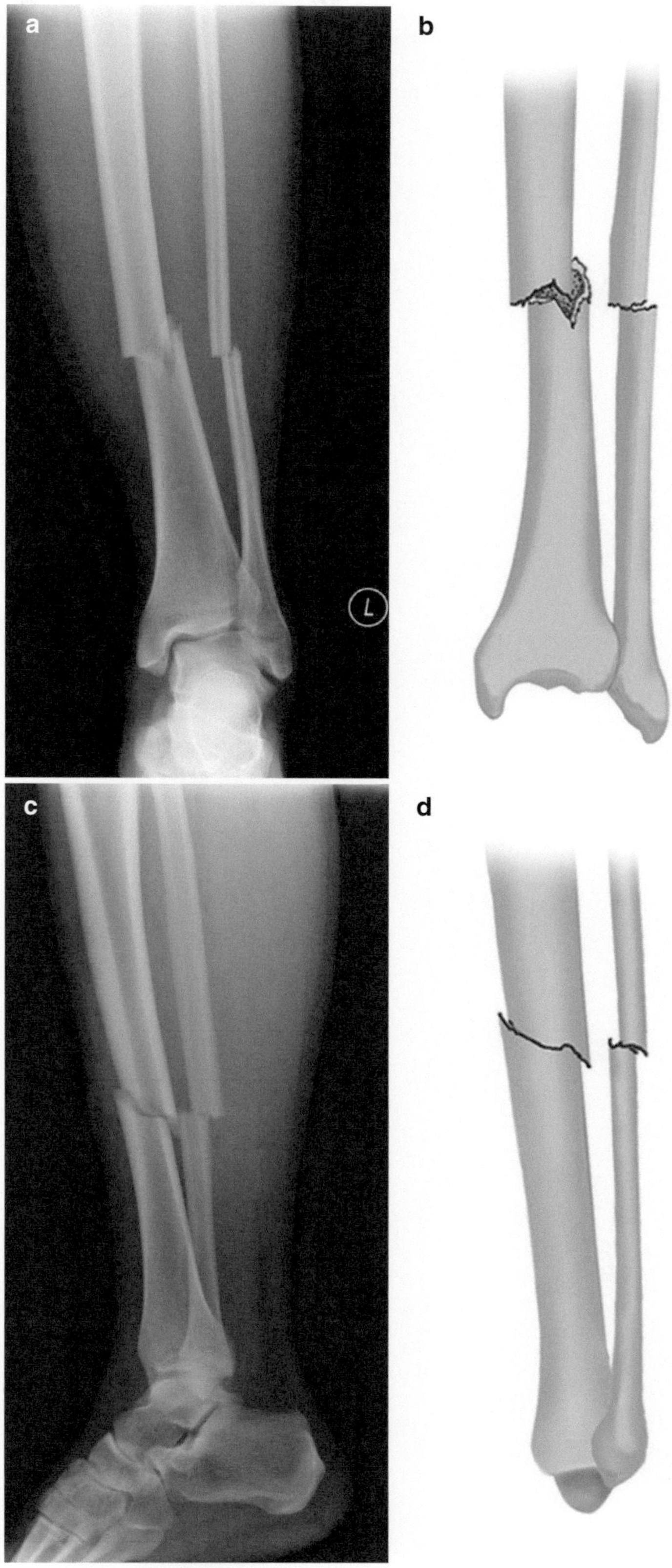

Fig. 12.15 (**a**, **c**) are respectively the lateral and anteroposterior (AP) views of the X-ray, showing a tibial oblique with fibular transverse fractures, and schematic diagram (**b**, **d**)

6. Differential diagnosis between oblique fracture and transverse fracture of the fibula
   6.1 X-ray (Fig. 12.16a–d)

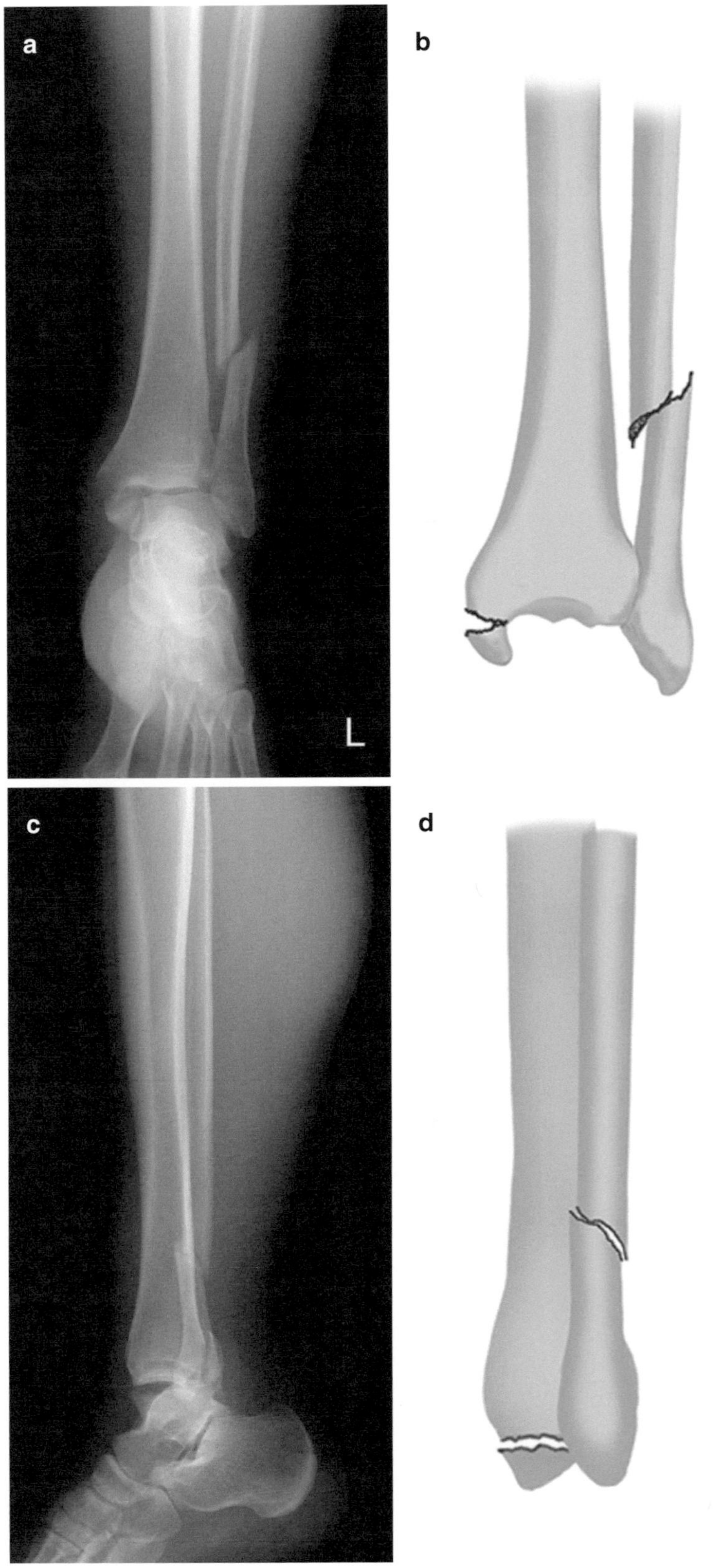

Fig. 12.16 (**a**, **c**) are respectively the lateral and anteroposterior (AP) views of the X-ray, showing a fibular oblique fracture with medial and posterior malleolus fractures, and schematic diagram (**b**, **d**)

7. Differential diagnosis between transverse fracture and oblique fracture of the tibia
   7.1 X-ray (Fig. 12.17a–d)

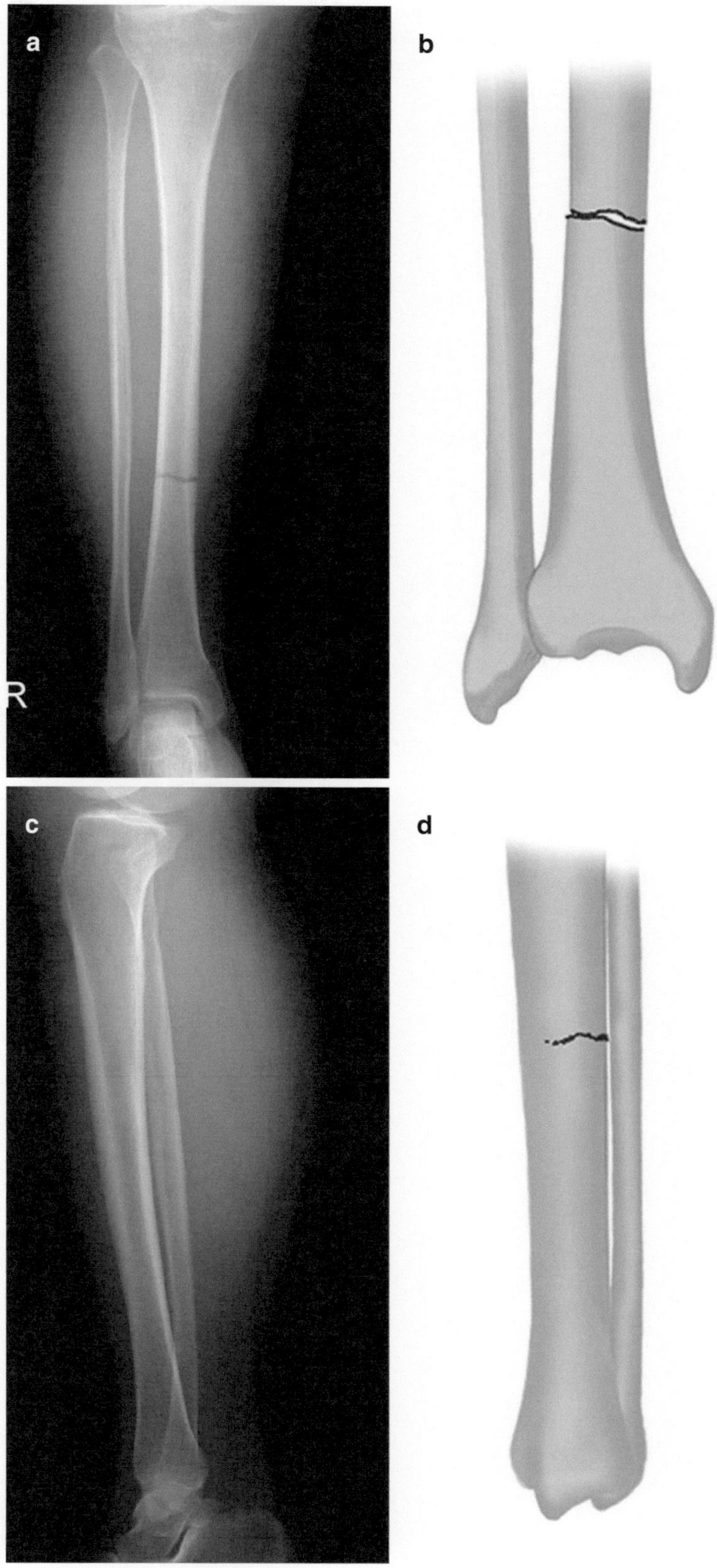

Fig. 12.17 (**a**, **c**) are respectively the lateral and anteroposterior (AP) views of the X-ray, showing a tibial transverse fracture without fibular fracture, and schematic diagram (**b**, **d**)

8. Differential diagnosis between transverse fractures and oblique fractures of the tibiofibular at the same level
   8.1 X-ray (Fig. 12.18a–d)

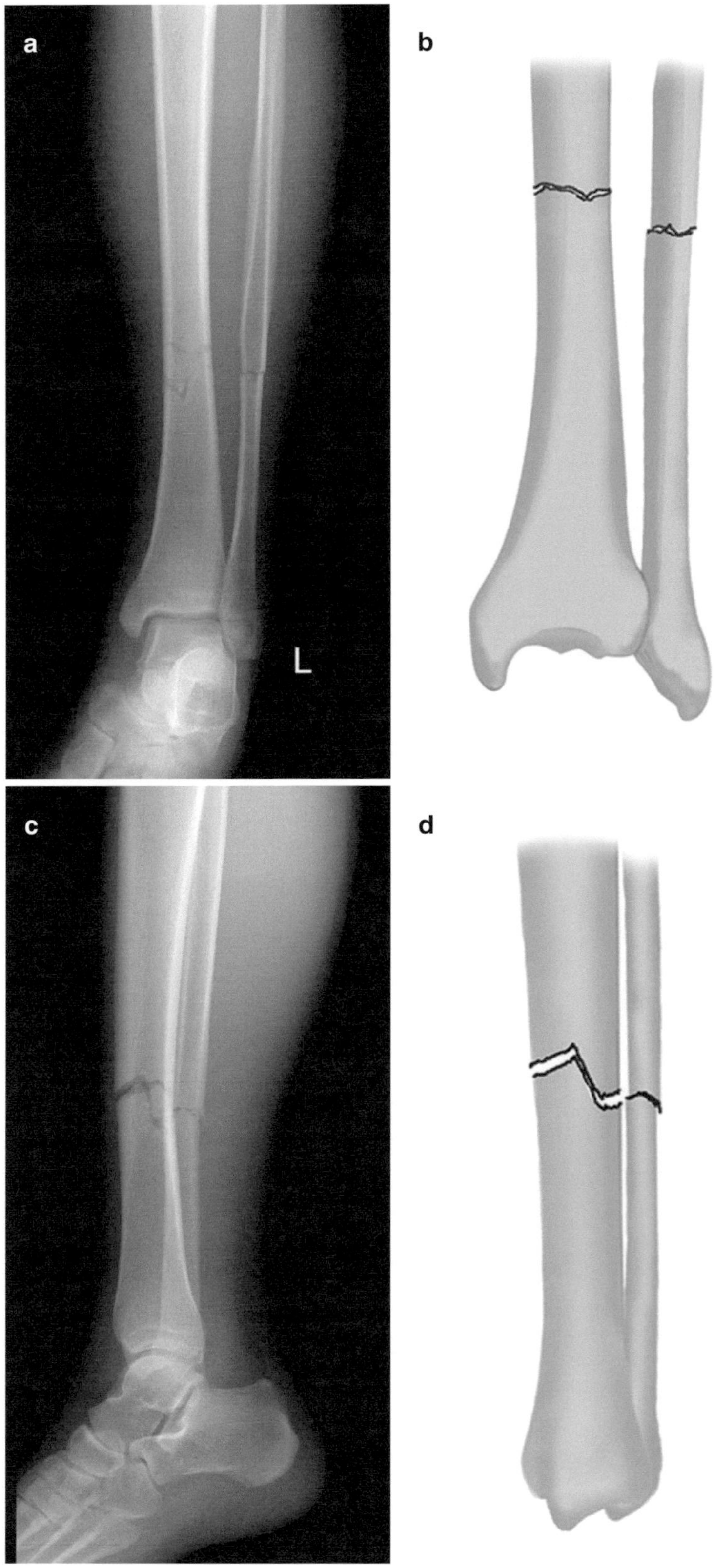

Fig. 12.18 (**a**, **c**) are respectively the lateral and anteroposterior (AP) views of the X-ray, showing a tibiofibular transverse fractures at the same level, and schematic diagram (**b**, **d**)

12.2.3.2 Type B Wedge Fracture

Wedge fractures are divided into spiral wedge fractures, curved fractures, and comminuted wedge fractures.

9. Differential diagnosis between spiral wedge fractures and simple spiral tibiofibular fractures
   9.1 X-ray (Fig. 12.19a–d)

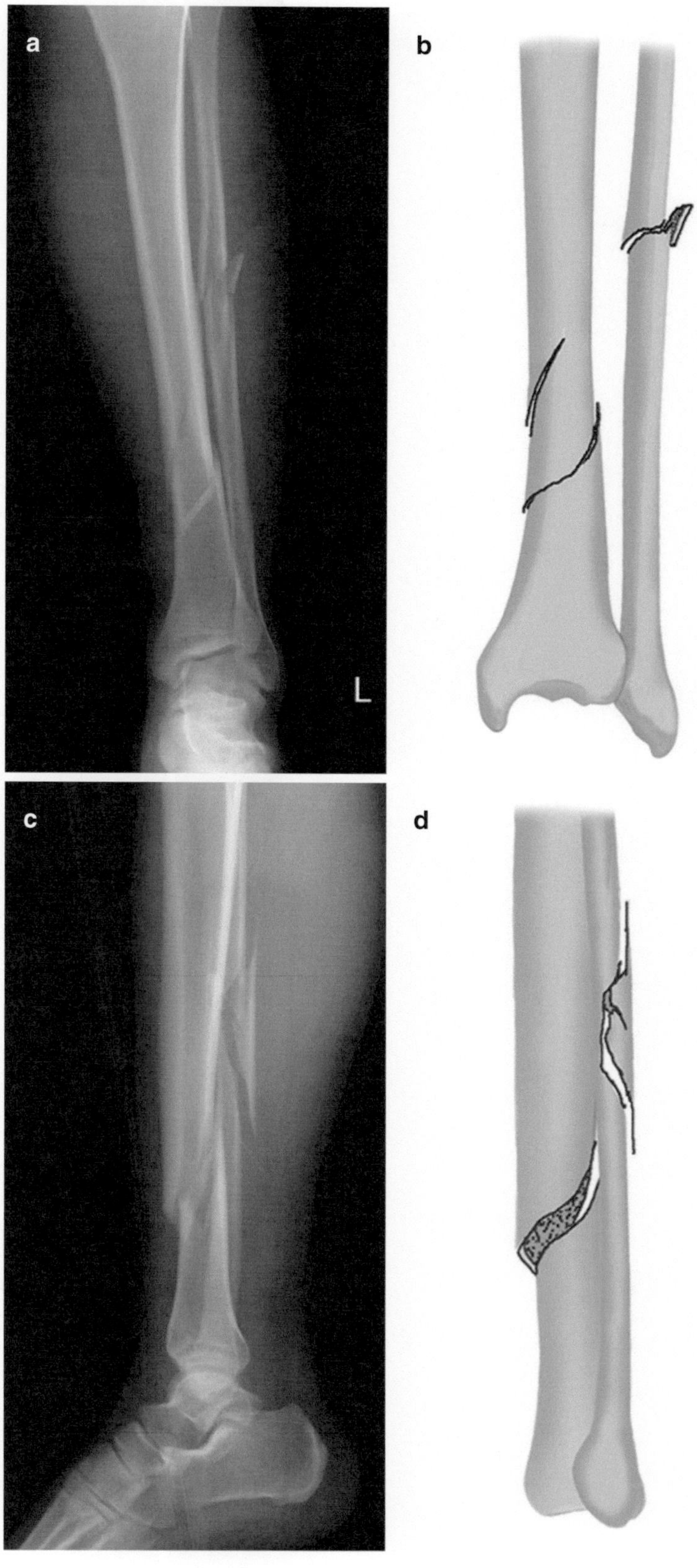

Fig. 12.19 (**a**, **c**) are respectively the lateral and anteroposterior (AP) views of the X-ray, showing a tibiofibular spiral wedge fractures, and schematic diagram (**b**, **d**)

10. Differential diagnosis between wedge fracture and oblique fracture of fibula with a tibial curved wedge fracture at the same level
    10.1 X-ray (Fig. 12.20a–d)

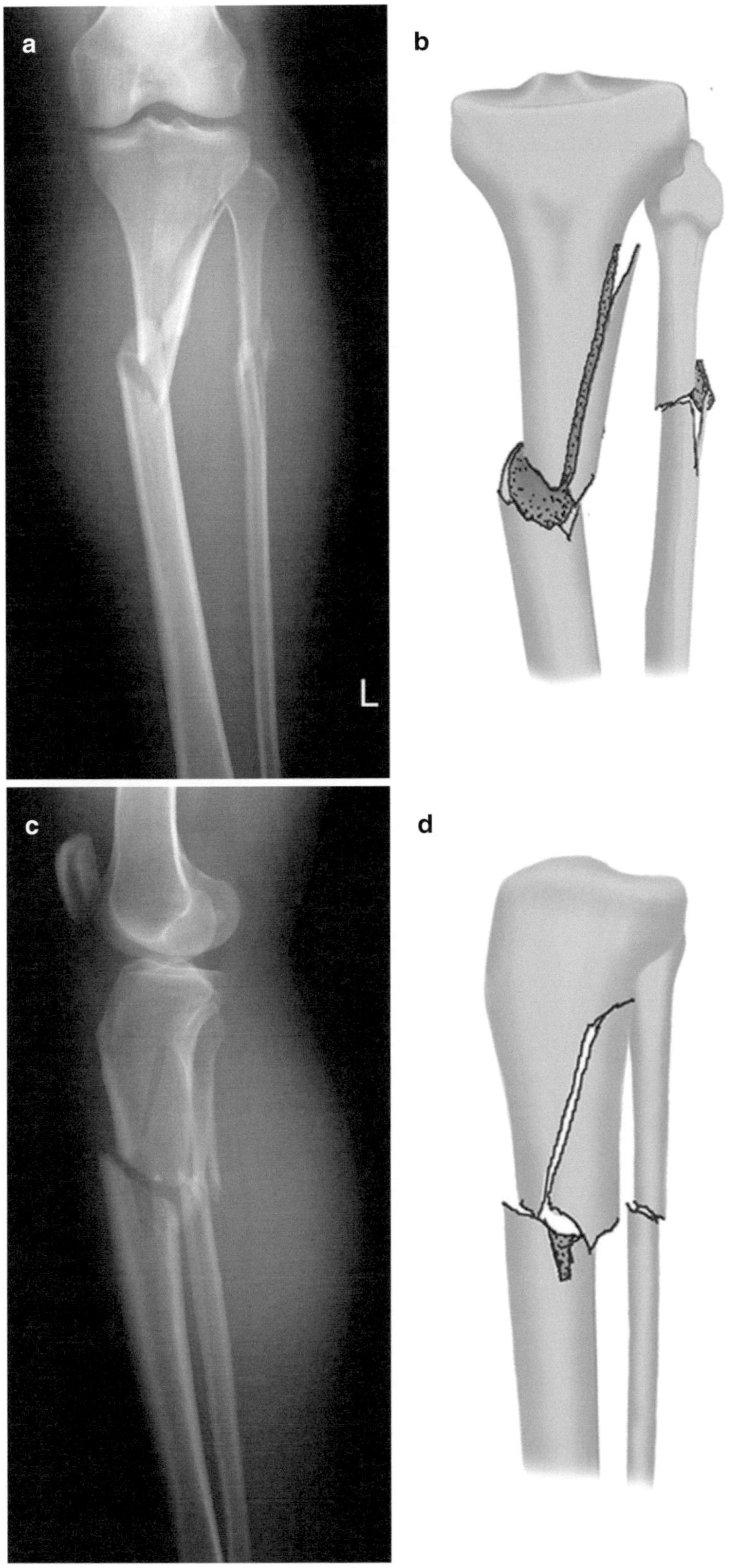

Fig. 12.20 (**a**, **c**) are respectively the lateral and anteroposterior (AP) views of the X-ray, showing a fibular wedge fracture with a tibial curved wedge fracture at the same level, and schematic diagram (**b**, **d**)

11. Tibial comminuted wedge fracture with fibular fracture at the same level

    11.1 X-ray (Fig. 12.21a–d)

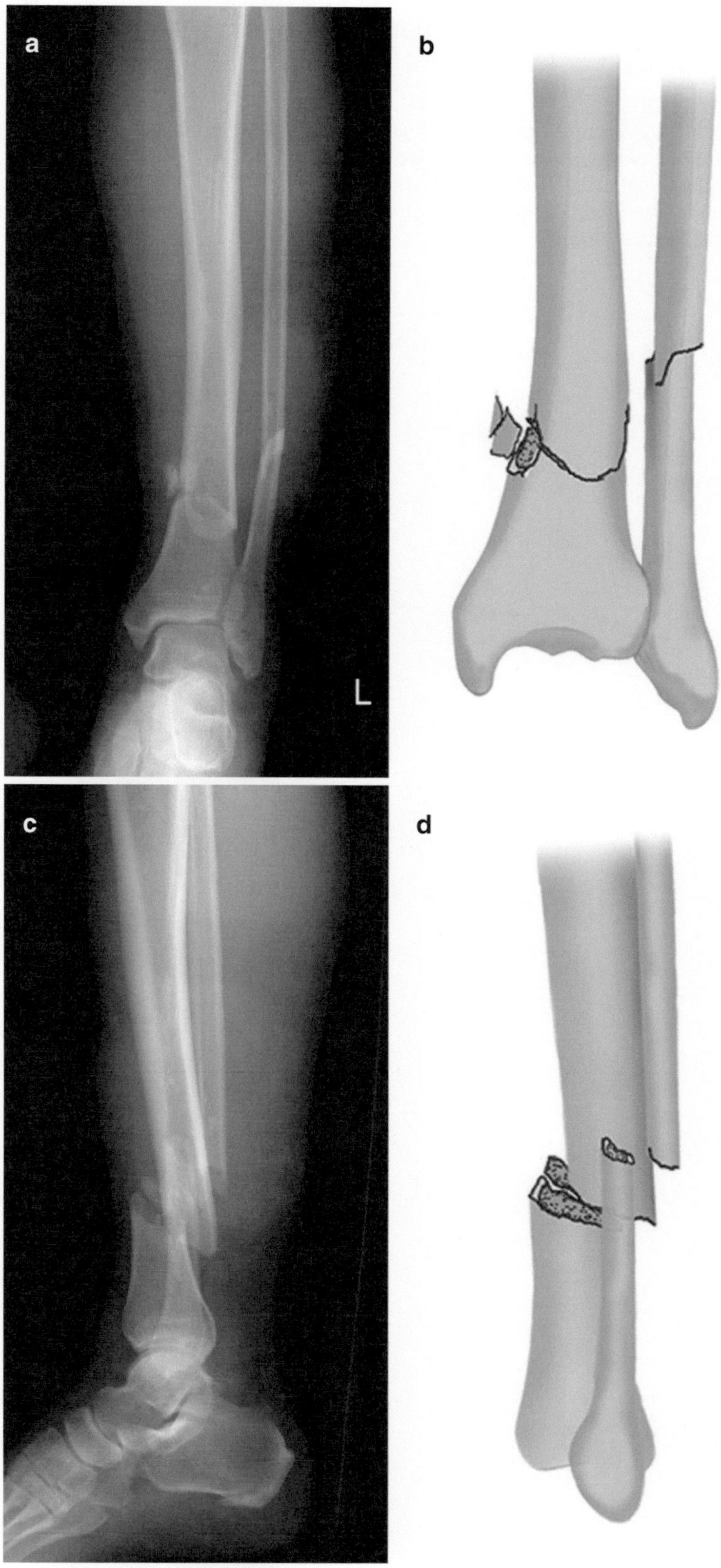

Fig. 12.21 (**a**, **c**) are respectively the lateral and anteroposterior (AP) views of the X-ray, showing a tibial comminuted wedge fracture with a fibular fracture at the same level, and schematic diagram (**b**, **d**)

12.2.3.3 Type C Comminuted Fracture

Comminuted fracture can be divided into: comminuted spiral fracture, multisegment comminuted fracture, and irregular comminuted fracture.

12. Lower tibial comminuted spiral fracture with fibular transverse fracture at the same level
    12.1 X-ray (Fig. 12.22a–d)

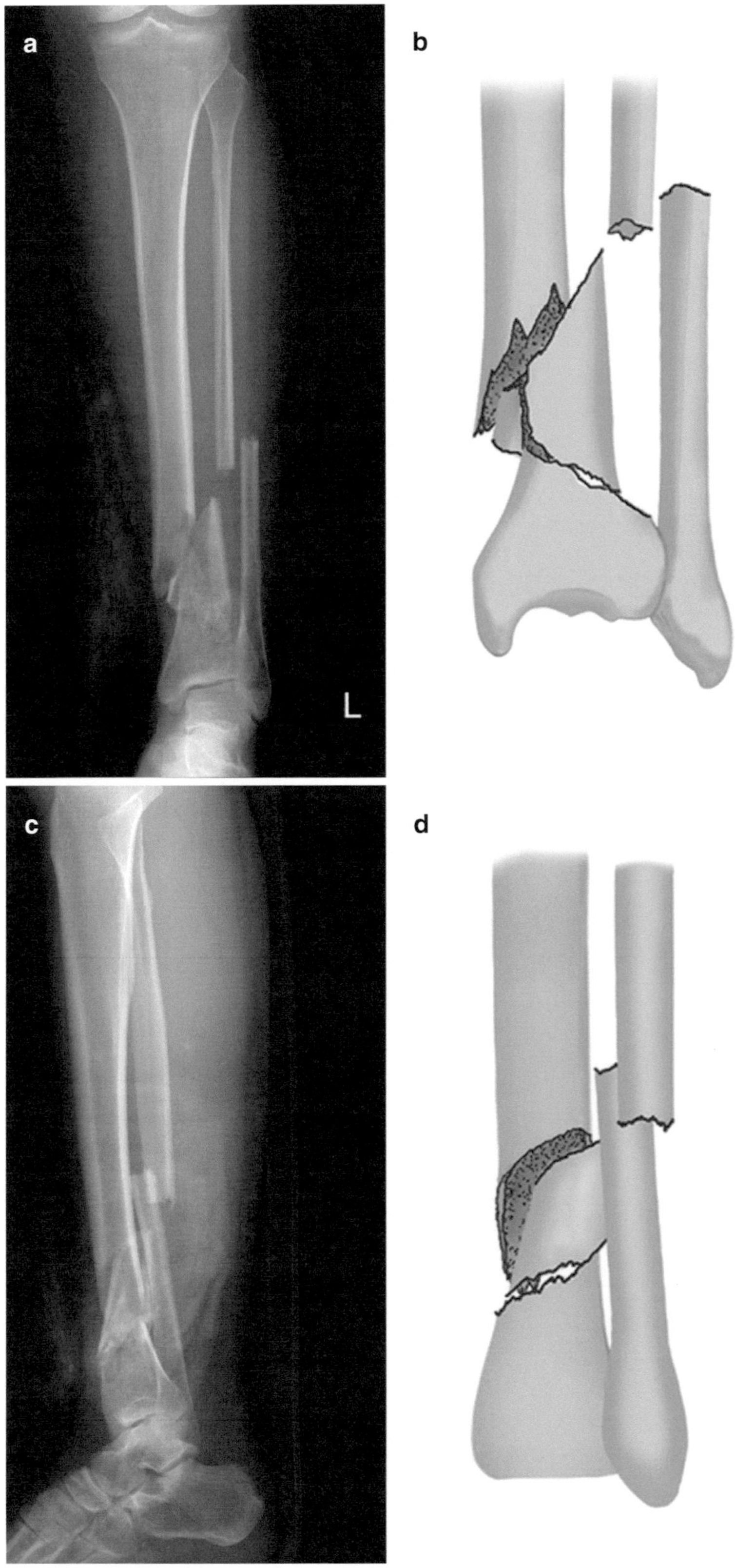

Fig. 12.22 (**a**, **c**) are respectively the lateral and anteroposterior (AP) views of the X-ray, showing a lower tibial comminuted spiral fracture with a fibular transverse fracture at the same level, and schematic diagram (**b**, **d**)

13. Lower tibial comminuted spiral fracture with fibular oblique fracture at the same level
    13.1 X-ray (Fig. 12.23a–d)

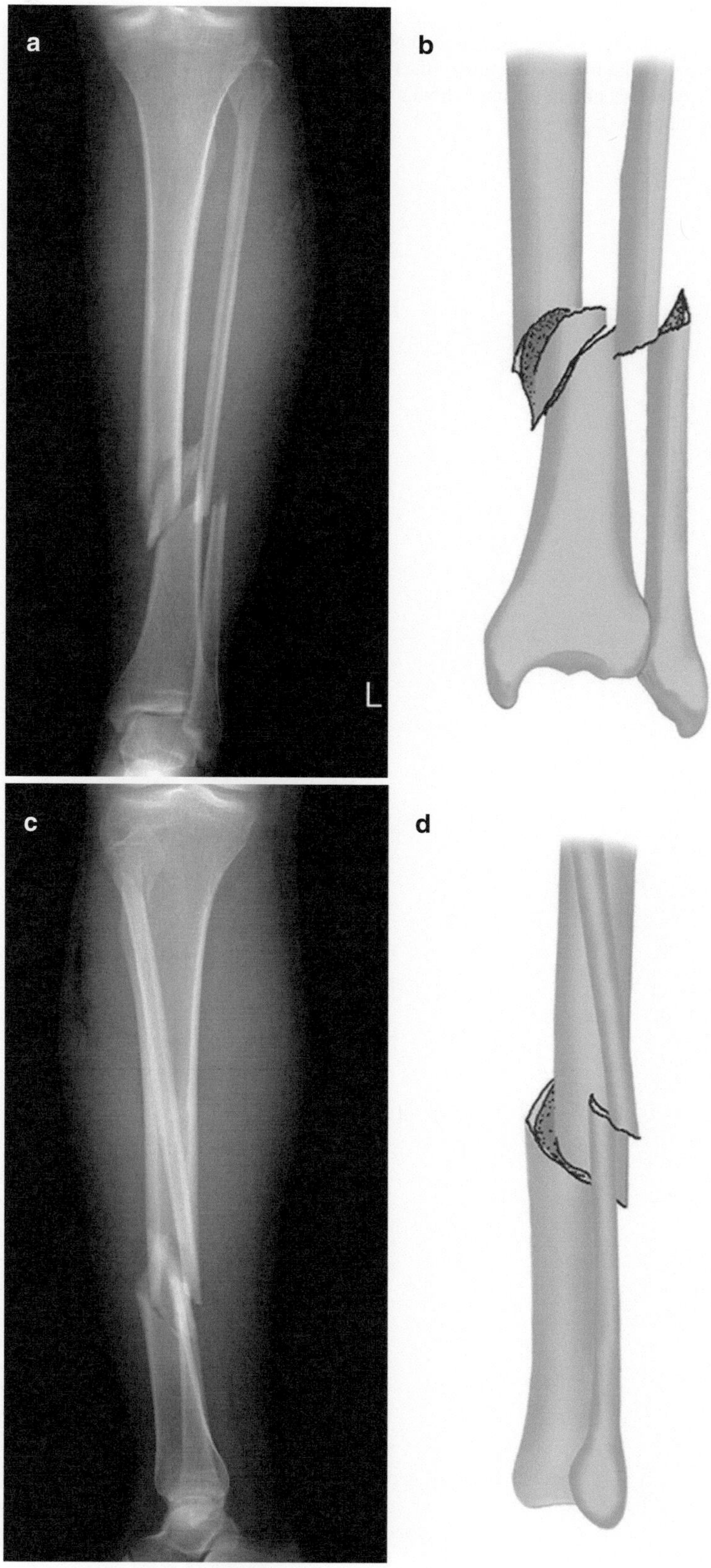

Fig. 12.23 (**a**, **c**) are respectively the lateral and anteroposterior (AP) views of the X-ray, showing a lower tibial comminuted spiral fracture with fibular oblique fracture at the same level, and schematic diagram (**b**, **d**)

14. Multisegment comminuted fracture of the tibial shaft with spiral fracture of the upper fibula
    14.1 X-ray (Fig. 12.24a–d)

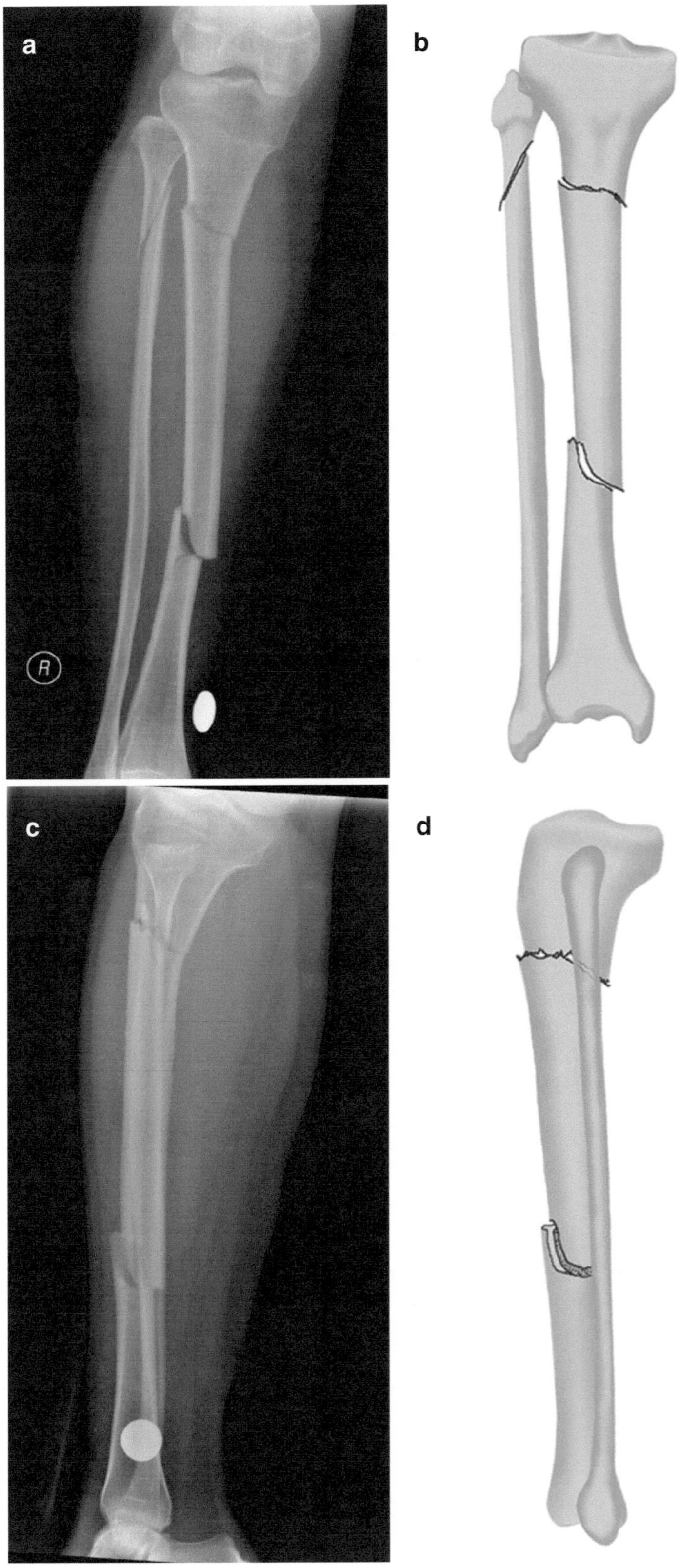

Fig. 12.24 (**a**, **c**) are respectively the lateral and anteroposterior (AP) views of the X-ray, showing a multisegment comminuted fracture of the tibial shaft with spiral fracture of the upper fibula, and schematic diagram (**b**, **d**)

15. Irregular comminuted fracture of the tibial shaft with upper fibula fracture
    15.1 X-ray (Fig. 12.25a–d)

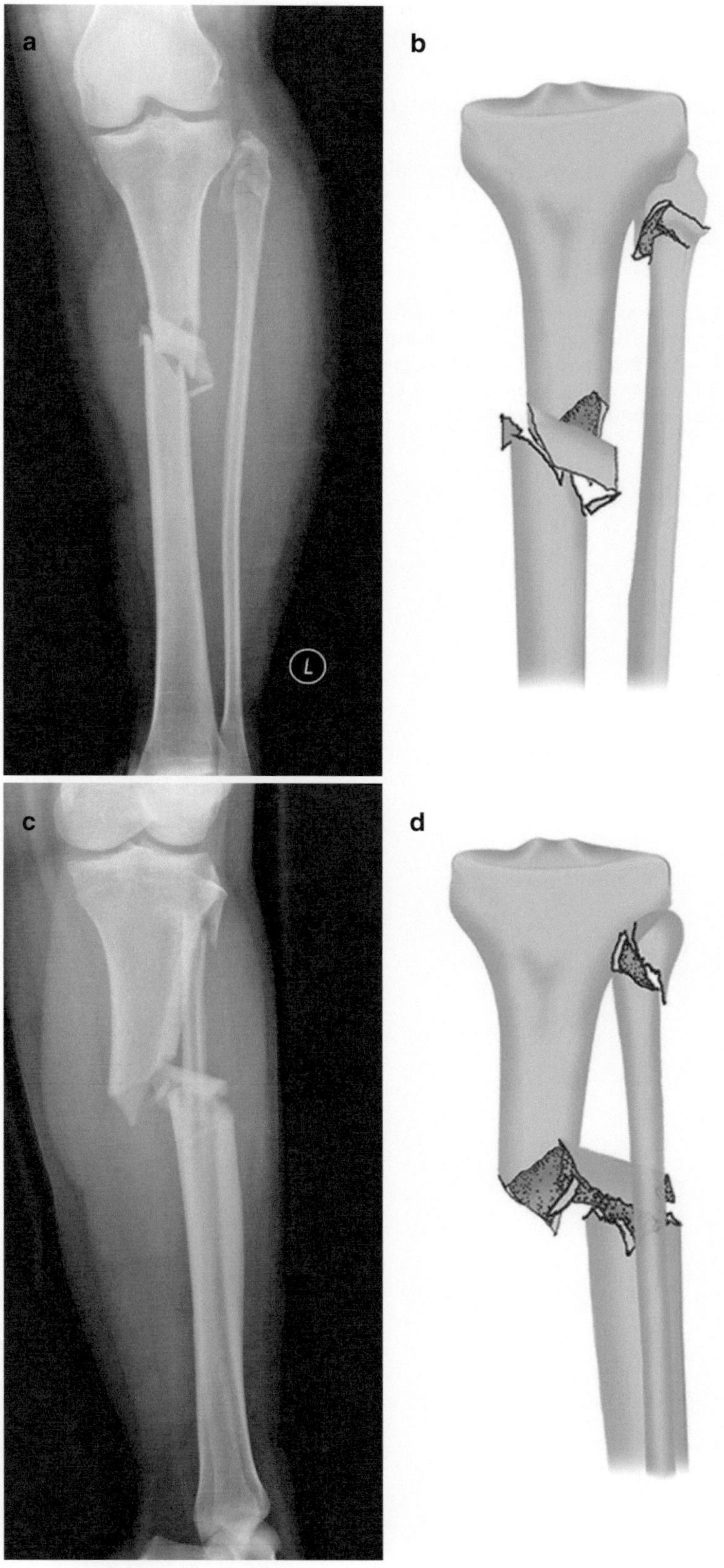

Fig. 12.25 (**a**, **c**) are respectively the lateral and anteroposterior (AP) views of the X-ray, showing an irregular comminuted fracture of the tibial shaft with upper fibula fracture, and schematic diagram (**b**, **d**)

12.2.3.4 Distal 1/3 Tibia Spiral Fracture Combined with Posterior Malleolus Fracture

According to Zhang Yingze classification, distal 1/3 tibia spiral fracture combined with posterior malleolus fracture can be divided into 4 types.

Type I: MRI shows posterior malleolus fracture, while X-ray or CT failed. Type II: CT and MRI show posterior malleolus fracture, while X-ray failed. Type III: X-ray, CT, and MRI all show posterior malleolus fracture, and X-ray shows no displacement or displacement ≤2 mm. Type IV: X-ray, CT, and MRI all show posterior malleolus fracture, and posterior malleolus fragment is significantly displaced or separated >2 mm.

16. Differential diagnosis between distal 1/3 tibia spiral fracture combined with posterior malleolus fracture and nonposterior malleolus fracture
    16.1 X-ray (Fig. 12.26a–d)

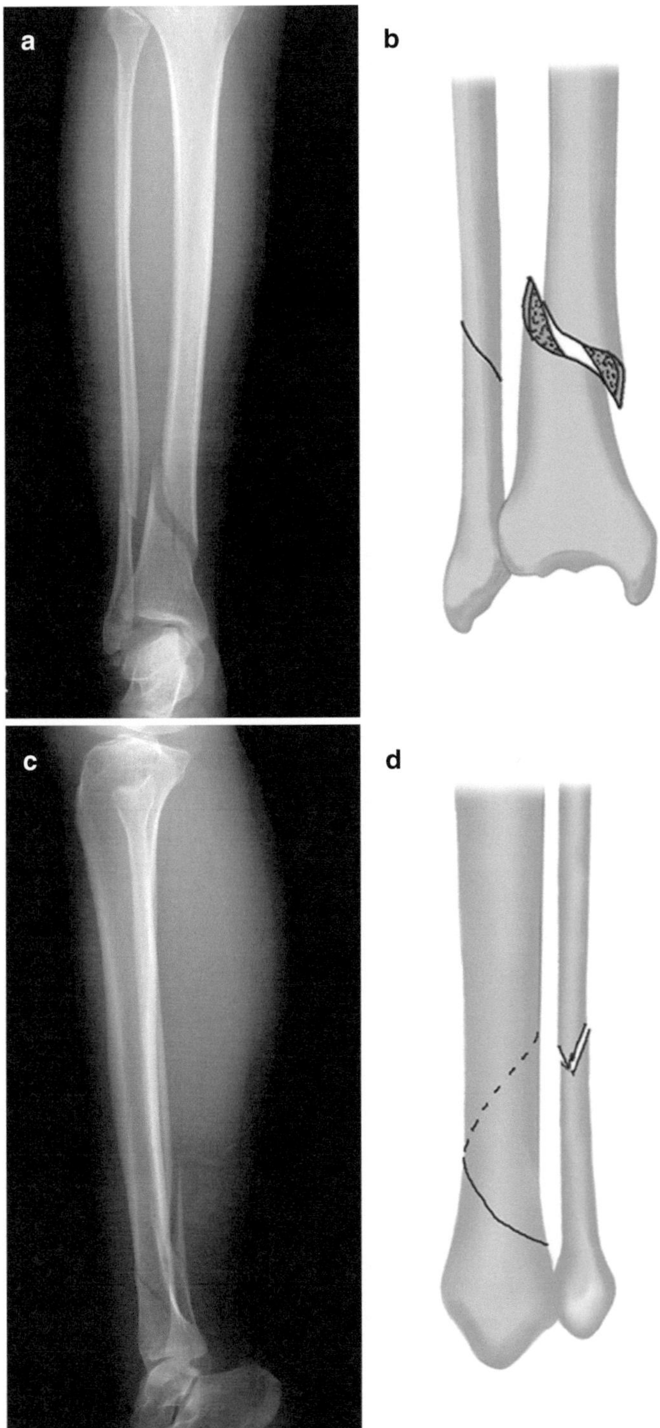

Fig. 12.26 (**a**, **c**) are respectively the lateral and anteroposterior (AP) views of the X-ray, showing a distal 1/3 tibia spiral fracture, and the posterior malleolus fracture is not obvious. Therefore, further CT scan was conducted. Schematic diagram (**b**, **d**)

16.2 CT scan (Fig. 12.26e–h)

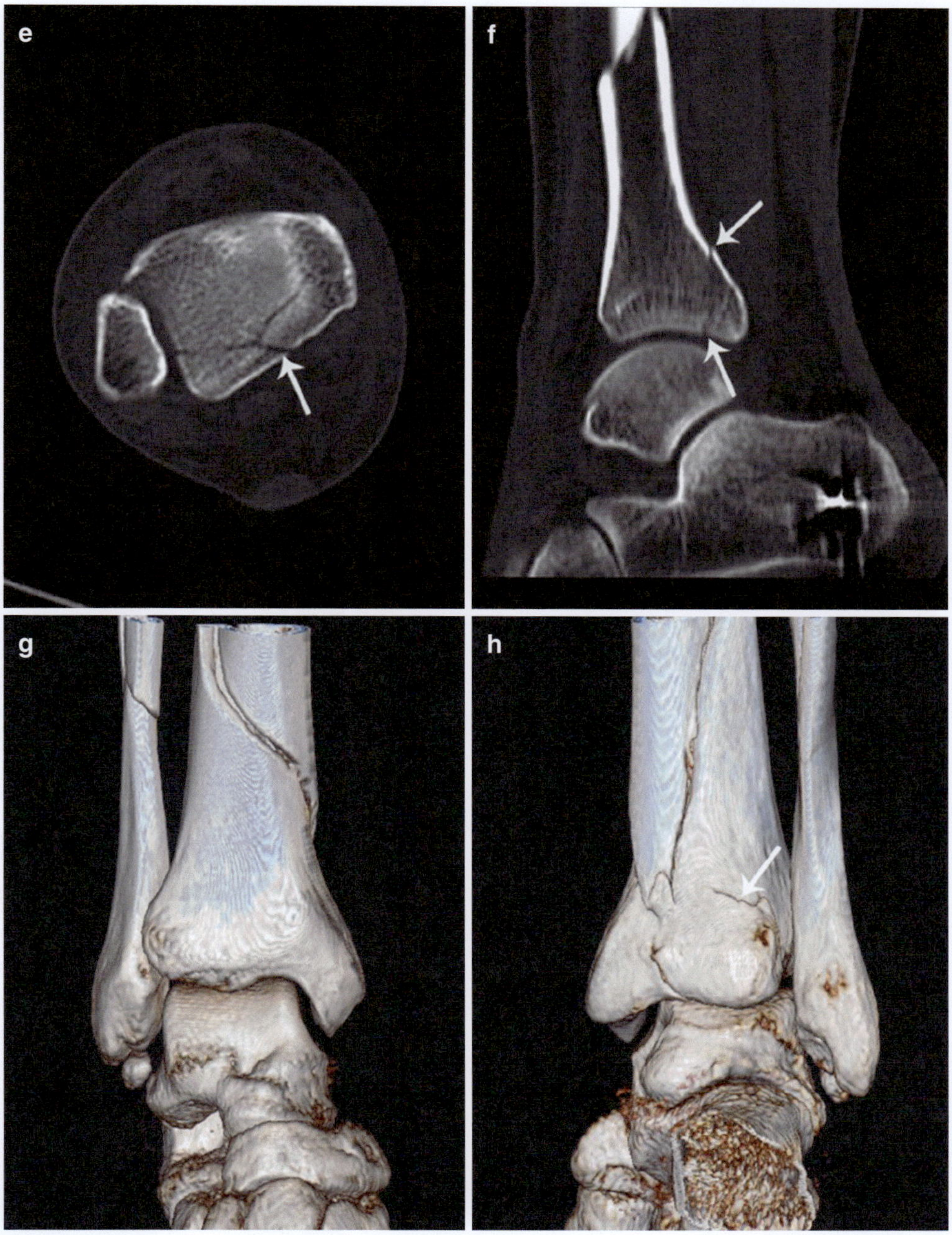

Fig. 12.26 (**e**–**h**) are CT reconstructions of transverse and sagittal planes, anterior and posterior views of CT 3d reconstruction, respectively, showing a distal 1/3 tibia spiral fracture combined with posterior malleolus fracture (white arrow)

17. Differential diagnosis between tibiofibular spiral fractures combined with posterior malleolus fracture and nonposterior malleolus fracture
    17.1 X-ray (Fig. 12.27a–d)

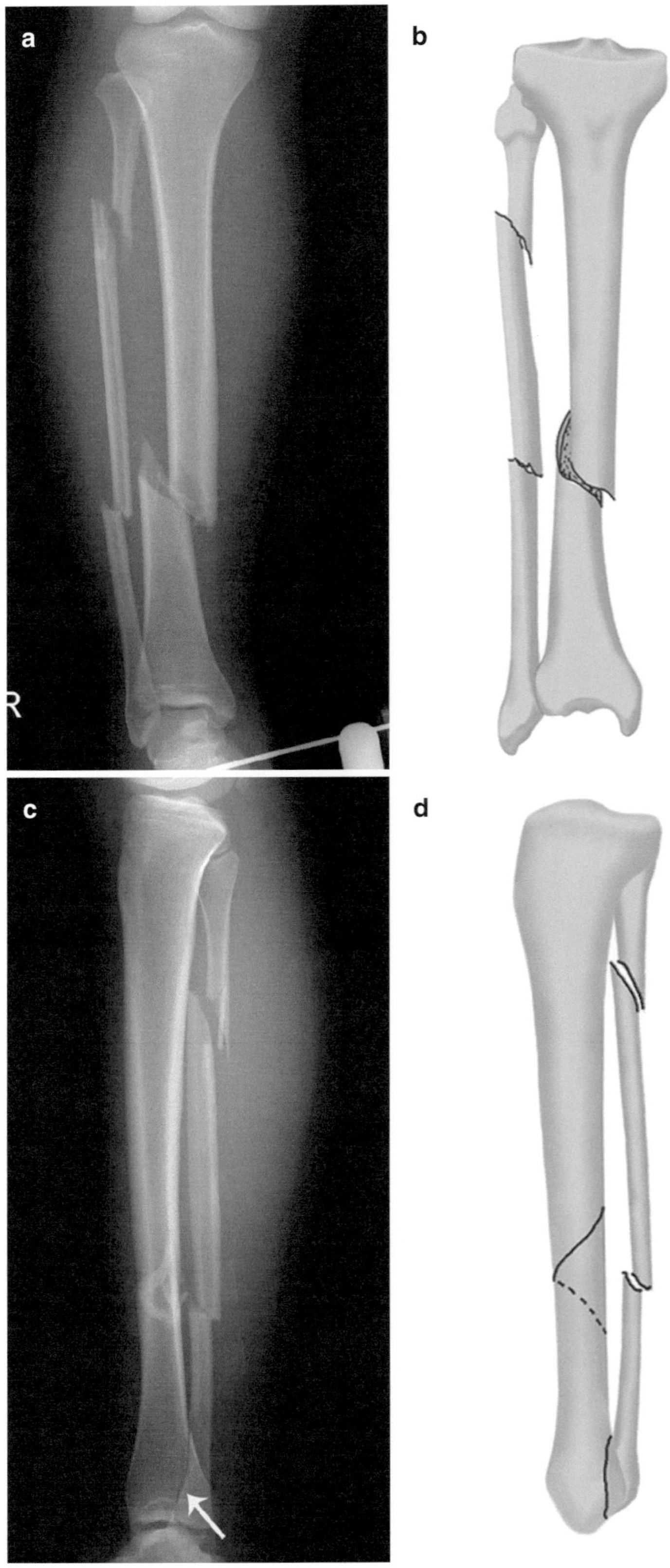

Fig. 12.27 (**a**, **c**) are respectively the lateral and anteroposterior (AP) views of the X-ray, showing lower tibiofibular spiral fractures, upper fibula spiral fracture combined with posterior malleolus fracture (white arrow), and schematic diagram (**b**, **d**)

17.2 CT scan (Fig. 12.27e–h)

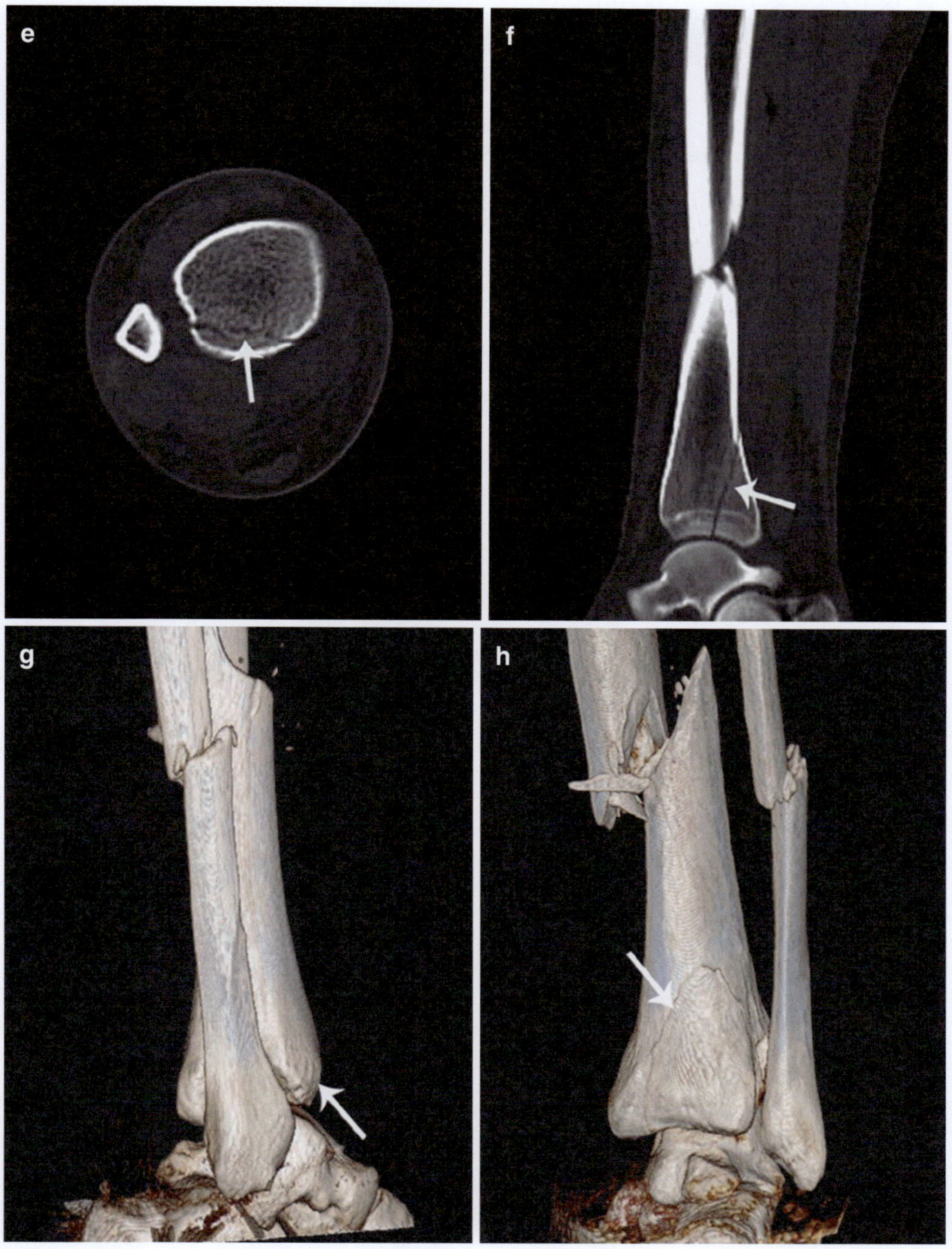

Fig. 12.27 (**e**–**h**) are CT reconstructions of transverse and sagittal planes, lateral and posterior views of CT 3D reconstruction, respectively, showing tibiofibular spiral fractures combined with posterior malleolus fracture (white arrow)

12.2.3.5 Vascular Groove and Growth Retardation Line

18. Identification of normal vascular groove and fracture
    18.1 CT scan (Fig. 12.28a, b)

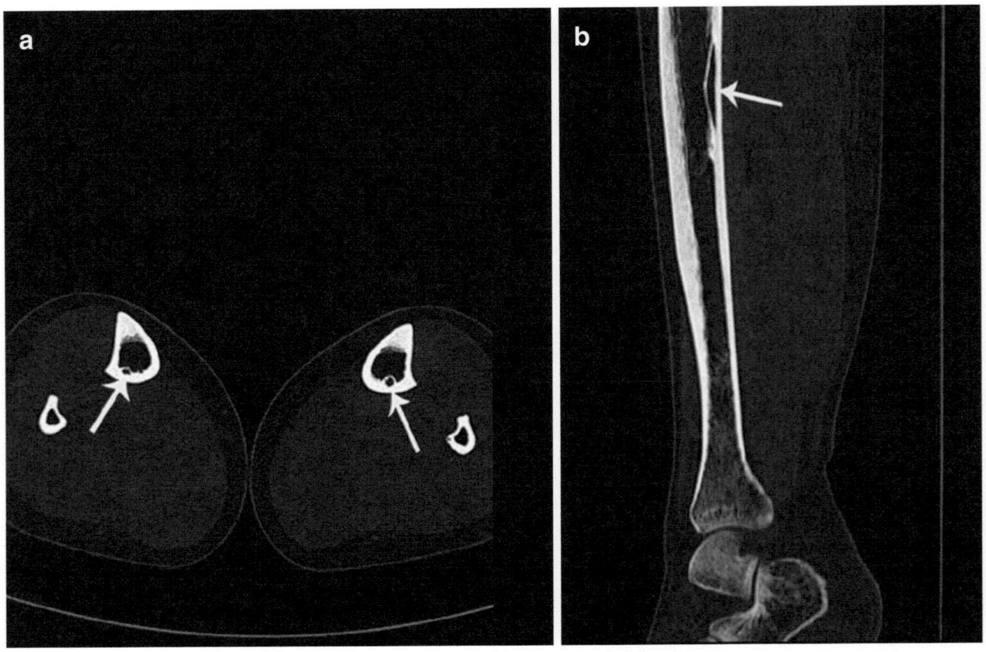

Fig. 12.28 (**a**) is the transverse plane of CT, showing the circular low-density shadow under the posterior cortex of bilateral tibia with clear boundaries. (**b**) shows the CT sagittal plane reconstruction, showing the striated low-density vascular groove

    18.2 MRI scan (Fig. 12.28c, d)

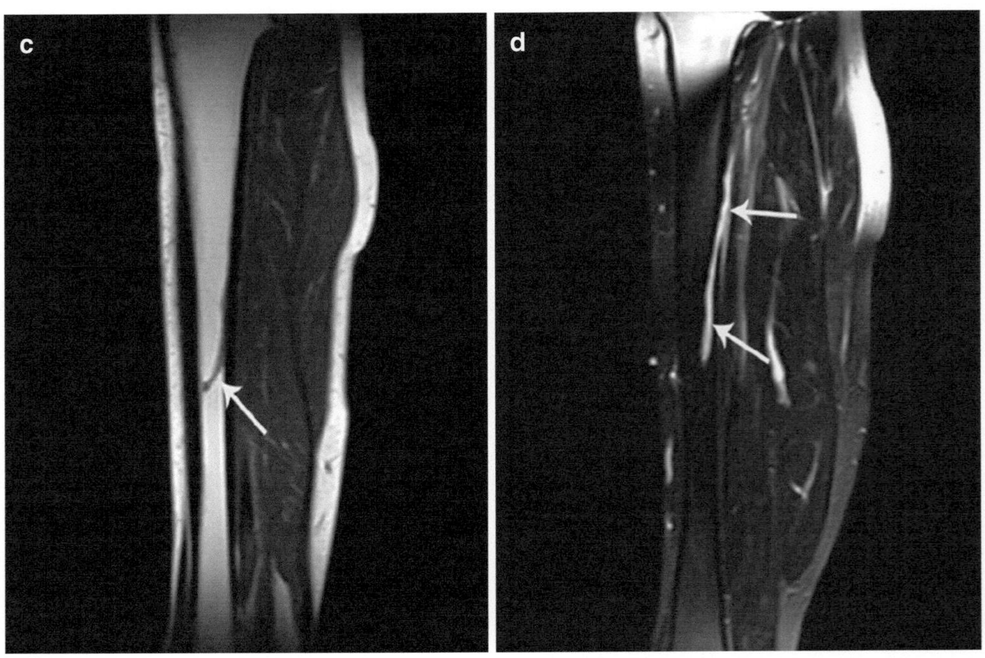

Fig. 12.28 (**c**, **d**) are respectively T1WI and T2WI in the sagittal plane of MRI, indicating that T1WI shows low signal and T2WI shows high signal in the vascular groove of the tibia (white arrow)

19. Identification of growth retardation line and fracture
    19.1 X-ray (Fig. 12.29a–d)

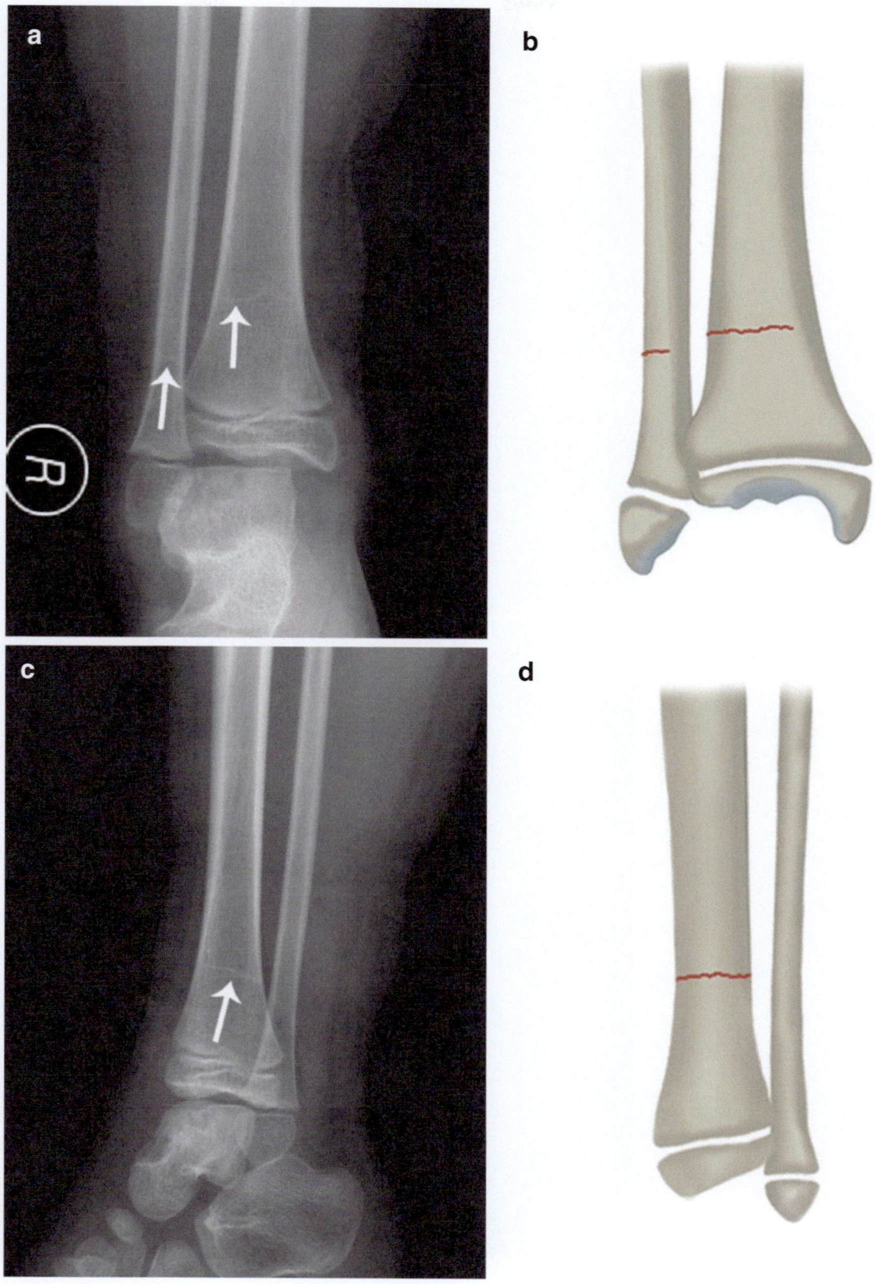

Fig. 12.29 (**a**, **c**) are respectively the lateral and anteroposterior (AP) views of the X-ray, showing transverse high-density shadow of metaphyseal in distal tibia and fibula (white arrow), and schematic diagram (**b**, **d**)

19.2 MRI scan (Fig. 12.29e–h)

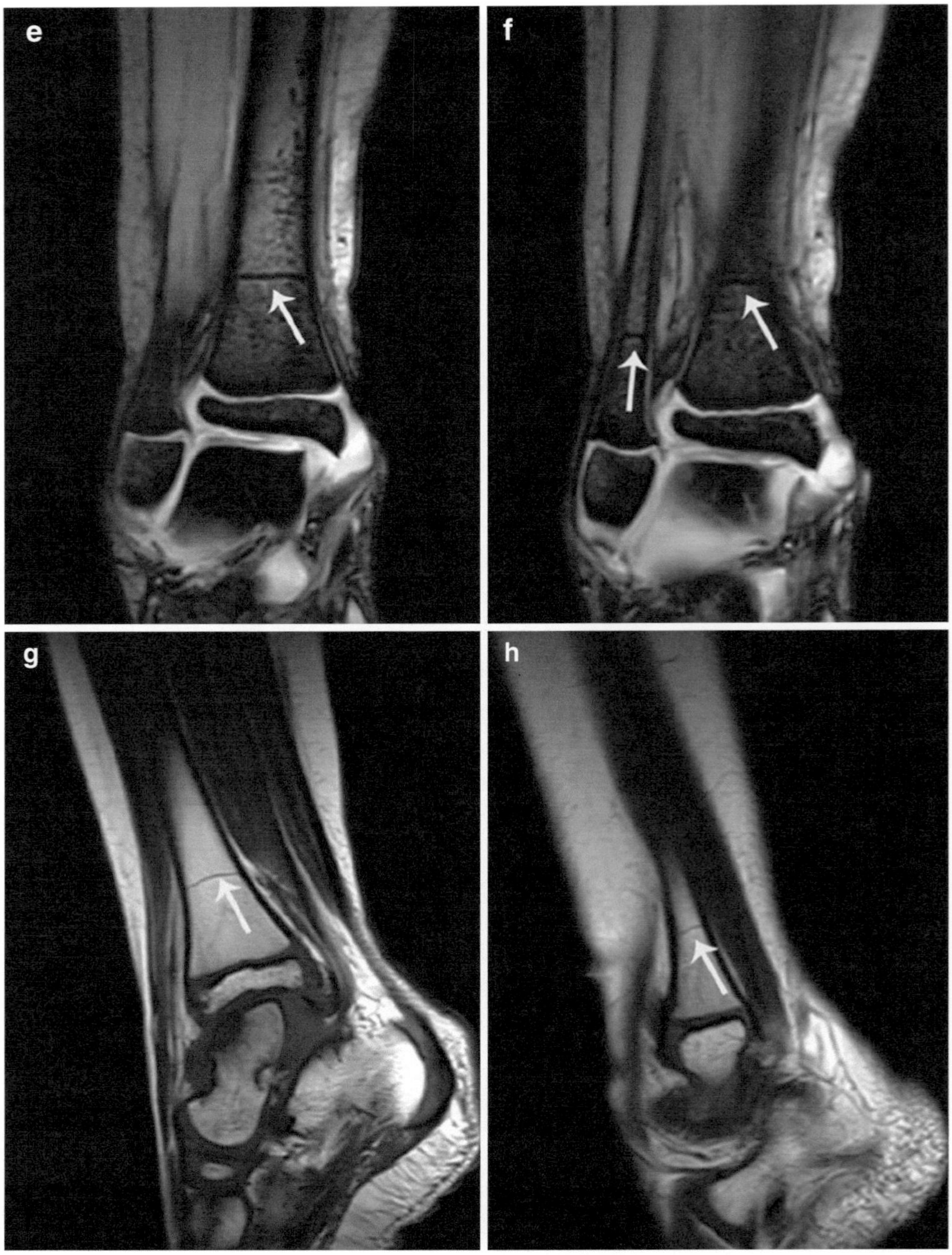

Fig. 12.29 (**e**–**h**) are respectively T2WI in coronal plane and T1WI in sagittal plane of MRI, indicating that growth retardation line shows low signal in both T1WI and T2WI, with smooth edge and without edema of surrounding bone (white arrow)

12.3 Stress Fracture of the Long Bone in Lower Limbs

Stress fractures include fatigue fractures and insufficiency fractures. Fatigue fracture is caused by repeated force loading on normal bone. Insufficiency fracture results from normal stress load on abnormal bone tissue with reduced bone mineral or decreasing elastic resistance. The fatigue fracture of the lower extremities mainly occurs in the upper tibia, the lower fibula (above the lateral malleolus), and the lower 1/3 femur.

12.3.1 Identification of Injury Mechanism

Fatigue fracture is caused by long-time nonphysiological stress on the skeletal system. It is often seen in soldiers' weight-bearing marching and running training.

12.3.2 Identification of Symptoms and Signs

The clinical symptoms are mainly local pain and swelling, which aggravates after activity and relieves when rest. Severe symptoms can lead to bone fracture and affect normal life. Without a history of typical trauma, early X-rays are usually negative and prone to missed diagnosis or misdiagnosis.

12.3.3 Imaging Differential Diagnosis

The X-ray manifestations of fatigue fractures are: (1) Early stage: Mostly no significant X-ray changes or only mild periosteal hyperplasia. (2) Middle stage: Plenty of periosteal proliferation and callus formation. (3) Late stage: Healing period, a large number of callus is gradually absorbed and became smooth, fused with the hyperplastic periosteum and the diaphysis. The evolution of periosteal response from wide to limited, from parallel to hilly, and gradually fused with cortical bone is an important indirect sign of fatigue fracture. Fracture line is a reliable evidence for diagnosis of fatigue fracture, mostly incompletely transverse or oblique. X-ray is often unable to show the thin fracture line in the early stage. If the stress is not continued, the X-ray can show no fracture, which is also an important reason for clinical misdiagnosis.

CT manifestations of fatigue fracture: CT can more accurately show the fracture line and the proliferation of the inner and outer periosteum of bone. The "notch sign" is characteristic in periosteal reaction of the fatigue fracture, which lays in the middle of the posterior margin of hemilateral multilayer or lace periosteum proliferation with smooth edge. The mechanism is that the intermuscular fascia, which firmly adheres to the diaphysis, influences the formation of the periosteum.

MRI manifestations of fatigue fracture: MRI has obvious advantages for the diagnosis of early fatigue fracture (in 2 weeks) with strong specificity. MRI can clearly display the fracture lines and edema or bleeding in medullary cavity and surrounding soft tissue. It shows low signal in T1WI, high signal in T2WI and fat-suppression T2WI. Especially, T1WI and fat-suppression T2WI images have the most diagnostic value. Bone marrow edema around the fracture represents a microfracture of the trabecular bone, which is the earliest manifestation of fatigue fracture. MRI can detect early changes, rather than X-rays and CT. The low-signal band in the bone marrow edema region associated with the bone cortex, representing the formation of internal callus after fracture, is an important sign for the diagnosis of fatigue fracture.

12.3.3.1 Fatigue Fracture of the Femur

1. Identification of bilateral femoral neck fatigue fracture and nonfracture
   1.1 X-ray (Fig. 12.30a, b)

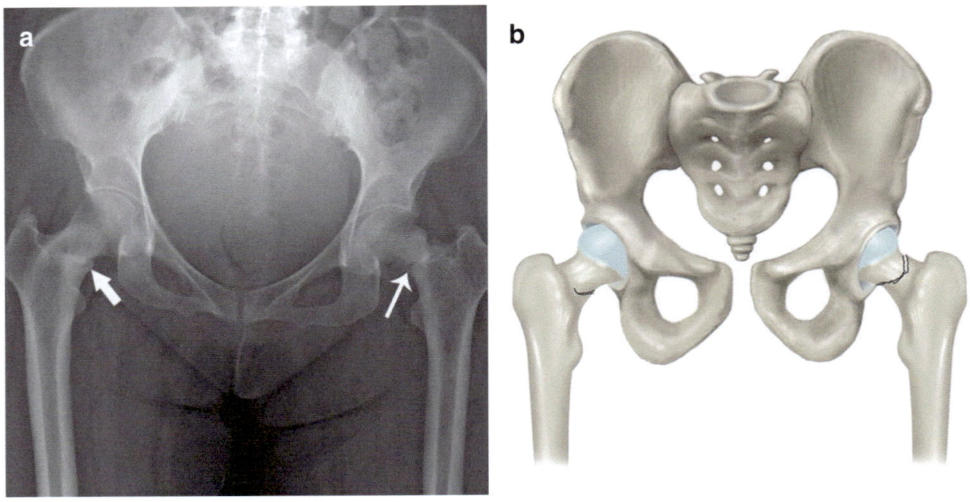

Fig. 12.30 (**a**) is the anteroposterior (AP) view of the X-ray, showing the linear low-density shadow of the right femoral neck, with bone sclerosis, and the fracture line does not run through the right femoral neck (thick white arrow). On the left side, edge sclerosis is showed around the fracture, with the fracture line throughout the femoral neck (thin white arrow), schematic diagram (**b**)

   1.2 CT scan (Fig. 12.30c–e)

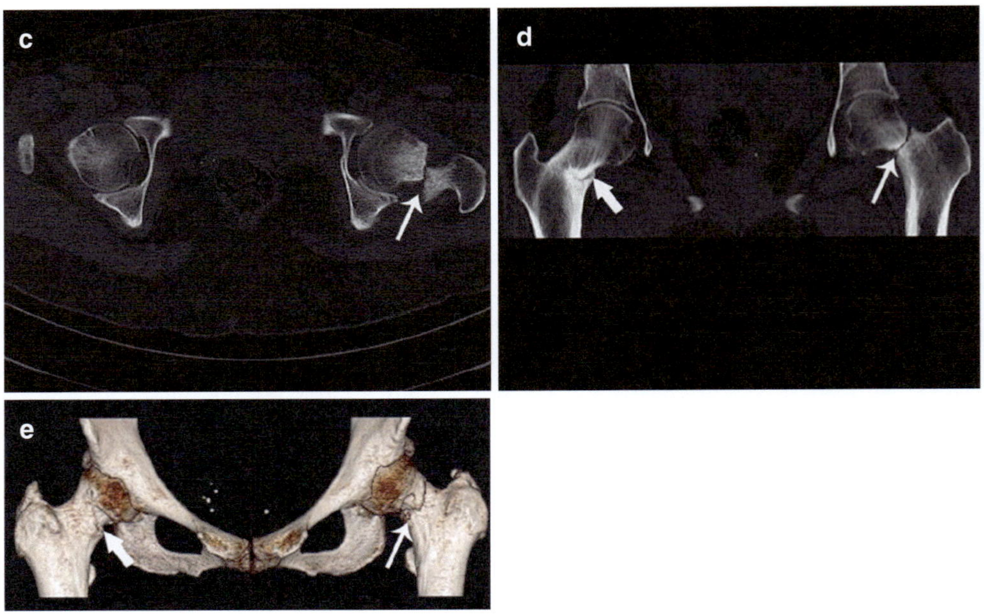

Fig. 12.30 (**c**, **d**, **e**) are respectively CT transverse plane, coronal plane reconstruction and 3D reconstruction images, showing the linear low-density shadow of the right femoral neck, with bone sclerosis, and the fracture line does not run through the right femoral neck (thick white arrow). On the left side, edge sclerosis is showed around the fracture, with the fracture line throughout the femoral neck (thin white arrow)

1.3 MRI scan (Fig. 12.30f–i)

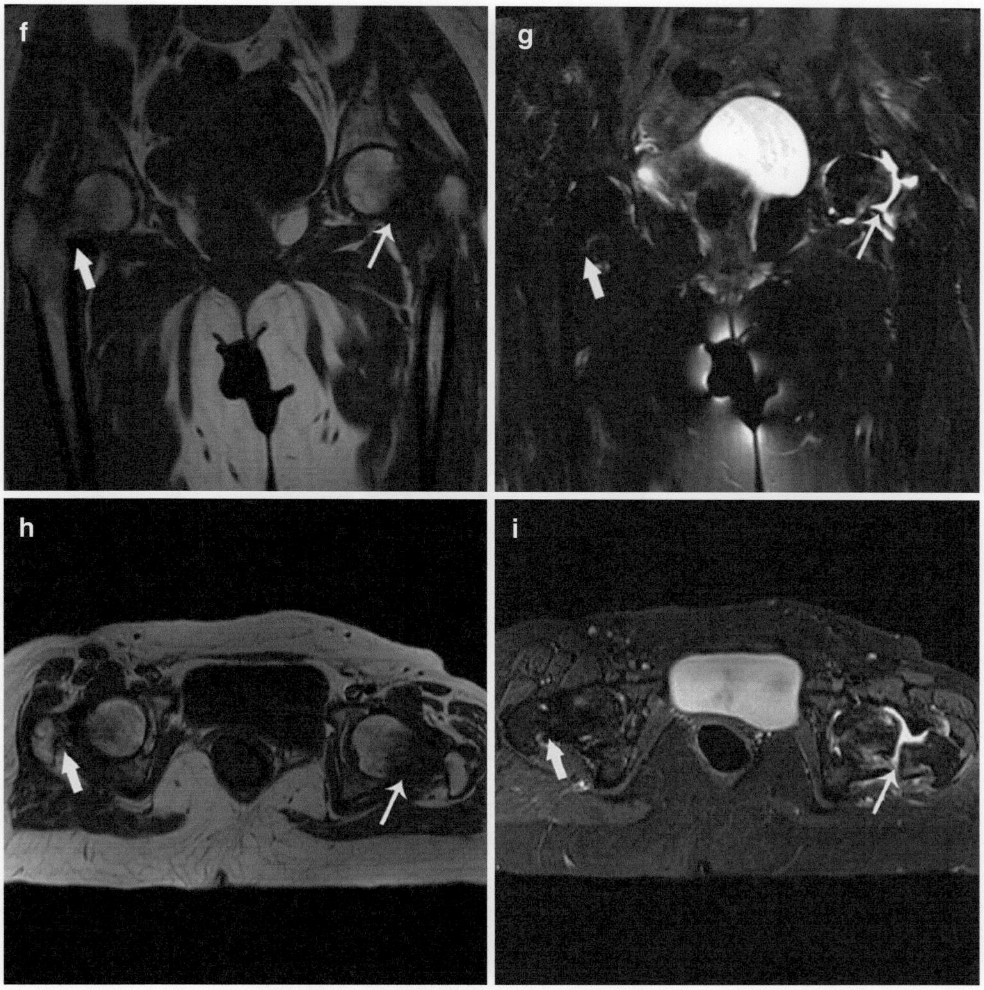

Fig. 12.30 (**f–i**) are respectively T1W and fat-suppression T2WI of coronal plane, T1WI and fat-suppression T2WI of transverse plane, showing the linear low-density shadow of the right femoral neck, with bone sclerosis, and the fracture line does not run through the right femoral neck (thick white arrow). On the left side, edge sclerosis is showed around the fracture, with the fracture line throughout the femoral neck (thin white arrow)

2. Identification of right femoral neck fatigue fracture and nonfracture
    2.1 X-ray (Fig. 12.31a–d)

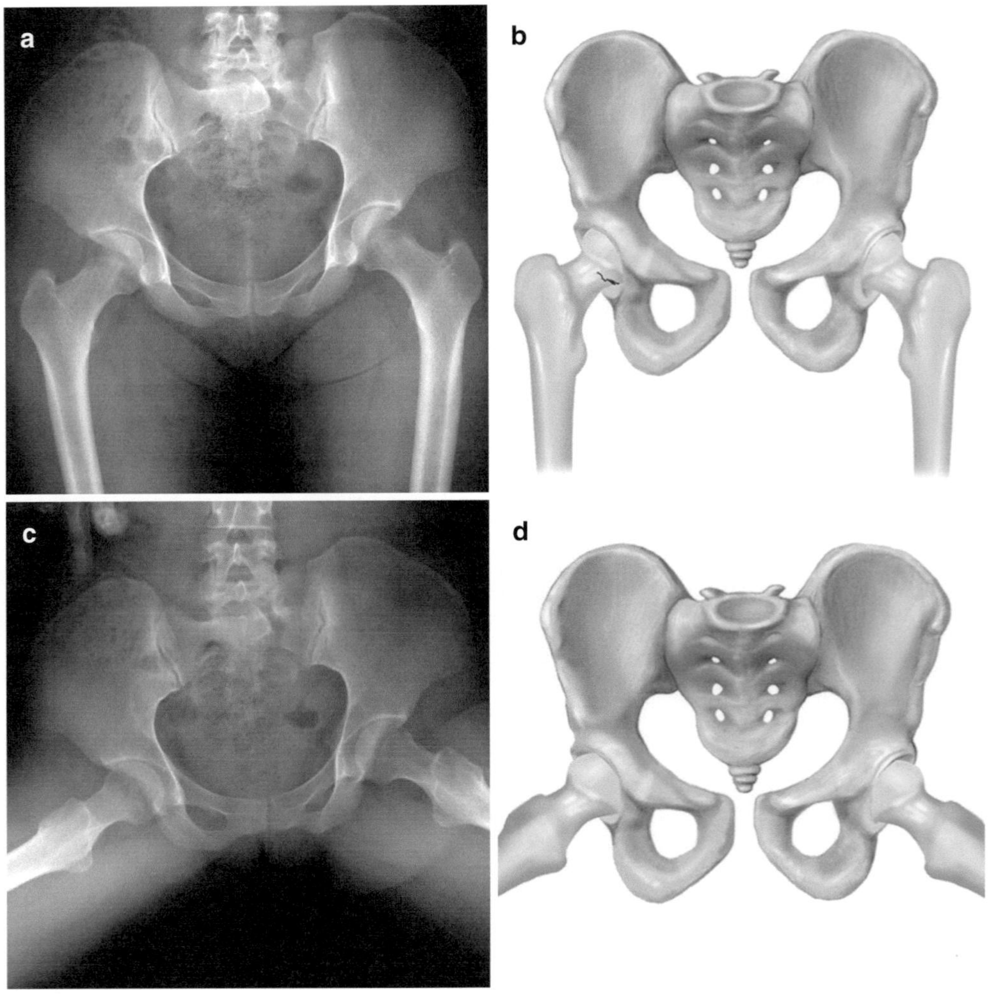

Fig. 12.31 (**a**, **c**) are respectively the anteroposterior (AP) and frog position views of the X-ray. No obvious fracture sign is seen in femoral neck on both sides, and further CT scan was performed for the purpose of definite diagnosis. Schematic diagram (**b**, **d**)

    2.2 CT scan (Fig. 12.31e, f)

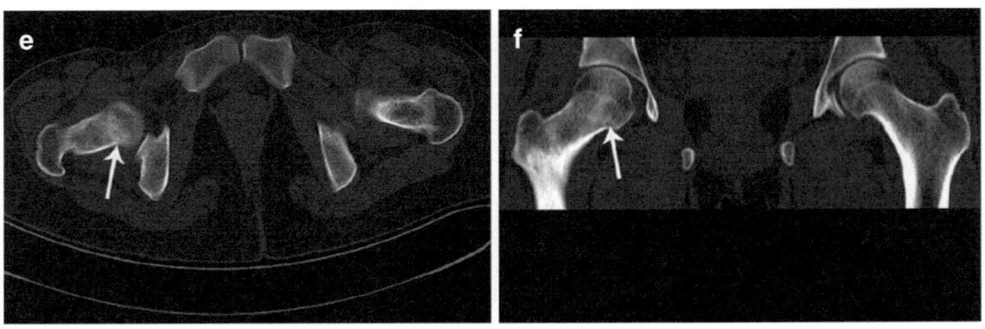

Fig. 12.31 (**e**, **f**) are respectively the reconstruction images of the transverse and coronal plane of CT, showing the slightly high-density linear shadow (white arrow) of the right femoral neck, and no abnormality in the left femoral neck

2.3 MRI scan (Fig. 12.31g–j)

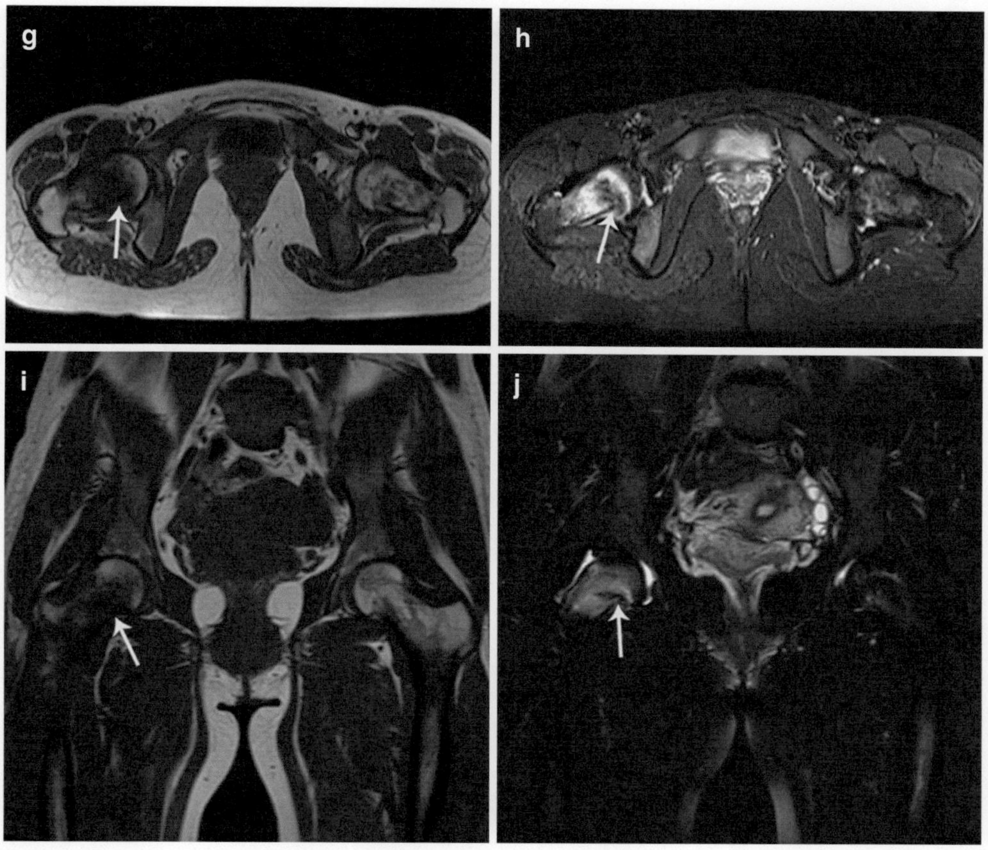

Fig. 12.31 (g–j) are respectively MRI T1WI and fat-suppression T2WI of transverse plane, T1WI and fat-suppression T2WI of coronal plane, showing low signal in T1WI and fat-suppression T2WI of right femoral neck (thin white arrow), and the surrounding patchy edema presented low signal in T1WI and high signal in fat-suppression T2WI with unclear edge

3. Identification of left upper femoral fatigue fracture and nonfracture
   3.1 X-ray (Fig. 12.32a, b)

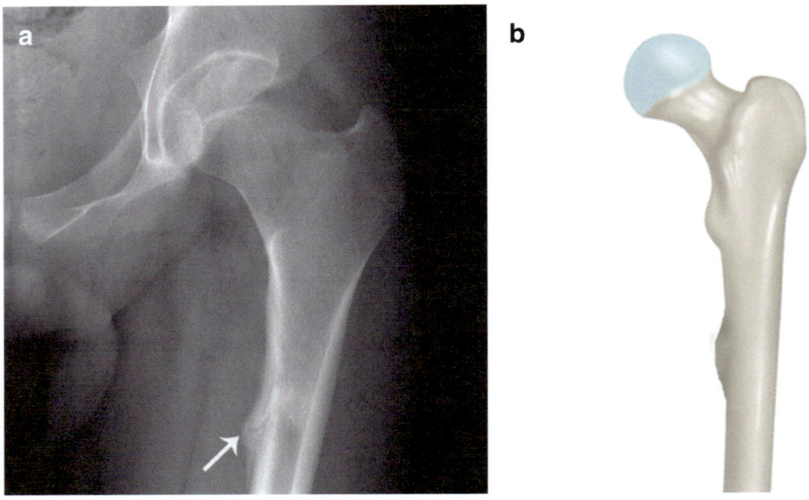

Fig. 12.32 (**a**) is the anteroposterior (AP) view of the X-ray, showing the linear low-density shadow (white arrow) in the upper part of the left femur, with bone sclerosis, indicating the periosteal reaction, and schematic diagram (**b**)

   3.2 CT scan (Fig. 12.32c)

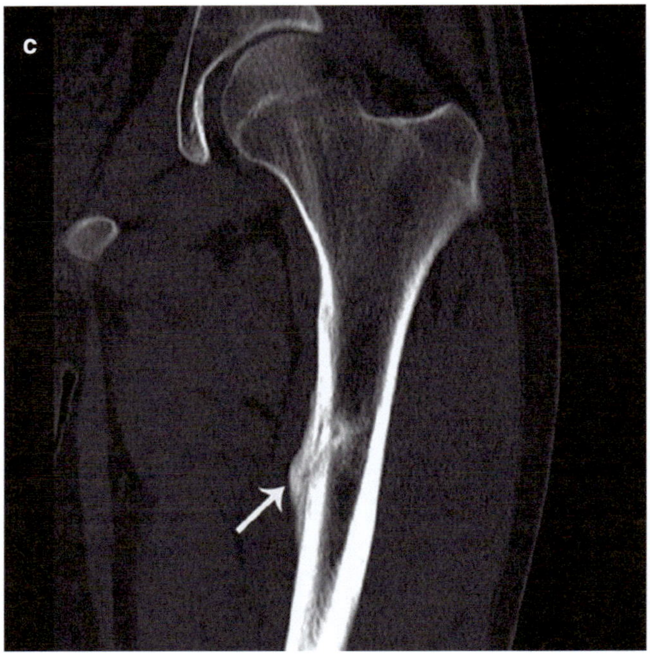

Fig. 12.32 (**c**) shows the coronal plane reconstruction of CT, showing the linear low-density shadow (white arrow) in the upper part of the left femur, with bone sclerosis, indicating the periosteal reaction

3.3 MRI scan (Fig. 12.32d, e)

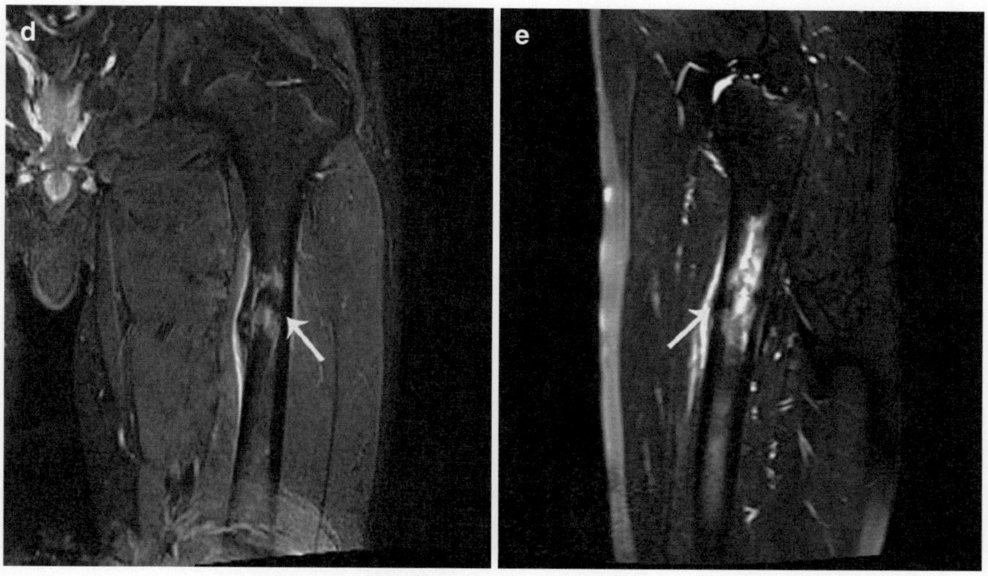

Fig. 12.32 (**d**, **e**) are respectively MRI fat inhibition T2WI of coronal and sagittal plane, showing the linear low-density shadow (white arrow), with surrounding patchy high-signal edema area, indicating the periosteal reaction and surrounding soft tissue swelling

4. Identification of left femoral shaft fatigue fracture and nonfracture
   4.1 X-ray (Fig. 12.33a–d)

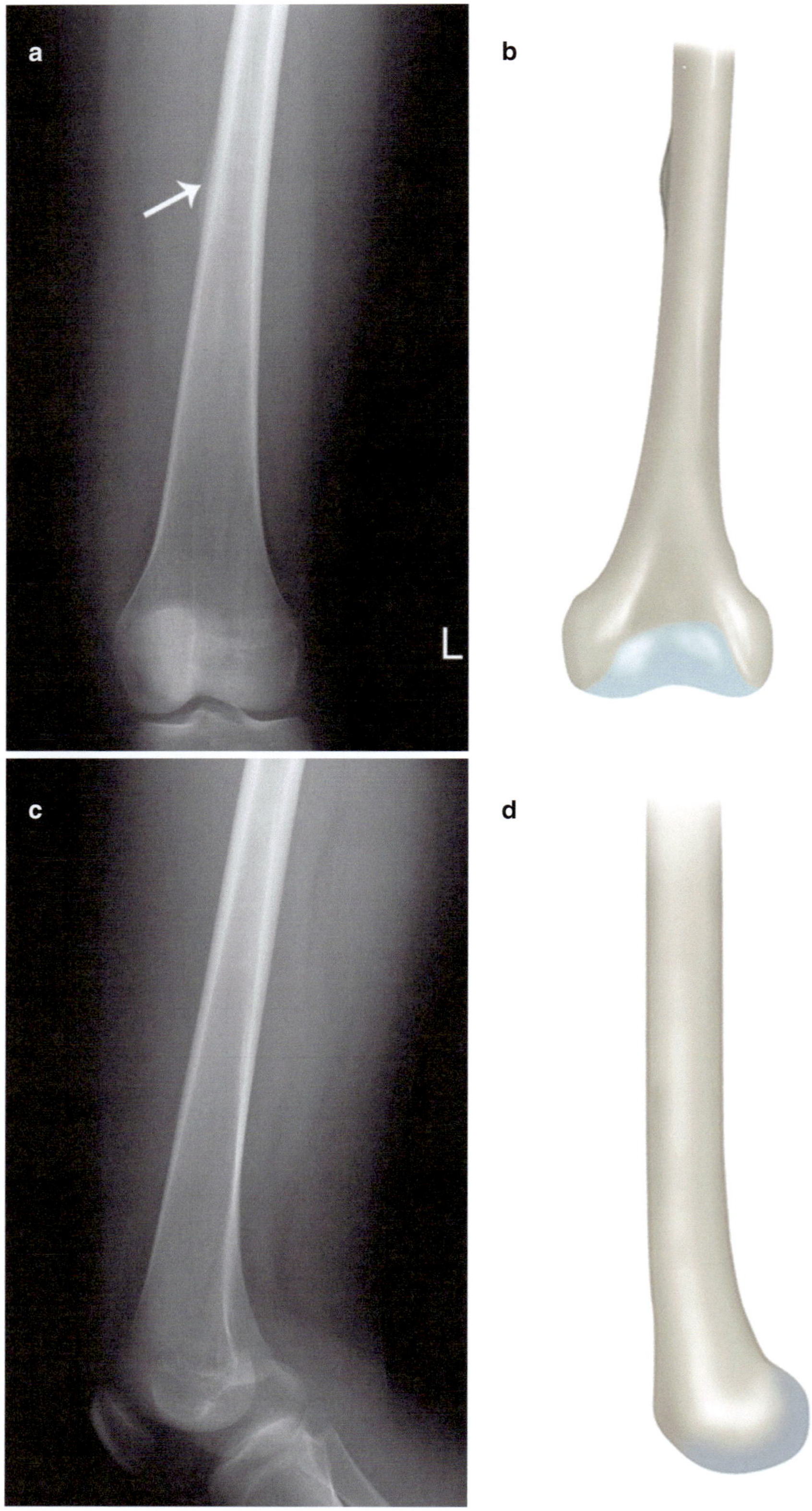

Fig. 12.33 (**a**, **c**) are respectively the lateral and anteroposterior (AP) views of the X-ray, showing local periosteal reaction (white arrow) in the middle part of the left femur without obvious fracture line. For the purpose of definite diagnosis, further MRI scan was performed, and the schematic diagram (**b**, **d**)

4.2 MRI scan (Fig. 12.33e, f)

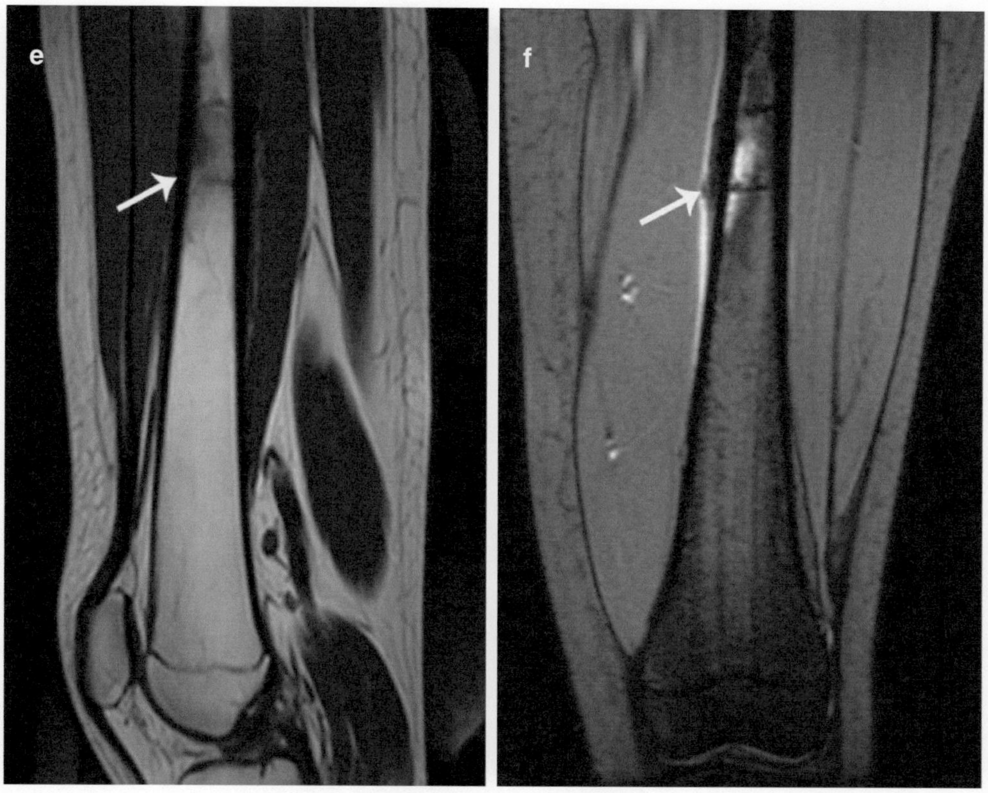

Fig. 12.33 (**e**, **f**) are respectively T1WI and T2WI of sagittal plane, showing linear low-density signal (white arrow), with surrounding patchy high-signal edema area, indicating the periosteal reaction and surrounding soft tissue swelling

5. Identification of lower femur fatigue fracture and nonfracture
   5.1 X-ray (Fig. 12.34a–d)

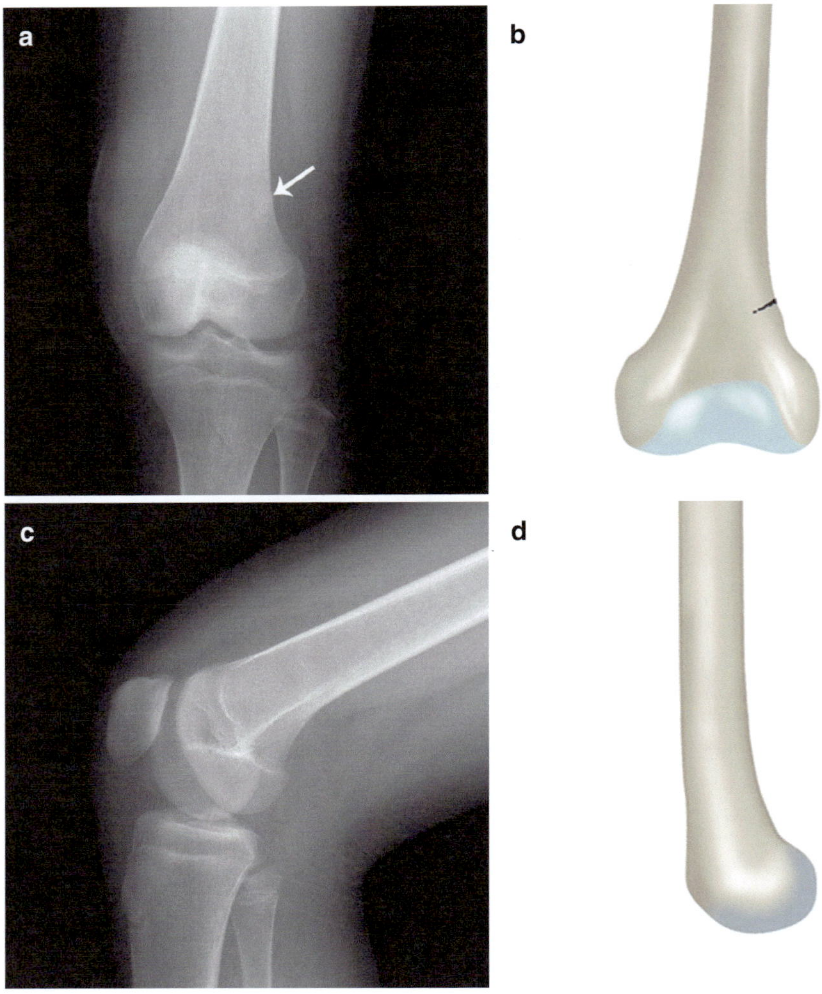

Fig. 12.34 (**a**, **c**) are respectively the lateral and anteroposterior (AP) views of the X-ray, showing linear high-density shadow (white arrow) in the distal part of the femur without obvious periosteal reaction. For the purpose of definite diagnosis, further MRI scan was performed, and the schematic diagram (**b**, **d**)

   5.2 MRI scan (Fig. 12.34e, f)

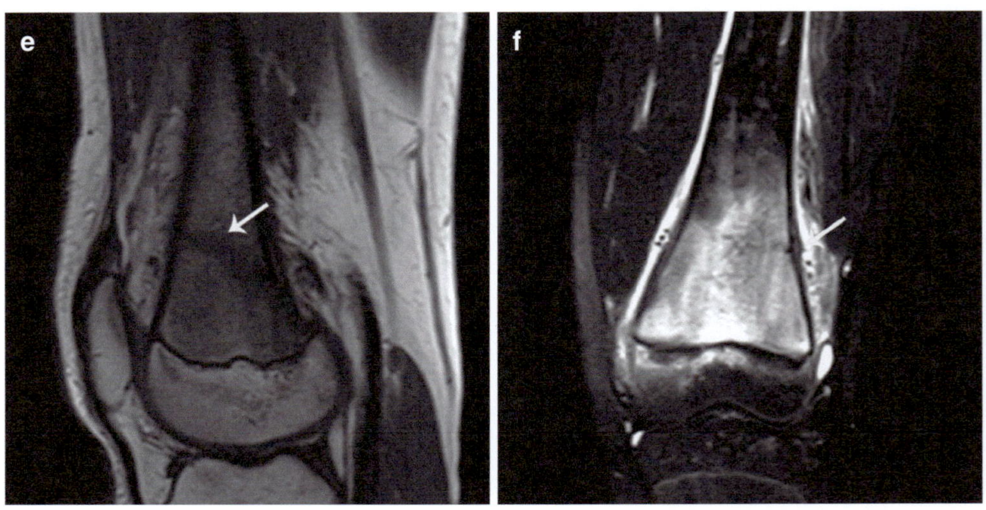

Fig. 12.34 (**e**, **f**) are respectively sagittal plane T1WI and coronal plane fat inhibition T2WI, showing linear low signal (white arrow), with surrounding patchy high-signal edema area, indicating the periosteal reaction and surrounding soft tissue swelling

12.3.3.2 Fatigue Fracture and Insufficiency Fracture of the Tibia

6. Identification of upper tibia fatigue fracture and nonfracture
   6.1 X-ray (Fig. 12.35a–d)

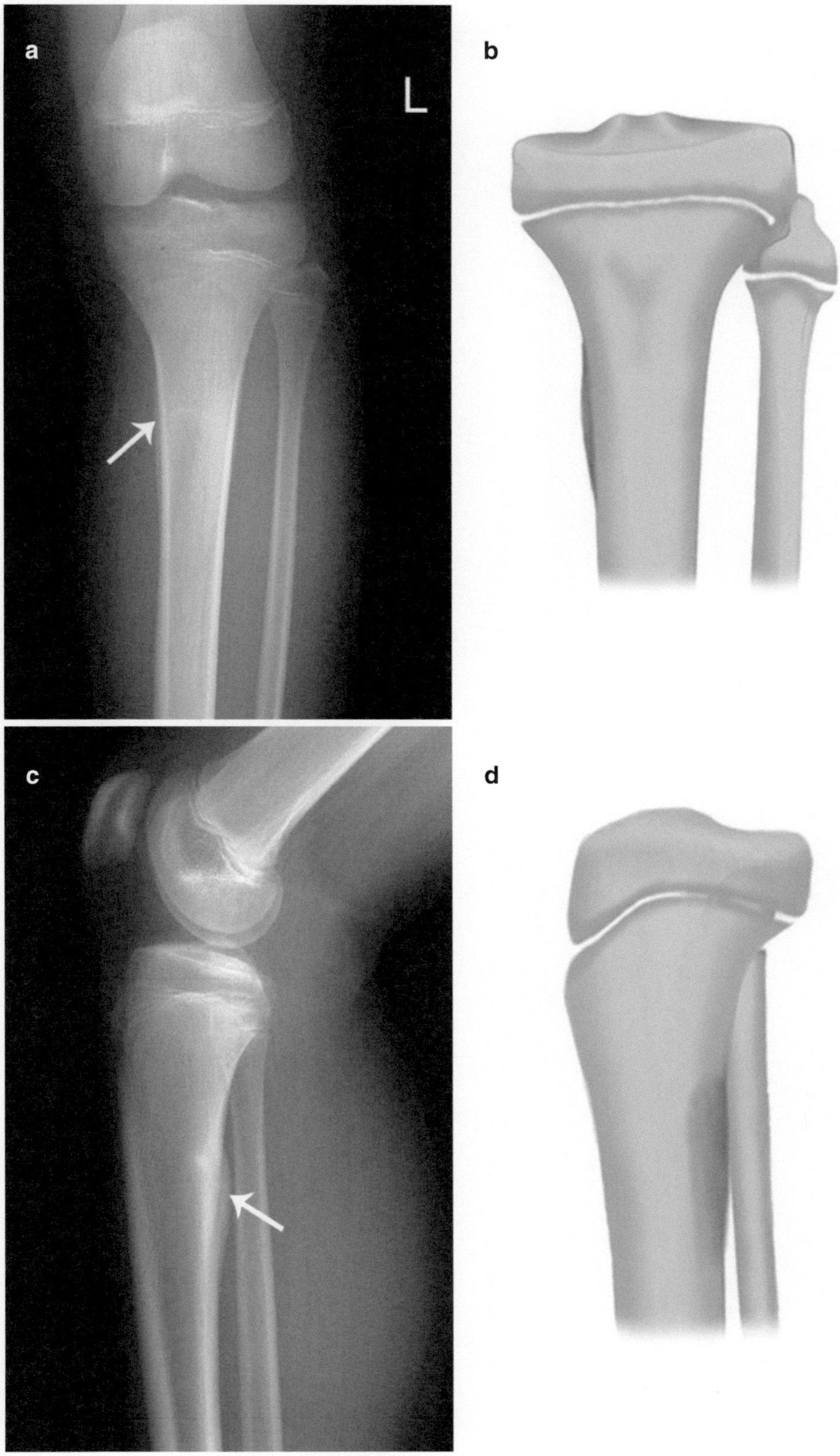

Fig. 12.35 (**a**, **c**) are respectively the lateral and anteroposterior (AP) views of the X-ray, showing linear low-density shadow in upper tibia with bone sclerosis, indicating the periosteal reaction(white arrow) and the schematic diagram (**b**, **d**)

6.2 MRI scan (Fig. 12.35e, f)

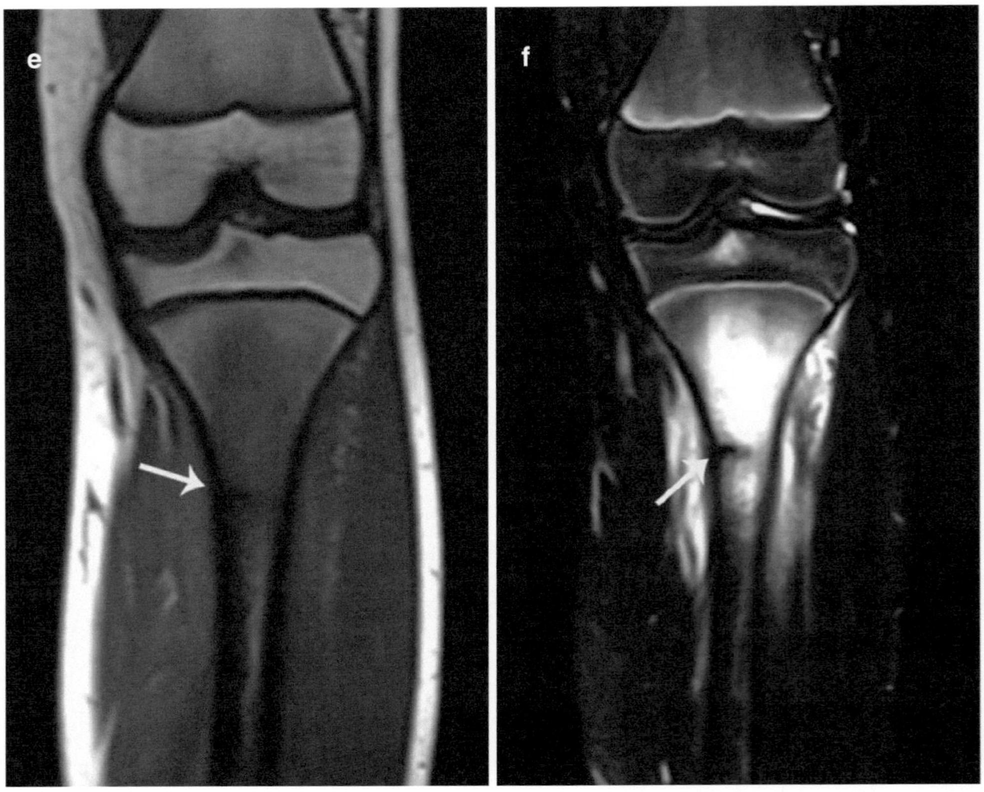

Fig. 12.35 (**e**, **f**) are respectively T1WI and fat inhibition T2WI of coronal plane, showing linear low signal (white arrow), with surrounding patchy high-signal edema area, indicating the periosteal reaction and surrounding soft tissue swelling

7. Identification of upper tibia fatigue fracture and bone tumors
   7.1 CT scan (Fig. 12.36a–d)

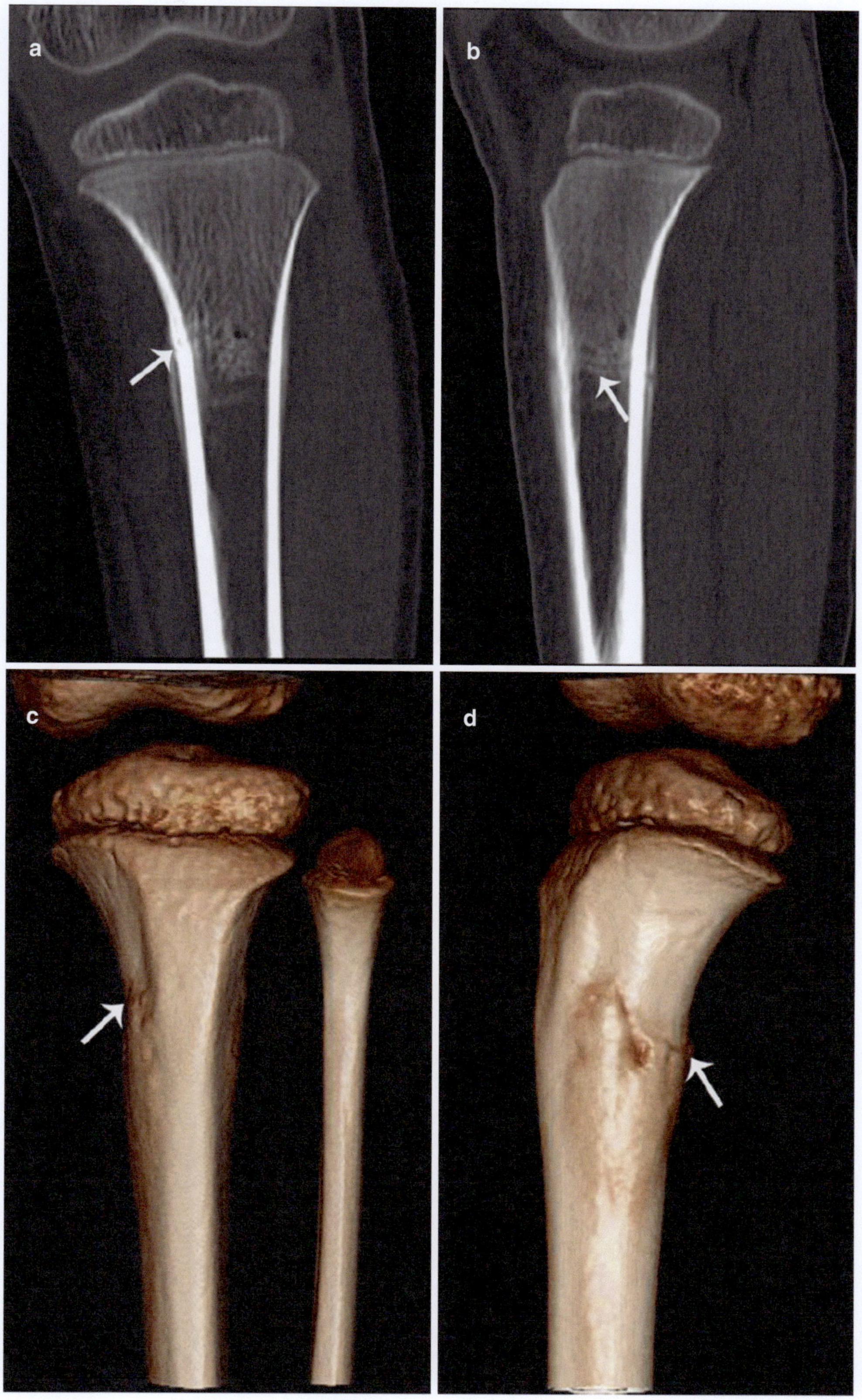

Fig. 12.36 (**a**, **b**) are respectively CT reconstruction of coronal and sagittal plane, showing linear high-density shadow of upper tibia and peripheral sclerosis, indicating periosteal reaction (white arrow). (**c**, **d**) are respectively anterior and anterolateral views of CT 3d reconstruction, showing the cortical discontinuity (white arrow) and the surrounding periosteal reaction

7.2 MRI scan (Fig. 12.36e, f)

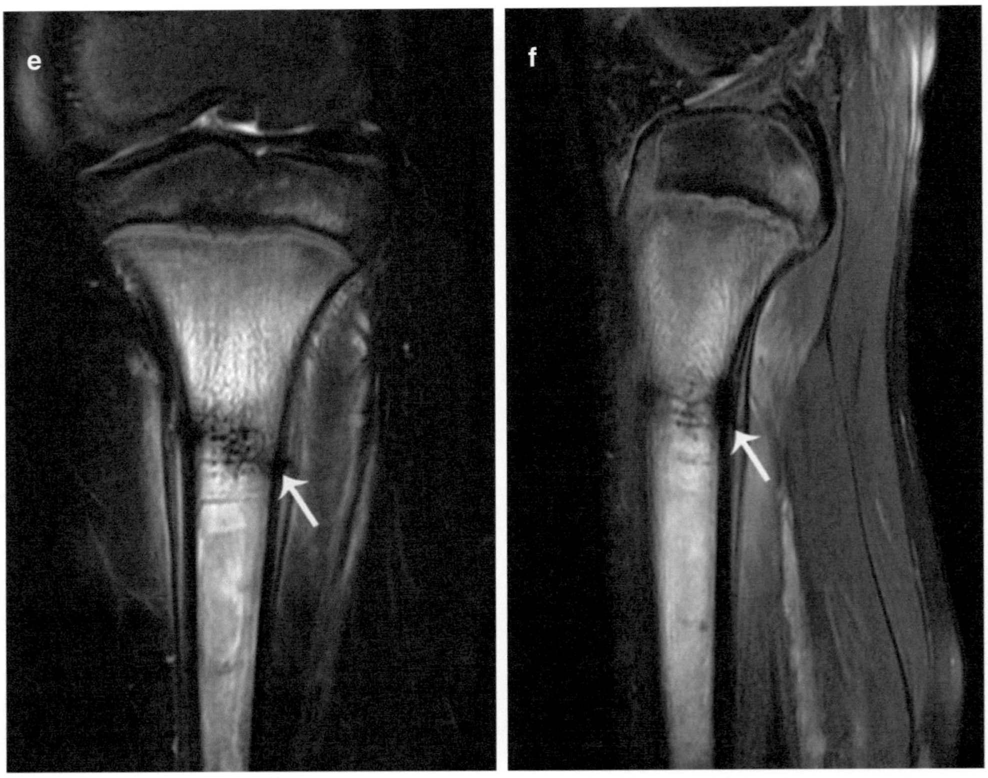

Fig. 12.36 (**e**, **f**) are respectively fat inhibition T2WI of coronal and sagittal plane, showing linear low signal (white arrow), with surrounding patchy high-signal edema area, indicating the periosteal reaction and surrounding soft tissue swelling

8. Identification of upper tibia fatigue fracture and nonfracture
   8.1 X-ray (Fig. 12.37a–d)

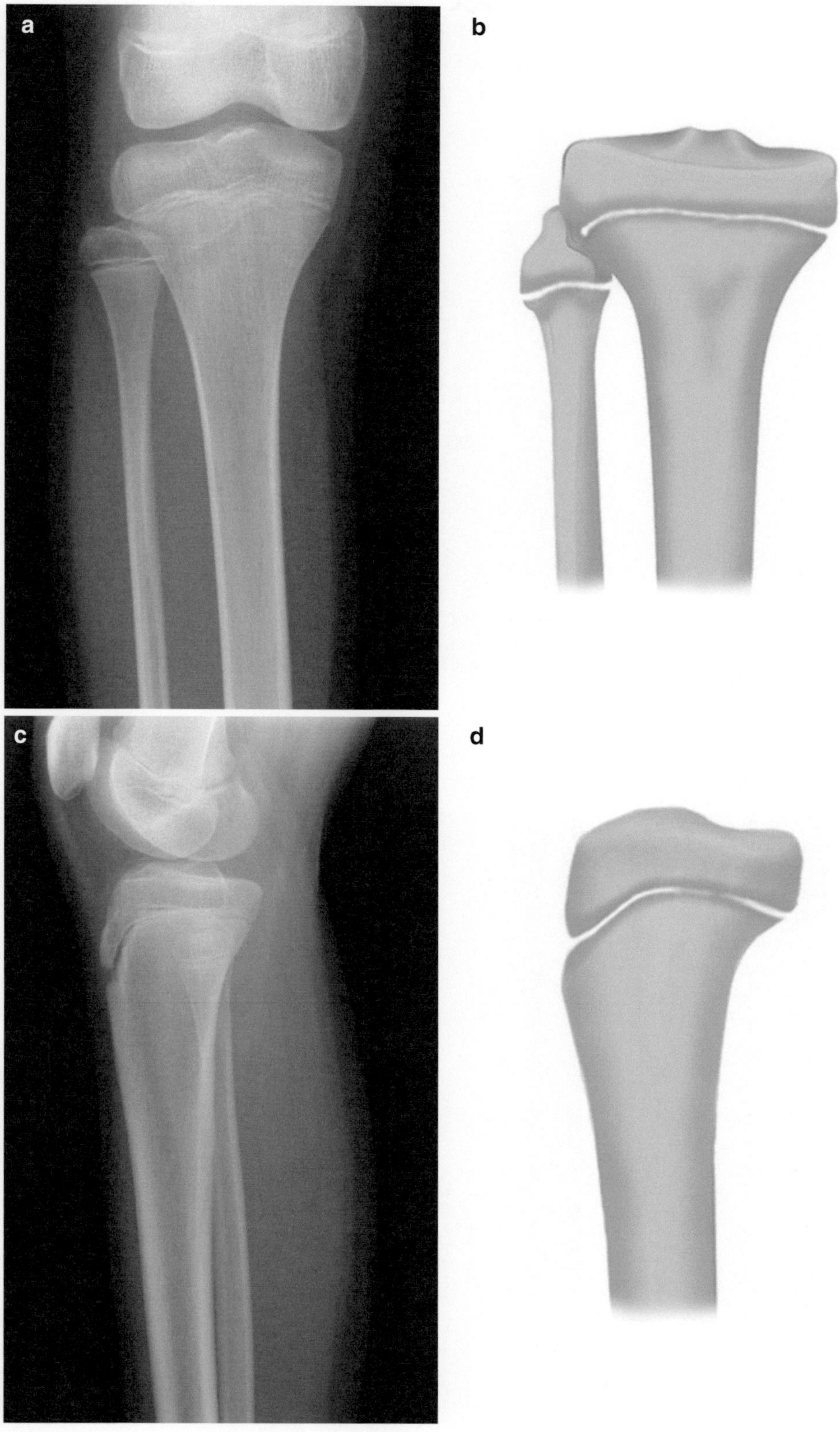

Fig. 12.37 (**a**, **c**) are respectively the lateral and anteroposterior (AP) views of the X-ray, showing no abnormalities observed in bone. For the purpose of definite diagnosis, further CT scan was performed, and the schematic diagram (**b**, **d**)

8.2 CT scan (Fig. 12.37e, f)

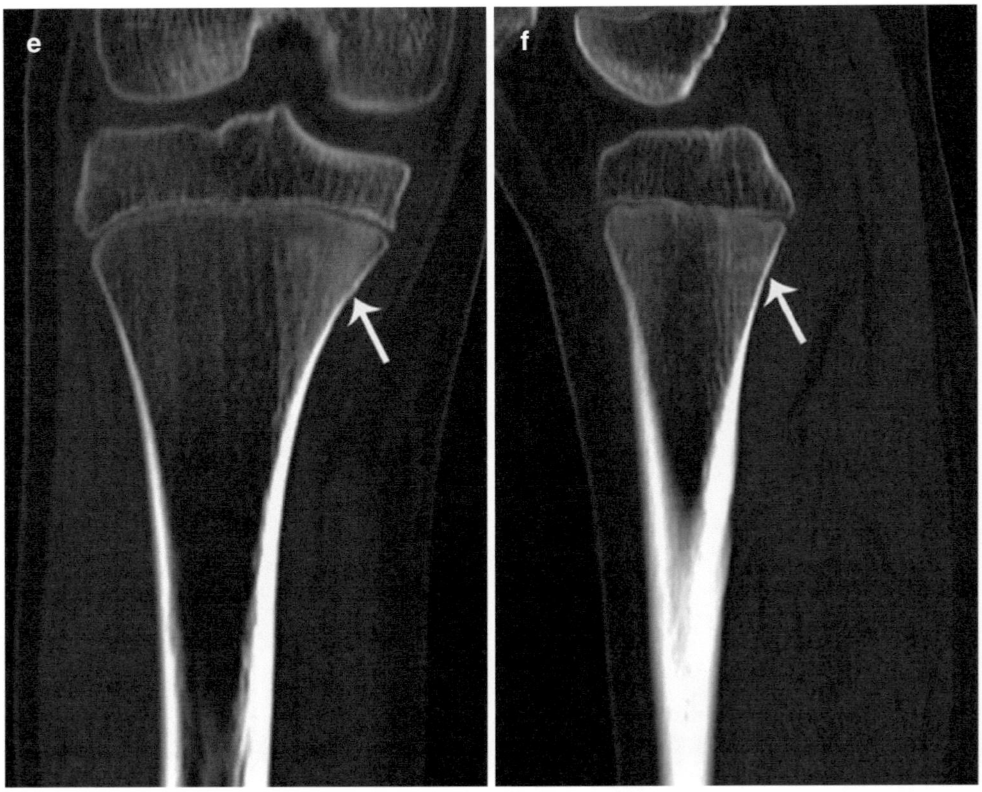

Fig. 12.37 (**e**, **f**) are respectively CT reconstruction of coronal and sagittal plane, showing discontinuity in the upper part of the right tibia (white arrow). For the purpose of definite diagnosis, further MRI scan was performed

8.3 MRI scan (Fig. 12.37g, h)

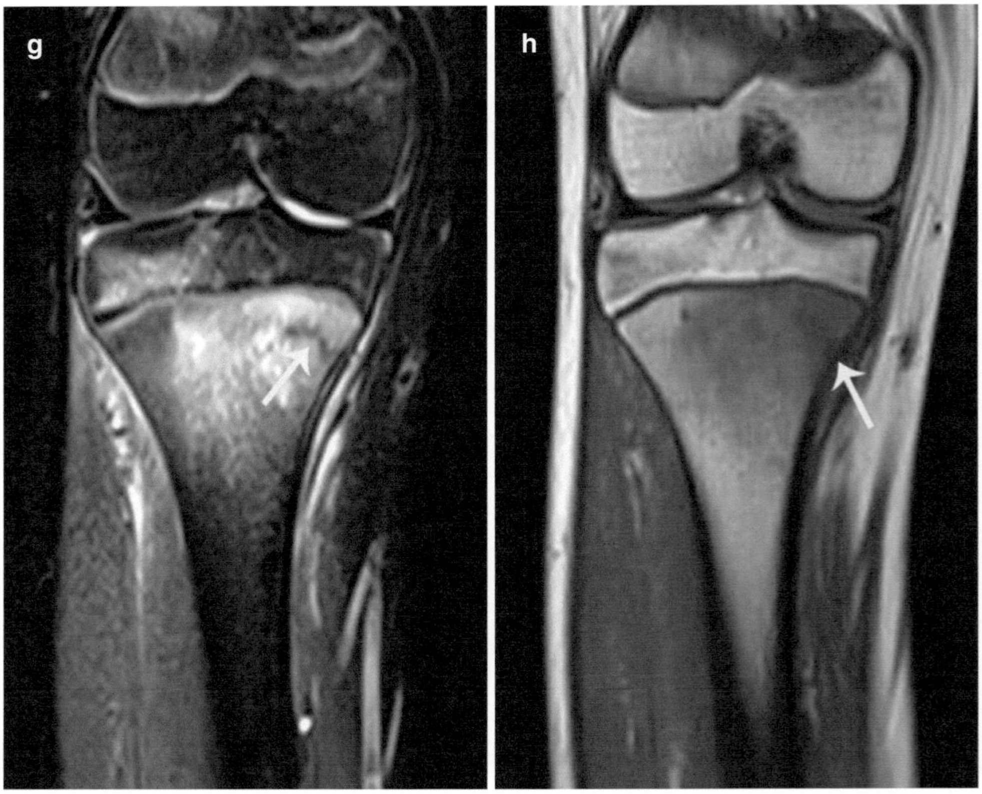

Fig. 12.37 (**g**, **h**) are respectively T1WI and fat inhibition T2WI of coronal plane, showing a low-signal fracture line shadow in upper right tibia (white arrow), with surrounding bone marrow edema and soft tissue swelling

9. Identification of tibial insufficiency fracture and nonfracture
   9.1 X-ray (Fig. 12.38a–d)

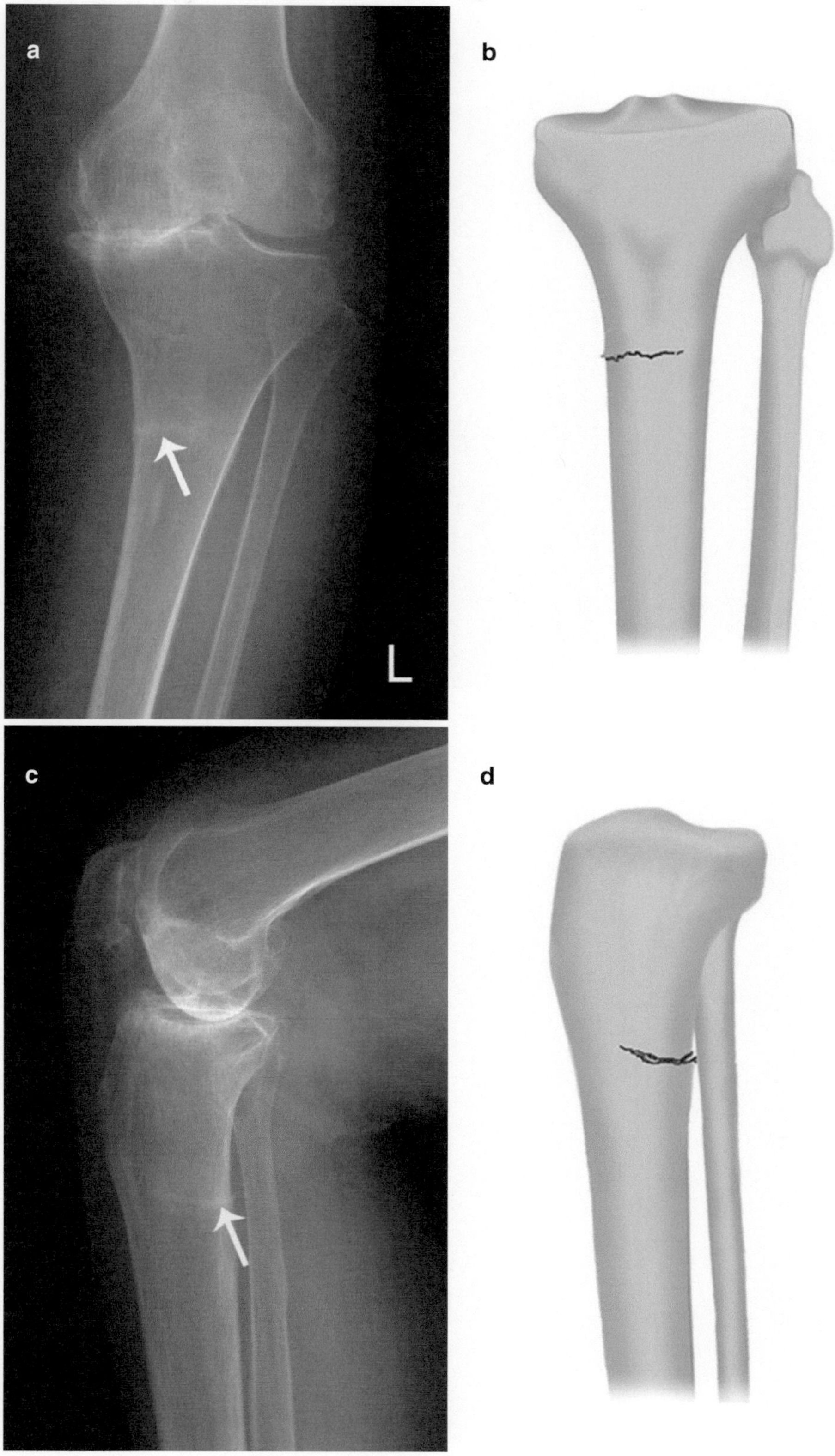

Fig. 12.38 (**a**, **c**) are respectively the lateral and anteroposterior (AP) views of the X-ray, showing linear high-density shadow of upper tibia (white arrow), varus deformity, osteoarthritis, and osteoporosis of the left knee joint. Schematic diagram (**b**, **d**)

9.2 MRI scan (Fig. 12.38e, f)

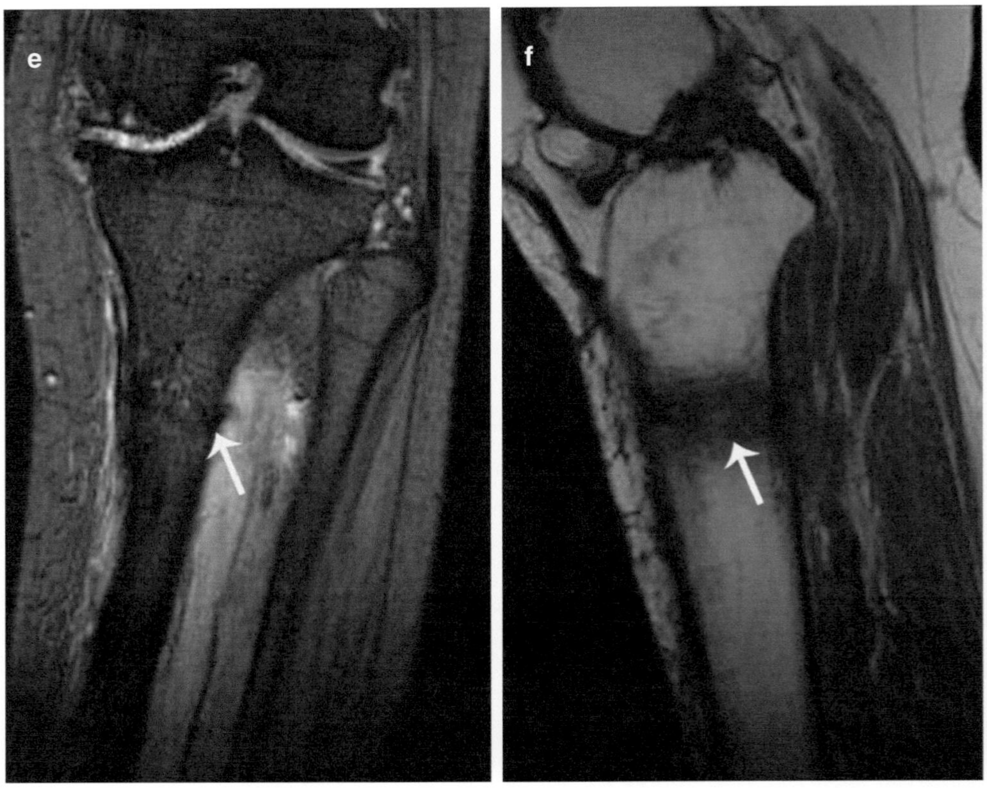

Fig. 12.38 (**e**, **f**) are respectively coronal plane T2WI and sagittal plane T1WI, showing linear low-density shadow in upper tibia (white arrow), with surrounding bone marrow and soft tissue edema

12.3.3.3 Fatigue Fracture of the Fibula

10. Identification of lower fibula fatigue fracture and nonfracture
    10.1 X-ray (Fig. 12.39a–d)

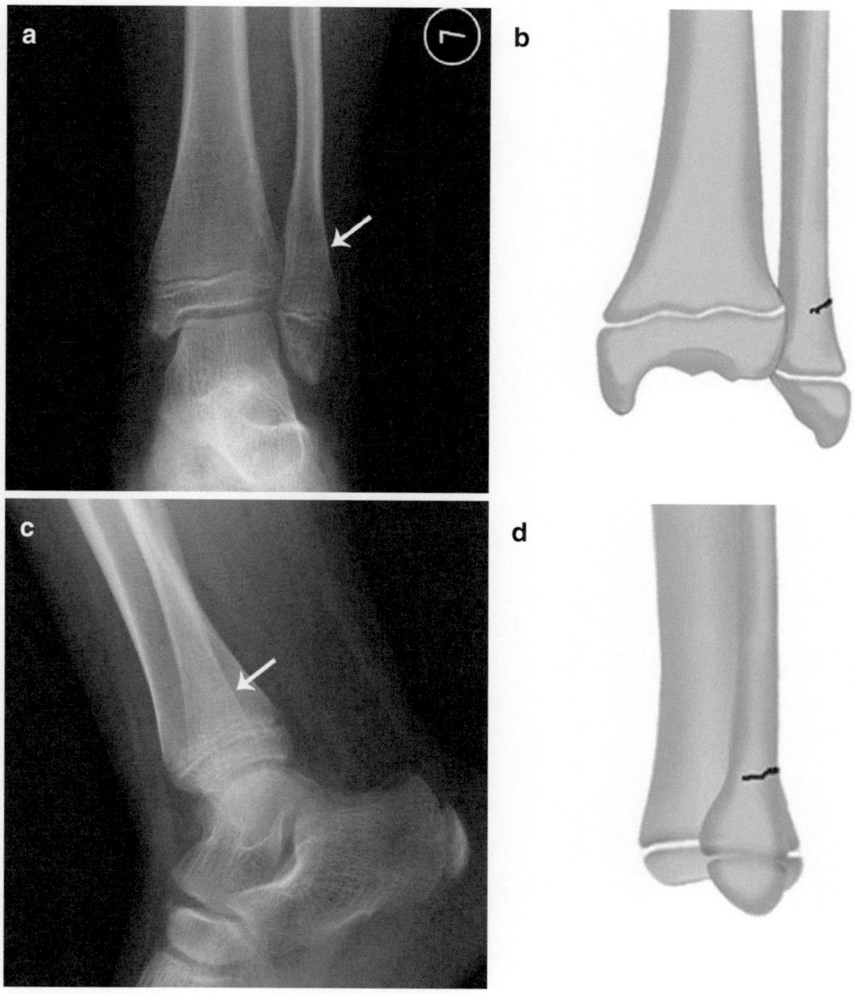

Fig. 12.39 (**a**, **c**) are respectively the lateral and anteroposterior (AP) views of the X-ray, showing linear high-density shadow of lower fibula (white arrow). For the purpose of definite diagnosis, further MRI scan was performed, and the schematic diagram (**b**, **d**)

10.2 MRI scan (Fig. 12.39e–h)

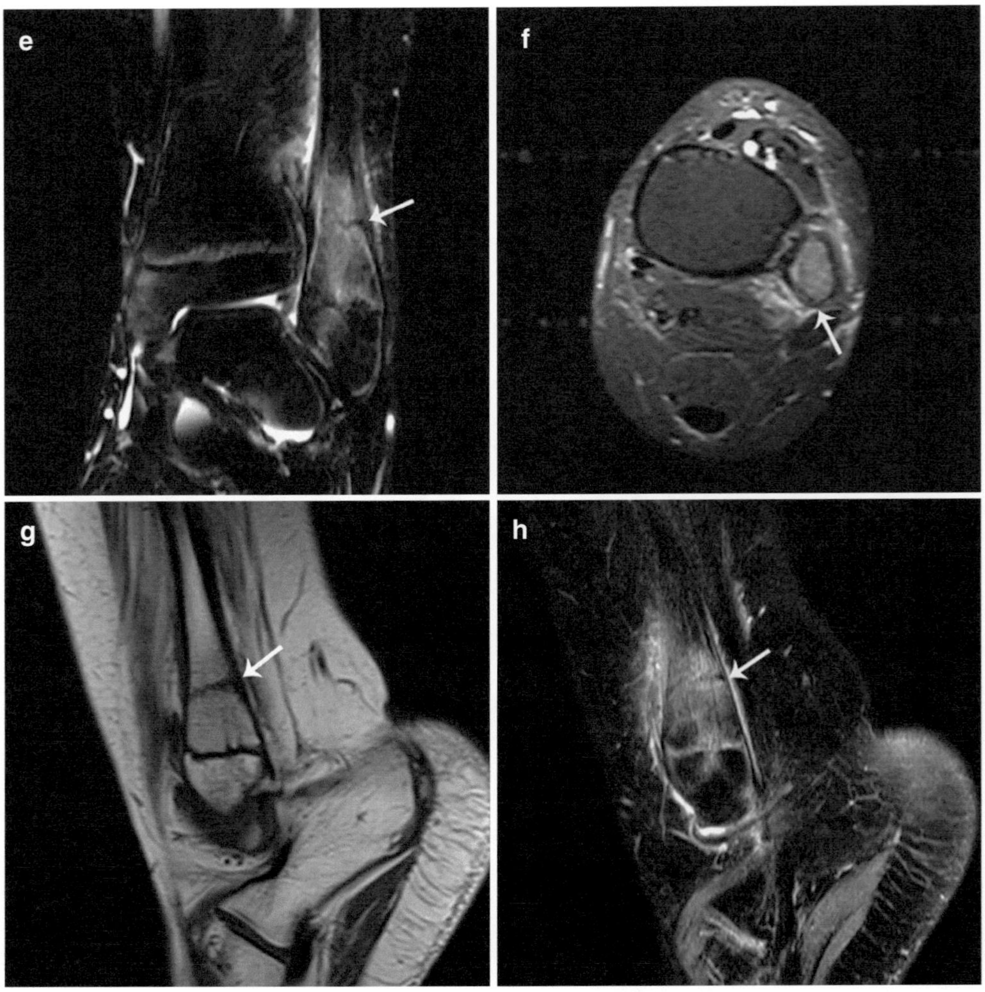

Fig. 12.39 (**e**–**h**) are respectively coronal plane fat inhibition T2WI, transverse plane fat inhibition T2WI, sagittal planeT1WI, and sagittal plane fat inhibition T2WI, showing linear low-density fracture line of lower fibula (white arrow), with surrounding bone marrow and soft tissue edema

12.4 Summary

1. X-ray can meet the diagnosis of lower limb shaft fracture. Attention should be paid to the adjacent joints to prevent missing fractures.
2. In cases of distal 1/3 tibia spiral fracture, the ankle joint should be examined by CT or MRI to confirm the presence of posterior malleolus fracture.
3. The lower limb shaft fracture should be identified with a diaphyseal vascular groove and growth retardation line. The fracture line is sharp, while the vascular groove is smooth and goes in the direction of the joint surface. Growth retardation line can be shown as transverse linear high-density shadow in X-ray and CT scans, while as low-signal line in MRI, perpendicular to the long axis of the diaphysis, without edema around the bone.
4. The lower limb diaphysis is a common site for stress fracture, and attention should be paid to the differential diagnosis. Often, there is no obvious history of trauma in stress fractures, and misdiagnosis is not uncommon. CT and MRI can help diagnose the fracture early.
5. Greenstick fractures in children often occur on the femoral condyle and proximal tibia and are prone to misdiagnosis and missed diagnosis.

Lower Limb Pathological Fractures

13

Xin Xing and Yingze Zhang

Pathological fractures refer to the fractures that occur on the basis of pathological changes to bone, which is usually seen in middle-aged and elderly patients. The older the patient is, the more likely the malignant lesion presents. Fractures caused by benign and malignant bone tumors in metaphysis of frequently occur the long bones, while those caused by non-neoplastic bone diseases mainly occur the in diaphysis. Furthermore, pathological fractures are more common in the lower limb than the upper limb, which is due to the higher morbidity of bone tumors in the lower limb and an increased weight-bearing. For instance, femoral and tibia are the most common areas for pathological fractures. In addition, benign bone tumors generally have no obvious symptoms, or only dull pain, intermittent discomfort, or pain after exertion.

Most patients are initially treated for pain, swelling, and dysfunction to improve the symptoms; they did not detect the pathological fracture until the imaging evaluation was investigated. The pathological fractures are often secondary to primary malignant tumor after taking a clinical history, which shows that these fractures are often caused by trivial trauma. Patients present with mild pain and limitation of motion; however, there are a small number of patients who have no obvious symptoms.

13.1 Identification of Injury Mechanism

Unlike simple traumatic fractures, the bones of pathological fractures are corroded, damaged, and cavitated by certain diseases in advance. They are then exposed to trivial external forces or even gravity, which causes the fracture. Therefore, if the external force causing the fracture is very mild, we should be alert to the possibility of pathological fractures.

13.2 Identification of Symptoms and Signs

The clinical manifestations are pain and limited motion at the fracture site, few patients have no obvious symptoms, and their clinical symptoms are not specific towards the diagnosis.

13.3 Imaging Differential Diagnosis

Imaging cannot only detect the presence of pathological fractures, but also provide clues for the diagnosis of primary bone diseases causing these pathological fractures. The imaging information displayed by CT and MRI has an important reference value for the treatment. Through the spiral CT 3D reconstruction, the three-dimensional condition of pathological fracture can be interpreted more comprehensively and providing more reliable data for surgery.

X. Xing · Y. Zhang (✉)
Department of Orthopaedics, The Third Hospital of Hebei Medical University, Shijiazhuang, Hebei, China

Y. Zhang (ed.), *Differential Diagnosis of Fracture*, https://doi.org/10.1007/978-981-13-8339-7_13

X-ray manifestations: Presence of fractures can be detected, more importantly, the diagnosis of primary bone disease can be obtained through meticulous scrutiny of the radiograph details, for example, whether there is a bony lesion with unclear boundaries, penetration and expansion of bone cortex, irregular nodules and calcifications, and periosteal reaction.

In general, benign bone tumors rarely have periosteal reactions, but exceptionally in eosinophilic granuloma, osteomyelitis, and fatigue fractures, they may have the periosteal reaction which needs to be identified differentially with malignant tumors. However, the shapes of the periosteal reaction are various in different malignant tumors: the most common ones are Codman triangle, onion skin, and spicules of periosteal bone. Codman triangle often appears in osteosarcoma, Ewing's sarcoma, and chondrosarcoma. Whereas the onion skin periosteal reaction is a feature of Ewing's sarcoma, but in fact it can also occur in a few cases of osteosarcoma or osteomyelitis. Spicules of periosteal reactions are more common in osteosarcoma.

CT manifestations: the cortical fracture of the bone in benign lesions is sharp and regular. On the other hand, the fracture of the bony cortex of malignant tumors is irregular and incomplete, often forming soft tissue masses. The irregular bone structure becomes flat, fractured, or partially impacted.

MRI manifestations: hemorrhage or hematoma at the fracture site form short T1, long T2 or long T1, and long T2 signals. The margin of bone destruction of benign tumor is regular, while that of malignant tumor is irregular. Small calcification and bone tissue showed low signal on T1WI and T2WI, which was not easy to identify with other tissues.

1. Differential diagnosis of femoral shaft osteofibrous dysplasia with fractures and normal fractures
   1.1. X-ray (Fig. 13.1a–d)

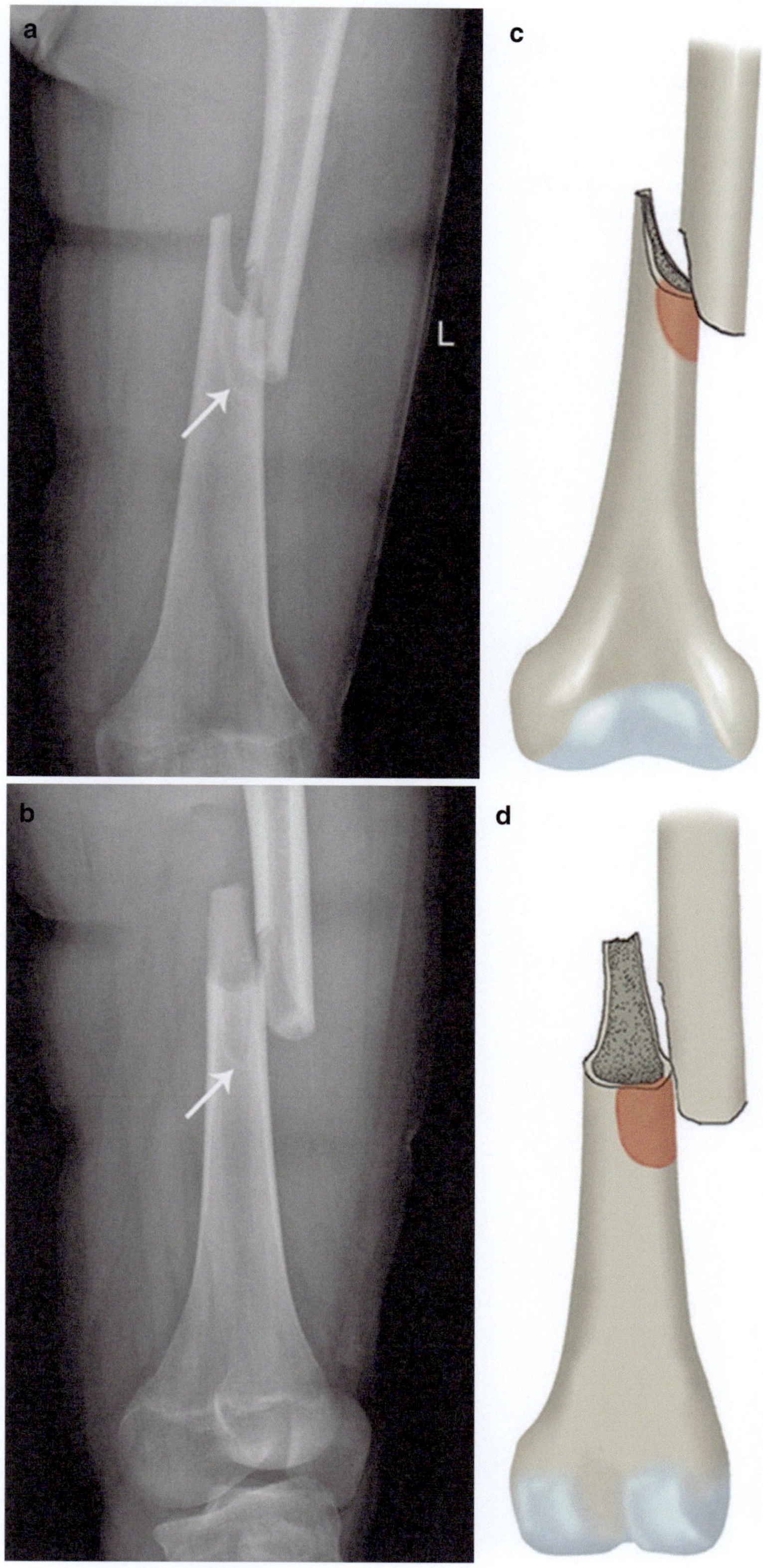

Fig. 13.1 (**a**, **c**) the lateral and anteroposterior (AP) views of the X-ray, showing a circular high-density shadow in distal side of the fracture, with a clear border and a hardened edge (white arrow). Further CT scan was ordered for the purpose of definite diagnosis. Schematic diagram (**b**, **d**)

1.2. CT scan (Fig. 13.1e, f)

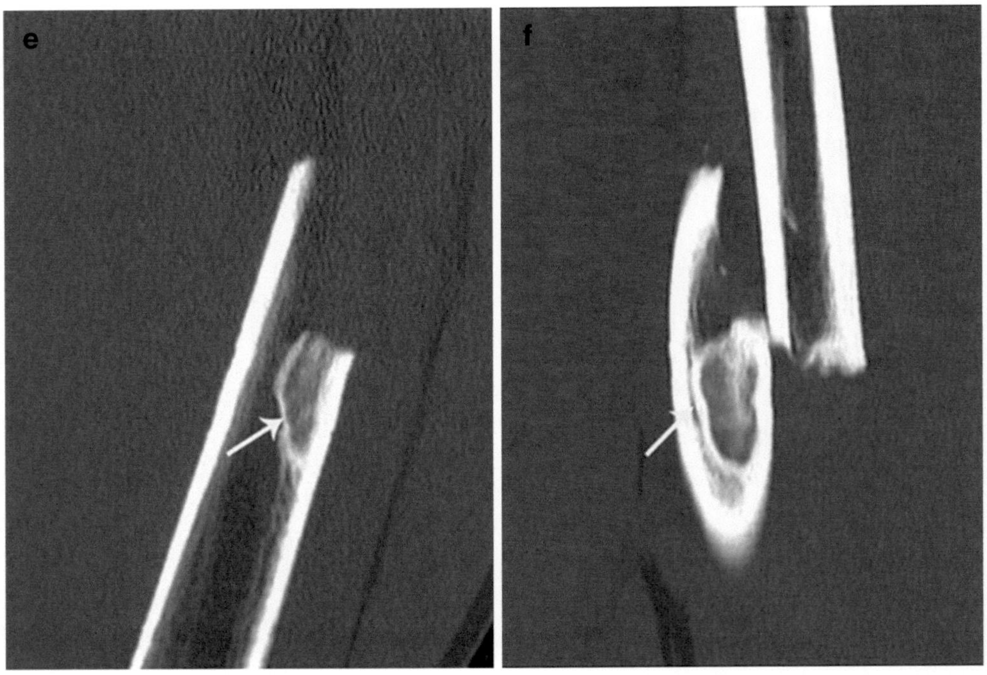

Fig. 13.1 (**e**, **f**) are CT reconstruction of sagittal and coronal plane, showing a round sclerotic lesion with a clear border and a hardened edge (white arrow) in the distal side of the fracture. Surgical biopsy confirmed osteofibrous dysplasia with pathological fracture

2. Identification of giant cell tumors of the distal femur with fracture and normal fracture
   2.1. X-ray (Fig. 13.2a–d)

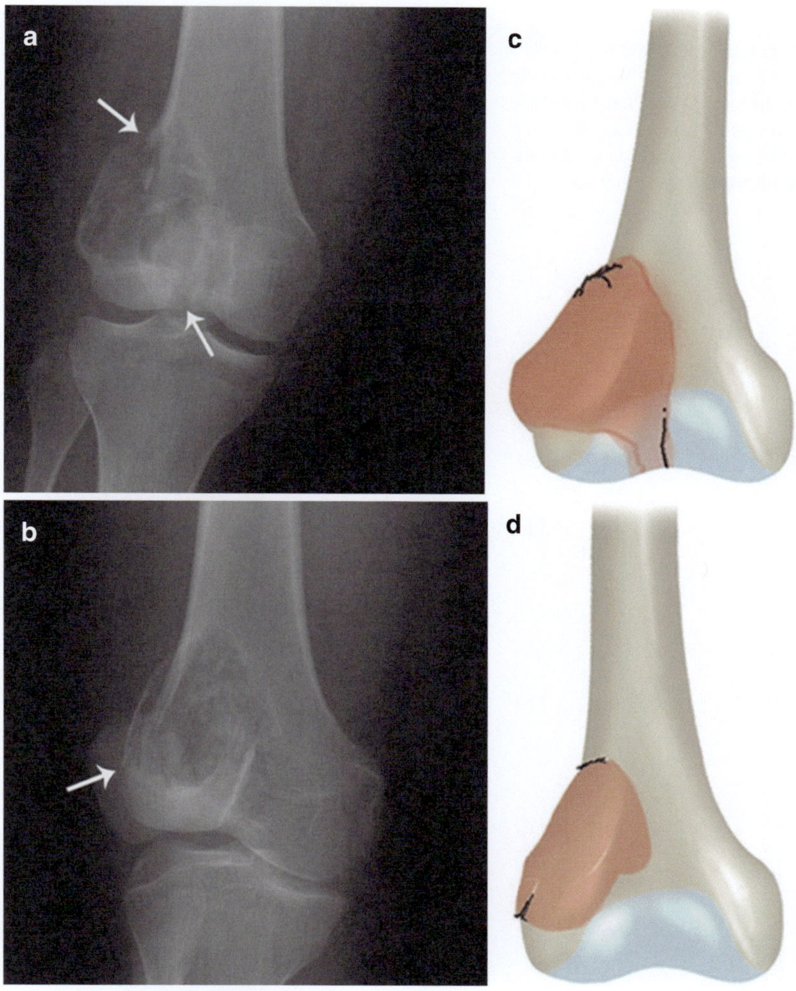

Fig. 13.2 (**a**, **c**) are the lateral and anteroposterior (AP) views of the X-ray, showing osteolytic destruction, swelling, cortical fracture (white arrow) in distal femur. Further CT scan was performed for the purpose of definite diagnosis. Schematic diagram (**b**, **d**)

   2.2. CT scan (Fig. 13.2e, f)

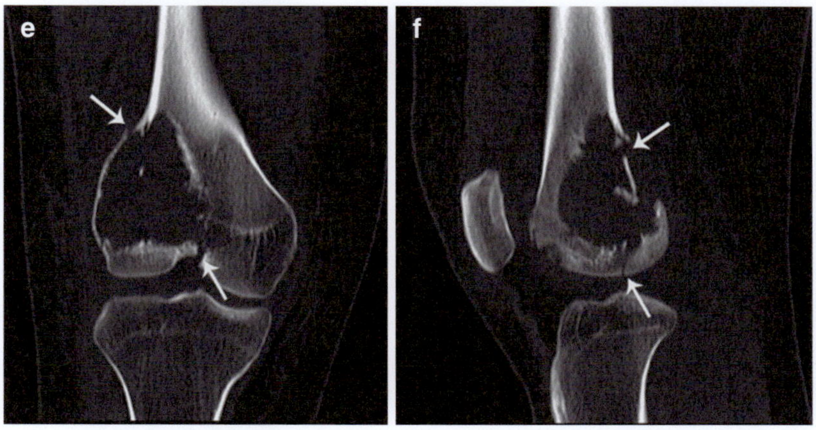

Fig. 13.2 (**e**, **f**) CT reconstruction of coronal and sagittal plane, showing osteolytic swelling bone destruction with a clear border and cortical fracture (white arrow) in distal femur

3. Identification of the femoral bone cyst with fracture and normal fracture
   3.1. X-ray (Fig. 13.3a–d)

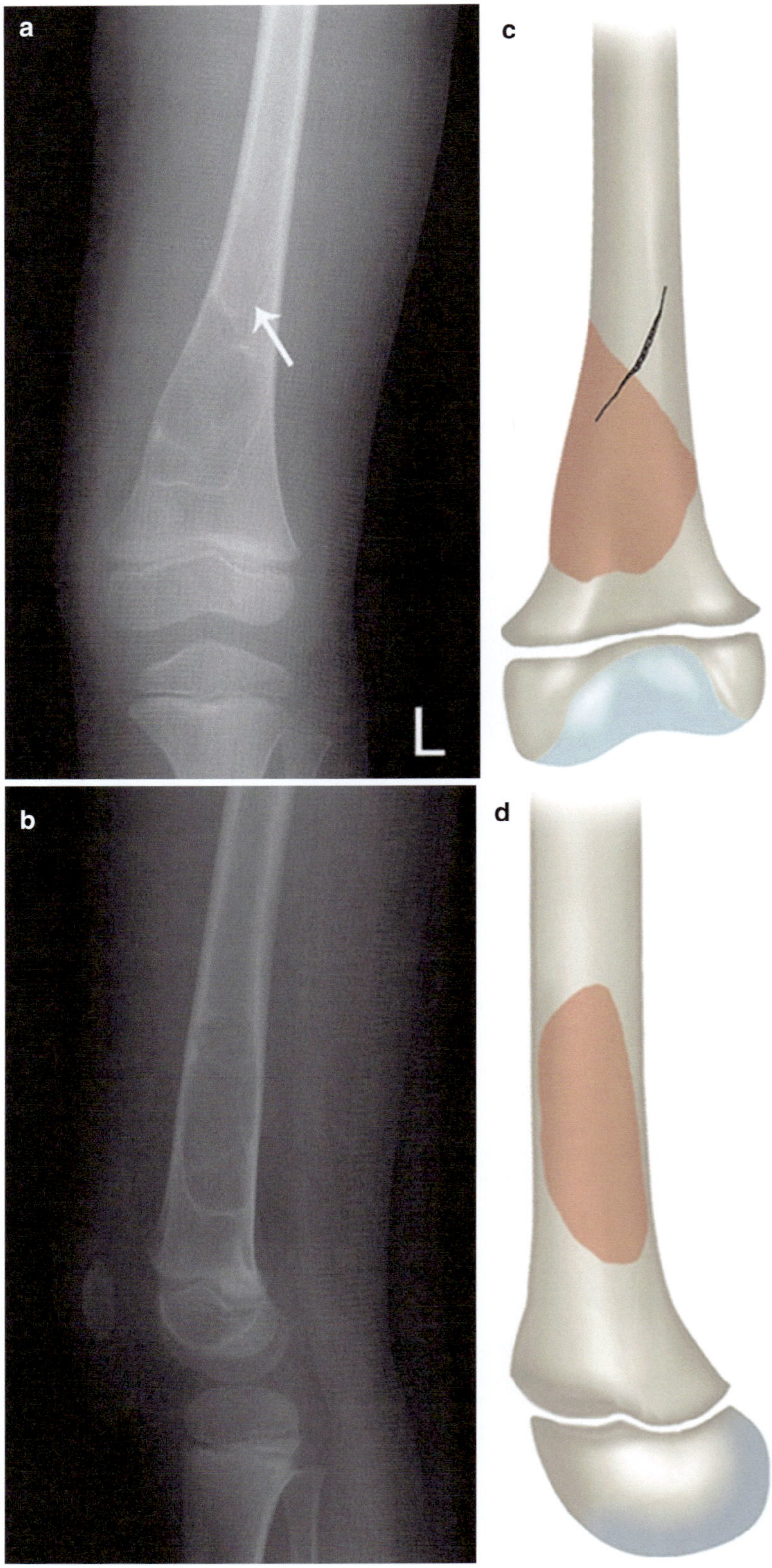

Fig. 13.3 (**a**, **c**) are the lateral and anteroposterior (AP) views of the X-ray, showing swelling, bone destruction with clear boundaries. Fracture line (thin white arrow) can be seen in anteroposterior (AP) view, while it is unclear in lateral view. Schematic diagram (**b**, **d**)

3.2. CT scan (Fig. 13.3e, f)

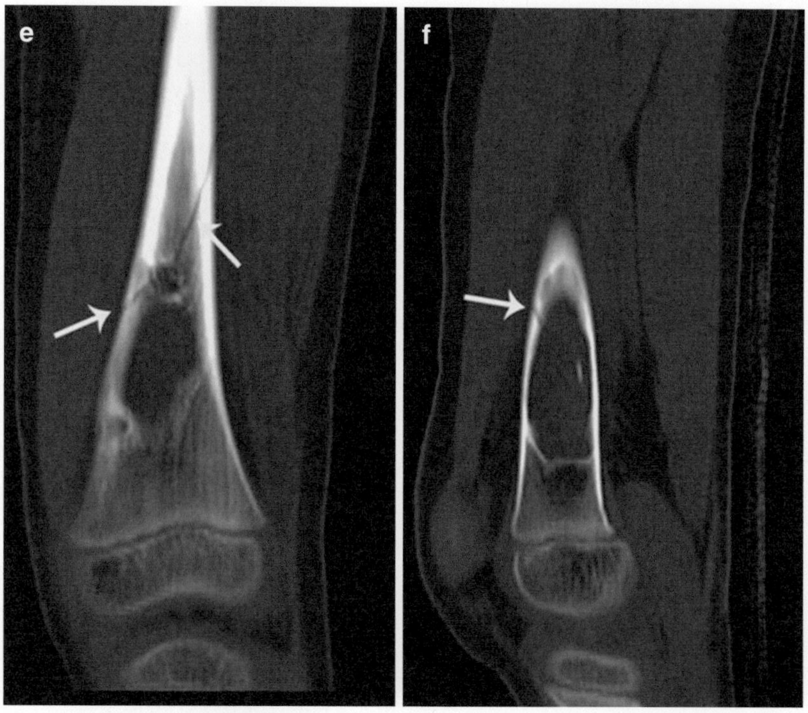

Fig. 13.3 (**e**, **f**) are respectively CT reconstruction of coronal and sagittal plane, showing a clear fracture line (thin arrow)

3.3. MRI scan (Fig. 13.3g, h)

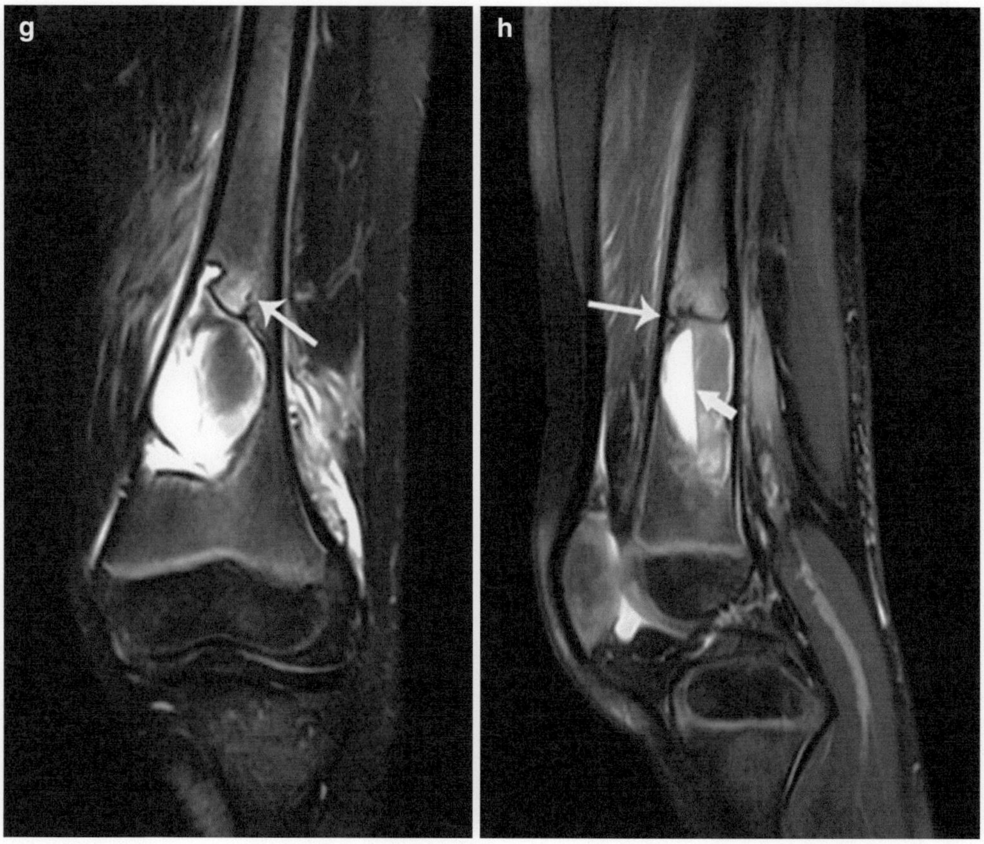

Fig. 13.3 (**g**) is MRI coronal plane fat-suppression T2WI, showing an uneven high signal with clear boundaries and fracture line (thin white arrow). (**h**) is MRI sagittal plane fat-suppression T2WI, showing a large liquid–liquid plane (thick white arrow) and the fracture line (thin white arrow) above

4. Identification of femoral bone cyst with fracture and normal fracture
   4.1. X-ray (Fig. 13.4a–d)

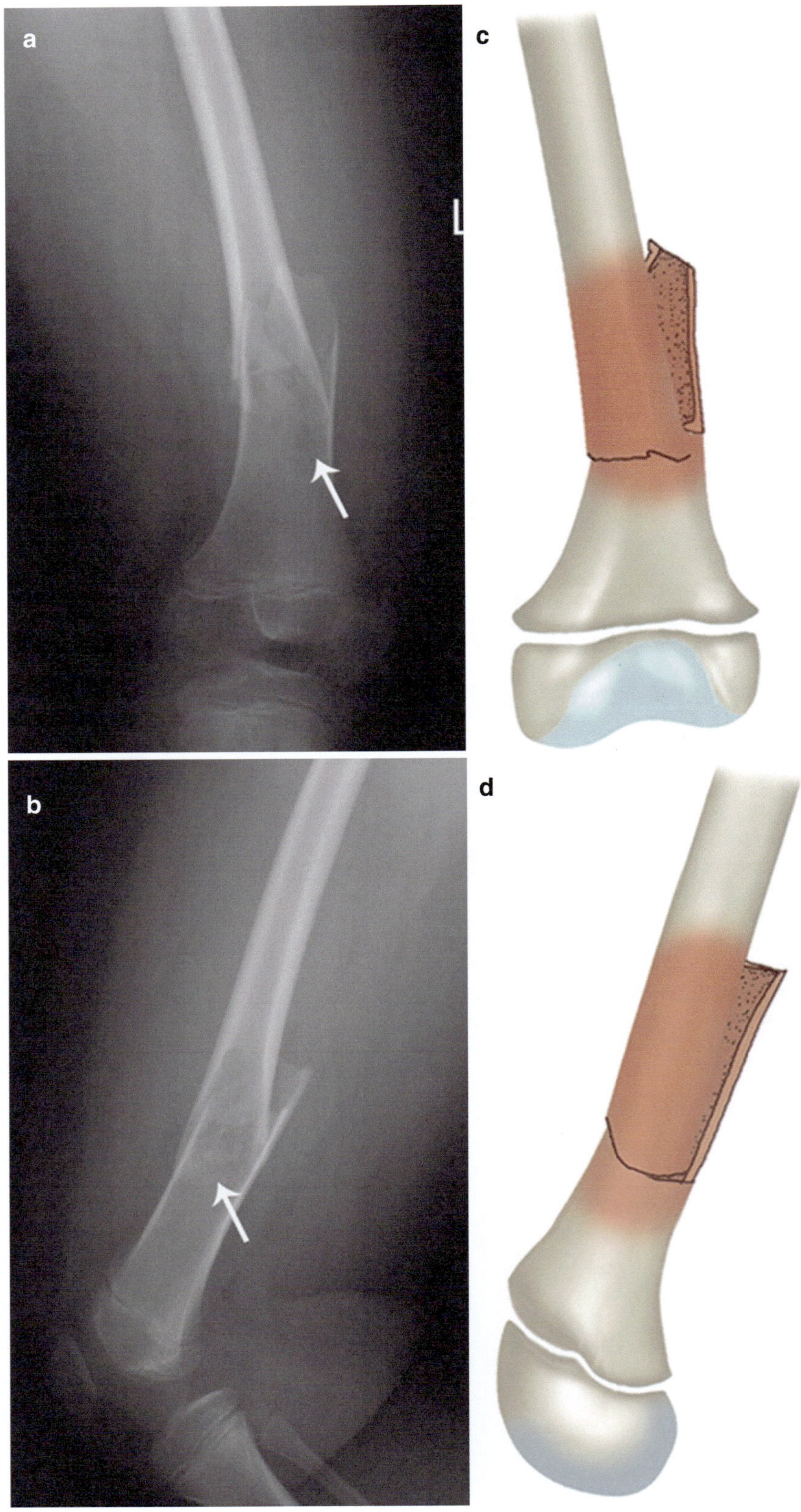

Fig. 13.4 (**a**, **c**) are respectively the lateral and anteroposterior (AP) views of the X-ray, showing swelling, bone destruction with fracture and dislocation. Schematic diagram (**b**, **d**)

4.2. CT scan (Fig. 13.4e, f)

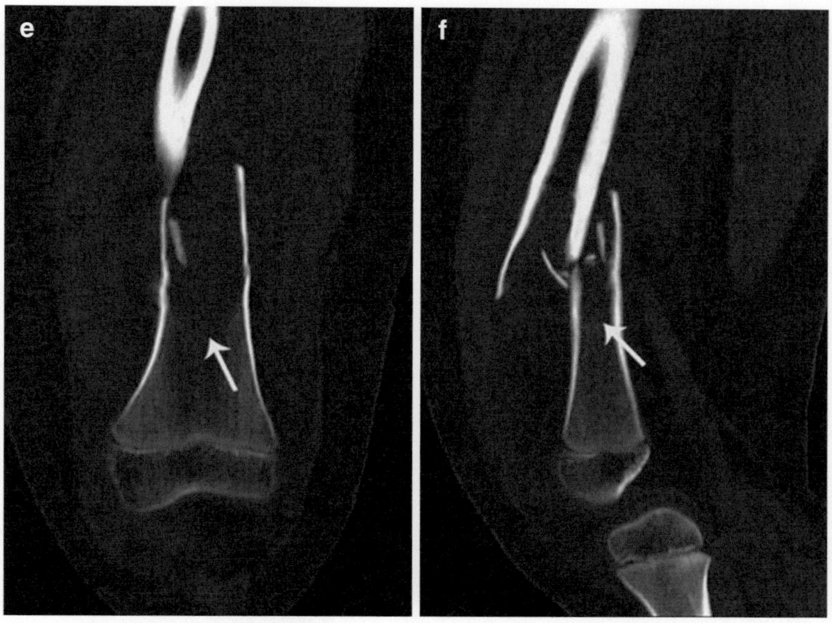

Fig. 13.4 (**e**, **f**) are respectively CT reconstruction of coronal and sagittal plane, showing bone destruction, clear border (white arrow), fracture dislocation, and fracture plate collapse

4.3. MRI scan (Fig. 13.4g, h)

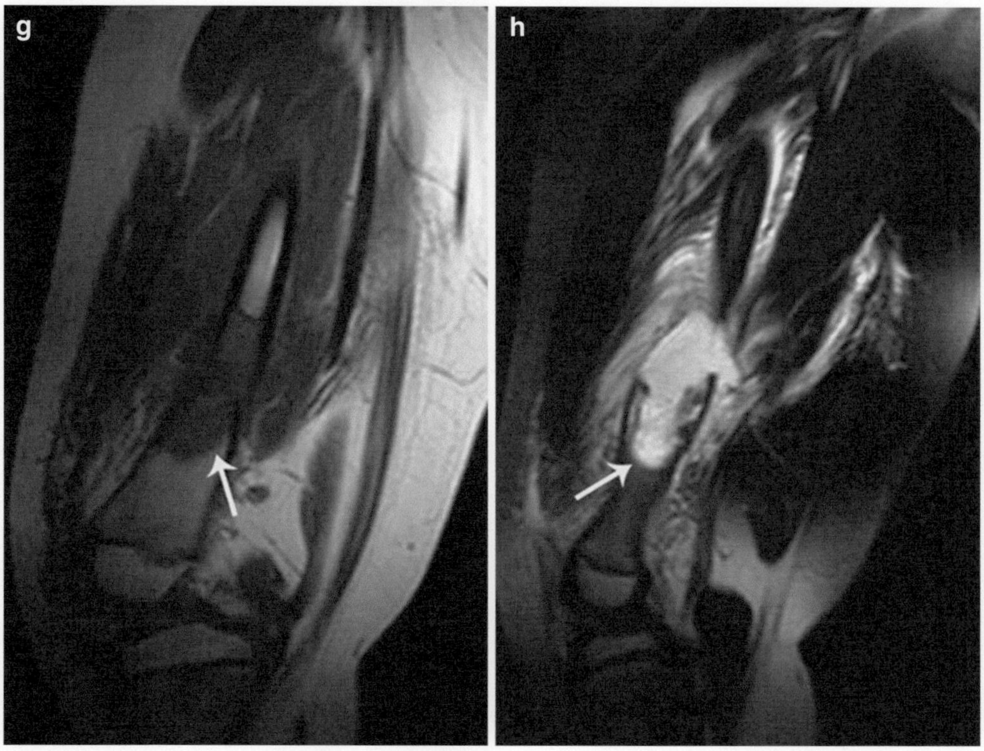

Fig. 13.4 (**g**, **h**) are respectively MRI T1WI and fat-suppression T2WI of sagittal plane, showing bone destruction, low signal in T1WI, and high signal in fat-suppression T2WI. The boundaries are clear (white arrow), with visible fracture line and surrounding soft tissue diffuse swelling

5. Identification of femoral giant cell tumor with fracture and normal fracture
   5.1. X-ray (Fig. 13.5a–d)

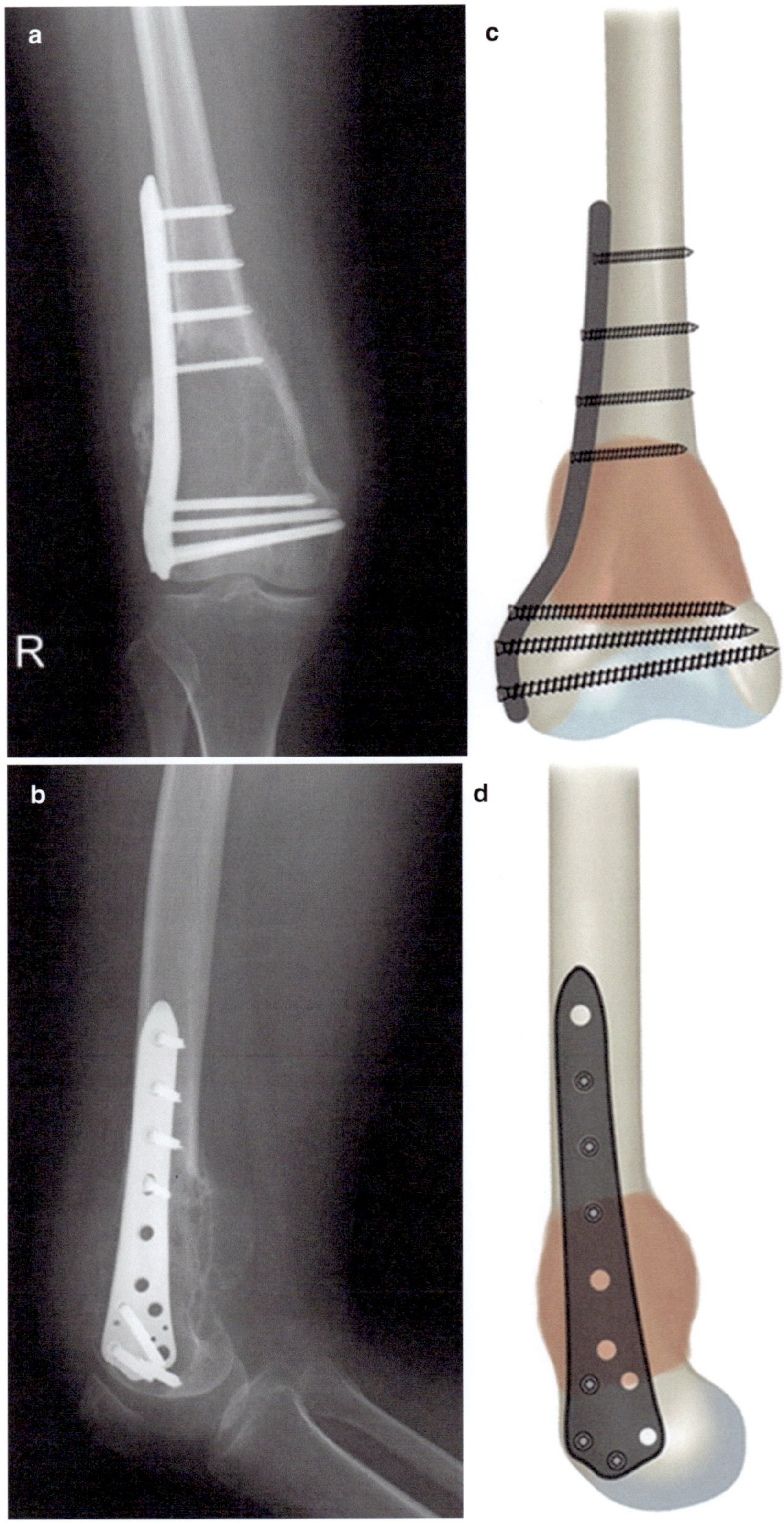

Fig. 13.5 (**a**, **c**) are respectively the lateral and anteroposterior (AP) views of the X-ray, showing swelling, bone destruction in distal right femur with uniform density. There is no calcification, and the femoral fixation shadow can be seen. Further CT scan was performed for the purpose of definite diagnosis. Schematic diagram (**b**, **d**)

5.2. CT scan (Fig. 13.5e, f)

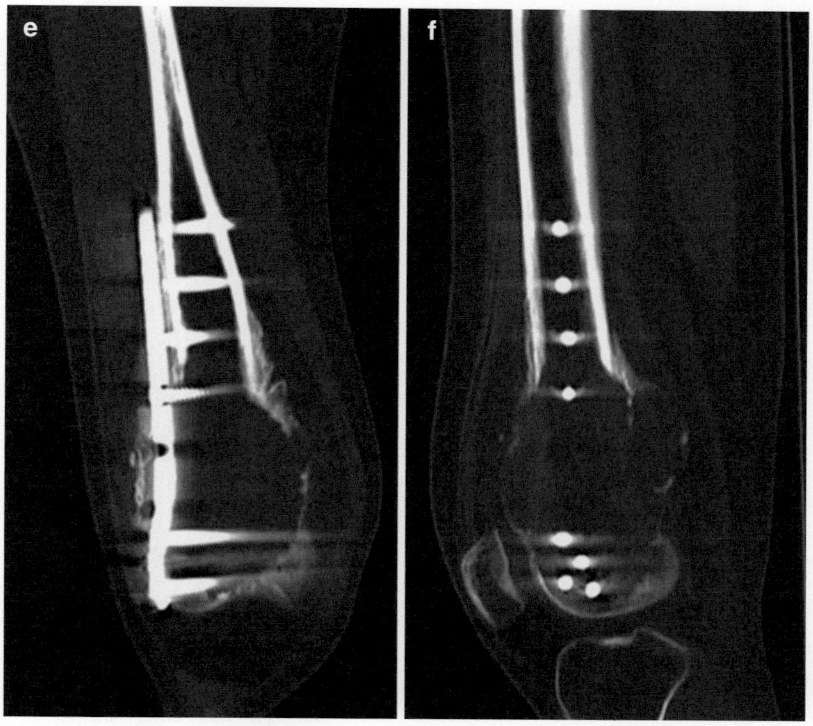

Fig. 13.5 (**e**, **f**) are respectively CT reconstruction of coronal and sagittal plane, showing swelling bone destruction in distal right femur with uniform density. There is no calcification, and the femoral fixation shadow can be seen

6. Identification of fibular nonossifying fibroma with fracture and normal fracture
   6.1. X-ray (Fig. 13.6a–d)

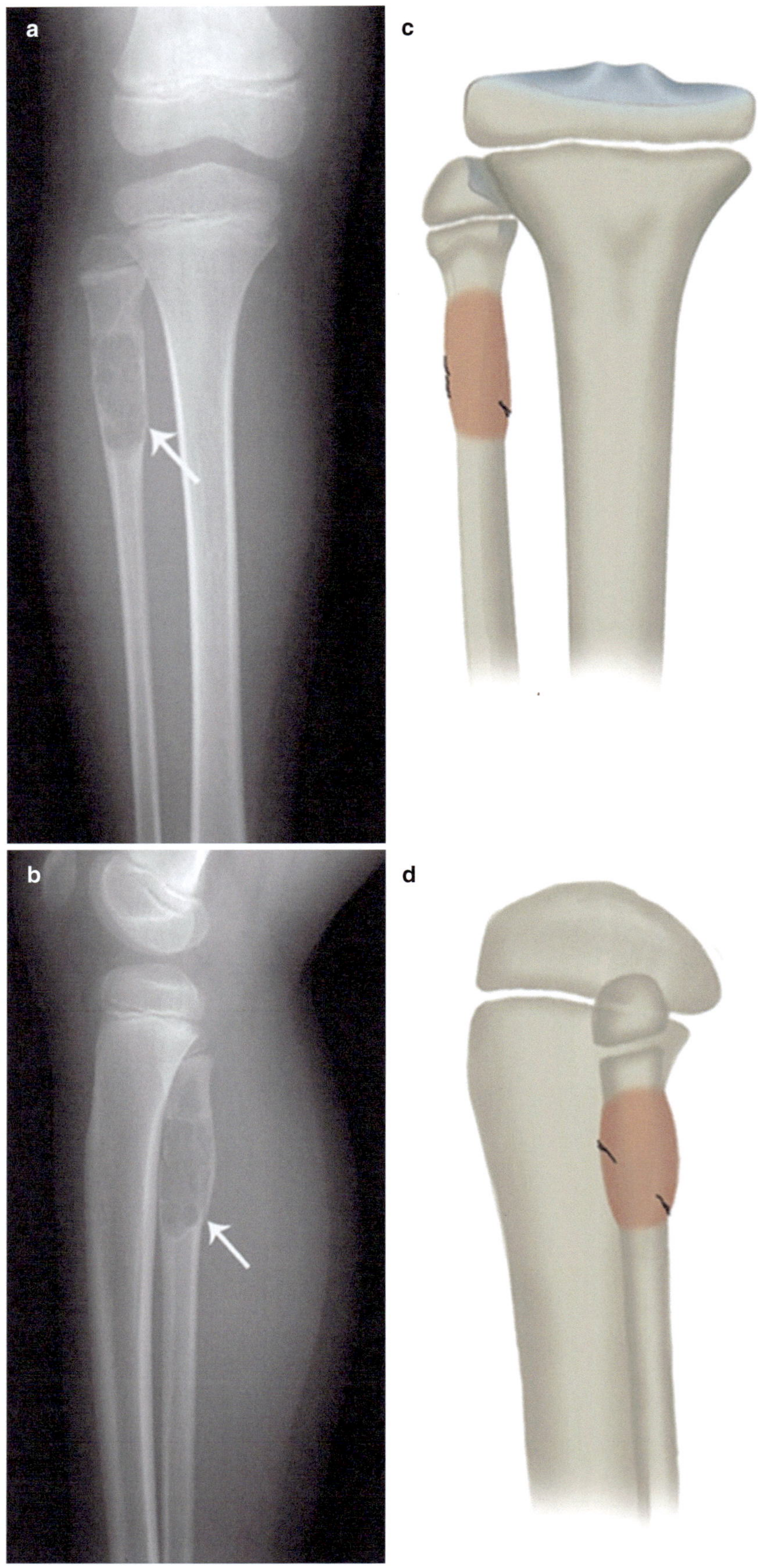

Fig. 13.6 (**a**, **c**) are respectively the lateral and anteroposterior (AP) views of the X-ray, showing swelling bone destruction in upper fibula with clear border and uniform density. There is no calcification, and the fracture line (white arrow) can be seen. Schematic diagram (**b**, **d**)

6.2. CT scan (Fig. 13.6e–h)

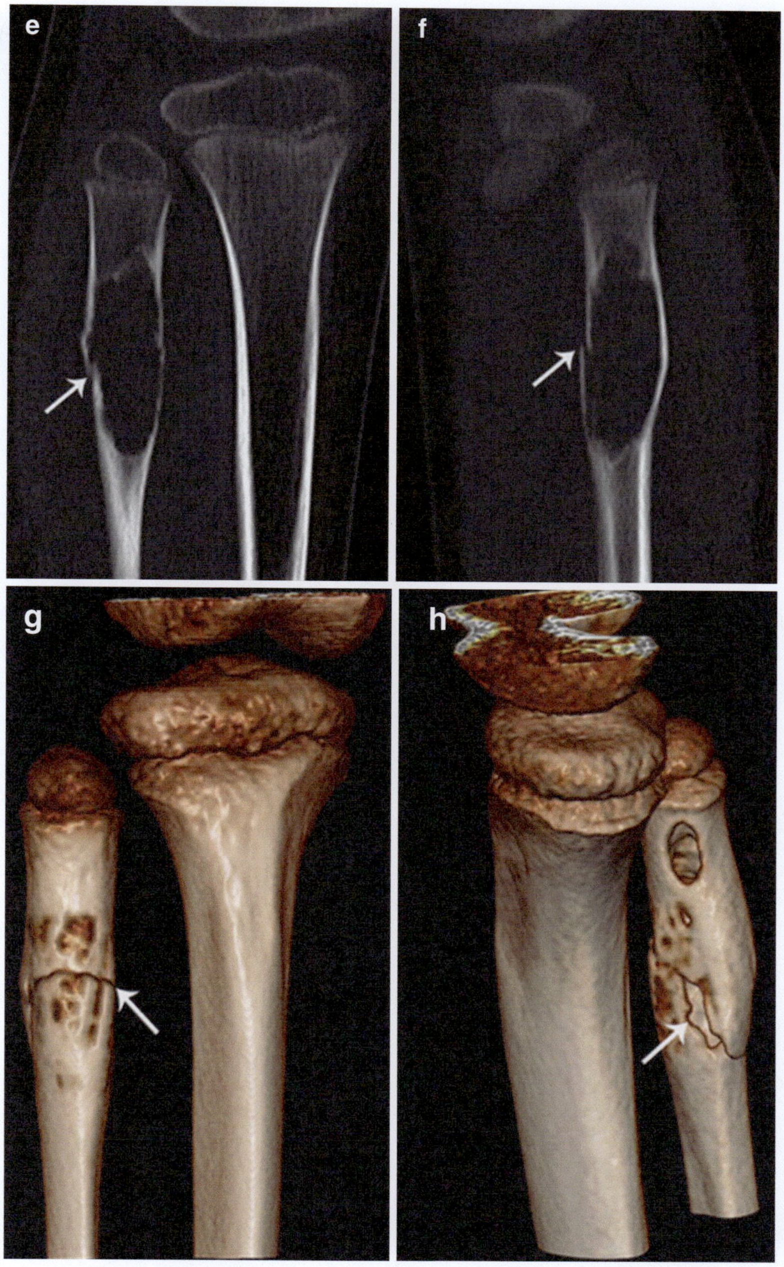

Fig. 13.6 (**e–h**) are respectively CT reconstruction of coronal and sagittal plane, anterior and anterolateral views of CT 3D reconstruction, showing bone destruction in the upper fibula with clear border and uniform density. There is no calcification, and the fracture line (white arrow) can be seen

6.3. MRI scan (Fig. 13.6i, j)

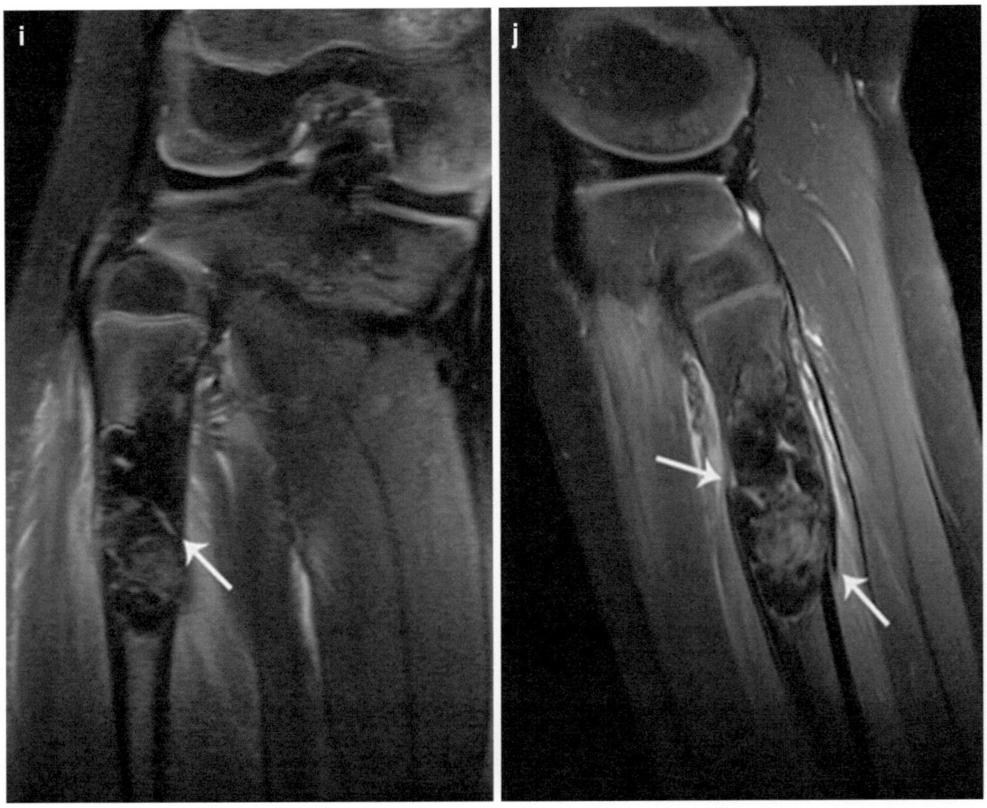

Fig. 13.6 (**i**, **j**) are respectively MRI fat-suppression T2WI of coronal and sagittal plane, showing uneven low signal with visible fracture line (white arrow) and the surrounding soft tissue swelling

7. Identification of metastatic tumors in left femoral neck with fracture and normal fracture
   7.1. X-ray (Fig. 13.7a, b)

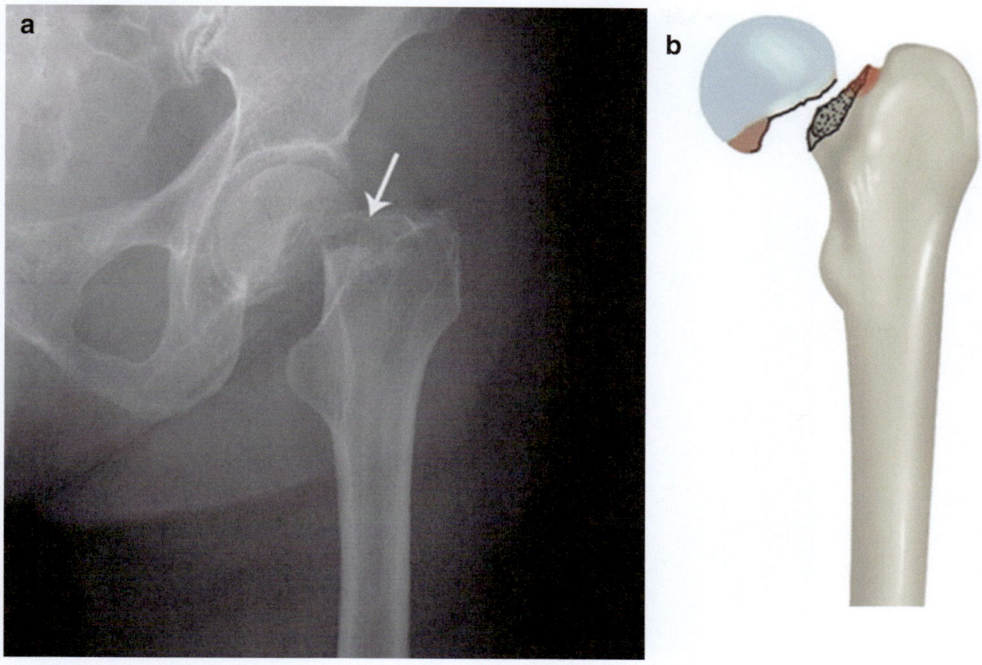

Fig. 13.7 (**a**) is the anteroposterior (AP) view of the X-ray, showing left femoral neck fracture, dislocation, uneven fracture end density, and less sharp fracture line (white arrow). Schematic diagram (**b**)

   7.2. CT scan (Fig. 13.7c–e)

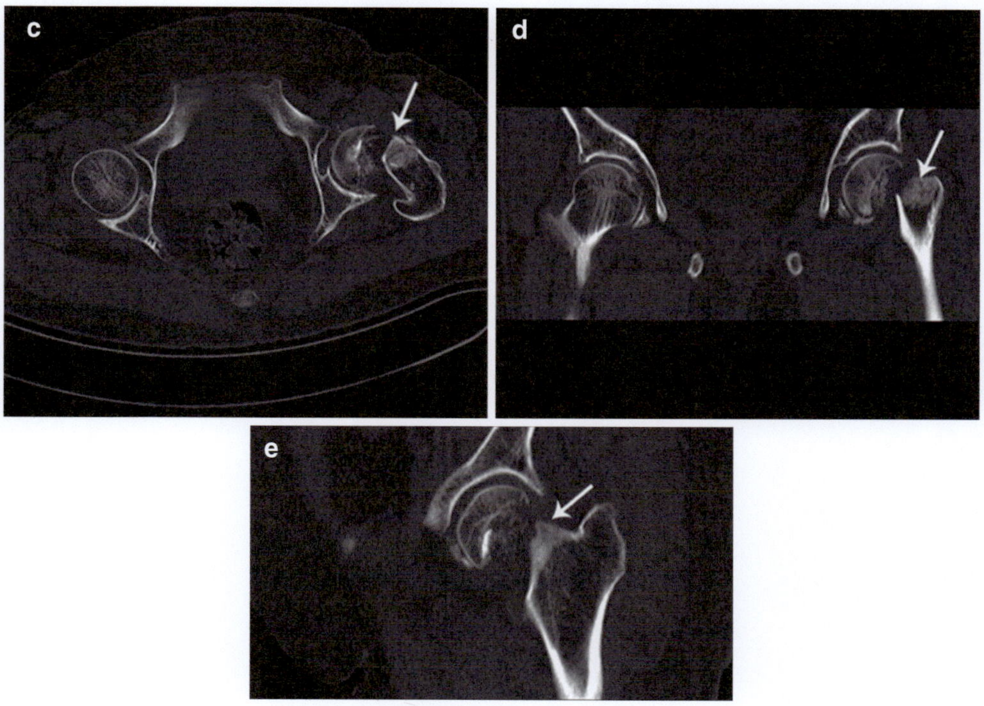

Fig. 13.7 (**c**–**e**) are respectively CT reconstruction of transverse, coronal, and sagittal plane, showing left femoral neck fracture with uneven sclerosis in fracture ends (white arrow)

7.3. MRI scan (Fig. 13.7f–i)

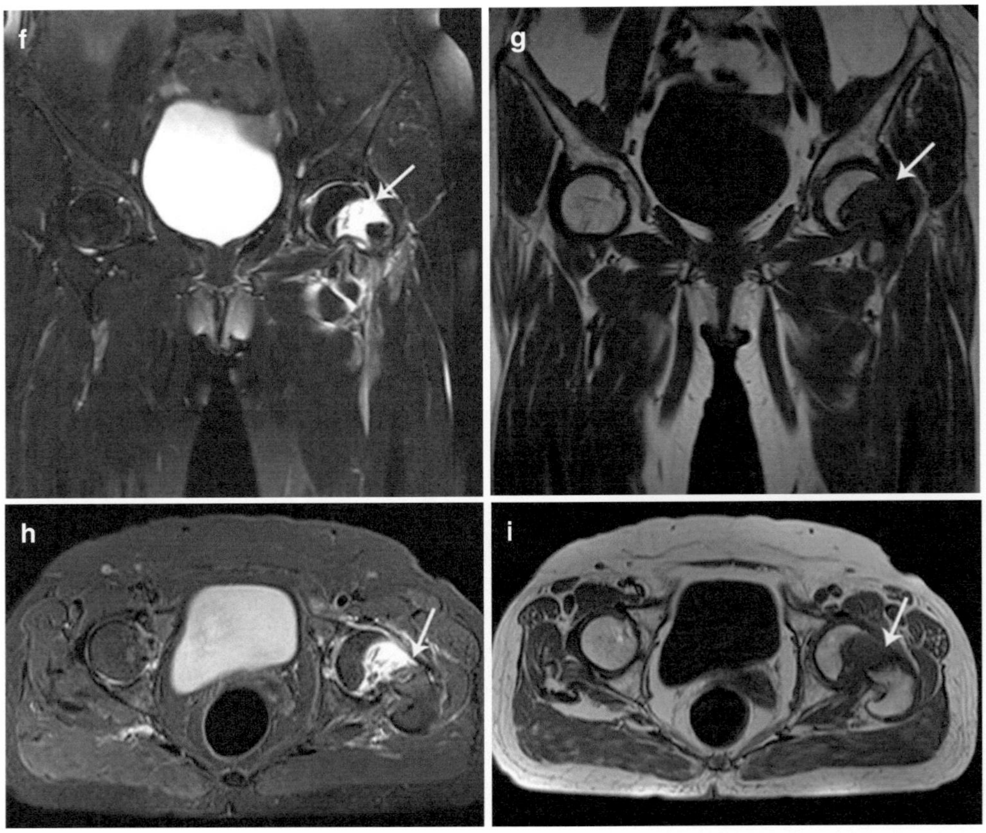

Fig. 13.7 (**f–i**) are respectively MRI fat-suppression T2WI and T1WI of the coronal plane, fat-suppression T2WI and T1WI of transverse plane, showing a left femoral neck fracture, dislocation, nonuniform signal at the fracture end, circular low signal in T1WI, and high signal in fat-suppression T2WI (white arrow)

8. Identification of small cell malignant tumor of femur with fracture and normal fracture
   8.1. X-ray (Fig. 13.8a–d)

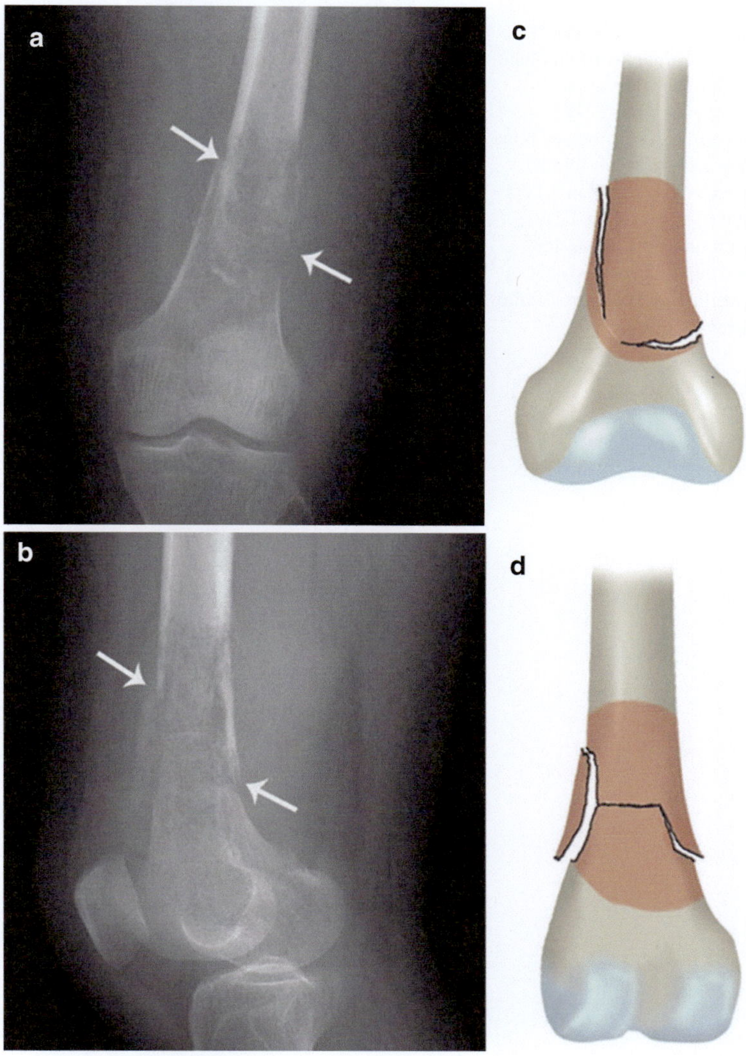

Fig. 13.8 (**a**–**c**) are respectively the lateral and anteroposterior (AP) views of the X-ray, showing a large area of osteolytic destruction in the lower part of the left femur with unclear boundaries and uneven density. The bone shows freeze-thaw change and fracture line (white arrow). Schematic diagram (**b**, **d**)

8.2. MRI scan (Fig. 13.8e–h)

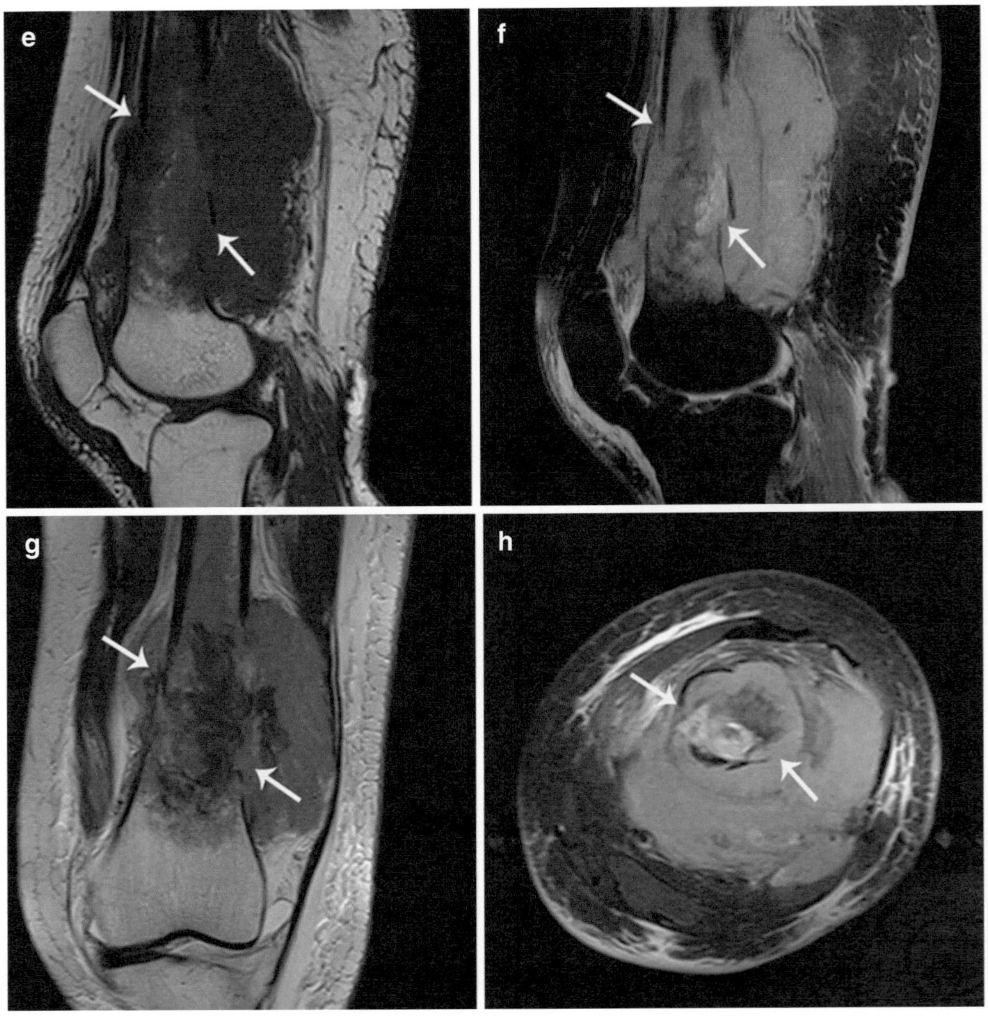

Fig. 13.8 (**e**–**h**) are respectively MRI T1WI and fat-suppression T2WI of sagittal plane, coronal plane T2WI and transverse fat-suppression T2WI, showing a large area of bone destruction in left femur, uneven low signal in T1WI and high signal on T2WI, with unclear boundaries, surrounding soft tissue swelling and fracture (white arrow)

9. Identification of multiple myeloma with right femur fracture and normal fracture
   9.1. CT scan (Fig. 13.9a, b)

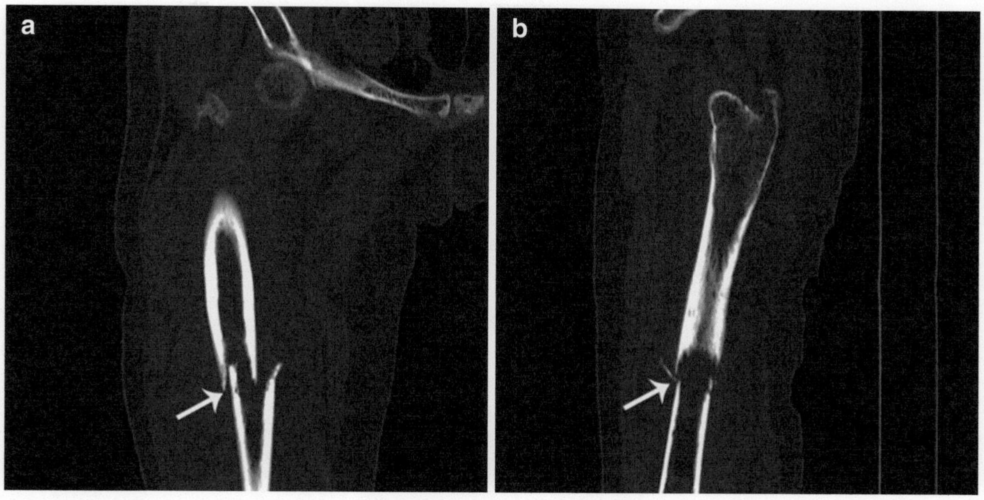

Fig. 13.9 (**a**, **b**) are respectively CT reconstruction of coronal and sagittal plane, showing osteolytic bone destruction in the right femoral shaft, with fracture and dislocation (white arrow)

   9.2. MRI scan (Fig. 13.9c, d)

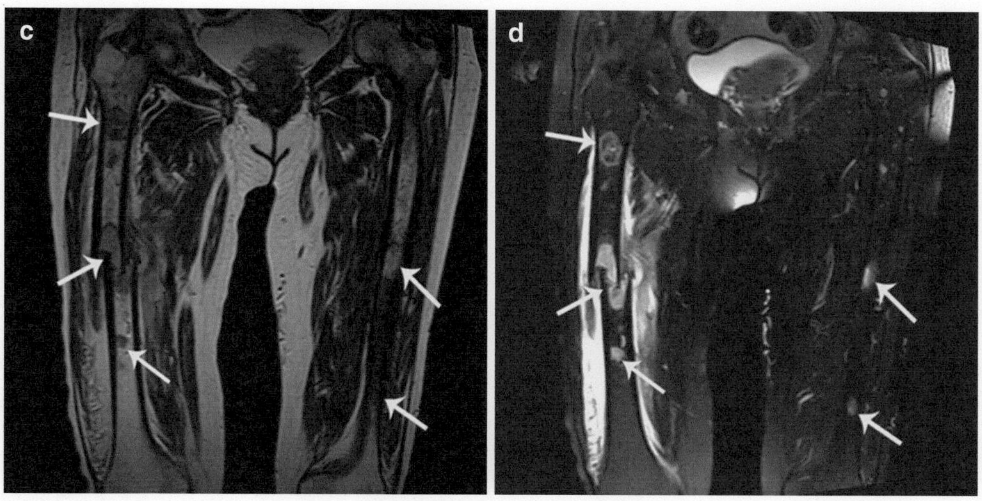

Fig. 13.9 (**c**, **d**) are respectively MRI T1WI and fat-suppression T2WI of the coronal plane, showing multiple destruction in bilateral femur, low signal in T1WI and high signal in fat-suppression T2WI (white arrow). The lesion edge is clear and the signal is not uniform. It also shows right femur fracture, dislocation, and surrounding soft tissue swelling

10. Identification of pathological fracture of left femur and normal fracture
    10.1. X-ray (Fig. 13.10a, b)

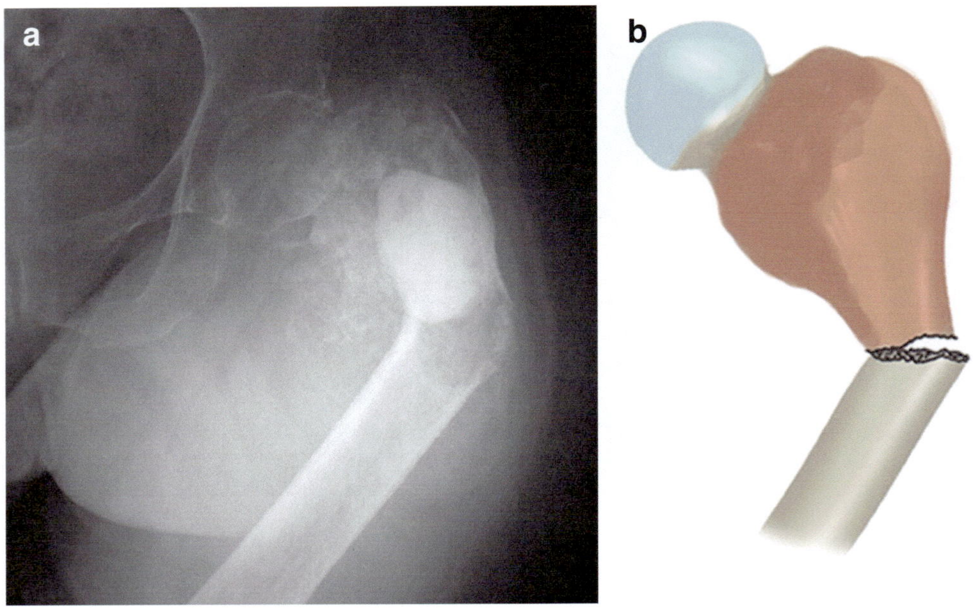

Fig. 13.10 (**a**) is the anteroposterior (AP) view of the X-ray, showing the destruction and expansion of proximal left femur, with high-density shadow and fracture visible in it, and schematic diagram (**b**)

    10.2. CT scan (Fig. 13.10c)

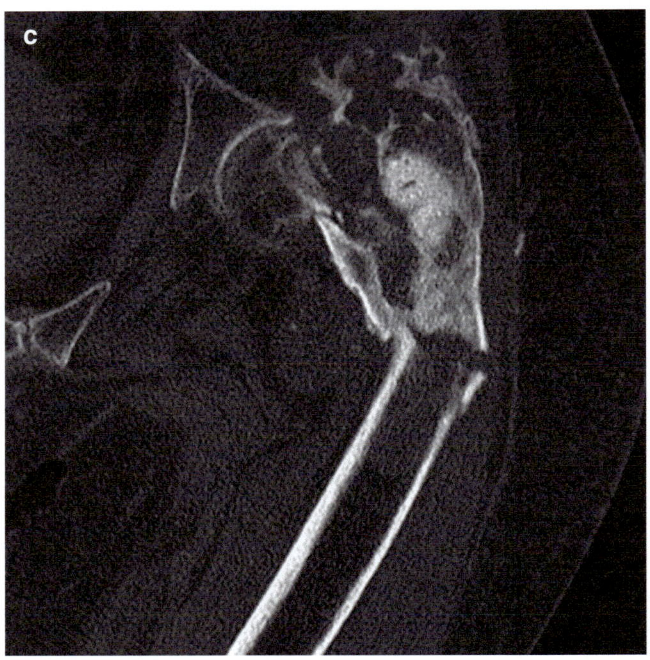

Fig. 13.10 (**c**) is CT coronal plane reconstruction, showing destruction and expansion of the proximal left femur, with high-density shadow and fracture visible in it

10.3. MRI scan (Fig. 13.10d, e)

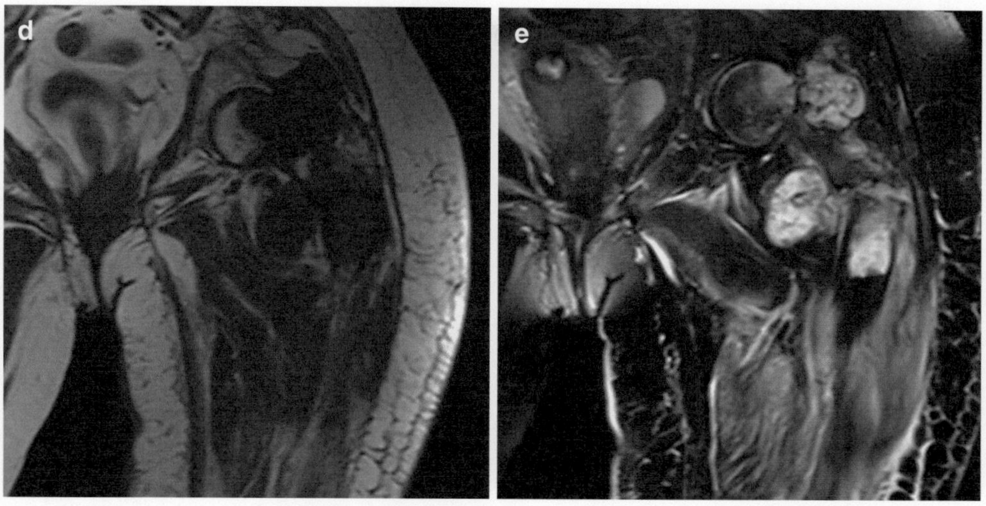

Fig. 13.10 (**d**, **e**) are respectively MRI T1WI and fat-suppression T2WI of the coronal plane, showing bone destruction of proximal left femoral shaft, uneven low signal in T1WI and high signal in fat-suppression T2WI, indicating soft tissue mass, and fracture line presented long T1 and long T2 signal shadow

11. Identification of right femoral metastatic tumor of lung cancer with fracture and normal fracture
    11.1. X-ray (Fig. 13.11a–d)

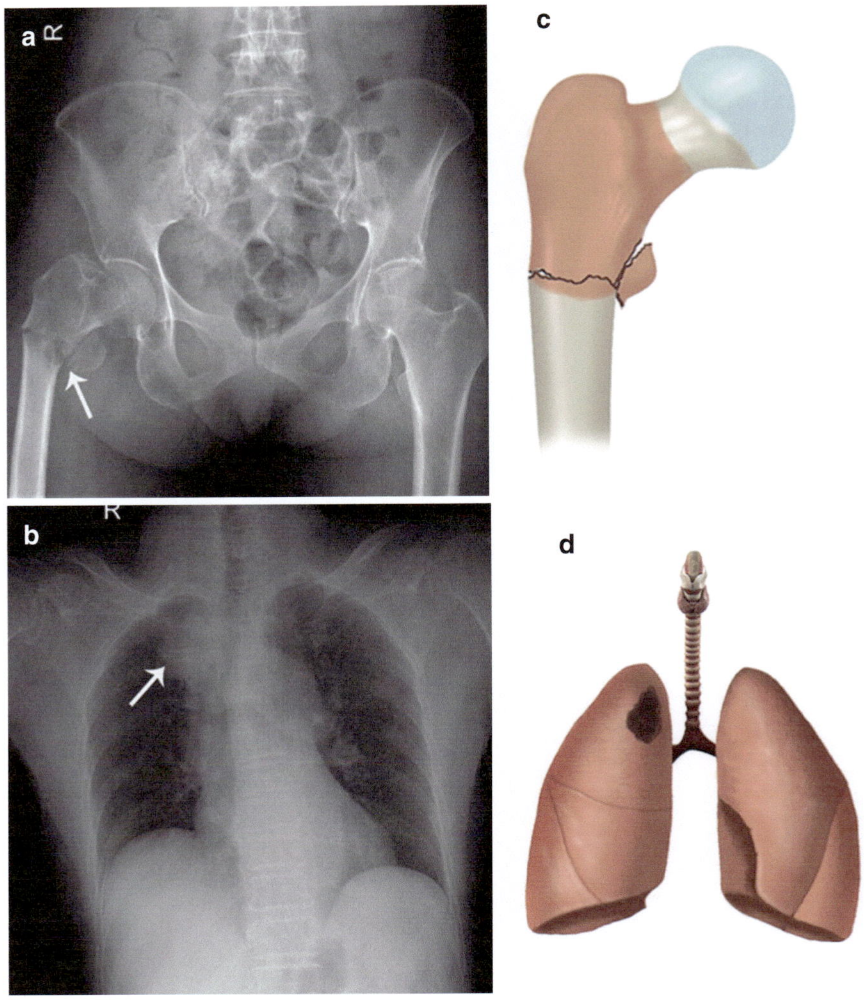

Fig. 13.11 (**a**) is the pelvic anteroposterior (AP) view of the X-ray, showing the osteolytic destruction in upper right femur with unclear boundary, visible fracture line, and angulated dislocation (white arrow). (**c**) is a chest anteroposterior (AP) view of the X-ray, showing a mediastinal mass (white arrow) in the upper right lung. Schematic diagram (**b**)

    11.2. CT scan (Fig. 13.11e, f)

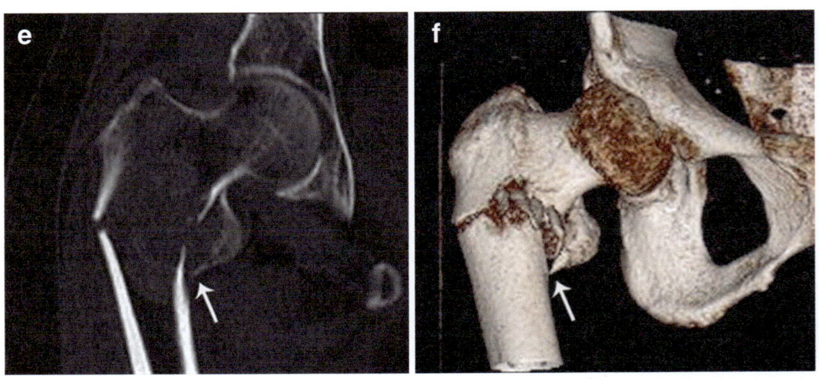

Fig. 13.11 (**e**, **f**) are respectively CT coronal plane reconstruction and front view of 3D reconstruction, showing osteolytic destruction in upper right femur with unclear boundary, visible fracture line and angulated dislocation (white arrow)

11.3. MRI scan (Fig. 13.11g, h)

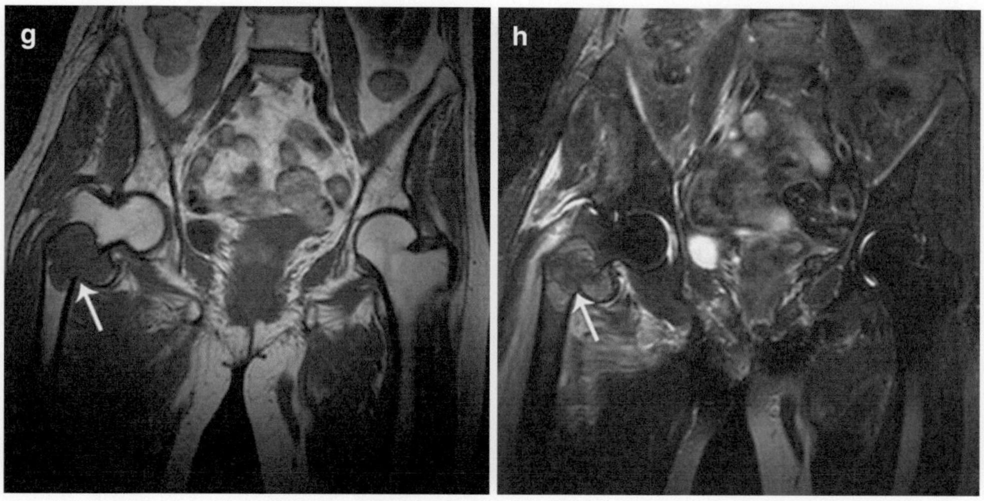

Fig. 13.11 (**g**, **h**) are respectively MRI T1WI and fat-suppression T2WI of the coronal plane, showing osteolytic destruction in upper right femur, uniform low signal in T1WI, and high signal in fat-suppression T2WI with clear boundary, indicating a fracture (white arrow) and surrounding soft tissue swelling

12. Identification of femoral telangiectasia osteosarcoma with fracture and normal fracture
    12.1. X-ray (Fig. 13.12a–d)

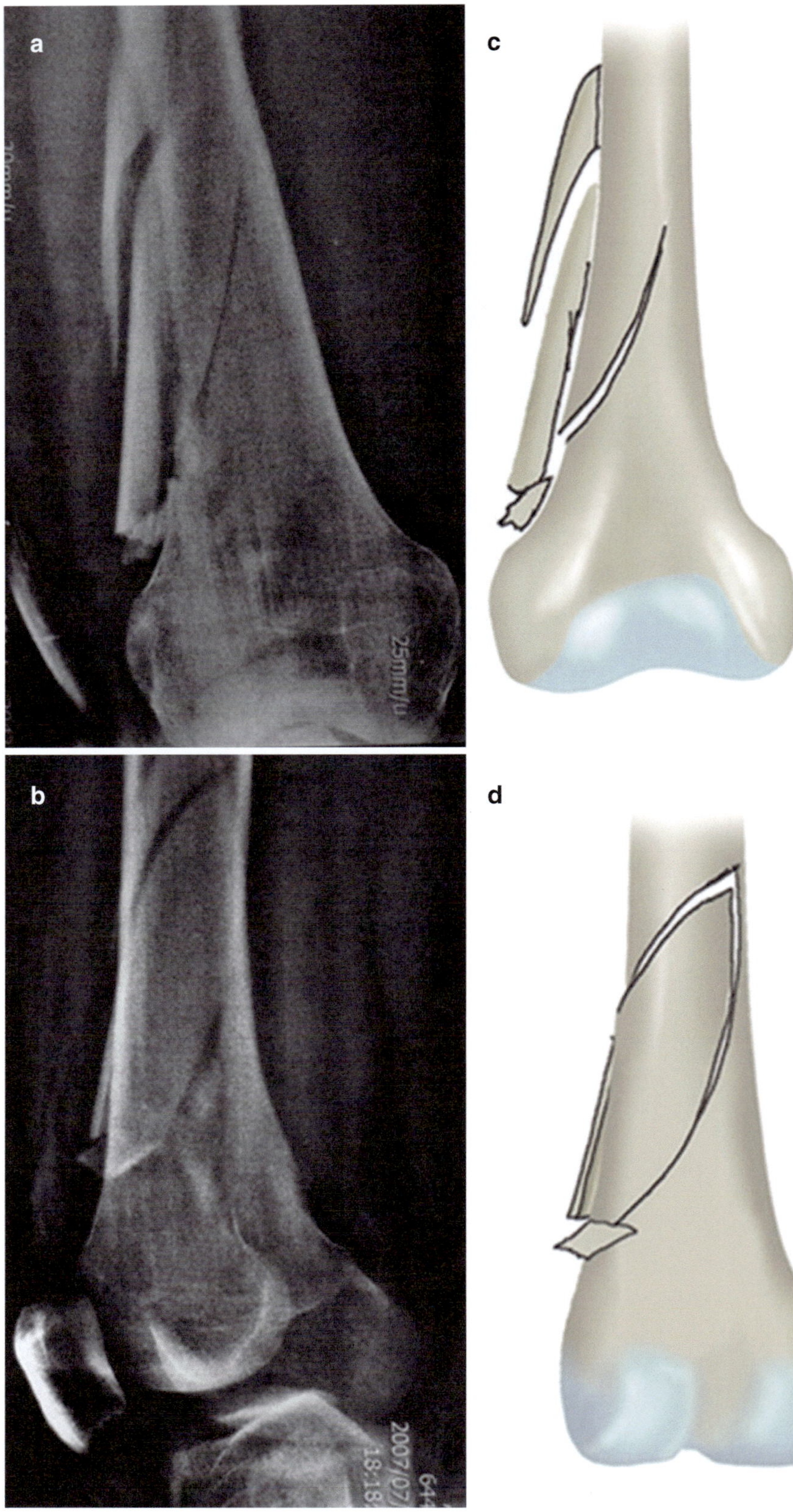

Fig. 13.12 (**a**, **c**) are respectively the lateral and anteroposterior (AP) views of the X-ray took in local hospital after injury, showing a femoral fracture and inconspicuous bone damage. Schematic diagram (**b**, **d**)

12.2. CT scan (Fig. 13.12e–i)

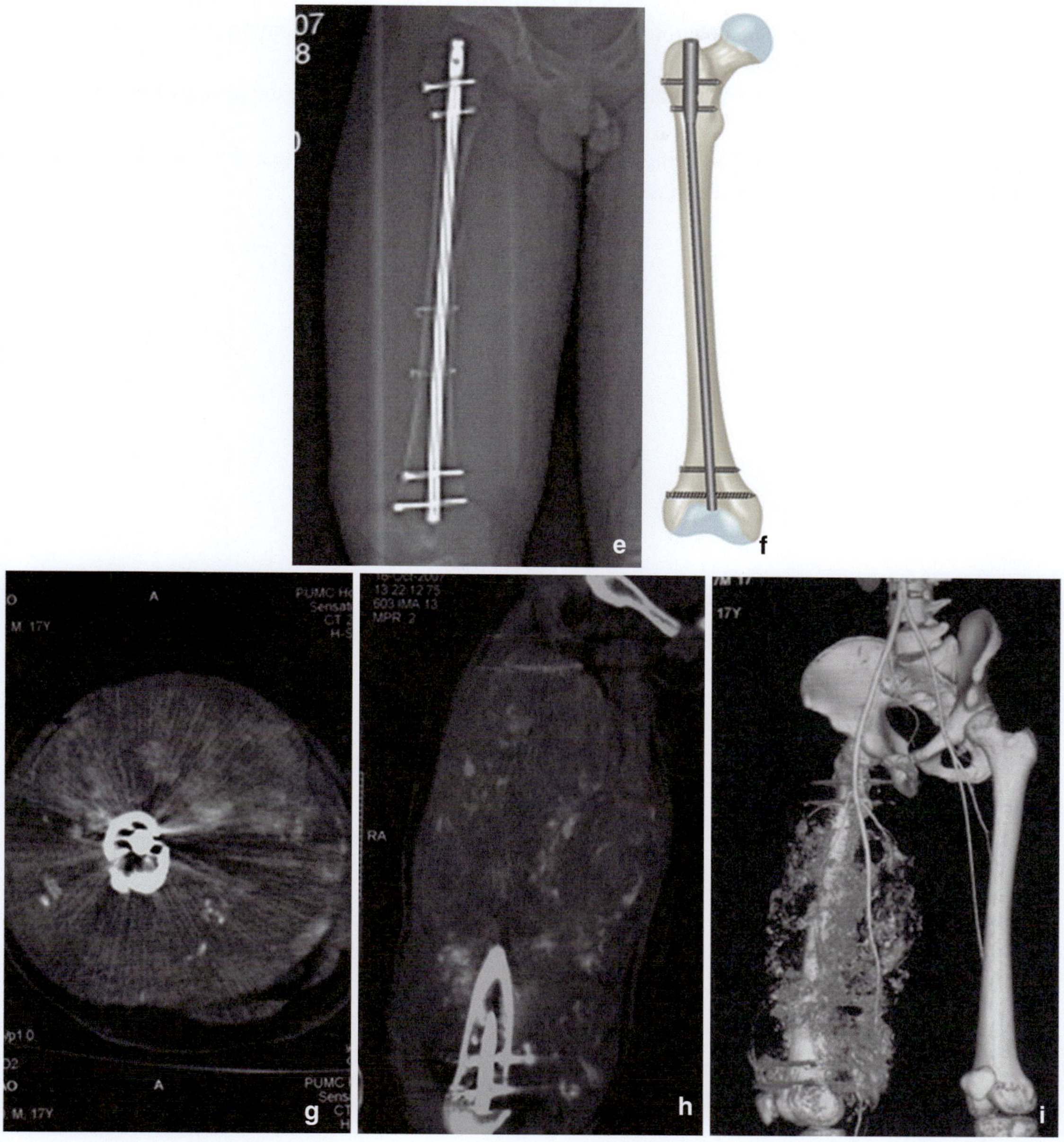

Fig. 13.12 (**e**) is the CT scanning image after surgery (schematic diagram **f**). (**g**, **h**) are the CT transverse plane and coronal plane reconstruction, respectively, showing a large soft tissue mass in the right thigh, with high-density shadow scattered in. (**i**) is CT angiography, showing multiple blood supply vessels of the tumor

13.4 Summary

1. Attention should be paid to pathological fracture of lower limbs. In the case of mild external force or without external force, the fracture should be suspected a pathological fracture. In addition to X-ray, multiple imaging methods of CT and MRI are conducive to identification.
2. In addition to diagnosing the fracture itself, imaging should also detect and evaluate the primary bone disease causing the pathological fracture.
3. In general, the cortical fracture of bone in benign lesions is sharp and orderly, whereas the fracture caused by malignant tumors is often accompanied by soft tissue masses.

Part IV

Fracture of Axial Skeleton

Cervical Spine Fracture

14

Yingcai Sun and Yingze Zhang

The first cervical vertebra is called the atlas, and the second cervical vertebra is called the axis. The atlas is an irregular ring with no actual vertebral body. It consists of bilateral lateral masses, transverse processes and anterior-posterior arches. The atlas articulates upper with the occipital condyles and the lateral masses of the axis below form the atlantoaxial joint. The anterior part of the axis is composed of vertebral bodies and odontoid process. The roots of the odontoid processes are thin and easy to fracture and dislocate. The lower cervical vertebral bodies are composed of C3-7, and the vertebrae structures are similar. It consists of vertebral body, bilateral pedicle, bilateral transverse processes, bilateral superior and inferior articular processes, lamina and spinous processes. Every vertebral body has a hook-shaped protrusion on each side of the upper edge, which forms Luschka joints with the upper vertebral body. The spinous processes of the cervical spine are bifurcated.

Y. Sun
CT/MRI Center, The Third Hospital of Hebei Medical University, Shijiazhuang, Hebei, China

Y. Zhang (✉)
Department of Orthopaedics, The Third Hospital of Hebei Medical University, Shijiazhuang, Hebei, China

Y. Zhang (ed.), *Differential Diagnosis of Fracture*, https://doi.org/10.1007/978-981-13-8339-7_14

1. Plain film and MR features of normal cervical vertebrae
   1.1 X-ray film (Fig. 14.1a–f)

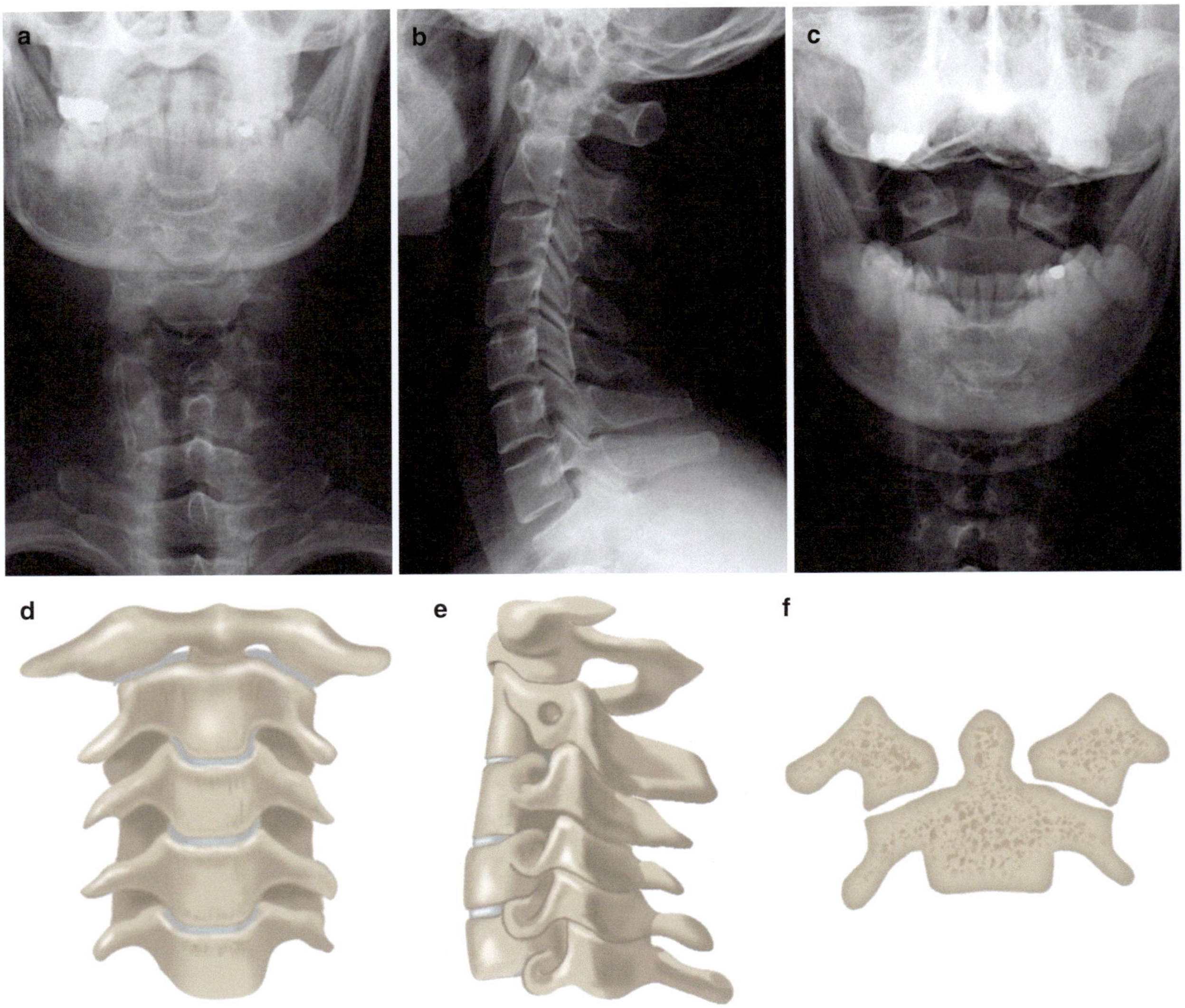

Fig. 14.1 (**a**, **b** and **c**) are the X-ray images of cervical vertebrae anteroposterior, lateral and opening position, respectively (schematic diagrams **d**, **e**, **f**)

1.2 MR imaging (Fig. 14.1g–i)

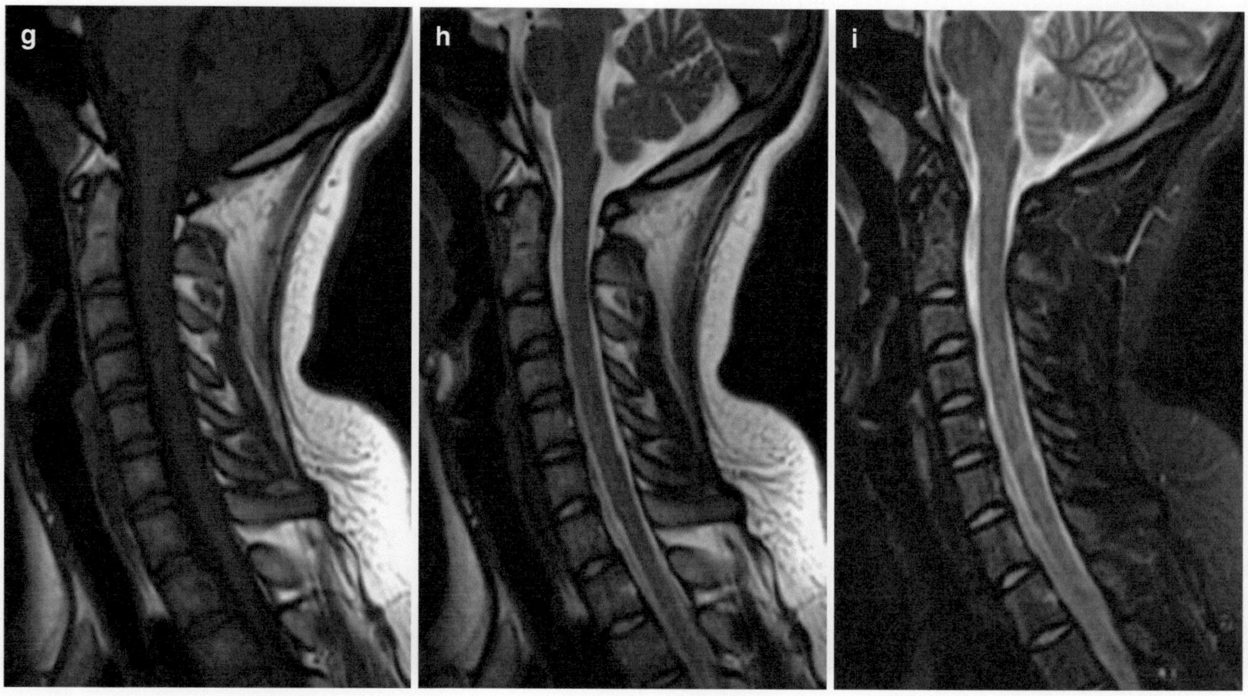

Fig. 14.1 (**g**, **h**, and **i**) are MR T1WI, T2WI, and STIR sequences of the cervical spine, respectively

14.1 Atlas Fracture

14.1.1 Identification of Injury Mechanism

Most are due to trauma, such as falling from a height or the neck violently flexing and retro-stretching in a traffic accident (whiplash injury); direct trauma is less common. According to the AO classification, it is divided into three types: type A is an anterior or posterior arch fracture, most caused by indirect traumatic injury. Type B is burst fracture (also known as Jefferson fracture). The axial trauma which attacks the top of the head is symmetrically transmitted to the lateral part of the atlas through the skull and the occipital condyle and pushes the lateral mass outward, causing anterior and posterior arch symmetry fractures. Type C is atlantoaxial dislocation. The head over flexion, head and neck subjected to violent impact, causes the atlantoaxial joint injury, odontoid fracture or/and the transverse ligament tear that restricts the odontoid posterior movement. Some patients may have spontaneous dislocation, often due to repeated infection of the upper respiratory tract, chronic inflammation of the neck and pharynx or mastoid leading to relaxation of the ligaments around the atlantoaxial joint, mostly resulting in rotational subluxation.

14.1.2 Identification of Symptom and Sign

The clinical manifestations are upper neck pain and limited mobility. It is easy to miss diagnosis and clinical examination lacks specificity. The atlantoaxial dislocation can manifest head tilted, stiff neck, limited rotation and paraplegia combined with spinal cord injury.

Some patients only show neck pain, limited mobility, and can present to the hospital on their own. With these patients, it is easy to misdiagnose as a sprain and not offer the patients any imaging, which may result in serious fracture dislocation.

14.1.3 Imaging Differential Diagnosis

Type A: X-ray lateral and opening position cannot diagnose this fracture. CT cross-sectional scans or reconstructed images can show fractures. This is due to the fact that the patient is in a passive position after trauma, the original image of the CT scan often does not show the overall atlas well. It is necessary to reconstruct the standard cross-sectional image by MPR.

Type B: X-ray opening position can indirectly diagnose the burst fracture of the atlas. The normal X-ray opening position of the lateral part of the atlas and the lateral edge of the atlantoaxial joint should be on the same line. When the bilateral lateral masses are displaced outward beyond the distances greater than 6.9 mm of the outer edge of the atlantoaxial joint, it indicates a rupture of the transverse ligament of the atlas and a fracture of the atlas. Due to the pain caused by the cervical spine injury, it is hard to get a proper open mouth position imaging. In addition, it is difficult to detect the atlantoaxial fracture via X-ray if there is no marked displacement. The axial imaging of CT reconstruction is the best method for the diagnosis of atlas fracture. MR is not as useful as CT in atlas fracture, but can show the ligament and spinal cord injury.

Type C: The X-ray lateral position can show that the atlas is displaced forward, and the distance between the odontoid and the posterior edge of the anterior arch of the atlas is increased. The child's distance exceeds 4 mm and the adult's distance exceeds 3 mm. The X-ray mouth opening position and the CT and MRI coronal position show the distances between the odontoid process and the lateral masses of the atlas are not equal; MRI shows the continuous interruption and signal abnormality of the transverse ligament and pterygoid ligament, and the corresponding planar spinal show high signals on T2WI when combined with the spinal cord injury.

The main imaging features of spontaneous dislocations are that the distance between the odontoid process and the lateral mass of the atlas is asymmetrical, and the posterior pharyngeal wall can be thickened.

Simple traumatic atlantoaxial joint dislocation is rare. It is always accompanied with vertebrae and ligament injuries. Attention should be paid to odontoid fracture or (and) transverse ligament tear, atlantoaxial joint rotatory subluxation. CT coronal reconstruction and MRI coronal plane can accurately measure the distance between the odontoid of the axis and the lateral mass of the atlas.

14.1.3.1 Atlas Fracture Type A

1. Atlas anterior arch and lateral block transition zone fracture and no fracture identification
   1.1 X-ray film (Fig. 14.2a, b)

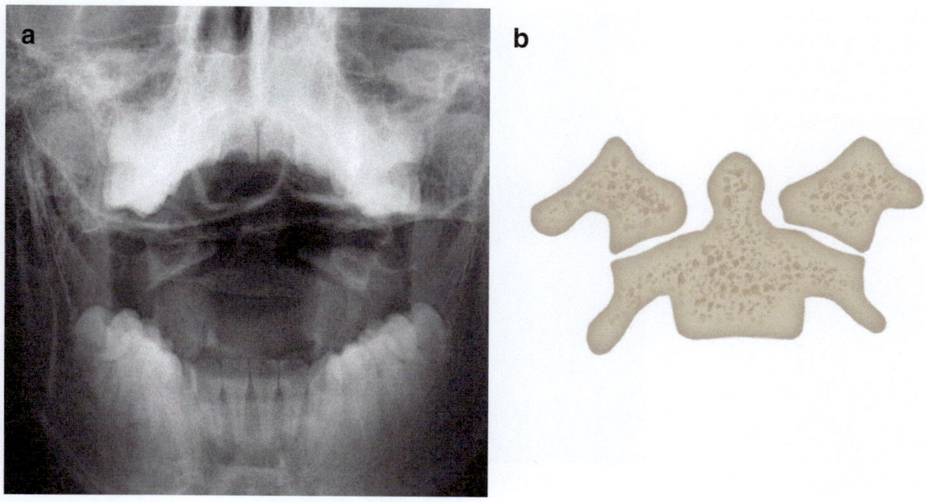

Fig. 14.2 (**a**) There is no abnormality in the opening position of the cervical vertebrae (**b**)

   1.2 CT scan (Fig. 14.2c)

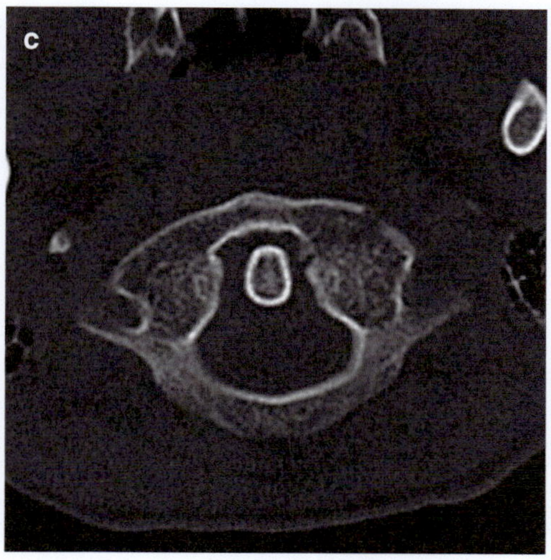

Fig. 14.2 (**c**) CT axial image shows bone fracture near the left side of the anterior arch, no obvious dislocation

2. Atlas anterior arch fracture and no fracture identification
   2.1 CT scan (Fig. 14.3a, b)

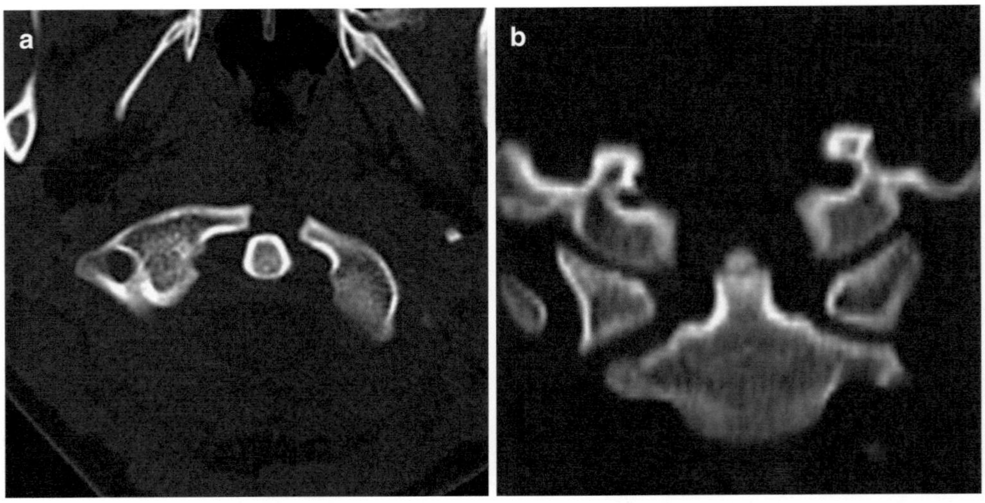

Fig. 14.3 The CT axial plane (**a**) image shows an anterior arch fracture, and the coronal reconstruction (**b**) shows a widening space between the lateral block and the odontoid

3. Identification of the posterior arch fracture with no fracture of the atlas
   3.1 X-ray film (Fig. 14.4a, b)

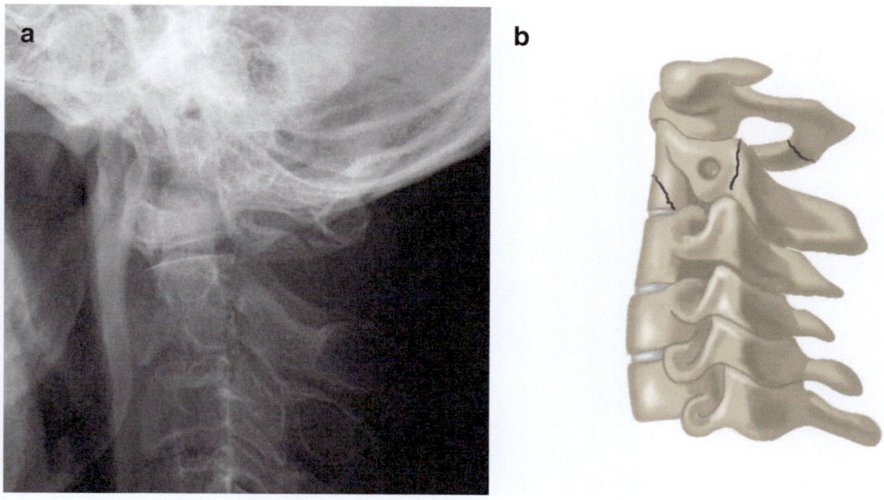

Fig. 14.4 The cervical lateral radiograph (**a**) shows the posterior arch fracture lines of the atlas (**b**)

   3.2 CT scan (Fig. 14.4c, d)

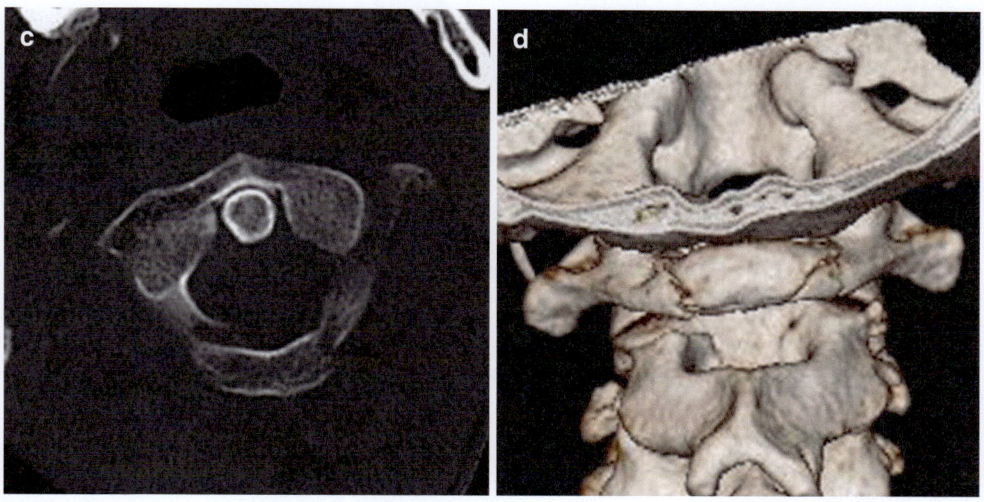

Fig. 14.4 CT axial plane (**c**) and VR reconstruction (**d**) show posterior arch bone fracture of the atlas

14.1.3.2 Atlas Fracture B Type

4. Identification of anterior and posterior arch fractures of the atlas and suspicious fractures
   4.1 X-ray film (Fig. 14.5a–d)

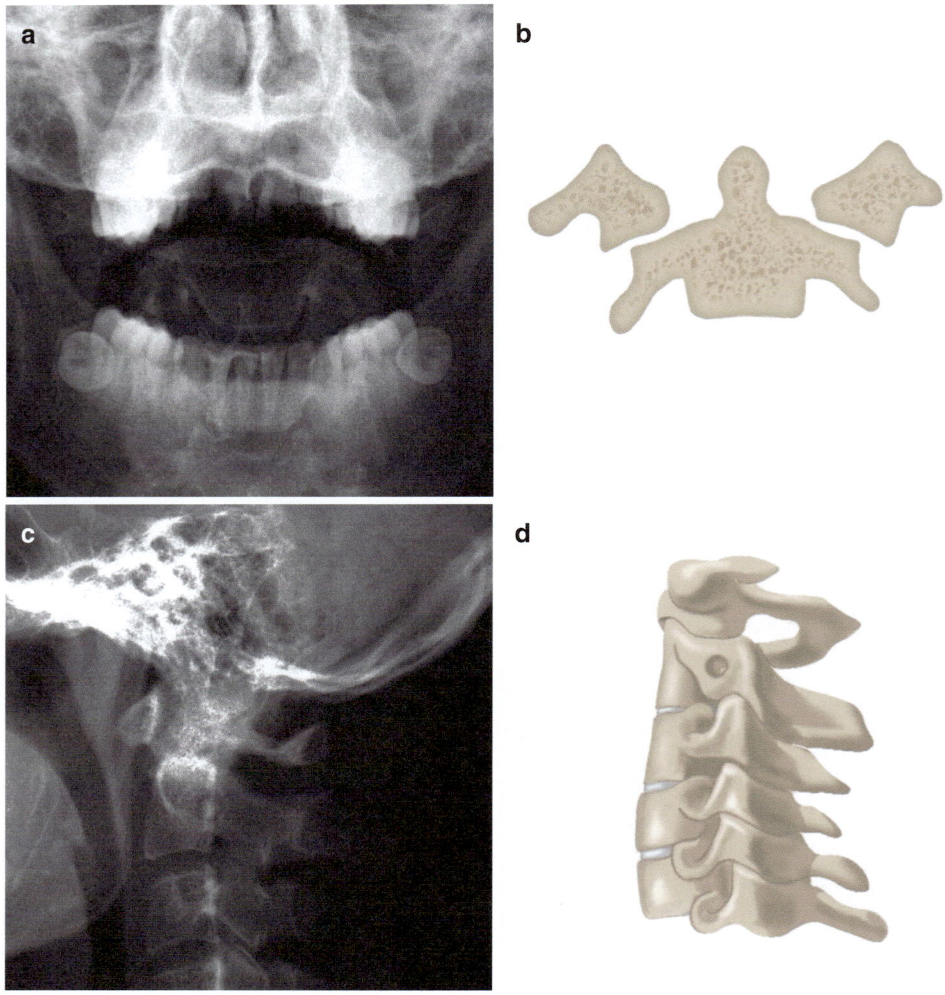

Fig. 14.5 The opening position of the cervical vertebrae (**a**) cannot be completely displayed due to the covering of the teeth, and the lateral mass are displaced to two sides. The lateral position of the cervical vertebra (**c**) shows no abnormality. (**b**, **d**)

   4.2 CT scan (Fig. 14.5e, f)

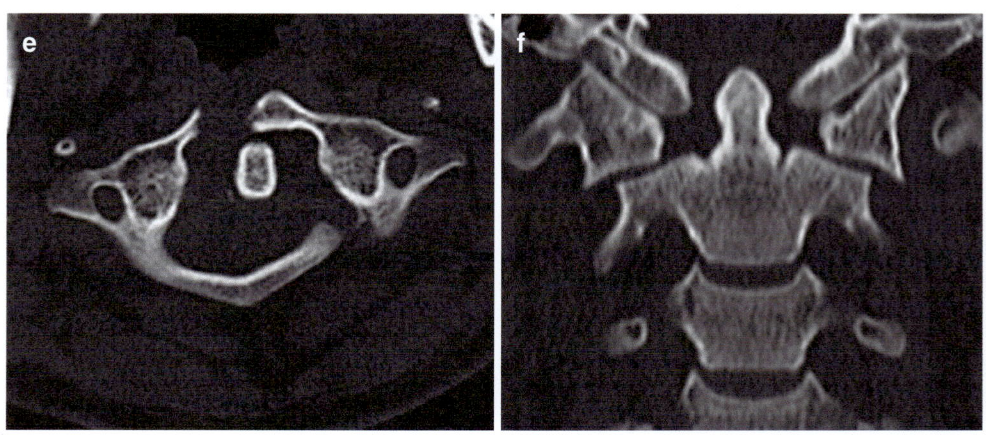

Fig. 14.5 The CT axial image (**e**) shows anterior and posterior arch fractures of the atlas, with the fracture ends are separated. The CT coronal plane (**f**) shows that the space between lateral mass and the odontoid is widened, and the bilateral lateral masses are displaced outward

5. CT and MR contrast of comminuted fractures of the atlas lateral mass
   5.1 CT scan (Fig. 14.6a, b)

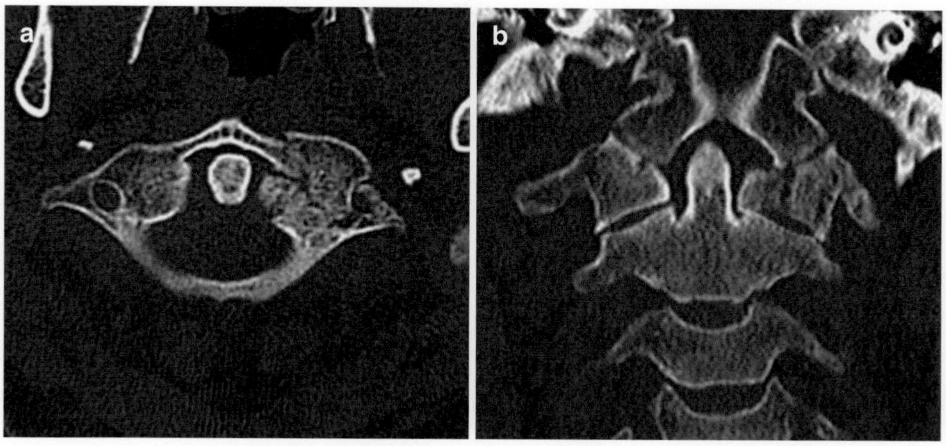

Fig. 14.6 The CT axial plane (**a**) and the coronal plane (**b**) show the lateral mass of the atlas fracture, the fracture block is displaced to the medial side, and the space of the left lateral mass and the vertebral odontoid is narrowed

   5.2 MR imaging (Fig. 14.6c)

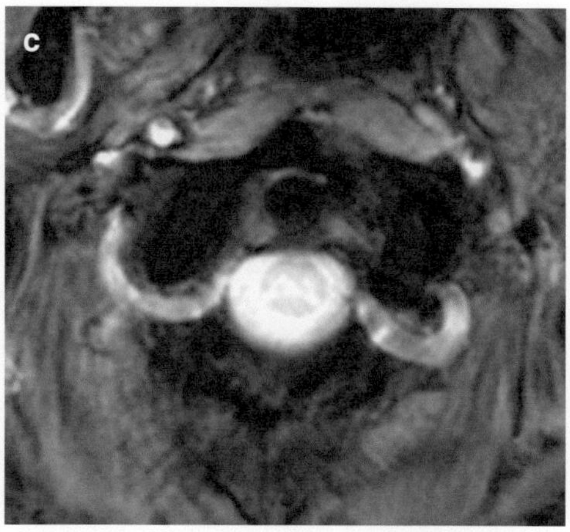

Fig. 14.6 MRI-T2WI axial surface (**c**) cannot be accurately diagnosed

14.1.3.3 The Atlantoaxial Dislocation

6. The flat film, CT and MR comparison of the atlantoaxial anterior dislocation
   6.1 X-ray film (Fig. 14.7a–d)

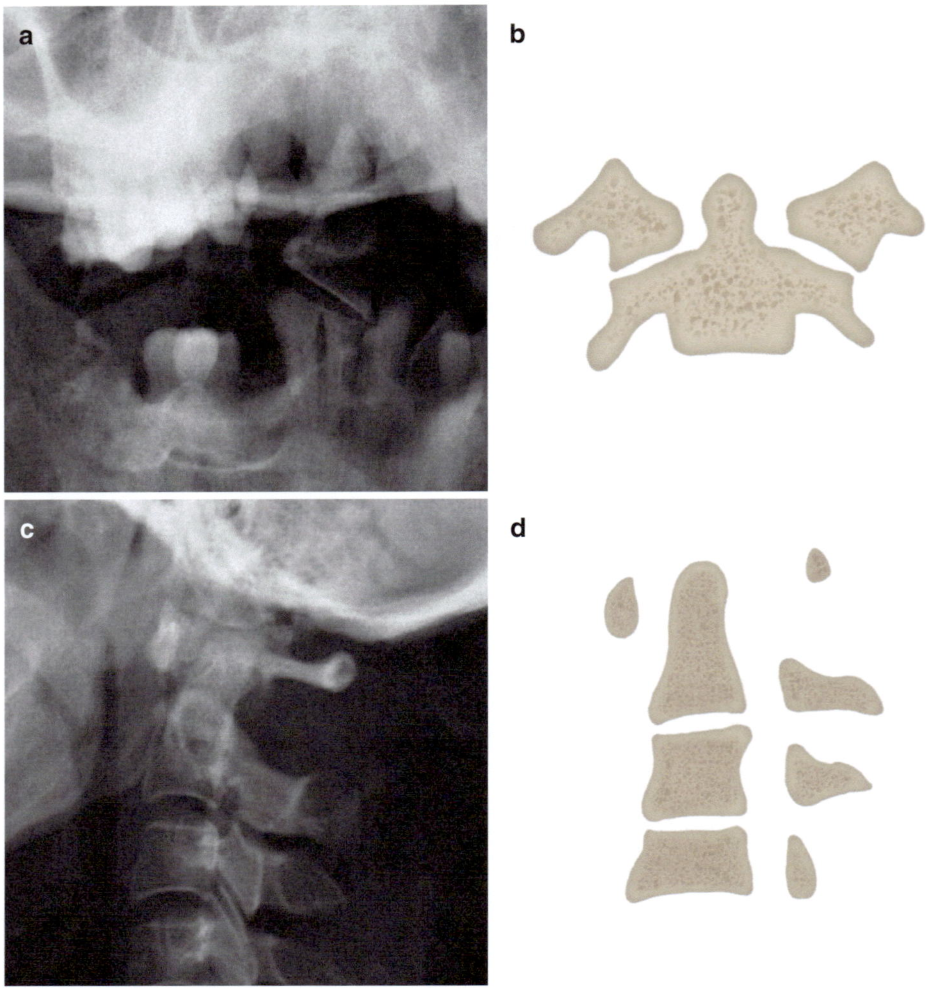

Fig. 14.7 The opening position X-ray film of the cervical vertebrae shows that the lateral space of the atlas, and the dentate process of the vertebral process were not equal width, and the right side was narrowed (**a**); Lateral radiographs of the cervical spine shows widening of the anterior arch of the atlas and the dentate process of the vertebral process (**b**–**d**)

   6.2 CT scan (Fig. 14.7e, f)

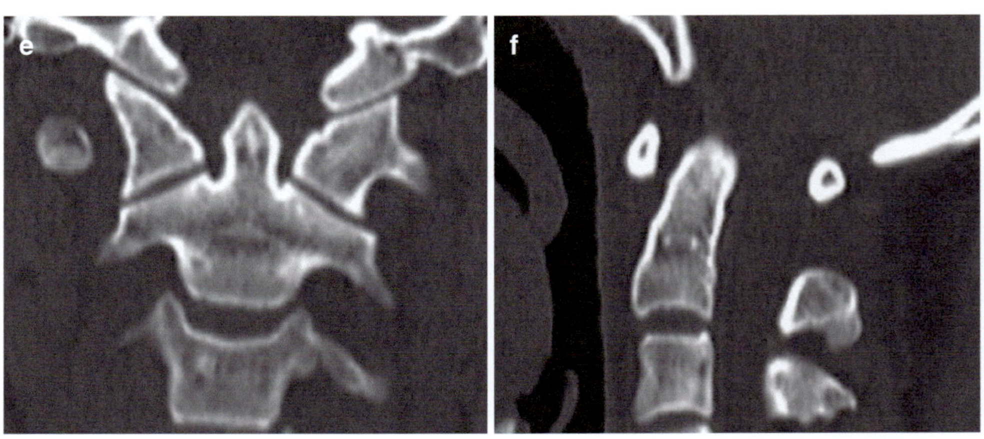

Fig. 14.7 CT coronal reconstruction (**e**) shows normal interstitial space between the lateral mass of the atlas and the odontoid of the axis, and sagittal reconstruction (**f**) shows widening interstitial space of the atlas anterior arch and the axis odontoid

6.3 MR imaging (Fig. 14.7g–i)

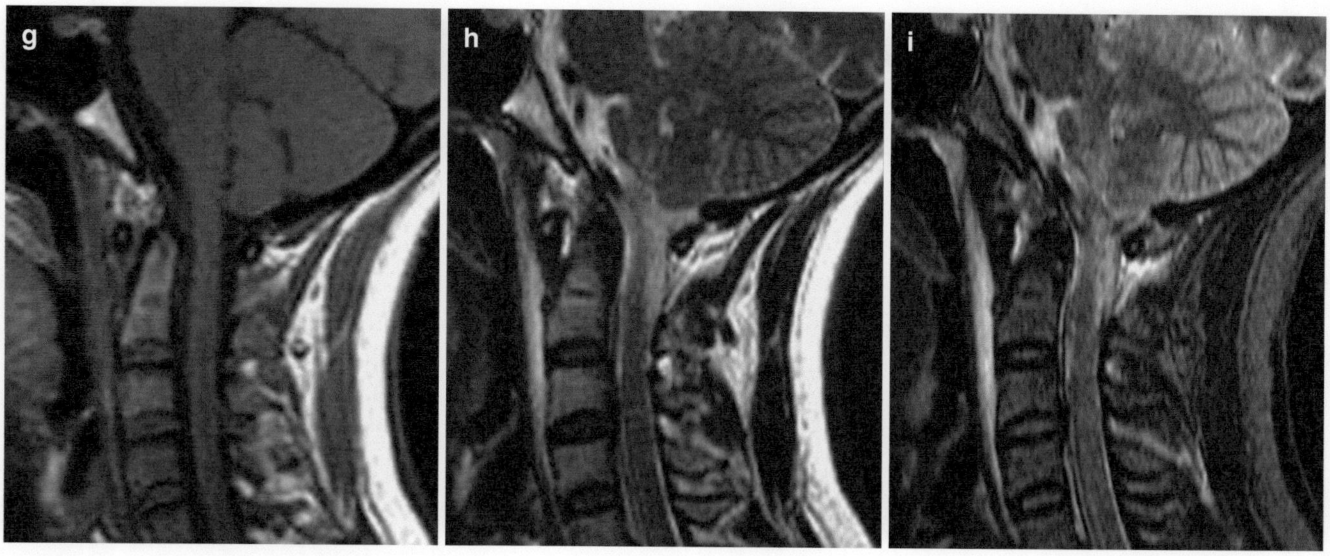

Fig. 14.7 The MRI images (**g–i**) show high signal of the alar ligaments in T2WI

7. Contrast of atlantoaxial anterior dislocation over-flexion plain film and CT
   7.1 X-ray film (Fig. 14.8a, b)

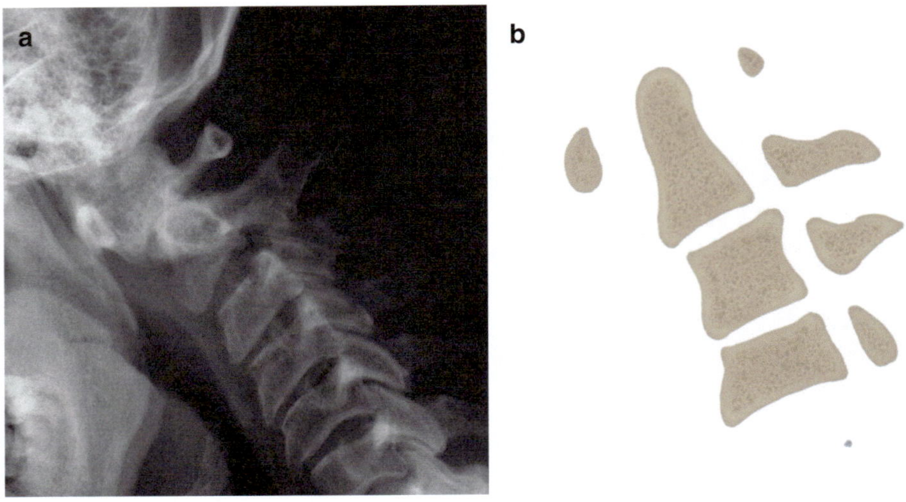

Fig. 14.8 Cervical vertebrae flexion flat (**a**) shows the atlas moving forward (**b**)

   7.2 CT scan (Fig. 14.8c, d)

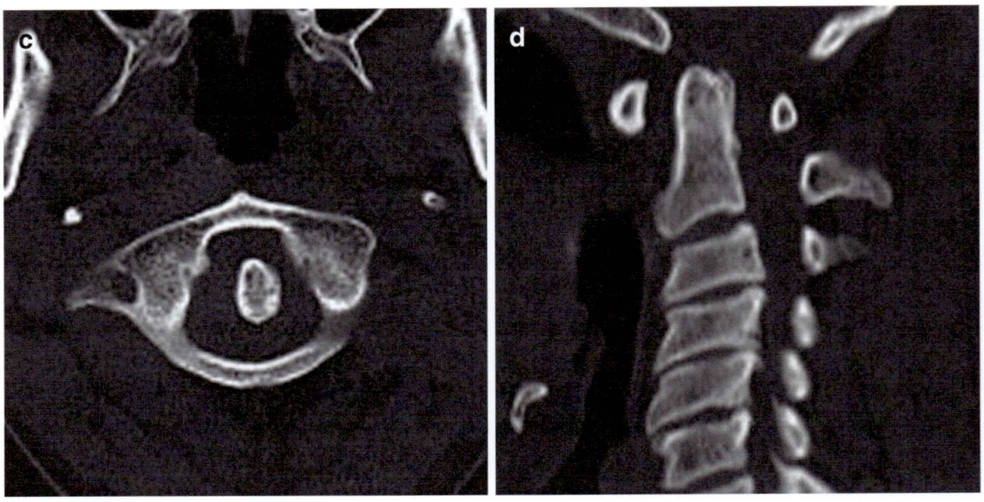

Fig. 14.8 CT axial plane (**c**) and sagittal plane (**d**) show widening space of odontoid process of axis and anterior arch of atlas

8. Atlantoaxial rotation and dislocation flat film compared with CT
   8.1 X-ray film (Fig. 14.9a, b)

Fig. 14.9 The flat section of the cervical vertebrae (**a**) shows that the right-side distance between the odontoid process of axis and the lateral mass of the atlas is wider than the left side, and the right side lateral mass of the atlas is moved outward (**b**)

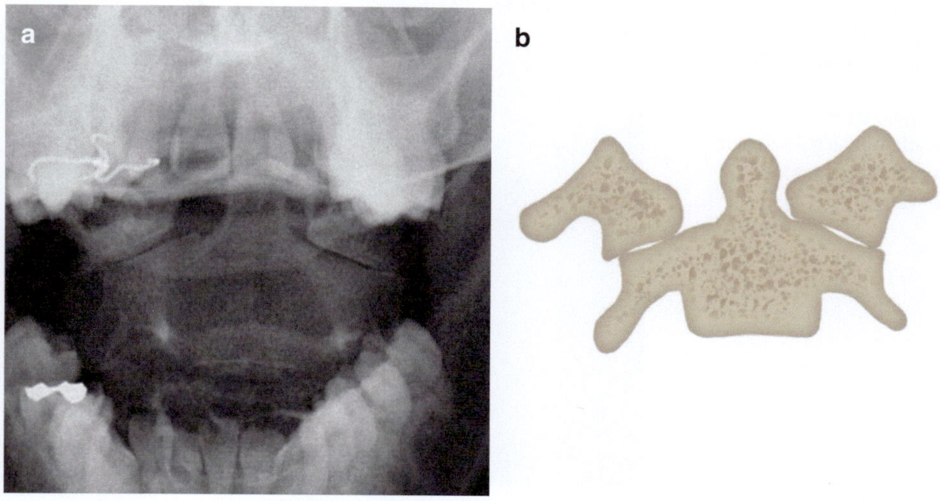

   8.2 CT scan (Fig. 14.9c–f)

Fig. 14.9 The CT axial position (**c**) and the coronal reconstruction (**d**) show that the distance between the odontoid process and the lateral masses of the atlas are not equal, and the sagittal reconstruction (**e**) shows the distance is slightly increased between the odontoid process and the anterior arch of the atlas; VR reconstruction (**f**) shows the left side block of the atlantoaxial as the axis, and the right-side block of the atlas is rotated backward

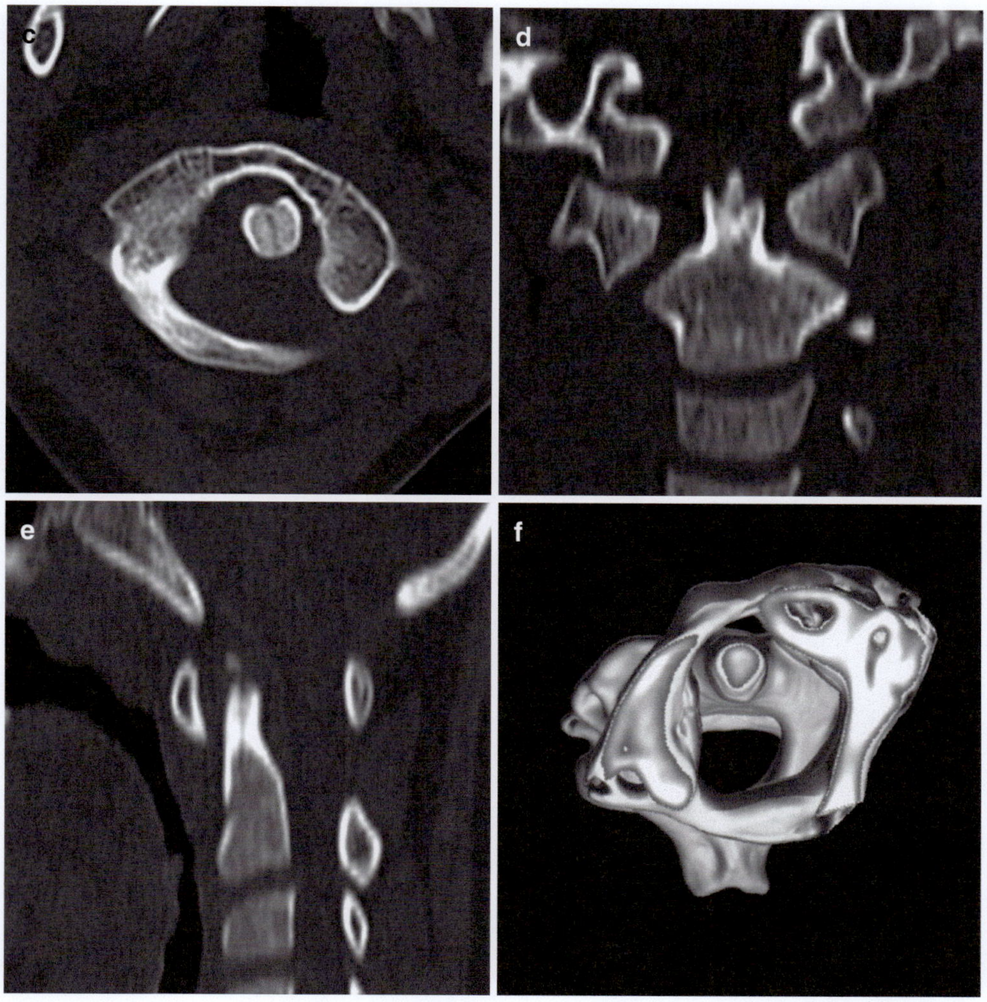

9. Atlantoaxial rotation and dislocation flat film compared with CT
   9.1 X-ray film (Fig. 14.10a, b)

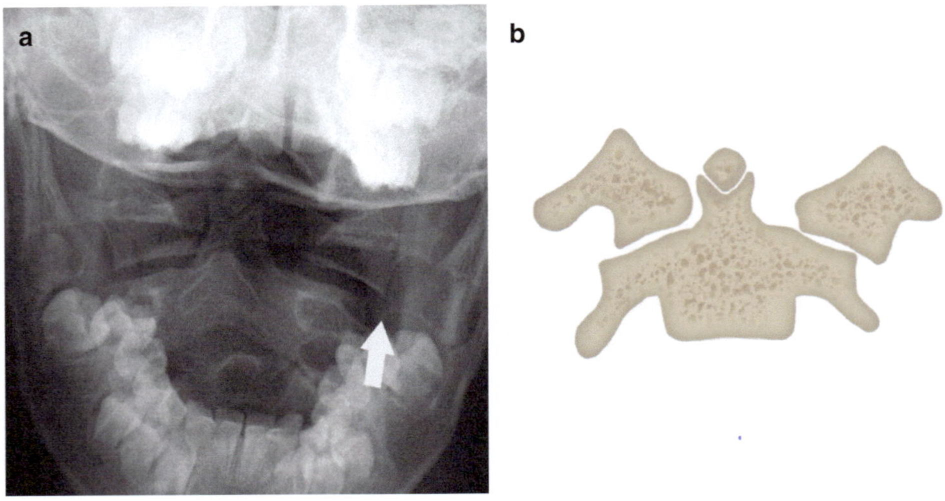

Fig. 14.10 The mouth opening flat film of cervical vertebrae (**a**) shows the right side distance of the odontoid process and the lateral mass of the atlas are narrowed, and the lateral side of the atlas moves laterally (**b**)

   9.2 CT scan (Fig. 14.10c, d)

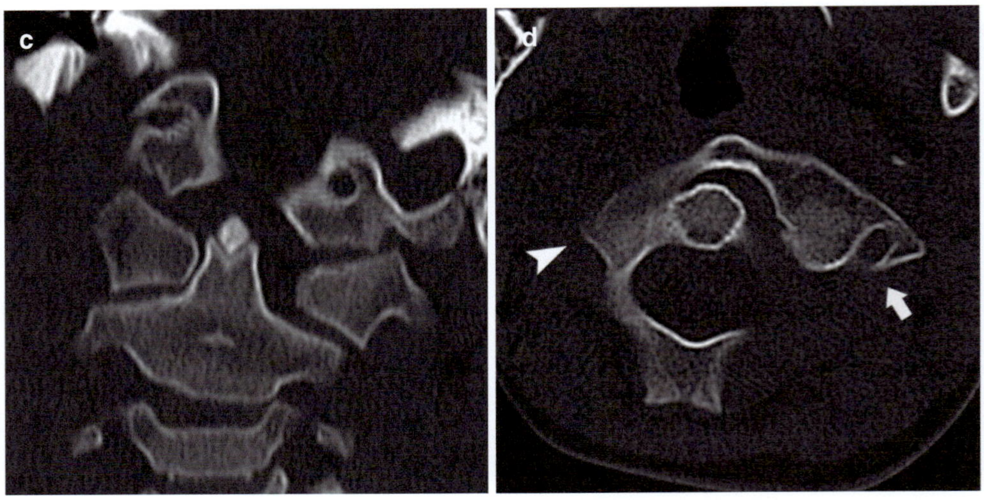

Fig. 14.10 Atlantoaxial rotation and dislocation, CT coronal reconstruction (**c**), the right space between the odontoid process and the lateral side of the atlas is narrowed, and the lateral side of the atlas is displaced laterally; CT axial image (**d**) shows the atlas takes the right-side block (arrow) as the axis, the left-side block (white arrow) rotates forward

14.2 The Axial Fracture

According to the AO classification method, the axial fractures are divided into three types: type A is the fracture of the isthmus; type B is the odontoid fracture; and type C is the fracture of the isthmus with odontoid fracture.

14.2.1 Identification of Injury Mechanism

Most are due to indirect injury. Type A is called Hangman fracture, the injury mechanism is mostly caused by bilateral vertebral pedicle fracture due to over-extension and traction, with the anterior dislocation of the vertebral body and the secondary tear of the spinal cord. Type B odontoid fractures are mostly over-flexion injuries. Type C fractures are mostly caused by mixed severe violence, often accompanied by at antoaxial joint dislocation.

14.2.2 Identification of Symptom and Sign

The clinical manifestations are upper neck pain and limited mobility. It is easy to miss diagnosis and clinical examination lacks specificity. Some patients only show neck pain, limited mobility, and can walk to the hospital on their own. The clinic is subject to misdiagnose as a sprain and not give patients filming, which may result in serious fracture dislocation.

14.2.3 Imaging Differential Diagnosis

Type A Hangman fracture, the larger displacement can be confirmed by the lateral position of the cervical vertebrae, and the smaller displacement requires CT for diagnosis. *Type B* is divided into three subtypes. *Type I*: The fracture above the middle of odontoid process, accounting for 9.6% of these fractures. The oblique fracture through the odontoid cusps are formed by avulsion of the pterygoid ligament. Most of them are stable fractures. These are not often shown of lateral position and mouth opening X-rays, but it can be clearly displayed on coronal and sagittal CT reconstructions. *Type II*: It is the fracture of the odontoid middle region, accounting for 58.9% of fractures. This type of fracture is located in conjunction with the odontoid process and the transverse ligament. The blood supply is poor, and prognostically, it is prone to fracture nonunion. *Type III*: The basal fracture of the odontoid process, accounting for 31.5%, occurs in the conjunction of the odontoid and the vertebral body of the axis, which is a type of unstable fracture. The fracture is displaced to the front and the C2–3 intervertebral discs are abnormal. The fracture displacement is small, but the angle is severe. The lateral position of the cervical vertebrae can show the fracture line. This type of fracture can be diagnosed definitively by CT, which is the most unstable with the displacement of the facet joint and flexion displacement of the anterior part fracture of vertebral. This type of fracture can be diagnosed by X-ray and CT. MRI should be further examined to observe the spinal cord injury. *Type C* isthmus fracture combined with odontoid fracture, often need CT for diagnosis.

1. The pedicle of the dentata and the anterior-inferior edge of vertebral fracture and suspected fracture identification
   1.1 X-ray film (Fig. 14.11a, b)

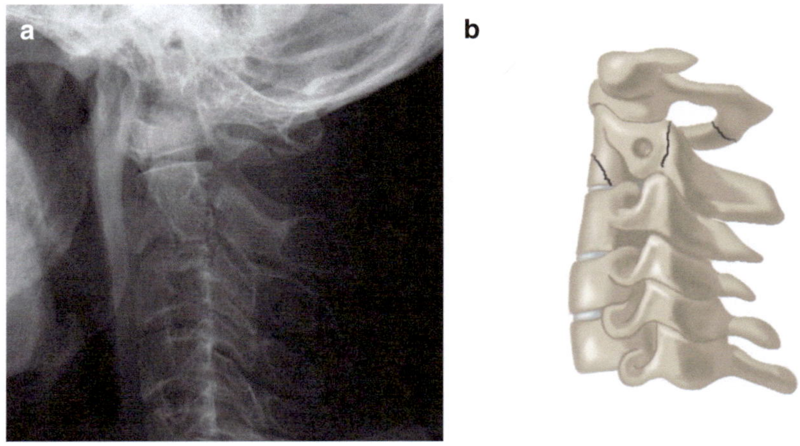

Fig. 14.11 The cervical lateral radiograph (**a**) shows the vertebral pedicle bone discontinuity, schematic (**b**)

   1.2 CT scan (Fig. 14.11c, d)

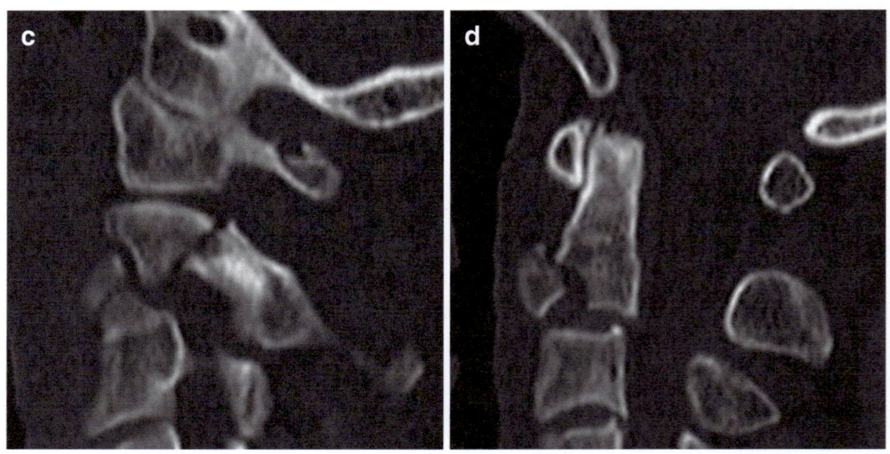

Fig. 14.11 CT sagittal reconstruction (**c**, **d**) shows vertebral pedicle and body fracture

2. Bilateral transverse process fracture and no fracture identification
   2.1 X-ray film (Fig. 14.12a, b)

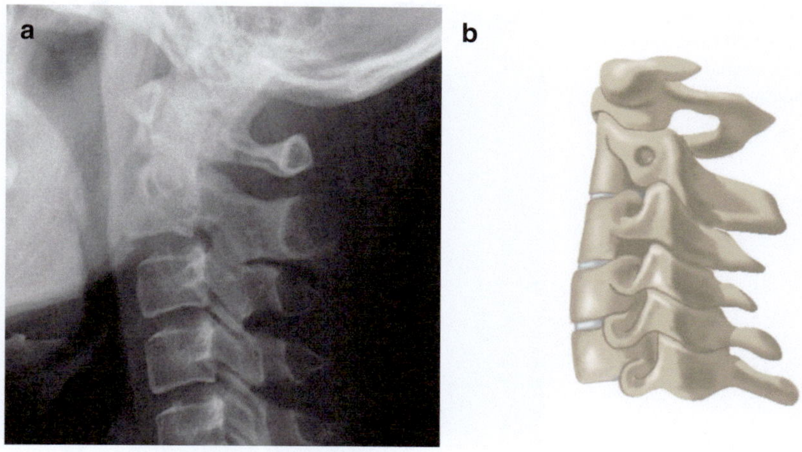

Fig. 14.12 There is no clear fracture sign in the lateral radiograph of the cervical vertebra (**a**). Schematic diagram (**b**)

   2.2 CT scan (Fig. 14.12c, d)

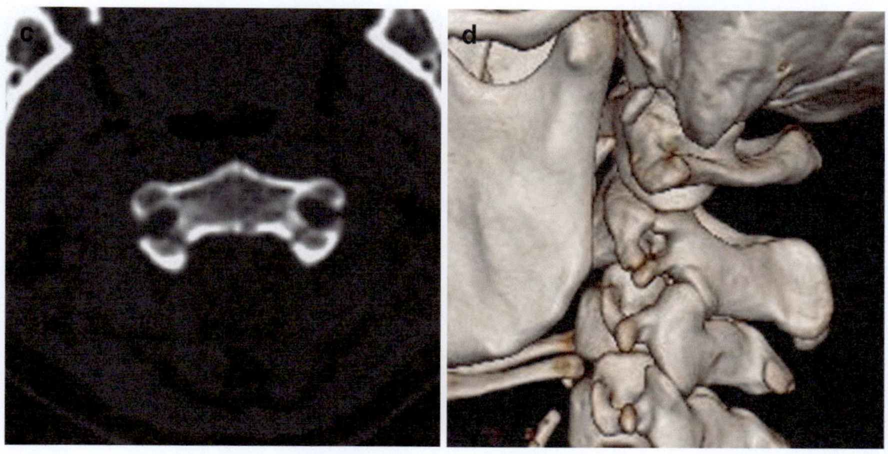

Fig. 14.12 CT axial plane (**c**) and VR image (**d**) show fractures of bilateral attachments, and the fracture line involved bilateral transverse protrusions

3. Identification of the odontoid fracture and the suspected fracture
   3.1 X-ray film (Fig. 14.13a, b)

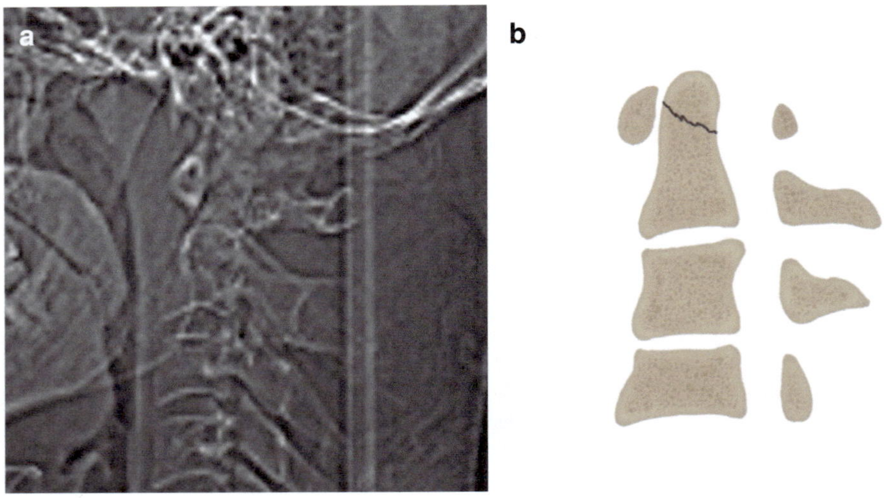

Fig. 14.13 The cervical lateral radiograph (**a**) shows the dentate line-like low-density shadow, schematic (**b**)

   3.2 CT scan (Fig. 14.13c, d)

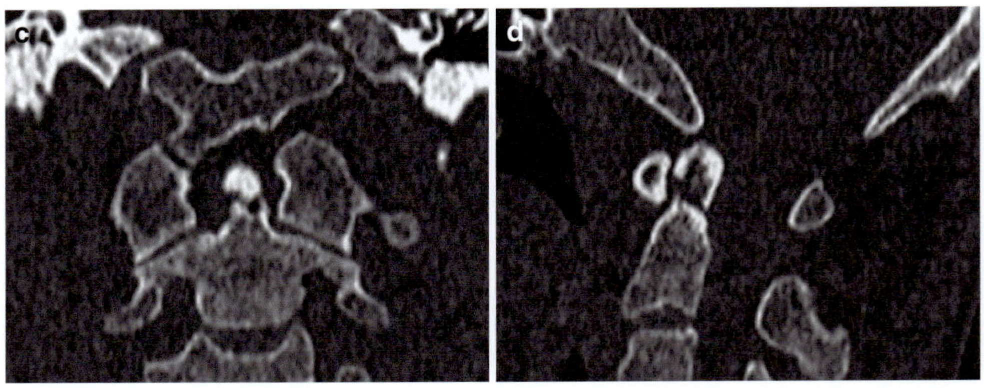

Fig. 14.13 CT coronal and sagittal reconstruction of type I of the odontoid fracture can show oblique line above the middle of dentate

4. The odontoid fracture and no fracture identification
   4.1 X-ray film (Fig. 14.14a, b)

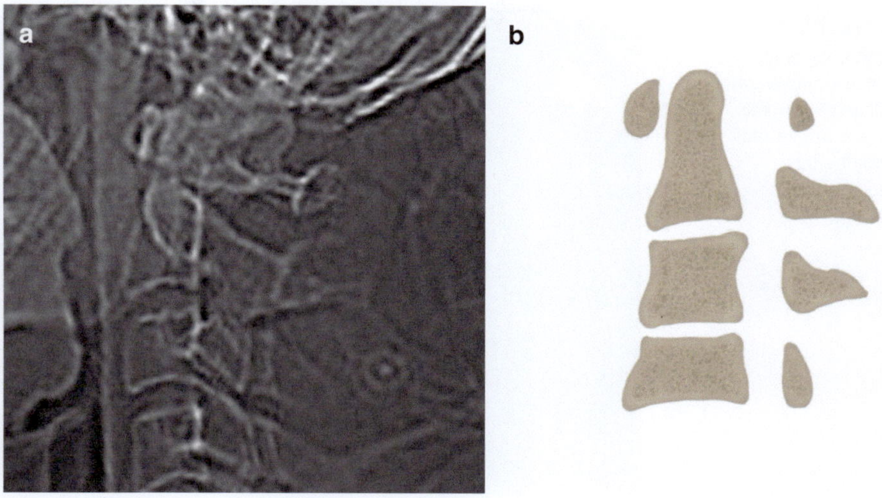

Fig. 14.14 Cervical lateral radiograph (**a**) failed to diagnose odontoid fracture, schematic (**b**)

   4.2 CT scan (Fig. 14.14c, d)

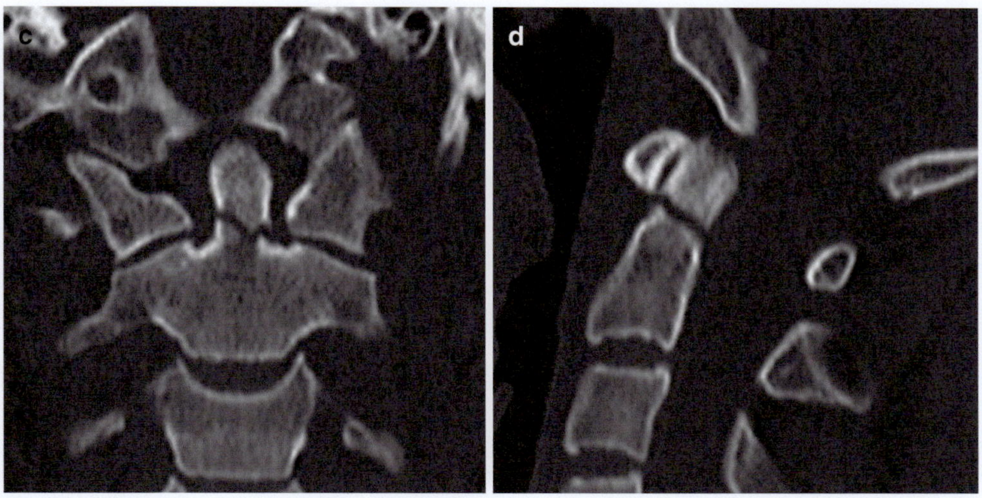

Fig. 14.14 Type I of the odontoid fracture, CT coronal plane (**c**) and sagittal reconstruction (**d**) show the fracture line

5. CT and MR comparison of the odontoid fracture
   5.1 CT scan (Fig. 14.15a, b)

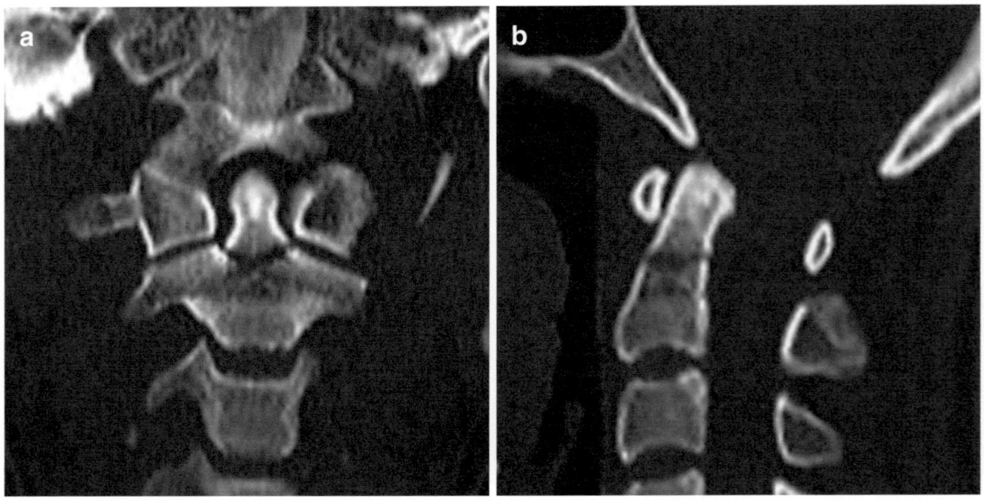

Fig. 14.15 The CT reconstructed images of coronal plane (**a**) and sagittal plane (**b**) clearly show the middle fracture line of the odontoid, no obvious dislocation

   5.2 MR imaging (Fig. 14.15c–e)

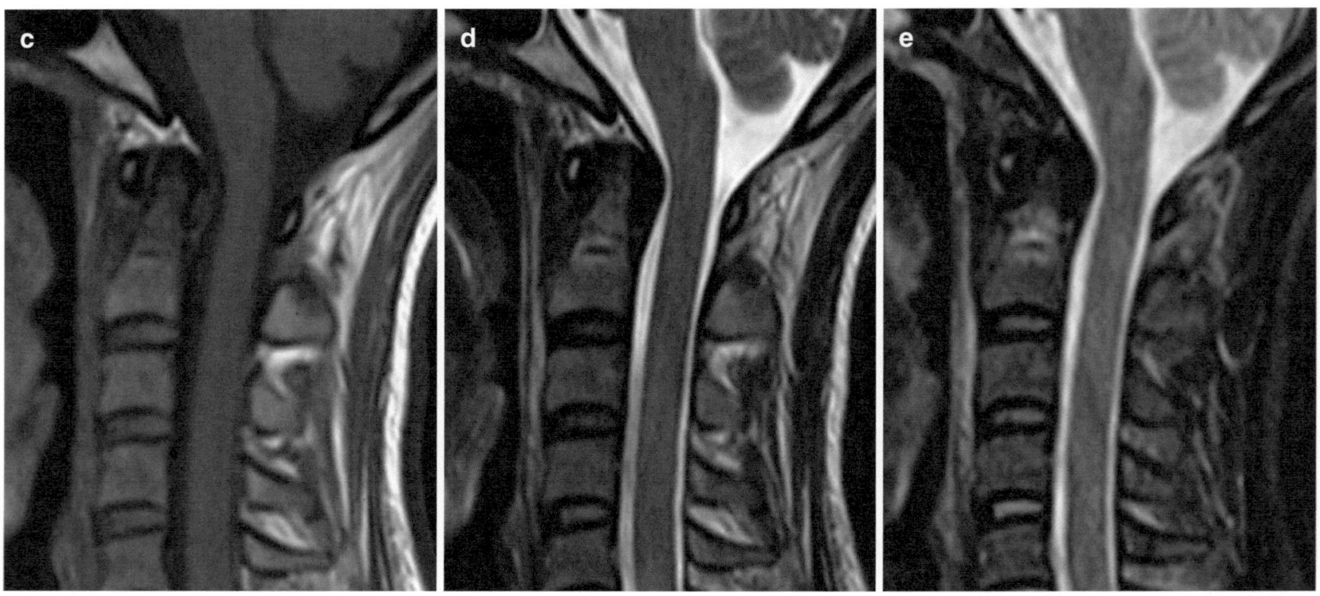

Fig. 14.15 Type II of the odontoid fracture, MRI (**c**–**e**) shows abnormal odontoid signal and the fracture line was not obvious

6. Comparison of plain film, CT and MR of the odontoid fracture
   6.1 X-ray film (Fig. 14.16a–d)

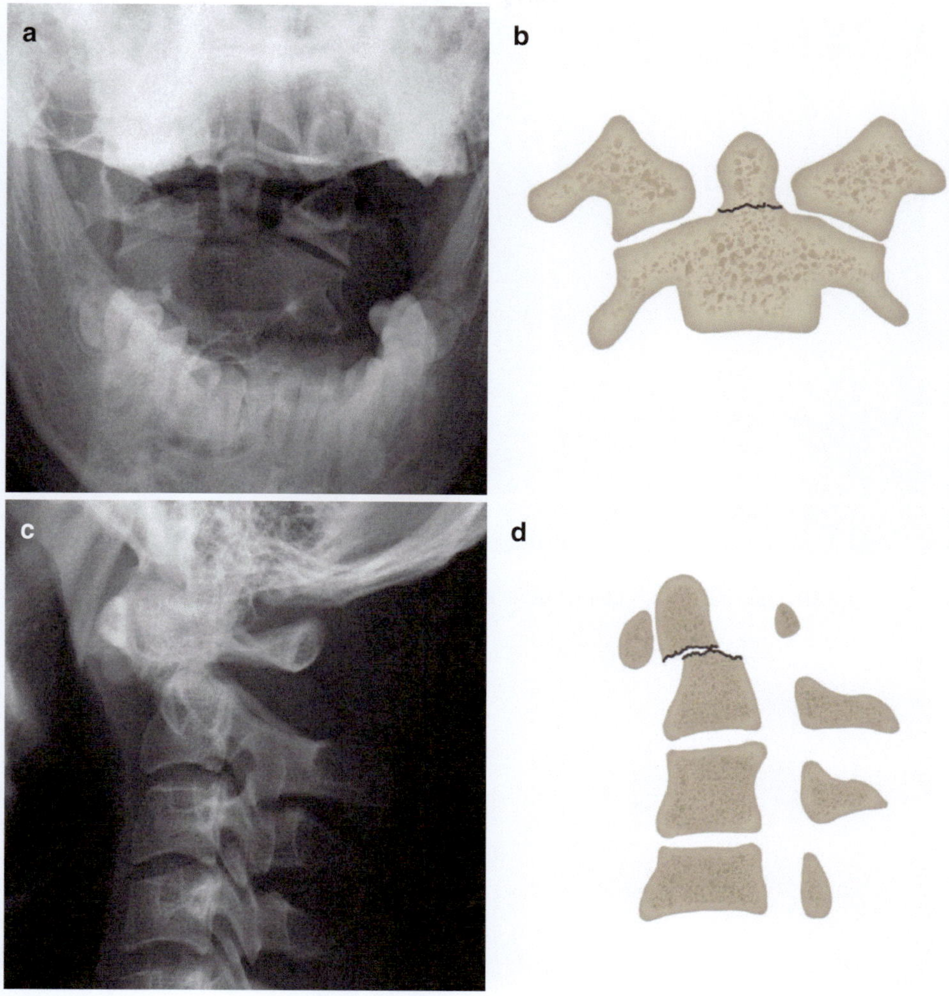

Fig. 14.16 There was no fracture in the mouth opening film of cervical vertebrae (**a**), and the cervical lateral radiograph (**c**) shows odontoid middle fracture, dentate process and atlas flexion displacement, schematic (**b**, **d**)

   6.2 CT scan (Fig. 14.16e, f)

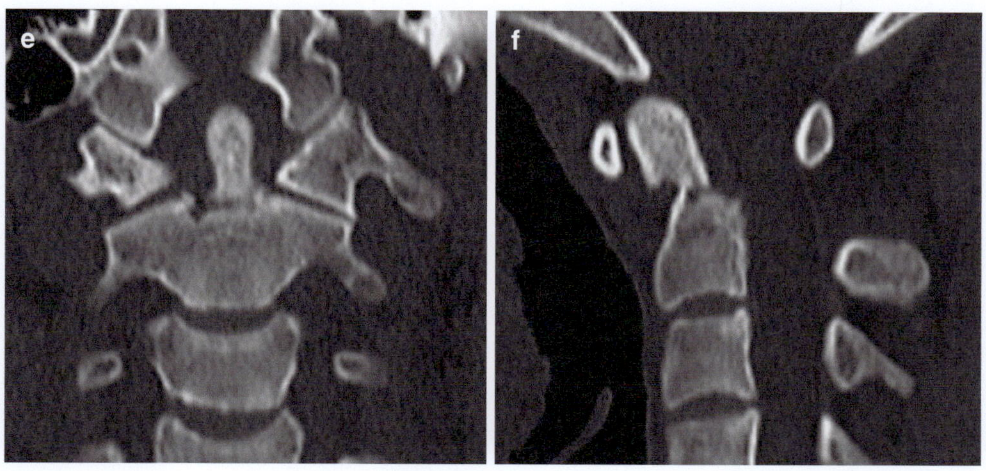

Fig. 14.16 CT sagittal plane (**e**) and coronal plane (**f**) reconstructions show so dontoid middle fracture, dentate process and atlas flexion displacement

6.3 MR imaging (Fig. 14.16g–i)

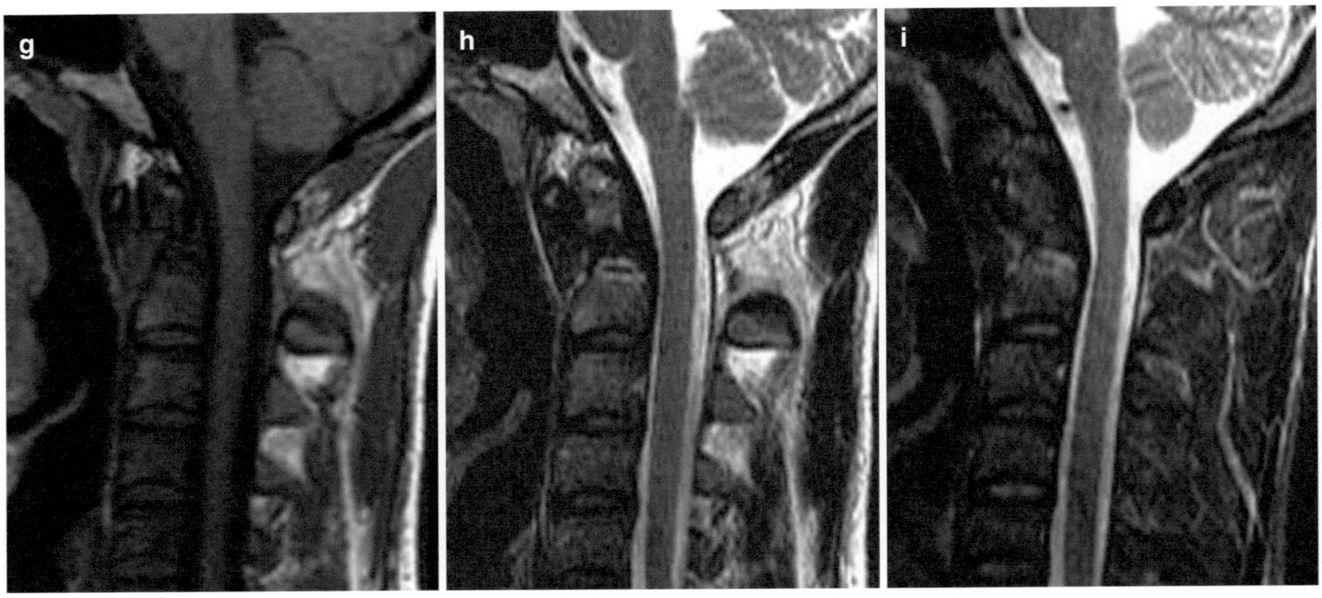

Fig. 14.16 Type III of the odontoid fracture, MR image (**g**–**i**) shows odontoid middle fracture, the odontoid and atlas flexion displacement

7. Contrast of plain film and CT of odontoid base fractures
   7.1 X-ray film (Fig. 14.17a, b)

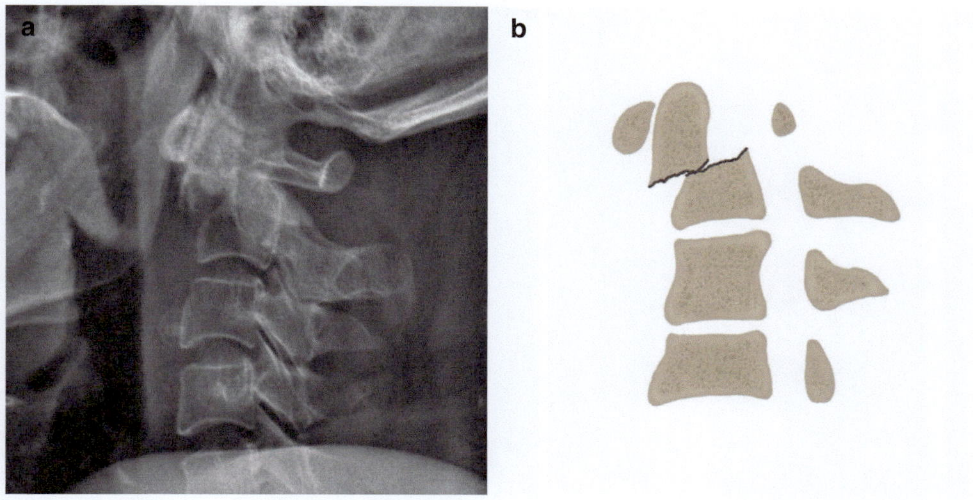

Fig. 14.17 The cervical lateral radiograph (**a**) shows the odontoid basal fracture and dislocation of the broken end, schematic view (**b**)

   7.2 CT scan (Fig. 14.17c, d)

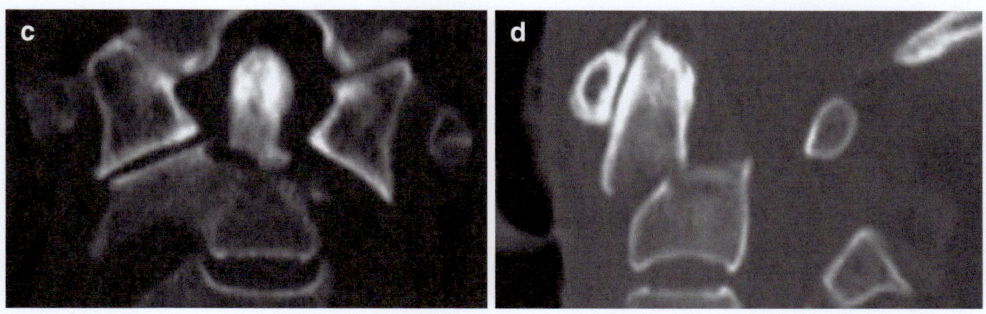

Fig. 14.17 CT coronal reconstruction (**c**) shows odontoid base fracture with a significant forward displacement of the fracture block. CT sagittal reconstruction (**d**) shows spinal stenosis

8. The plain film and CT contrast of old odontoid fractures
   8.1 X-ray film (Fig. 14.18a–f)

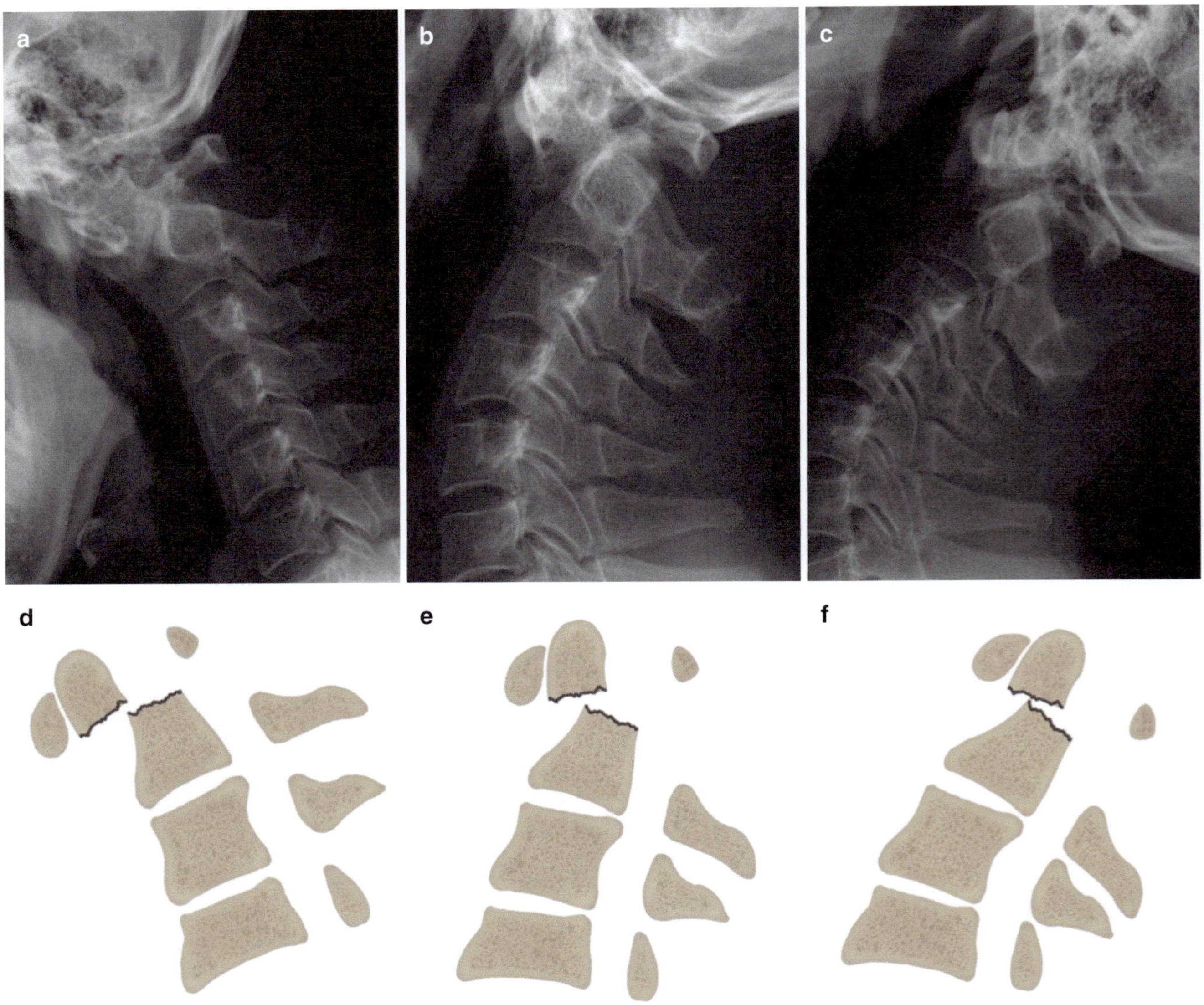

Fig. 14.18 The plain film of lateral and over-flexion position of the cervical vertebrae (**a**) shows a significant advancement of the atlas, the neutral plane (**c**) was centered, and the plain film of over-extension position (**e**) had the least advancement, schematic view (**b**, **d**, **f**)

8.2 CT scan (Fig. 14.18g, h)

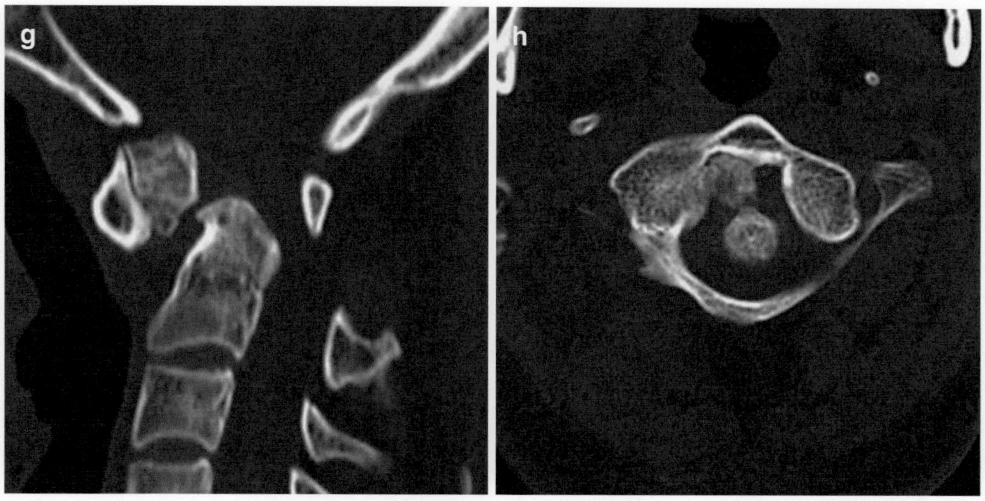

Fig. 14.18 Odontoid fracture III (old), odontoid free CT sagittal reconstruction (**g**) shows odontoid free, free odontoid edge sclerosis, spinal stenosis, cross-sectional image (**h**) shows spinal canal narrow

9. The plain film and CT contrast of the odontoid fractures
   9.1 X-ray film (Fig. 14.19a, b)

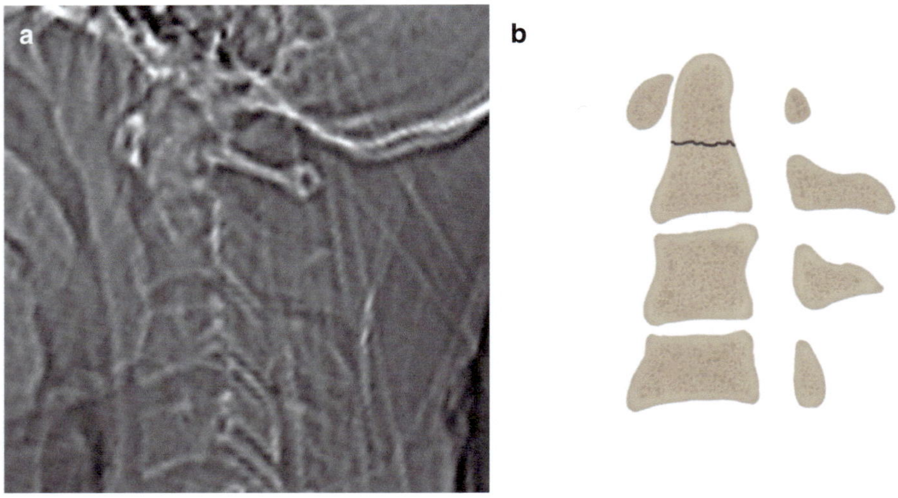

Fig. 14.19 The lateral radiograph of the cervical vertebra (**a**) shows the odontoid fracture, schematic view (**b**)

   9.2 CT scan (Fig. 14.19c, d)

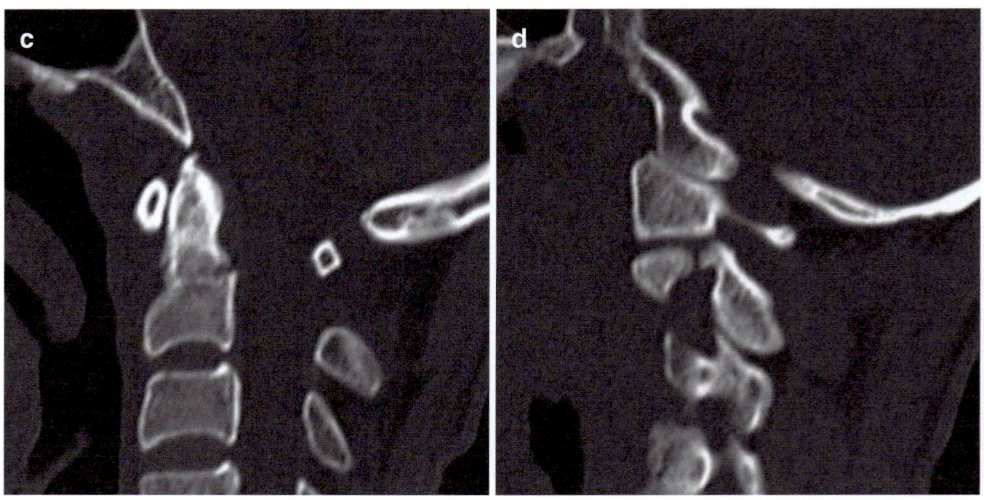

Fig. 14.19 CT sagittal reconstruction (**c**, **d**) shows odontoid fractures, and the front edge of the left pedicle was discontinuous

10. Identification of the axis fracture and suspected fracture
    10.1 X-ray film (Fig. 14.20a–d)

Fig. 14.20 The mouth opening plain film (**a**) shows a suspected line-like low density on the right side of the odontoid base. The lateral plain film of the cervical vertebra (**c**) does not show the axial fracture line, schematic view (**b**, **d**)

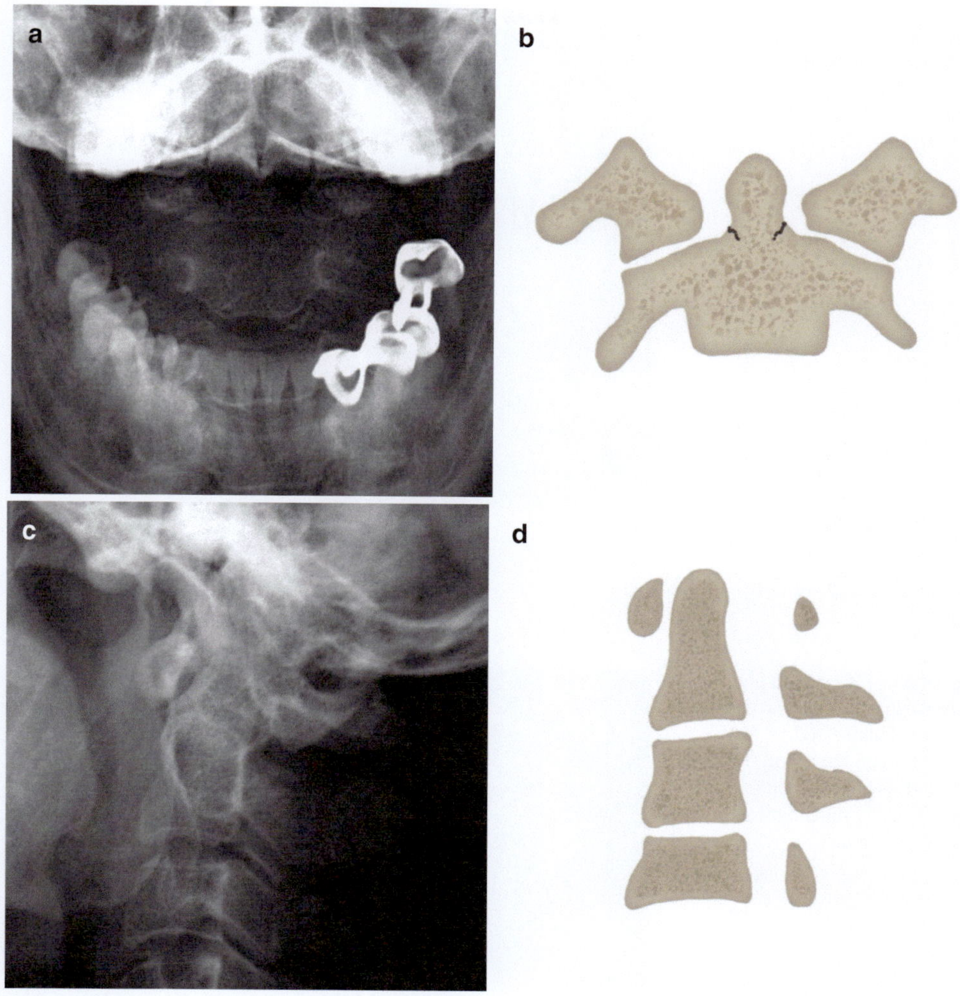

    10.2 CT scan (Fig. 14.20e)

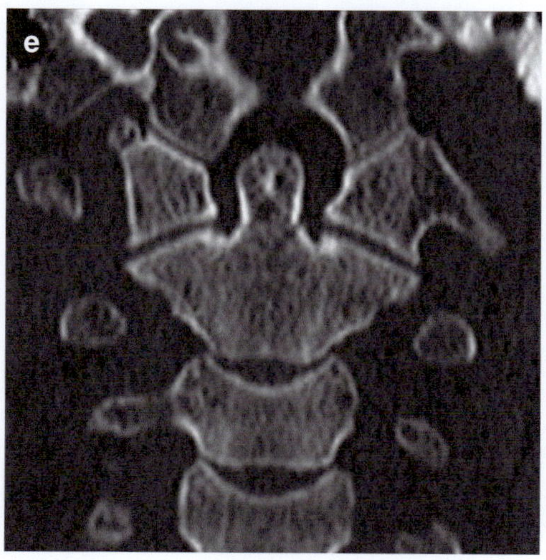

Fig 14.20 (**e**) CT coronal reconstruction confirmed the fracture line through the odontoid base to the vertebral body

11. Identification of sesamoid bone and fracture of the odontoid process
    11.1 X-ray film (Fig. 14.21a, b)

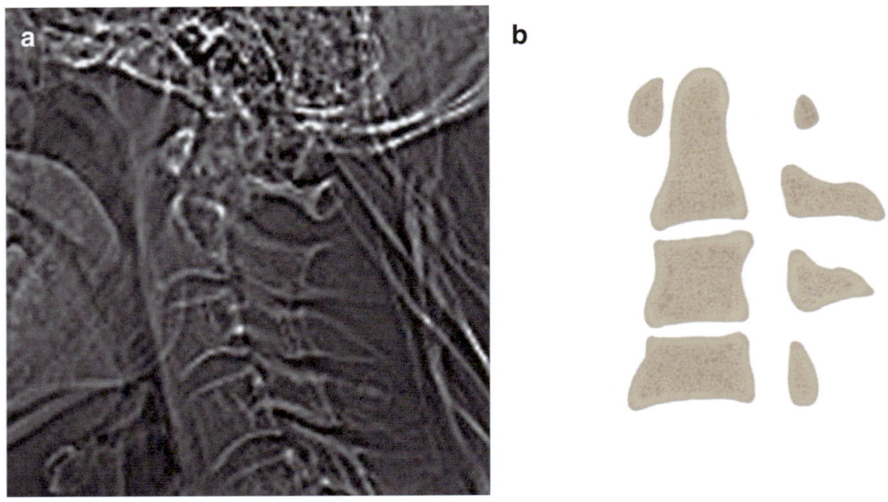

Fig. 14.21 There is no abnormality in the lateral radiograph of the cervical vertebra (**a**), schematic view (**b**)

    11.2 CT scan (Fig. 14.21c, d)

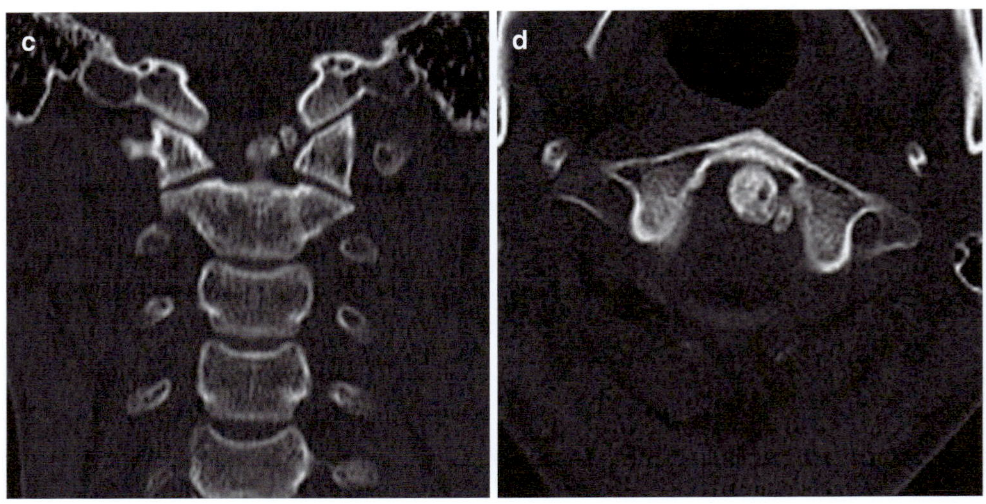

Fig. 14.21 CT coronal plane (**c**) reconstruction and cross section (**d**) show free ossification on the tip of odontoid, visible cortical shadow, easily misdiagnosed as a fracture block

14.3 Lower Cervical Spine Fracture

14.3.1 Identification of Injury Mechanism

Most are indirect traumatic injury, such as falling from a height or the neck violently front-flexing and retro-stretching in a traffic accident (whiplash injury); direct trauma is less common. According to the external force of injury, it is divided into flexion type and overextension type. Specifically, it can be divided into vertebral compression fracture, Clay-Shoveler fracture, vertebral burst fracture, teardrop fracture, cervical anterior dislocation, facet joint dislocation, twist lock and so on.

14.3.2 Identification of Symptom and Sign

The clinical manifestations are upper neck pain and limited mobility. It is easy to miss diagnosis and clinical examination lacks specificity. Some patients only show neck pain, limited mobility, and can present to the hospital on their own. It can often be misdiagnosed as a sprain with imaging not offered, which may result in serious fracture dislocation.

14.3.3 Imaging Differential Diagnosis

In the injury of the cervical vertebrae, if the shape or position of the vertebral body is not clearly dislocated, the fracture appears in the attachment area. X-ray plain film often does not show the correct diagnosis, as does MRI. The most accurate examination method is thin-layer CT and CT reconstruction, which play an important role in the diagnosis of cervical vertebrae attachment fractures. Due to the occlusion of the lower neck, the X-ray often cannot show the C6-7 and spinous process fractures. CT sagittal reconstruction or MRI sagittal plane is required. In addition, the fracture and dislocation of the facet joints of the vertebral body, especially unilateral dislocation, X-ray plain film often cannot be correctly diagnosed, and CT sagittal reconstruction is needed.

1. C3 pedicle fracture and no fracture identification
   1.1 X-ray film (Fig. 14.22a–d)

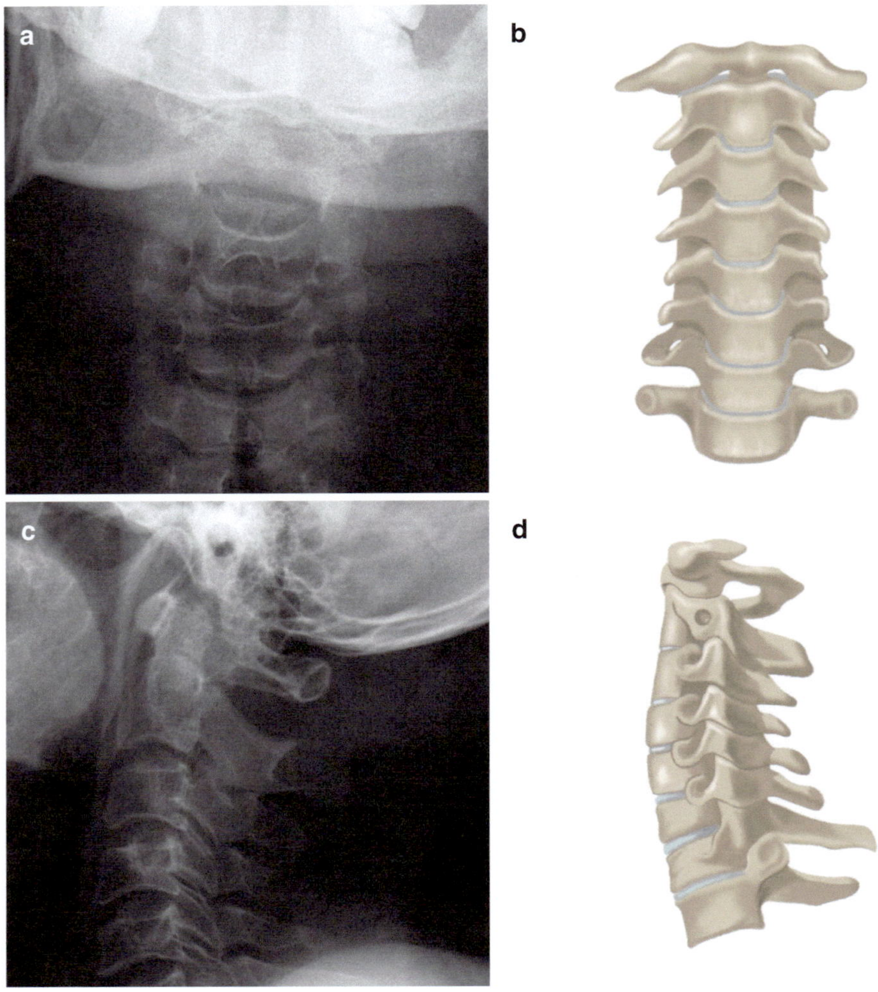

Fig. 14.22 The cervical vertebra anterior-posterior (**a**) and lateral (**c**) plain film shows no fracture, schematic view (**b**, **d**)

   1.2 CT scan (Fig. 14.22e)

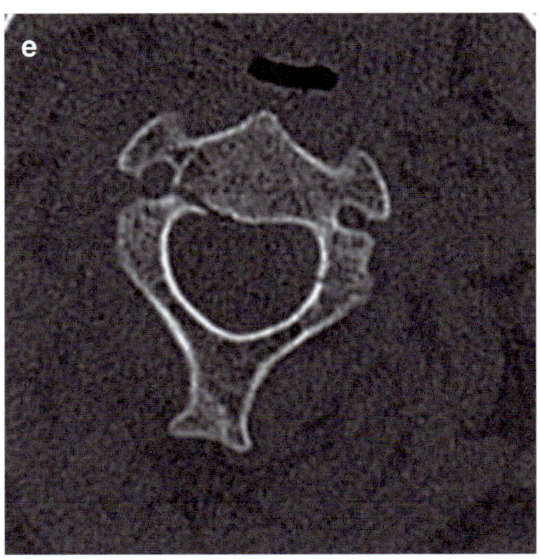

Fig. 14.22 The CT axial plane (**e**) image shows the fracture line passing through the right transverse foramen and posterior edge of the left pedicle of C3

2. Identification of the cervical spinous process fractures and suspected fractures
   2.1 X-ray film (Fig. 14.23a–d)

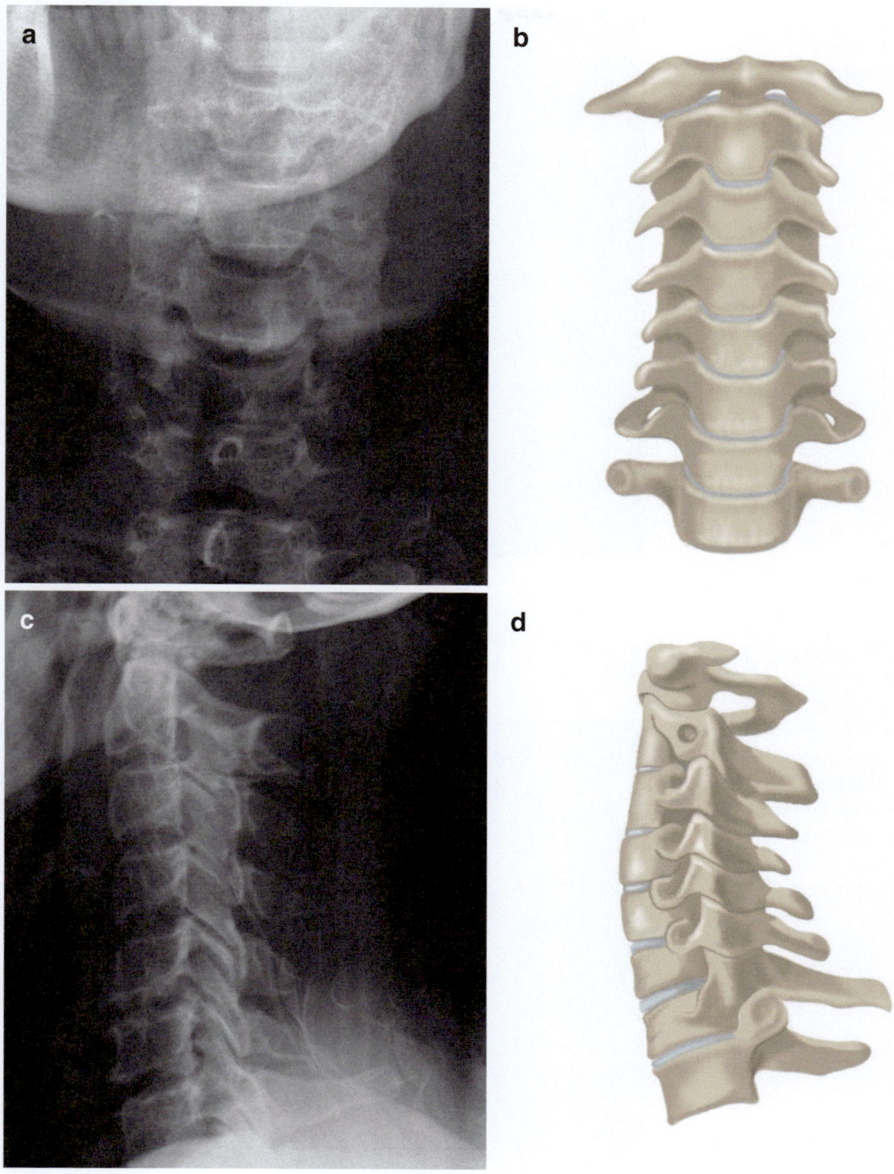

Fig. 14.23 The cervical anterior-posterior (**a**) and lateral plain film (**c**) show no fracture, schematic view (**b**, **d**)

2.2 CT scan (Fig. 14.23e, f)

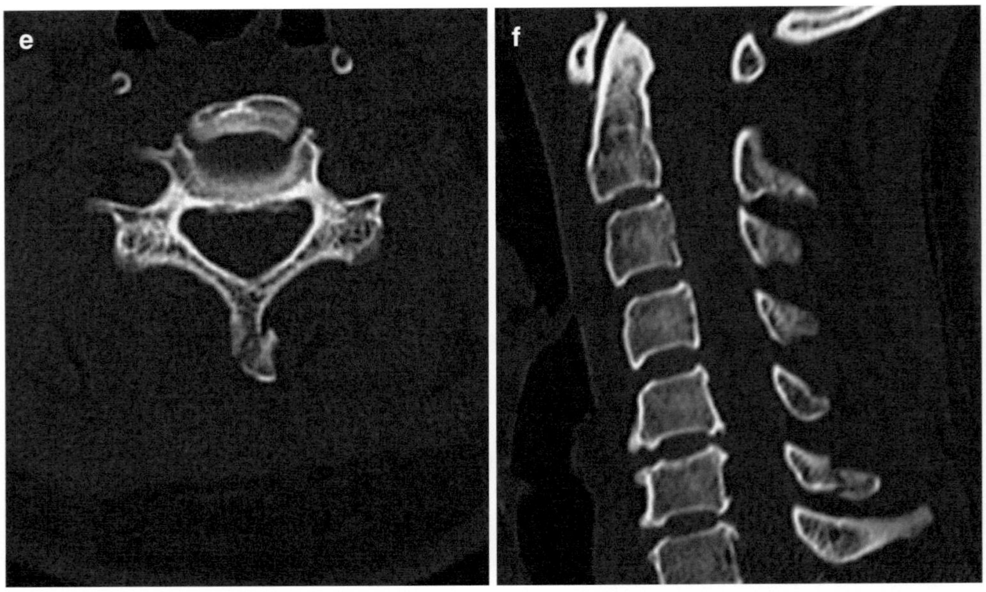

Fig. 14.23 CT axial position (**e**) image and sagittal plane (**f**) reconstruction show C6 spinous process fracture

2.3 MR imaging (Fig. 14.23g, h)

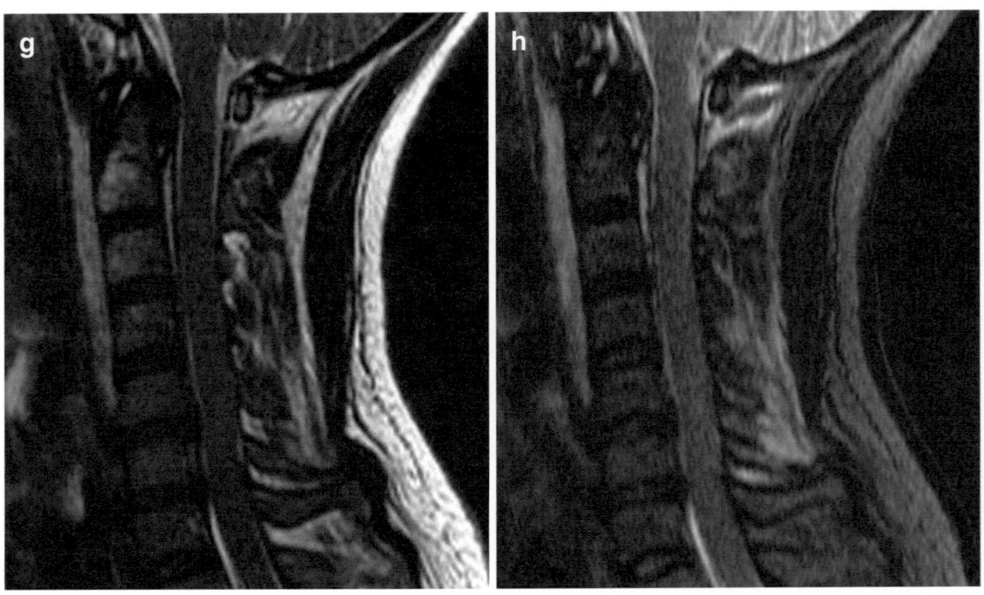

Fig. 14.23 No signs of fracture were seen in MRI T2WI (**g**), and the STIR sequence (**h**) shows an increase signal of the soft tissues around spinous process of C4-6

3. Identification of multiple spinous process fractures and suspected fractures of the cervical vertebra
   3.1 X-ray film (Fig. 14.24a–d)

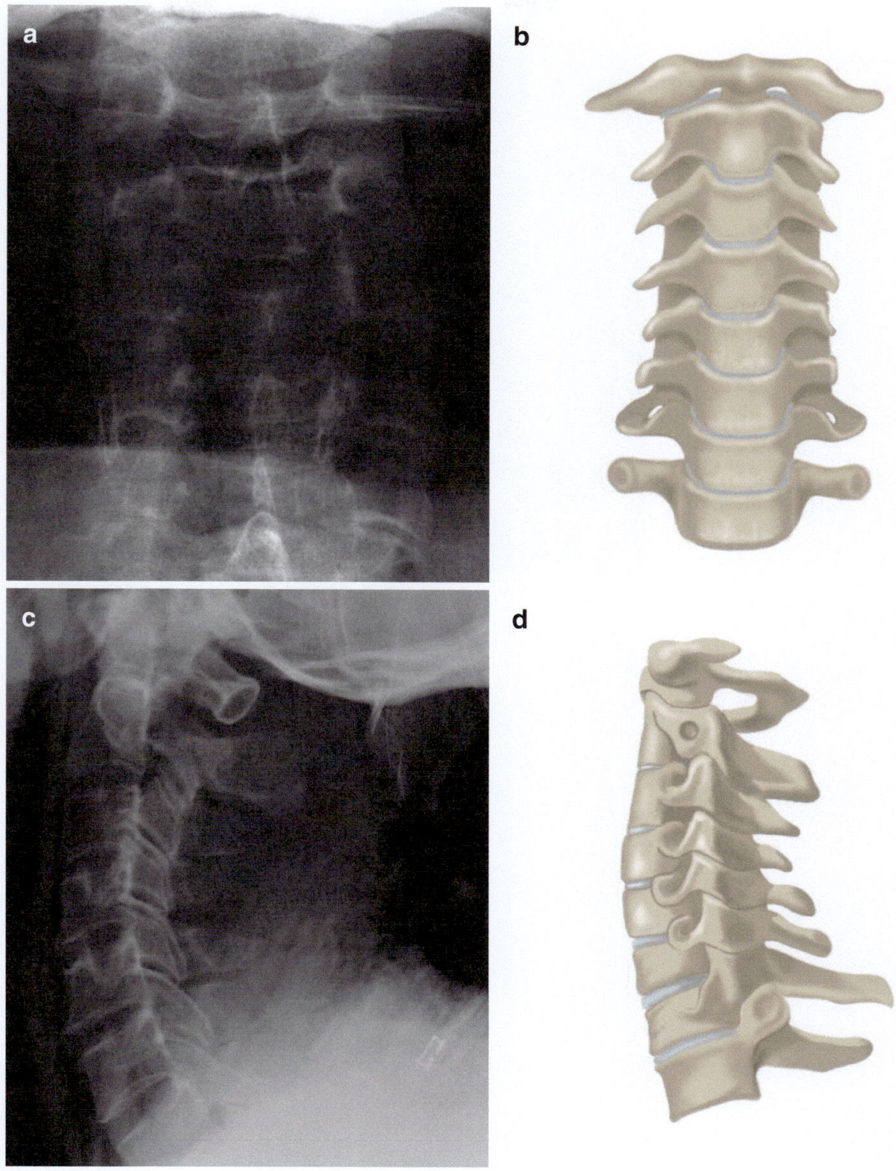

Fig. 14.24 The cervical spine PA (**a**) shows that the "ghost sign" is visible in C7 and T1 spinous processes, and the cervical lateral film (**c**) has no fractures. (**b**, **d**)

3.2 CT scan (Fig. 14.24e, f)

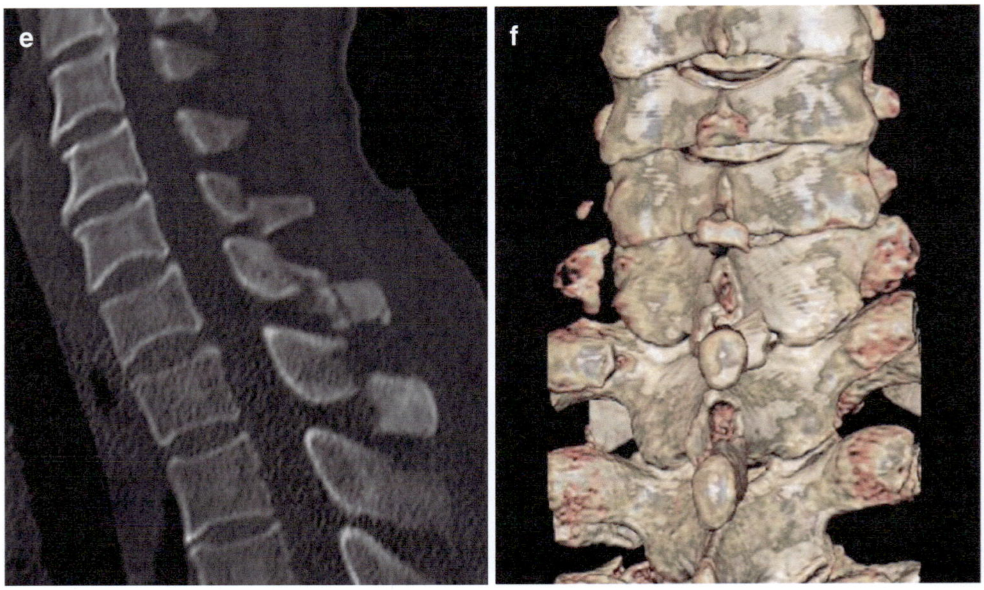

Fig. 14.24 CT sagittal plane (**e**) reconstruction and VR reconstruction (**f**) show spinous process fractures of C6-T1

4. Identification of multiple spinous process fractures and no fracture of cervical vertebra
   4.1 X-ray film (Fig. 14.25a–d)

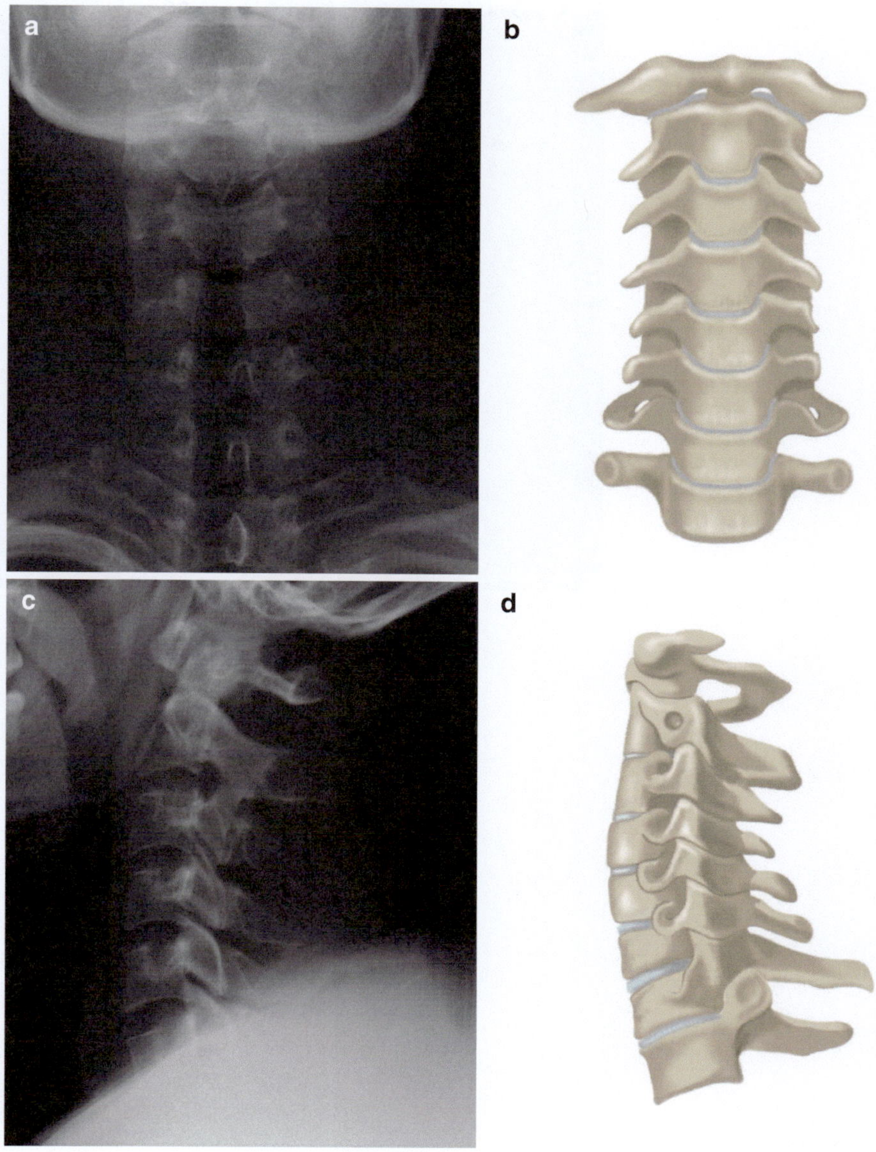

Fig. 14.25 The cervical vertebra PA (**a**)-LAT (**c**) plain film shows no fractures, schematic view (**b**, **d**)

4.2 MR imaging (Fig. 14.25e, f)

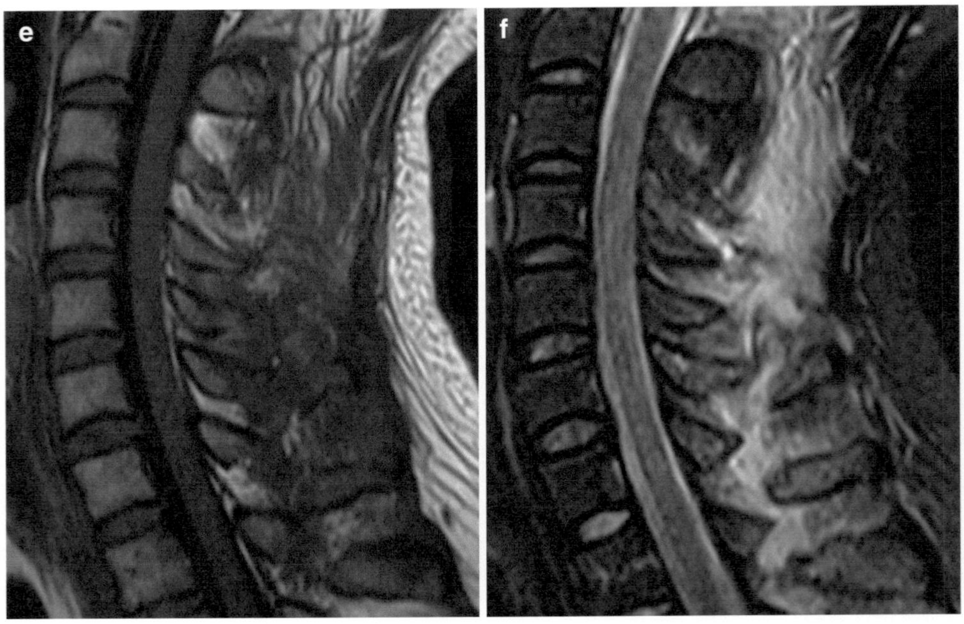

Fig. 14.25 MRI shows spinous process fractures of C6-T1 (**e**, **f**)

5. Cervical vertebral endplate inferior fracture and no fracture identification
   5.1 X-ray film (Fig. 14.26a, b)

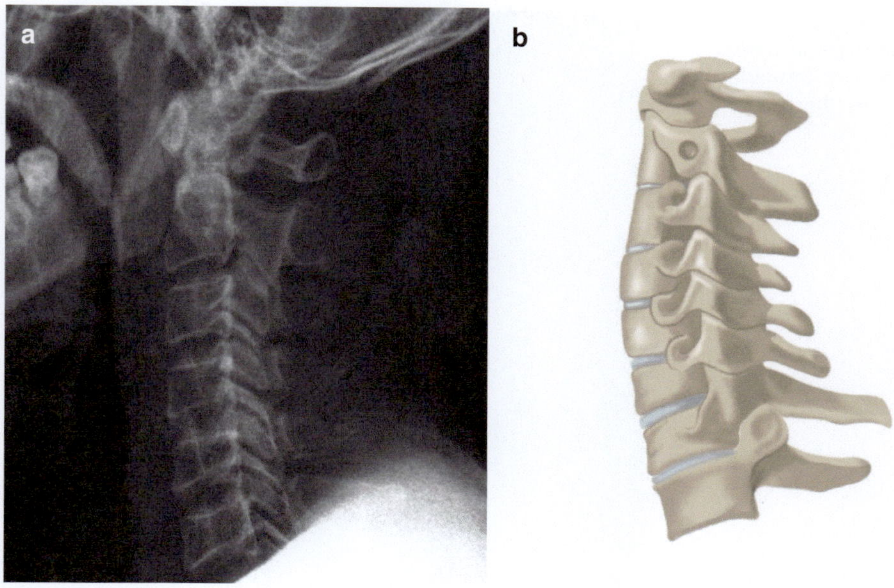

Fig. 14.26 No fractures were found in the lateral radiograph of the cervical vertebra (**a**), and the soft tissue was thickened anterior the vertebrae, schematic view (**b**)

   5.2 MR imaging (Fig. 14.26c, d)

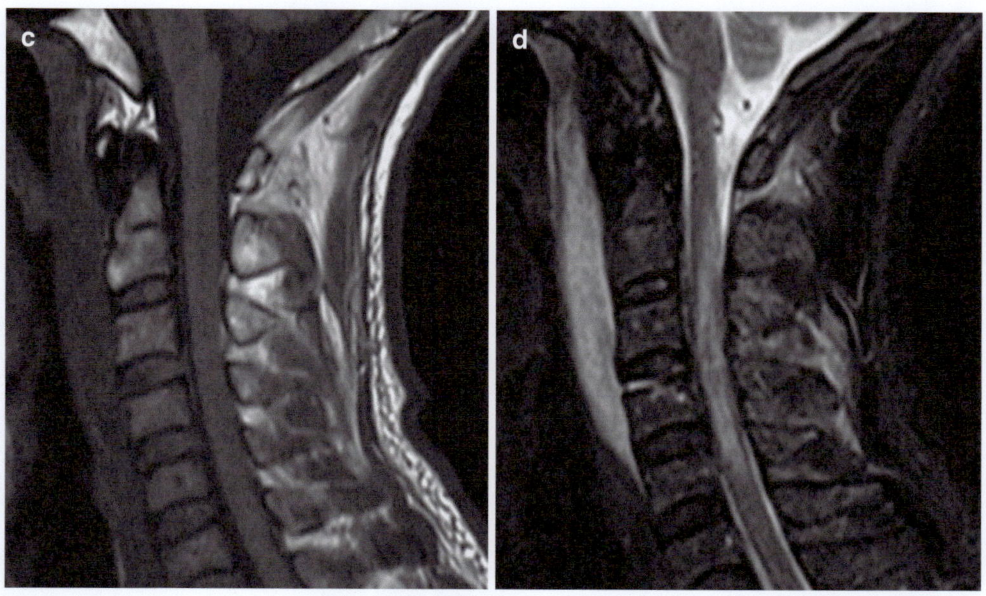

Fig. 14.26 MRI images show C4 inferior vertebral endplate and vertebrae fractures, cervical anterior hematoma, cervical interspinous ligament injury, and C2-5 spinal cord injury (**c**, **d**)

6. Comparison of X-ray film and MR of the cervical intervertebral disc and interspinous ligament injury
   6.1 X-ray film (Fig. 14.27a, b)

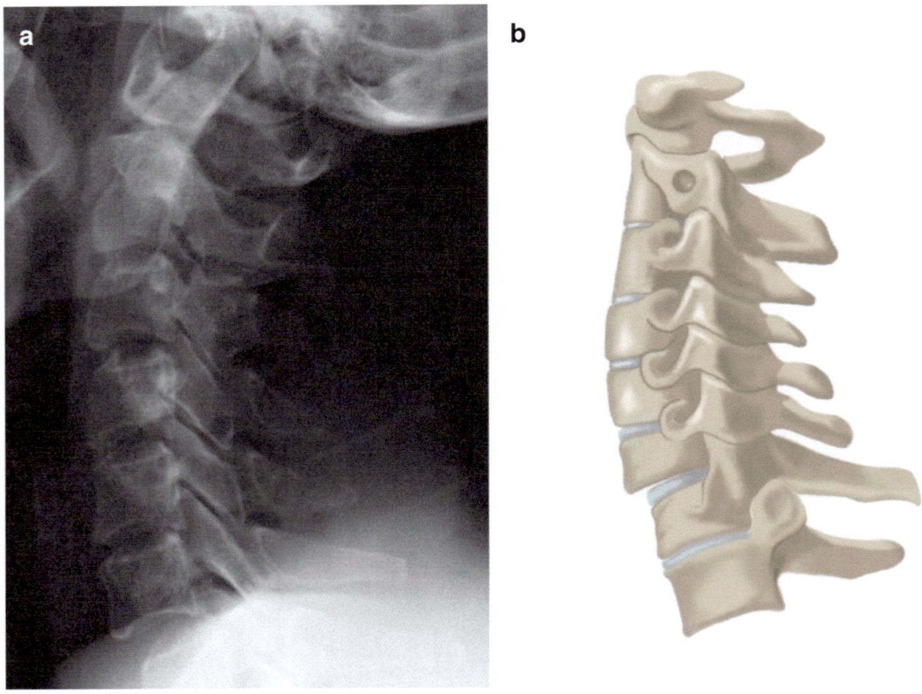

Fig. 14.27 The cervical lateral radiograph (**a**) shows C6 vertebral body forward, schematic view (**b**)

   6.2 MR imaging (Fig. 14.27c–e)

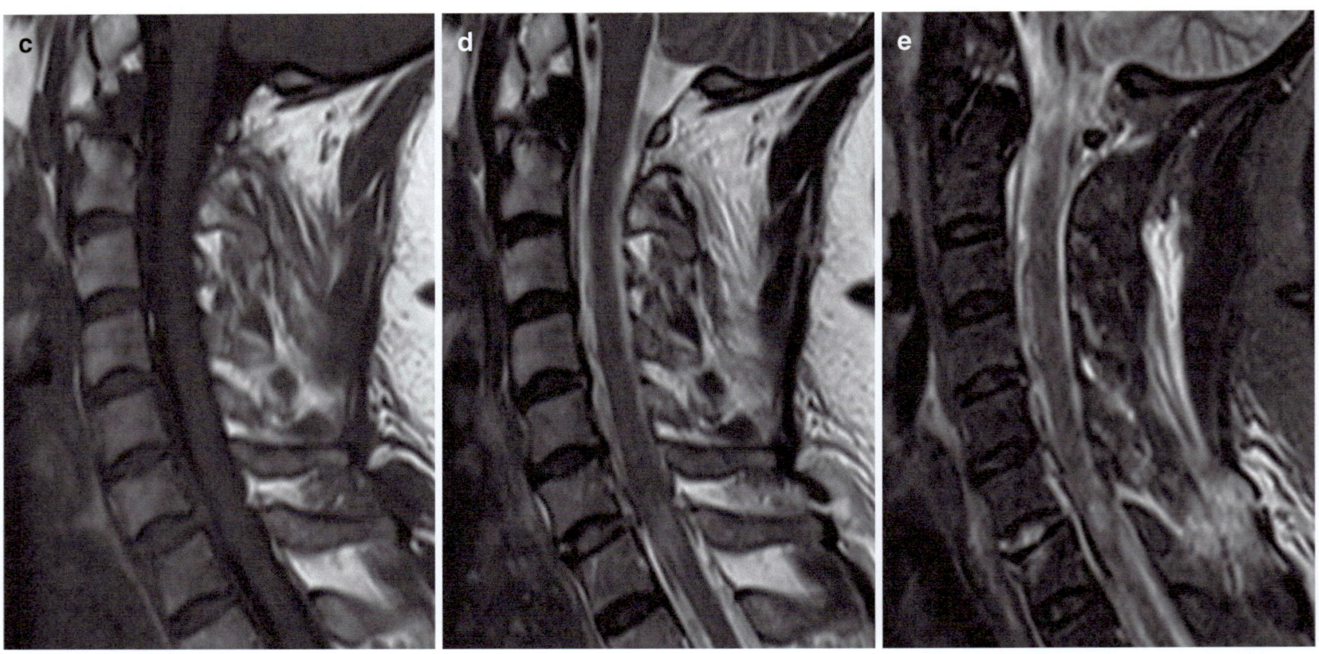

Fig. 14.27 MRI images show that the arrangement of cervical vertebrae was well, and anterior longitudinal ligament, intervertebral disc and interspinous ligament of C6-7 were injured (**c–e**)

7. Comparison between X-ray film and CT of cervical facet joint dislocation
   7.1 X-ray film (Fig. 14.28a, b)

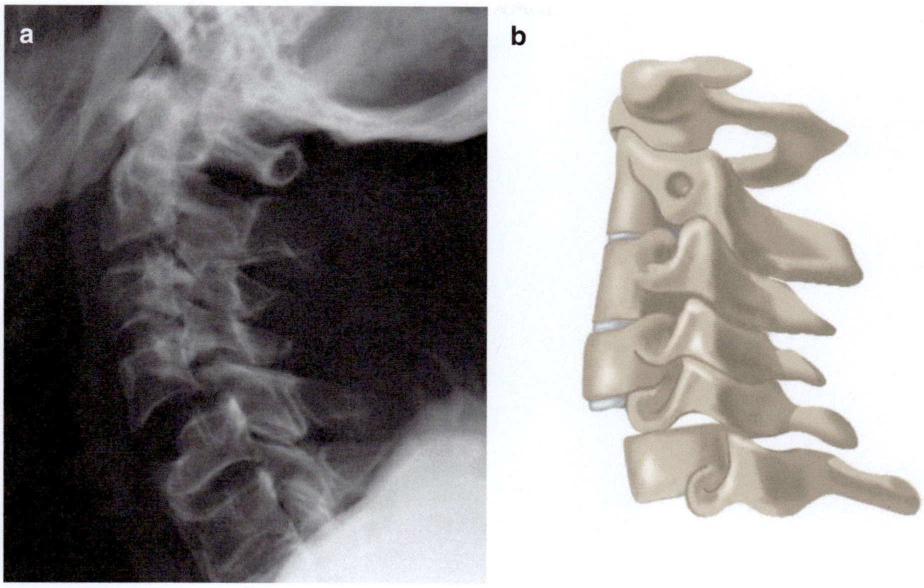

Fig. 14.28 The cervical lateral radiograph (**a**) shows that C4 vertebral body is displaced forward, and the small joints correspond well. Schematic view (**b**)

   7.2 CT scan (Fig. 14.28c, d)

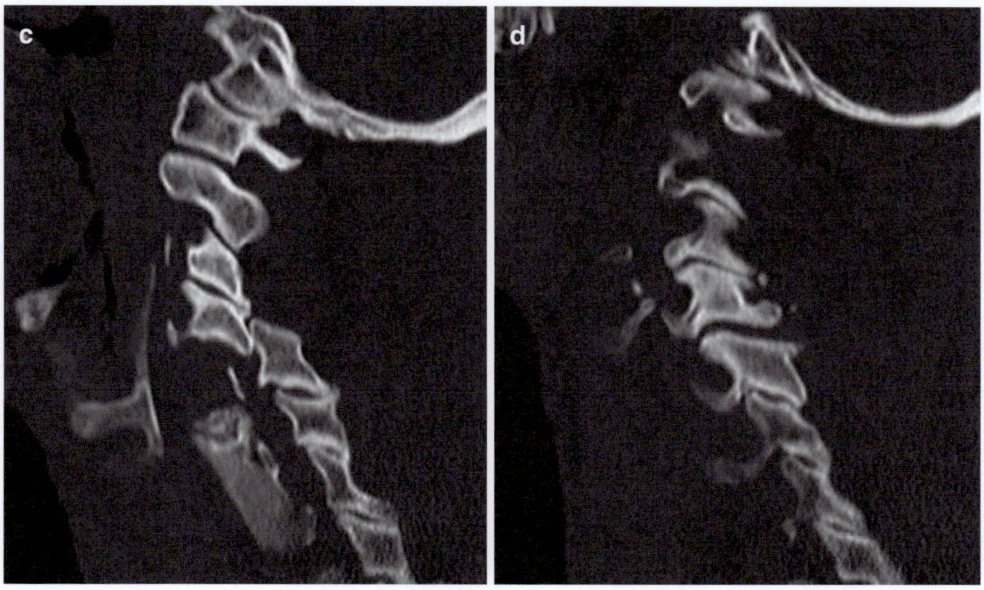

Fig. 14.28 CT sagittal reconstruction shows dislocation of the right vertebral facet joint, and the left facet joint space was slightly widened (**c**, **d**)

8. Comparison between plain film, CT and MR of multiple anterior-inferior margin teardrop fractures of cervical vertebrae
   8.1 X-ray film (Fig. 14.29a, b)

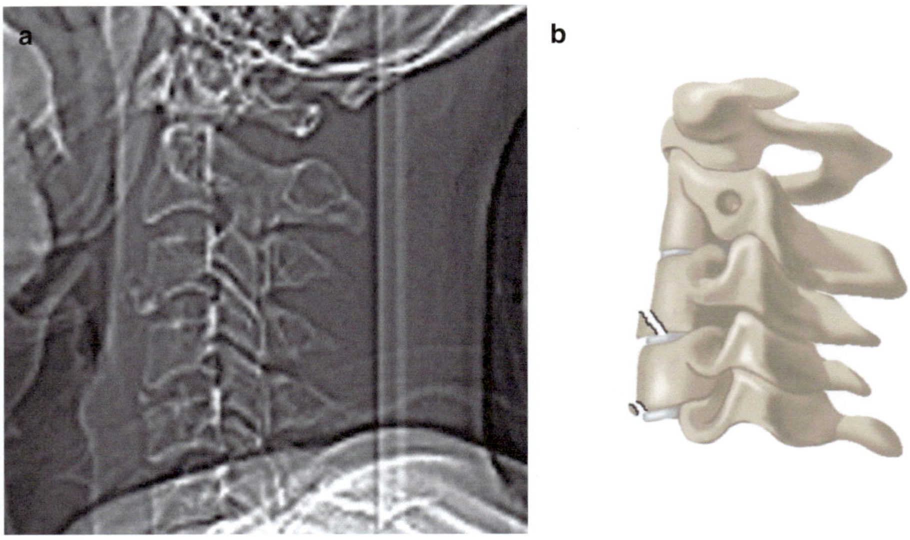

Fig. 14.29 Cervical lateral radiograph (**a**) shows the anterior-inferior border bone fracture of C3 and C4, and fracture blocks dislocation of C3, schematic view (**b**)

   8.2 CT scan (Fig. 14.29c, d)

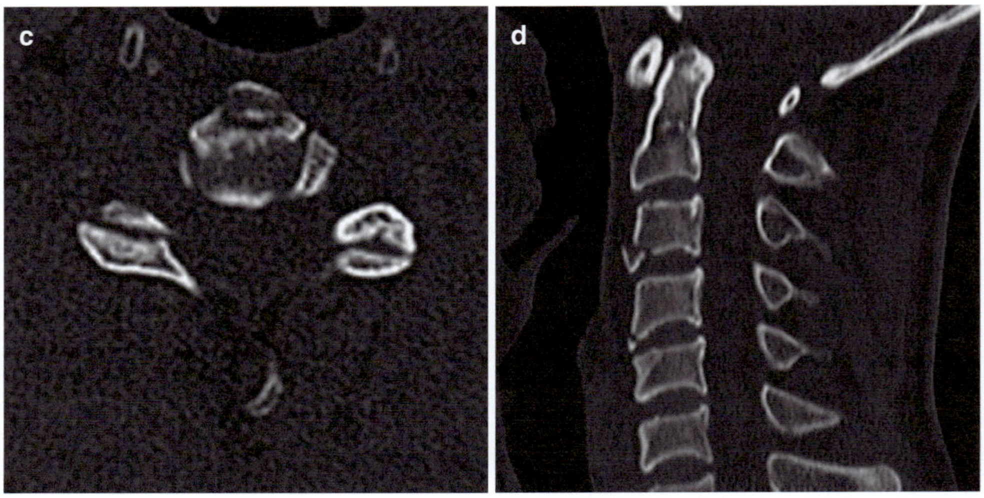

Fig. 14.29 CT cross-sectional and sagittal reconstruction shows the anterior-inferior border fracture of C3-4, and the dislocation of C3 fracture block (**c**, **d**)

8.3 MR imaging (Fig. 14.29e–g)

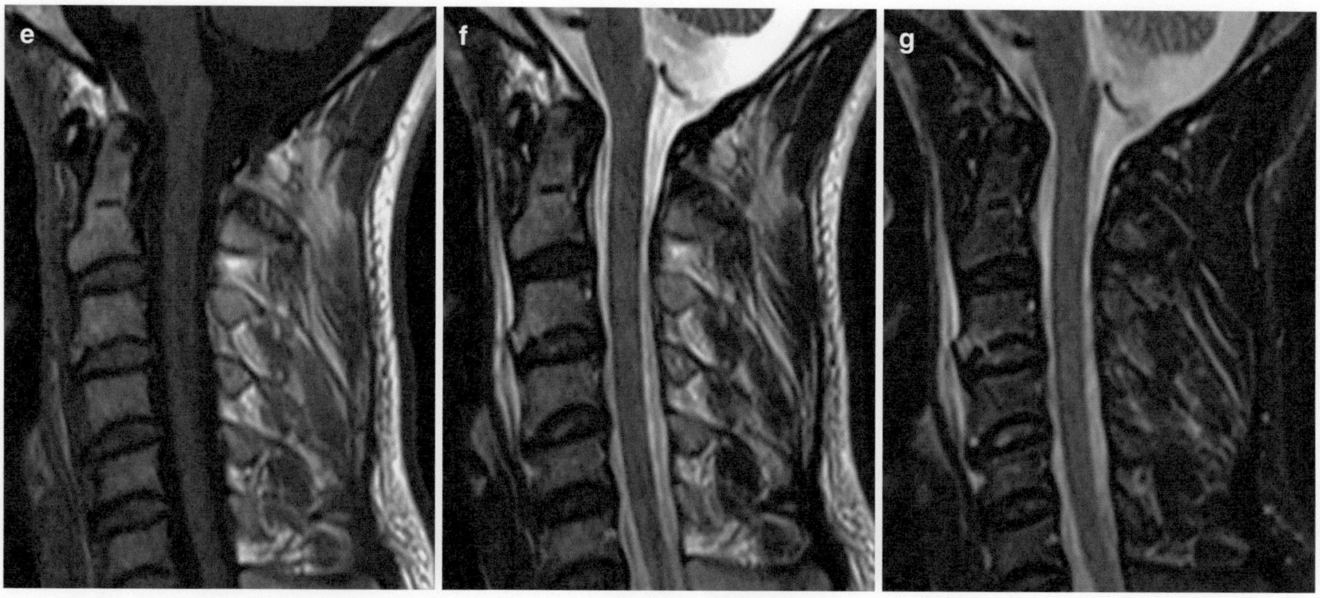

Fig. 14.29 MRI can show the fracture block of C3, but the fractures of C4 is unclear (**e**, **f**)

9. Cervical spine compression fracture and no fracture identification
   9.1 X-ray film (Fig. 14.30a–d)

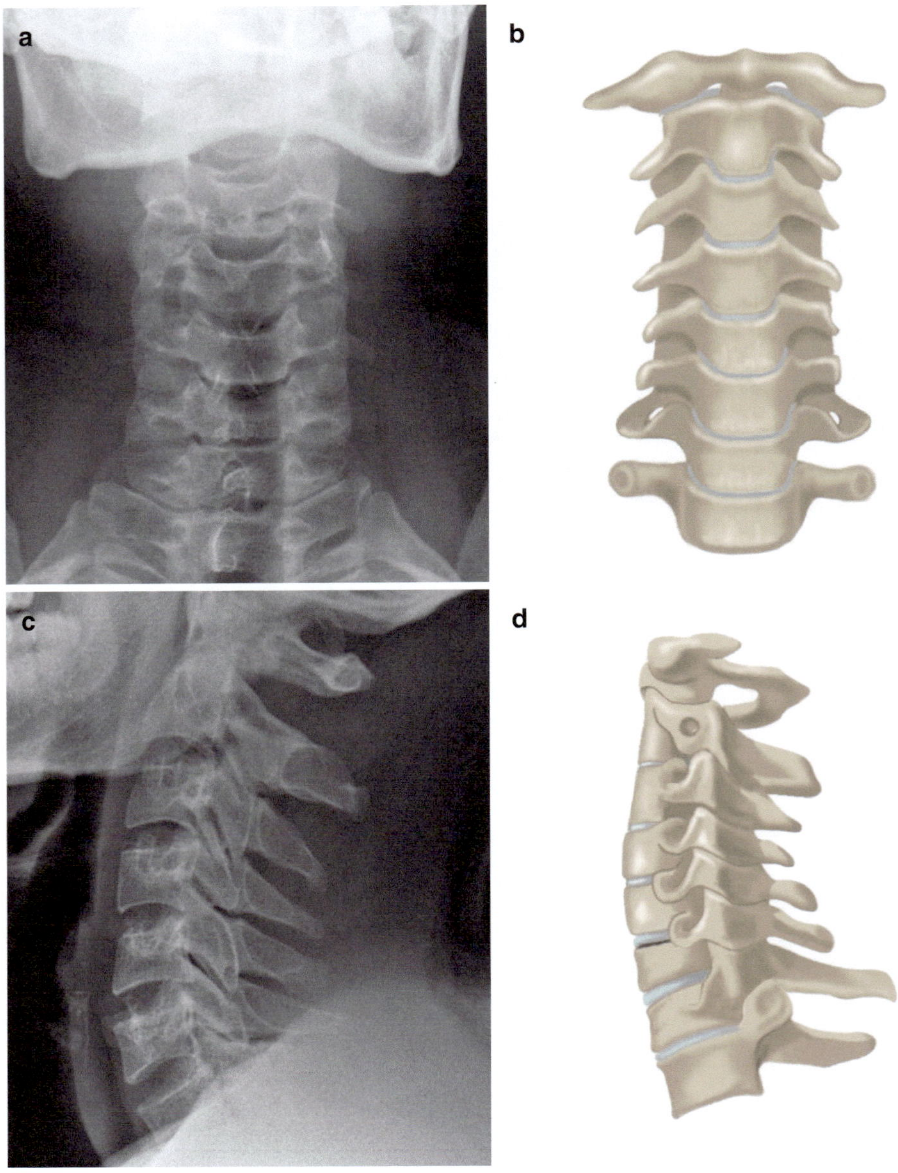

Fig. 14.30 The cervical vertebra anterior-posterior (**a**) and lateral (**c**) plain films show the cervical vertebrae have no clear fracture signs, schematic view (**b**, **d**)

9.2 CT scan (Fig. 14.30e, f)

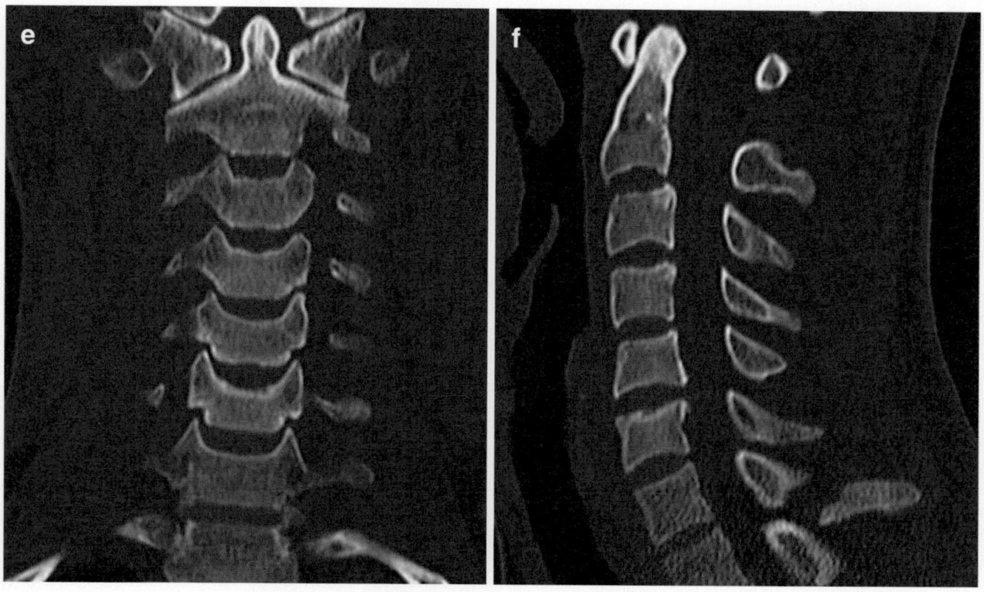

Fig. 14.30 CT coronal reconstruction (**e**) and sagittal reconstruction (**f**) show that the upper edge of C6 was slightly depressed, and the spinous process of C7 was broken and the fracture block was dislocated

9.3 MR imaging (Fig. 14.30g–i)

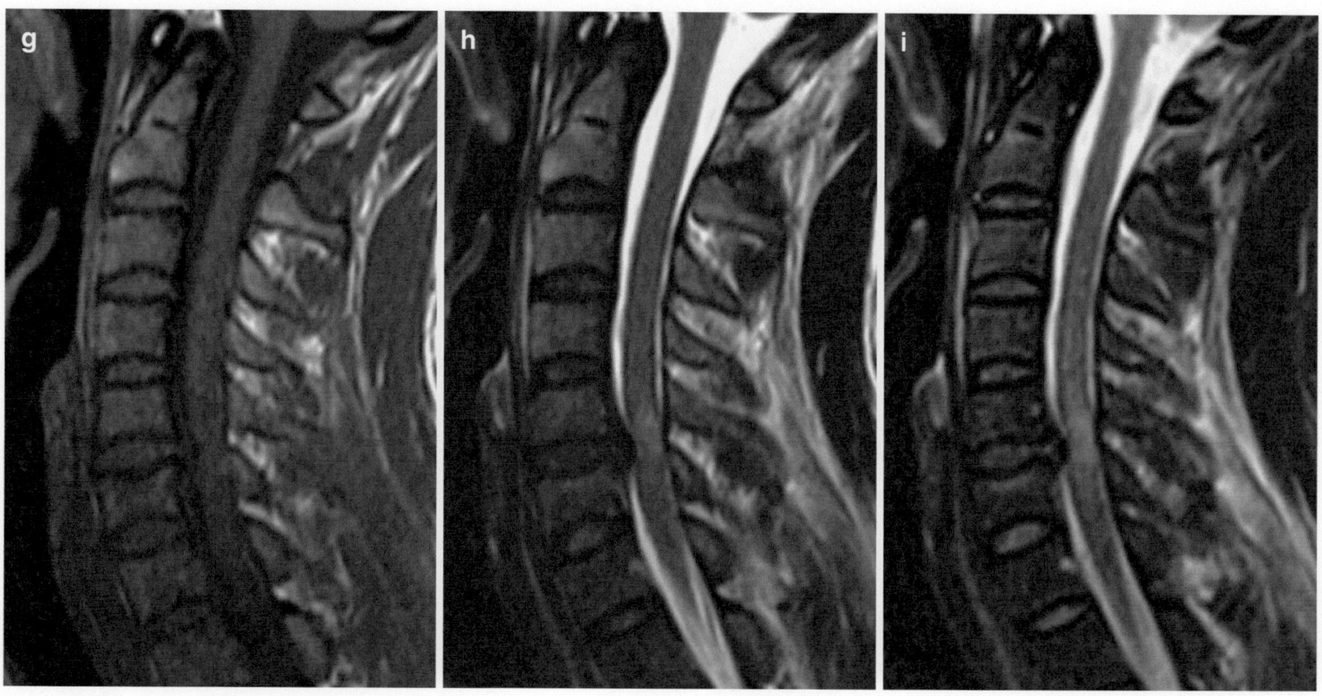

Fig. 14.30 MRI sagittal plane T1WI (**g**) T2WI (**h**) T2WI-FS (**i**) show compression fracture of the upper edge of C6, with a line-like long T1 long T2 signal, C5/6 intervertebral disc protruding backward, local spinal canal narrowed, the spinal cord compressed, and a patchy T2 high signal in the spinal cord

10. Identification of cervical burst fractures and compression fractures
    10.1 X-ray film (Fig. 14.31a–d)

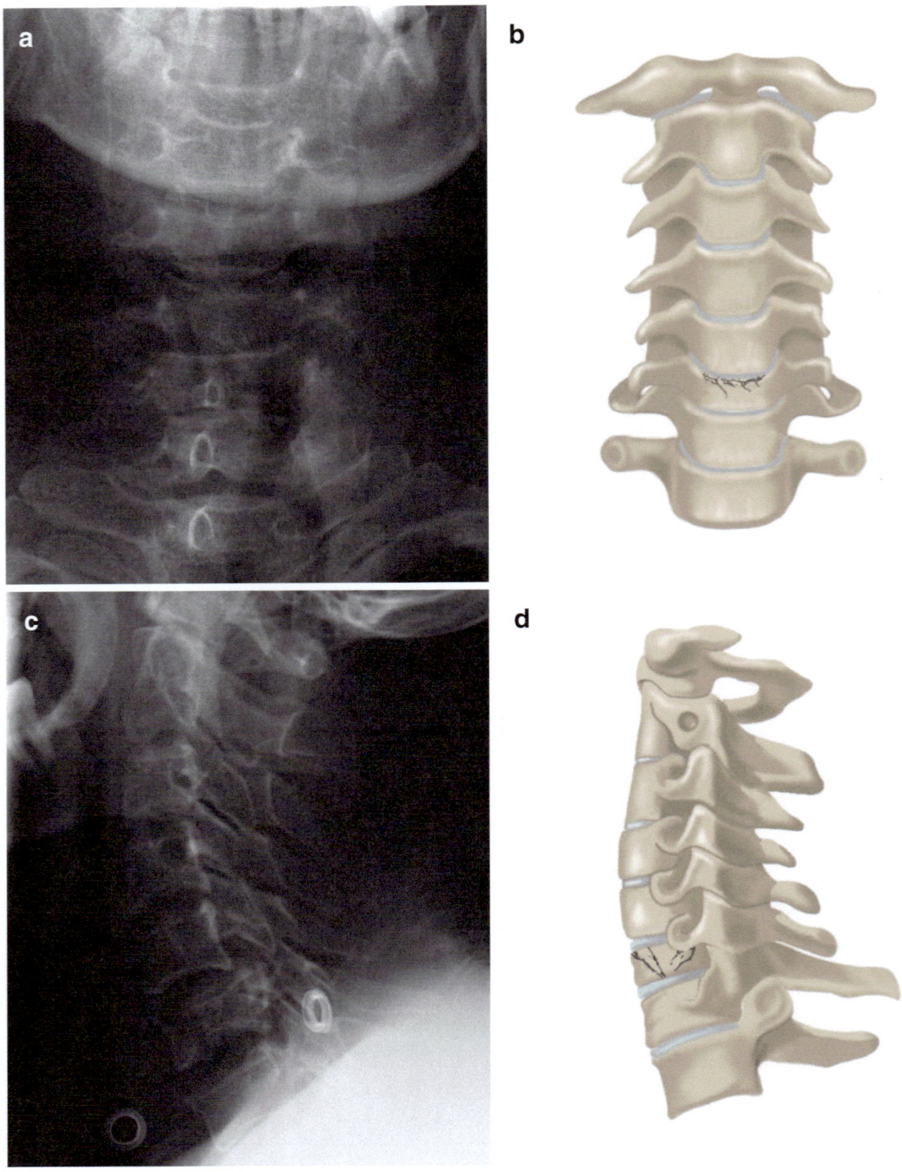

Fig. 14.31 The cervical vertebra anterior-posterior (**a**) and lateral (**c**) plain films show that the cervical vertebral body of C6 is flattened, the bone is fragmented, the anteroposterior diameter is enlarged, and the spinal canal is narrowed, schematic view (**b**, **d**)

10.2 CT scan (Fig. 14.31e–h)

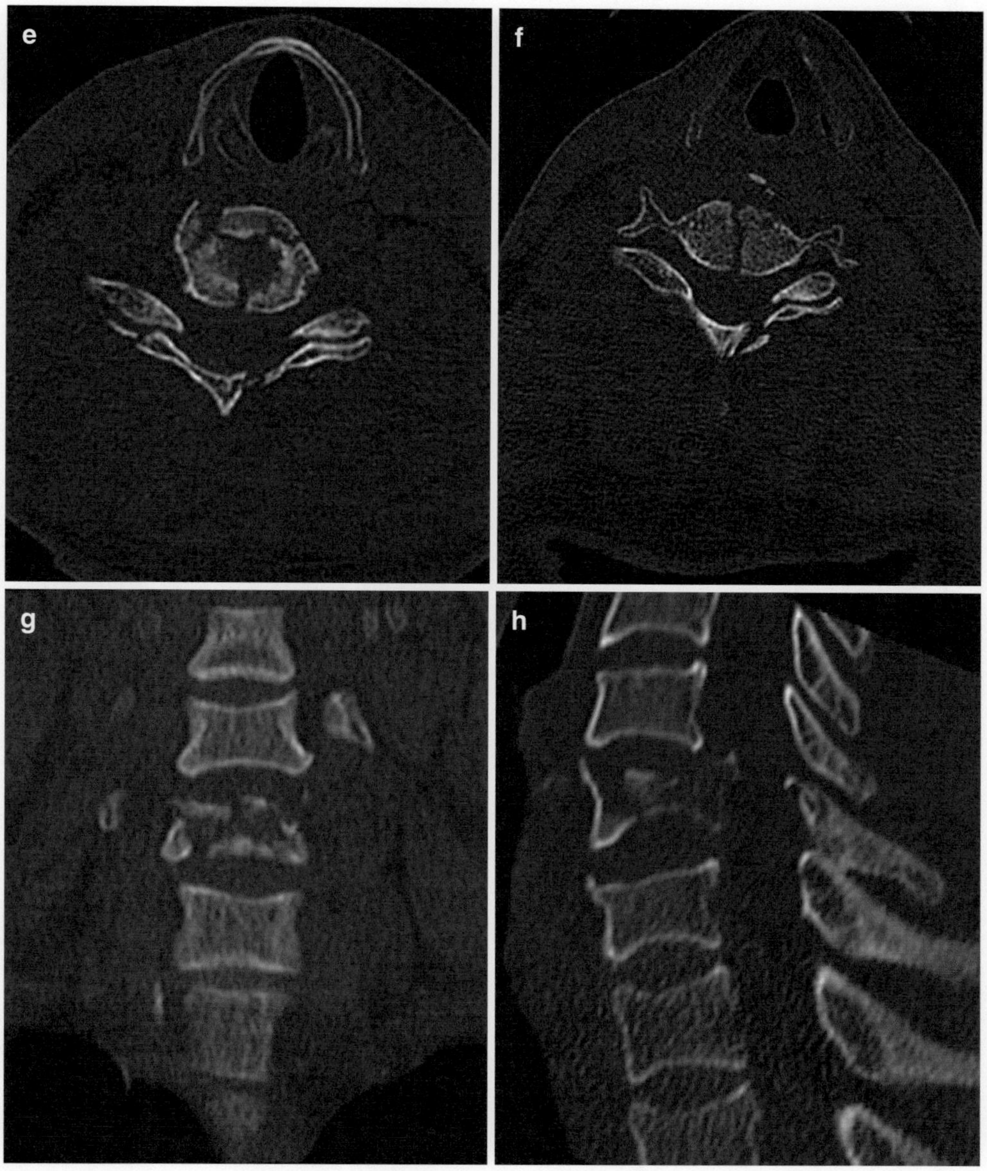

Fig. 14.31 CT cross-section (**e**, **f**), coronal reconstruction (**g**) and sagittal reconstruction (**h**) show that C6 vertebral body became flattened obviously, companied with the fracture block protruding backward into the narrowing spinal canal

10.3 MR imaging (Fig. 14.31i–l)

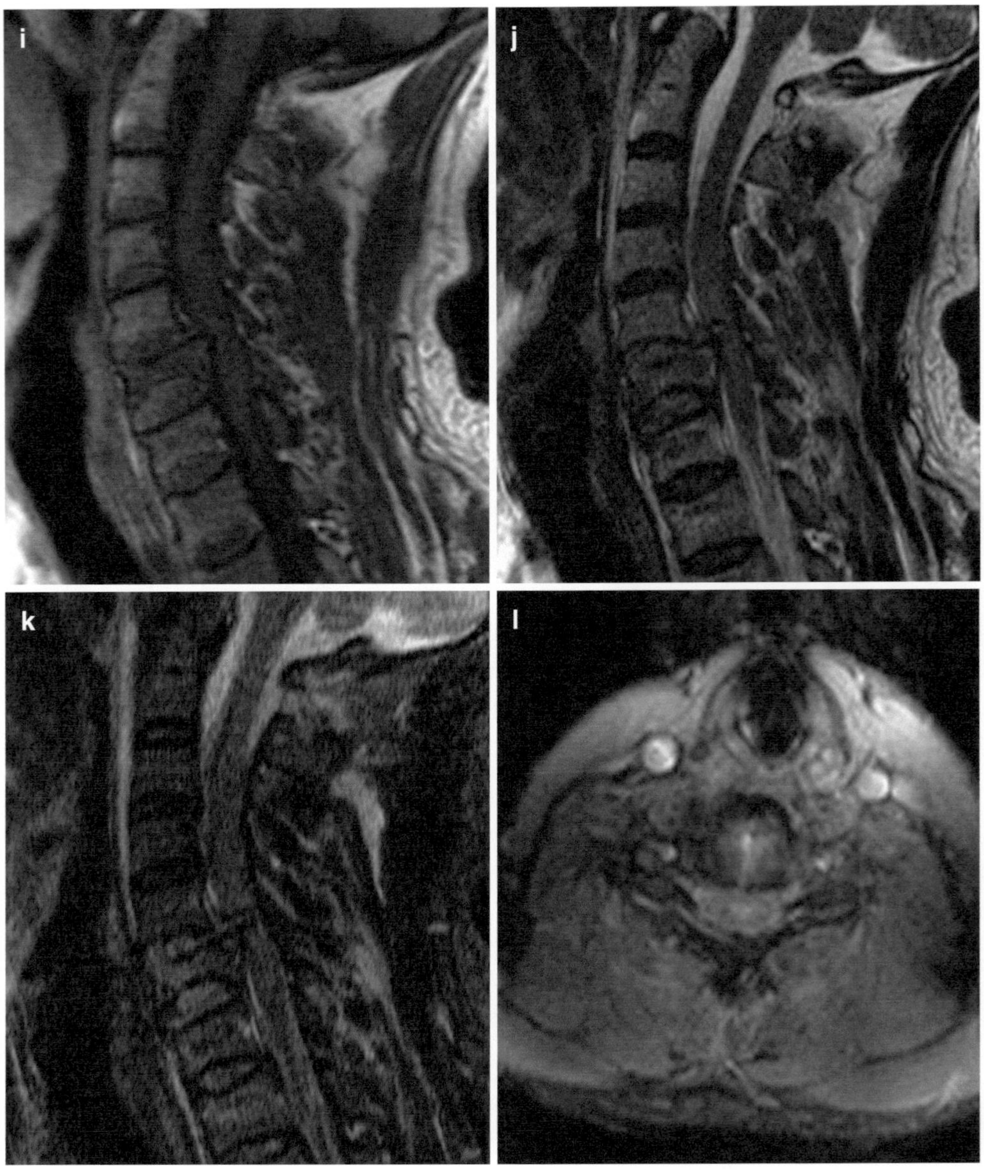

Fig. 14.31 MRI sagittal plane T1WI (**i**) T2WI (**j**) T2WI-FS (**k**) and axial T2WI-FS (**l**) show that C6 vertebral body is flattened, the bone is broken, and the posterior margin of the vertebral body backward, the spinal canal narrowed, the spinal cord is compressed, and the spinal cord is partially contiguous, showing T2 high signal

14.4 Summary of the Points

1. X-ray plain film is the most basic method for diagnosing cervical spine fracture and dislocation. However, due to the overlapping structure, the imaging of fine structures is not optimal, and it cannot show the damage of spinal cord and soft tissue.
2. The examination value of CT scan of vertebral fractures, appendix fractures, bony spinal canal is higher than X-ray and MRI, such as atlanto-occipital injury, atlantoaxial injury, cervicothoracic fracture, facet joint dislocation. Multi-planar reconstruction can comprehensively interpret the spinal canal condition and fracture fragment displacement. CT scan for ligaments and spinal cord around the vertebral body also has limitations.
3. MRI imaging can show bone contusion. It is the best method to observe the damage of the spinal cord, intervertebral disc and ligament. MRI is commonly used to identify fresh and old fractures of the vertebral body, but for the fracture itself it is not as good as CT.

Thoracic and Lumbar Vertebral Fractures

15

Zhigang Peng and Yingze Zhang

1. Features of thoracic X-Ray and MR (Fig. 15.1)

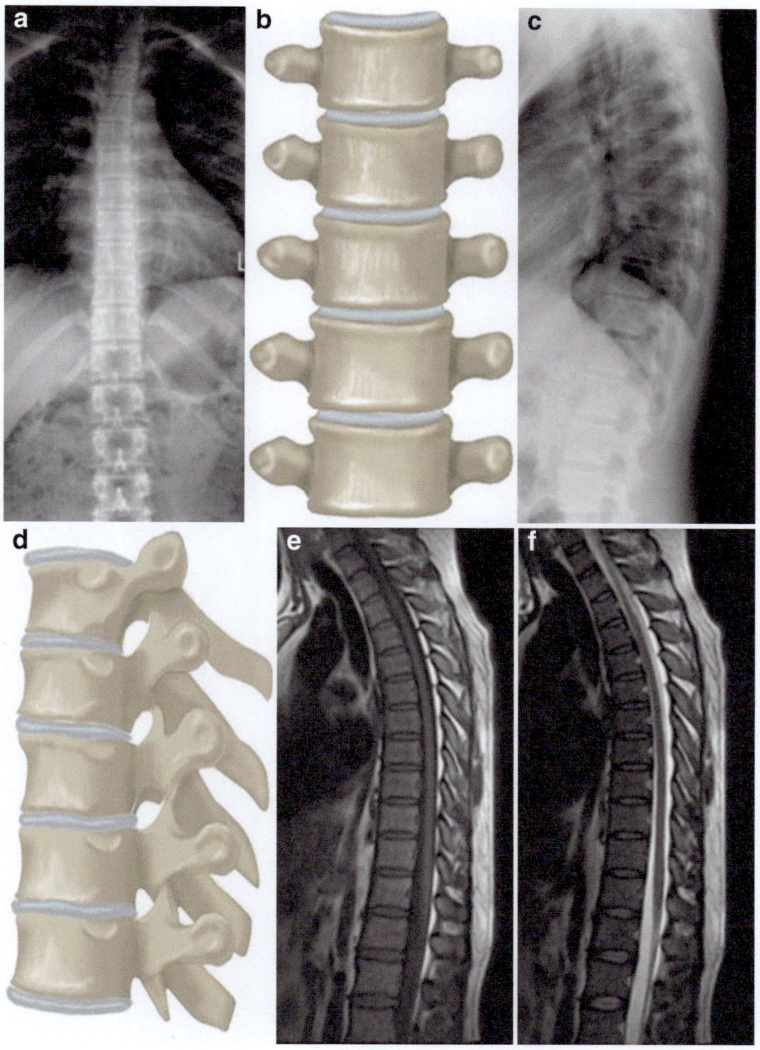

Fig. 15.1 The thoracic X-ray (**a**, **c**) shows that the vertebral bodies were neatly arranged, the physiological curvature was present, and no obvious abnormalities were found in the vertebral bodies and the appendix. (**b**, **d**); Sagittal MR T1WI (**e**) and T2WI (**f**) can clearly show the structure of the vertebral body, intervertebral disc, spinal cord, and the spinal canal

Z. Peng
CT/MRI Center, The Third Hospital of Hebei Medical University, Shijiazhuang, Hebei, China

Y. Zhang (✉)
Department of Orthopaedics, The Third Hospital of Hebei Medical University, Shijiazhuang, Hebei, China

Y. Zhang (ed.), *Differential Diagnosis of Fracture*, https://doi.org/10.1007/978-981-13-8339-7_15

2. Features of a normal lumbar spine X-Ray and MR (Fig. 15.2)

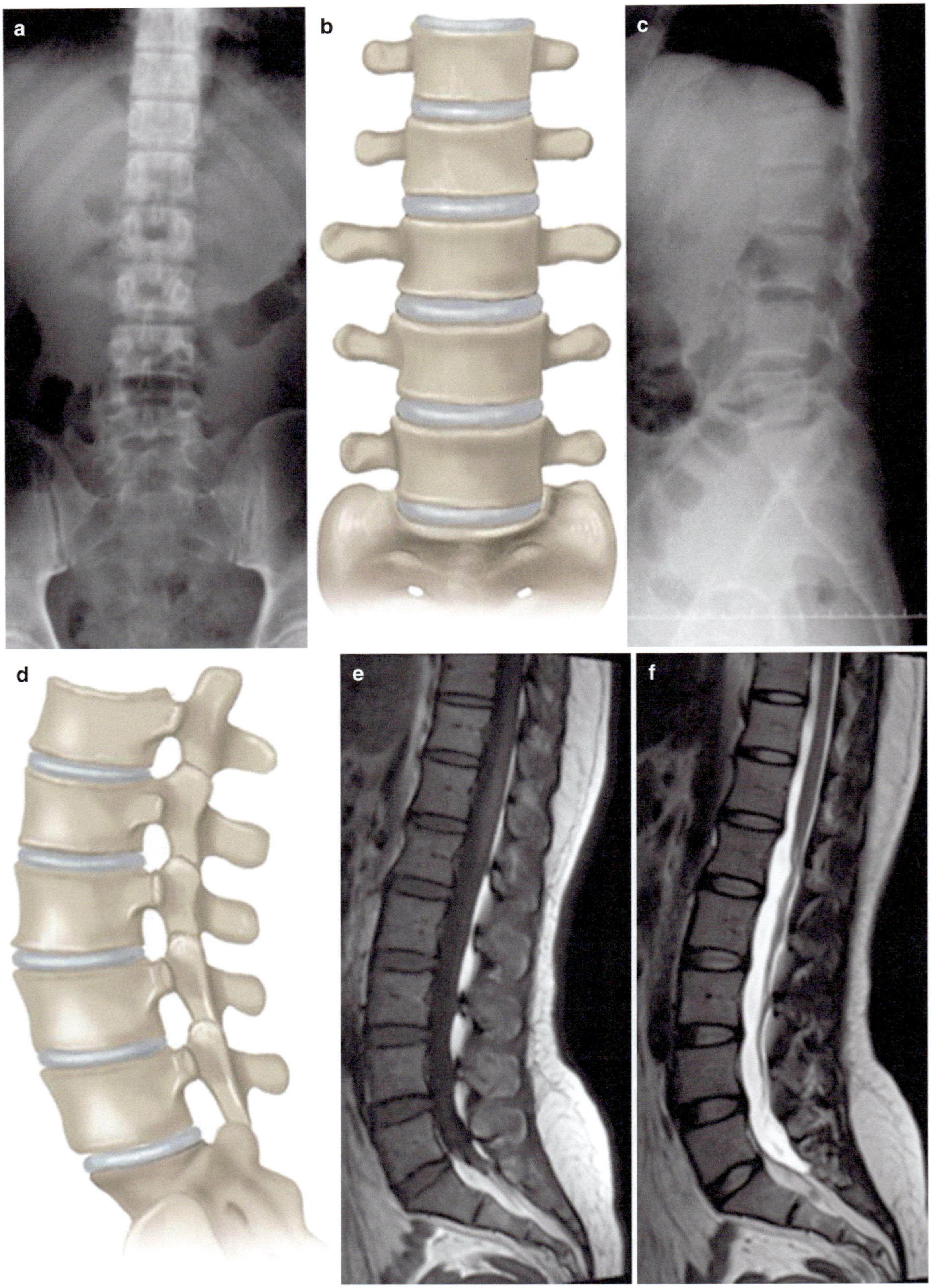

Fig. 15.2 Lumbar spine PA & LAT (**a**, **c**) shows neat vertebral body arrangement, physiological curvature, no obvious abnormalities in the vertebral body and appendix (**b**, **d**); sagittal MR T1WI (**e**) and T2WI (**f**) can clearly show the structure of the vertebral body, intervertebral disc, and the spinal cord

3. Plain film and MR features of the lumbar vertebral permanent epiphysis (Fig. 15.3)

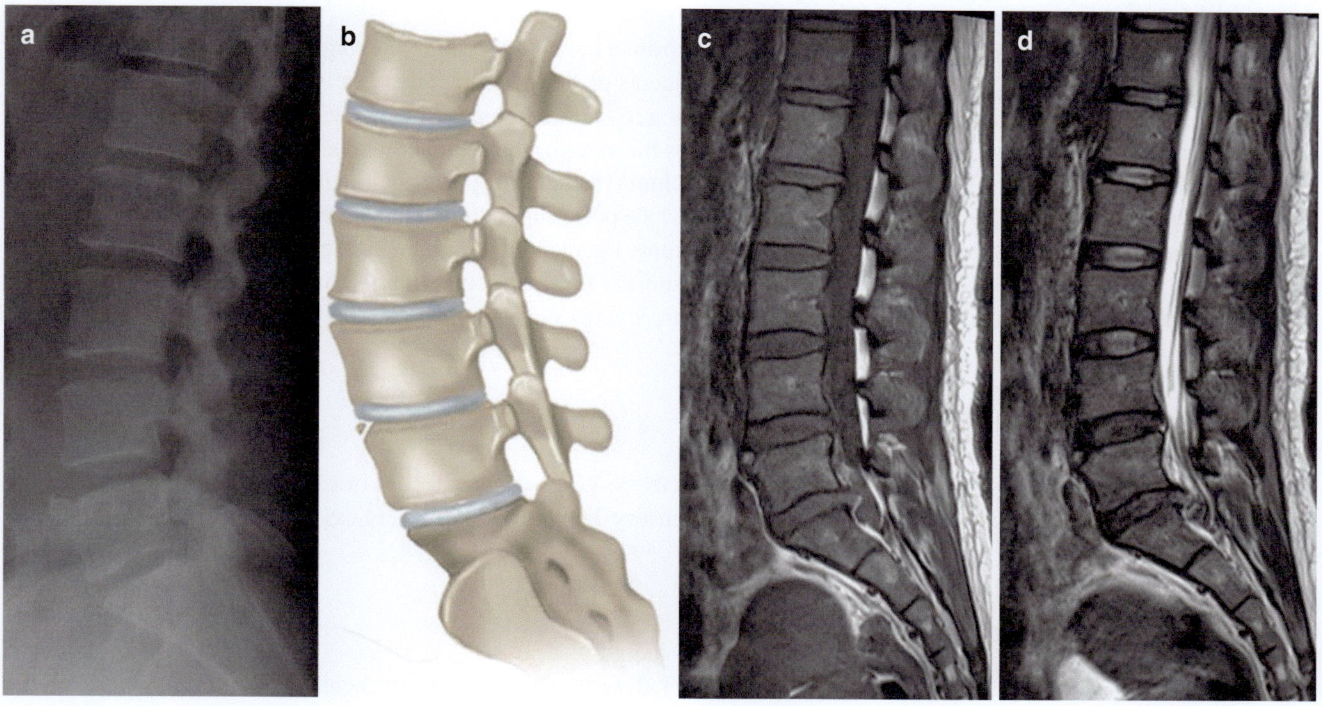

Fig. 15.3 Lateral lumbar X-ray (**a**) shows the anterior superior margin of L5 vertebral body, rounded, blunt, local vertebral osteosclerosis (**b**); sagittal MR T1WI (**c**) and T2WI (**d**) clearly shows the permanent epiphysis of the anterior superior edge of the L5 vertebral body

15.1 Vertebral Fracture

15.1.1 Injury Mechanism Identification

Most of them are caused by indirect trauma, such as falling from a height or violently flexing their torso; direct trauma can happen less often, with things such as impacts of traffic accidents or sharp contraction of muscles leading to avulsion fractures or transverse process fractures. The injury type according to the fracture position can be divided into anterior, middle, and posterior column fractures. The anterior column includes the anterior longitudinal ligament, the anterior 1/2 of the vertebral body, and the anterior portion of the disc; the middle column includes the posterior longitudinal ligament, the posterior 1/2 of the vertebral body, and the posterior portion of the disc; the posterior column includes the vertebral arch, the ligamentum flavum, and the intervertebral facet joints and interspinous ligaments. According to the injury mechanism, it can be divided into: (1) flexion compression fracture, (2) burst fracture, (3) flexion traction injury (chance fracture, also known as a seat belt fracture), (4) flexion and rotation fracture dislocation, and (5) shear-type dislocation.

15.1.2 Symptom and Sign Identification

The typical clinical features are low back pain and limited activity. When the spinal cord or cauda equina is damaged, there will also be neurological symptoms, such as movement or sensory disturbances. In severe cases, paraplegia exists.

15.1.3 Image Differential Diagnosis

Thoracic and lumbar vertebral compression fractures can be judged by the change of the height of the vertebral body in the X-ray film. If the height change of the vertebral body is not obvious, especially the microcompression of multiple vertebral bodies, the X-ray film often cannot be taken. A complete diagnosis requires a CT or MRI to confirm the diagnosis. The cervical and thoracic positions are affected by the shoulder joint. The X-ray of this position is often incapable of diagnosing such cases. The upper thoracic vertebral body is affected by the thoracic gas. The vertebral fracture is not easily shown and may even be misjudged due to factors such as osteophytes and intestinal gas, meaning that these sites often require CT or MRI for diagnosis.

1. Identification of thoracic spine burst fracture and fracture
   1.1. X-ray film (Fig. 15.4a–d)

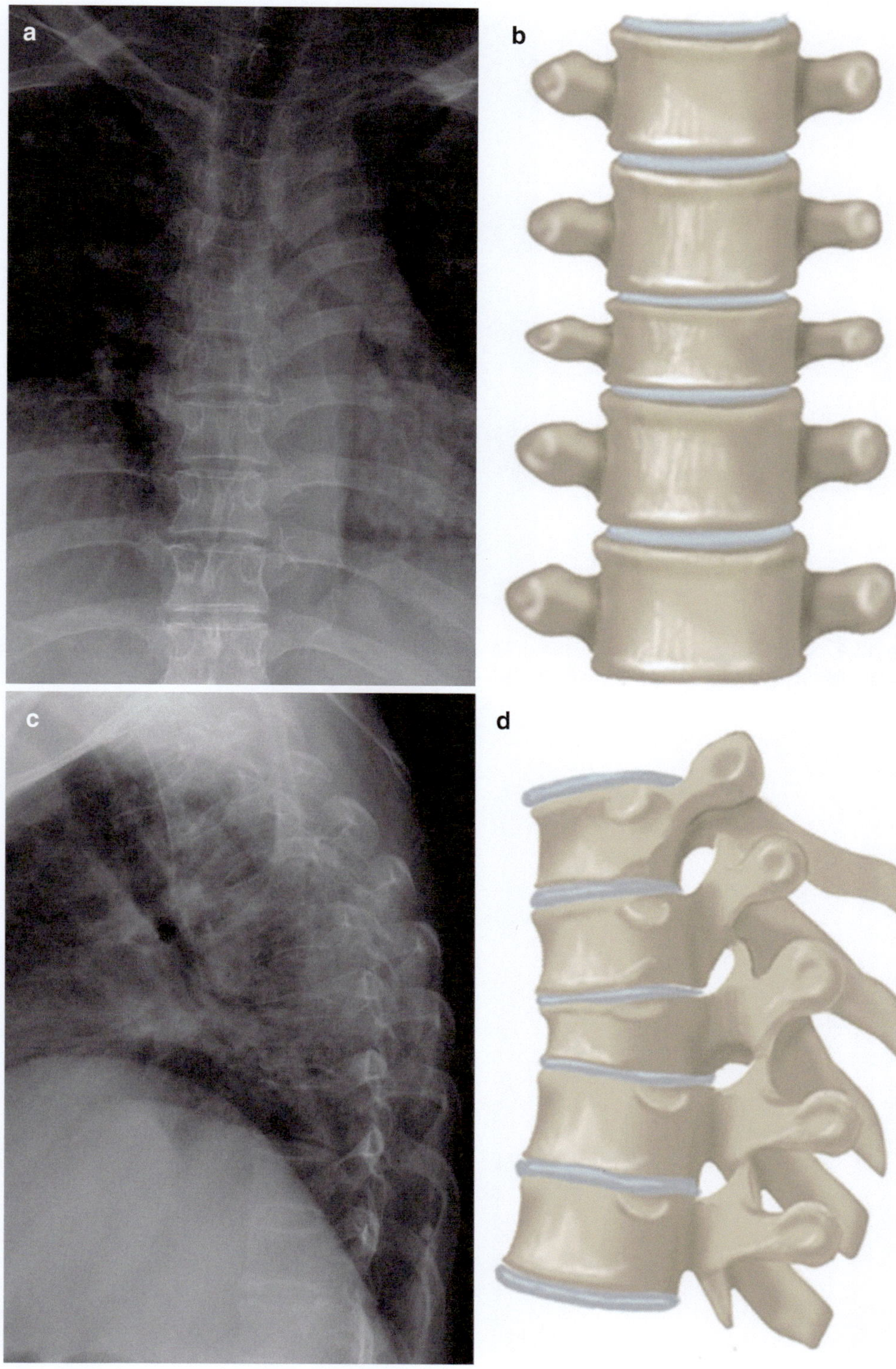

Fig. 15.4 The thoracic vertebrae lateral plain film (**a**, **c**) shows T6 vertebral body wedge deformation (**b**, **d**)

1.2. CT scan (Fig. 15.4e)

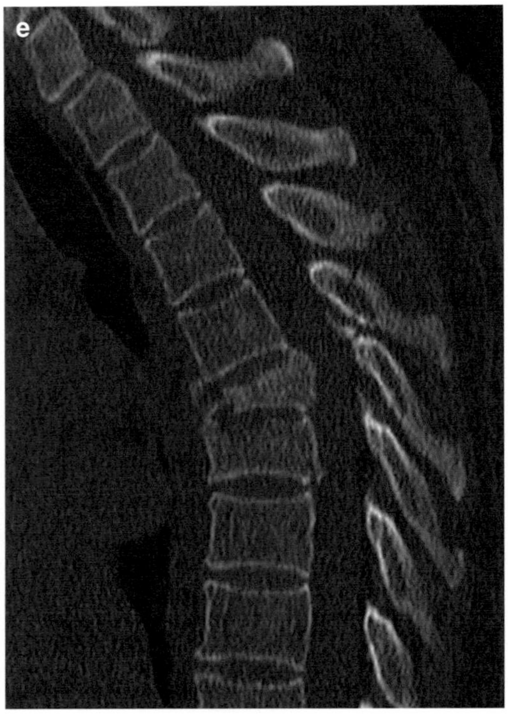

Fig. 15.4 Sagittal CT reconstruction (**e**) shows T6 vertebral compression and flattening, anterior and posterior vertebral body diameter increasing, spinal stenosis, T7 vertebral fracture, upper margin endplate incomplete, T5 and T6 appendices fractures

2. Identification of multiple compression fractures and wedge deformation in the thoracolumbar segment
   2.1. X-ray film (Fig. 15.5a, b)

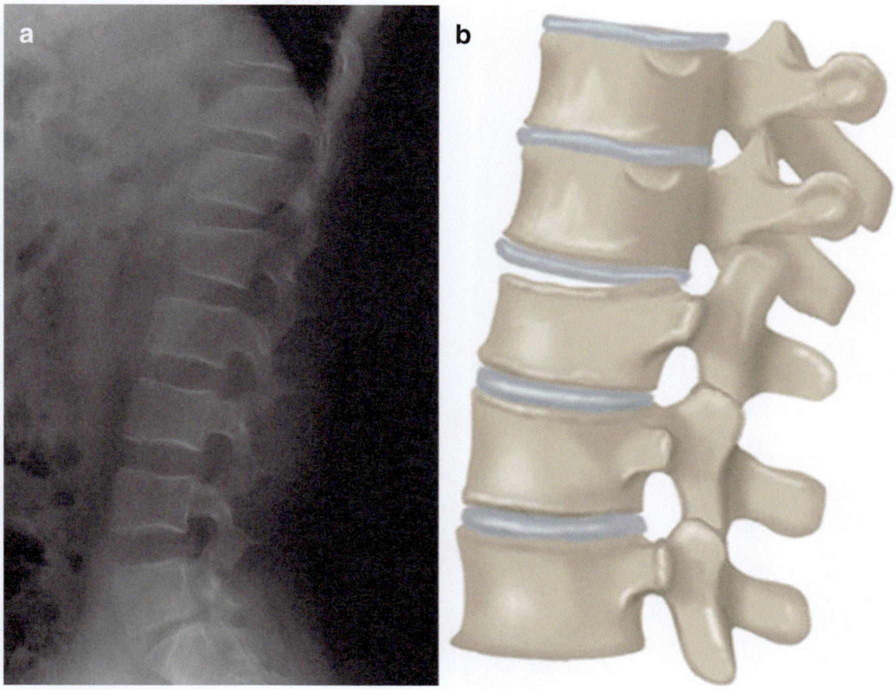

Fig. 15.5 The thoracolumbar lateral X-ray (**a**) shows T11 and L1 vertebral wedge deformation (**b**)

   2.2. MR imaging (Fig. 15.5c–e)

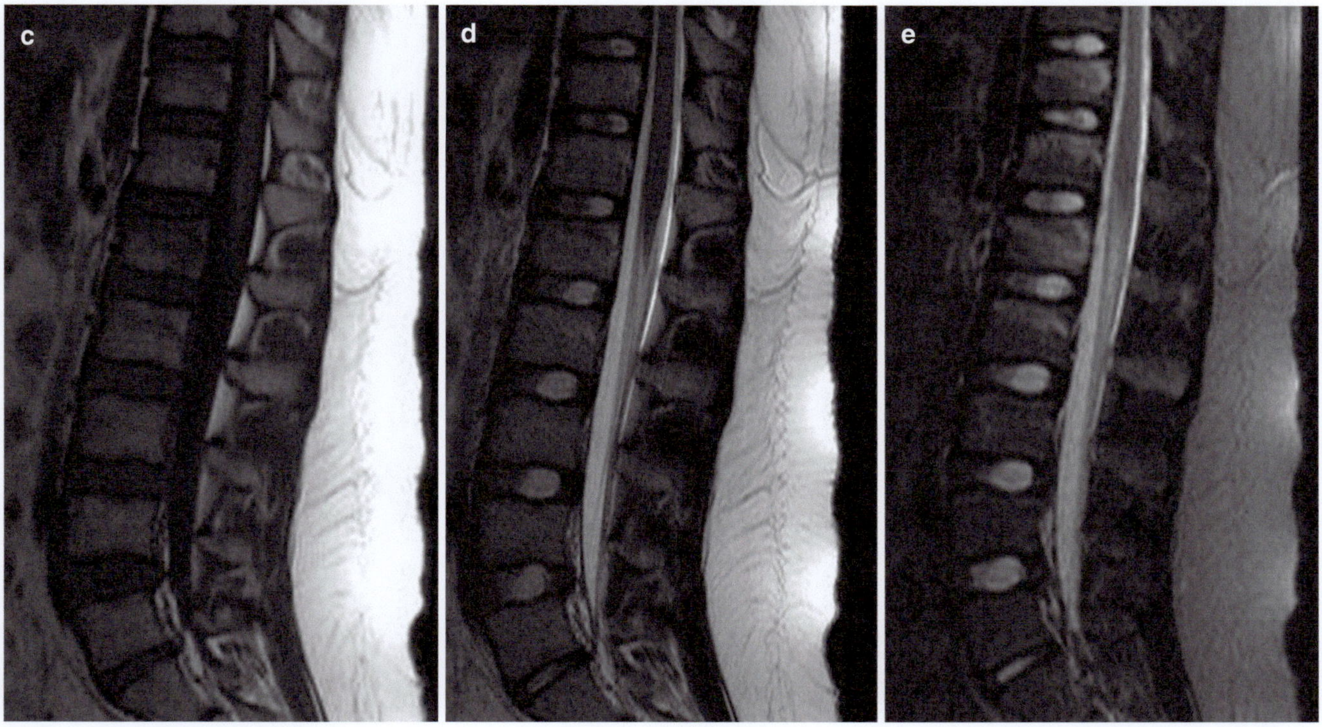

Fig. 15.5 MRI T1WI (**c**) shows strip and lamellae low signal in T11-L2 vertebral body; T2WI (**d**) shows slightly lower signal in L1 vertebral body; STIR (**e**) image shows high signal intensity T11-L2 vertebral body, suggesting a fresh compression fracture

3. Identification of multiple fractures of thoracic spine and suspicious fractures
   3.1. X-ray film (Fig. 15.6a, b)

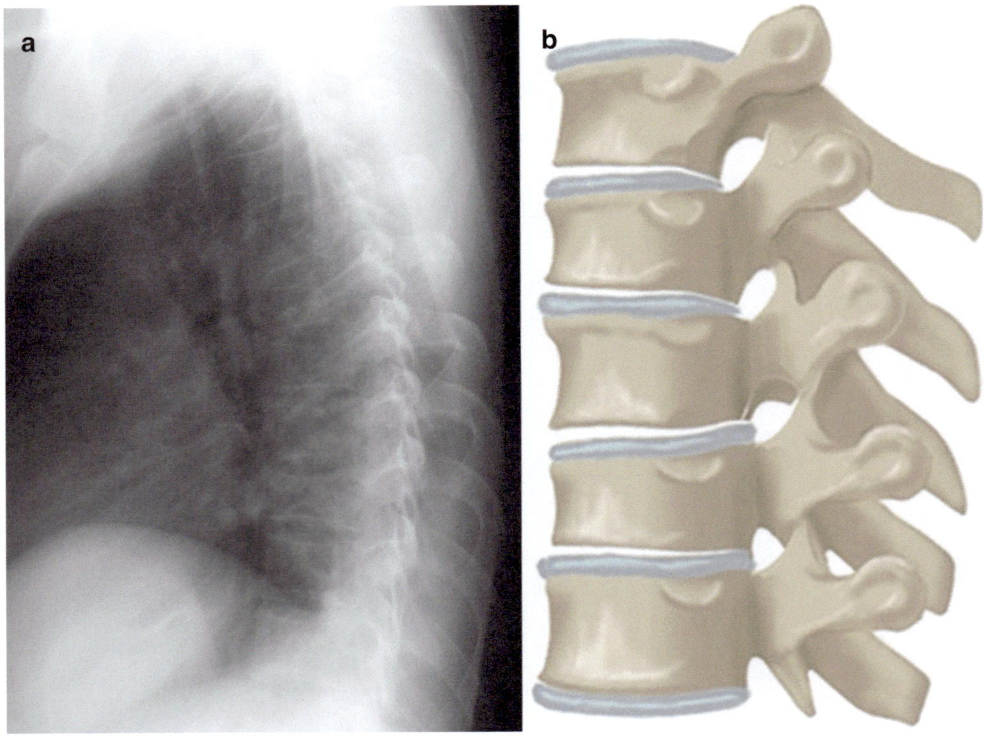

Fig. 15.6 The lateral thoracic X-ray (**a**) shows that the vertebral body is slightly flattened; the details are unclear (**b**)

3.2. CT scan (Fig. 15.6c)

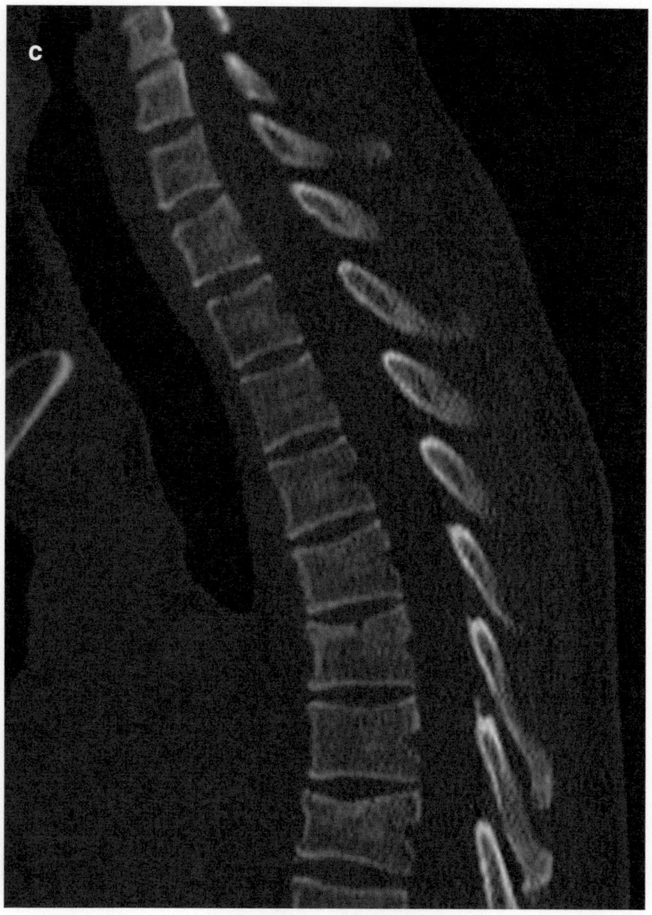

Fig. 15.6 Sagittal CT reconstruction (**c**) shows T6 and T8 vertebral compression fractures

3.3. MR imaging (Fig. 15.6d, e)

Fig. 15.6 MRI (**d**, **e**) shows a mild compression fracture of T5-8 vertebral body with no stenosis in the spinal canal

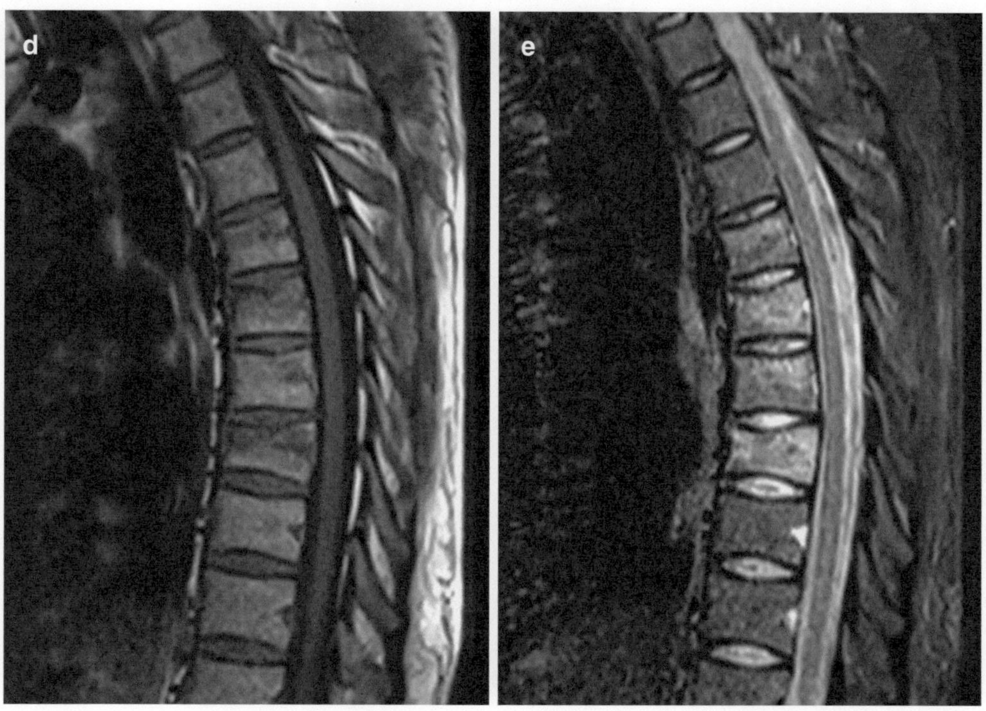

4. Identification of lumbar burst fractures and compression fractures
   4.1. X-ray film (Fig. 15.7a–d)

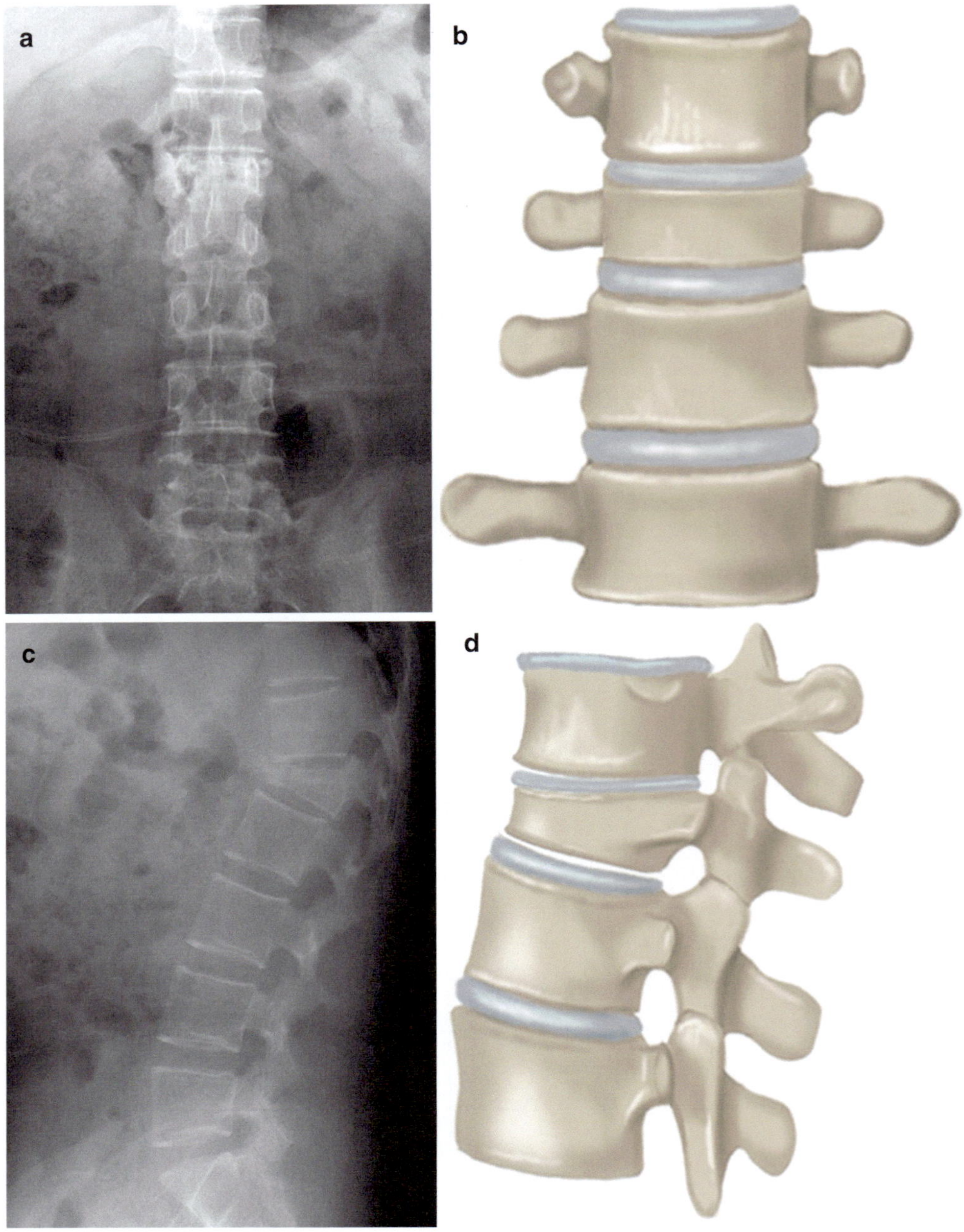

Fig. 15.7 Lumbar spine PA & LAT (**a**, **c**) shows L1 vertebral compression fracture, posterior margin of the vertebral body protrudes backward (**b**, **d**)

4.2. MR imaging (Fig. 15.7e–g)

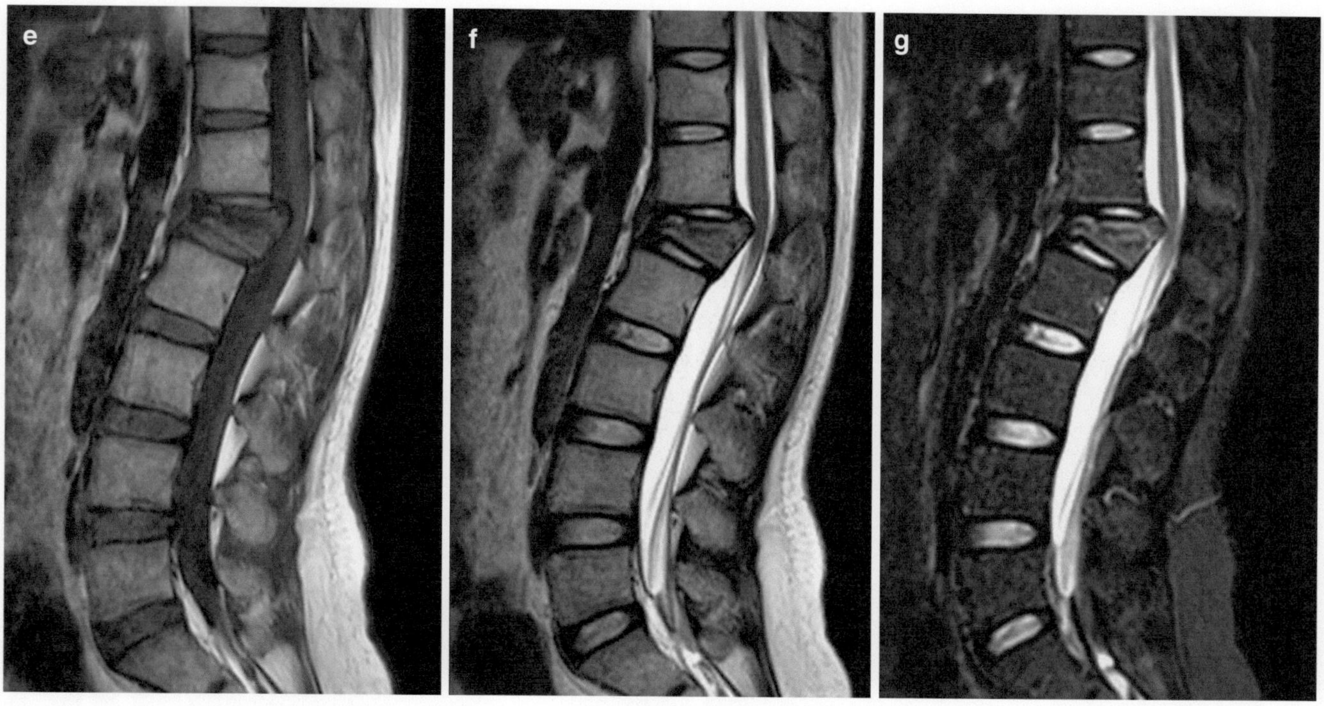

Fig. 15.7 MRI (**e**–**g**) shows a compression fracture of the lumbar vertebral body. The posterior margin of the vertebral body was protruded, the spinal canal was narrowed, and no abnormal signal was seen in the spinal cord

5. Comparison of plain film and CT for lumbar compression fracture
   5.1. X-ray film (Fig. 15.8a–d)

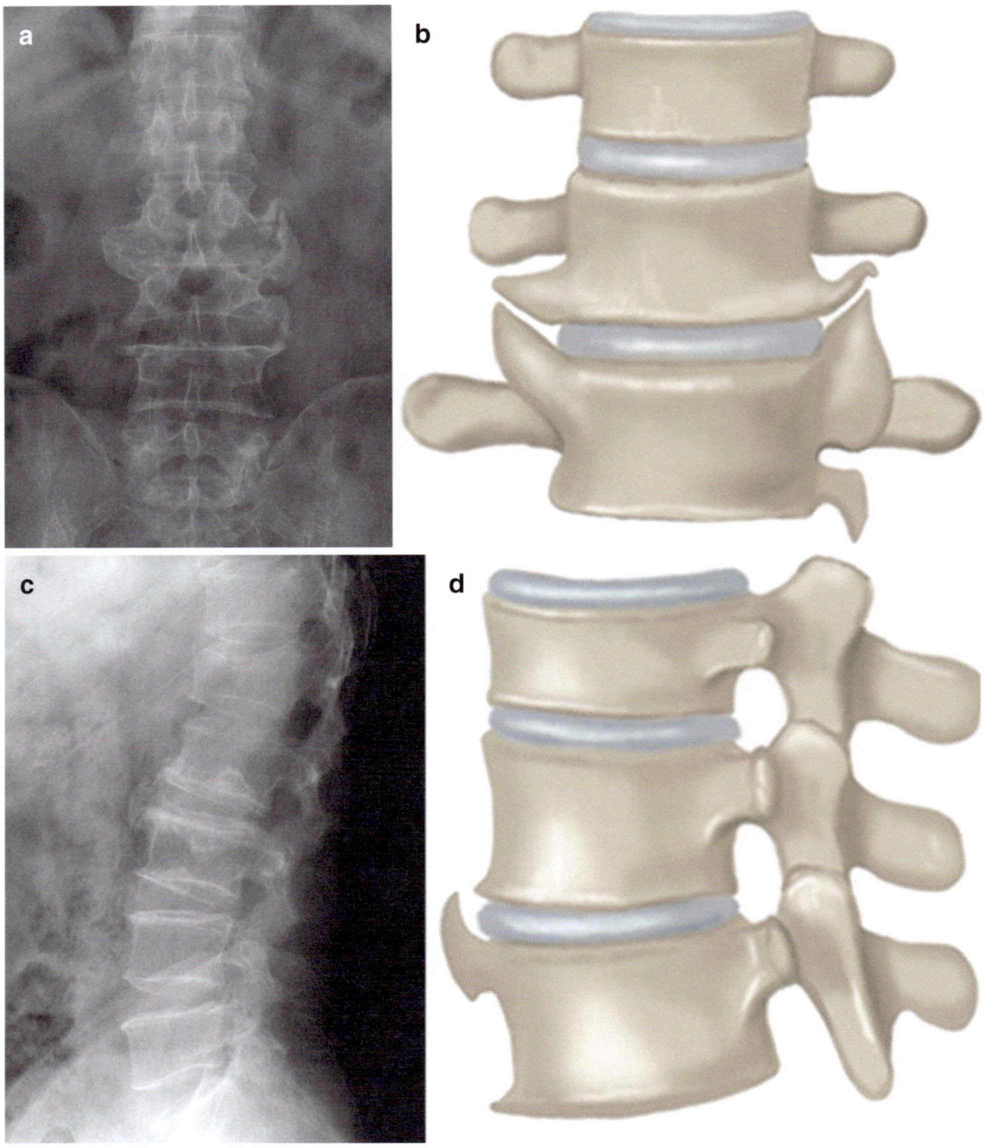

Fig. 15.8 Lumbar spine PA & LAT (**a**, **c**) shows L1 vertebral compression fracture, L2 vertebral body Schmorl's nodule, L3 vertebral compression fracture or Schmorl's nodule (**b**, **d**)

   5.2. CT scan (Fig. 15.8e, f)

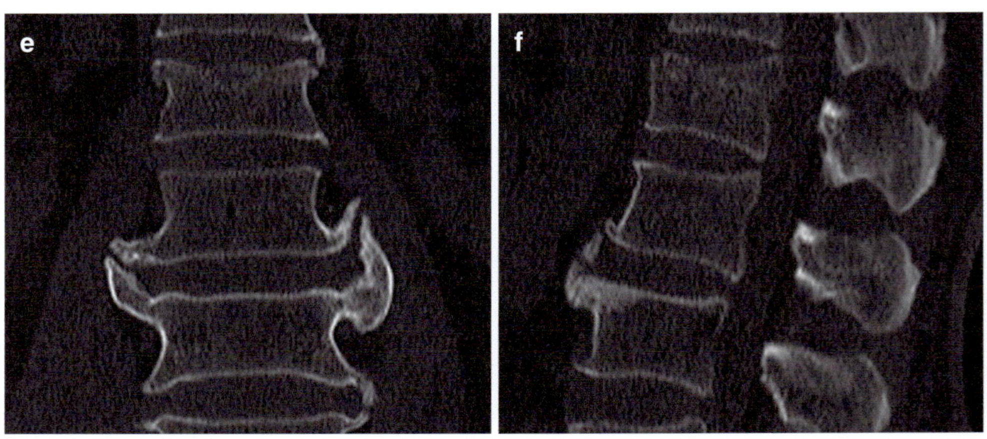

Fig. 15.8 CT reconstruction images (**e**, **f**) show L1 vertebral compression fractures, and L2, 3 vertebral body osteophytes

6. Identification of lumbar compression fractures and suspicious fractures
    6.1. X-ray film (Fig. 15.9a, b)

Fig. 15.9 The lumbar lateral plain film (**a**) shows the compression of the L1 vertebral body, but the X-ray lateral image of the injured L1 was affected by the intestinal gas and cannot determine the extent of the fracture accurately. (**b**)

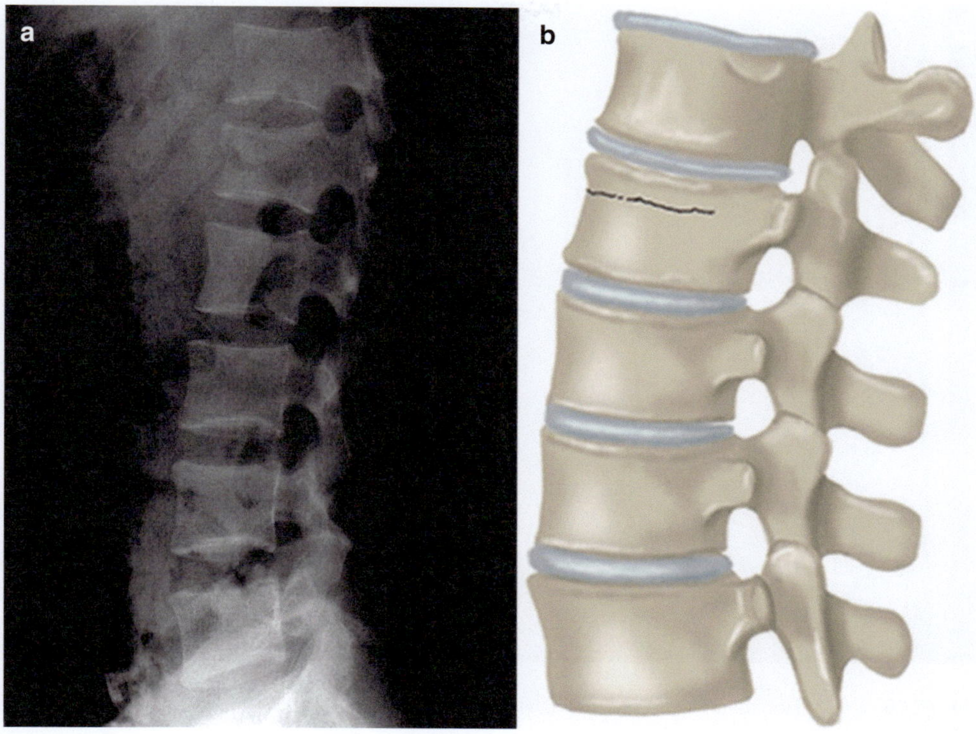

    6.2. CT scan (Fig. 15.9c)

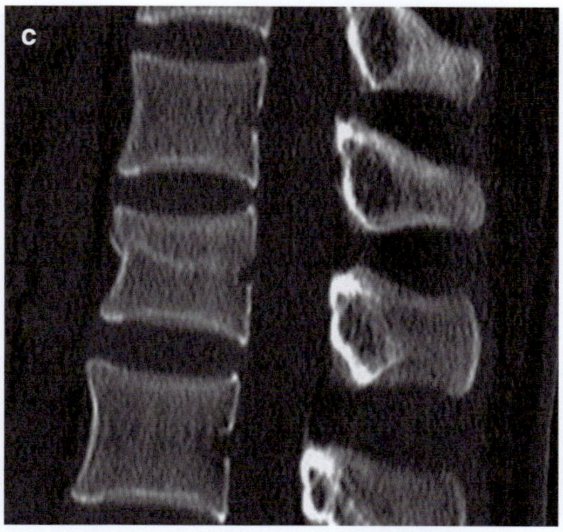

Fig. 15.9 Sagittal CT reconstruction (**c**) shows compression of the L1 vertebral body with a discontinuous anterior vertebral body

7. Identification of thoracic fractures and suspected fractures
   7.1. CT scan (Fig. 15.10a, b)

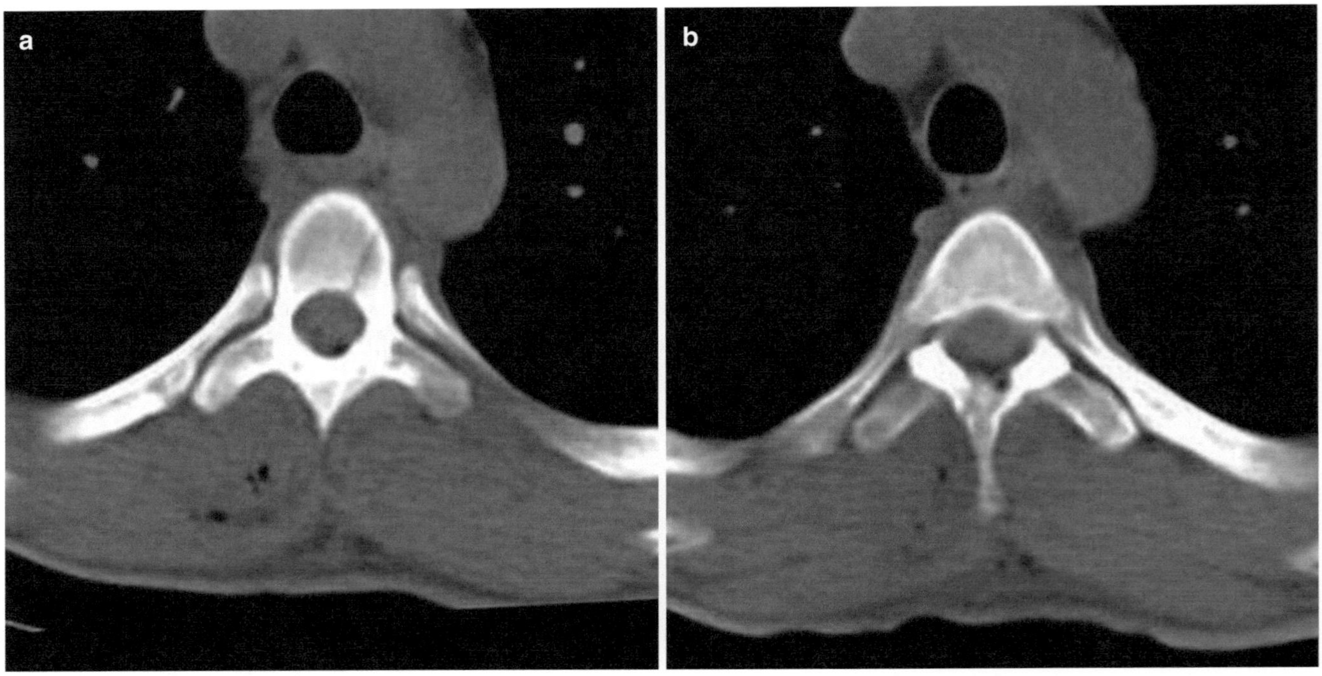

Fig. 15.10 Knife stabbing injury, CT (**a**, **b**) shows the T4 vertebral body and laminar line low density, visible gas density signal in the posterior soft tissue

   7.2. MR imaging (Fig. 15.10c–e)

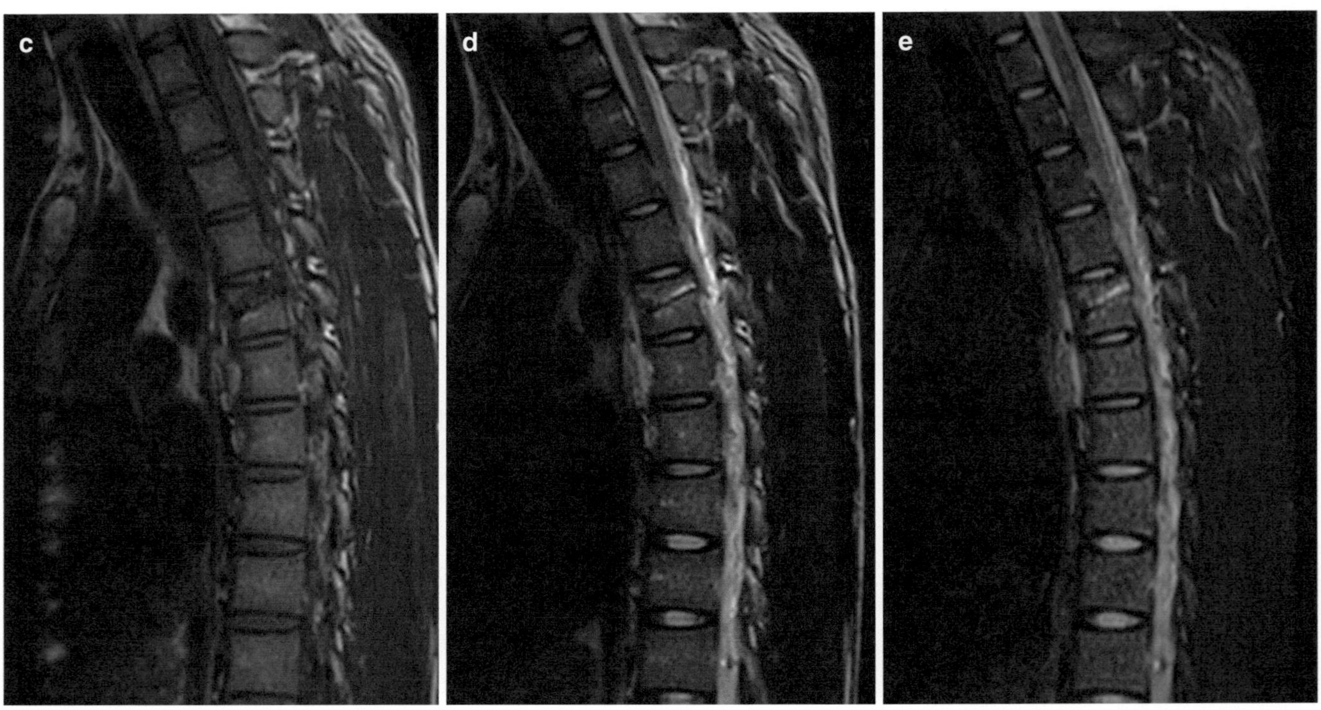

Fig. 15.10 The MR T1WI shows (**c**) the line-like and punctate low signals in the T4 vertebral body. The T2WI (**d**) and STIR (**e**) show a high signal intensity in the vertebral body

8. Identification of multiple old fractures and fresh fractures of the thoracic spine
   8.1. MR imaging (Fig. 15.11a–c)

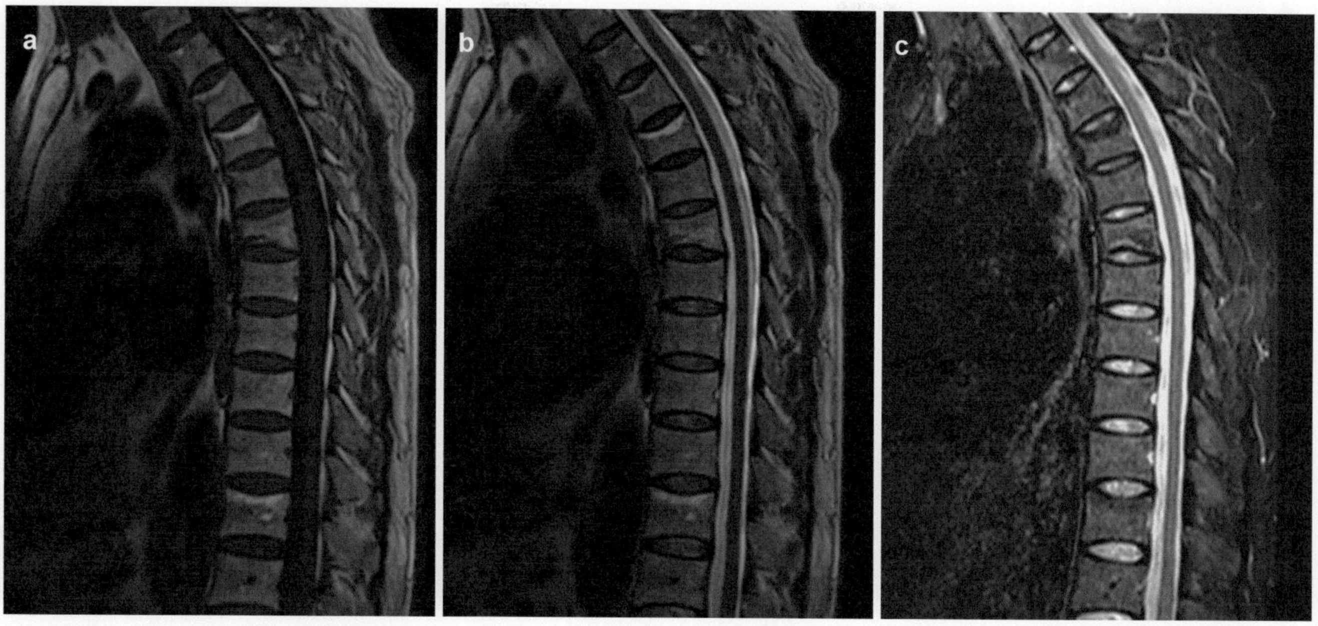

Fig. 15.11 The multiple thoracic vertebrae compression fractures, and the vertebral bodies of the T3, 4, 6, and 11 were flattened; STIR shows no obvious high signal

9. Identification of thoracic wedge deformation with gas and compression fracture
   9.1. X-ray film (Fig. 15.12a, b)

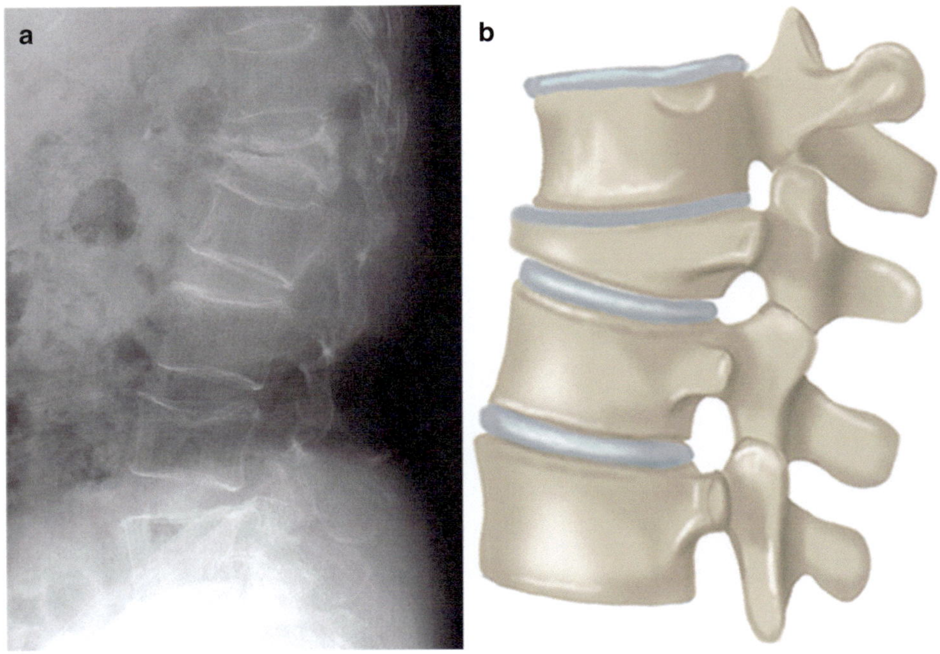

Fig. 15.12 The lumbar lateral plain film (**a**) shows that L1 vertebral body is compressed and flattened, and the vertebral body has a slightly low-density shadow (**b**)

   9.2. CT scan (Fig. 15.12c, d)

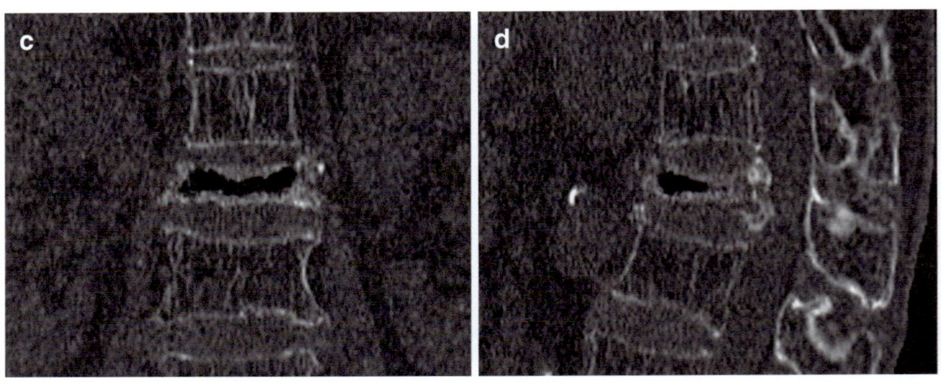

Fig. 15.12 CT (**c**, **d**) shows that the lumbar vertebral body is obviously flattened, with gas density in the vertebral body, the posterior margin of the vertebral body is protruded backward, and the spinal canal is narrowed

9.3. MR imaging (Fig. 15.12e, f)

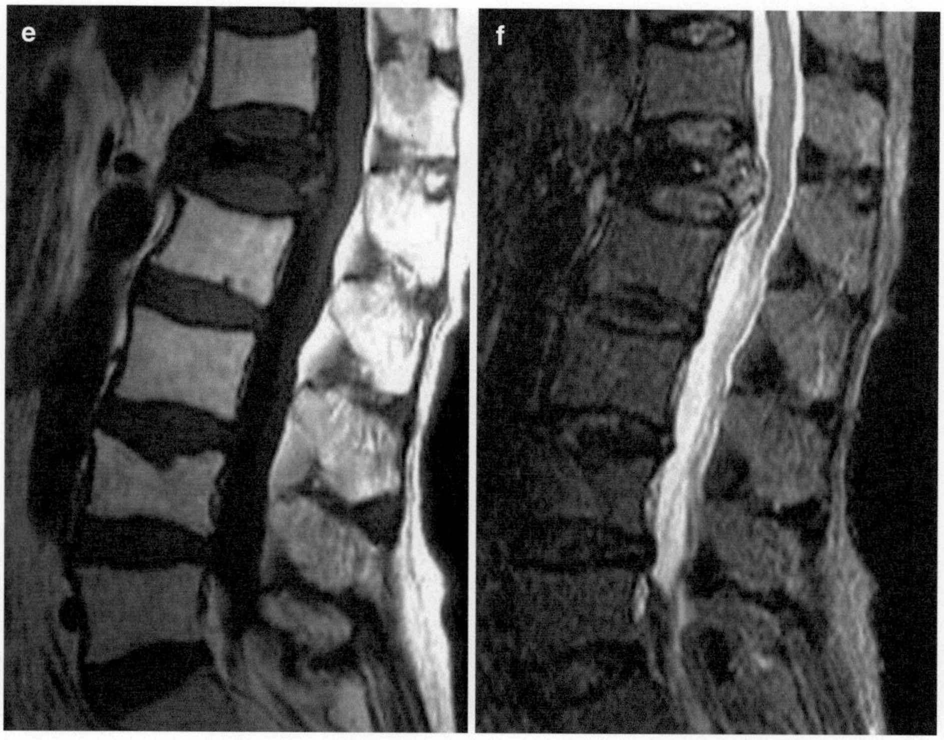

Fig. 15.12 MR shows low signal intensity in the L1 vertebrae, increased anteroposterior diameter of the vertebral body, and the spinal canal stenosis (**e**, **f**)

10. Identification of old fractures and fresh fractures of the thoracic spine
    10.1. X-ray film (Fig. 15.13a, b)

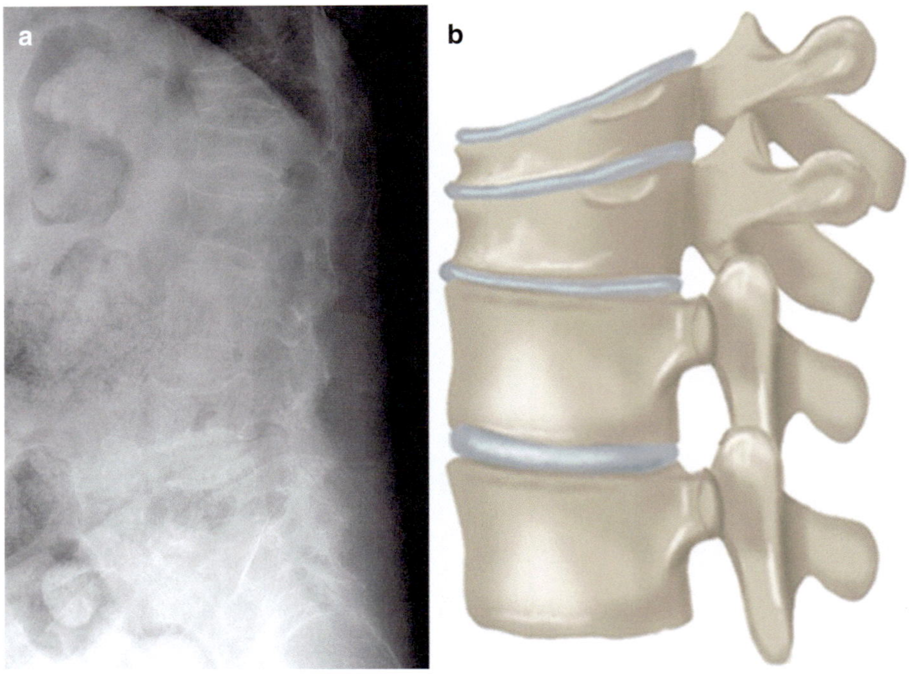

Fig. 15.13 Lumbar lateral X-ray (**a**) shows T11 and T12 vertebral body flattening (**b**)

10.2. CT scan (Fig. 15.13c)

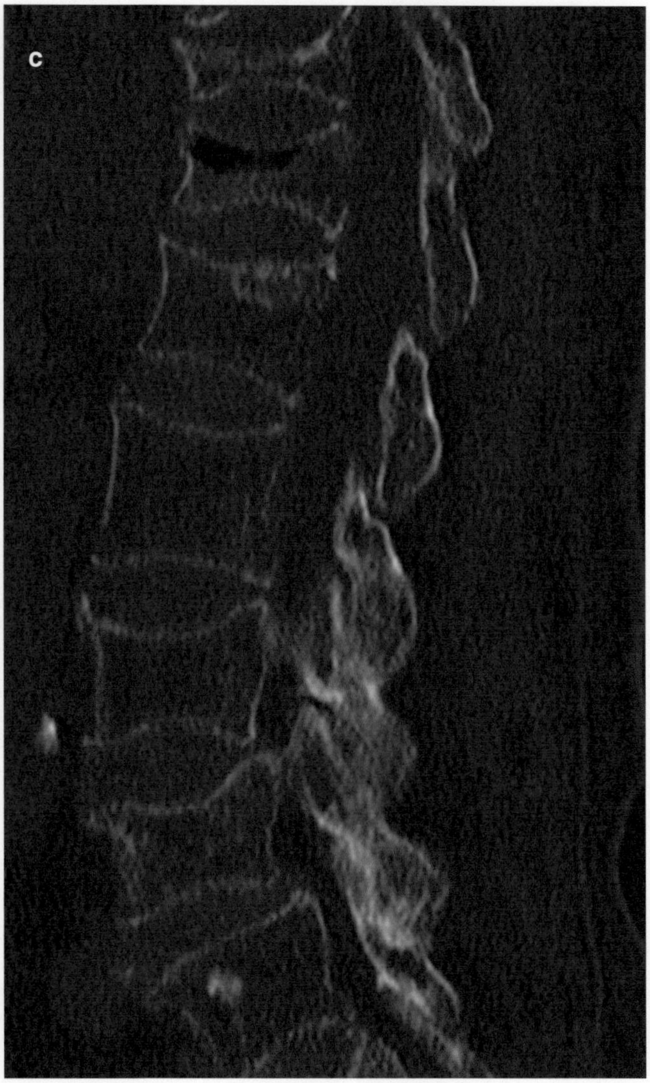

Fig. 15.13 CT (**c**) shows the visible gas density in the T12 vertebral body

10.3. MR imaging (Fig. 15.13d, e)

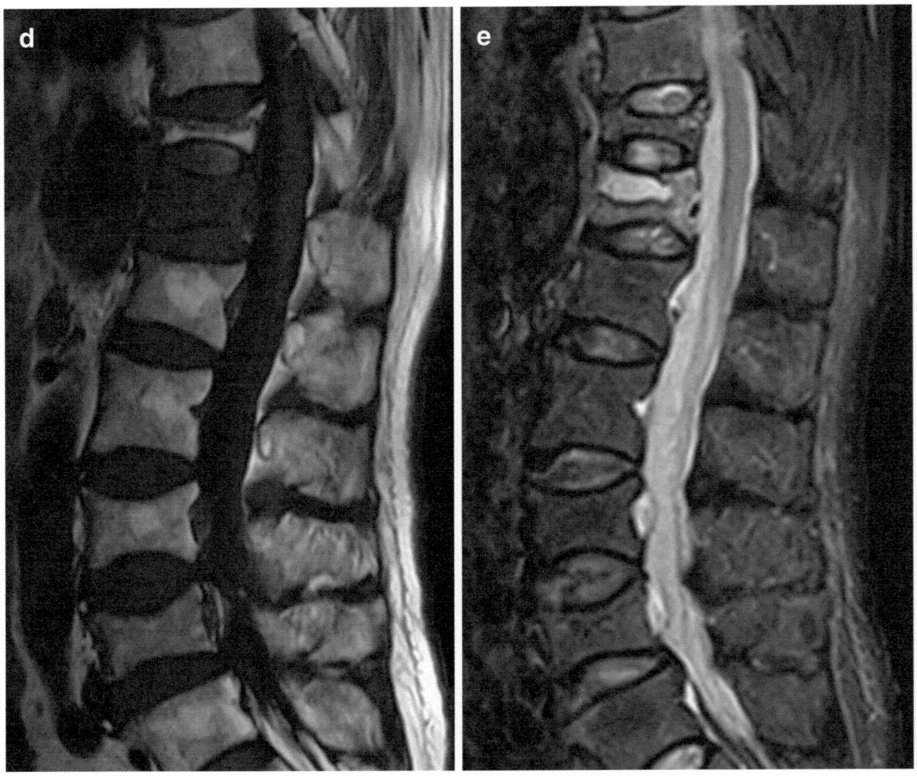

Fig. 15.13 MR: T11 has an old compression fracture, T1WI of T12 vertebral body shows a low signal; STIR of vertebral body inferior edge shows a high signal, where CT scan shows vacuum (**d**, **e**)

11. Identification of lumbar burst fractures and pathological fractures
    11.1. X-ray film (Fig. 15.14a, b)

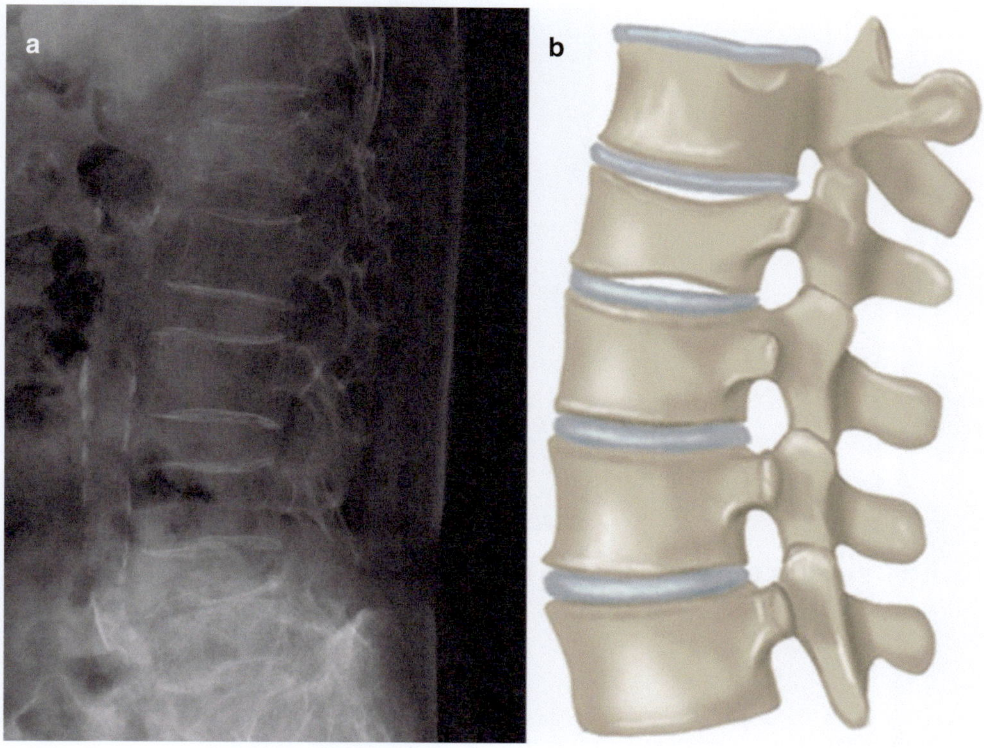

Fig. 15.14 Lumbar lateral film (**a**) shows L1 vertebral wedge deformation, vertebral bone density is slightly increased, and the remaining vertebral body bone density is reduced (**b**)

11.2. CT scan (Fig. 15.14c)

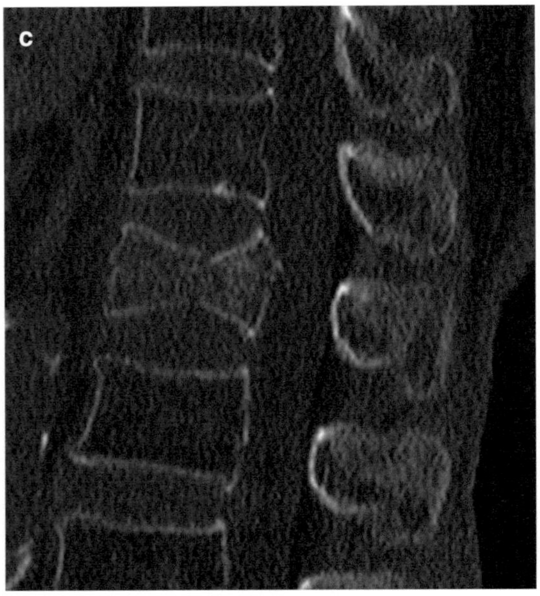

Fig. 15.14 Sagittal CT (**c**) reconstruction shows the upper and lower margin fracture line of the L1 vertebral body

11.3. MR imaging (Fig. 15.14d, e)

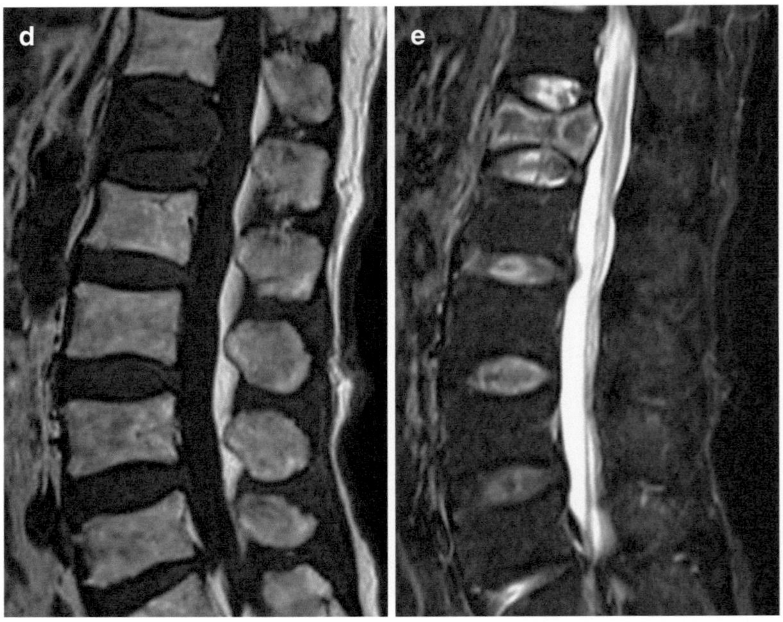

Fig. 15.14 MR T1WI (**d**) shows a significant decreased signal in the L1 vertebrae, and the STIR (**e**) was slightly higher

15.2 Thoracolumbar Spine Fracture and Facet Joint Dislocation

15.2.1 Injury Mechanism Identification

Most of them are due to indirect trauma, such as falling from a height or violently flexing the torso; direct trauma happens less often, with the examples of traffic accidents and sharp contraction of muscles leading to avulsion fractures or transverse process fractures.

15.2.2 Symptom and Sign Identification

The typical clinical feature of lumbar spine appendix fracture is lateral pain in the midline of the lower back, but this finding lacks specificity.

15.2.3 Image Differential Diagnosis

Thoracic and lumbar transverse processes and spinous processes are discontinuous, mostly in the thoracolumbar segment. The forward or backward movement of the vertebral body often indicates an abnormality of the facet joints. X-ray is often indistinguishable from facet joint fractures and dislocations. CT sagittal plane reconstruction plays an important role in the diagnosis of appendix fractures and dislocation of the facet joints, whereas MRI imaging often has misjudgments in the diagnosis of appendix fractures. However, the dislocation of the facet joints can be clearly presented in MRI scan. Moreover the MRI has more clear displays of ligament injury and intervertebral disc injury which can make up for the deficiency of CT scan in diagnosis of soft tissue injury.

1. (Lumbar fracture) Identification of thoracic spinous process fracture and no fracture
   1.1. X-ray film (Fig. 15.15a–d)

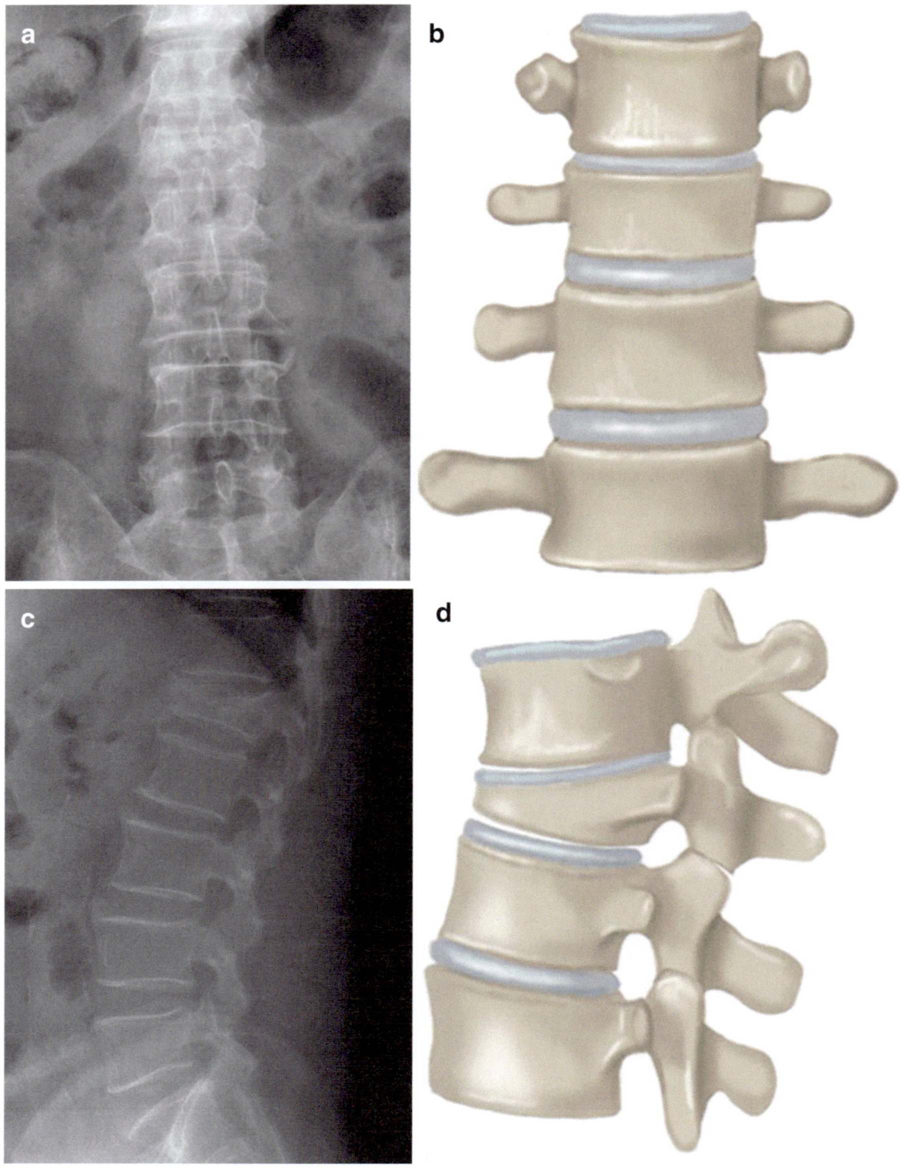

Fig. 15.15 Lumbar spine PA & LAT (**a**, **c**) shows L1 vertebral compression fracture (**b**, **d**)

1.2. CT scan (Fig. 15.15e)

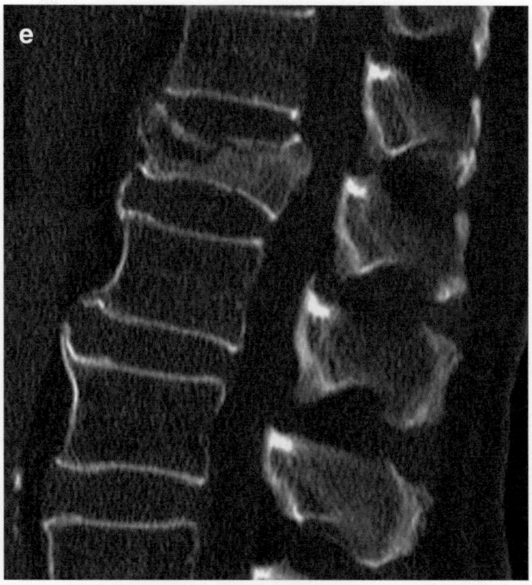

Fig. 15.15 CT (**e**) shows compression of the L1 vertebral body, the vertebral body protruded backward, the spinal canal narrowing, and the T12 spinous process fracture

1.3. MR imaging (Fig. 15.15f–h)

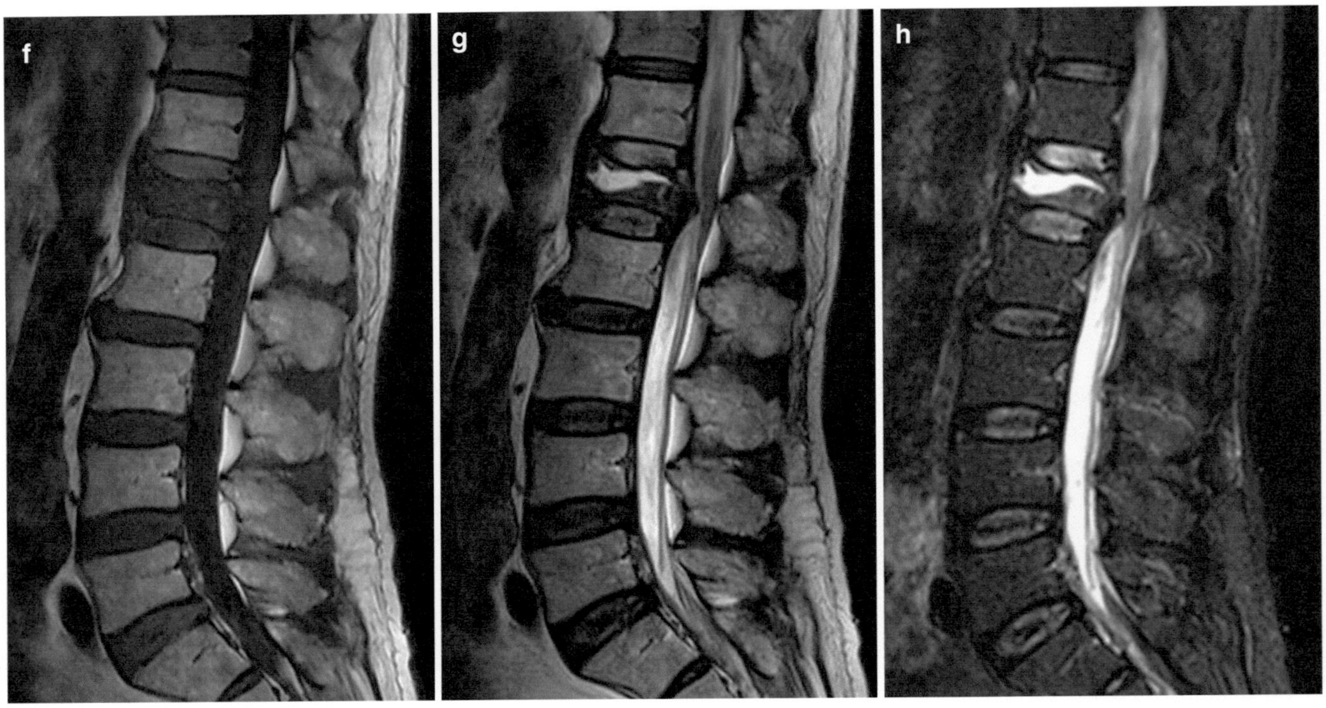

Fig. 15.15 MRI shows L1 compression fracture, the vertebral body protruded backward, the spinal canal narrowing, and the T12 spinous process fracture (**f**–**h**)

2. Comparison of X-ray and CT of thoracic vertebral burst fracture with multiple fractures of the appendix
   2.1. X-ray film (Fig. 15.16a–d)

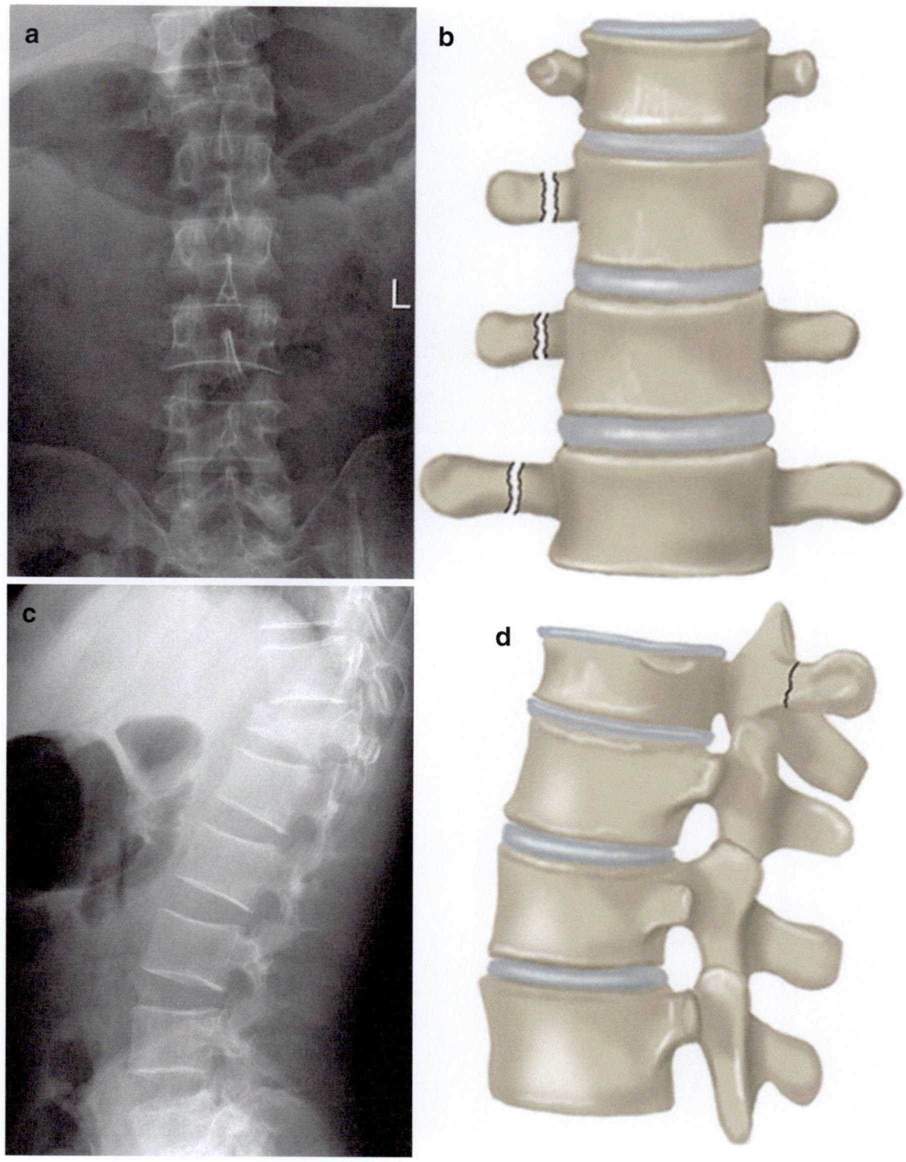

Fig. 15.16 Lumbar spine PA & LAT (**a**, **c**) shows T12 vertebral compression fracture (**b**, **d**)

2.2. CT scan (Fig. 15.16e, f)

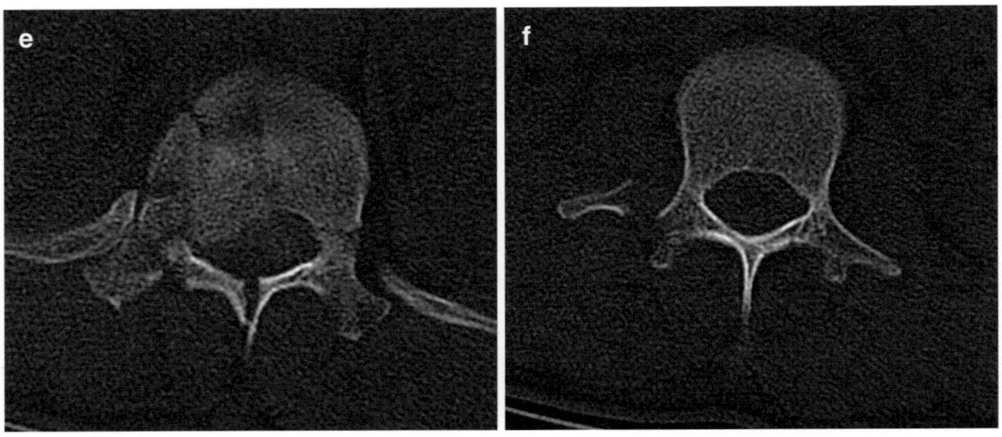

Fig. 15.16 CT images (**e**, **f**) show T12 lamina, spinous process, and L1 transverse process fracture

3. Comparison of plain film and CT of thoracic vertebral body fracture with a facet joint dislocation or fracture
   3.1. X-ray film (Fig. 15.17a–d)

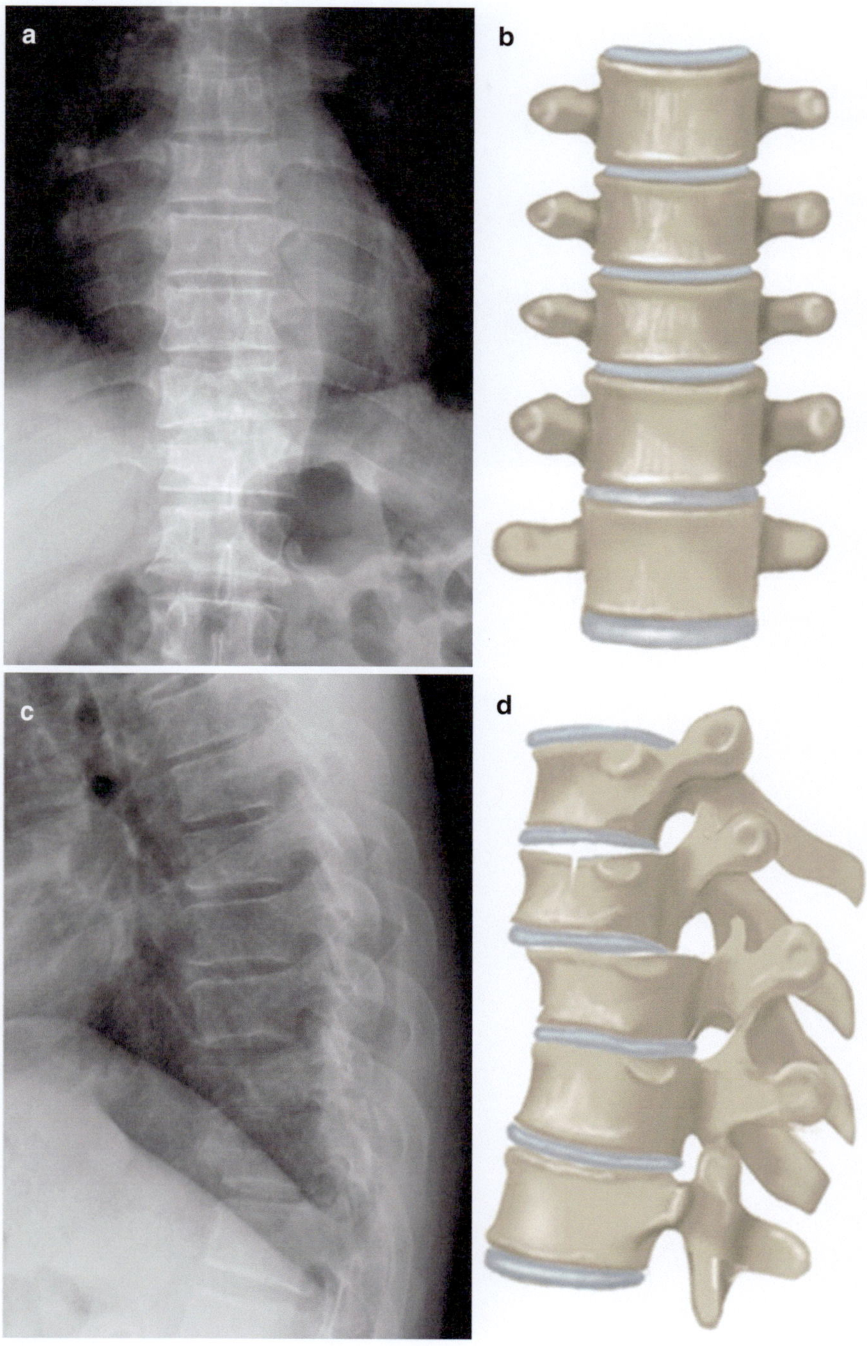

Fig. 15.17 The thoracic spine PA & LAT (**a**, **c**) shows that T10 vertebral body is moved forward, and T10, 11 vertebral bodies are compressed and flattened (**b**, **d**)

3.2. CT scan (Fig. 15.17e, f)

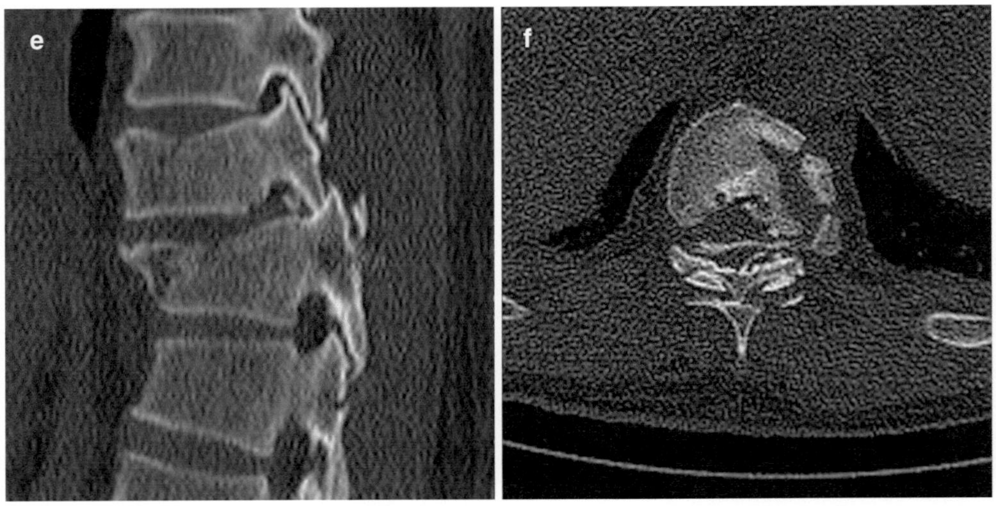

Fig. 15.17 CT sagittal reconstruction (**e**) shows dislocation of T10-11 facet joint, multiple facet joint fracture, and axial CT scan (**f**) showing backward movement of T11 vertebral compression fracture, spinal canal narrowing, the facet joints disorder, and the bone fragments are locally visible

4. Comparison of CT and MR of lumbar vertebral fracture with facet joint fracture
   4.1. CT scan (Fig. 15.18a, b)

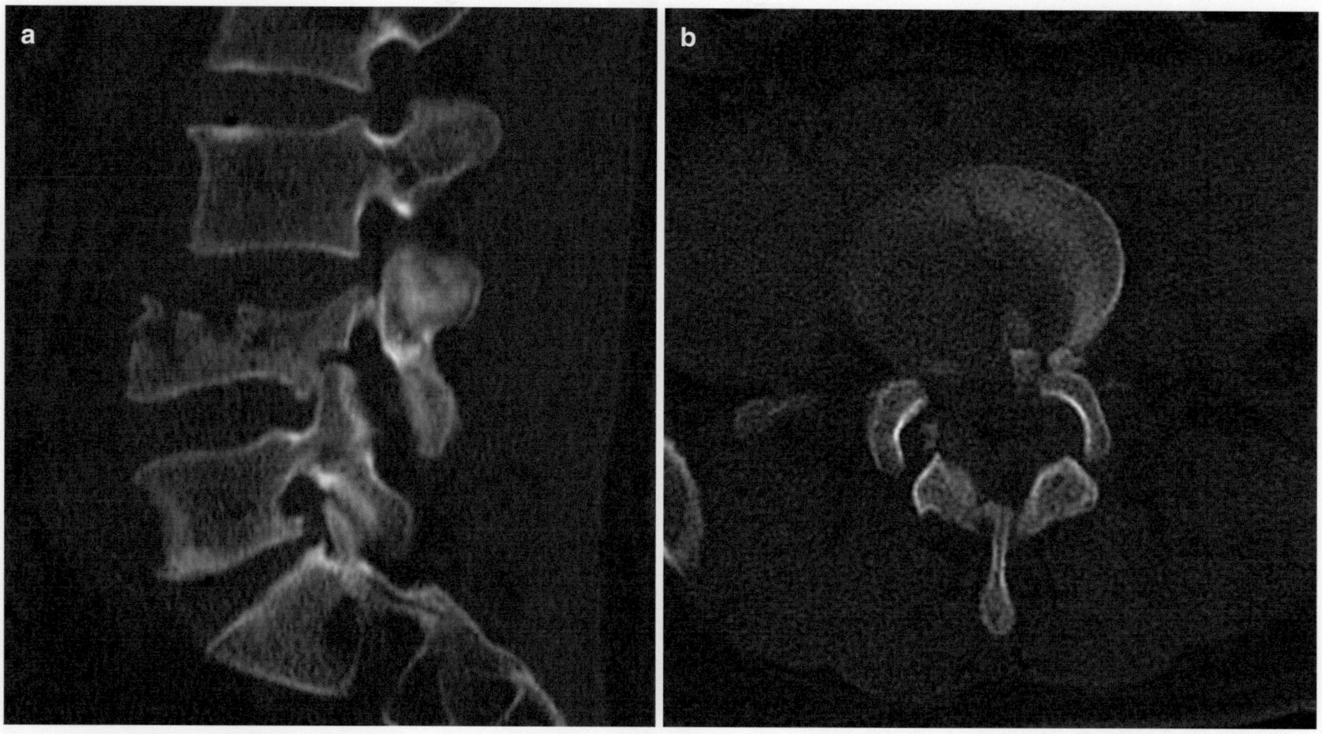

Fig. 15.18 Sagittal CT scan (**a**) shows that L4 vertebral body is compressed and flattened, the vertebral body fracture, L4 vertebral body moved backward, L4-5 intervertebral space widened, and the axial plane (**b**) shows interval between L4-5 facet joints widened, localized bone fragments

4.2. MR imaging (Fig. 15.18c, d)

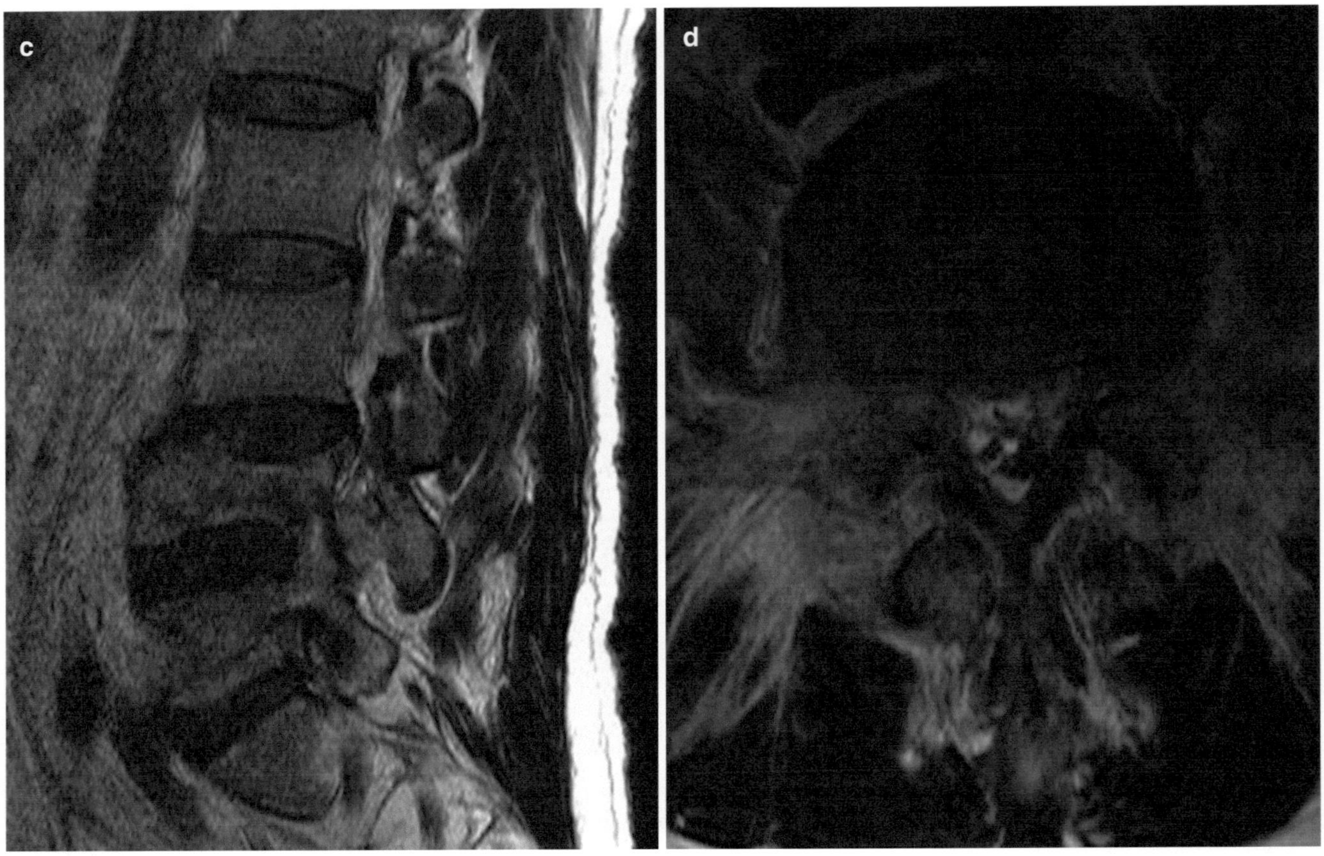

Fig. 15.18 Sagittal MRI (**c**) and axial plane (**d**) T2WI show that the L4 vertebral body was compressed and flattened, the vertebral body fracture, the L4 vertebral body moved backward, and the L4-5 vertebral joint space was widened. Soft tissue swelling

5. CT scan of lumbar vertebral fracture with a facet joint dislocation
   5.1. CT scan (Fig. 15.19a–c)

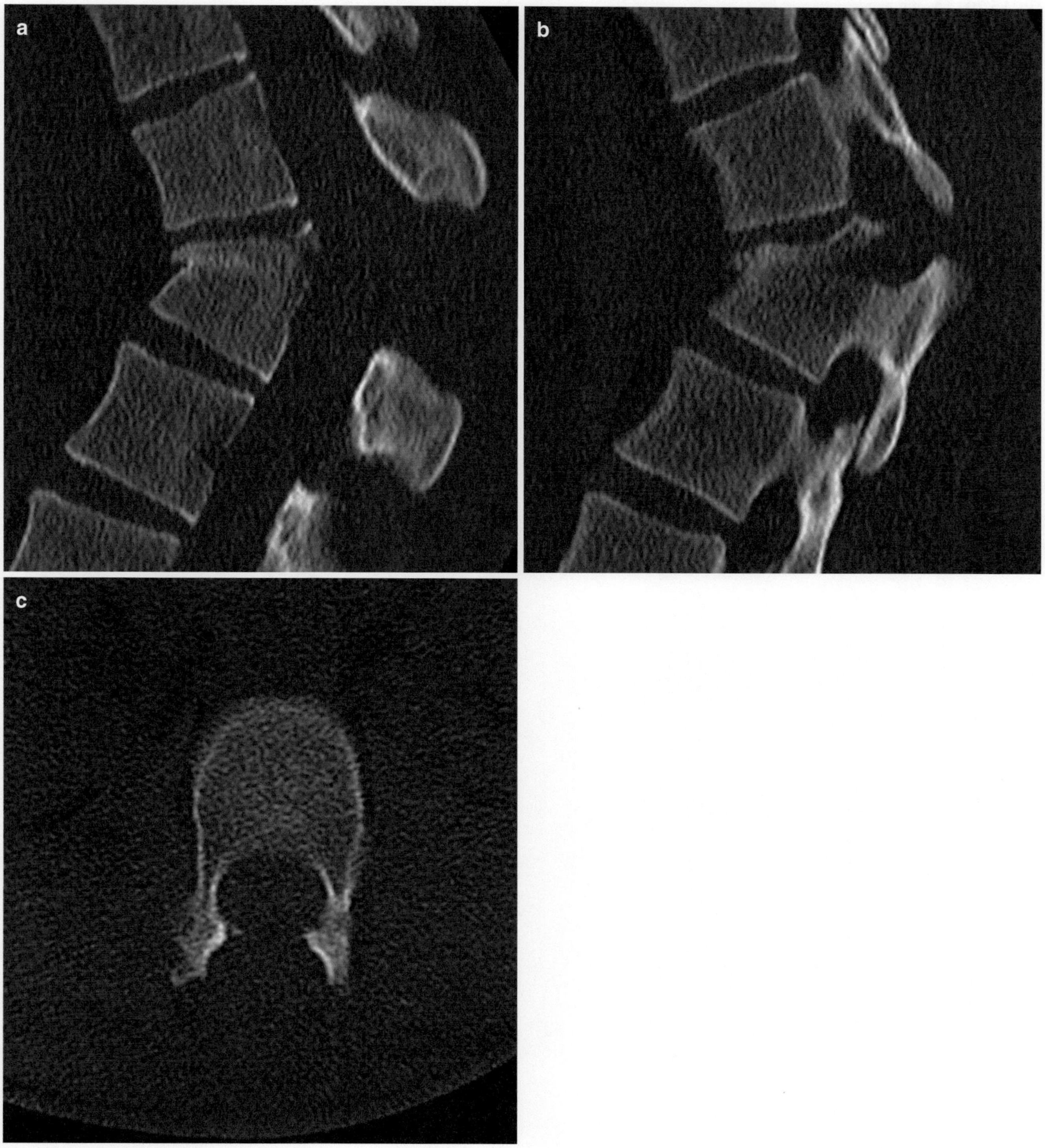

Fig. 15.19 CT sagittal reconstruction (**a**, **b**) and axial plane (**c**) shows compression of the anterior margin of the L1 vertebral body, fracture and separation of the posterior margin of the vertebral body, and dislocation of the T12-L1 facet joint

6. Identification of lumbar spondylolysis and suspicious fractures
   6.1. X-ray film (Fig. 15.20a–d)

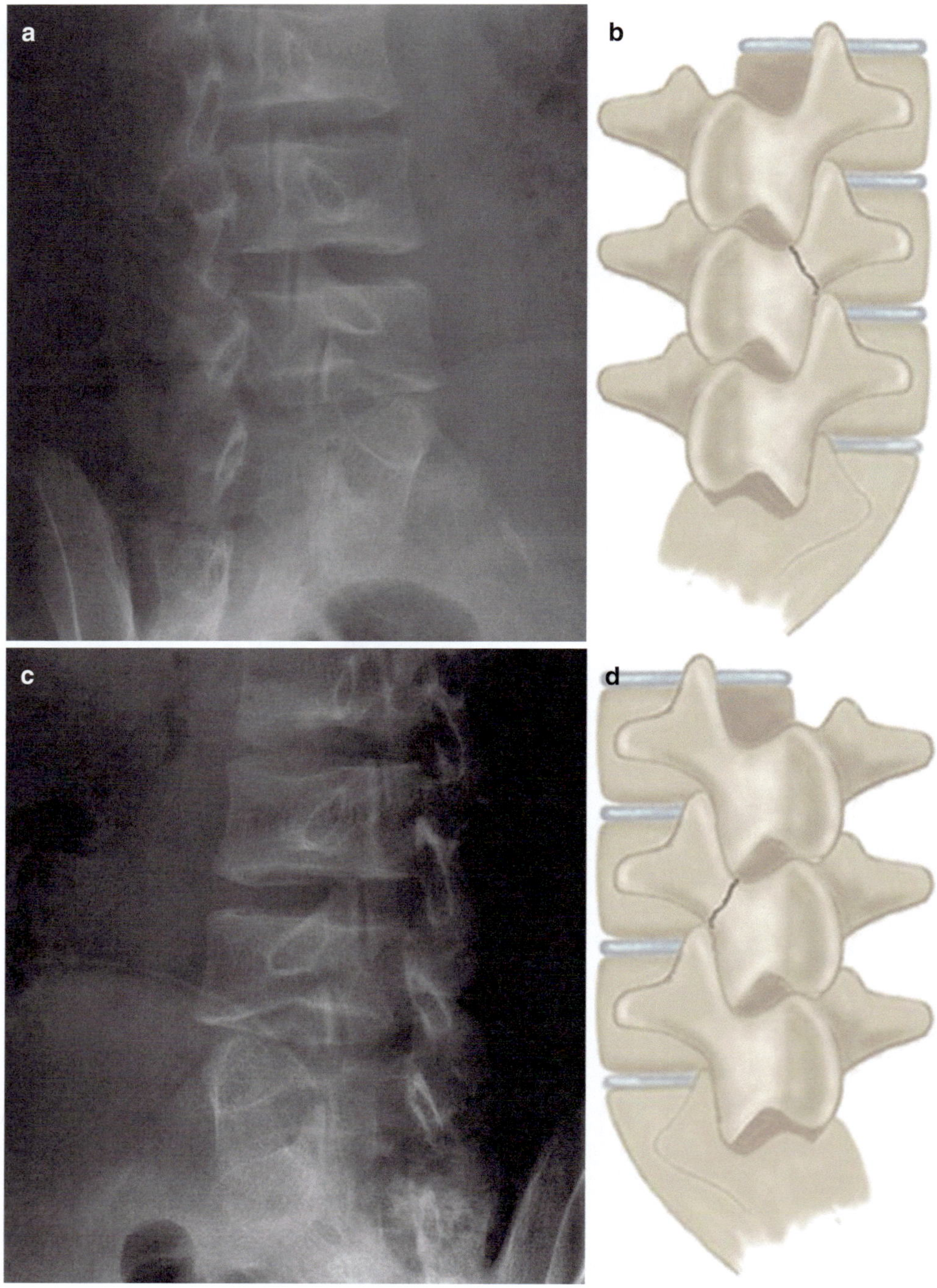

Fig. 15.20 The lumbar bilateral oblique plain film (**a**, **c**) shows the density reduction of the L4 vertebral isthmus (**b**, **d**)

6.2. CT scan (Fig. 15.20e–g)

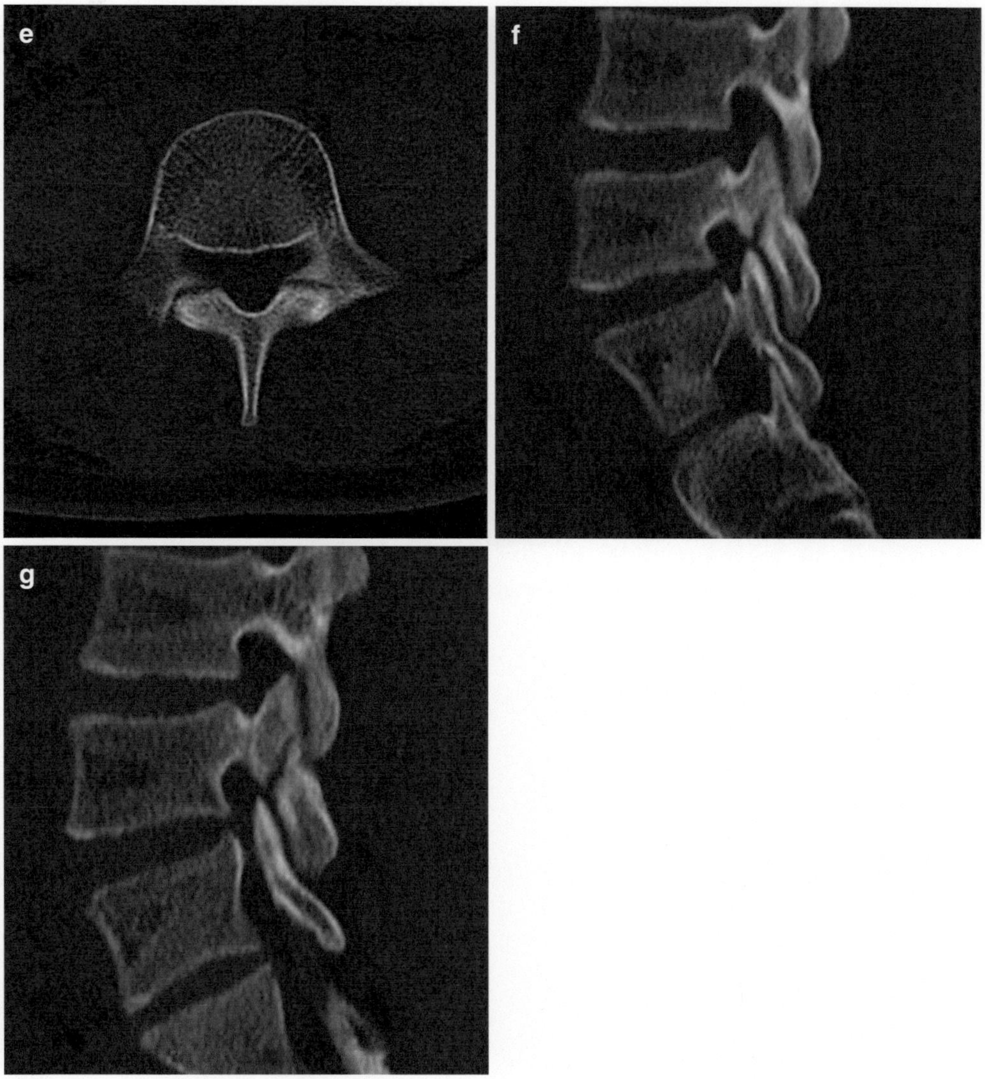

Fig. 15.20 CT axial (**e**) and sagittal reconstruction (**f**, **g**) shows that the bilateral vertebral isthmus was not connected, and the fracture site was not hardened

6.3. MR imaging (Fig. 15.20h)

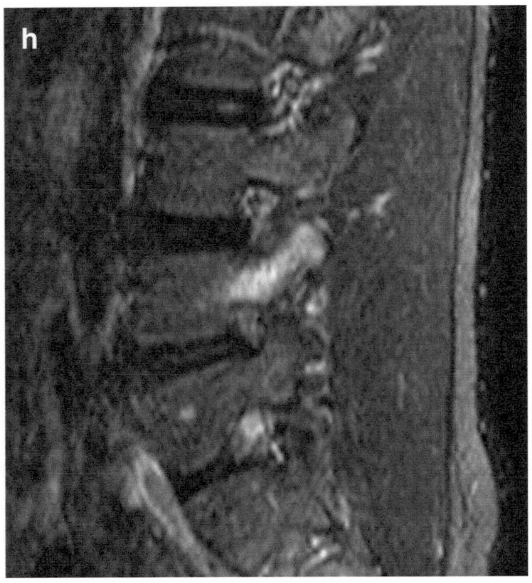

Fig. 15.20 The MRI sagittal plane (**h**) shows increasing signal in the L4 appendix

7. Identification of lumbar spondylolysis and fracture
   7.1. X-ray film (Fig. 15.21a–f)

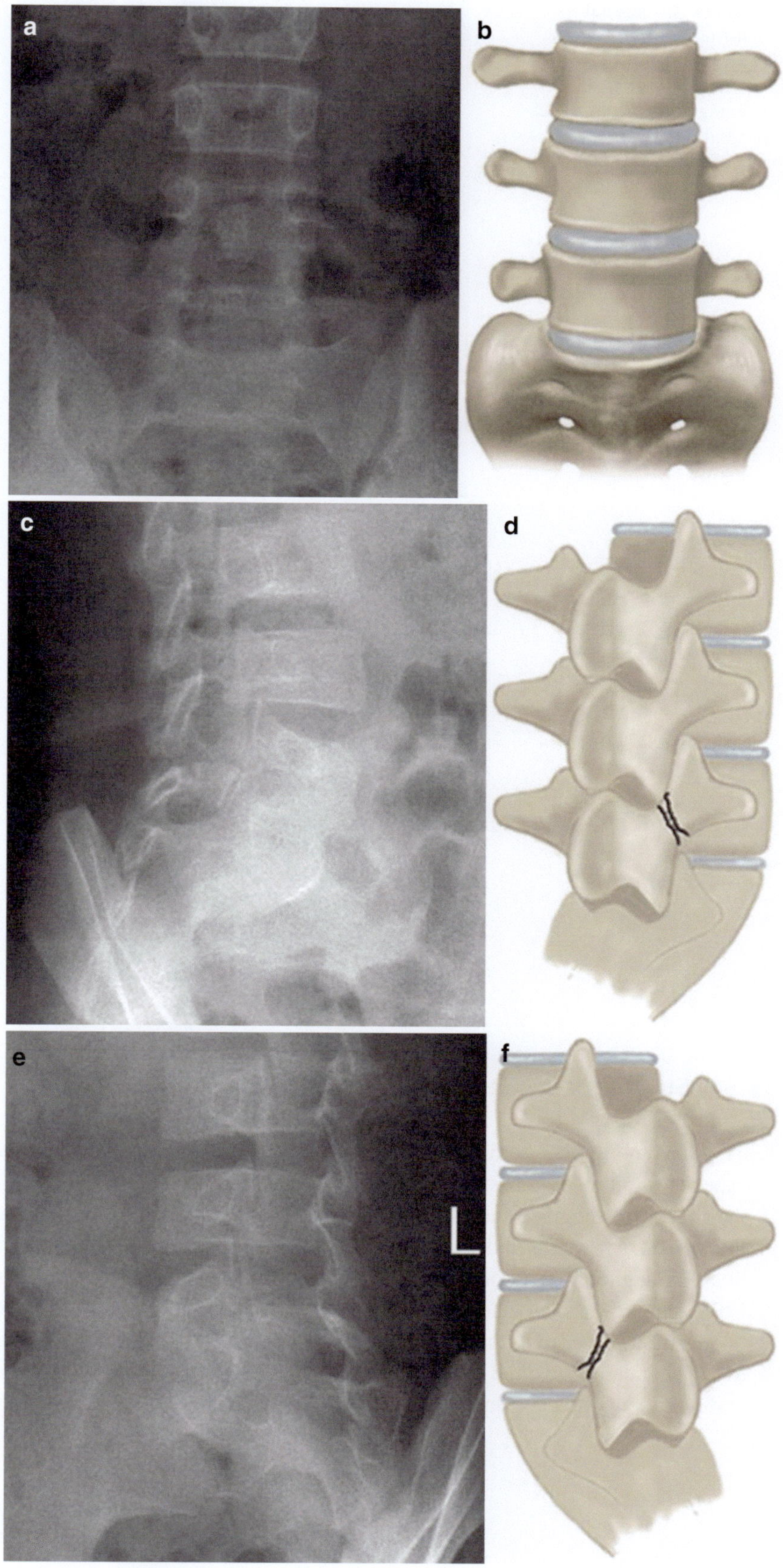

Fig. 15.21 Lumbar spine PA (**a**) and bilateral oblique plains (**c**, **e**) show that L5 bilateral isthmus is not connected (**b**, **d**, **f**)

7.2. CT scan (Fig. 15.21g–i)

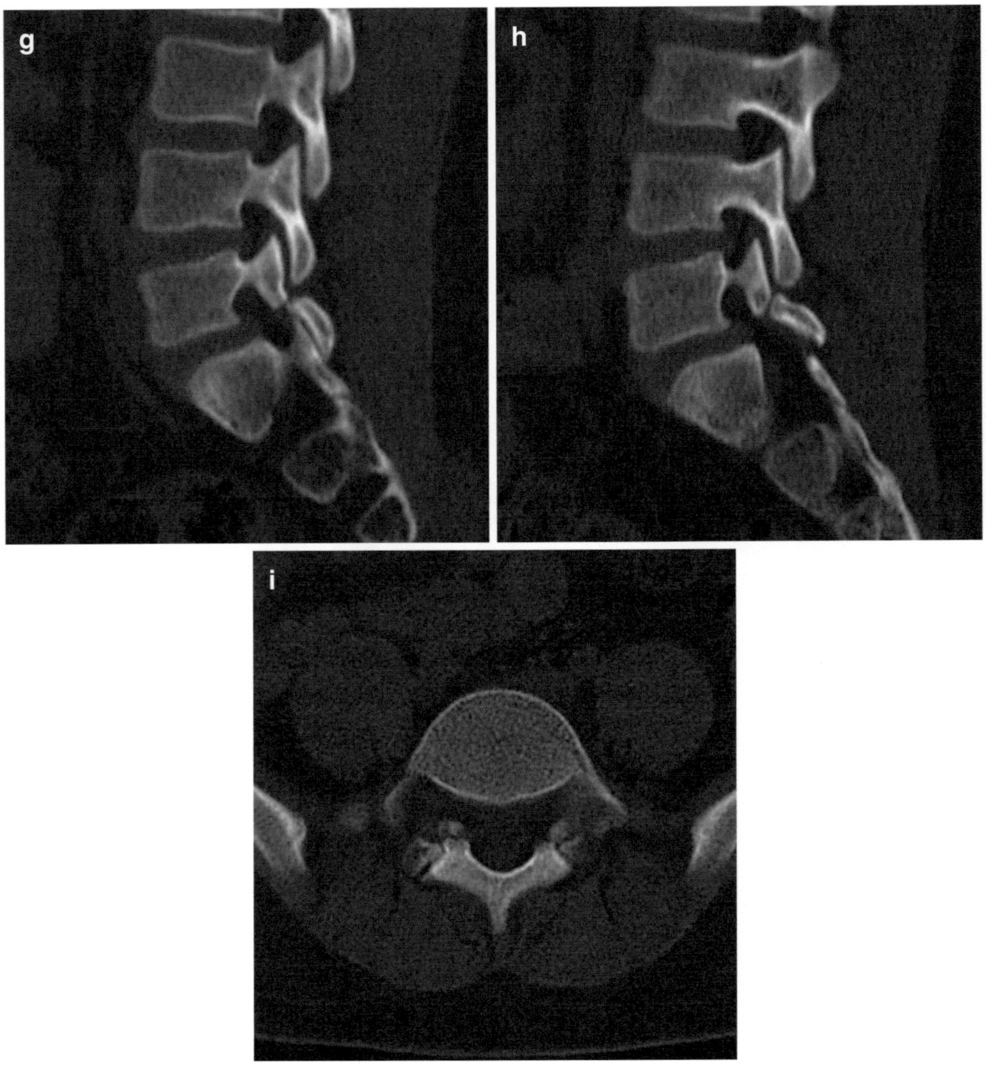

Fig. 15.21 CT sagittal reconstruction (**g**, **h**) shows that L5 isthmus was not connected, with apparent hardening of the fracture site. The axial CT (**i**) shows bilateral facet joint signs

15.3 Summary of the Points

1. Thoracic and lumbar compression fractures can be judged mostly by X-ray plain film, but minor compression fractures, especially microcompression of multiple vertebral bodies cannot be shown on X-ray films due to the X-ray plain films at the overlap of the neck and shoulder joints. CT and / or MRI imaging are needed to confirm the diagnosis.
2. For transverse process and spinous process fractures and small anomalies of the facet joints, X-ray films are often unclear; thus, CT sagittal and coronal reconstruction is required to confirm the diagnosis.
3. MRI imaging for diagnosis ligament and intervertebral disc injury can make up for the deficit of CT scans for diagnosis of soft tissue injury. On the other hand, there are limitations for MRI in diagnosing appendix fractures.
4. MRI can clearly show the location and extent of the spinal cord injury and can also identify fresh and old fractures of the vertebral body. It is currently a routine investigation method for spinal injuries.

16 Sacral and Coccygeal Vertebral Fractures

Wenjuan Wu and Yingze Zhang

16.1 Sacral vertebral Fracture

The sacral vertebra, also known as sacrum, is composed of five vertebral bodies, which are articulate with L5 and coccygeal vertebral body. The anterosuperior apophysis is called sacral promontory, and there are four pairs of anterior sacral foramina on both sides. The middle part of the dorsal sacrum is central sacral crest, with the intermediate sacral crest on the side. Laterally to the intermediate sacral crest are the posterior sacral foramina and lateral sacral crest. The anterior and posterior foramina directly communicate with the sacral canal, and the anterior and posterior branches of the sacral nerves cross the foramina. The extremitas inferior of the sacral canal is sacral hiatus, and the two sides protrude downward is called sacral cornu. The lateral surface of the sacrum and the auricular surface of the hip compose sacroiliac joint.

1. CT features of normal sacrum (Fig. 16.1a, b)
   1.1. CT scan

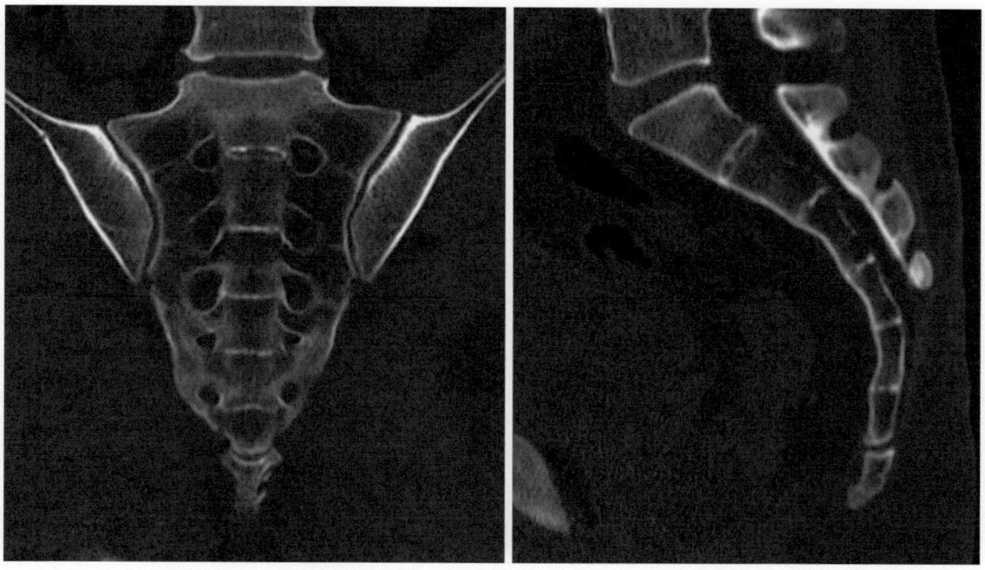

Fig. 16.1 Coronal and sagittal reconstruction of the normal sacrum

W. Wu
Department of Radiology, The Third Hospital of Hebei Medical University, Shijiazhuang, Hebei, China

Y. Zhang (✉)
Department of Orthopaedics, The Third Hospital of Hebei Medical University, Shijiazhuang, Hebei, China

Y. Zhang (ed.), *Differential Diagnosis of Fracture*, https://doi.org/10.1007/978-981-13-8339-7_16

16.1.1 Injury Mechanism Identification

Fracture of the sacrum can occur alone or in combination with other parts of the pelvis. (1) The transverse fractures are mostly caused by direct landing when falling. (2) Longitudinal fractures are caused by trauma and often occur with iliac or pubic fractures. The fractures mostly result from car accidents and falling injury. (3) Comminuted fractures are mainly caused by localized severe trauma, forming stellate or irregular comminuted fractures. (4) Avulsion fractures are easily mistaken for the sacrotuberous ligament avulsion, which occur in the inferolateral sacrum. Differential diagnosis with pathological fractures: when fractures with mild injury happen, sacral tumors should be highly suspected.

16.1.2 Symptom and Sign Identification

The manifestations of sacrum fractures always lack specificity, including pain, swelling, and limited lumbosacral range of motion, the patient cannot sit normally. It is difficult to diagnose through these manifestations. Therefore, when the fracture is suspected, further X-ray or CT scan is needed. In addition, a pelvic separation and compression test may help to clarify the diagnosis.

16.1.3 Imaging Differential Diagnosis

In Routine X-ray films, sacral fractures are often missed; and it is difficult to differentiate between old and new displaced fractures. Therefore, a CT scan has become an effective method for diagnosing sacral fractures.

16.1.3.1 Transverse Fracture

X-ray lateral radiographs of the sacral vertebrae can show the fracture with a dislocation, while fractures without dislocation happens, CT scan with sagittal reconstruction should be required.

2. Identification of sacral fractures and suspected fractures
   2.1. X-ray film (Fig. 16.2a, b)

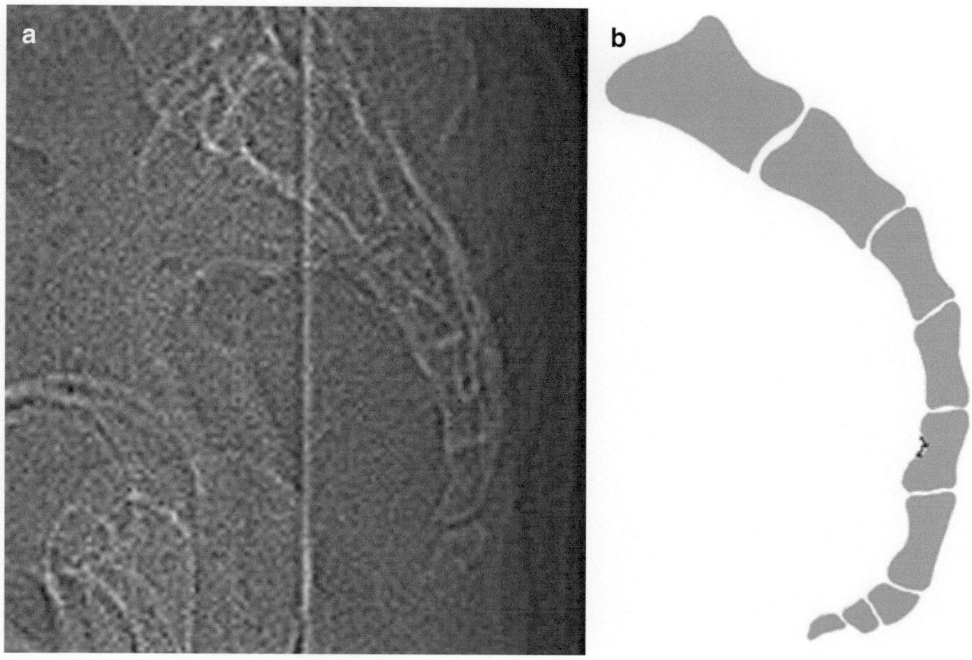

Fig. 16.2 The lateral radiograph of the sacrum (**a**) shows that the S5 vertebral anterior line is not smooth (**b**)

   2.2. CT scan (Fig. 16.2c, d)

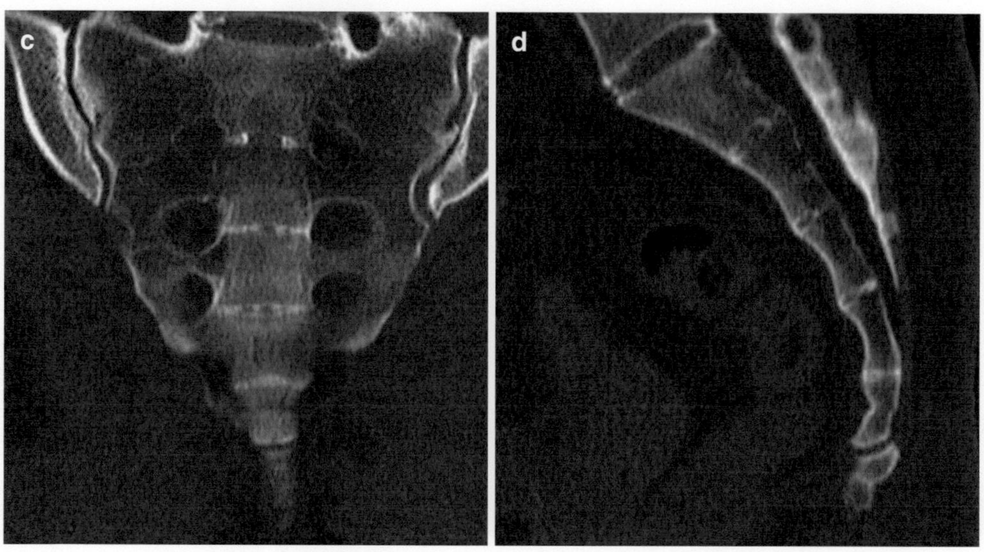

Fig. 16.2 (**c**, **d**) Coronal reconstruction shows a transverse fracture line crossing the S5 vertebral body. Sagittal reconstruction shows the anterior cortex distortion and posterior cortical fracture

3. Identification of old fractures and suspected fractures of the sacrum
   3.1. X-ray film (Fig. 16.3a, b)

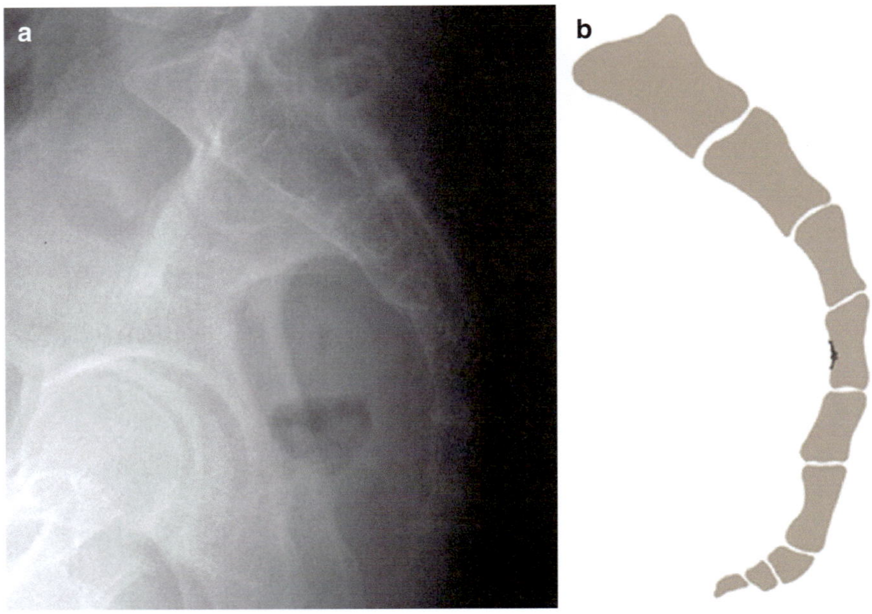

Fig. 16.3 Lateral radiograph of the sacrum (**a**) shows that the anterior cortex of S4 vertebral body is not smooth (**b**)

   3.2. CT scan (Fig. 16.3c)

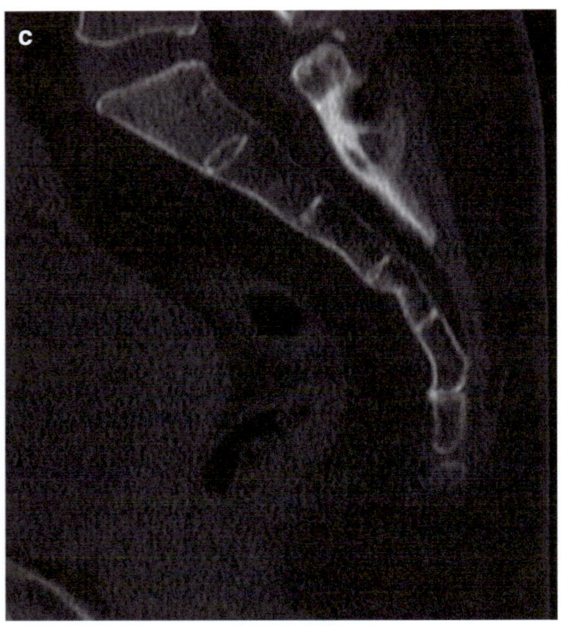

Fig. 16.3 (**c**) Sagittal reconstruction shows distortion of the anterior cortex, considering an old fracture

16.1.3.2 Longitudinal Fracture

Longitudinal fractures are often overlapped with intestinal contents and intestinal gas. Most of the X-rays cannot display these fractures, but on coronal and axial CT scans, they are clearly visible.

4. Comparison of X-ray and CT of the longitudinal sacral fracture
   4.1. X-ray (Fig. 16.4a, b)

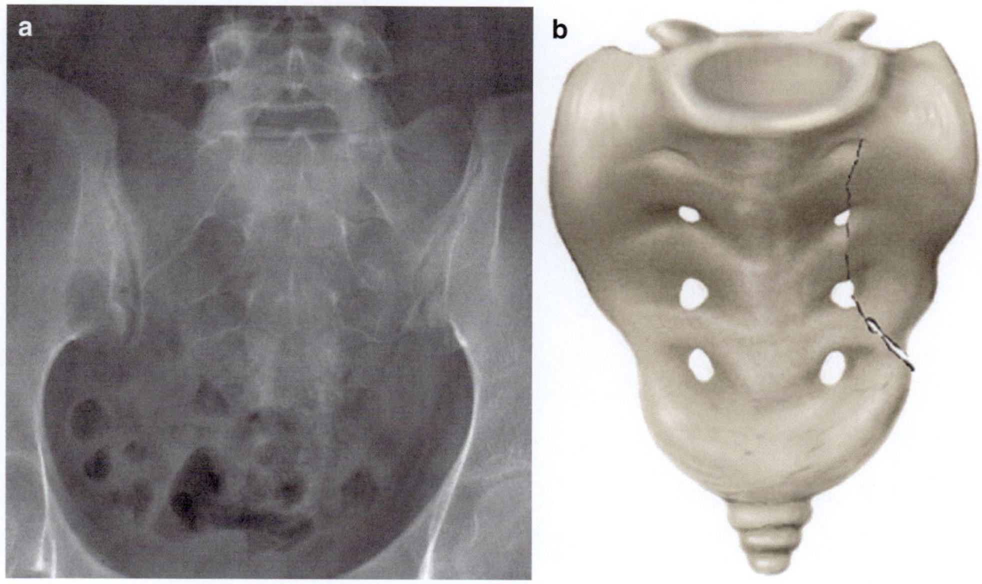

Fig. 16.4 The sacral vertebrae PA (**a**) shows a longitudinal fracture of the sacrum, and the fracture line involves the left sacral foramina (**b**)

   4.2. CT scan (Fig. 16.4c, d)

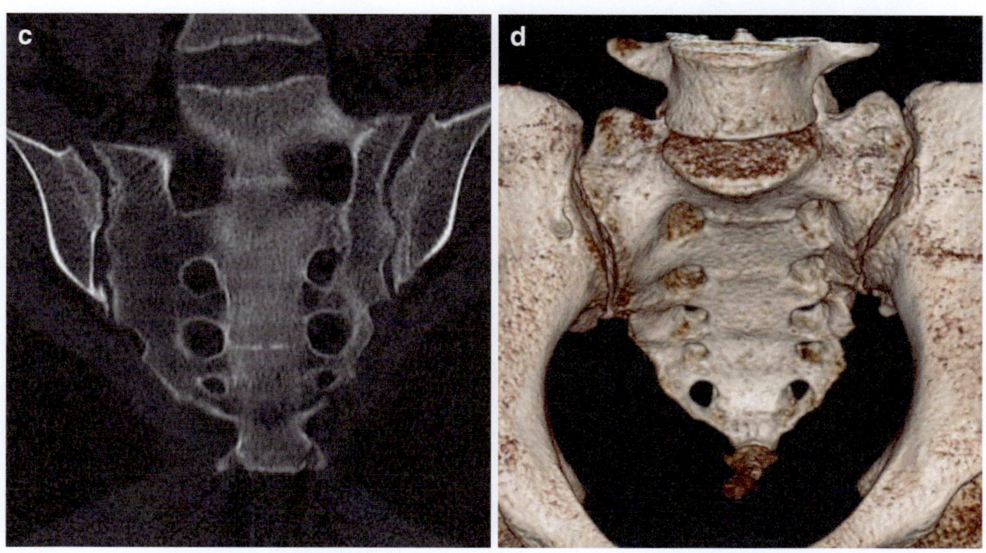

Fig. 16.4 (**c**, **d**) Coronal CT reconstruction (**c**) and VR image (**d**) clearly shows the left sacral foramina irregularity

5. Identification of sacral fracture and no fracture
   5.1. X-ray (Fig. 16.5a, b)

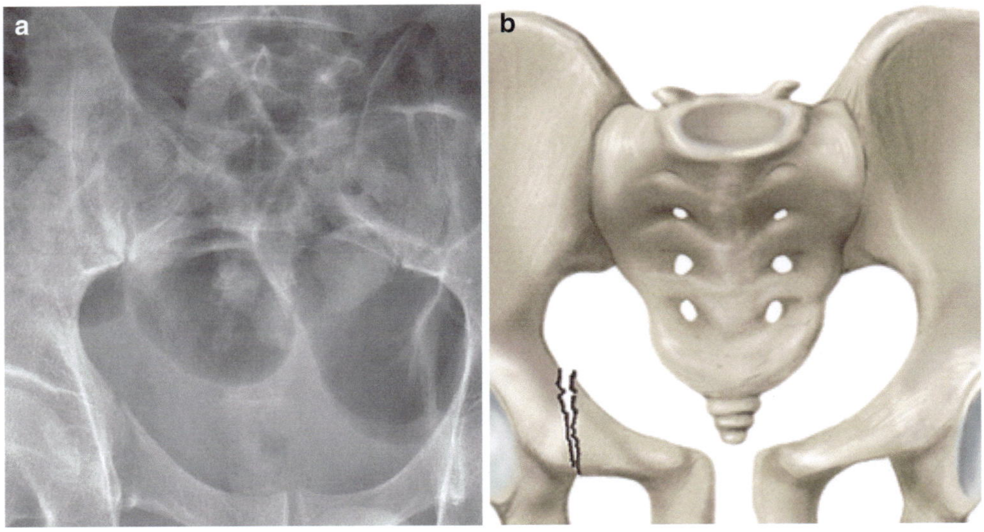

Fig. 16.5 The sacral PA (**a**) shows apparent intestinal pneumatosis, the sacrum structure is unclear, and the right superior ramus of pubis is also fractured (**b**)

   5.2. CT scan (Fig. 16.5c)

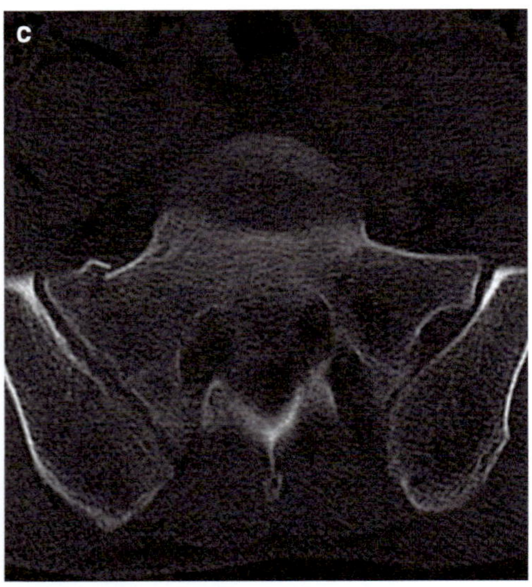

Fig. 16.5 (**c**) Axial CT shows right sacral wing fracture

16.1.3.3 Comminuted Fracture

6. Comparison of X-ray, CT, and MR of sacral comminuted fractures
   6.1. X-ray (Fig. 16.6a, b)

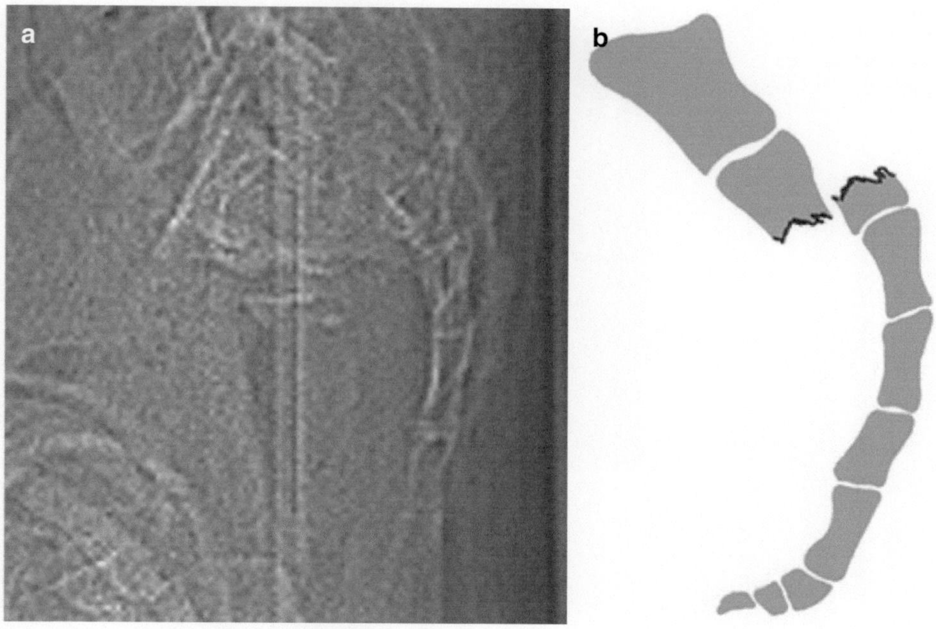

Fig. 16.6 Lateral X-ray of the sacrum (**a**) shows fracture of the sacrum, apparent dislocation (**b**)

6.2. CT scan (Fig. 16.6c–e)

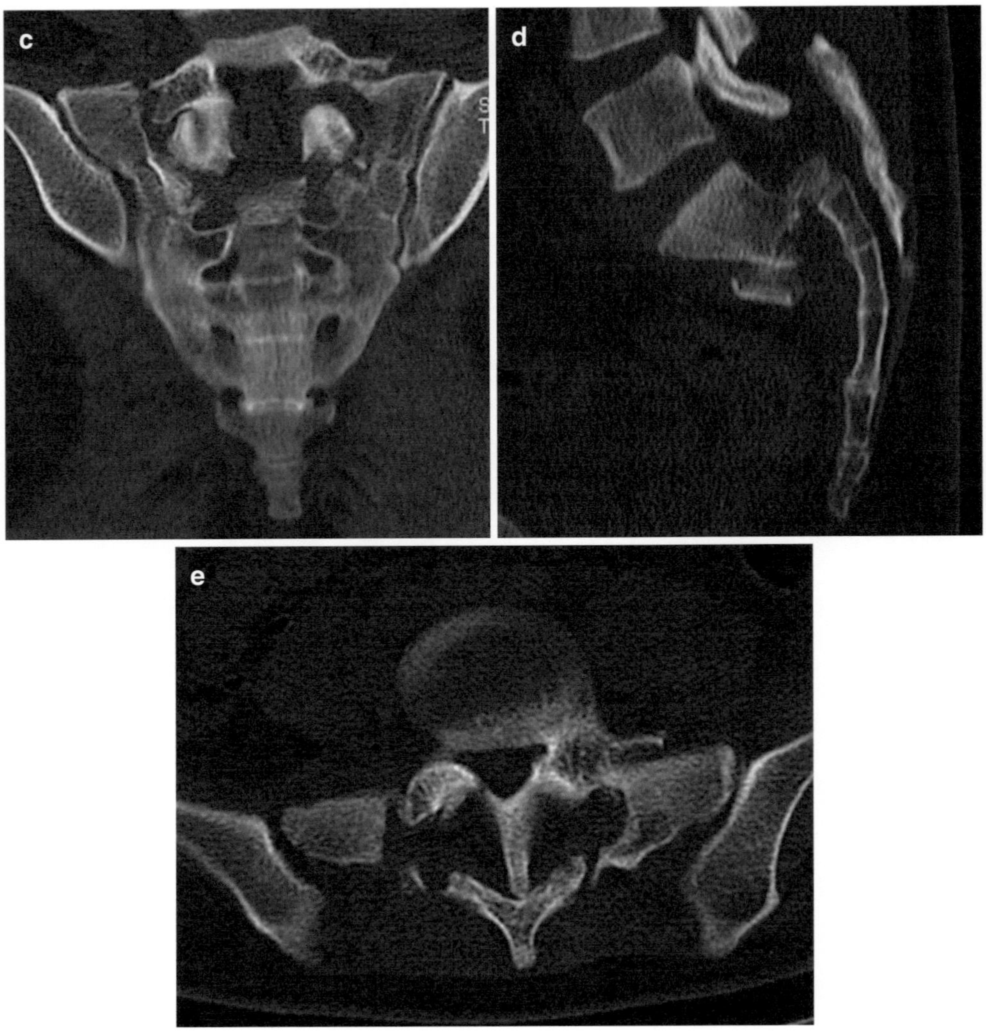

Fig. 16.6 (**c**, **d**) (coronal and sagittal CT reconstruction), (**e**) (axial CT): show that S1, S2 vertebral body and appendix fractures, are comminuted, and dislocated

6.3. MR imaging (Fig. 16.6f–h)

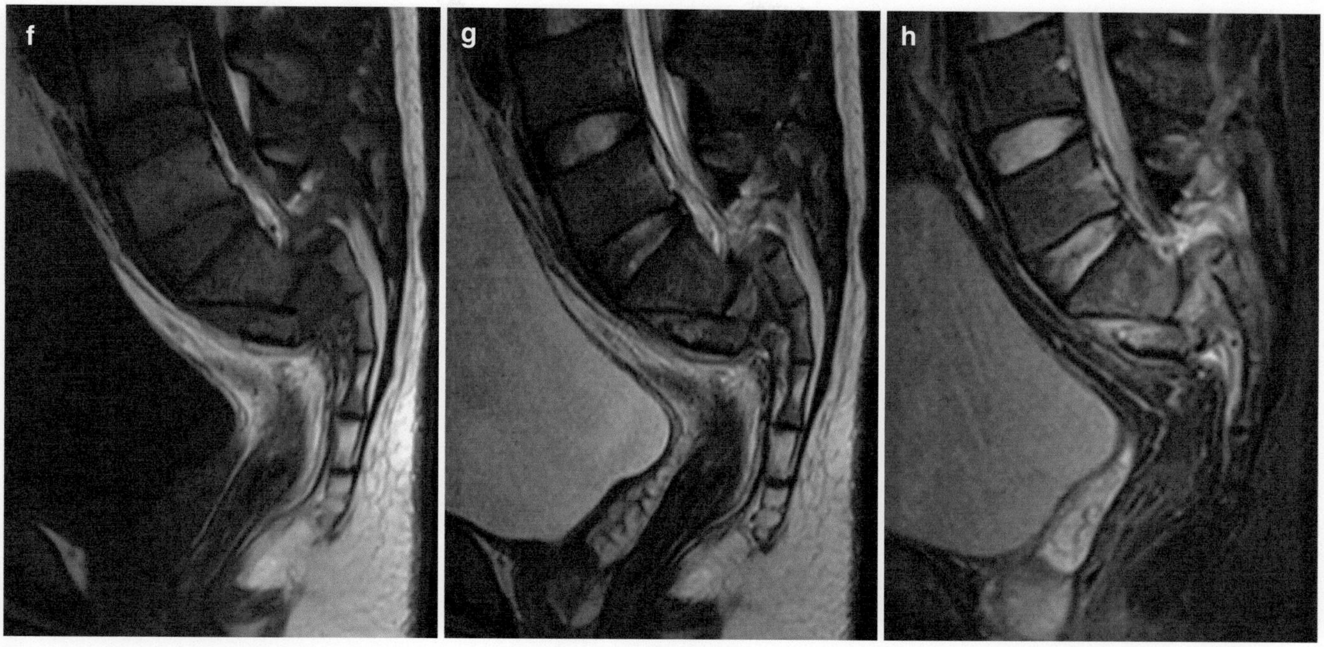

Fig. 16.6 (**f–h**) (MRTIWI, T2WI, STIR) clearly show S2 vertebral body and appendix fracture, sacral transverse fracture

7. Comparison of CT and MR of the sacral and coccygeal fracture
   7.1. CT scan (Fig. 16.7a, b)

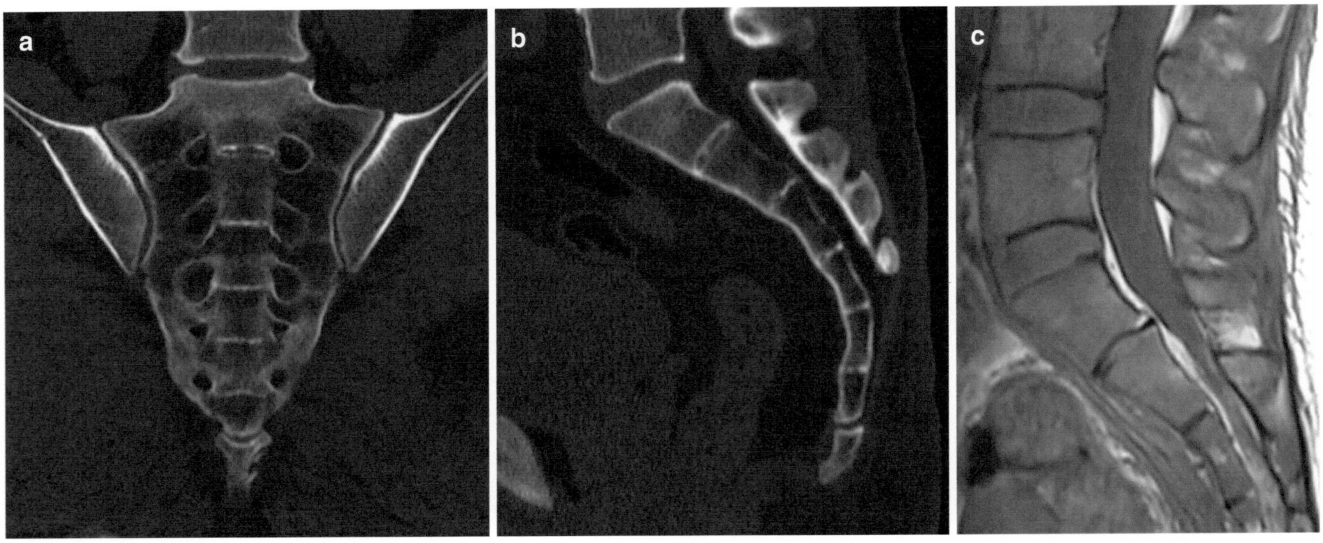

Fig. 16.7 (**a**, **b**) (coronal and sagittal CT reconstruction) show comminuted fractures of S5 and first coccygeal vertebra, and fracture of the left S3 foramina

   7.2. MR imaging (Fig. 16.7c–e)

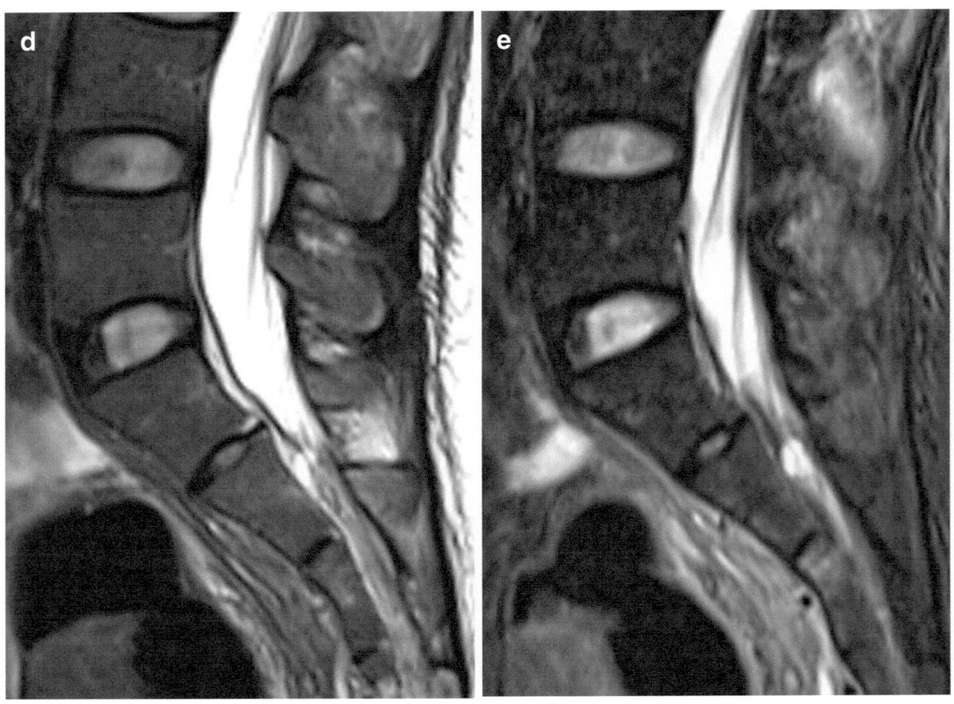

Fig. 16.7 (**c**, **d**) (TSE-T1WI and TSE-T2WI) show no abnormalities in S1-4, and (**e**) (STIR) shows S3 patchy high signal (bone contusion), soft tissue swelling before sacrum

16.2 Coccygeal Fracture

The coccygeal vertebrae, also known as coccyx, are located at the lower end of the sacrum and fused by 3–4 coccyges. There are two kinds of injury: coccygeal fracture and sacrococcygeal joint dislocation. After the injury, the distal bone fragment is mostly displaced forward.

16.2.1 Injury Mechanism Identification

The cause of coccygeal fracture is that the coccyx or its joint ligament has suffered from direct trauma, meaning that when falling injury occurs, the coccyx directly hits the ground.

16.2.2 Symptom and Sign Identification

The most apparent manifestation is sacrococcygeal pain. Severe coccygeal fractures can affect rectal function and defecation. There is a potential possibility for women to affect the bony birth canal.

16.2.3 Imaging Differential Diagnosis

The coccygeal fracture is not easy to be identified on X-ray film. The PA image is affected by the contents of intestine and the lower part of the sacrum, therefore, the coccyx cannot be clearly displayed. The lateral position view is ideal for showing the anterior cortex of sacrum, and the dislocation. However, X-ray film cannot provide a precise diagnosis. Sagittal and coronal CT reconstruction play an important role in the diagnosis of sacral fractures.

16.2.3.1 Coccygeal Fracture

1. Identification of coccygeal fracture and nonfracture
   1.1. X-ray (Fig. 16.8a, b)

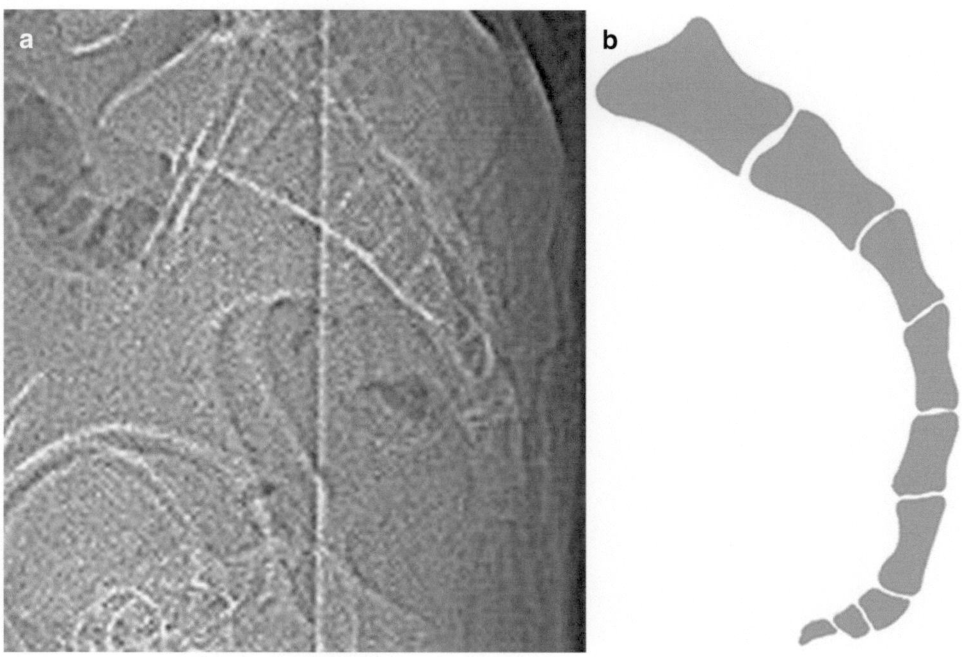

Fig. 16.8 The lateral position of the sacrococcygeal X-ray (**a**) shows the structure of coccyx unclear (**b**)

1.2. CT scan (Fig. 16.8c)

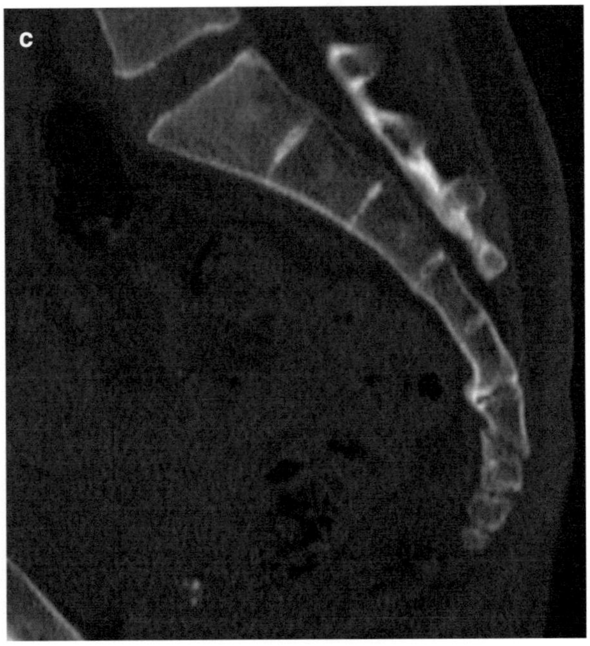

Fig. 16.8 (**c**) Sagittal CT reconstruction shows fracture and dislocation of the first coccyx and dislocation

2. Identification of coccygeal fractures and suspicious fractures
   2.1. X-ray (Fig. 16.9a, b)

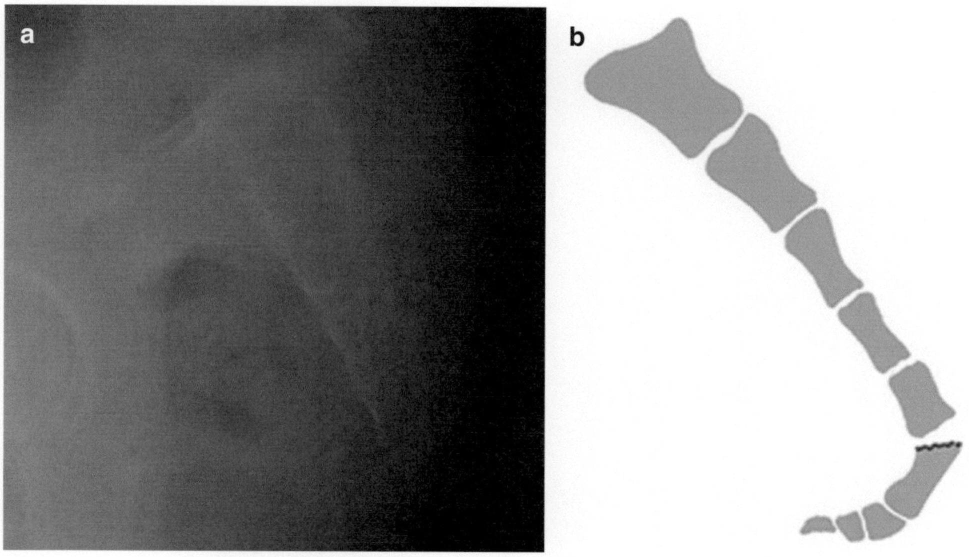

Fig. 16.9 The lateral position of sacrococcygeal X-ray (**a**) shows an increase in the anterior flexion angle of the coccyx (**b**)

   2.2. CT scan (Fig. 16.9c)

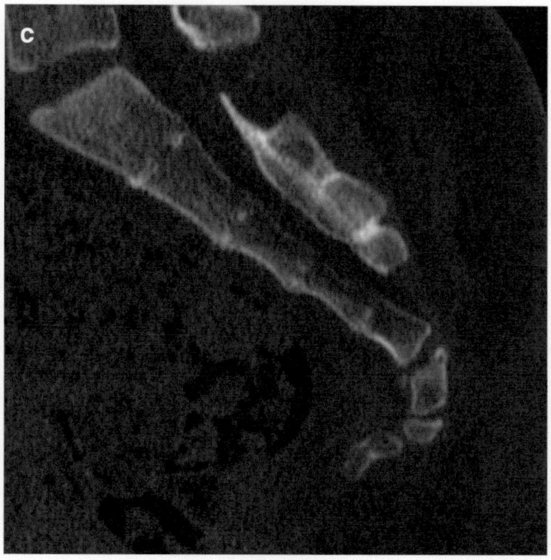

Fig. 16.9 (**c**) Sagittal CT reconstruction shows that the first coccygeal vertebral body with anterior edge dissociated

16.2.3.2 Sacrococcygeal Joint Dislocation

3. Comparison of X-Ray and CT for sacrococcygeal joint dislocation
   3.1. X-ray (Fig. 16.10a, b)

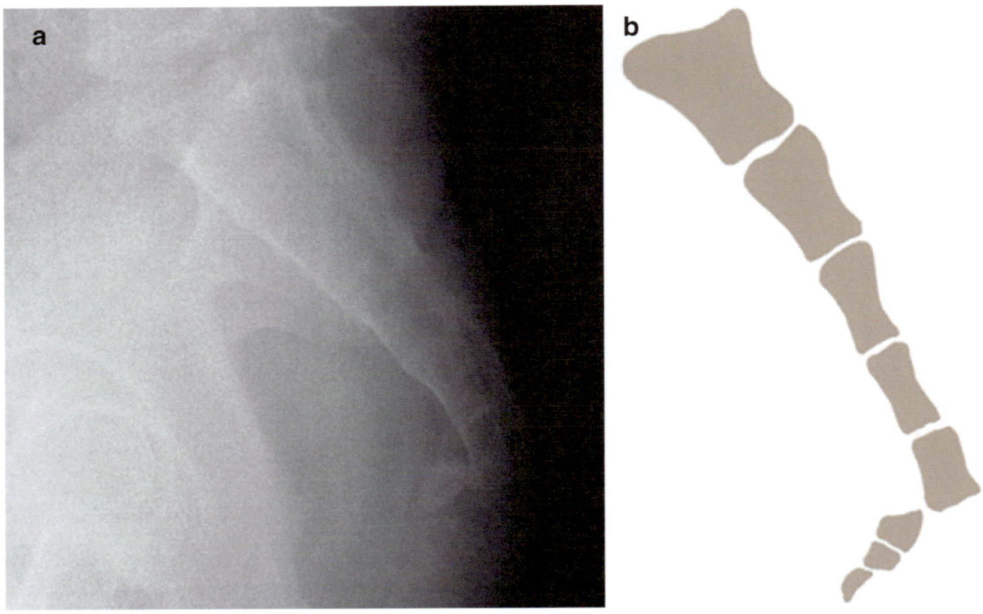

Fig. 16.10 Lateral sacrococcygeal X-ray (**a**) shows sacrococcygeal dislocation and coccyx forward (**b**)

   3.2. CT scan (Fig. 16.10c)

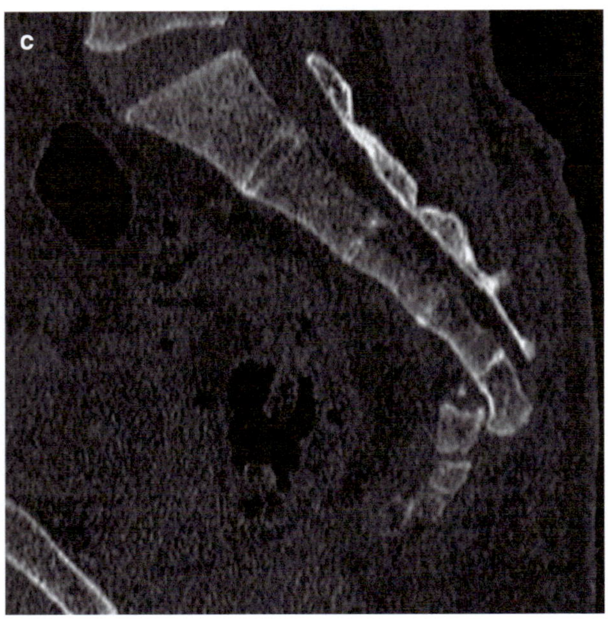

Fig. 16.10 (**c**) Sagittal CT reconstruction shows sacrococcygeal dislocation, and the coccyx has moved forward, the fragments are partially visible

4. Comparison of CT and MR for sacrococcygeal dislocation
   4.1. CT scan (Fig. 16.11a, b)

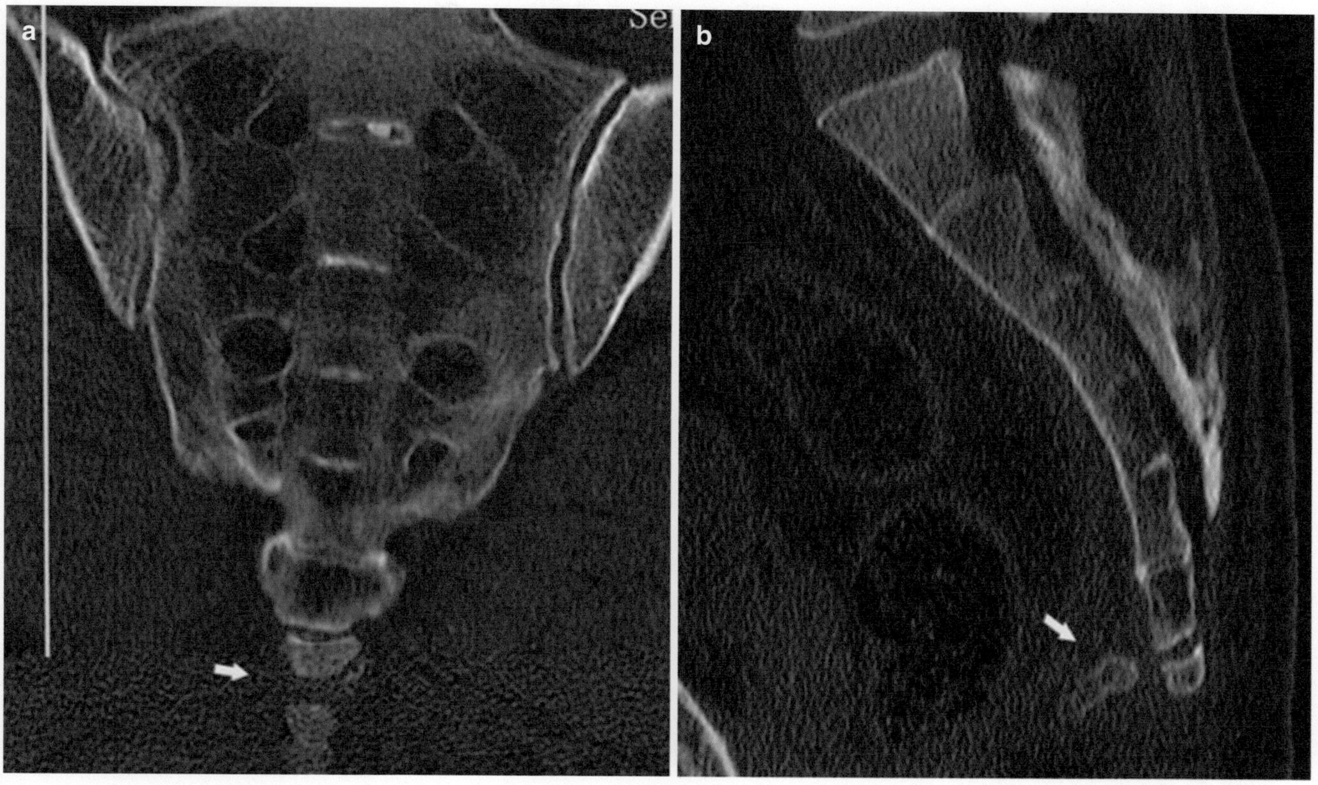

Fig. 16.11 (**a**) CT shows the interval between the second and third coccyx widening; (**b**) Sagittal CT shows the third coccyx moving forward

   4.2. MR imaging (Fig. 16.11c–e)

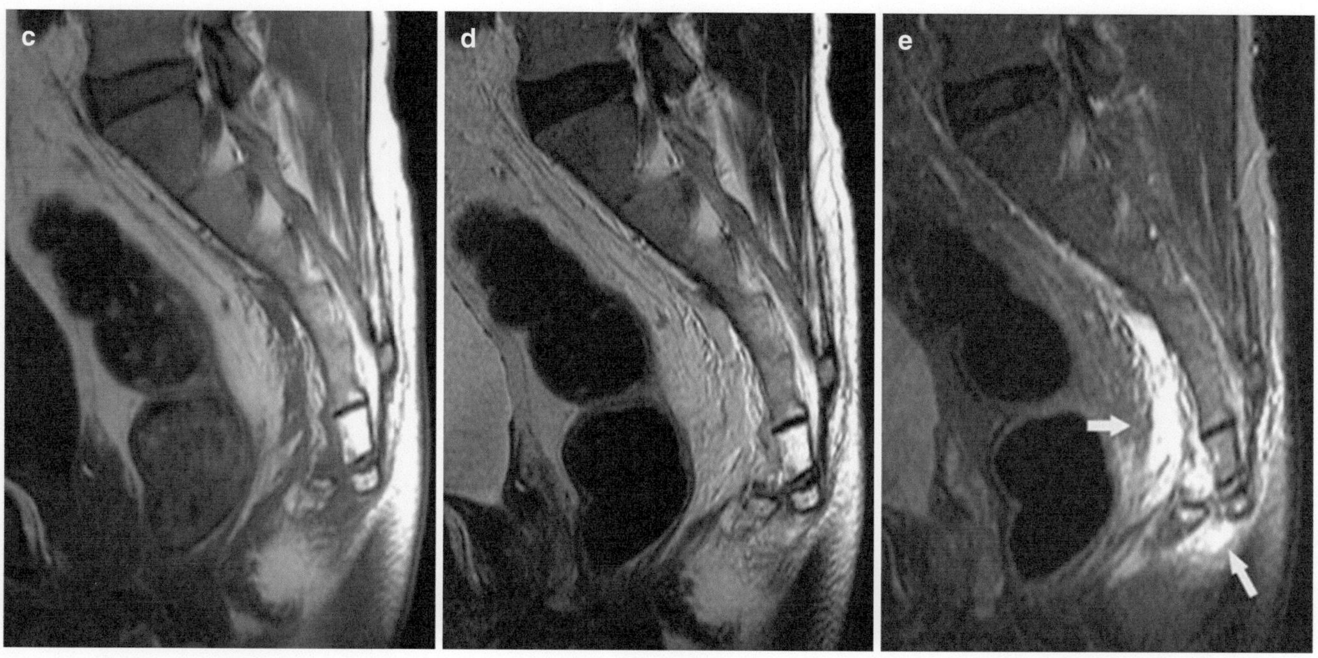

Fig. 16.11 (**c**, **d**) (TSE-T1WI and TSE-T2WI) show that the third and fourth coccyx has moved forward. (**e**) (STIR sequence) shows the third coccyx moving forward with soft tissue swelling

16.3 Summary of the Points

1. The sacrococcygeal fracture often has a direct injury mechanism. Both the sacral and coccygeal fractures are mostly caused by a fall onto the tailbone in the sitting position, against a hard surface.
2. Due to the contents of the intestine overlapping with the sacrococcygeal lesion, X-ray films can easily miss the diagnosis of sacrococcygeal fracture. It is also difficult to differentiate old fractures and new fractures. While CT scan with reconstruction images can show fractures and dislocations better.
3. According to the history of injury and clinical symptoms, the sacrococcygeal fracture can be highly suspected. If the fracture is not found on X-ray and CT scans, MRI can be performed. MRI can show fracture lines, bone marrow, and swelling soft tissue around the fracture and can identify fresh fractures and old fractures.

17 Pelvic Ring Fractures

Zhiyong Hou and Yingze Zhang

The pelvis is composed of the sacrum, bilateral ilia, pubes, and ischia. The pelvic ring could be divided into anterior and posterior rings. Anterior ring consists of bilateral ischial and pubic rami, which are connected by symphysis pubis (cartilage connection). Posterior ring is connected by the sacroiliac joint composed by bilateral ear surface of sacrum and ilium. The upper part of the sacroiliac joint is the ligament joint; however, the lower part is the synovial joint. Posterior pelvic ring, as a weight-bearing part, fracture line rarely involves this area because of its hard cortex. However, anterior ring may be easily displaced because of its weak bone stock. Multiple insertions of muscles of the torso and lower limbs are located in the pelvis; for example, the biceps femoris, semitendinosus, and semimembranosus attach to the ischial tuberosity; the sartorius arises from the anterior superior iliac spine; the rectus femoris reaches the anterior inferior iliac spine; and the psoas major reaches the iliac crest. Avulsion fracture and displacement of pelvic fragments may occur in areas of muscular attachment when relevant muscles contracted rapidly. In AO/OTA classification system, posterior ring injury is divided into stable fracture with integral posterior ring, partially stable fracture with interrupted posterior ring, and unstable fracture with complete posterior ring injury. Stable fractures with integral posterior ring can be subdivided into with avulsion fracture of the pelvis (accounting for 5.64% of pelvic ring injury), direct traumatic fracture in the pelvis (accounting for 42.81% of pelvic ring injury), and transverse sacral fracture (accounting for 21.21% of pelvic ring injury). Partially stable fracture with interrupted posterior ring could be subdivided into unilateral open book external rotation injury (accounting for 4.56% of pelvic ring injury), unilaterally lateral compression internal rotation injury (accounting for 2.45% of pelvic ring injury), and incomplete injury bilateral posterior ring (accounting for 0.47% of pelvic ring injury). Unstable fracture with complete posterior ring injury could be subdivided into unilaterally complete posterior ring injury (accounting for 1.68% of pelvic ring injury), unilaterally complete posterior ring injury associated with contralateral incomplete injury (accounting for 0.35% of pelvic ring injury), and complete injury of bilateral posterior rings (accounting for 0.30% of pelvic ring injury).

17.1 Identification of Injury Mechanisms

The majority of pelvic ring displacement is caused by car accidents, fall injuries, and sport injuries. The pelvic ring injury could be divided into avulsion, rotationally unstable, vertically unstable, and complex fractures.

17.2 Identification of Symptoms

Relevant symptoms that include pain, swelling, deformity, and shock may occur after pelvic ring fracture. Further X-ray, CT scans, and antishock treatment should be performed when a fracture is suspected.

Z. Hou · Y. Zhang (✉)
Department of Orthopaedics, The Third Hospital of Hebei Medical University, Shijiazhuang, Hebei, China

Y. Zhang (ed.), *Differential Diagnosis of Fracture*, https://doi.org/10.1007/978-981-13-8339-7_17

17.3 Identification of Radiograph

In general, displaced fractures could easily be diagnosed on the X-rays. Crack fracture and ligamentous injury could be diagnosed by CT and MRI, respectively. CT scans should be routinely conducted because injury always involves both the anterior and posterior pelvic rings.

1. Comparison of X-ray and CT scans in the integral posterior ring with avulsion fracture of anterior superior iliac spine
   1.1. X-ray (Fig. 17.1a, b)

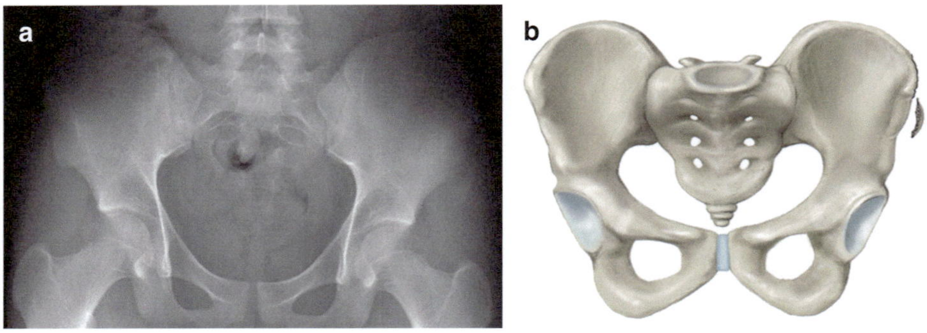

Fig. 17.1 X-ray shows that there is an avulsion fragment in the left anterior superior iliac spine (**a**). An inferolateral displaced fragment is observed in schematic diagram (**b**)

   1.2. CT scan (Fig. 17.1c–f)

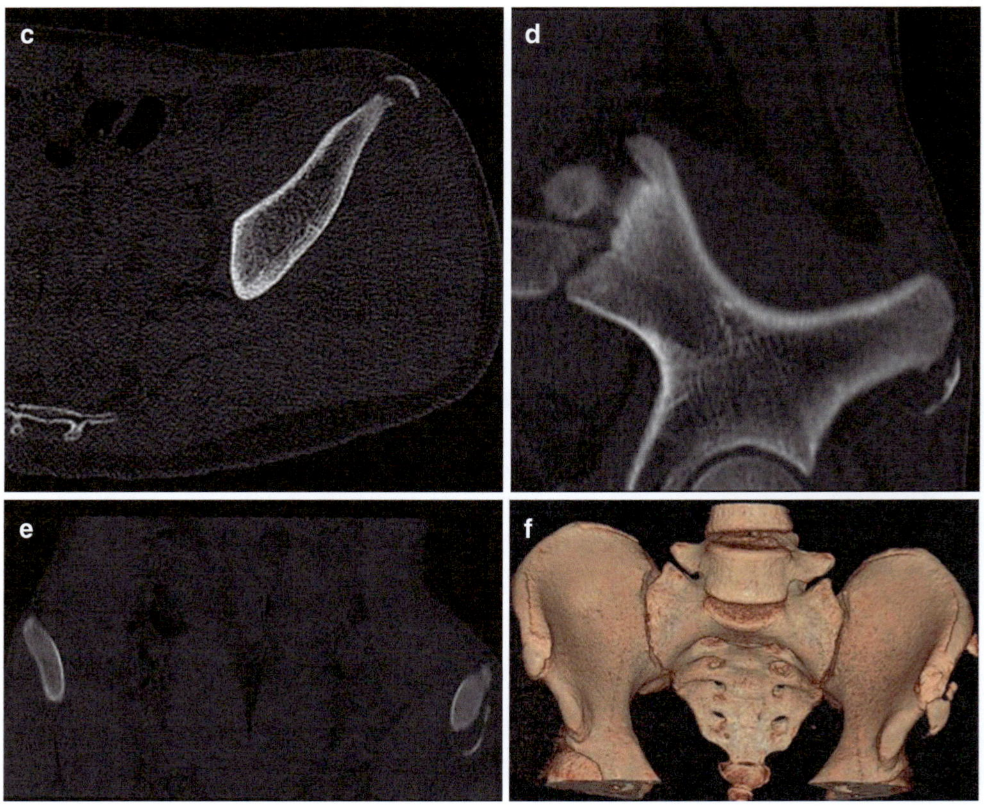

Fig. 17.1 Transverse section (**c**), Oblique sagittal section (**d**), Coronal section (**e**), and three-dimensional reconstruction (**f**) show that there are multiple inferolateral displaced fragments in the left anterior superior iliac spine

2. Comparison of X-ray and CT scans in the integral posterior ring with displaced fragment in iliac crest margin
   2.1. X-ray (Fig. 17.2a, b)

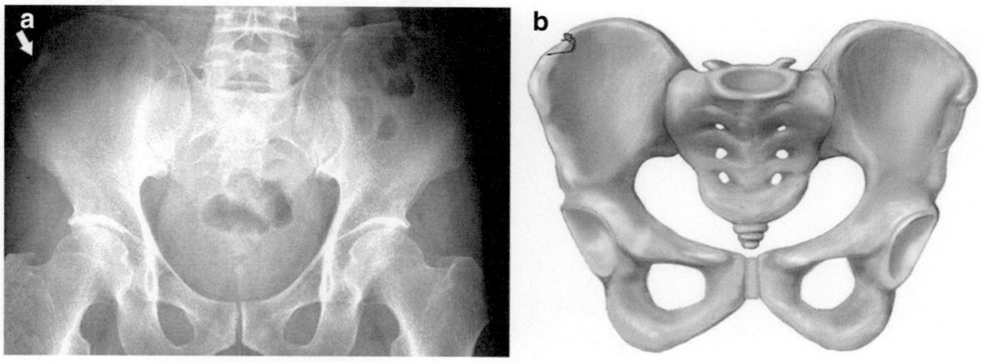

Fig. 17.2 X-ray (**a**) shows that there is a displaced, overlapped fragment in the right iliac crest (**b**)

   2.2. CT scan (Fig. 17.2c)

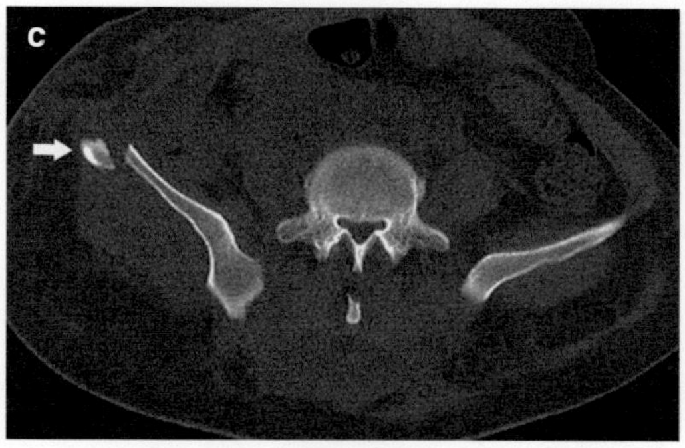

Fig. 17.2 CT cross section (**c**) shows that displaced fragments in the right iliac crest and fifth lumbar spinous process

3. Comparison of X-ray and CT scans in the integral posterior ring avulsion fracture of the anterior superior iliac spine
   3.1. X-ray (Fig. 17.3a, b)

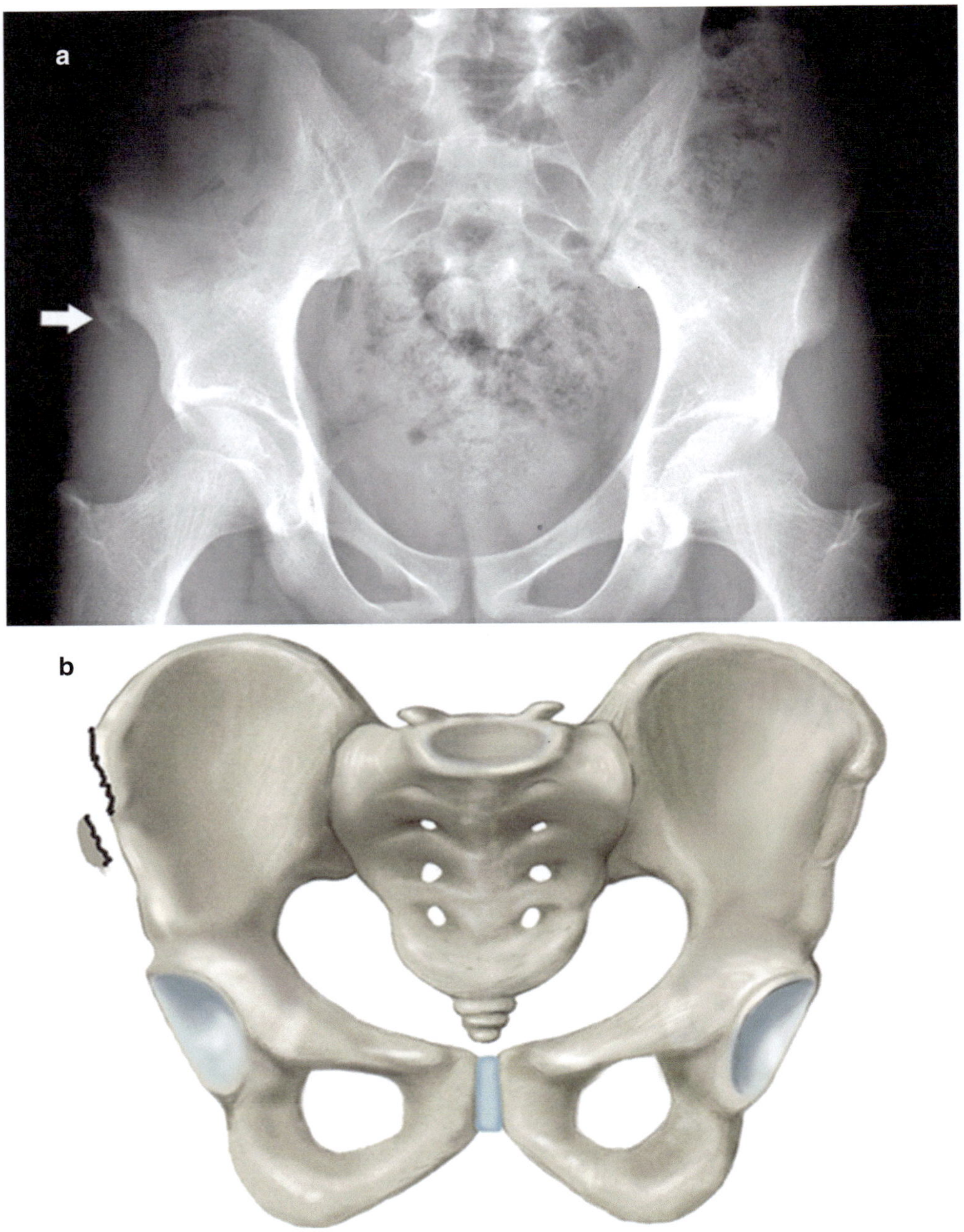

Fig. 17.3 X-ray (**a**) shows an inferolateral displaced fragment of the right anterior superior iliac spine (**b**)

3.2. CT scan (Fig. 17.3c)

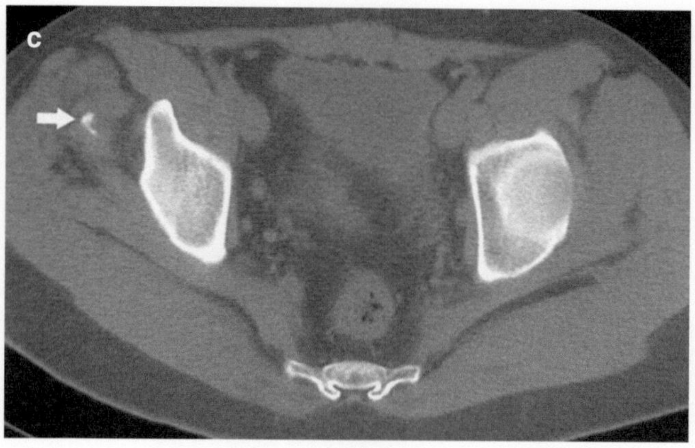

Fig. 17.3 CT cross section (**c**) shows an inferolateral displaced fragment of the right anterior superior iliac spine

4. Comparison of X-ray and CT scans in the integral posterior ring with displaced fragment in the iliac wing
   4.1. X-ray (Fig. 17.4a, b)

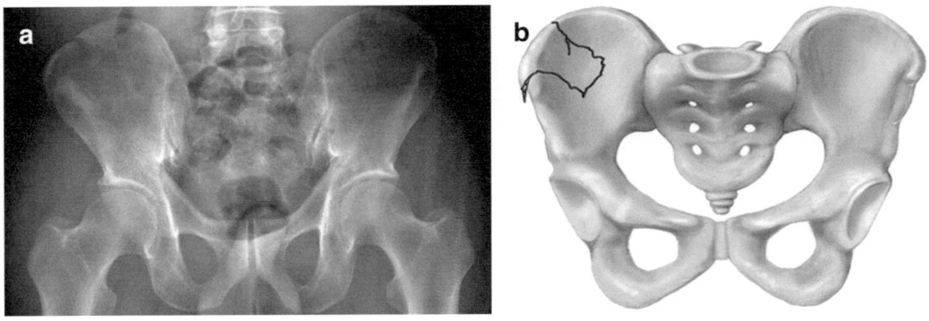

Fig. 17.4 X-ray and schematic diagram (**a**, **b**) show displaced comminuted fractures in iliac wing

   4.2. CT scan (Fig. 17.4c, d)

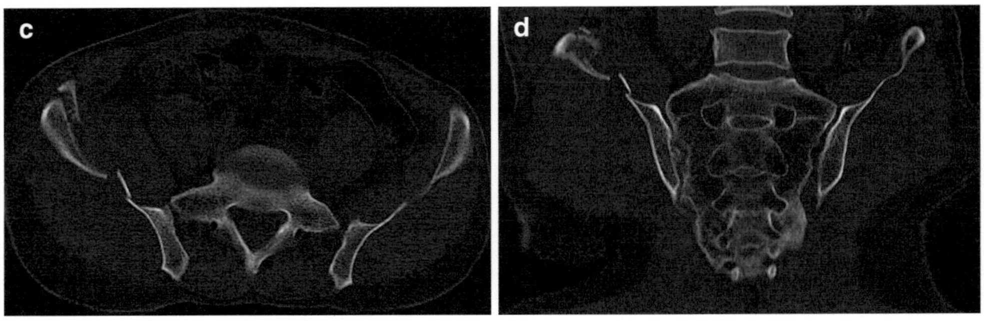

Fig. 17.4 CT cross section and coronal section (**c**, **d**) show multidisplaced comminuted fragments in the right iliac wing, swelling of the surrounding soft tissue accompanied

5. Comparison of X-ray and CT scans in the integral posterior ring with unilaterally displaced pubic rami fracture
   5.1. X-ray (Fig. 17.5a, b)

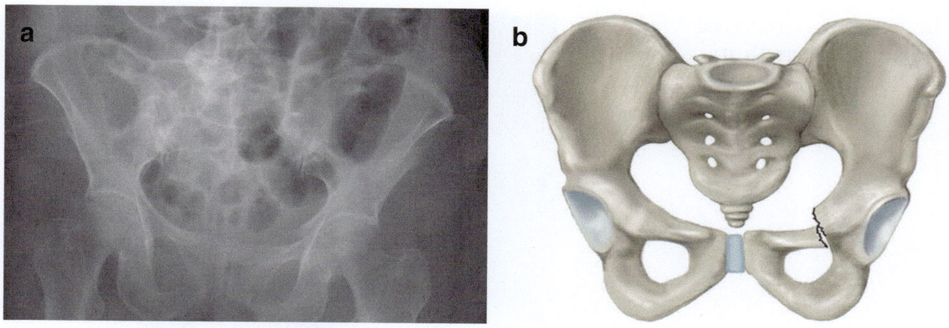

Fig. 17.5 X-ray and schematic diagram (**a**, **b**) show displaced fractures in the left superior ramus

   5.2. CT scan (Fig. 17.5c, d)

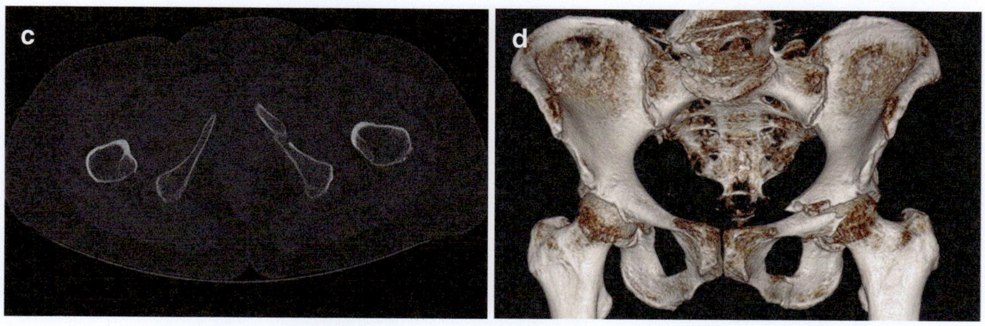

Fig. 17.5 CT cross section (**c**) and 3D reconstruction (**d**) show fracture line involves the pubic rami and acetabulum

6. Comparison of X-ray and CT scans in the integral posterior ring with transverse sacral fracture
    6.1. X-ray (Fig. 17.6a–d)

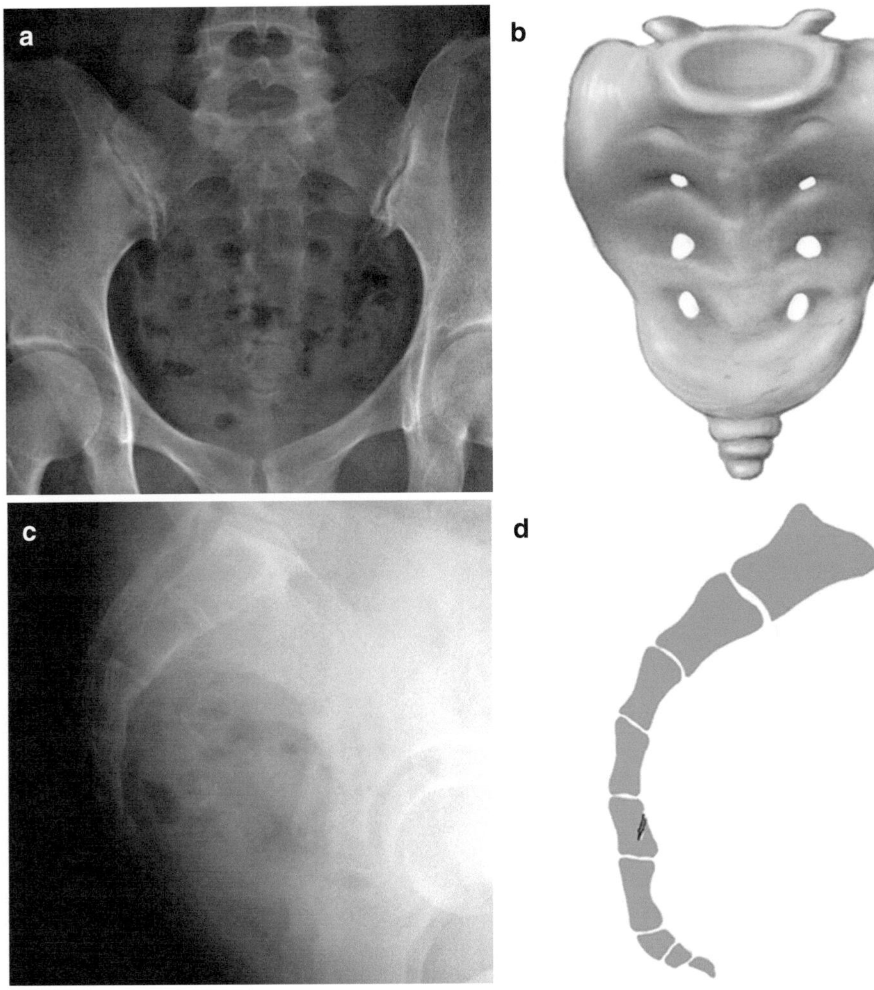

Fig. 17.6 X-rays (**a**, **c**) and schematic diagrams (**b**, **d**) show the breakage of the anterior border of the S5 vertebrae and trabecula

    6.2. CT scan (Fig. 17.6e, f)

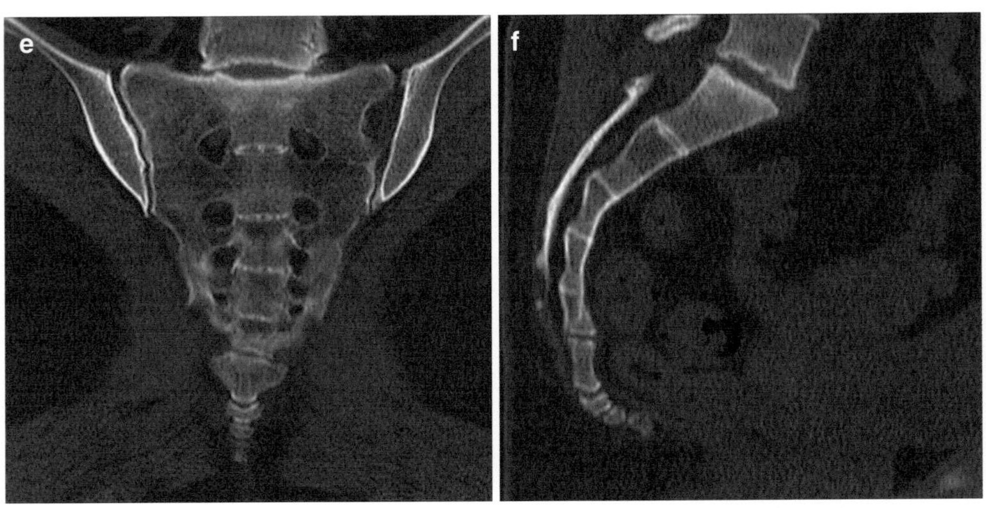

Fig. 17.6 CT coronal and sagittal section (**e**, **f**) show S5 vertebrae fracture with no dislocated fragment in the S5 vertebrae

7. CT features of the integral posterior ring with transverse sacral fracture
   7.1. CT scan (Fig. 17.7a–d)

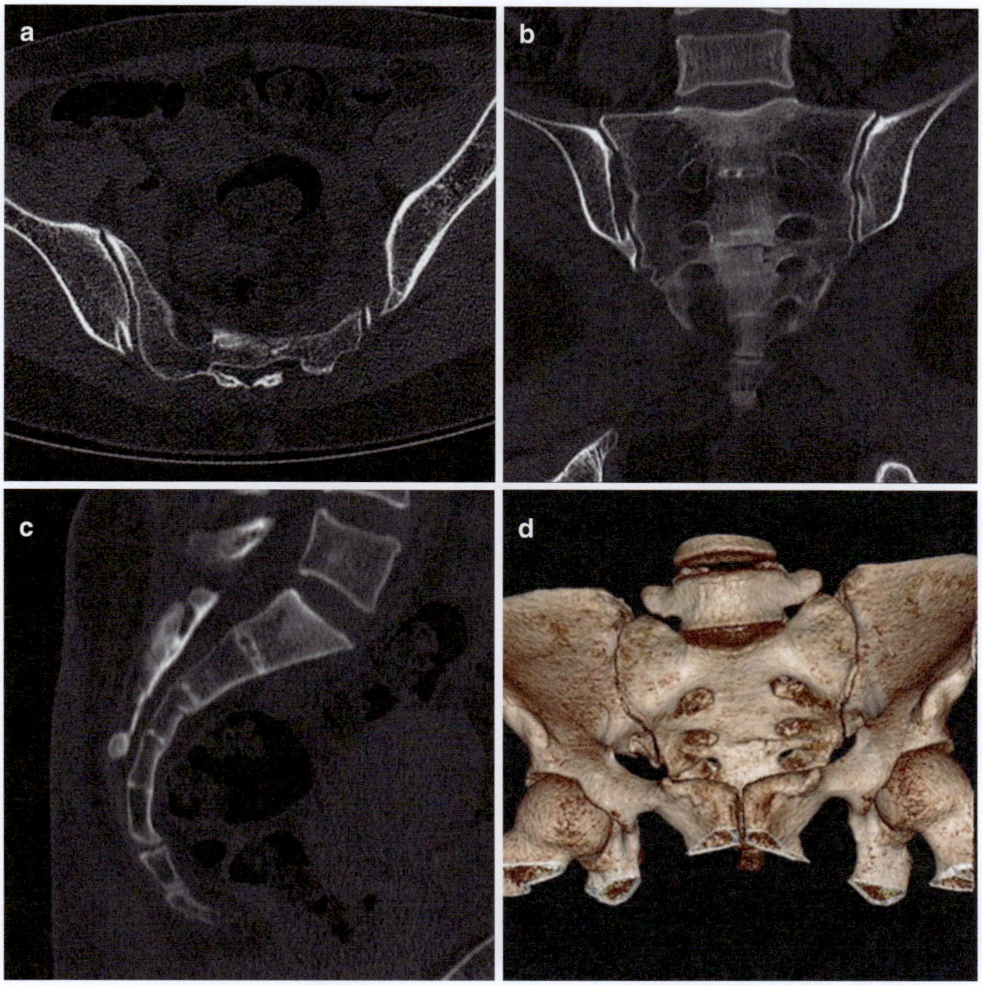

Fig. 17.7 CT sections and reconstruction (**a**–**d**) show transverse fragment of S3, and the fracture line involves the sacral foramina

8. Comparison of X-ray and CT scans in the integral posterior ring with completely displaced sacral fracture
   8.1. X-ray (Fig. 17.8a–d)

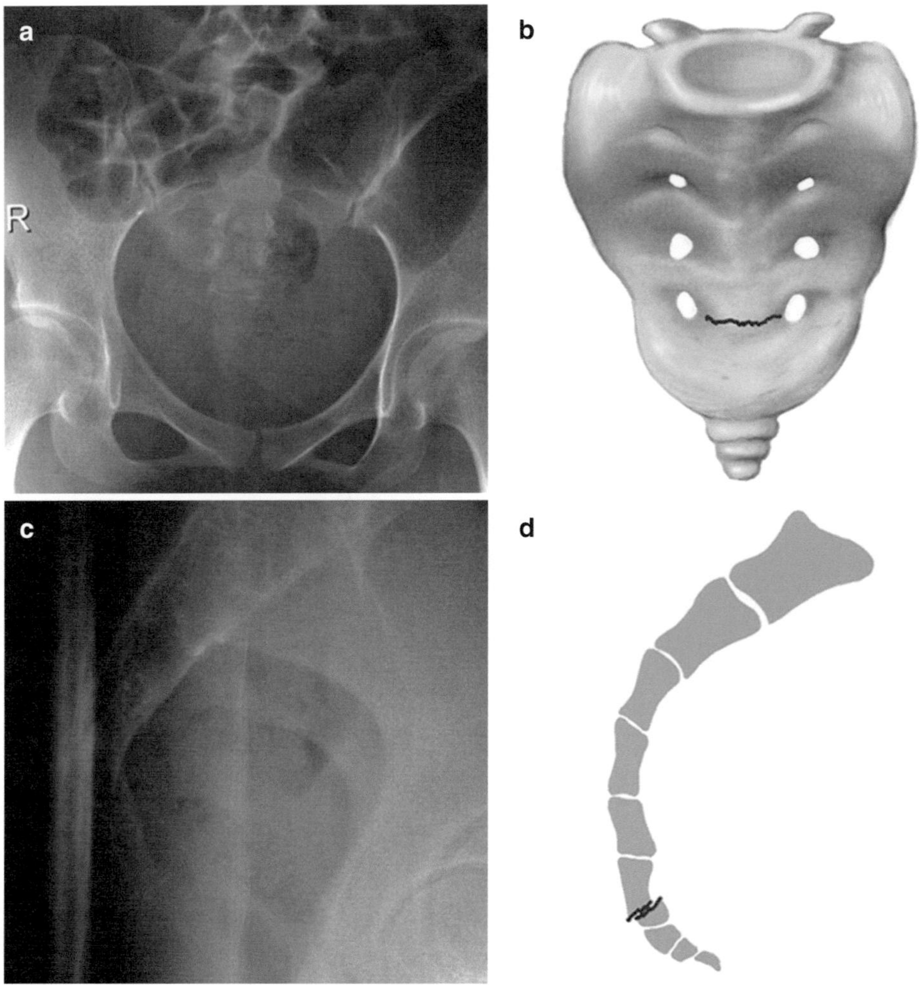

Fig. 17.8 X-rays (**a**, **b**) and schematic diagrams (**c**, **d**) show anteriorly displaced fragment in the distal S5 vertebrae

   8.2. CT scan (Fig. 17.8e, f)

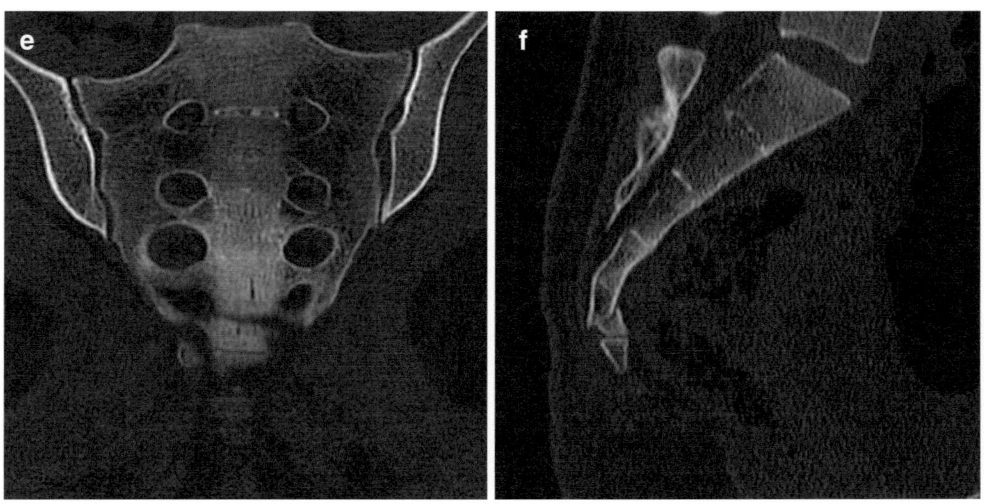

Fig. 17.8 CT coronal and sagittal sections (**e**, **f**) anterior displacement of distal S5 vertebrae

9. CT features of incomplete injury of posterior pelvic ring (unilateral open book external rotation injury pattern
   9.1. CT scan (Fig. 17.9a–d)

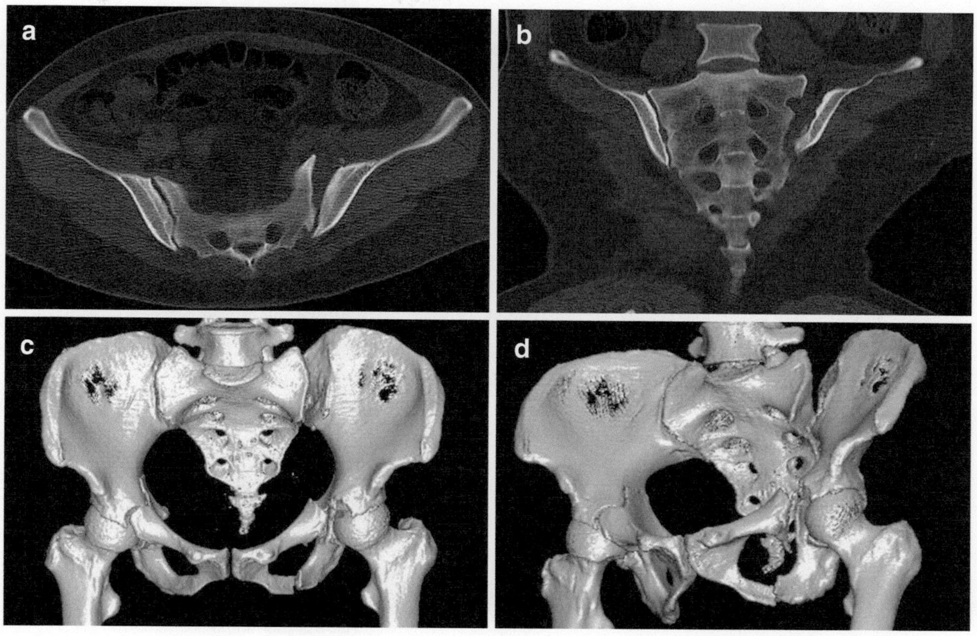

Fig. 17.9 CT scans and 3D reconstruction (**a**–**d**) show the dislocation of sacroiliac joint with posterior-laterally displaced ilium. The fracture lines involve the left pubic rami and acetabulum

10. Comparison of X-ray and CT scans for incomplete injury of posterior ring with unilateral open book external rotation injury
    10.1. X-ray (Fig. 17.10a–f)

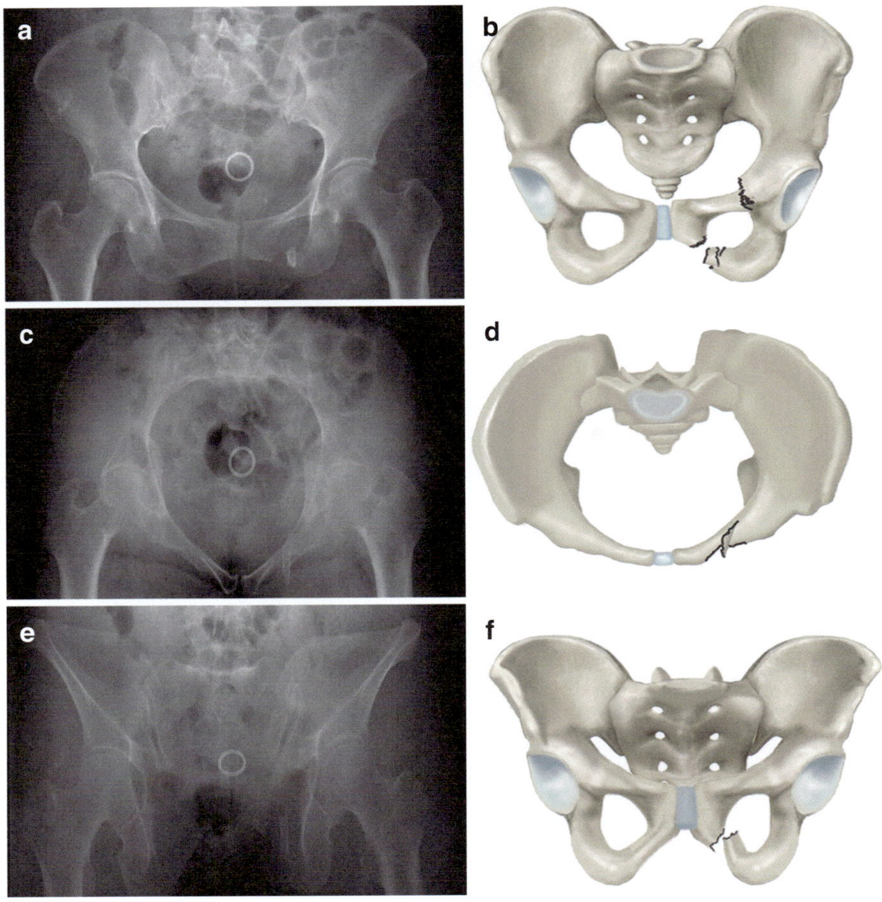

Fig. 17.10 Anteroposterior, inlet, and outlet projections combined with related diagram (**a**–**f**) show that the fracture lines involve the pubic rami and left sacrum

    10.2. CT scan (Fig. 17.10g–i)

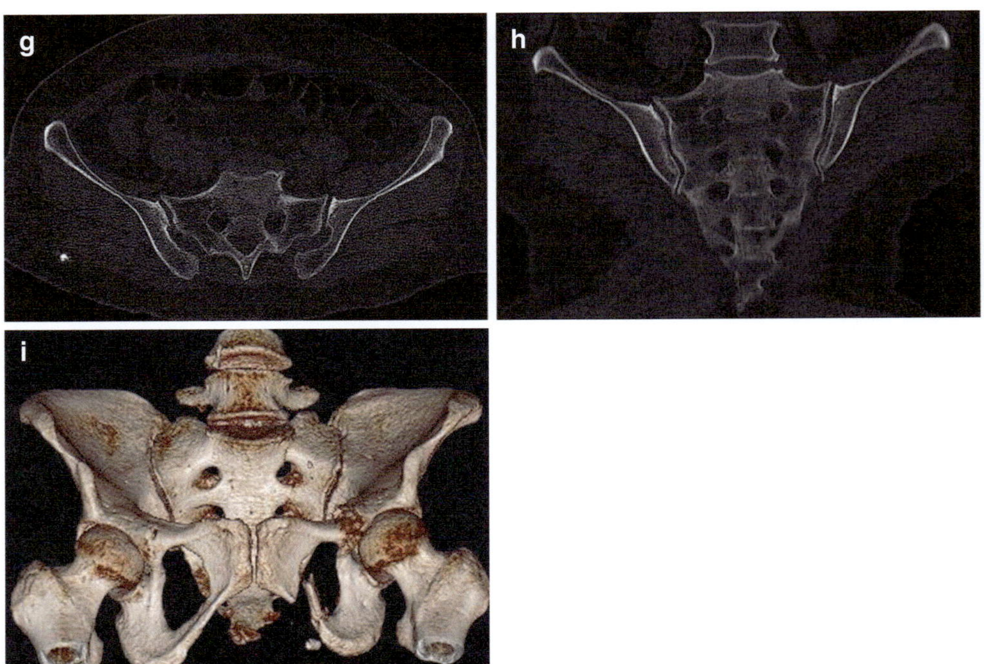

Fig. 17.10 CT scans (**g**, **h**) and 3D (**i**) reconstruction show that the fracture line involves the left sacral nerve foramen and pubic rami

11. Comparison of X-ray and CT scans for incomplete injury of posterior ring with unilateral lateral compression internal rotation damage
    11.1. X-ray (Fig. 17.11a, b)

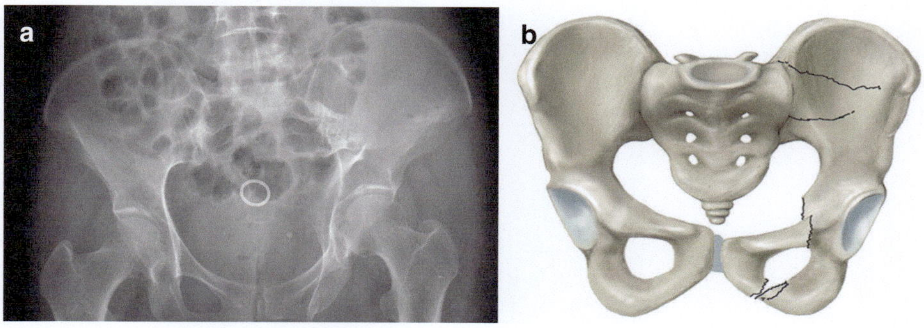

Fig. 17.11 X-ray and schematic diagram (**a**, **b**) show the comminuted fragments of the left ilium and the fracture line of the left pubic rami

    11.2. CT scan (Fig. 17.11c–f)

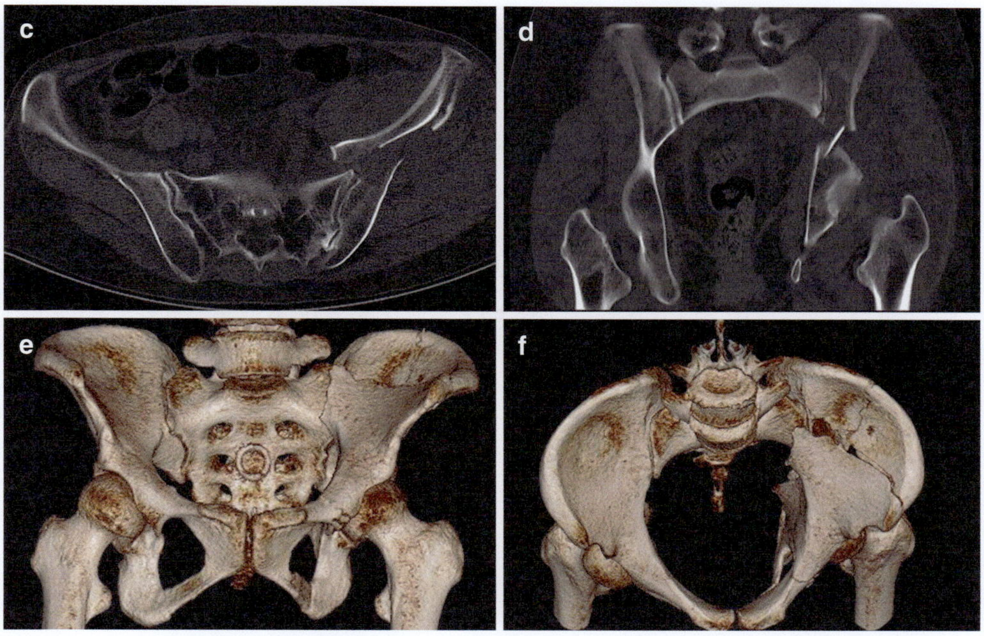

Fig. 17.11 CT scans and reconstruction (**c**–**f**) show displaced comminuted fractures of the left ilium. The fragment was medially displaced, and the fracture line involves the sacroiliac joint and left pubic rami

12. Comparison of X-ray and CT scans for incomplete injury of posterior ring with unilateral lateral compression internal rotation damage
    12.1. X-ray (Fig. 17.12a, b)

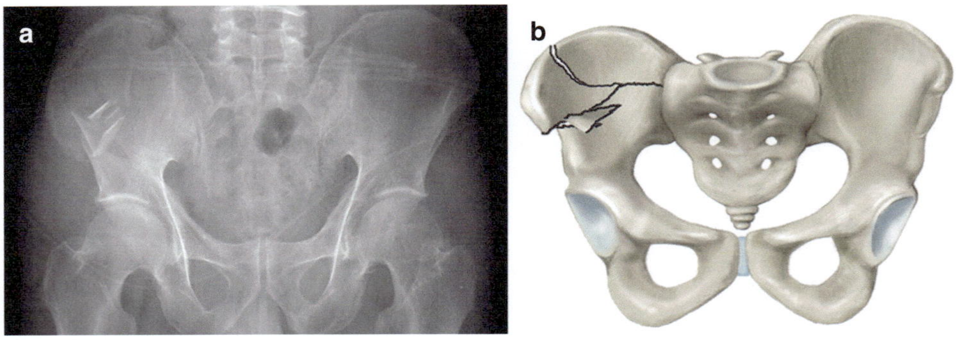

Fig. 17.12 X-ray and schematic diagram (**a**, **b**) show displaced fractures in the right ilium

    12.2. CT scan (Fig. 17.12c, d)

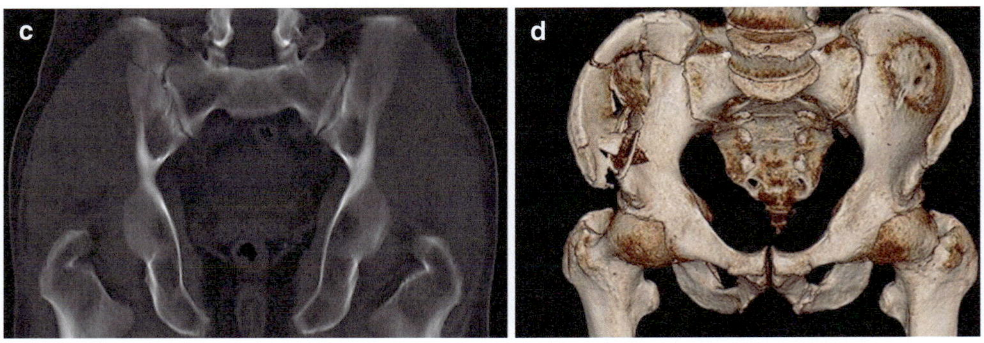

Fig. 17.12 CT cross section and reconstruction (**c**, **d**) show displaced comminuted fractures in the right ilium, and the fracture line involves the sacroiliac joint

13. Comparison of X-ray and CT scans for incomplete injury of posterior ring with unilateral lateral compression internal rotation damage
    13.1. X-ray (Fig. 17.13a–f)

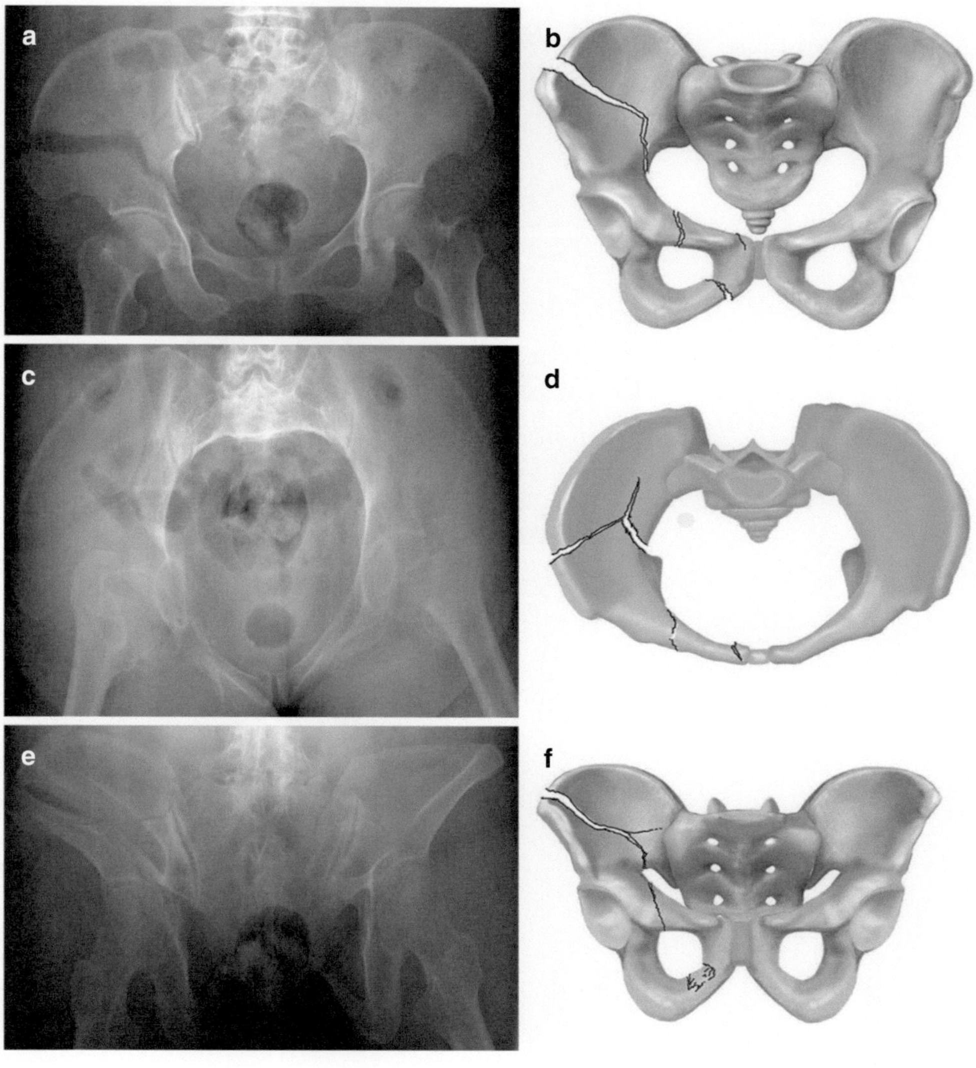

Fig. 17.13 Anteroposterior, inlet, and outlet projections combined with related diagram (**a**–**f**) show comminuted fractures of the ilium and fracture lines that involve the pubic rami and sacroiliac joint

13.2. CT scan (Fig. 17.13g–i)

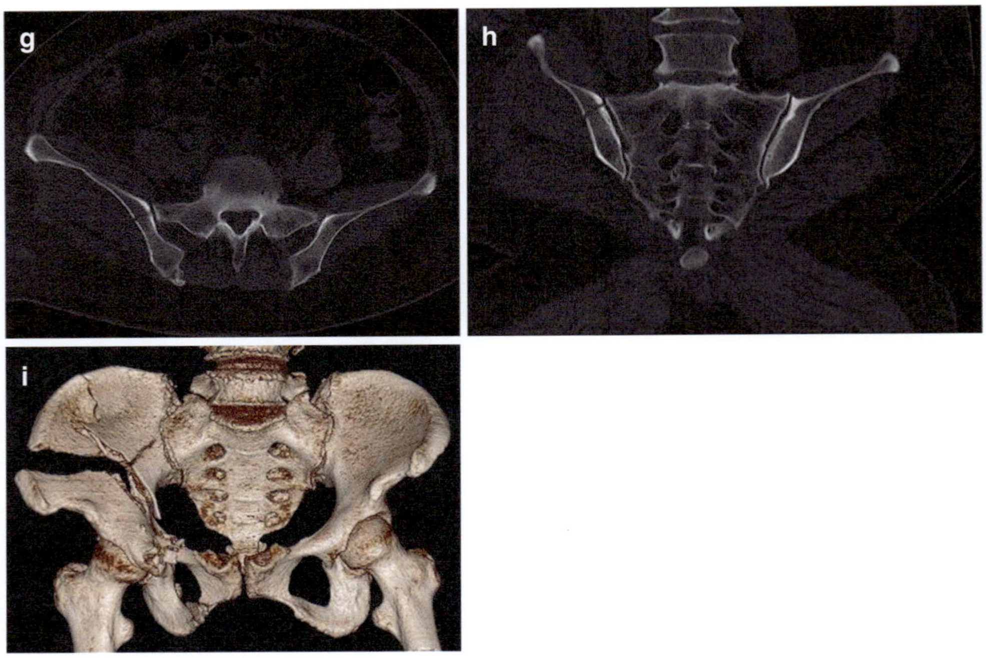

Fig. 17.13 CT scans and reconstruction (**g**–**i**) show the comminuted detachment of the right ilium and the fracture lines involve the sacroiliac joint, acetabulum, and right pubic rami

14. Comparison of X-ray and CT scans for bilaterally incomplete posterior pelvic ring injury (bilateral compression)
    14.1. X-ray (Fig. 17.14a, b)

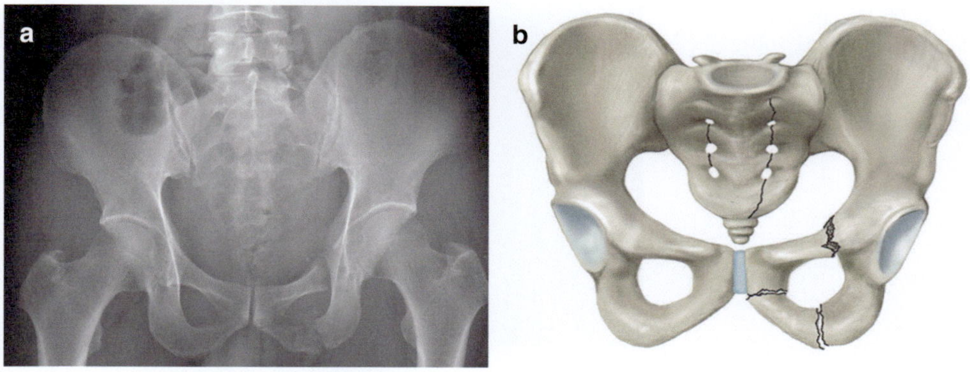

Fig. 17.14 X-ray and schematic diagram (**a**, **b**) show the comminuted sacral fragments, and the fracture lines involve the sacral foramen and left pubic rami

    14.2. CT scan (Fig. 17.14c–e)

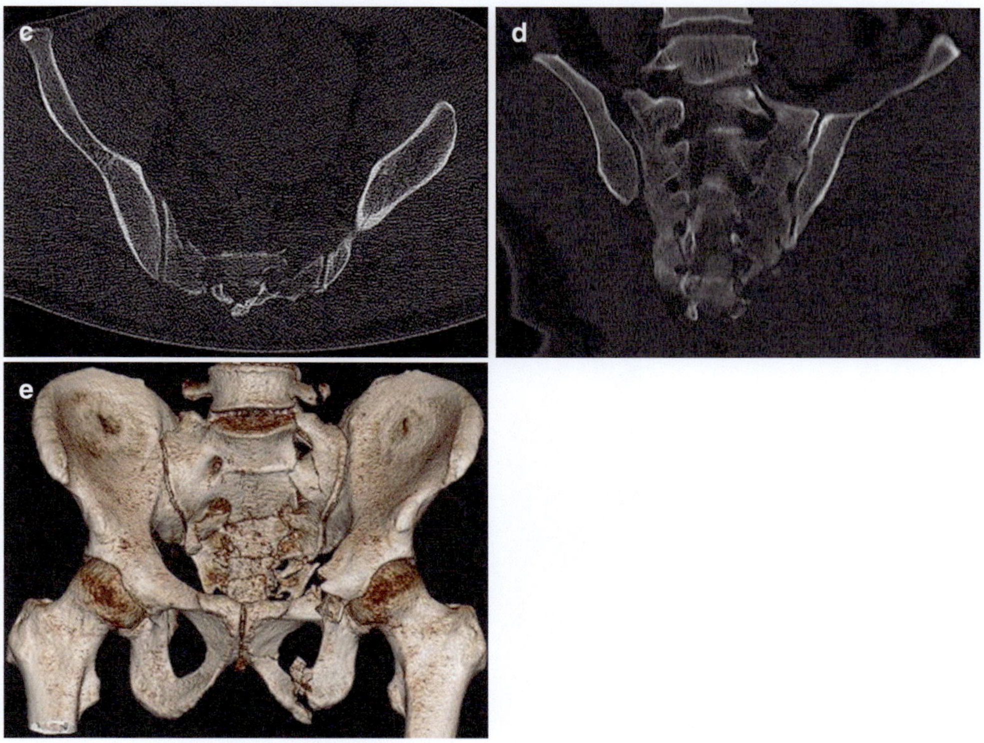

Fig. 17.14 CT scans and reconstruction (**c**–**e**) show the compression fragments of sacrum and left pubic rami. The fracture lines involve the left S1-5, right S3-5, and left superior and inferior rami

15. Comparison of X-ray and CT scans for bilaterally incomplete posterior pelvic ring injury (left compression and right open book)
    15.1. X-ray (Fig. 17.15a, b)

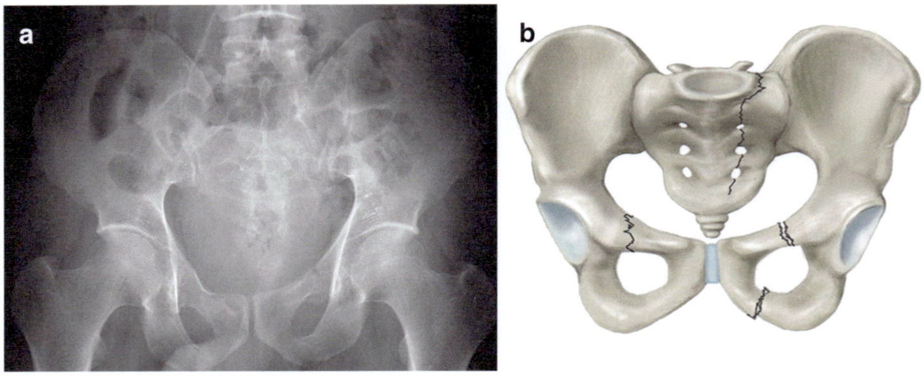

Fig. 17.15 X-ray and schematic diagram (**a**, **b**) show fracture lines involve the left pubic rami and sacrum and the broadening of the left sacroiliac joint

    15.2. CT scan (Fig. 17.15c–e)

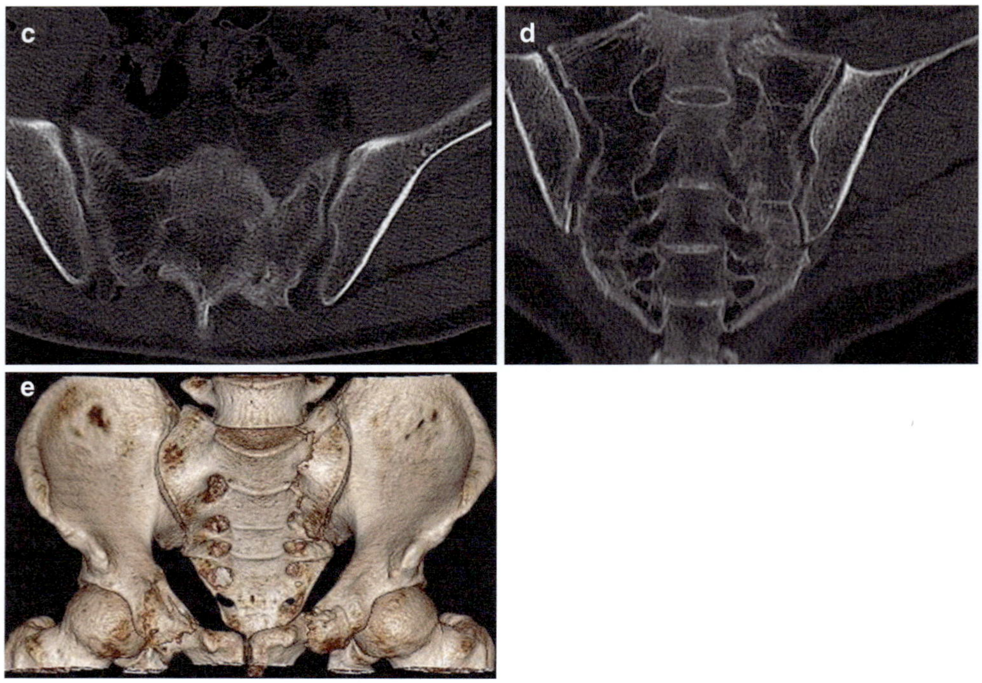

Fig. 17.15 CT scans and reconstruction (**c**–**e**) show the broadening of the right sacroiliac joint, and comminuted fractures involve the sacral foramen of the left S1-S3 and bilateral pubic rami

16. Comparison of X-ray and CT scans for unilateral complete posterior ring injury involving ilium
    16.1. X-ray (Fig. 17.16a–f)

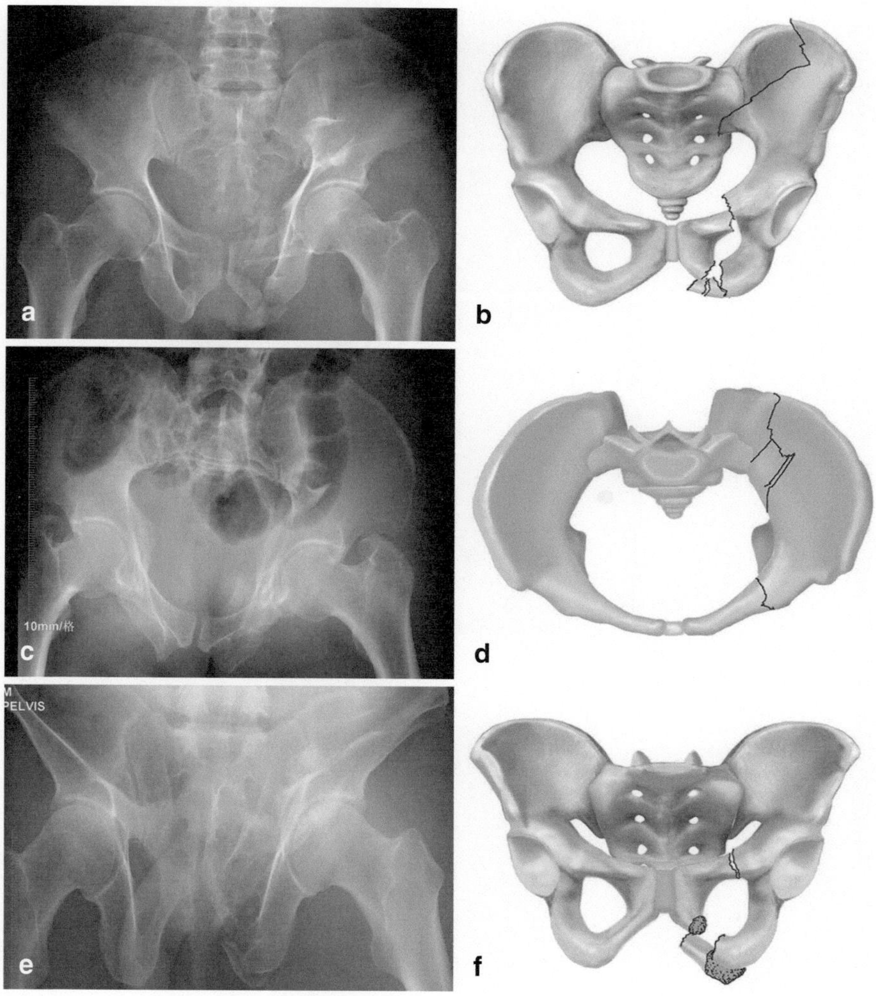

Fig. 17.16 X-ray and schematic diagram (**a**–**f**) show the displaced comminuted fragments in the left ilium and pubic rami, and the fracture lines involve the sacroiliac joint

16.2. CT scan (Fig. 17.16g–i)

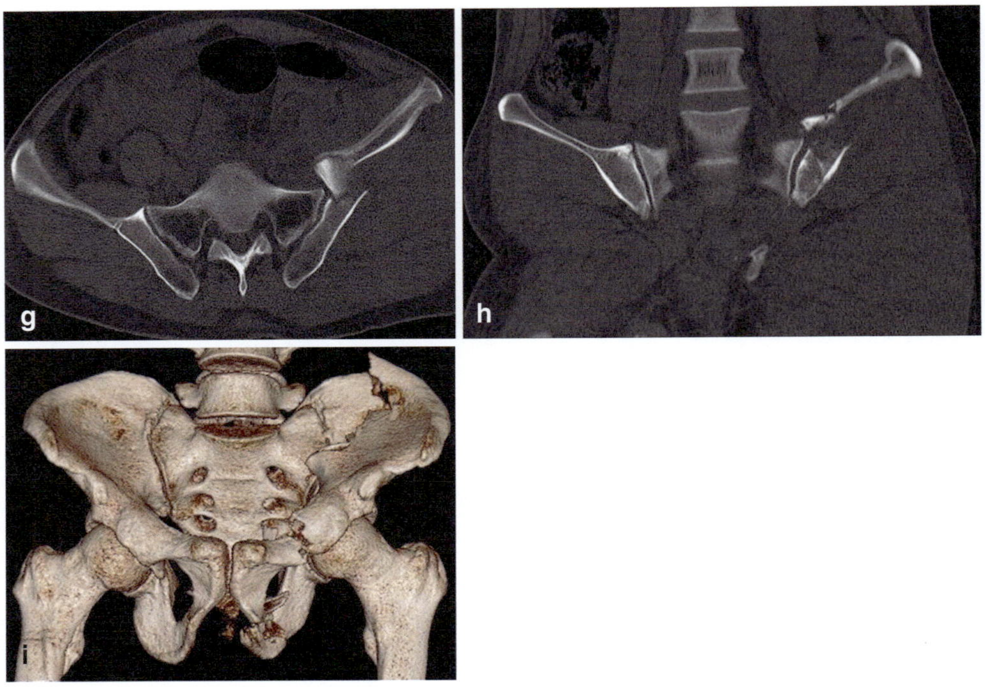

Fig. 17.16 CT scans and reconstruction (**g–i**) show there are displaced fractures in the left ilium and pubic rami. Fracture line involves the sacroiliac joint

17. Comparison of X-ray and CT scans of unilateral complete posterior pelvic ring injury involving sacroiliac joint dislocation

    17.1. X-ray (Fig. 17.17a–f)

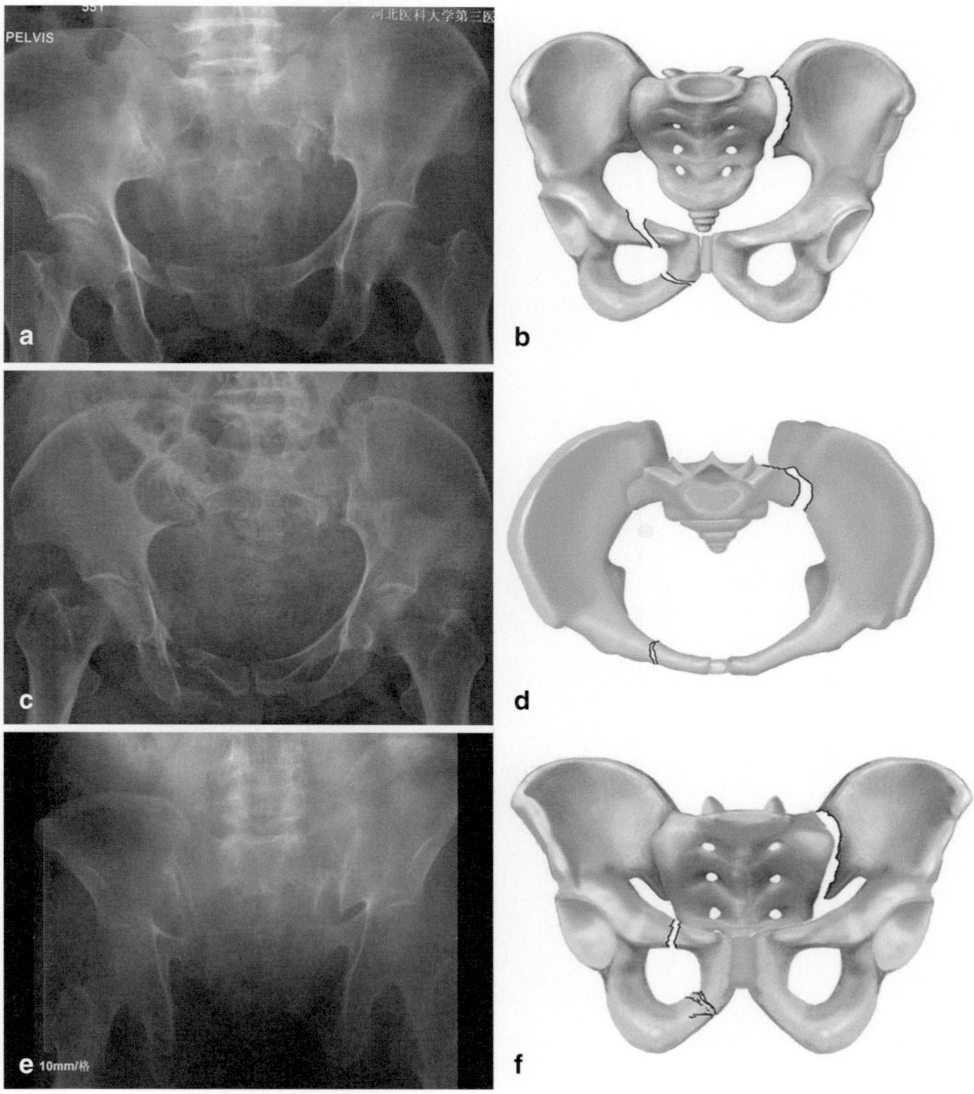

Fig. 17.17 X-rays and schematic diagrams (**a–f**) show the dislocation of the sacroiliac joint, comminuted fractures of the sacrum, proximally displaced ilium, and fractures of the right pubic rami

    17.2. CT scan (Fig. 17.17g, h)

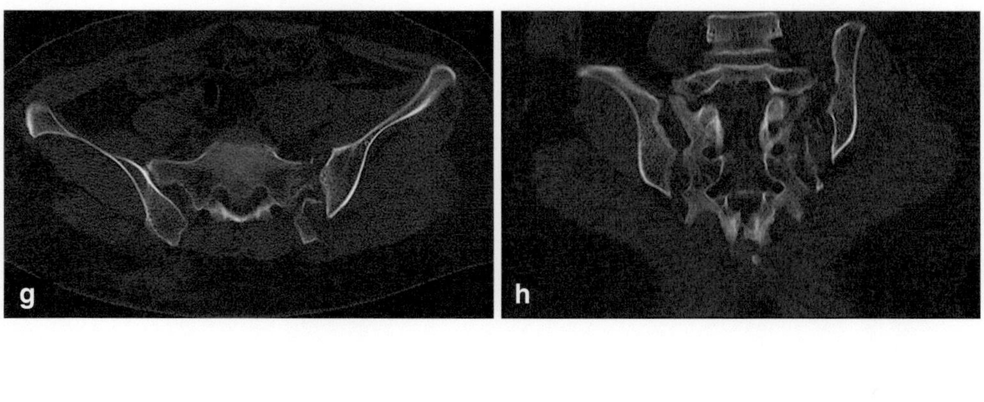

Fig. 17.17 CT cross (**g**) and coronal (**h**) sections show the dislocation of the left sacroiliac joint, the comminuted fragments of the left sacrum, and lateral-proximally displaced left ilium

18. Comparison of X-ray and CT scans of unilateral completely posterior pelvic ring injury involving sacrum
    18.1. X-ray (Fig. 17.18a–f)

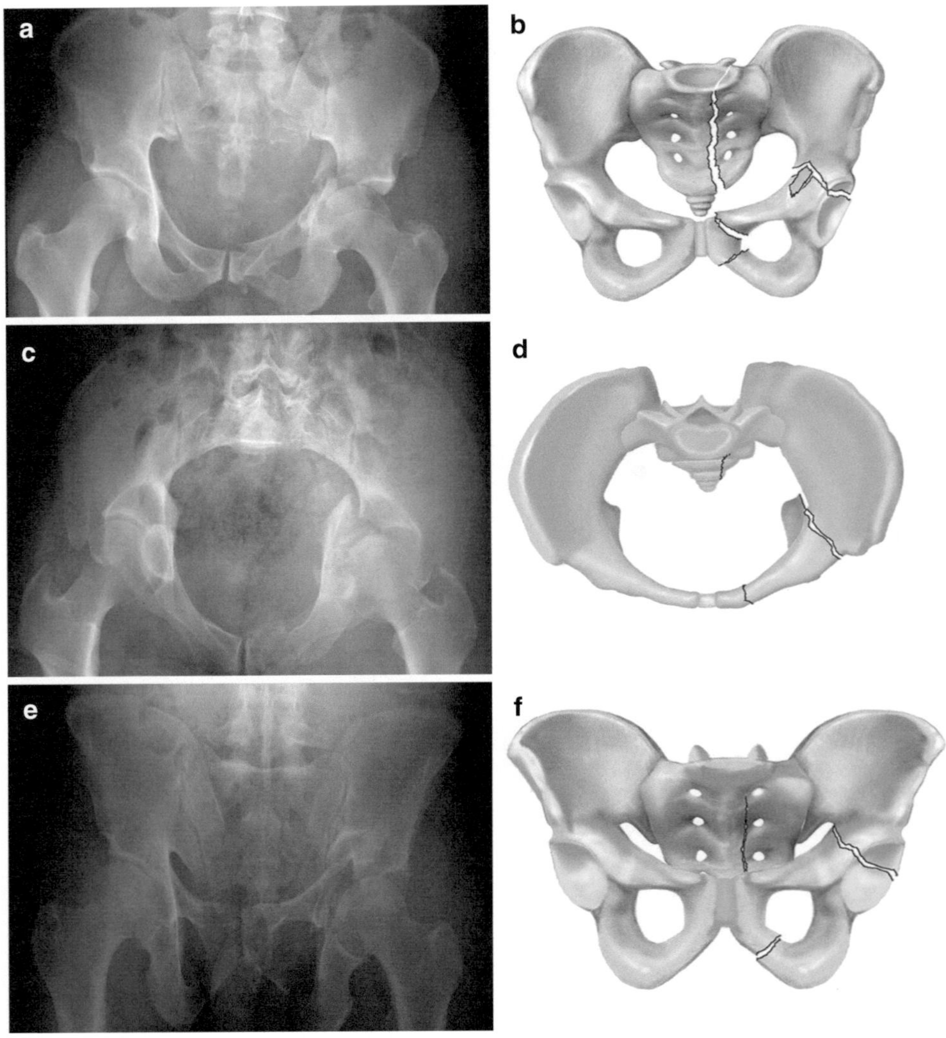

Fig. 17.18 X-ray and schematic diagram (**a**–**f**) show left sacral fractures involving the sacral foramen, displaced acetabular fractures, and displaced fragments of the left pubic rami

18.2. CT scan (Fig. 17.18g–i)

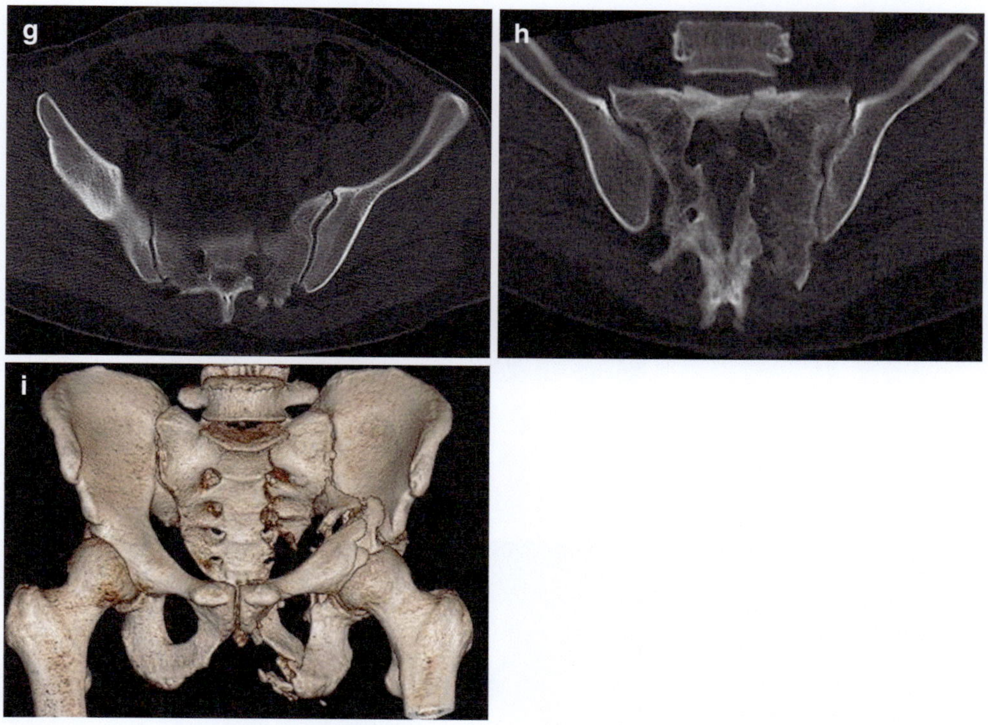

Fig. 17.18 CT scans and reconstruction (**g–i**) show a longitudinal fracture line involving sacral foramen, left acetabulum, and left pubic rami

19. Comparison of X-ray and CT scans of unilateral complete and contralateral incomplete posterior ring injury.
    19.1. X-ray (Fig. 17.19a, b)

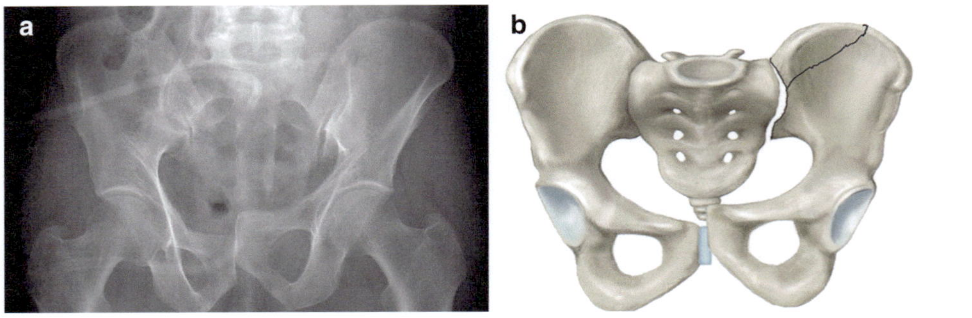

Fig. 17.19 X-ray and schematic diagram (**a**, **b**) show the disruption of the symphysis pubis, the broadening of the left sacroiliac joint and the morphological irregularity of the left ilium

    19.2. CT scan (Fig. 17.19c, d)

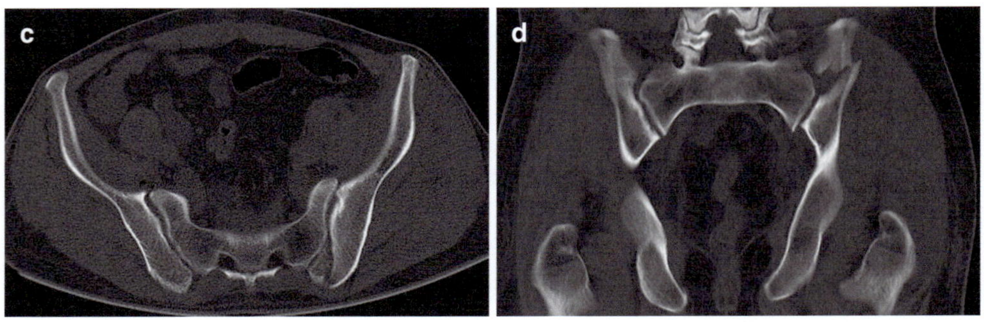

Fig. 17.19 CT cross section and coronal sections (**c**, **d**) show the dislocation of the left sacroiliac joint and the iliac fragments, those fracture line involves the sacroiliac joint. There is tissue swelling in the local area with gas density shadow

20. Comparison of X-ray and CT scans of unilateral complete and contralateral incomplete injury in the posterior ring injury.
    20.1. X-ray (Fig. 17.20a, b)

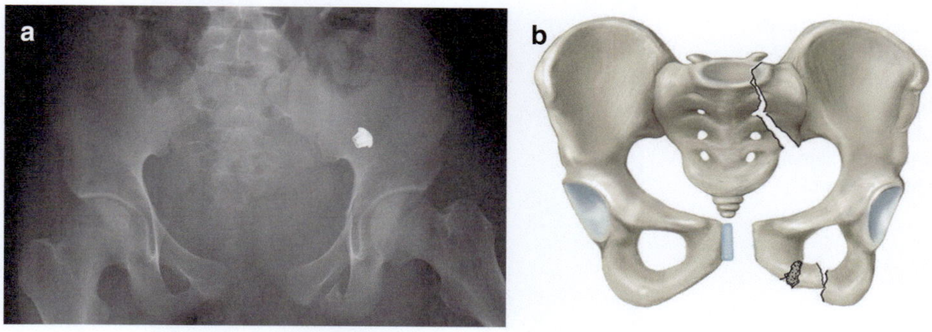

Fig. 17.20 X-ray and schematic diagram (**a**, **b**) show disruption of pubic symphysis, fractures of the left pubic rami, and morphological irregularity of sacrum

    20.2. CT scan (Fig. 17.20c–e)

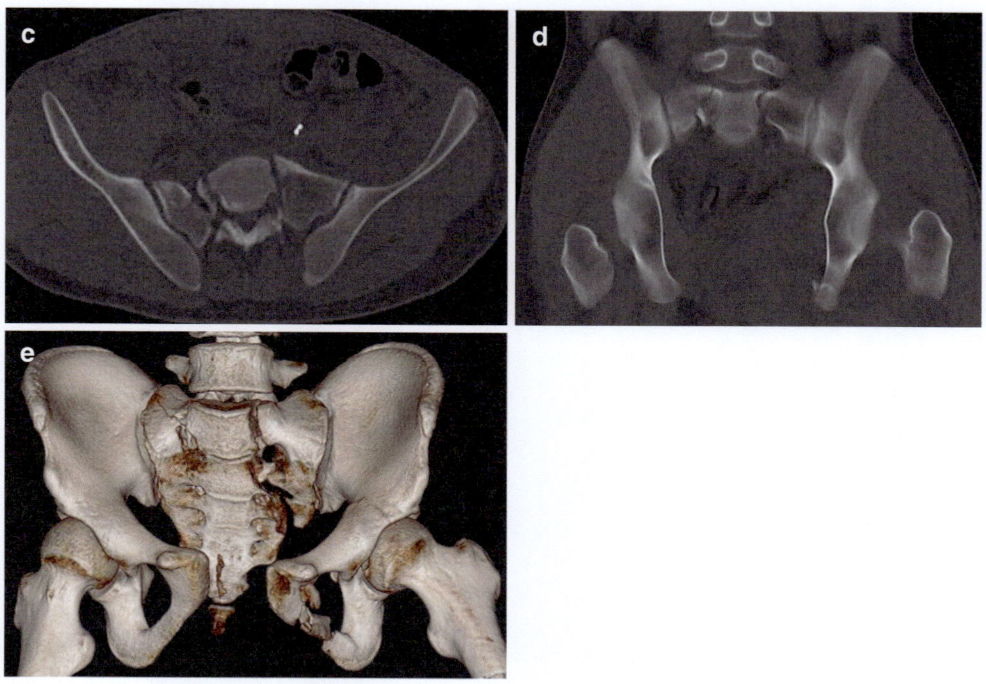

Fig. 17.20 CT scans and reconstruction (**c**–**e**) show longitudinal fracture lines of bilateral sacral foramen, distinct dislocation of pubic symphysis, and displaced fragments of the left pubic rami

21. Comparison of X-ray and CT scans unilateral completely posterior pelvic ring injury involving sacroiliac joint
    21.1. X-ray (Fig. 17.21a–d)

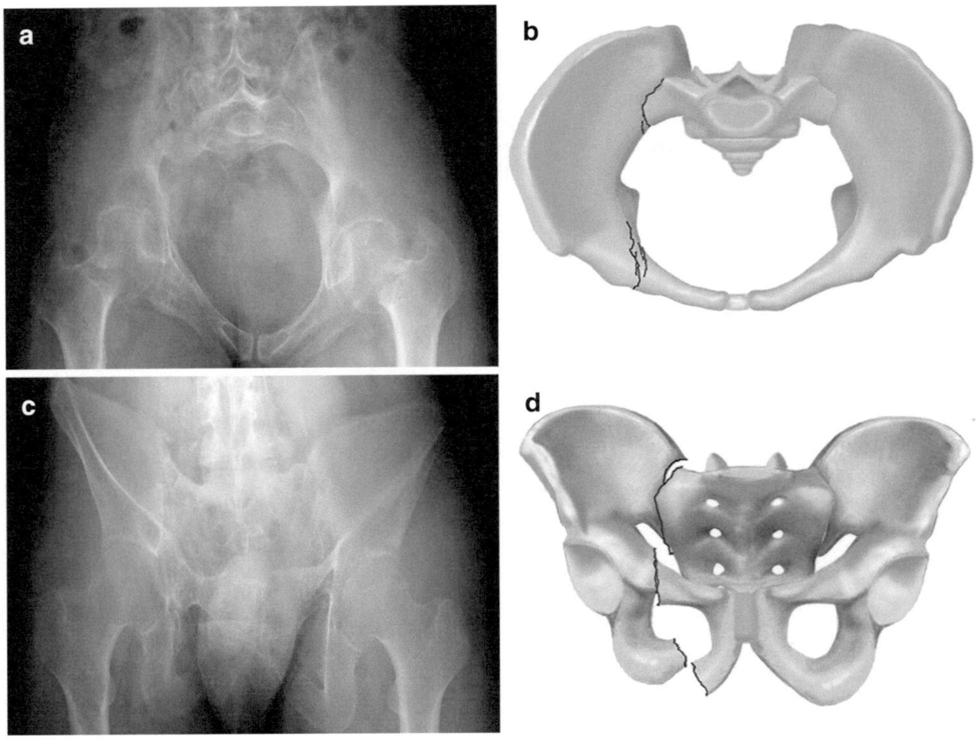

Fig. 17.21 X-ray and schematic diagram (**a**–**d**) show the dislocation of the right sacroiliac joint, morphological irregularity of the right ilium and sacrum, and displaced fragments of the right pubic rami

21.2. CT scan (Fig. 17.21e–g)

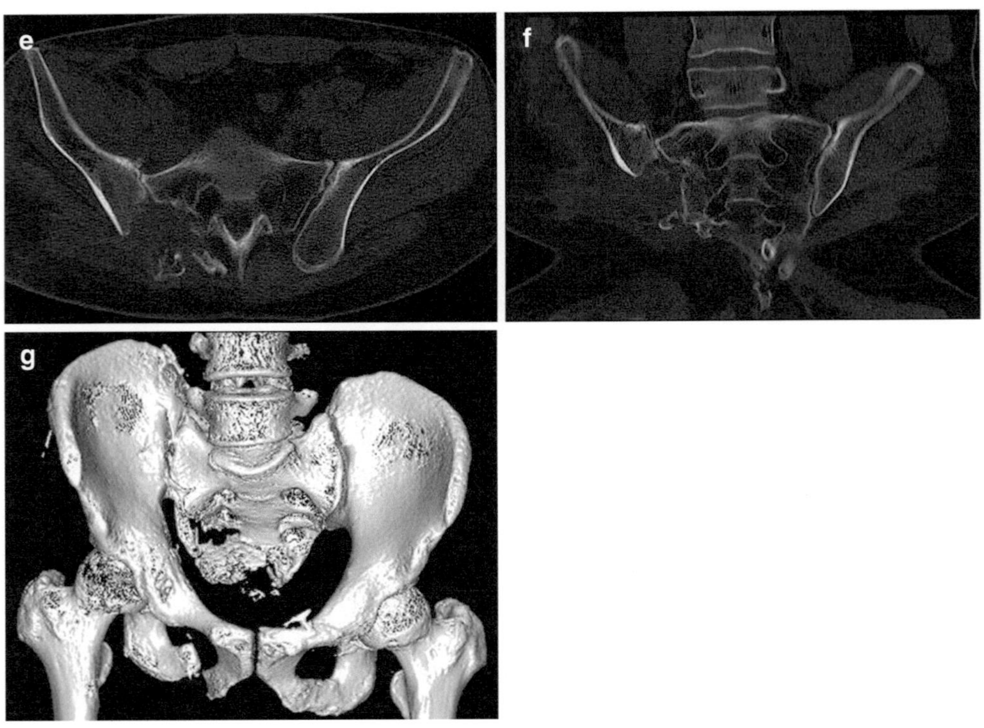

Fig. 17.21 CT scans and reconstruction (**e**–**g**) show the separated dislocation of sacroiliac joint, comminuted fragments in right sacral foramen and ilium, and displaced fractures of right pubic rami

22. Comparison of X-ray and CT scans for bilateral complete posterior ring injury
    22.1. X-ray (Fig. 17.22a–f)

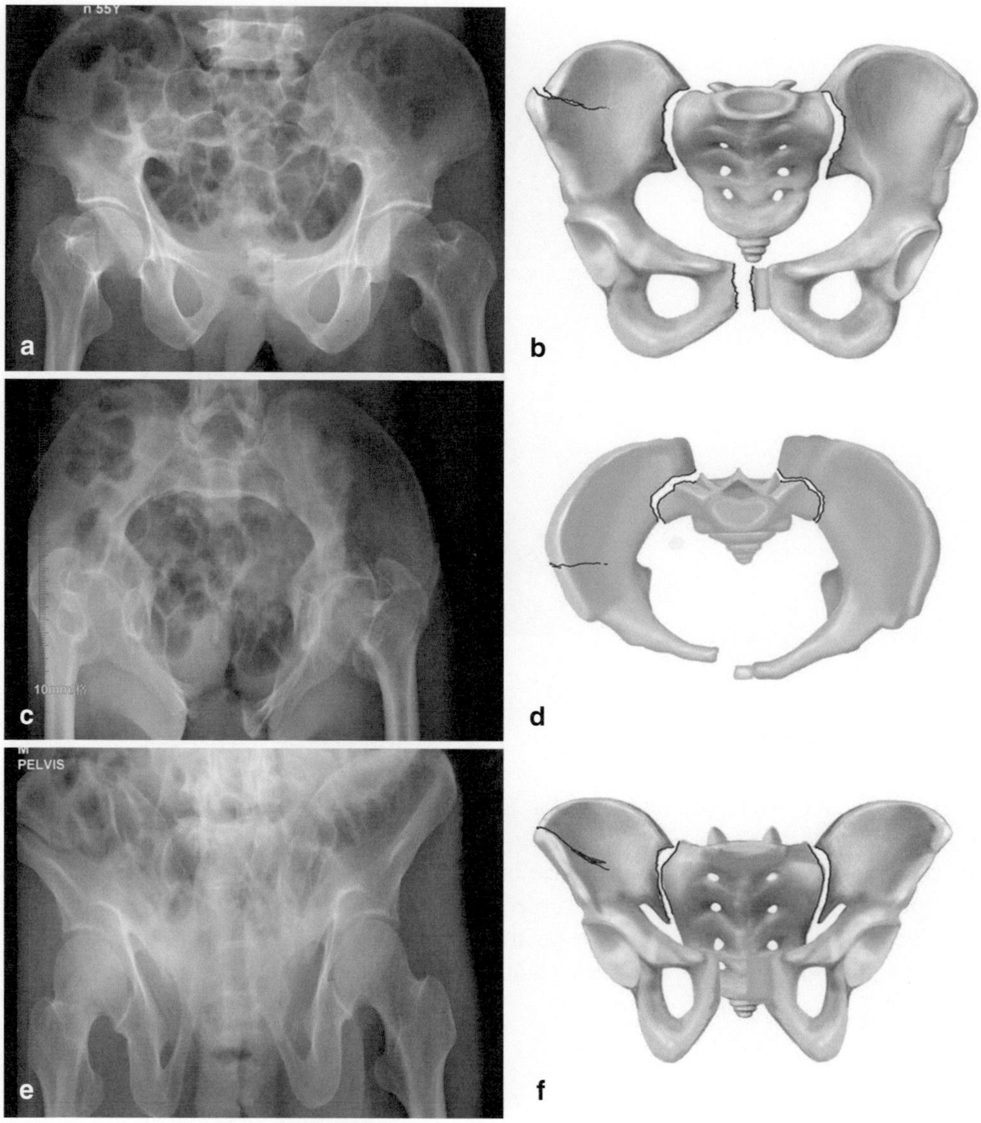

Fig. 17.22 X-ray and schematic diagram (**a**–**f**) show the disruption of pubic symphysis, bilateral sacroiliac joints, and fracture of the right ilium

22.2. CT scan (Fig. 17.22g–i)

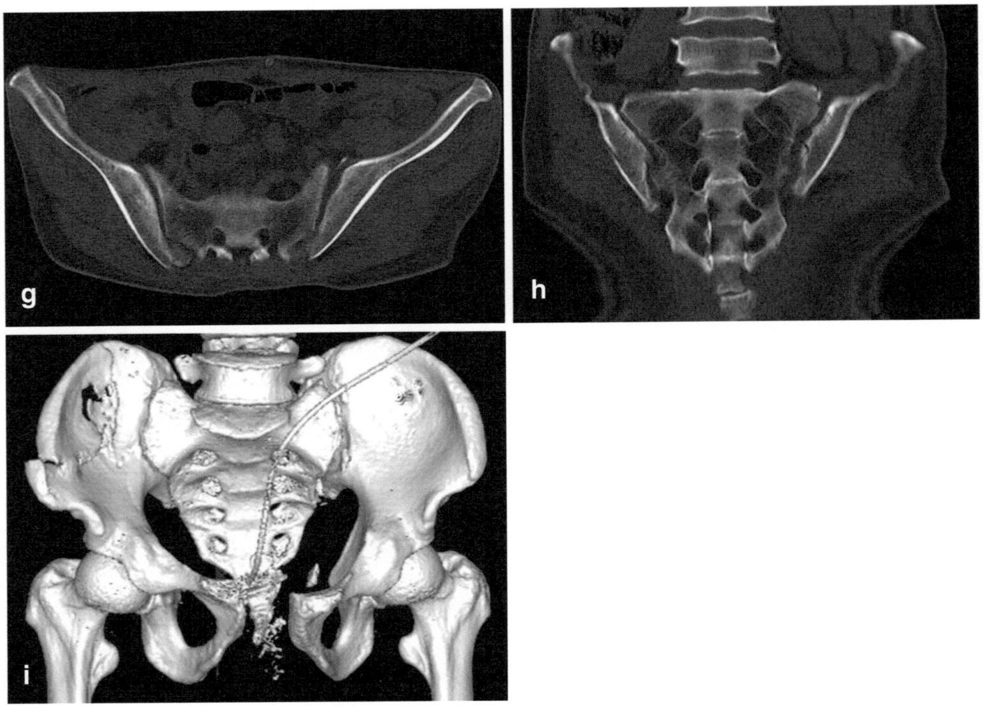

Fig. 17.22 CT scans and reconstruction (**g–i**) show separated dislocation of the bilateral sacroiliac joints, displaced fractures of the right ilium, and dislocation of the pubic symphysis

17.4 Summary

1. The pelvis is composed by anterior and posterior rings, whose stability is the key basis of the pelvic injury classification.
2. There are complex anatomic structures in the pelvis. The fracture traits in this area could be totally displayed by single projection. Inlet, outlet, and Judet projections are always performed to diagnose the fractures through different views, which could be applied in the intraoperative assessment of the positioning and reduction.
3. The entire pelvis and fine structures could be exposed through CT scans and three-dimensional reconstruction.

18 Axial Bone Fracture

Xin Xing and Yingze Zhang

18.1 Pathological Spine Fractures

18.1.1 Osteoporotic Fracture

18.1.1.1 Identification of Injury Mechanism

Bone loss due to senile or postmenopausal osteoporosis without definite trauma or minor trauma can result in fractures. Therefore, when elderly patients complain of lower back pain, even if there is no definite history of trauma, X-ray and other scans should be carried out to confirm the diagnosis.

18.1.1.2 Identification of Symptoms and Signs

The most obvious manifestations of osteoporotic fractures are pain, limited activity. A difficulty can be observed in clinical examination to obtain a definite diagnosis due to lack of specificity.

18.1.1.3 Imaging Differential Diagnosis

In senile osteoporosis with fractures, X-rays and CT show a general reduction in bone density in the spine. Typical manifestations are multiple vertebral body with double concave deformation. QCT can quantitatively analyze vertebral osteoporosis. MRI does not directly show bone density; however, vertebral osteoporosis can be predicted by the proportion of fat in vertebral bone; in addition, old and fresh compression fractures can be identified in many double-concaved deformed vertebral bodies.

X. Xing · Y. Zhang (✉)
Department of Orthopaedics, The Third Hospital of Hebei Medical University, Shijiazhuang, Hebei, China

Y. Zhang (ed.), *Differential Diagnosis of Fracture*, https://doi.org/10.1007/978-981-13-8339-7_18

1. Identification of old and fresh thoracic fractures with multiple thoracic body flattening due to osteoporosis
   1.1. X-ray plain film (Fig.18.1a–d)

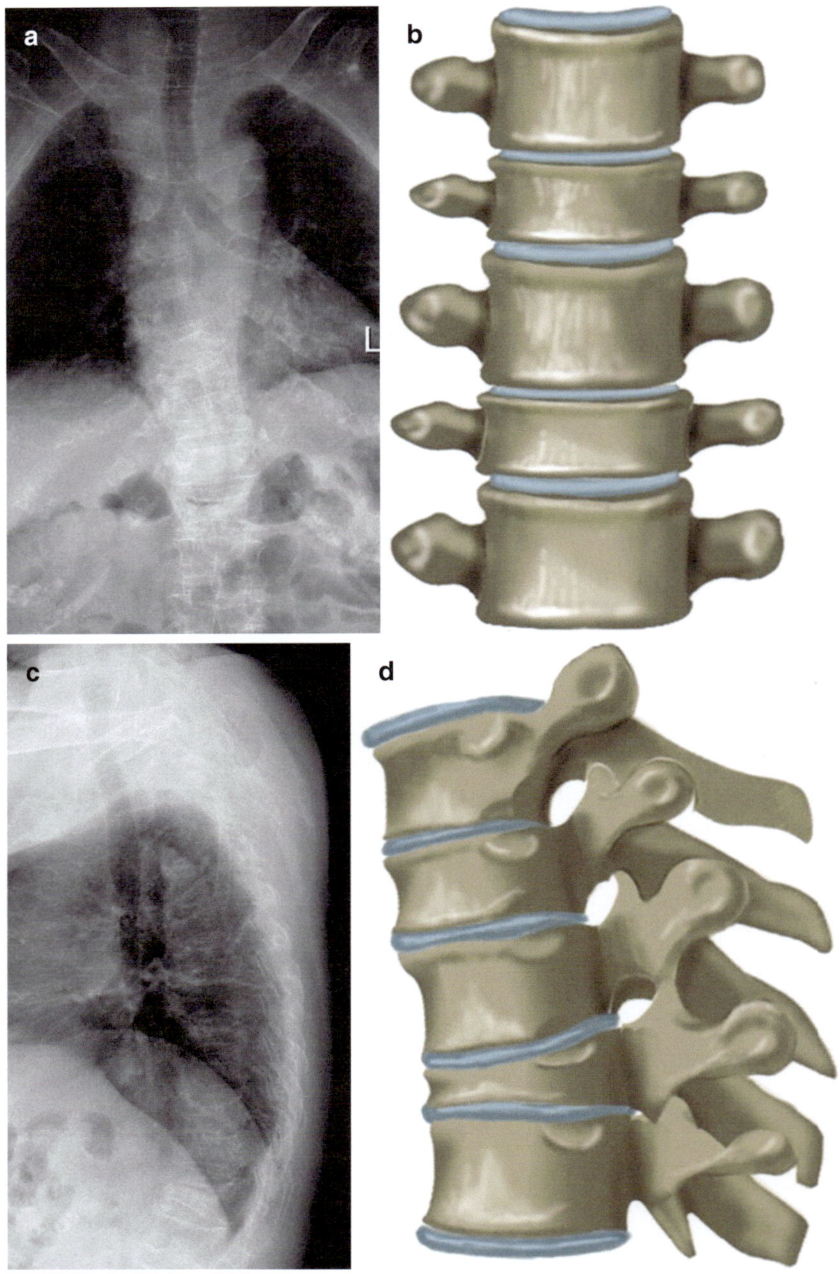

Fig. 18.1 The X-ray plain film (**a**, **c**) shows that the bone density of thoracic vertebra decreased and part of vertebral body which became flat, schematic diagram (**b**, **d**)

1.2. CT scan (Fig.18.1e)

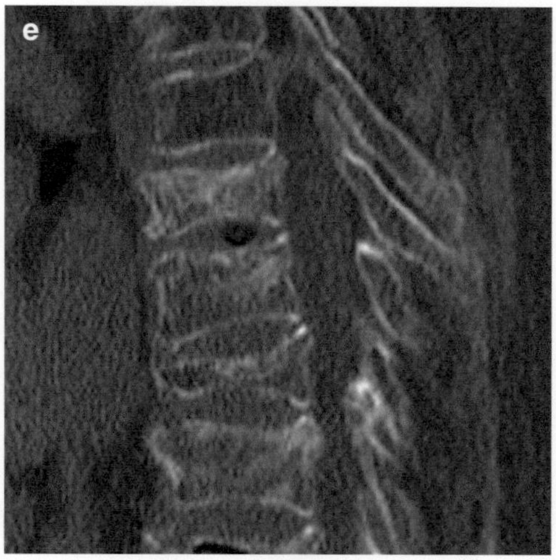

Fig. 18.1 CT sagittal plane reconstruction (**e**) shows the osteoporosis of various thoracic vertebrae, the flattening of multiple vertebral bodies, the disordered structure of the flattened vertebral bodies, and the compression zone

1.3. MRI scan (Fig.18.1f–h)

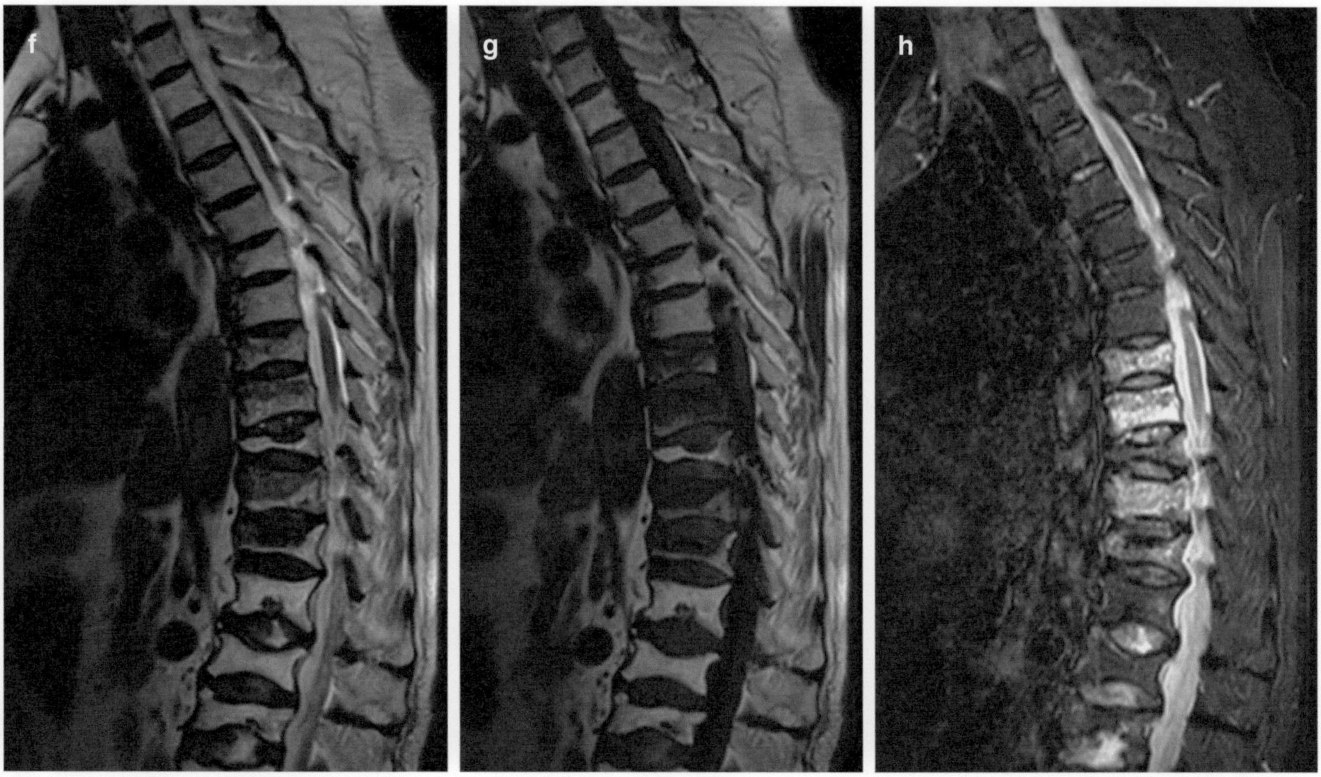

Fig. 18.1 MRI (**f**, **g**) shows that the lower thoracic and partial lumbar vertebrae were flattened, the intervertebral space was widened, and the STIR sequence (**h**) shows the high signal of the T8, T9, T11, and T12 vertebral bodies, indicating fresh compression fractures

2. Identification of old and fresh lumbar vertebrae fractures with multiple lumbar vertebral body flattening due to osteoporosis
   2.1. X-ray plain film (Fig. 18.2a–d)

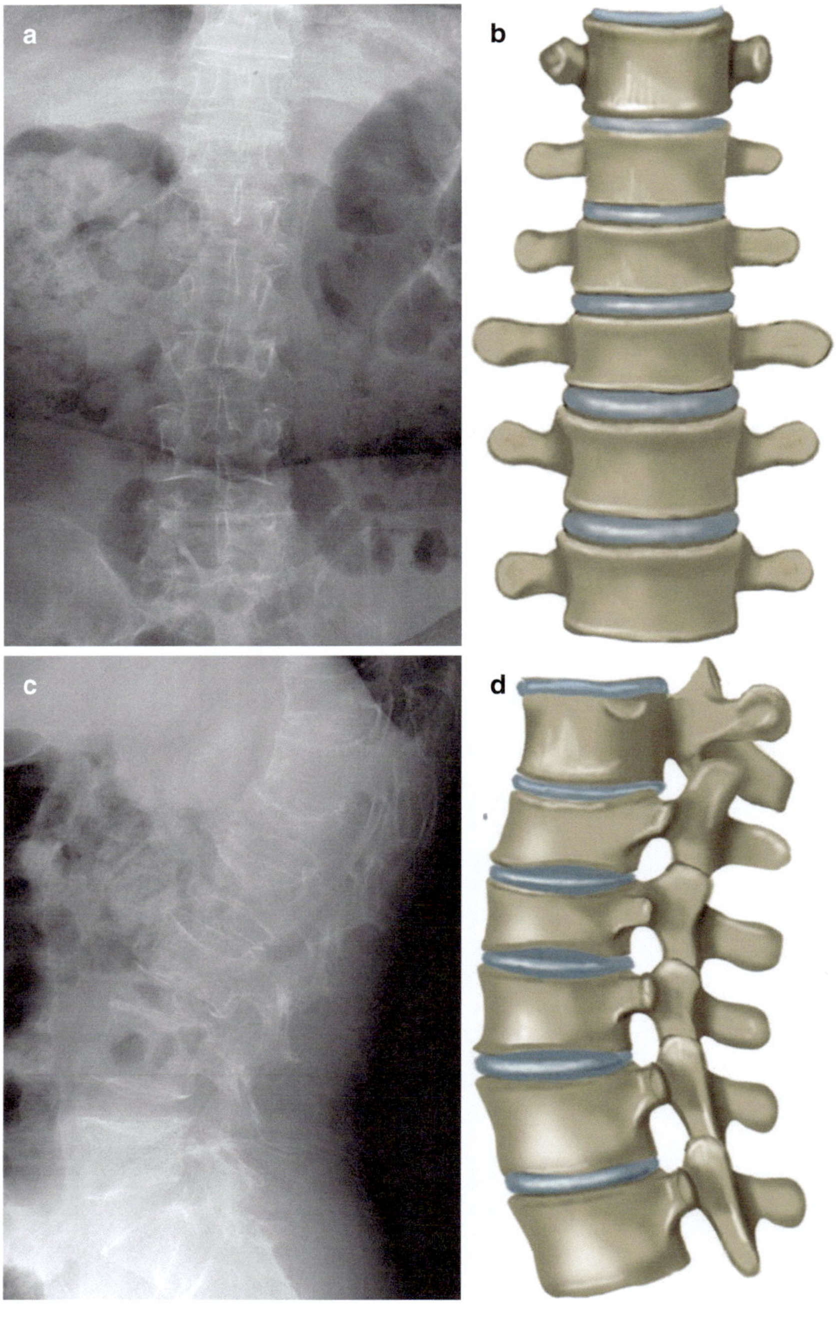

Fig. 18.2 X-ray plain film (**a**, **c**) shows the reduction of lumbar bone density and the double concave deformation of multiple vertebral bodies (**b**, **d**)

2.2. MRI scan (Fig. 18.2e, f)

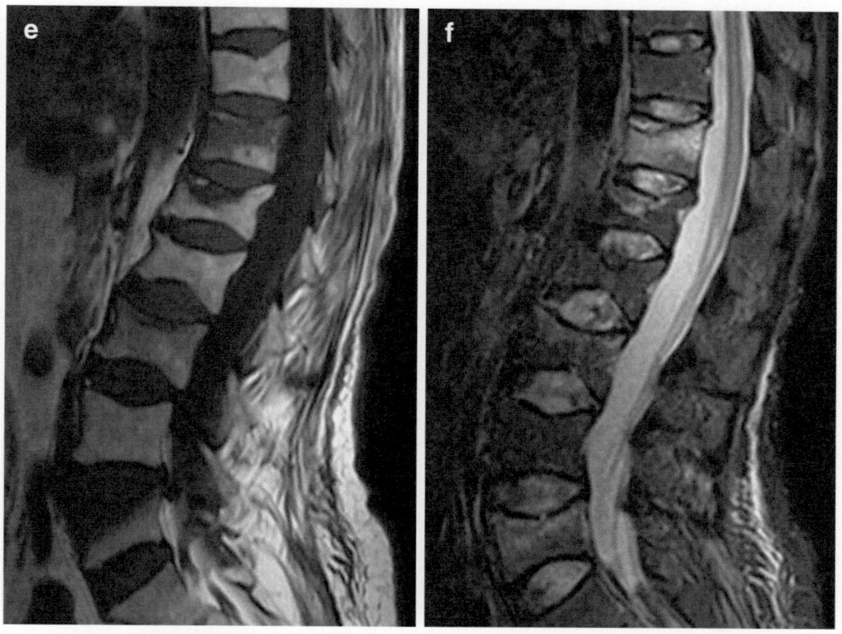

Fig. 18.2 MRI-TIWI (**e**) shows abnormal signals in T12, L1, L3, and L5; STIR sequence (**f**) shows high signal, indicating fresh fracture. T11 and L2 vertebral body T1WI (**e**) and STIR sequence (**f**) show the same signals, indicating old compression fractures

3. Identification of vertebral body flattening after lumbar multiple vertebral body reconstruction and fresh fracture
   3.1. X-ray plain film (Fig 18.3a–d)

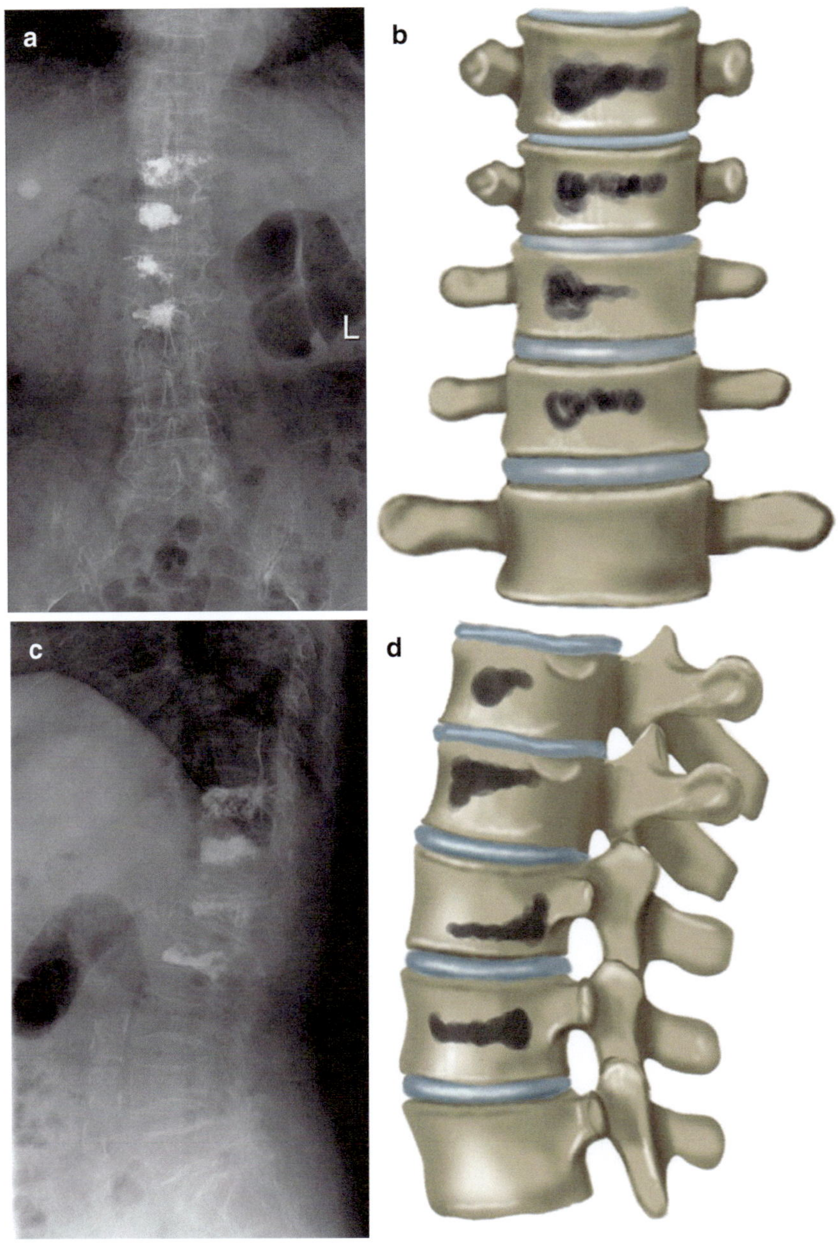

Fig. 18.3 Vertebroplasty was performed many years ago, Flat X-ray (**a**, **c**) shows the flattening of multiple vertebral bodies in the thoracolumbar spine, high-density bone cement in vertebral body, diagram (**b**, **d**)

3.2. CT scan (Fig 18.3e)

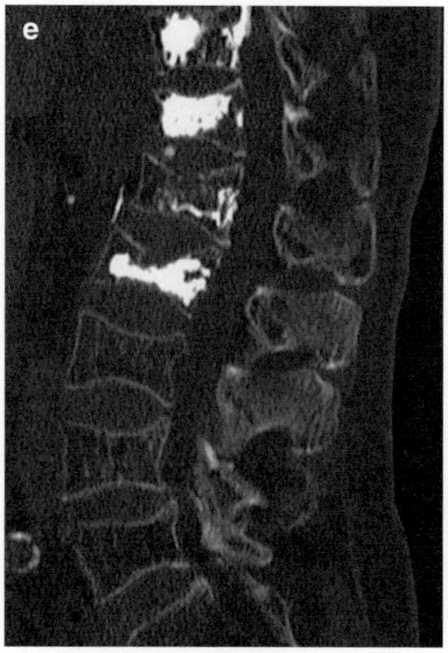

Fig. 18.3 CT sagittal reconstruction (**e**) shows a reduction in bone density in the thoracolumbar vertebral body, sparsity of trabecular bone, bone cement shadow can be seen in T11-L2 vertebrae

3.3. MRI scan (Fig 18.3f–h)

Fig. 18.3 MRI sagittal T1WI T2WI and STIR sequences (**f–h**) show L3 and L4 vertebral laminar high signal shadows; this suggests a fresh compression fracture

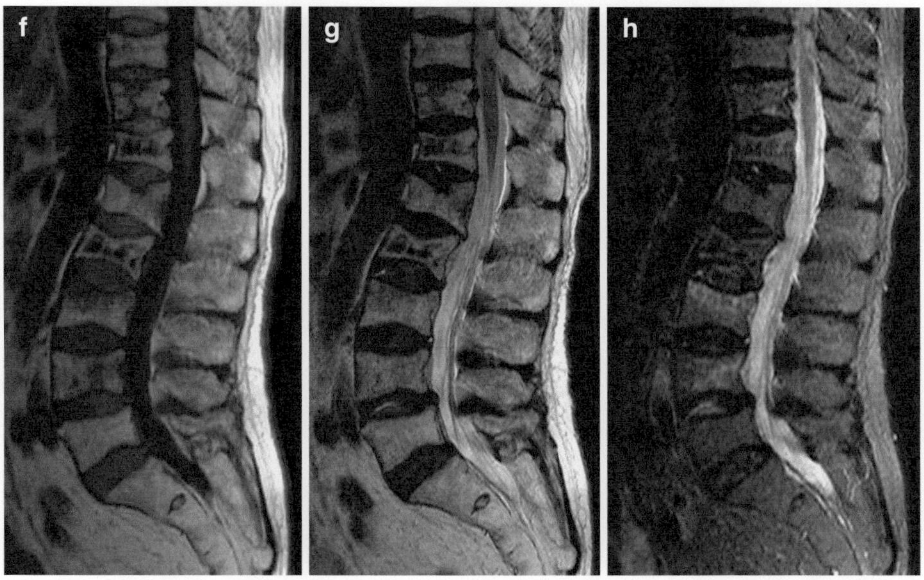

4. Identification of vertebral body flattening after lumbar multiple vertebral body reconstruction and vertebral fractures
    4.1. X-ray plain film (Fig 18.4a, b)

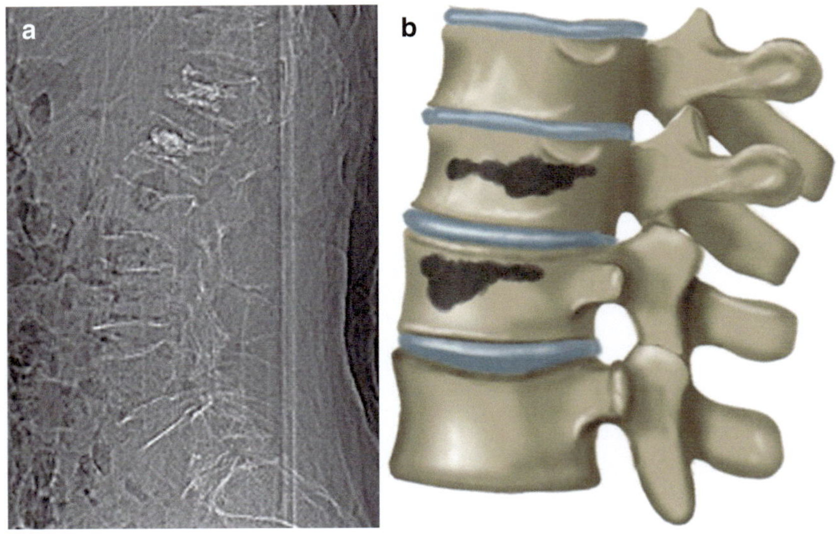

Fig. 18.4 X-ray (**a**) shows that many vertebral wedge changes occur after vertebroplasty, diagram (**b**)

    4.2. CT scan (Fig 18.4c, d)

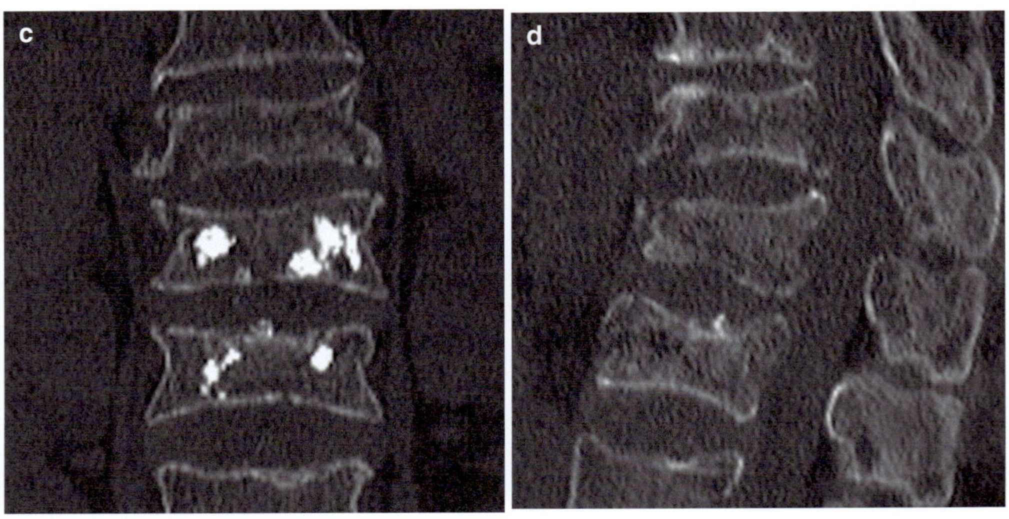

Fig. 18.4 CT reconstruction (**c**, **d**) shows the flattening of T11- L1 vertebral bodies; the vertebral body density decreases and breaks

4.3. MRI scan (Fig 18.4e–g)

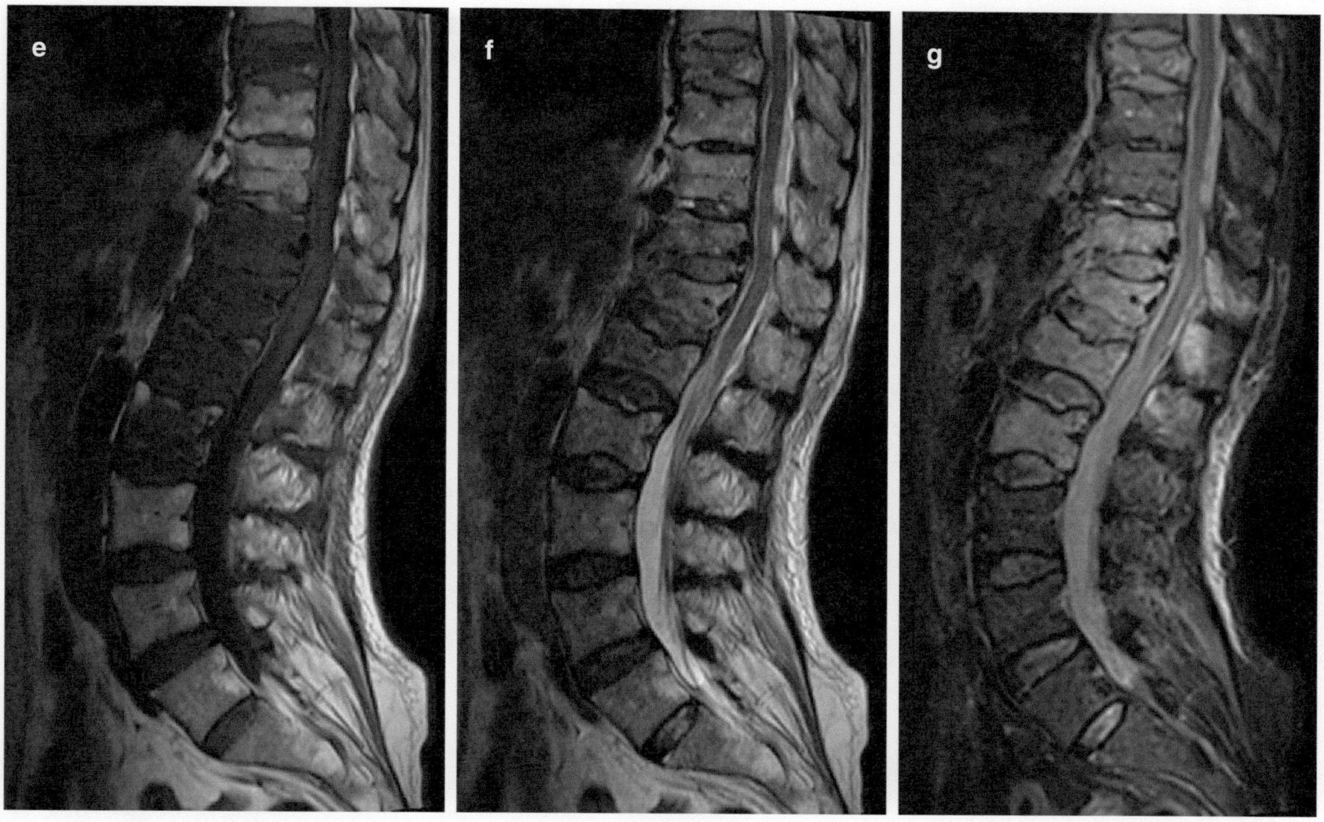

Fig. 18.4 MRI (**e–g**) shows abnormal signal of T8, T11- L2 vertebral body, multiple compression fractures

18.1.2 Spinal Tumors or Inflammatory Fractures

18.1.2.1 Identification of Injury Mechanism

Bone damage due to tumor, inflammation, and so on, without definite trauma or minor trauma, can result in fractures. When a patient complains of low back pain, an X-ray or other scan should be performed to confirm the diagnosis, even if the history of trauma is not clearly defined.

18.1.2.2 Identification of Symptoms and Signs

The most common manifestation after a tumor or inflammatory fracture is pain, limited activity, lack of specificity, and difficulty in definite diagnosis.

18.1.2.3 Imaging Differential Diagnosis

A pathological fracture of the spine causes the vertebral body to become flat. The edges of vertebral body are generally full and round. CT scan shows vertebral body or adnexal bone destruction, and the appearance of primary lesions can be seen. Paravertebral soft tissue masses are often seen in tumors, while paravertebral abscess is often seen in tuberculosis. Pathological fractures caused by metastases: Multiple damage, compression vertebral body, margin full swelling, the attachment often has the bone destruction, and the vertebral side common soft tissue tumor. Pathological fracture caused by tuberculosis present with: Adjacent vertebral body damages compression; the intervertebral disc is often involved; paravertebral abscess is common; and one side of the vertebral pedicle structure disappeared or blurred when the vertebral pedicle was involved on the positive position of the X-ray. The X-ray often cannot determine the nature of the lesion, but MRI scans play an important role in the identification of pathological compression and common compression fractures.

5. Identification of thoracic tuberculosis and vertebral body fracture
   5.1. X-ray plain film (Fig. 18.5a, b)

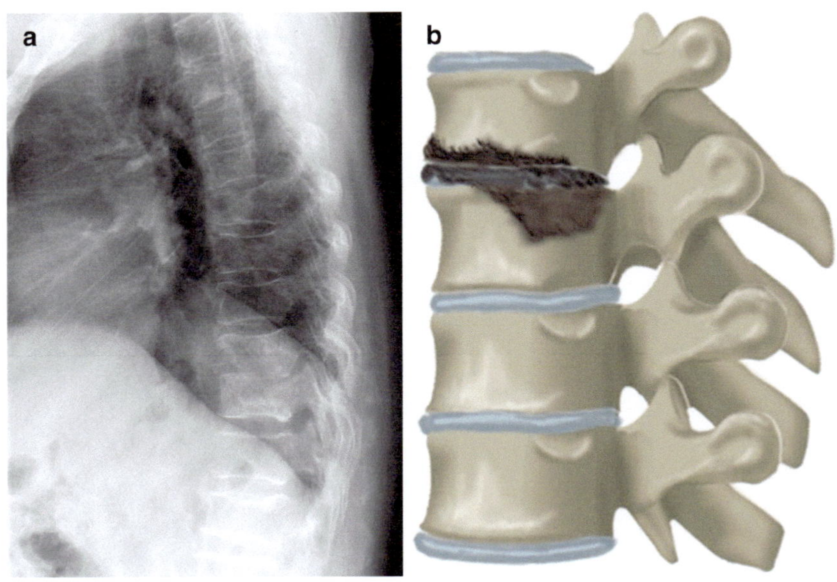

Fig. 18.5 The lateral position of the X-ray (**a**) shows that the T10 vertebral body was flat, and the T10-11 intervertebral space was not clear, diagram (**b**)

5.2. CT scan (Fig. 18.5c, d)

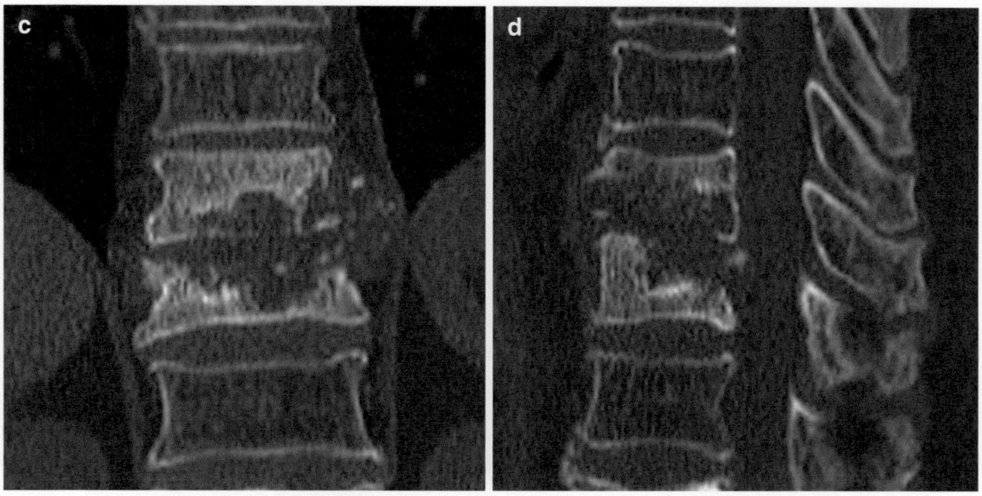

Fig. 18.5 CT reconstruction (**c**, **d**) shows bone destruction of the T10-11 vertebral body, thickening of the perivertebral soft tissue, and sandy dead bone shadow in the damaged area and the perivertebral tissue

5.3. MRI scan (Fig. 18.5e–g)

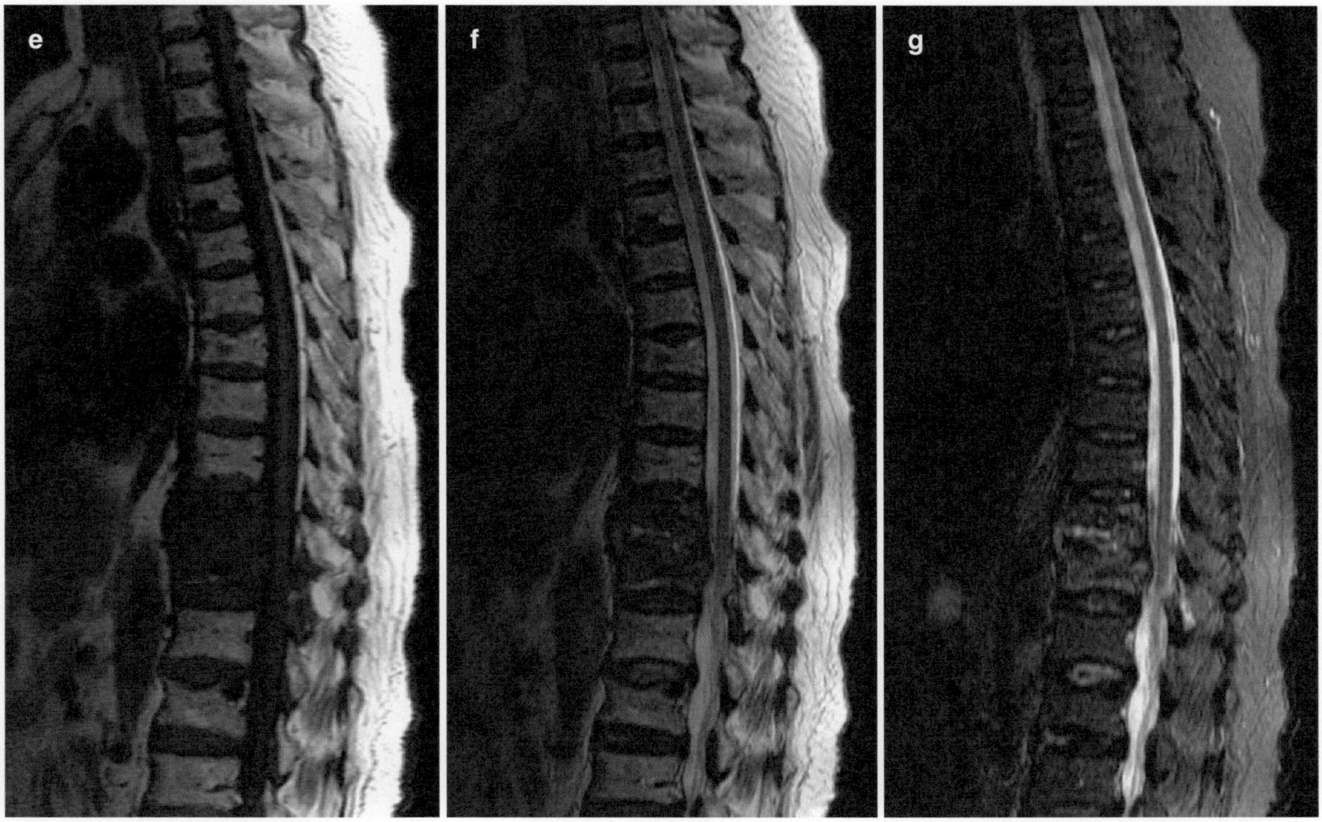

Fig. 18.5 MRI (**e**–**g**) shows abnormal signal of T10-11 vertebral body and thickening of soft tissue before vertebral body

6. Identification of cervical metastatic tumor flattening and vertebral body fracture
   6.1. X-ray plain film (Fig. 18.6a, b)

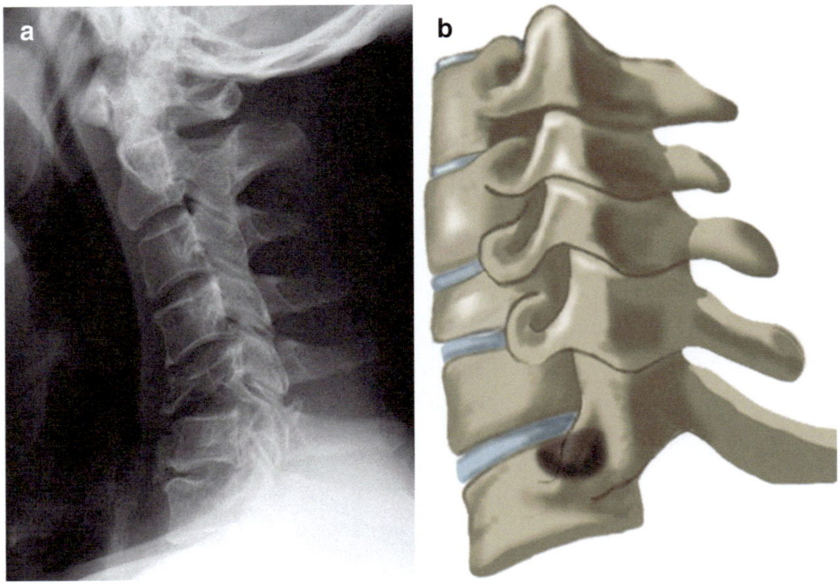

Fig. 18.6 Lung cancer cervical metastases tumor, X-ray lateral slice (**a**) shows C5 vertebral body flattening, cervical curvature reversed, diagram (**b**)

   6.2. CT scan (Fig. 18.6c, d)

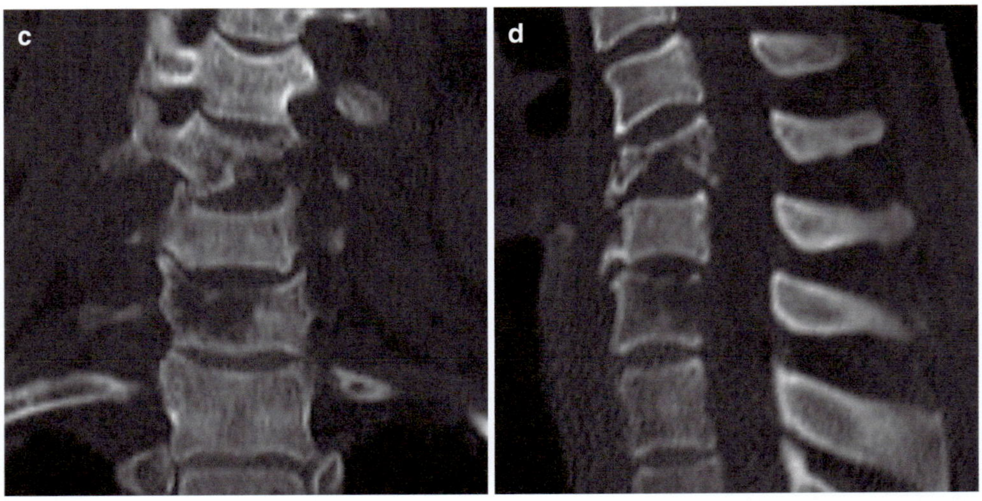

Fig. 18.6 CT coronal plane (**c**) and sagittal plane (**d**) reconstruction shows osteolytic destruction of C5, C7, and sagittal plane reconstruction shows wedge-shaped degeneration of C5

6.3. MRI scan (Fig. 18.6e–g)

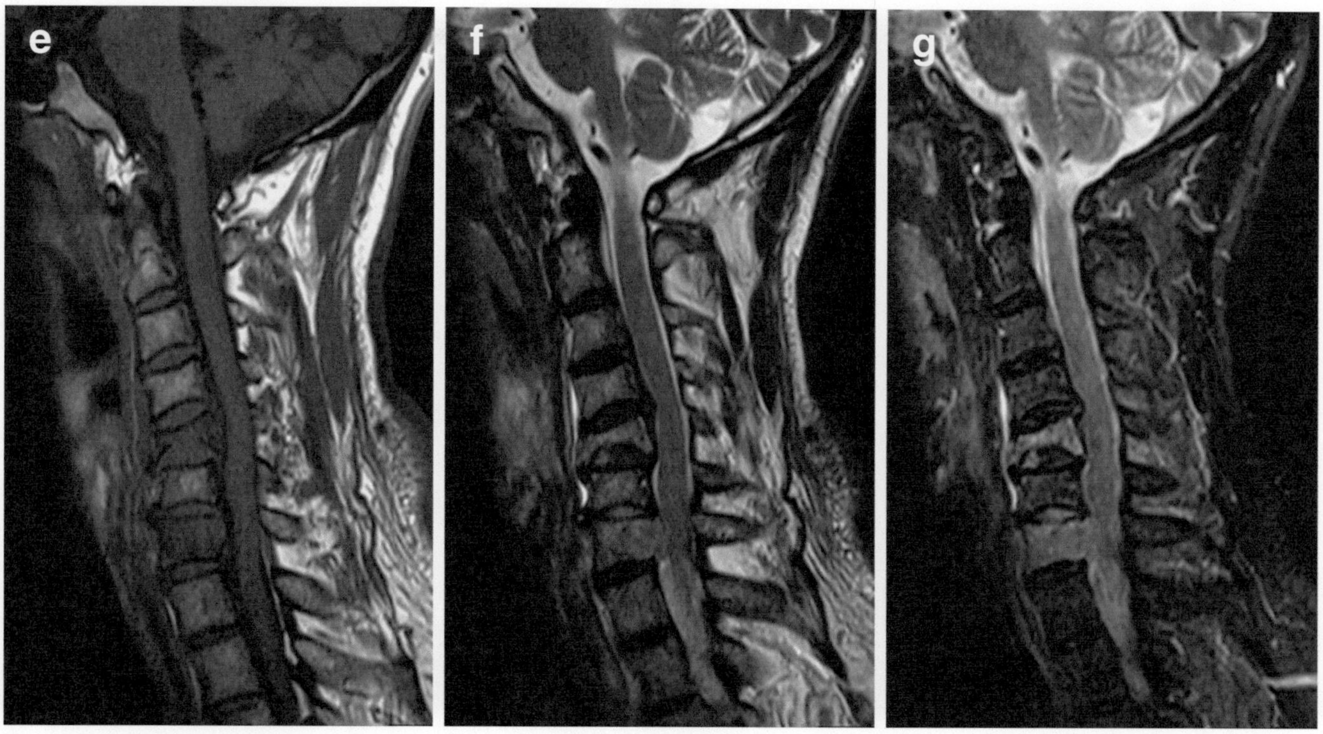

Fig. 18.6 MRI shows the flattening of the fifth cervical vertebral body. Compared with the adjacent vertebral body, T1WI (**e**) shows the decrease of the C 5-7 body signal, T2WI (**f**) shows the equal signal, and the STIR sequence (**g**) shows the high signal

7. Identification of vertebral body flattening in eosinophilic granuloma of thoracic spine and vertebral fracture
   7.1. X-ray plain film (Fig. 18.7a–d)

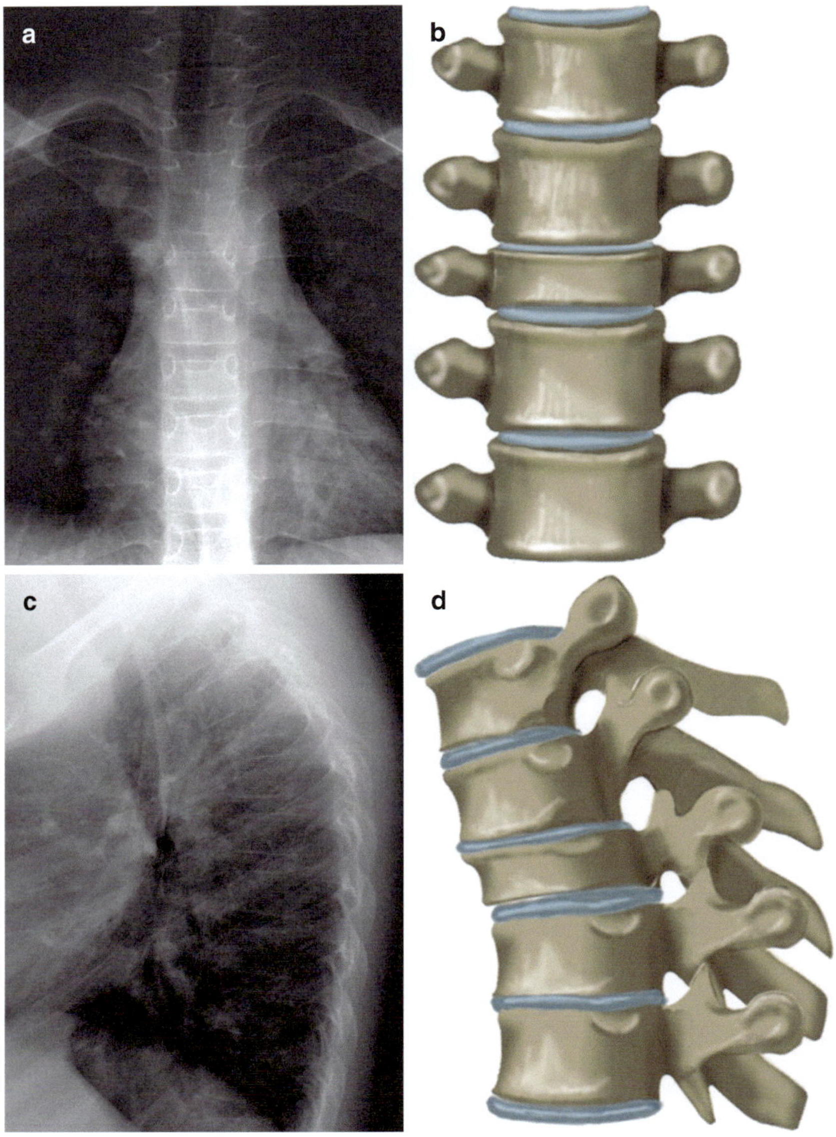

Fig. 18.7 X-ray (**a**, **c**) shows that the T4 vertebral body is flattened. Due to the overlapping of ribs and shoulders, the details are not clear, diagram (**b**, **d**)

7.2. CT scan (Fig. 18.7e)

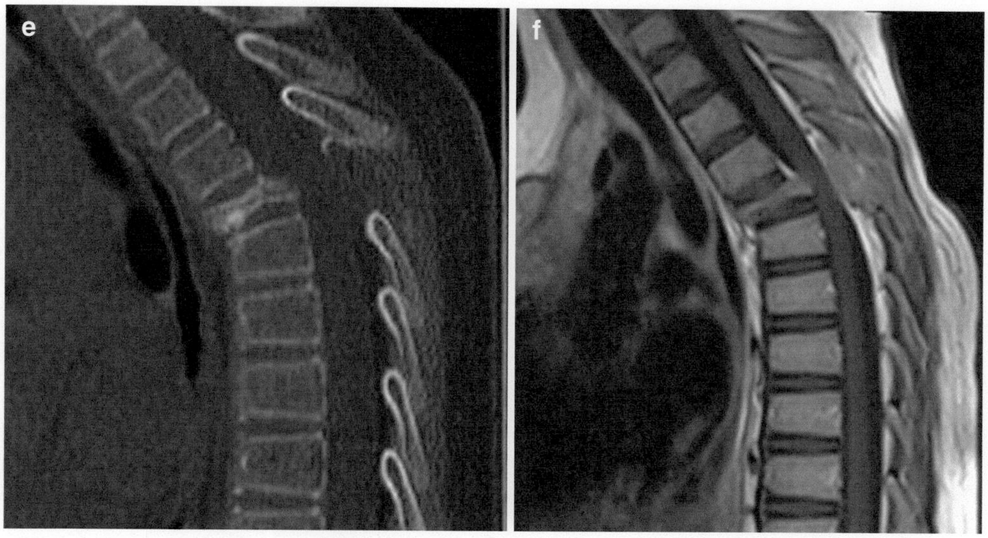

Fig. 18.7 CT sagittal plane (**e**), the T4 vertebral body is compressed and flattened, and the anterior and posterior diameters are enlarged, presenting a coin sign, with broken spine and narrow vertebral canal

7.3. MRI scan (Fig. 18.7f–h)

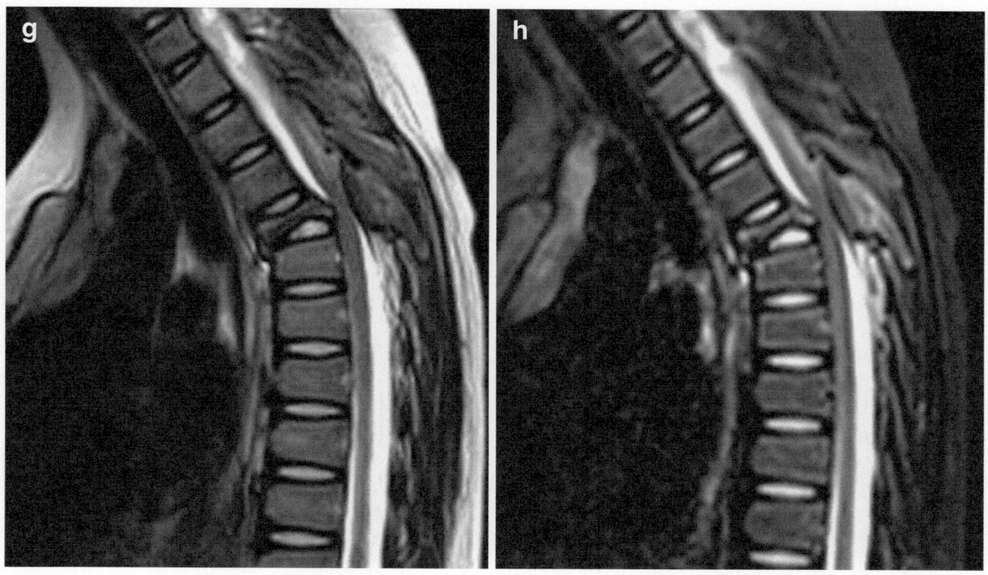

Fig. 18.7 MRI sagittal plane (**f**–**h**), the compression and flattening of the T4 vertebral body, presenting a coin sign, abnormal signals of vertebral body and attachment, tumor shadows around the attachment, and narrowing of the vertebral canal

8. Identification of vertebral body flattening due to thoracic infection and vertebral body fracture
   8.1. X-ray plain film (Fig. 18.8a–d)

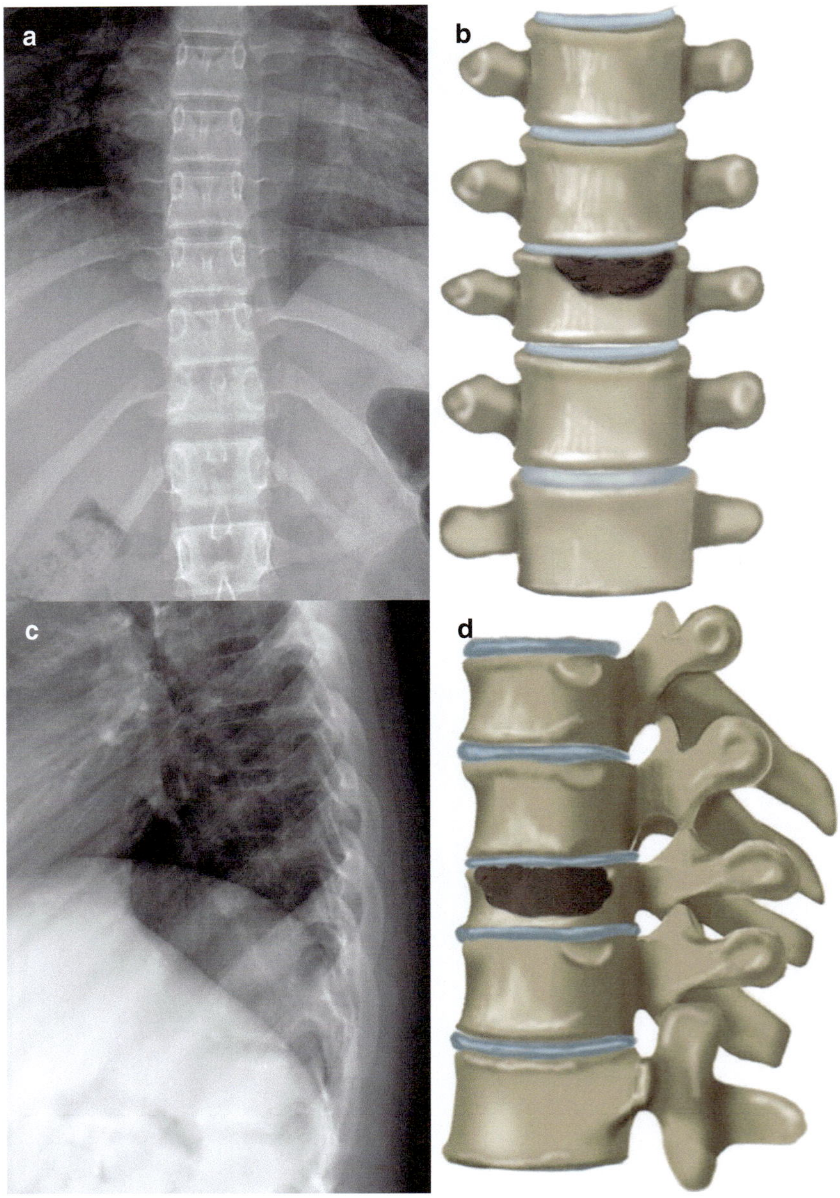

Fig. 18.8 Chronic inflammation of T11 vertebral body, the positive position of thoracic X-ray (**a**) shows that the upper margin endplate of T11 vertebral body is not clear, and the lateral position (**c**) shows the wedge-shaped change of T11 vertebral body diagram (**b**, **d**)

8.2. CT scan (Fig. 18.8e)

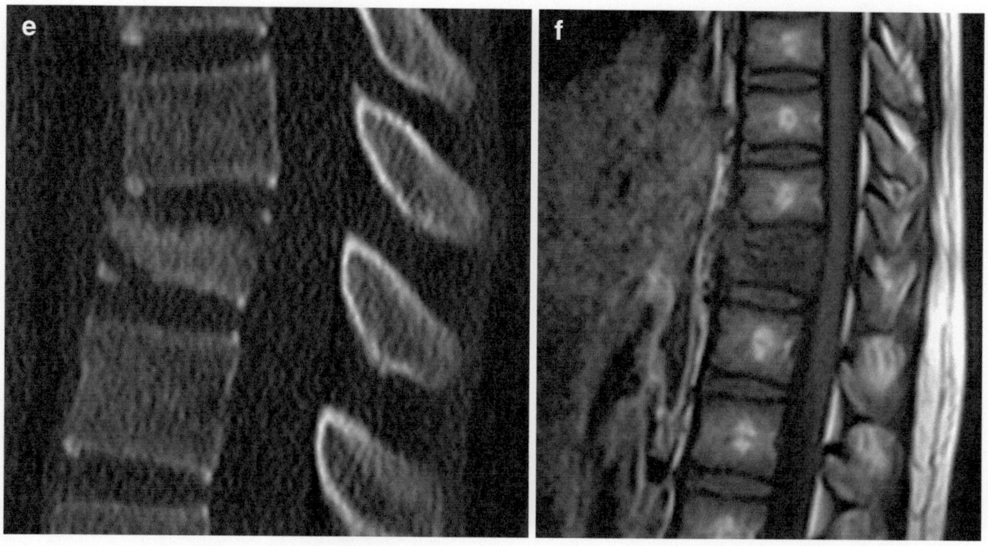

Fig. 18.8 CT sagittal plane reconstruction (**e**) shows that the T11 vertebral body was flattened, the bone density increased, and the edge bone was free

8.3. MRI scan (Fig. 18.8f–h)

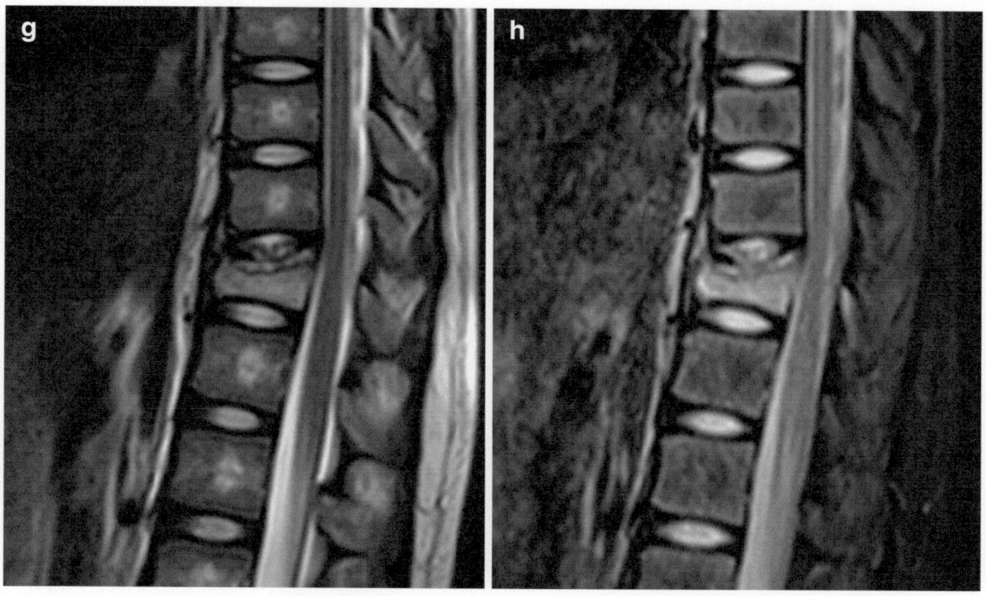

Fig. 18.8 MRI (**f–h**) shows that the T11 vertebral body was flattened, T1WI shows low signal, T2WI and STIR sequences show slightly higher signal, and the upper edge endplate of vertebral body was not clear

9. Identification of thoracic vertebral flattening in hematopathy and vertebral body fracture
   9.1. X-ray plain film (Fig. 18.9a–d)

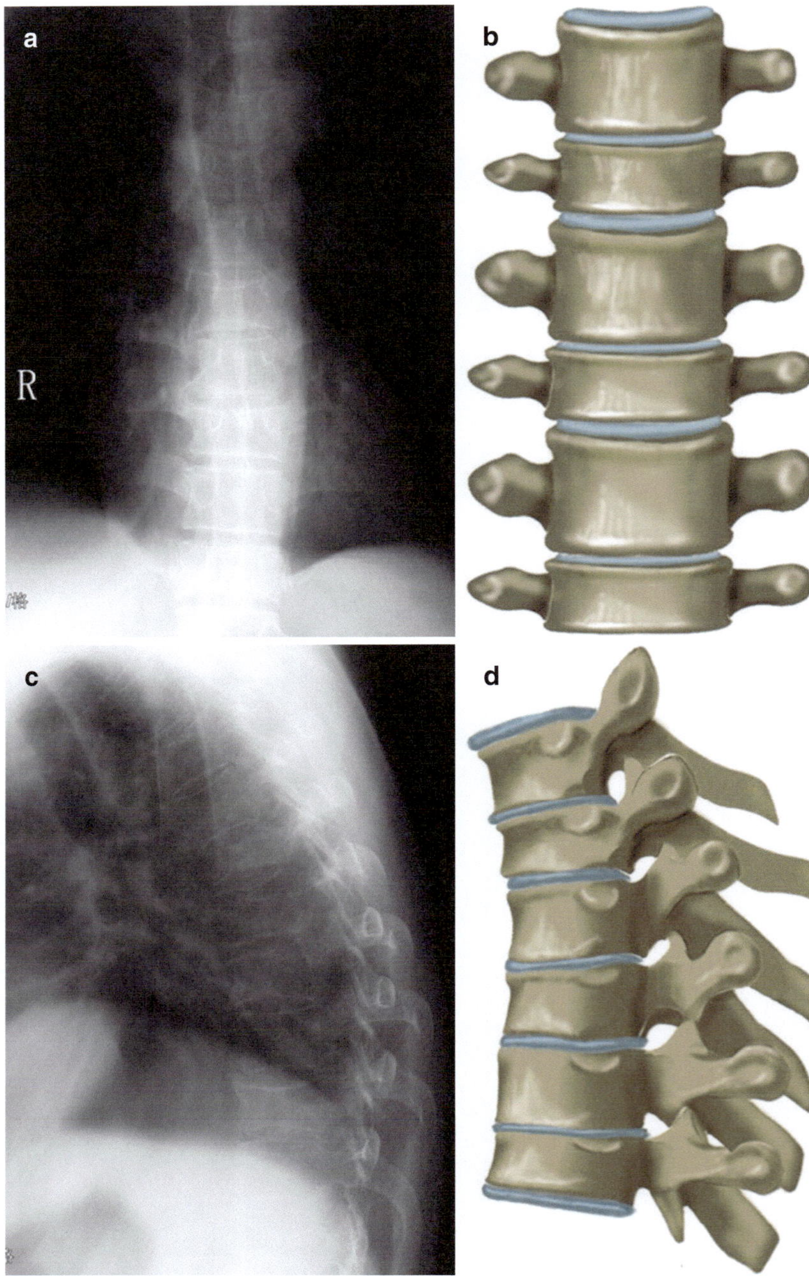

Fig. 18.9 X-ray plain film (**a**, **c**) shows that multiple vertebral bodies in the thoracic vertebra become flat and the density of the vertebral body is reduced unevenly, diagram (**b**, **d**)

9.2. CT scan (Fig. 18.9e)

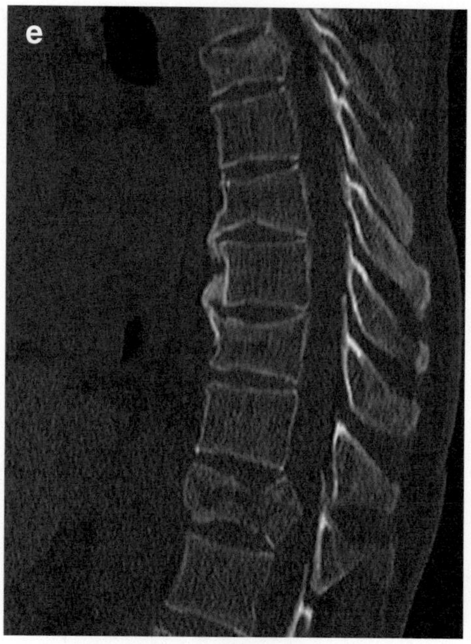

Fig. 18.9 CT sagittal plane reconstruction (**e**) shows compression fractures of multiple vertebral bodies in the thoracic spine, and uneven reduction of vertebral density

9.3. MRI scan (Fig. 18.9f–h)

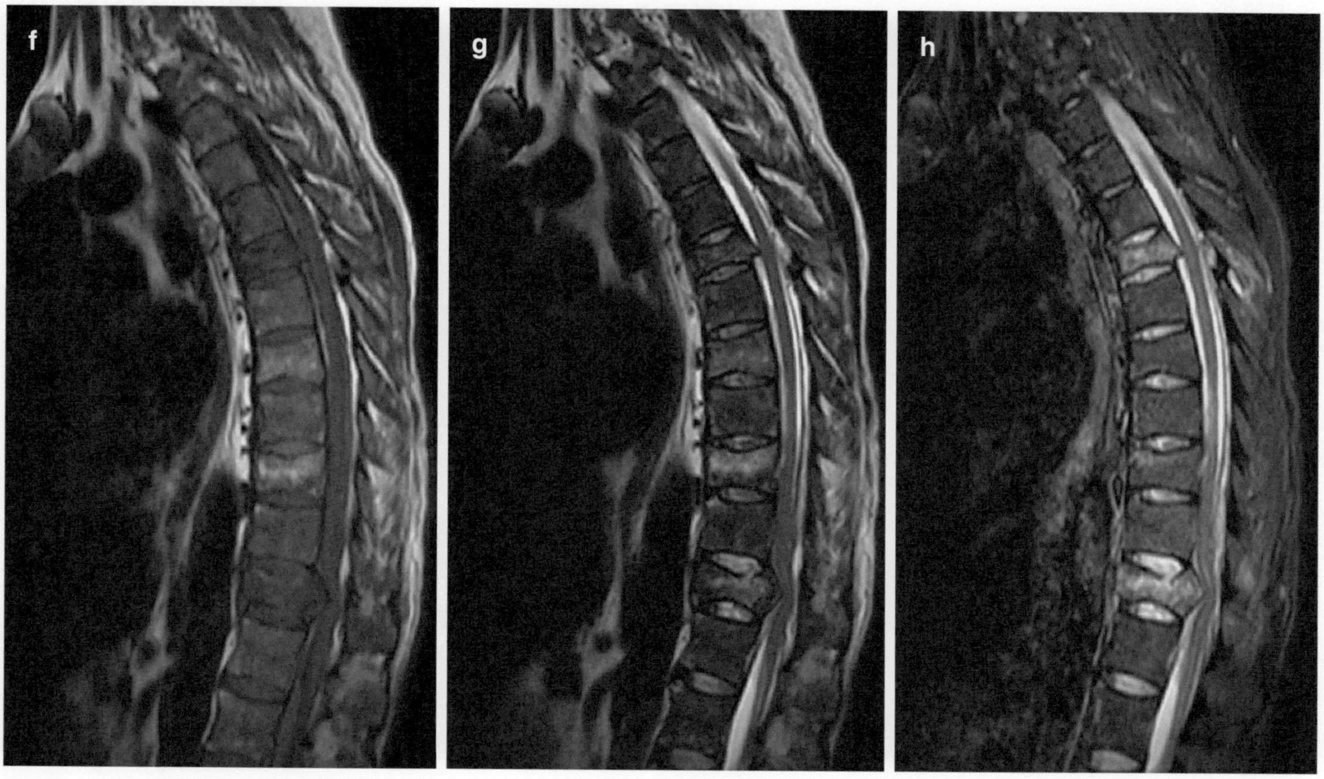

Fig. 18.9 MRI image (**f**–**h**) shows diffuse signal abnormality of thoracic vertebral body and attachment, and compression and flattening of multiple vertebral bodies

10. Identification of lumbar vertebral flattening in multiple myeloma and vertebral fracture
    10.1. X-ray plain film (Fig. 18.10a, b)

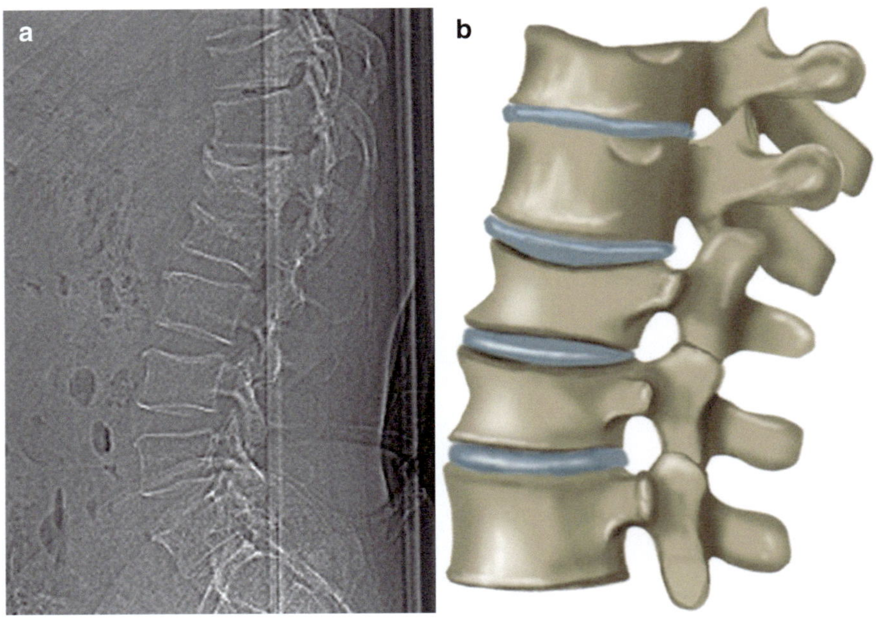

Fig. 18.10 The lateral position of the X-ray (**a**) shows wedge-shaped changes in the T11 and L1, L2 vertebral bodies, diagram (**b**)

    10.2. CT scan (Fig. 18.10c, d)

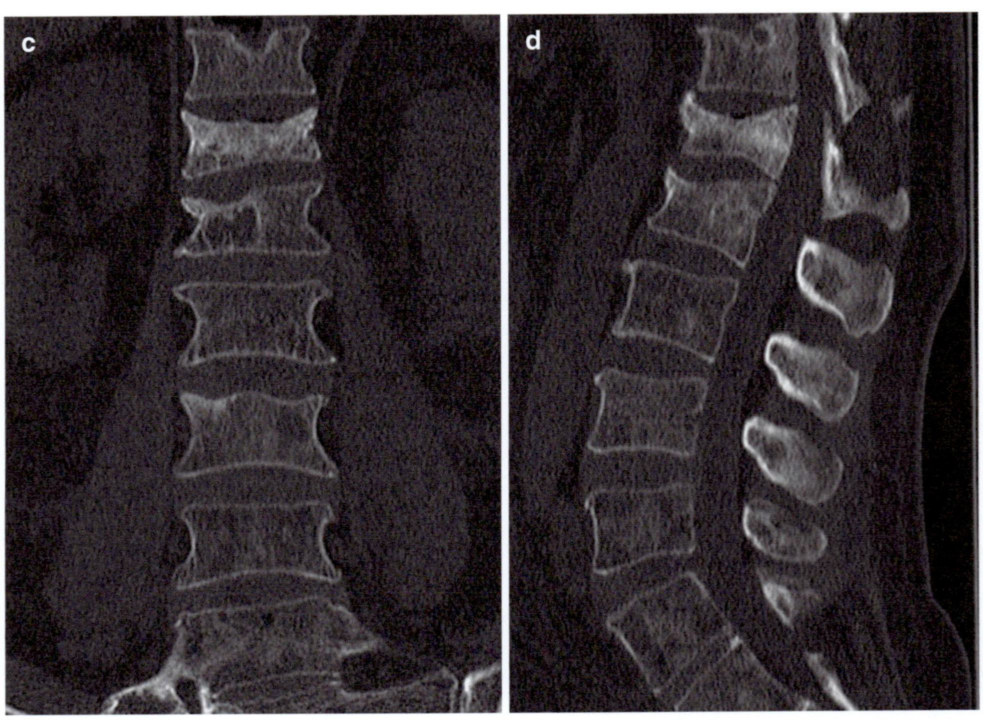

Fig. 18.10 CT reconstruction (**c**, **d**) shows L1 and 2 vertebral bodies were flattened, vertebral bone density increased, upper margin of T12 vertebral bodies was sunken, and speckle low-density shadows were seen in the rest vertebral bodies

10.3. MRI scan (Fig. 18.10e–g)

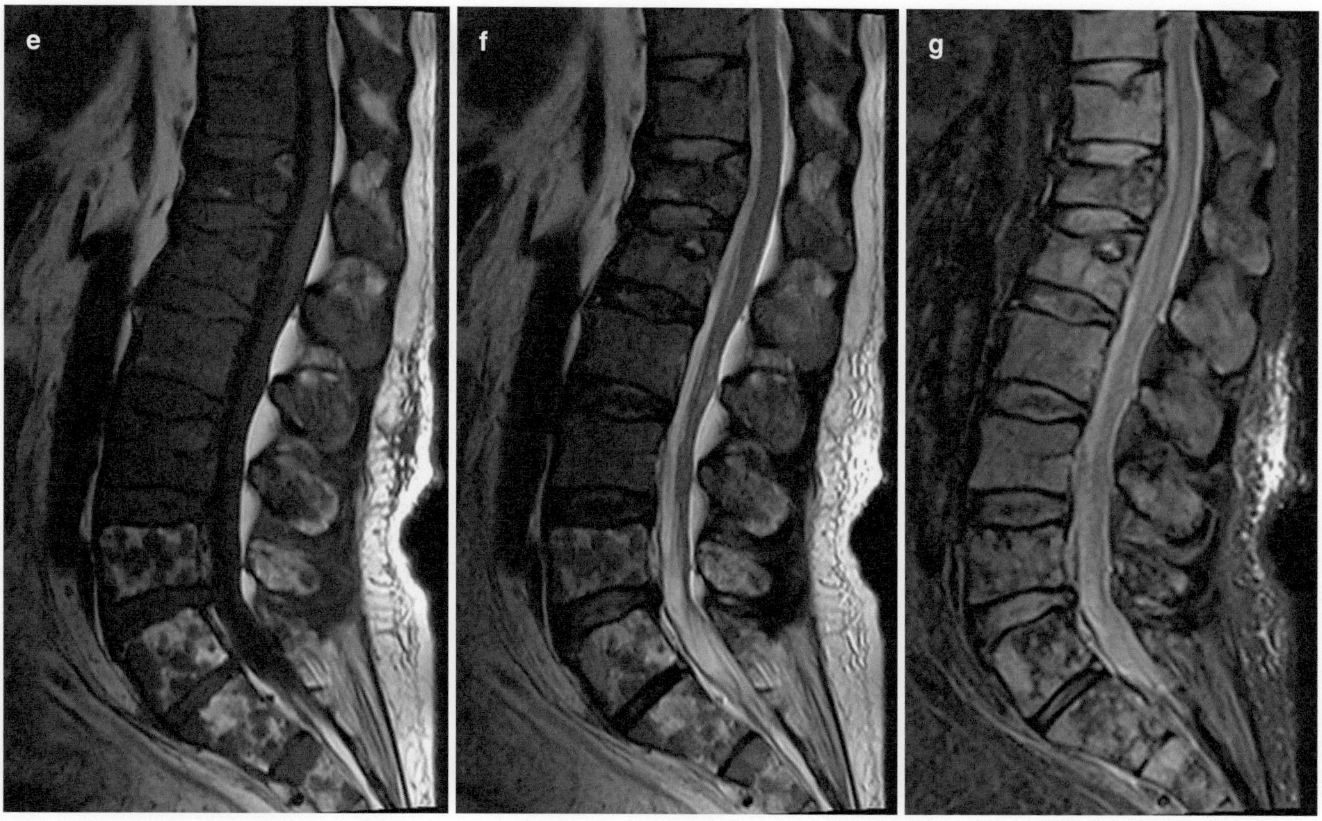

Fig. 18.10 MRI-T1WI (**e**) and T2WI (**f**) show abnormal thoracolumbar vertebral body signal, low lumbosacral punctate signal shadow, and STIR sequence (**g**) shows slightly higher signal universality

11. Differential diagnosis between pathological fracture of sacral giant cell tumor and vertebral body fracture
    11.1. X-ray plain film (Fig. 18.11a–d)

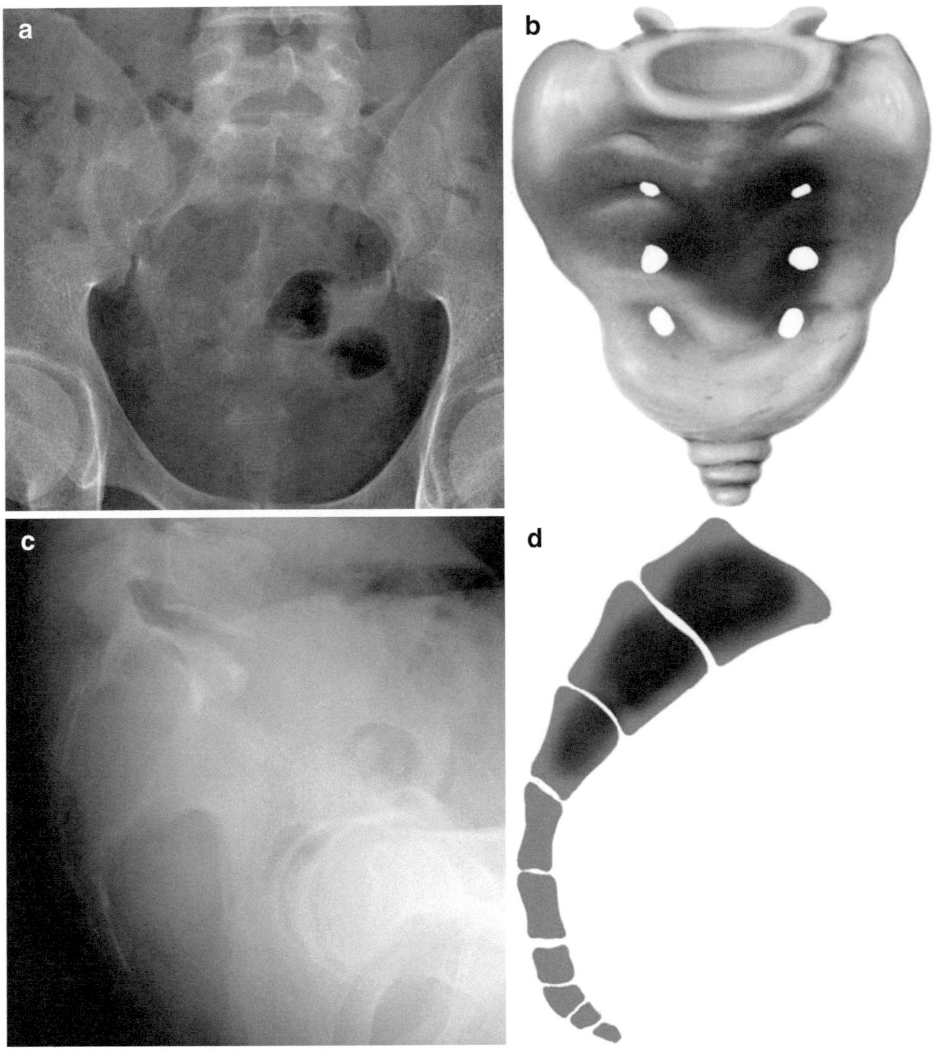

Fig. 18.11 The X-ray flat (**a**, **c**) shows the distended bony destruction of the upper sacrum and the thinning of the bony cortex, diagram (**b**, **d**)

    11.2. CT scan (Fig. 18.11e, f)

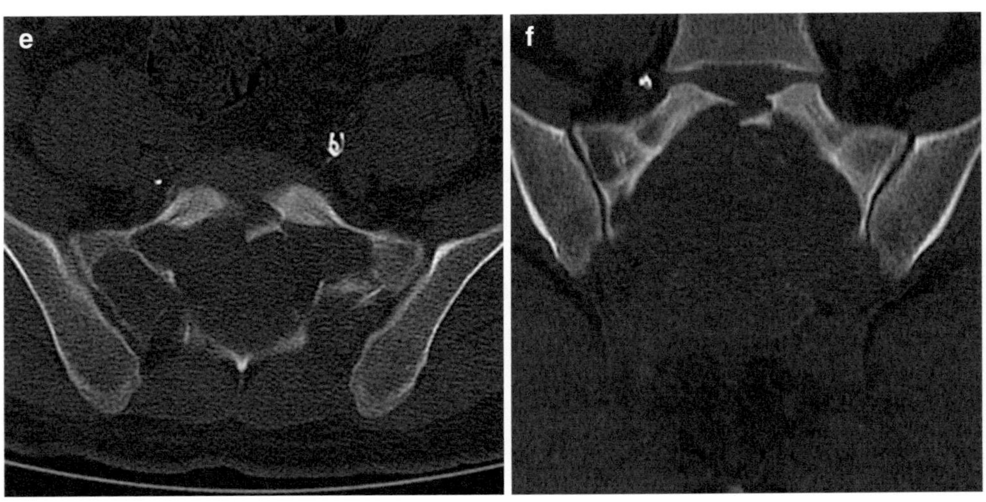

Fig. 18.11 CT cross section (**e**) coronal plane (**f**) shows the swelling fracture of sacral bone, the collapse of the upper margin of sacral 1 vertebral body, and the pathological fracture

12. Differential diagnosis between pathological fracture of sacral schwannoma and vertebral body fracture
    12.1. X-ray plain film (Fig. 18.12a–d)

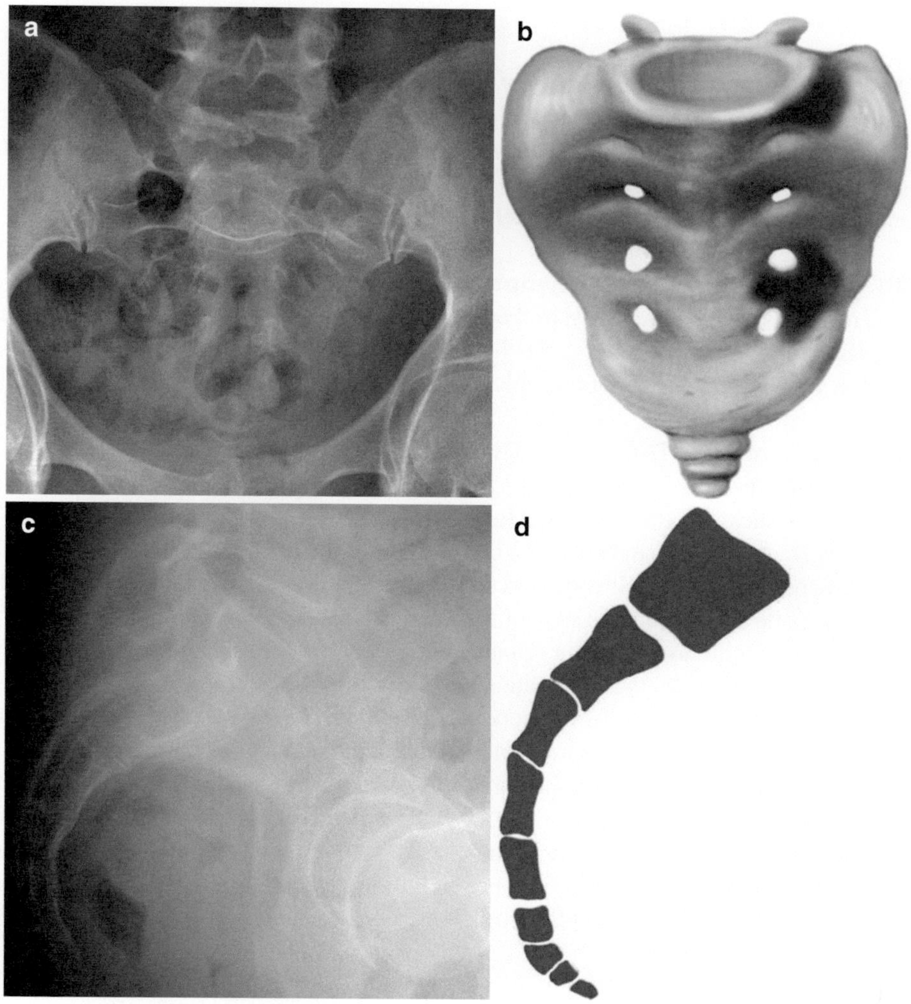

Fig. 18.12 The X-ray plain film (**a**, **c**) shows the decrease of bone density in the left flank of the sacrum, the destruction of distended expanded bone, the thinning of bone cortex, diagram (**b**, **d**)

    12.2. CT scan (Fig. 18.12e, f)

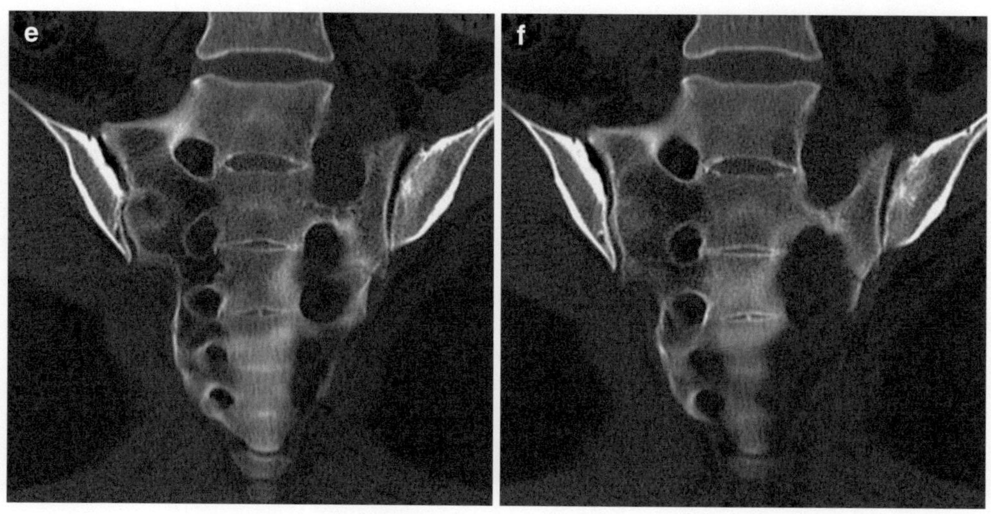

Fig. 18.12 CT cross section (**e**) coronal plane (**f**) shows the swelling fracture of sacral bone, the collapse of the upper margin of sacral 1 vertebral body, and the pathological fracture

18.1.3 Ankylosing Spondylitis and DISH Fractures

Patients with ankylosing spondylitis (AS) or diffuse idiopathic skeletal hyperostosis (DISH) form rigid, fixed deformities due to the ossification of ligaments, intervertebral discs, and paravertebral tissues, resulting in spinal fusion and reduced functional activity.

18.1.3.1 Identification of Injury Mechanism

Due to stiffness and osteoporosis of spinal motor segments, spinal fractures can be caused by mild trauma or even no external force. The incidence of AS combined with spinal fractures is 1.5% to 2.3%, 3.5 times higher than that of normal people, most commonly seen in the lower cervical spine, followed by the thoracolumbar and lumbar spine, respectively. Continuous movement of fracture segments is likely to be followed by functional prosthetic joint formation.

18.1.3.2 Identification of Symptoms and Signs

The most obvious manifestation of the patient after fracture is the pain in the fracture area. Severe fracture shows abnormal activity of the fracture segment, which can be used as a basis for diagnosis. When examining the body, attention should be paid to whether there is abnormal activity or bone grinding sound, which can be used for definite diagnosis.

18.1.3.3 Imaging Differential Diagnosis

The imaging features of AS penetrating fractures are classified according to Graham's classification and can be divided into three types: shear fracture (fresh fracture), stress fracture, and compression fracture.

Shear fracture occurs mostly in the cervical spine, and the fracture line is mostly extended through the intervertebral space and the posterior column. It is hard to see the fracture line in the intervertebral disc, but the fracture line can be seen on the vertebral plate and the joint process of the same or adjacent segments, and it can also be seen as the continuity interruption of the anterior longitudinal ligament or interspinous ligament of ossification fusion. X ray has a certain rate of missed diagnosis for fractures without obvious dislocation, but CT multiplanar reconstruction (MPR) has a high value for the diagnosis of cervical spine fracture with ankylosing spondylitis, and it can be found that the articular process injury of the posterior column and the fracture of the ossified anterior longitudinal ligament. Most of AS thoracolumbar fractures are stress fracture, i.e., the penetrating fracture that involves the three columns, with the fracture line through intervertebral disc or vertebral body. Viewed from X-ray and CT MPR images, there are characteristic changes for AS thoracolumbar fractures, i.e., existence of destructive vertebral body lesions (Andersson lesions) of the intervertebral disc at the fracture plane, and it is manifested as a wide range of subchondral bone destruction of upper and lower endplate of the adjacent vertebral bodies, ragged edge, partly accompanied by bone sclerosis and pseudarthrosis formation around.

13. Differential diagnosis between cervical endplate fracture with ankylosing spondylitis and nonfracture in ankylosing spondylitis
    13.1. X-ray plain film (Fig. 18.13a, b)

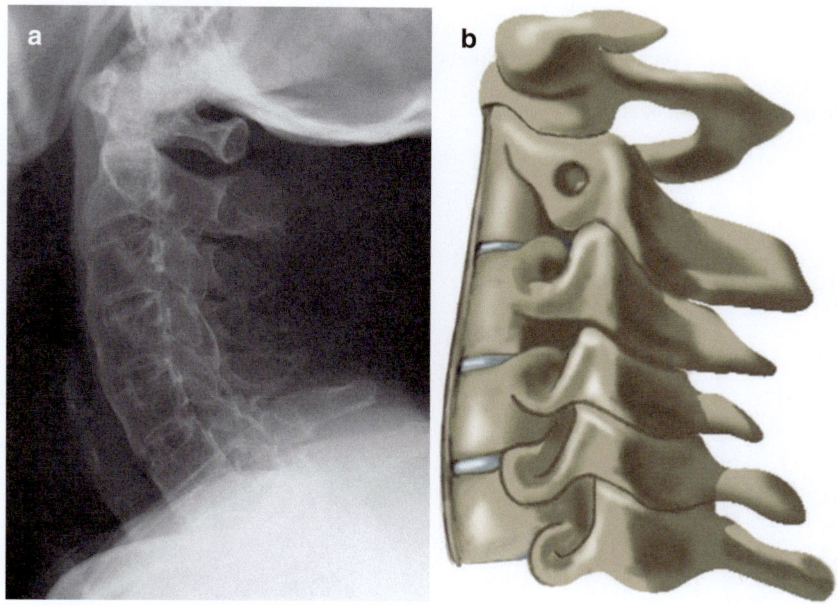

Fig. 18.13 The lateral position of the cervical spine (**a**) shows the anterior longitudinal ligament calcification of the cervical spine, no clear fracture shadow, ankylosing spondylitis, diagram (**b**)

    13.2. CT scan (Fig. 18.13c, d)

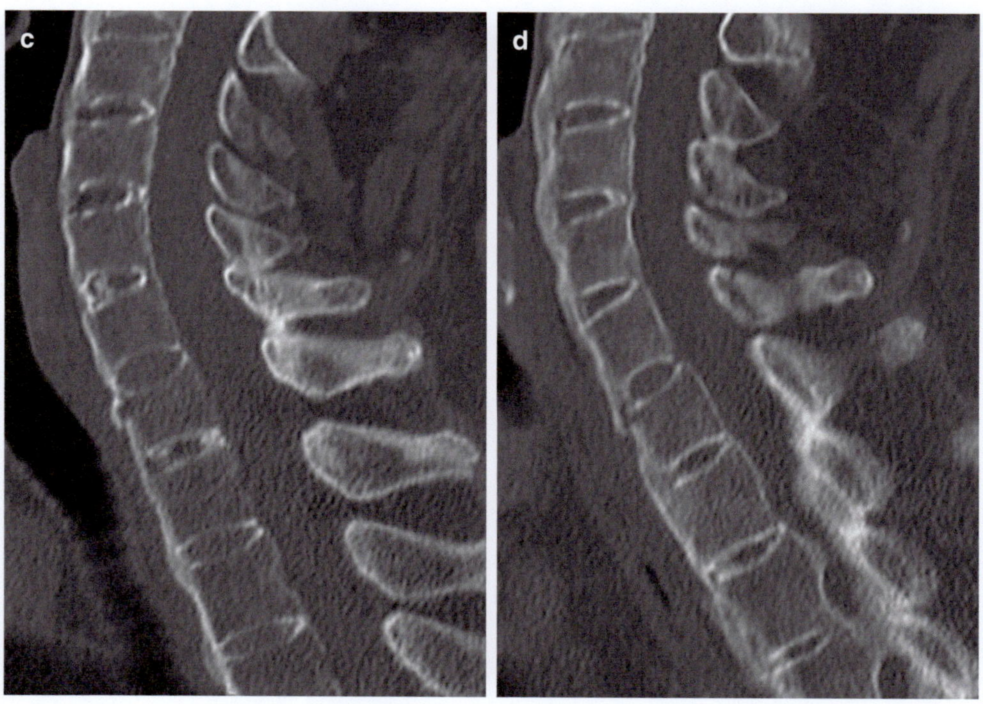

Fig. 18.13 CT sagittal reconstruction (**c**, **d**) shows calcification of the anterior and posterior longitudinal ligaments of the cervical vertebra. The fracture line passed through the anterior longitudinal ligament of the C6-7 ossification, the upper margin of the C7-7 vertebra, the C6-7 intervertebral disc, and the C6-6 vertebral plate

14. Differential diagnosis between lumbar endplate fracture with ankylosing spondylitis and nonfracture in ankylosing spondylitis
    14.1. X-ray plain film (Fig. 18.14a, b)

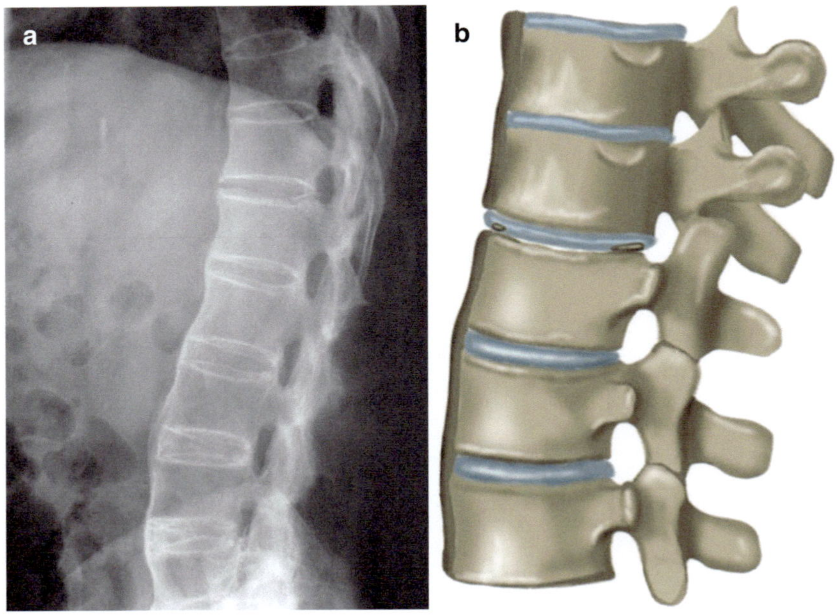

Fig. 18.14 X-ray (**a**) shows that the lumbar vertebra is A square cone, and no clear fracture signs are seen. The lateral position of T12 – L1 indicates that the anterior longitudinal ligament of ossified vertebral space is not continuous, diagram (**b**)

    14.2. MRI scan (Fig. 18.14c, d)

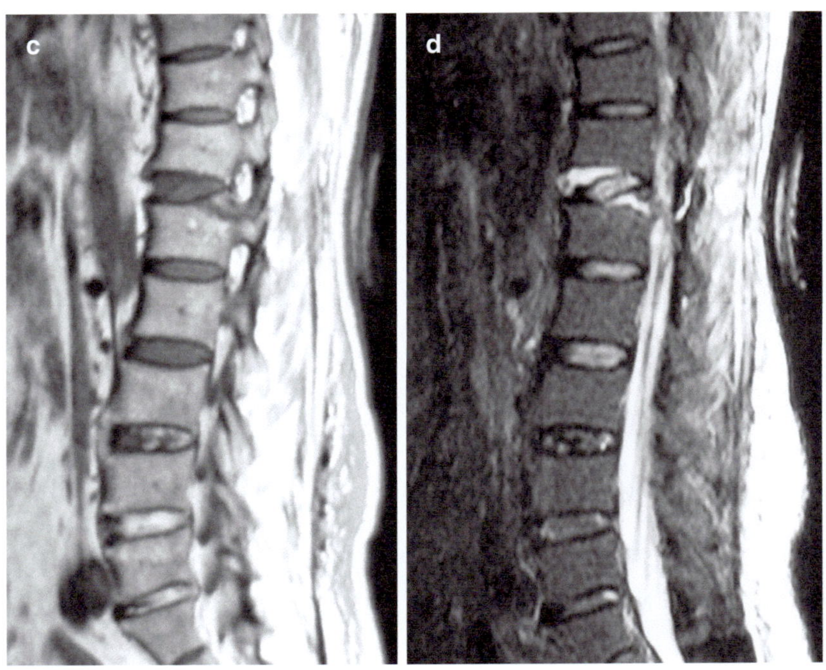

Fig. 18.14 MR image (**c**, **d**) shows that the fracture line passes through the posterior margin of T12- L1 intervertebral disc and L1 vertebral body

15. Differential diagnosis between false joint formation by an old fracture with ankylosing spondylitis and tumor
    15.1. X-ray plain film (Fig. 18.15a, b)

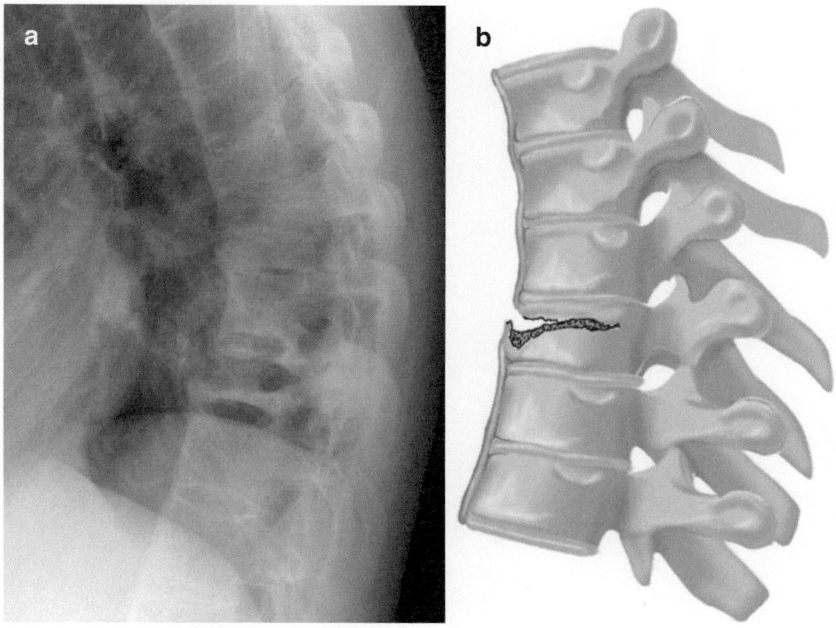

Fig. 18.15 Old thoracic spine fracture with ankylosing spondylitis, false joint formed, X-ray flat (**a**) showing discontinuity of bone in T10 vertebral bodies, local bone defect, and peripheral bone sclerosis, diagram (**b**)

    15.2. CT scan (Fig. 18.15c, d)

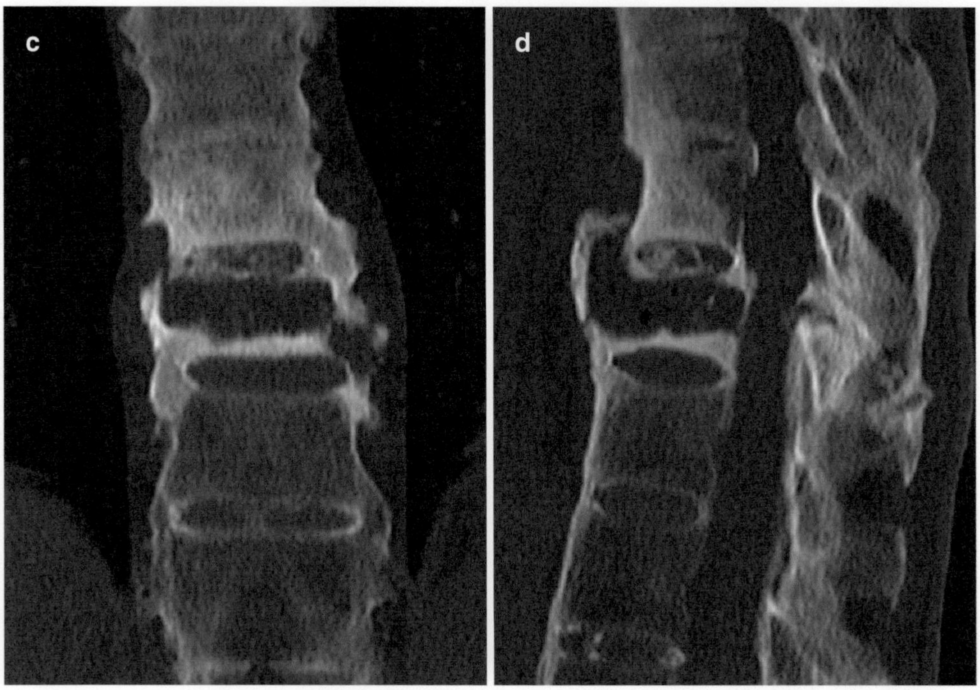

Fig. 18.15 The CT reconstruction image (**c**, **d**) shows that the thoracic vertebral body shows changes of bamboos and cones, discontinuity of the T10 vertebral body, local bone defects, bone sclerosis of the edge, and upper vertebral body

16. Differential diagnosis between lumbar vertebral body fracture with ankylosing spondylitis and nonfracture in ankylosing spondylitis
    16.1. X-ray plain film (Fig. 18.16a–d)

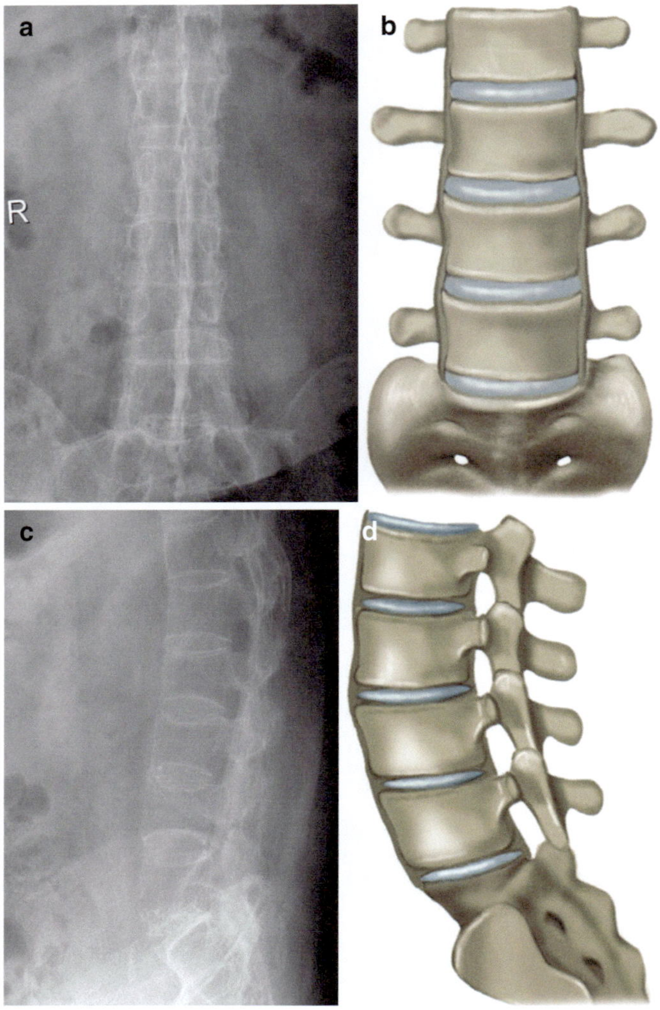

Fig. 18.16 Ankylosing spondylitis, the normal position of the X-ray (**a**) shows that the lumbar vertebra is in the shape of a bamboo node, the lateral position (**c**) shows the square vertebra, and no clear fracture line is seen, diagram (**b**, **d**)

16.2. CT scan (Fig. 18.16e)

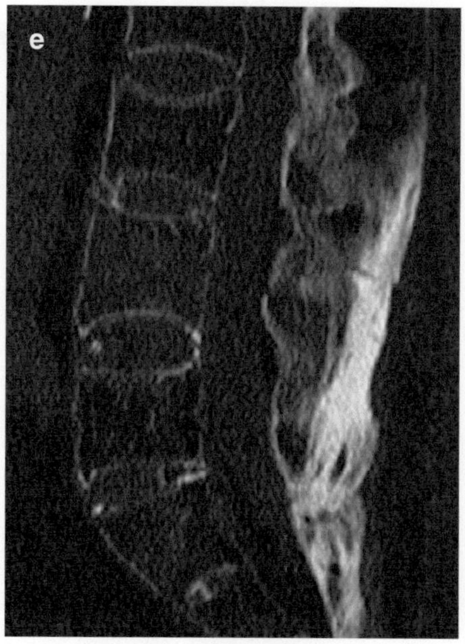

Fig. 18.16 CT (**e**) shows that L4 vertebral body front cortical discontinuity, lumbar spinous process fusion, visible fracture line shadow

16.3. MRI scan (Fig. 18.16f–h)

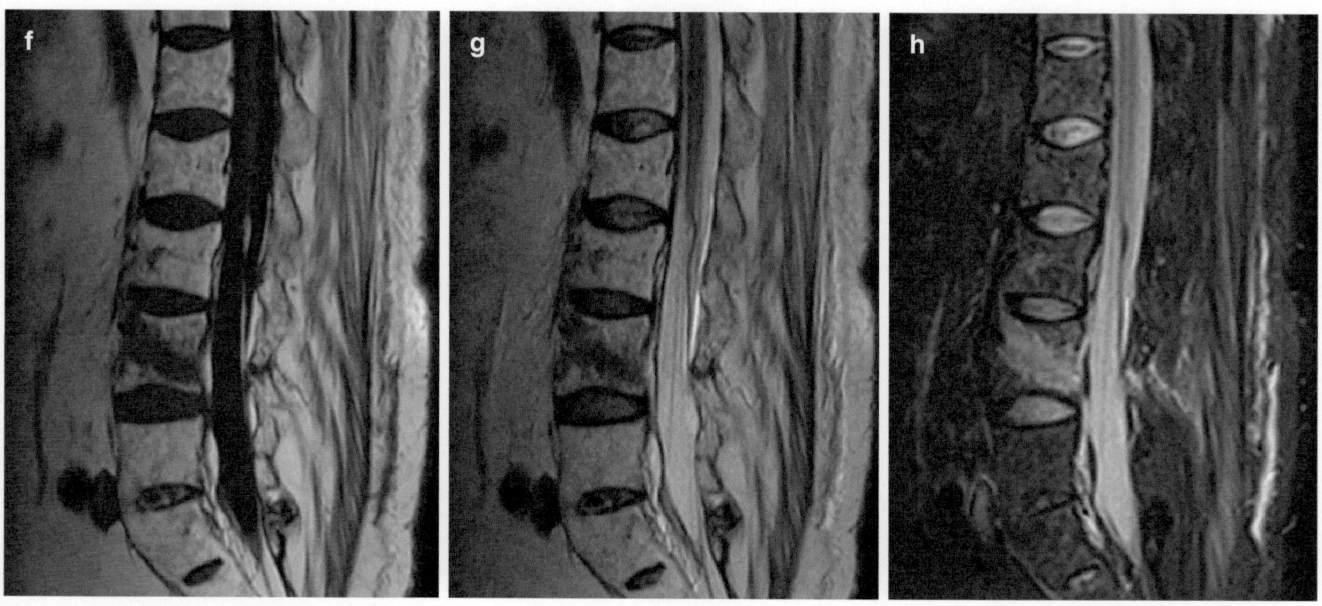

Fig. 18.16 MRI-T1WI **f**) and T2WI (**g**) shows oblique low signal shadows in the L4 vertebra, and the STIR sequence (**h**) shows patchy high signal, while the band high signal shadows were seen in the L4 spinous process. The subcutaneous tissue of the back is swollen

17. Differential diagnosis between Andersson lesions with ankylosing spondylitis and bone tumors
    17.1. X-ray plain film (Fig. 18.17a–d)

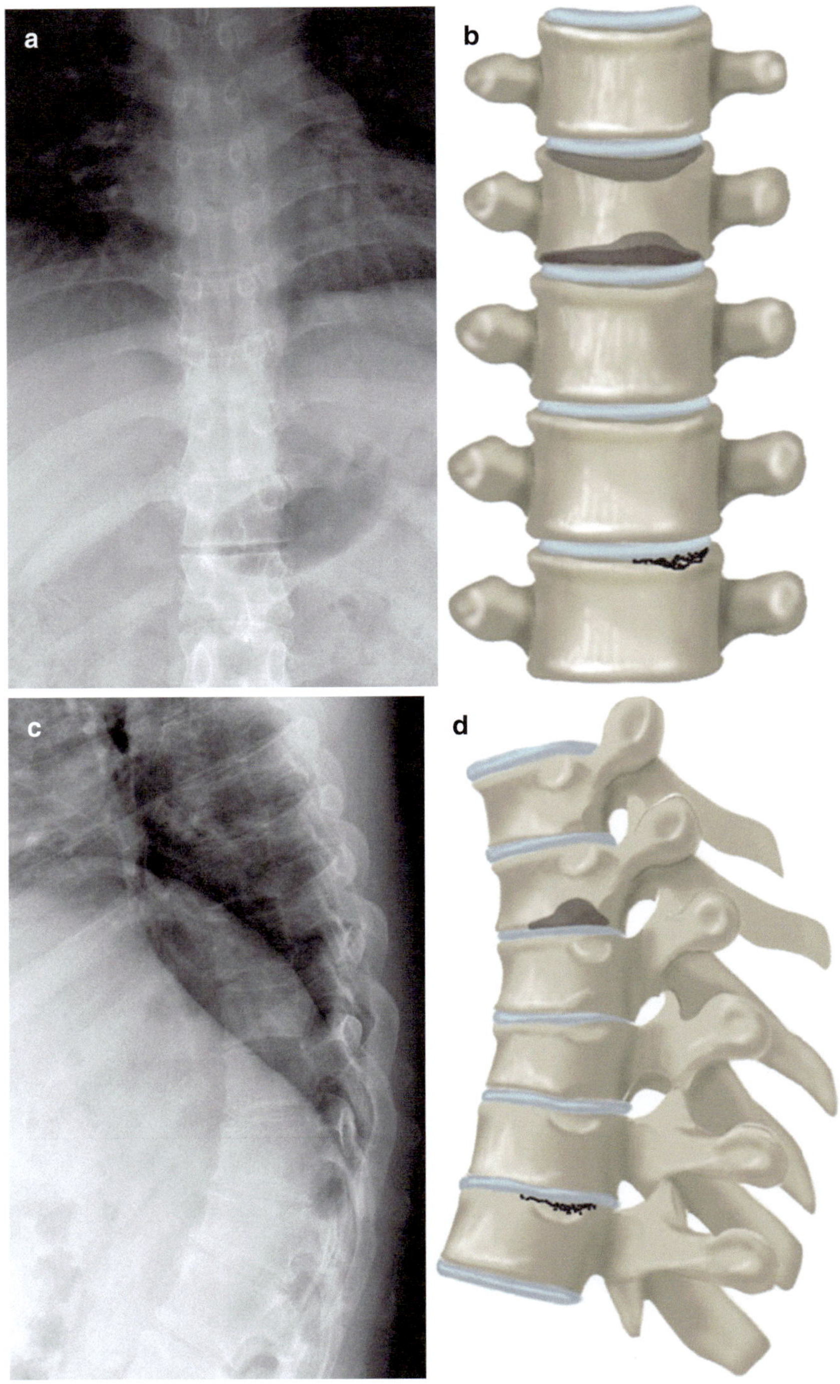

Fig. 18.17 Andersson lesions with ankylosing spondylitis, X-ray (**a**, **c**) shows posterior thoracolumbar processes, partial vertebral space narrowing, diagram (**b**, **d**)

17.2. CT scan (Fig. 18.17e, f)

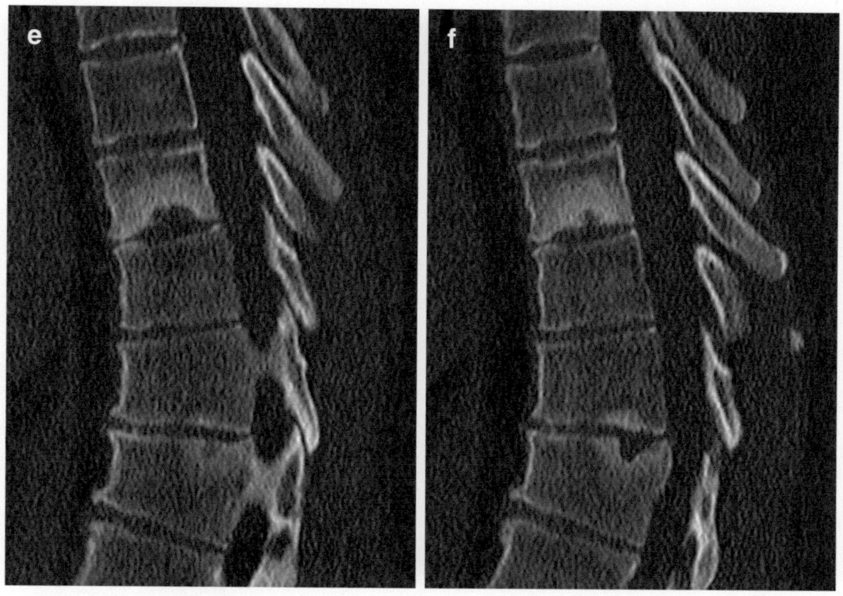

Fig. 18.17 CT reconstruction (**e**, **f**) shows localized depressions in the lower margin of T9 vertebral body and upper margin of T12 vertebral body, and edge osteosclerosis

17.3. MRI scan (Fig. 18.17g, h)

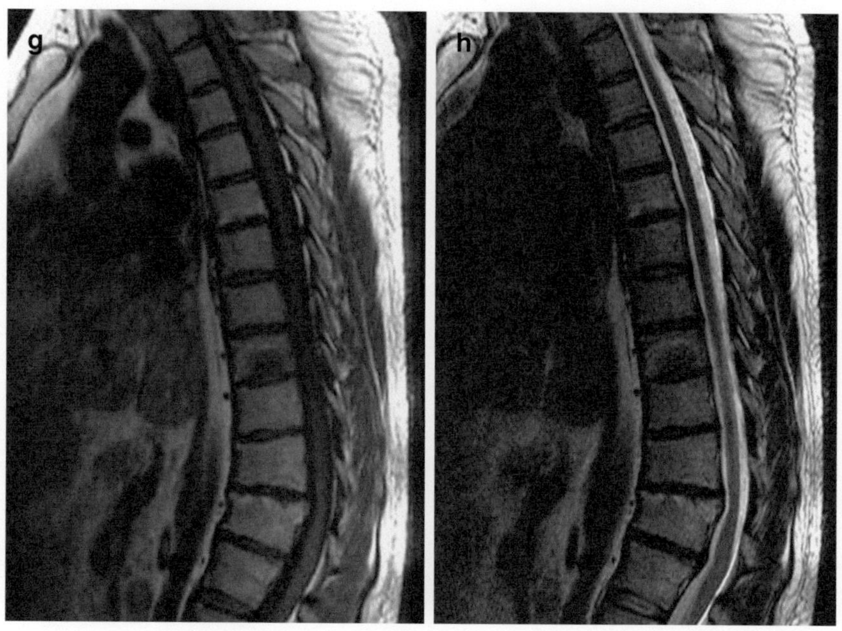

Fig. 18.17 MR images (**g**, **h**) show a narrowing of the multiple intervertebral space, irregular vertebral endplate, and low local signal

18. Differential diagnosis between vertebral body fracture of DISH lumbar vertebra and nonfracture
    18.1. X-ray plain film (Fig. 18.18a–d)

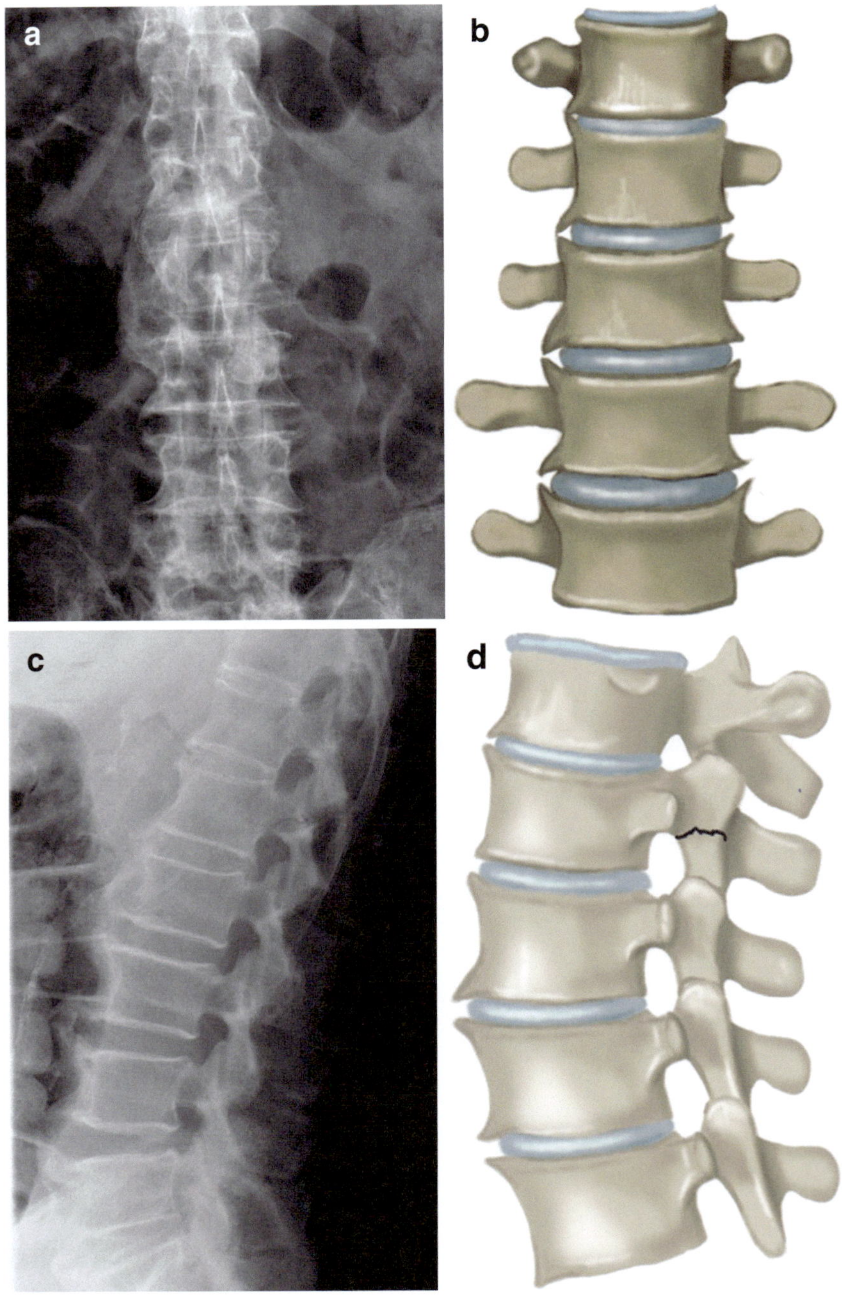

Fig. 18.18 DISH, the normal lateral position of lumbar vertebra (**a**, **c**), shows that lumbar vertebral body edge hyperplasia is significant, part of which forms bone bridge, low-density image of irregular line at the pedicle of L1, diagram (**b**, **d**)

18.2. CT scan (Fig. 18.18e)

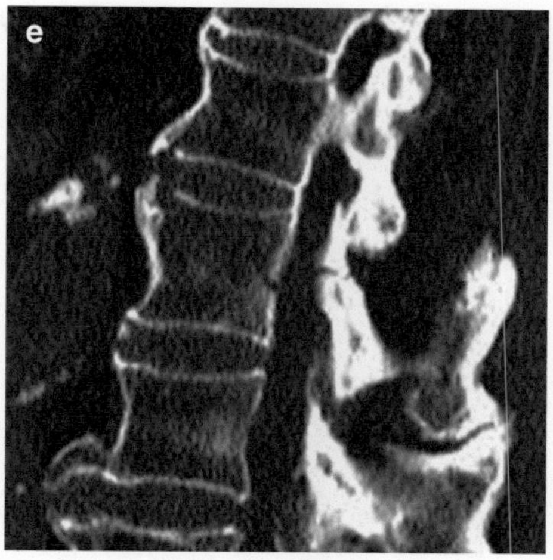

Fig. 18.18 CT sagittal reconstruction (**e**) shows that the vertebral body and spinous process of the lumbar spine had significant hyperosteogeny, the formation of bone bridge, and that L1 vertebral body and superior articular process were transverse fracture lines

19. Differential diagnosis between thoracic Kümmell disease and fracture
    19.1. X-ray plain film (Fig. 18.19a–d)

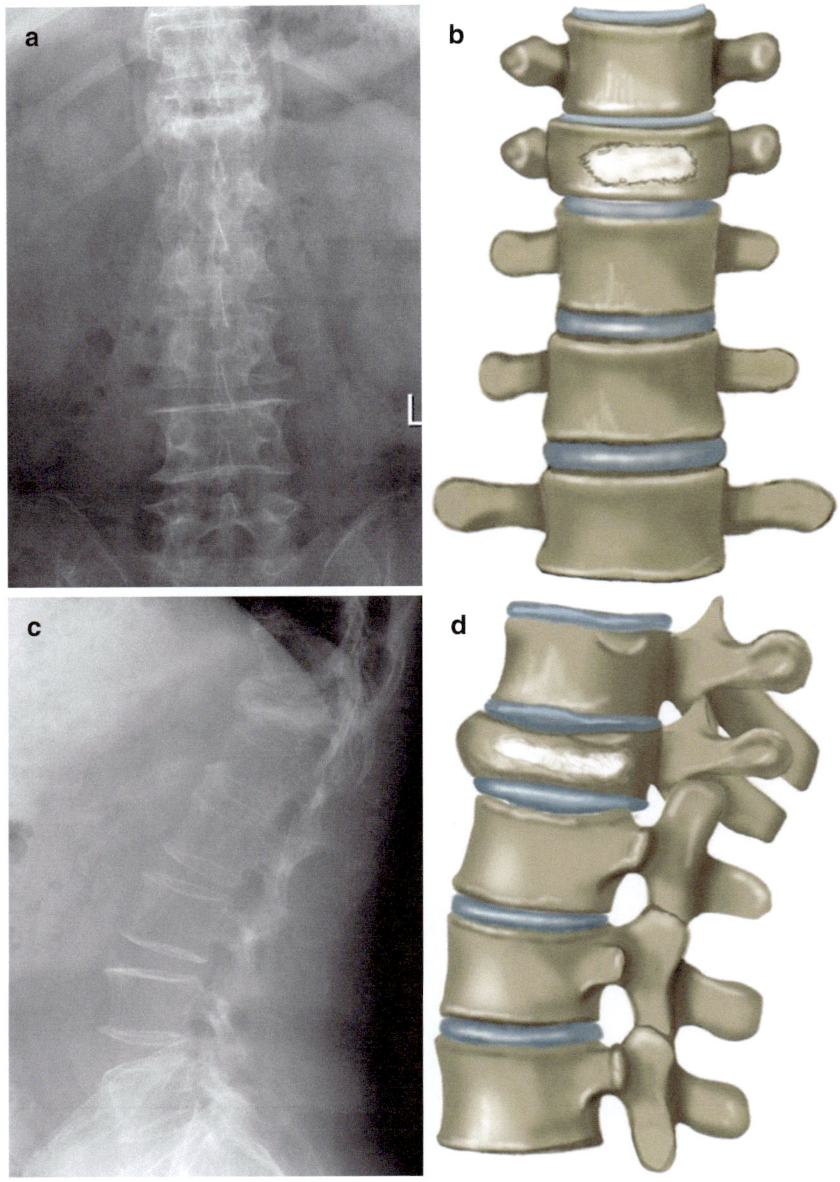

Fig. 18.19 X- ray (**a**, **c**) shows that the T12 vertebral body is flattened, and the local bone density is increased, diagram (**b**, **d**)

19.2. CT scan (Fig. 18.19e)

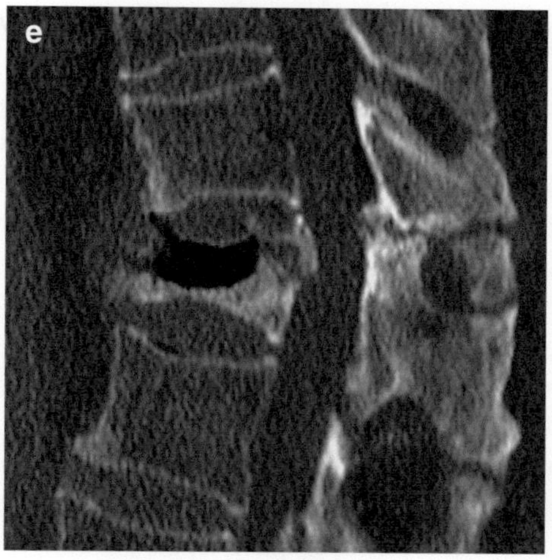

Fig. 18.19 CT (**e**) shows that the upper part of 12 vertebral bodies was a radiolucent density shadow, and the spinous process in the lumbar thoracic segment increased in volume, with obvious edge hyperplasia, a linear low-density shadow can be seen between the spines of T11-12, with increased bone density at the margin

19.3. MRI scan (Fig. 18.19f–h)

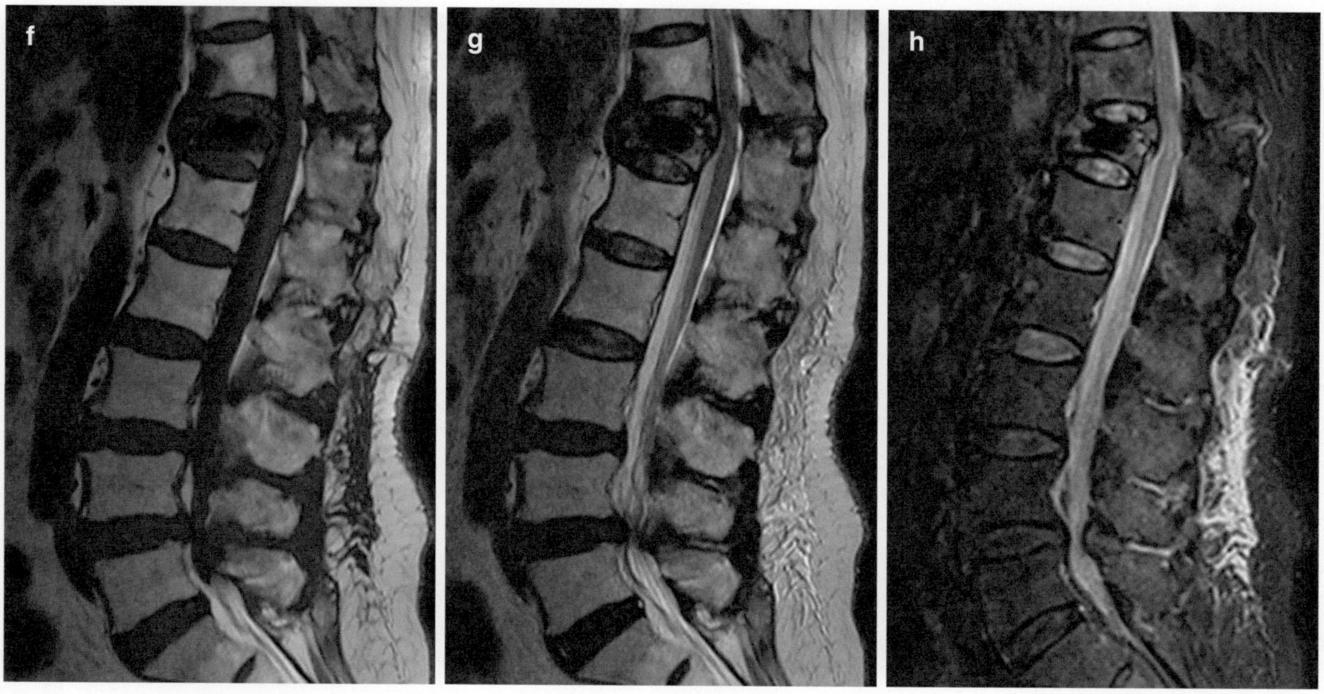

Fig. 18.19 MRI (**f**–**h**) shows low signal shadow (gas) in T12 vertebra

18.2 Pelvic Pathological Fractures

Pathological fractures are fractures that occurred on the basis of bone lesions. The most common causes are primary or metastatic tumors, and other factors including osteoporosis, endocrine disorders, and developmental disorders of bone and cartilage.

Pathological fractures caused by bone tumor refer to the fractures caused by bone tumor or tumor-like lesions. There are many kinds of bone tumors that lead to pathological fractures. Metastatic tumors are the most common, accounting for 37.85%, followed by myeloma, accounting for 14.64%, and poor fibrous structure, accounting for 13.81%.

Neoplastic pathological fractures occur at different ages and can vary in different locations. The proportion of pelvic pathological fractures is relatively low with only 9 out of 375 pathological fractures cases in our hospital, which account for 2.4% of pathological fractures (compared with metastatic tumors accounting for 55.6% at most).

The speed of bone erosion from neoplastic pathological fractures especially in malignant tumor exceeds the speed of osteoporosis. Neoplastic pathological fractures often cause dysfunction after pathological fracture. Moreover, the fractures not only cannot recover but can get worse with pathological circumstance changes. Therefore, we are supposed to comprehensively analyze the neoplastic pathological fractures according to gender, age, location of the tumor, and its imaging. The more reliable bases for clinical treatment we provide, the more precise diagnosis we will make.

Failure fracture, a type of pathological fractures, occurs under normal activity or when activity increases slightly, due to factors such as osteoporosis, reduced bone mineral content, and strength. Failure fracture is a normal stress that puts on abnormal bone tissues such as decreased bone mineral content or decreased elastic resistance. It often occurs on a number of diseases, including rheumatoid arthritis, osteoporosis, Paget's disease, osteomalacia, hormone therapy, hyperthyroidism, renal osteodystrophy, hypoplasia of cartilage, arthroplasty, osteomalacia, and fibrous dysplasia, among which the rheumatoid arthritis and osteoporosis are the commonest causes of failure fracture and deserve special attention.

The sacrum is the best site for failure fracture. Sacrum works to transmit the body's gravity to the lower extremities, and when bone mass of sacrum decreases to a certain inflection that is inadequate to bear the stress caused by body weight, insufficiency fracture will occur. Osteoporosis reduces bone mass and weakens bone structure. Therefore, sacral failure fractures are most common in old women. If the clinician fails to recognize the disease, he might think that the symptoms are caused by lumbar or intervertebral disc diseases, which will lead to unnecessary lumbar or intervertebral disc scan or even surgery. A study on the women over the age of 55 reported that incidence of sacral stress fractures was 1.8%. It is often seen in patients with rheumatoid arthritis treated with glucocorticoid or pelvic malignant tumor treated with radiotherapy. Furthermore, sacral failure fractures also occur in women at the time of 3 months after pregnancy or several weeks after birth. The main risk factors include overweight infants, increased anterior lumbar protrusion, overweight pregnant women, and vaginal births. Other triggers are vitamin D deficiency, heparin anticoagulation therapy, transient osteoporosis during pregnancy, and lactation.

The two sacral wings are located outside the sacrum triangle, which is highly active and has concentrated stress. Therefore, stress fracture usually occurs in the 1st area of sacrum, which is parallel to the sacroiliac joint. Further stress results in transverse sacral fractures.

It is important to note that sacral stress fractures are not supposed to be treated with ice compress or nonsteroidal anti-inflammatory and analgesic drugs, as it can prolong healing time. Attention should be paid to treatment plan—rest and restricted mobility. After 2 weeks of feeling no pain, the patients can carry heavy load to walk and gradually return to normal activity within 12–14 weeks. Other conservative treatments include pain relief and physical therapy. According to the above points, fracture healing time depends on the fracture severity. Vitamin D and calcium supplements are recommended for healing process.

Failure fractures in other parts of the pelvis include the ramus of the pubis, near the symphysis pubis and around the acetabulum.

18.2.1 Identification of Injury Mechanism

Unlike simple traumatic fractures, the pathological fractures are eroded, destructive, or decayed by certain diseases, and when exposed to a slight external force or even due to its own gravity, pathological bones have a tendency to break spontaneously. Therefore, when a fracture occurs with a slight external force and there exists pains around this part before the fracture or there has been a fracture in the same part or other parts in the past, the possibility of pathological fracture should be accounted for.

18.2.2 Identification of Symptoms and Signs

The clinical symptoms are lower back pain or pelvic pain or pain from hip and inguinal area while other clinical symptoms are not specific.

18.2.3 Identification of Imaging Diagnosis

Pathological fractures, especially the fractures due to a slight external force, should be highly identified, and CT or MRI should be performed when necessary. If the X-ray shows that the fracture is round and blunt or the surrounding bone structure is disordered, CT or MRI scan should be carried out to determine whether there is a pathological fracture. Due to osteoporosis, overlap of intestinal contents and other factors, X-ray is not sensitive to the display of sacral stress fracture. A control study on X-ray, CT, and MRI showed that X-ray could only identify 3.8% of sacral stress fractures, presenting a sacral pterygoid sclerotic zone parallel to the sacroiliac joint. Compared with MRI, the sensitivity of CT in diagnosing sacral failure fracture was 74.6%, and CT also showed sclerotic zones and fracture lines. CT can also provide bone details. The uptake of nuclide at the stress fracture site of radionuclide bone scanning was increased, which showed the letter "H" or its variant. It was reported that the sensitivity and specificity of this sign in the diagnosis of stress fracture were 96% and 92%, respectively. Among them, the complete type accounts for 63%, and the incomplete type (variation type) accounts for 33%. The vertical part of the letter "H" is located in the sacrum wing, and the transverse part is located in the sacrum body, which exists about 8–10 months. A diagnosis sign of stress fracture by MRI is bone marrow edema, which may show a low signal fracture line. There are also abnormal signal distributions: similar to the letter "H" for both complete and incomplete types. Scanning sequences include transverse and coronal T1WI and lipid T2WI/ STIR. Seventy-eight percent of sacral stress fractures are complicated with stress fractures of the pubic ramus. It may be that the incomplete pelvic ring increases stress in other areas. The clinical symptoms are pains in the hip or inguinal region. It may also be considered that the pain is caused by the spine and a spine scan is initiated. The image can also be shown as a linear sclerotic area, and it is more obvious on CT than X-ray. MR can show bone marrow edema and is associated with a low signal fracture line. When a failure fracture is found, other predilection sites should be carefully examined. Pelvic stress fracture is a process of repeated injury and repair. Generally, there is no obvious displacement of fractures, which may show irregular fracture lines or a large number of calluses. These with the condition may be misdiagnosed with tumors or infections, which lead to unnecessary aggressive treatment. Its treatment is mainly non-weight-bearing rest so as not to continue the activity and delay the healing of the fracture.

1. Comparison between X-ray and CT of iliac pathological fractures due to multiple metastatic tumors of the pelvis
   1.1. X-ray (Fig. 18.20a, b)

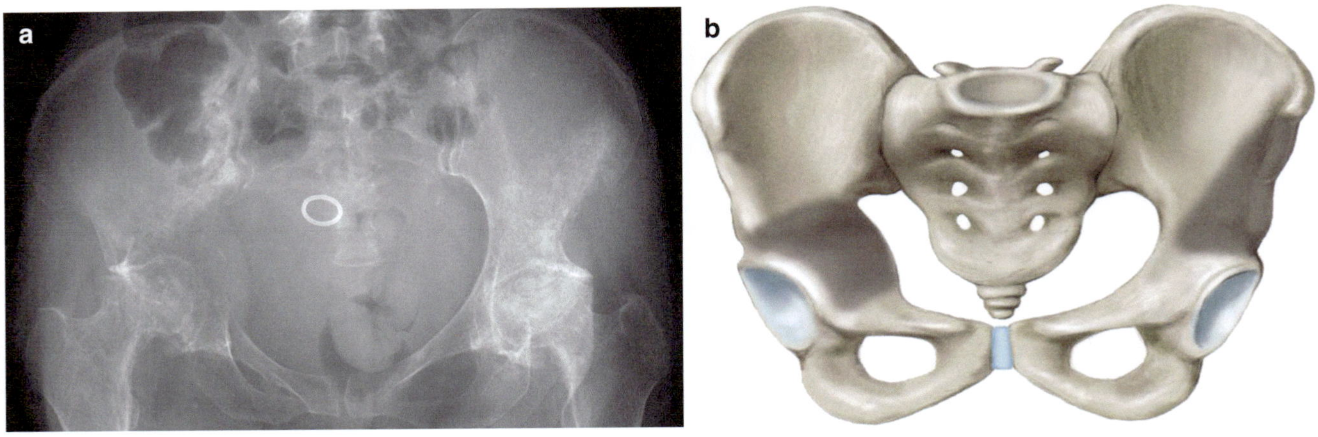

Fig. 18.20 The X-ray (**a**) shows the osteolytic destruction of the right acetabulum. With the insertion of the broken ends, the fracture is above the acetabulum. With the narrowing hip joint space, the left ilium shows sclerosis and bilateral femoral head become compressed. (**b**)

   1.2. CT (Fig. 18.20c, d)

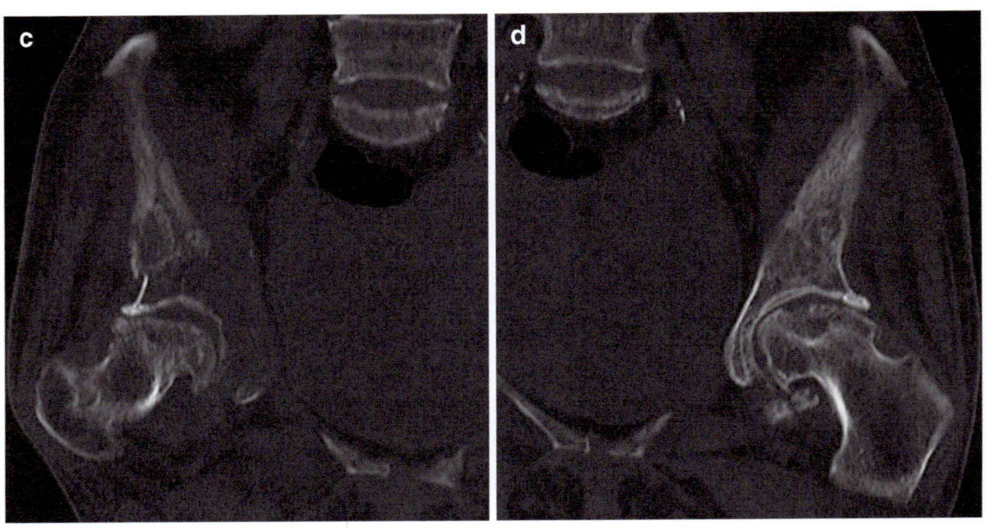

Fig. 18.20 Coronal surface of CT (**c**) shows the right acetabular osteolytic destruction, pathological fracture of the ilium, slightly dislocation of the broken ends, soft tissue mass inside, flattening femoral head, and osteophytes on the margin of the acetabulum. Coronal surface of CT (**d**) shows the left iliac sclerosis with uneven density, flattening left femoral head, and narrowing hip joint space

2. Comparison between X-ray and CT of iliac metastatic tumors with pathological fractures
   2.1. X-ray (Fig. 18.21a, b)

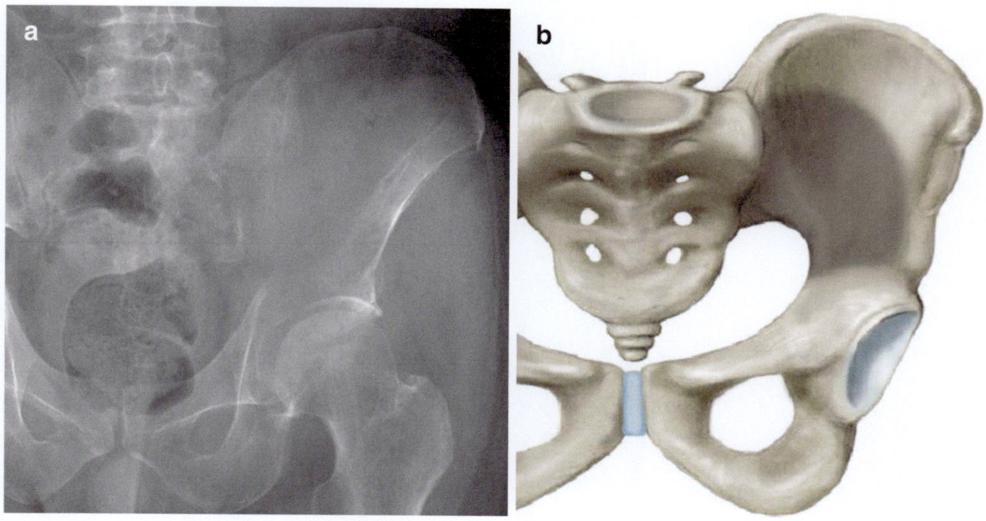

Fig. 18.21 X-ray (**a**) shows the osteolytic destruction of the left ilium, the irregular outer margin of the iliac cortex, and the defect of the inner iliac cortex (**b**)

   2.2. CT (Fig. 18.21c)

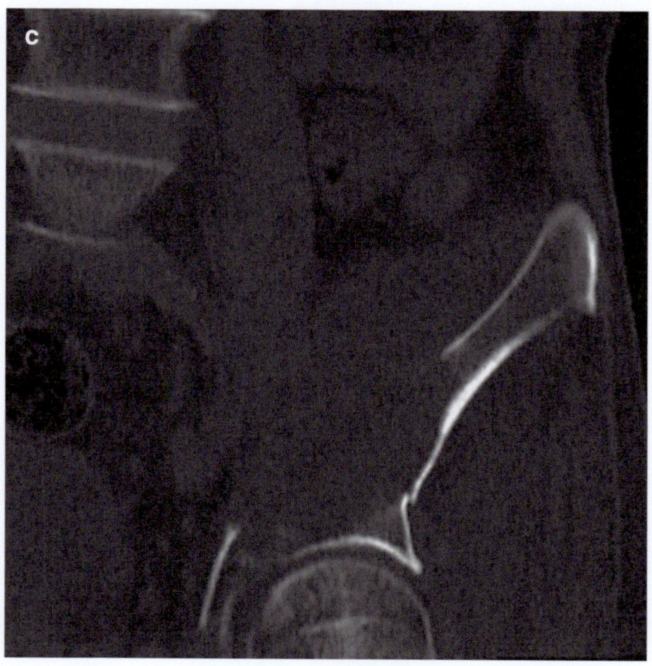

Fig. 18.21 The coronal surface of CT (**c**) shows the osteolytic destruction of the left ilium, the defect of the medial cortex, the soft tissue mass, the pathological fracture outside the iliac cortex, and slight dislocation of the broken ends

3. Comparison between X-ray and CT of iliac osteosarcoma with pathological fractures
   3.1. X-ray (Fig. 18.22a, b)

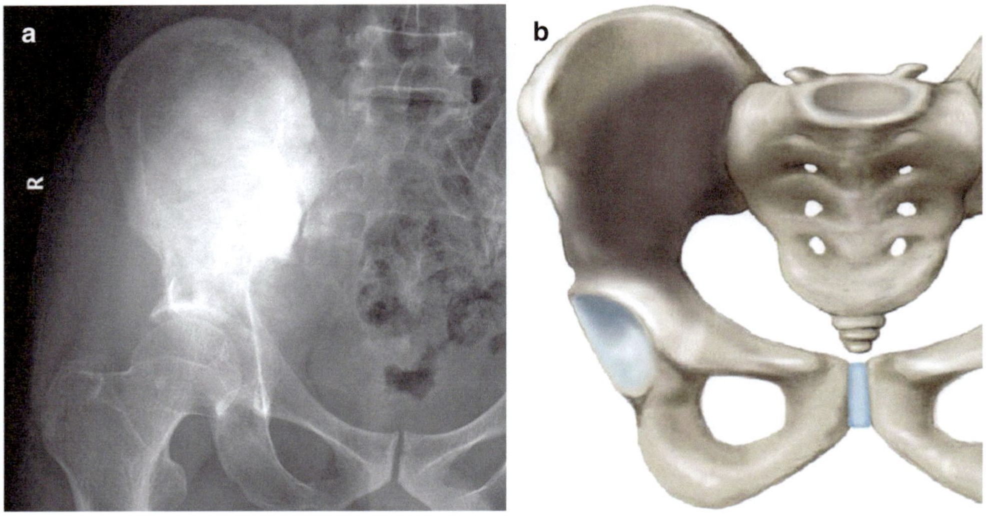

Fig. 18.22 X-ray (**a**) shows the osteogenic destruction of the right ilium, increased osteal density, unclear boundary, and radial periosteal reaction (**b**)

   3.2. CT (Fig. 18.22c)

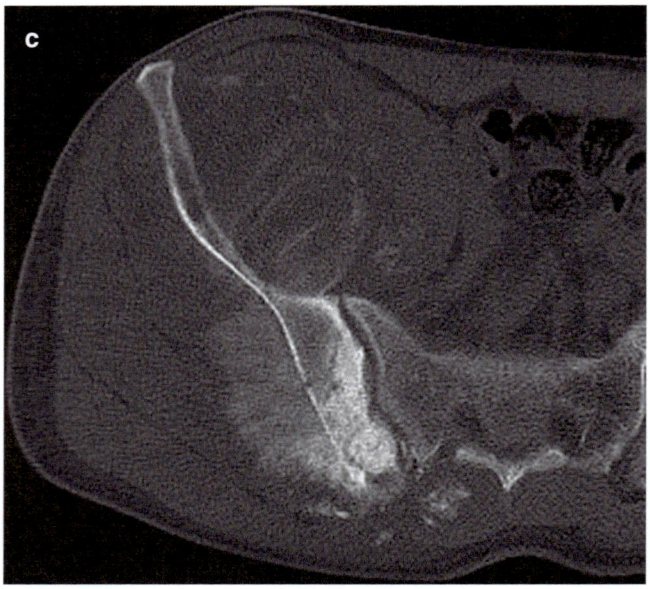

Fig. 18.22 The cross section of CT (**c**) shows the mixed osteoid destruction of the right ilium. The iliac ala shows punctiform osteolytic destruction. The sacroiliac joint of the ilium is mainly osteoblast, and the lateral osteocortex is broken. Shadow with low linear density, radial periosteal reaction, and the soft tissue mass can be seen

4. Comparison between X-ray and CT of superior ramus of the pubis with pathological fracture
   4.1. X-ray (Fig. 18.23a, b)

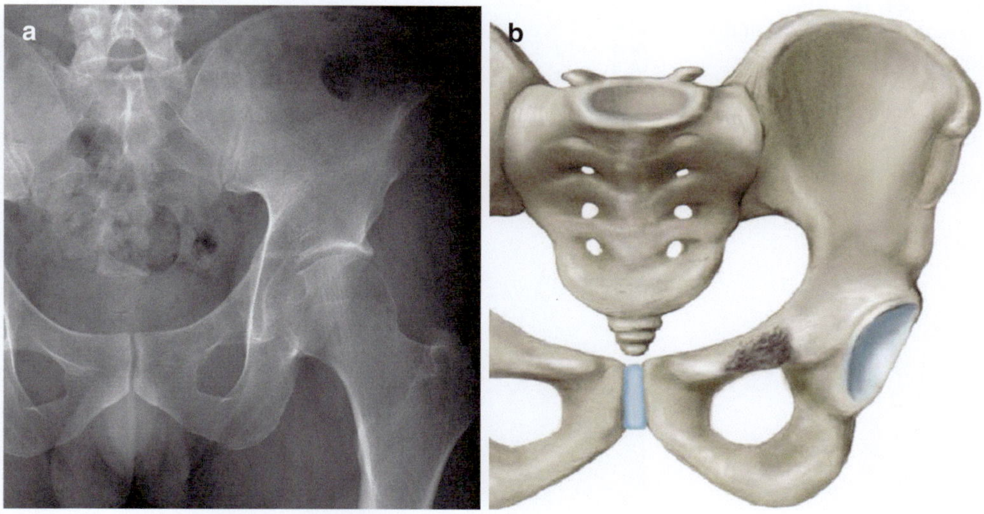

Fig. 18.23 X-ray (**a**) shows infiltrative osseous destruction of the left superior ramus of the pubis (**b**)

   4.2. CT (Fig. 18.23c–e)

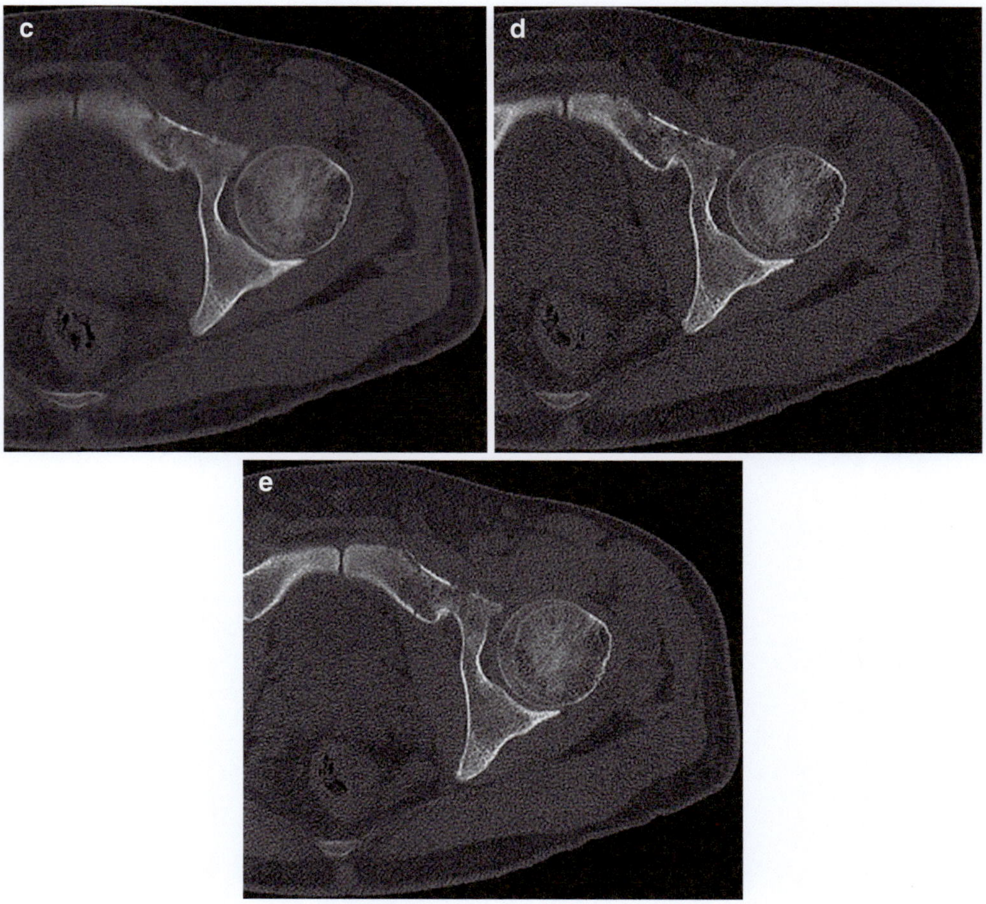

Fig. 18.23 Cross-section of CT (**c–e**) shows infiltrative osseous destruction of the left superior ramus of the pubis, uneven density, disordered structure, fractures of the anterior and posterior cortical bone, and no obvious dislocation of the broken ends

5. Comparison of X-ray, CT, and MR of sacral failure fractures
   5.1. X-ray (Fig. 18.24a, b)

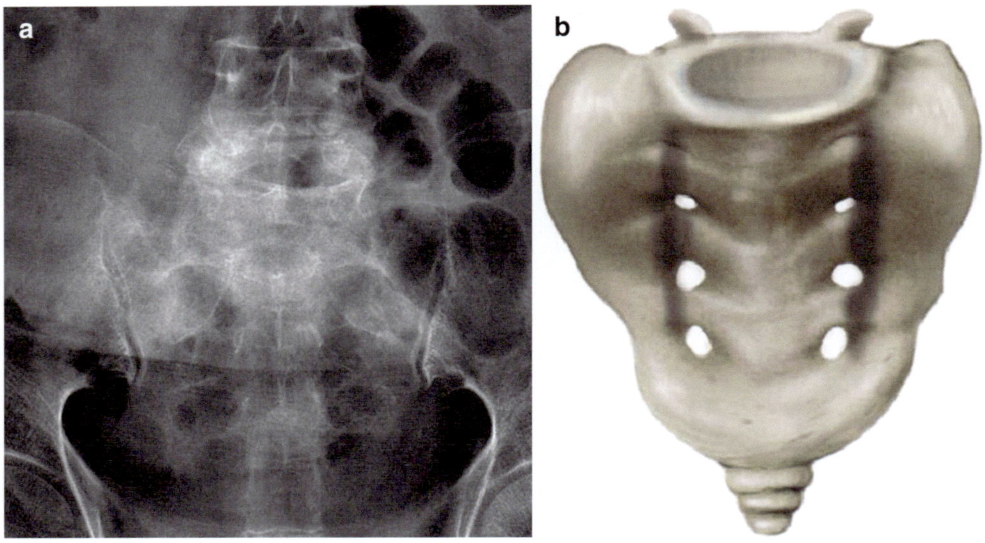

Fig. 18.24 (**a**) In the anteroposterior position of the lumbosacral junction and sacrum, bone structure is messy with increased density. (**b**)

5.2. CT (Fig. 18.24c–f)

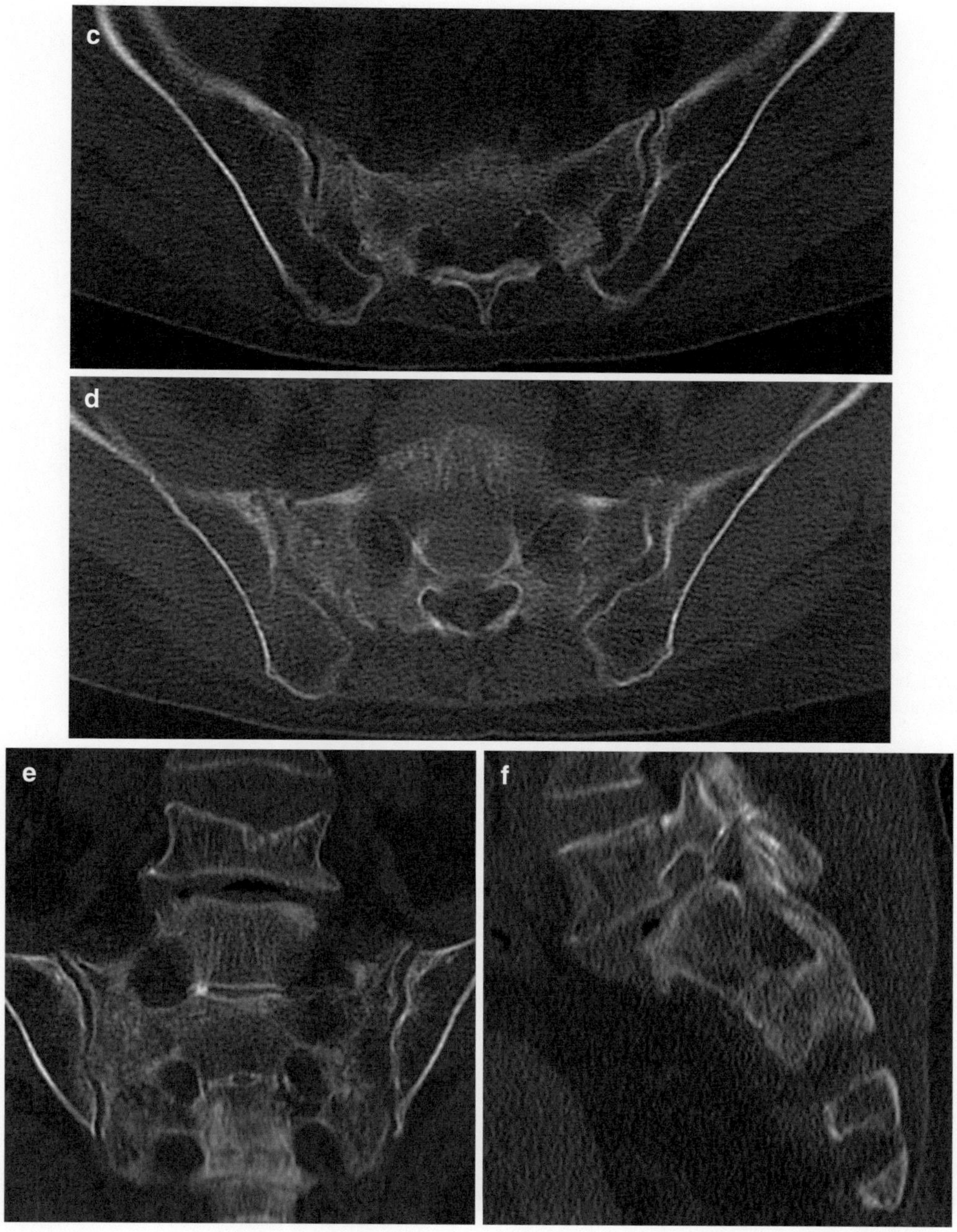

Fig. 18.24 (**c**, **d**) Horizontal axis of CT shows dense high-density lines in bilateral sacrum 1st region and fractures on the right side. (**e**) Reconstruction of coronal CT shows irregular high-density lines walking along the bilateral sacroiliac joint in sacrum I region. The upper margin of the bilateral sacrum is discontinuous, and the right side is obvious. (**f**) Reconstruction of sagittal CT shows the L5 vertebral body's slipping forward (II degrees), defect of vertebral arch isthmus, and vacuum signs between lumbar and sacral intervertebral disc

5.3. MR (Fig. 18.24g)

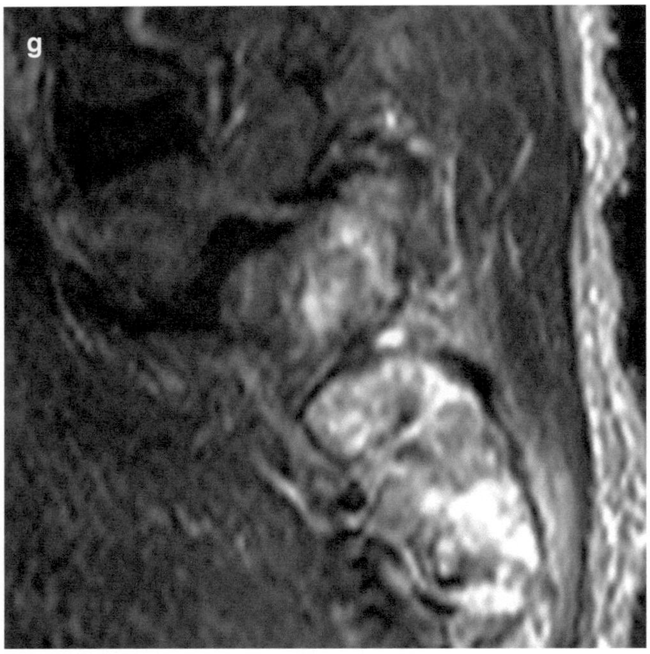

Fig. 18.24 (**g**) In fat-suppression T2WI sequence, sagittal MR shows L5 vertebral body's sliding forward (II degrees) and high signal of sacral vertebra in the bone marrow edema region. In this case, it is the fifth lumbar (II degree) slip with failure fractures of bilateral sacrum 1st area. Failure fractures of the sacrum can be better characterized by MR scanning on the coronal or oblique position

6. Comparison of X-ray, CT, and MR on pubic failure fractures
   6.1. X-ray (Fig. 18.25a, b)

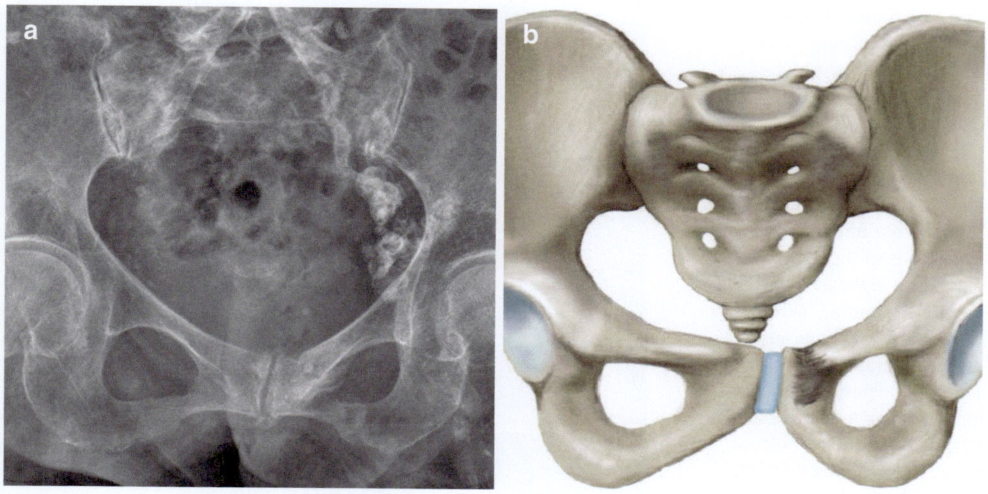

Fig. 18.25 (**a**) In the anteroposterior position, the pelvis is slightly deformed. With increased density, the upper and lower ramus of the left pubis and the symphysis of the pubis are irregularly deformed. The lower ramus of the pubis shows a low-density region and bilateral sclerosis. The lower lumbar spine degenerates and the density of sacrum is not uniform with overlapping high density in the 1st and 2nd right sacrum areas. Calcified image aggregates on the left side of pelvis (**b**)

   6.2. CT (Fig. 18.25c, d)

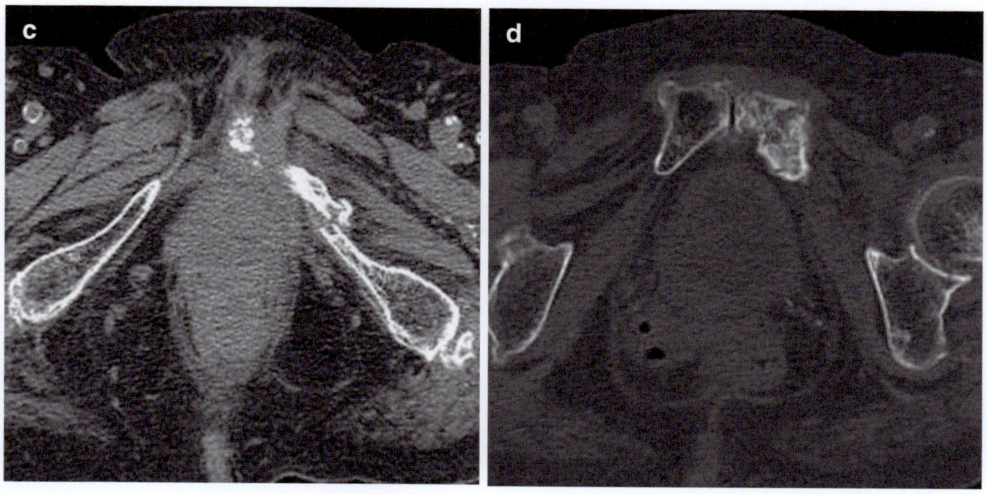

Fig. 18.25 (**c**, **d**) Horizontal axis of CT shows discontinuity of the left lower ramus and symphysis of the pubis as well as high osseous density

6.3. MR (Fig. 18.25e–i)

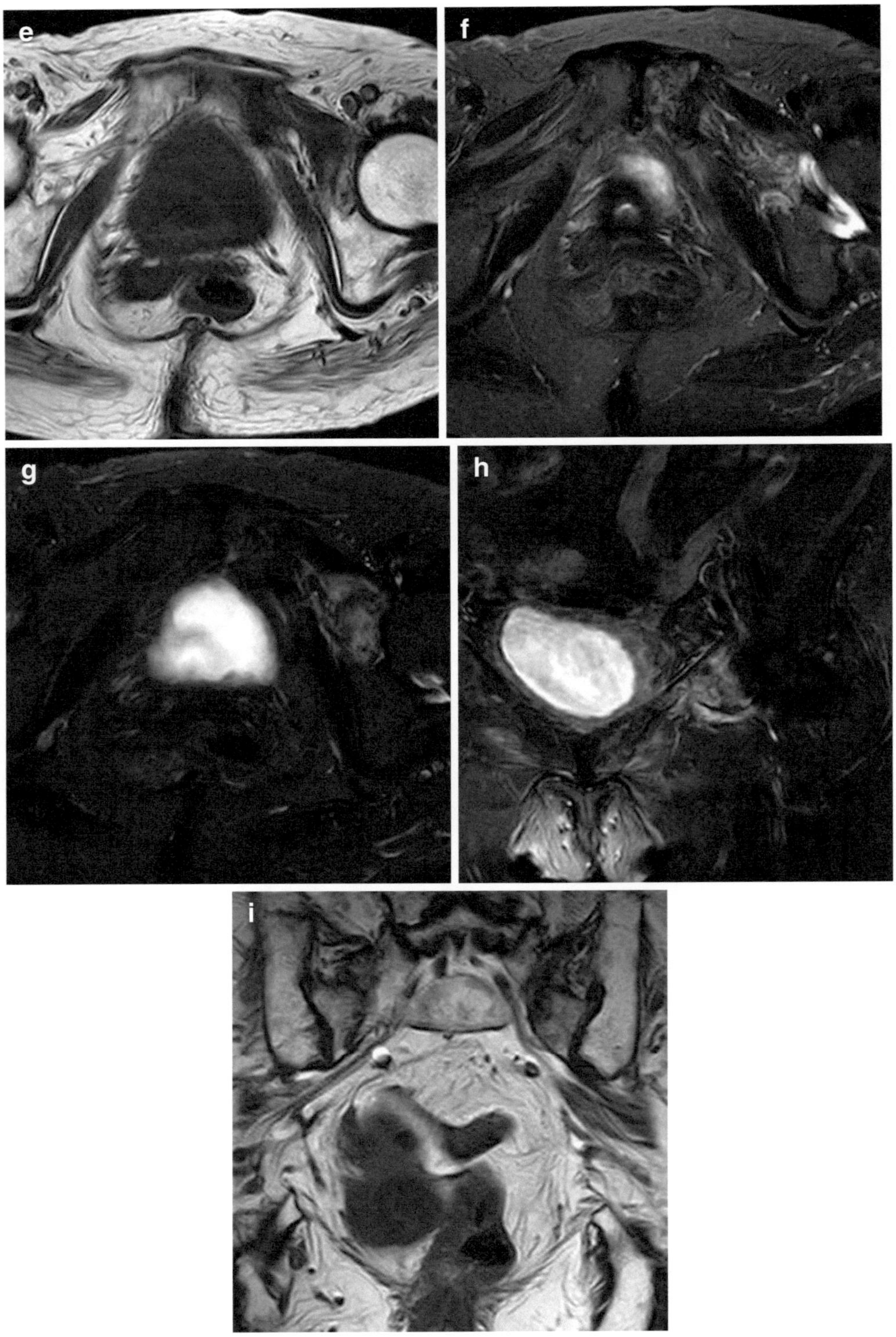

Fig. 18.25 (**e**) (T1WI) and (**f**) (T2WI+FS): the horizontal axis MR shows abnormal bone signal of long T1 and T2 in the left lower ramus and the symphysis of the pubis. (**g**) (T1WI) and (**h**) (T2WI+FS): the coronal MR also shows abnormal long T1 and T2 bone signal at the left lower ramus and the symphysis of the pubis extending to the acetabulum. (**i**) (T1WI) coronal MR shows bone marrow edematous signal in bilateral sacral alar region. The patient was an elderly woman with extensive osteoporosis and no soft tissue mass in the abnormal signal area, which was consistent with the characteristics of multiple failure fractures of the sacrum and pubic bone

7. Comparison between X-ray and CT of pubic failure fractures
   7.1. X-ray (Fig. 18.26a, b)

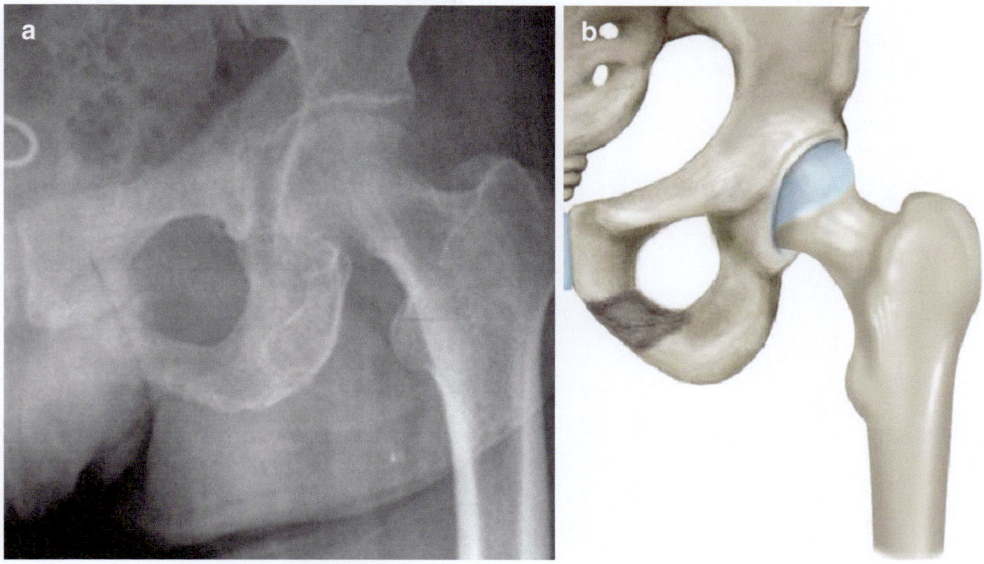

Fig. 18.26 (**a**) In the anteroposterior position of the left inferior and the superior ramus of the pubis, the acetabulum are all discontinuous and locally irregular (**b**)

   7.2. CT (Fig. 18.26c, d)

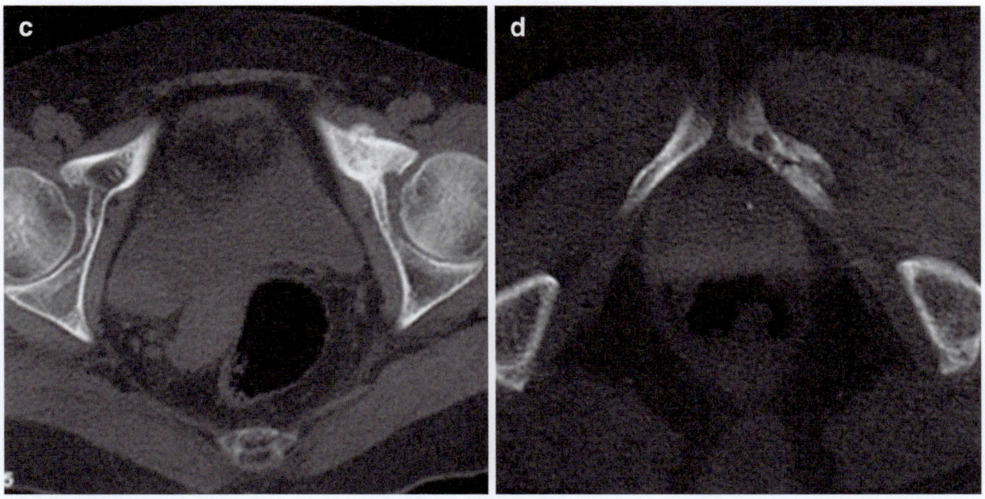

Fig. 18.26 (**c**, **d**) horizontal axis of CT shows discontinuity of the left inferior ramus of the pubis near the symphysis pubis, cystic changes, increased local osseous density, and uneven osseous density near the acetabulum and clumpy callus at the local site. The patient is an elderly woman with a history of rheumatoid arthritis, extensive osteoporosis, and a failure pubic fracture. The fracture line is irregular, and the general shift is not obvious, which can form a large number of callus

8. Comparison between X-ray and CT of pubic failure fractures
   8.1. X-ray (Fig. 18.27a–d)

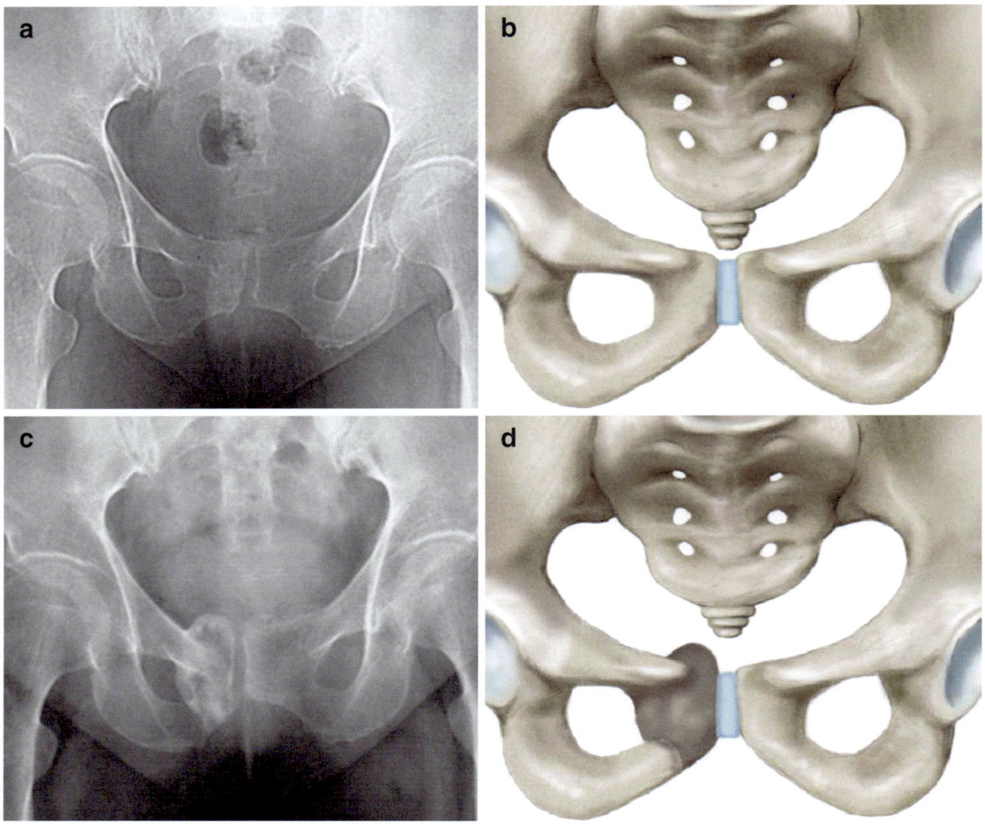

Fig. 18.27 (**a**) the bone density of the normal pelvis is low, and no obvious abnormal structural area is seen (**b**). (**c**) several months later, reexamination of the orthotopic pelvis shows significant bone deformation at the right symphysis pubis (**d**)

   8.2. CT (Fig. 18.27e, f)

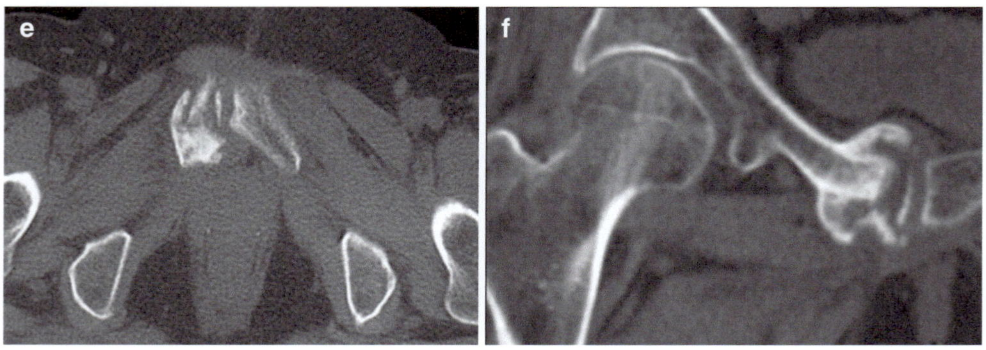

Fig. 18.27 (**e**) Horizontal axis of CT shows discontinuity of bone at the right pubic symphysis, fragmentary bones, and high local bone density. (**f**) Reconstruction of coronal CT shows deformation, discontinuity of bone, and callus at the right symphysis pubis. The patient felt pains in the right inguinal region for 5 months. She was an elderly woman with a history of rheumatoid arthritis and extensive osteoporosis. No abnormalities were found in the first tablet, while MR scan may detect signs of bone marrow edema early. They are features of pubic failure fracture

9. Comparison between X-ray and CT of pubic failure fractures
   9.1. X-ray (Fig. 18.28a, b)

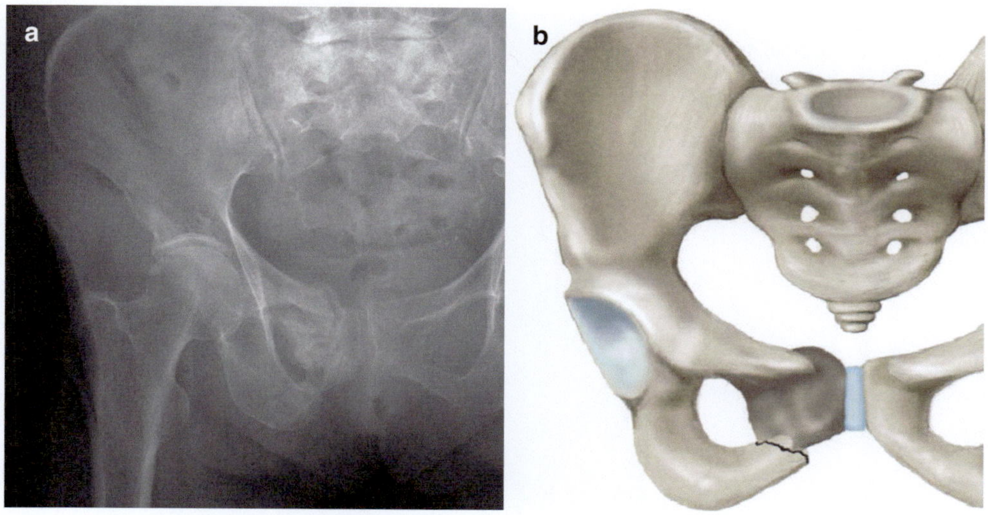

Fig. 18.28 X-ray (**a**) shows the bone deformation of right pubic symphysis, discontinuous fracture of bone as well as dislocation and insertion of broken ends. Schematic diagram (**b**)

   9.2. CT (Fig. 18.28c–e)

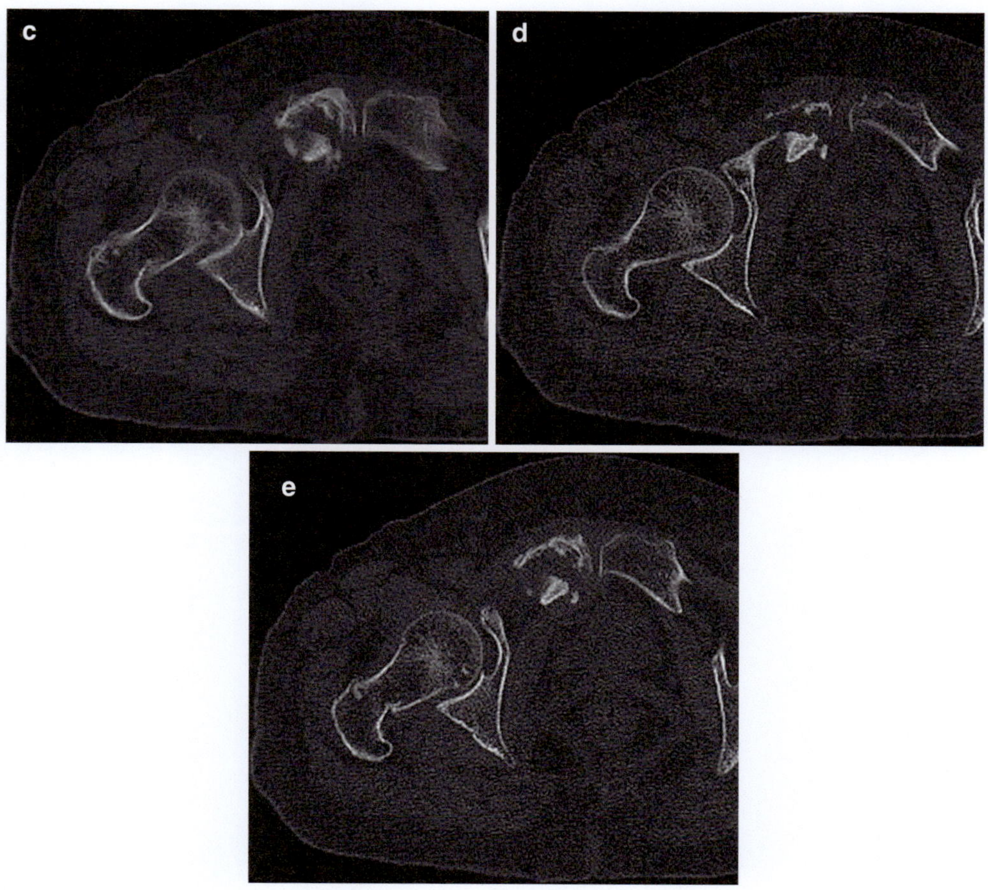

Fig. 18.28 Cross section of CT (**c**–**e**) shows the deformation of the symphysis pubis at the right side, fragmentary and discontinuous bone, and formation of callus

10. Comparison between X-ray and CT of sacral failure fractures
    10.1. X-ray (Fig. 18.29a, b)

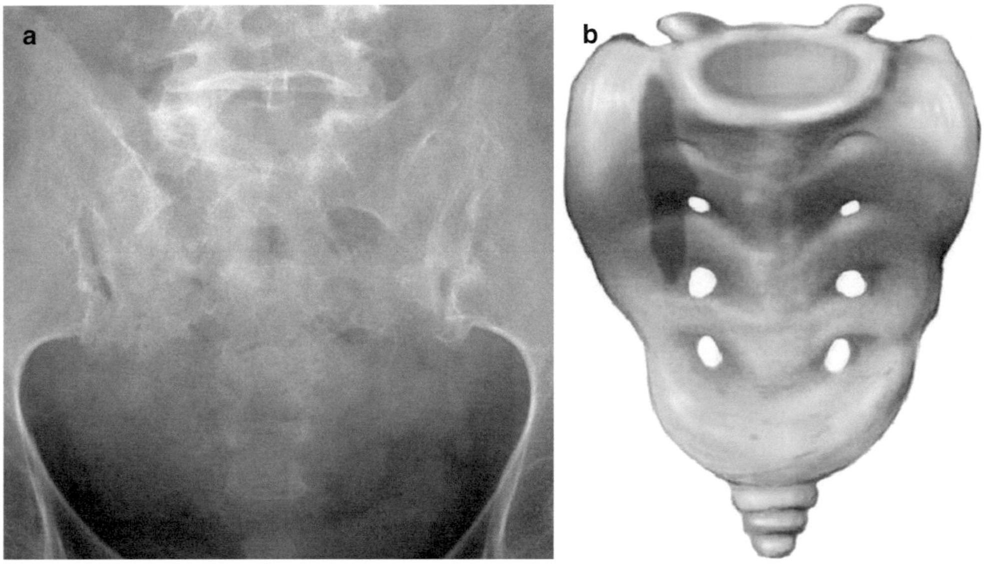

Fig. 18.29 (**a**) In the anteroposterior position, it shows the disordered structure and increased density of the right sacrum ala (**b**)

10.2. CT (Fig. 18.29c–e)

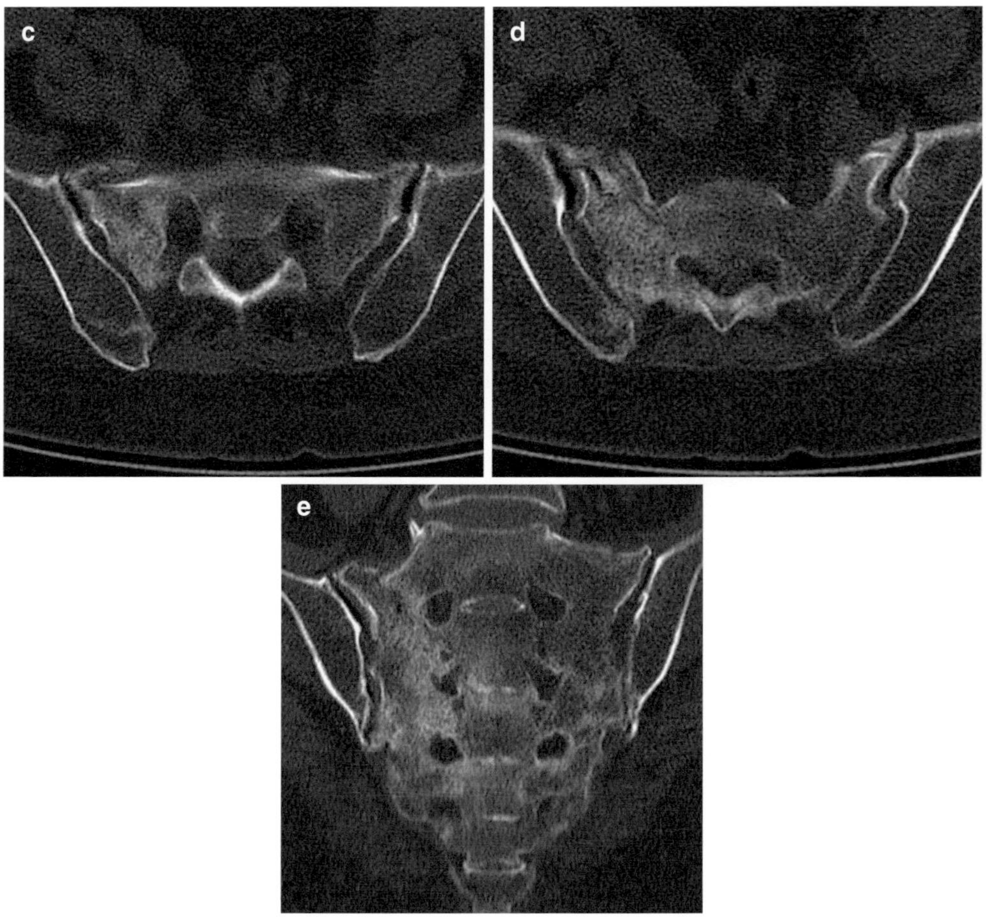

Fig. 18.29 (**c**, **d**) In horizontal axis, CT shows dense high-density lines in the I region of the right sacrum. (**e**) Reconstruction of coronal CT shows that irregular high-density lines in bilateral sacrum I region walking along the bilateral sacroiliac joint. The upper margin of the bilateral sacrum was discontinuous, and it was more obvious the right side

11. Comparison of X-ray and CT of sacral failure fracture
    11.1. X-ray (Fig. 18.30a, b)

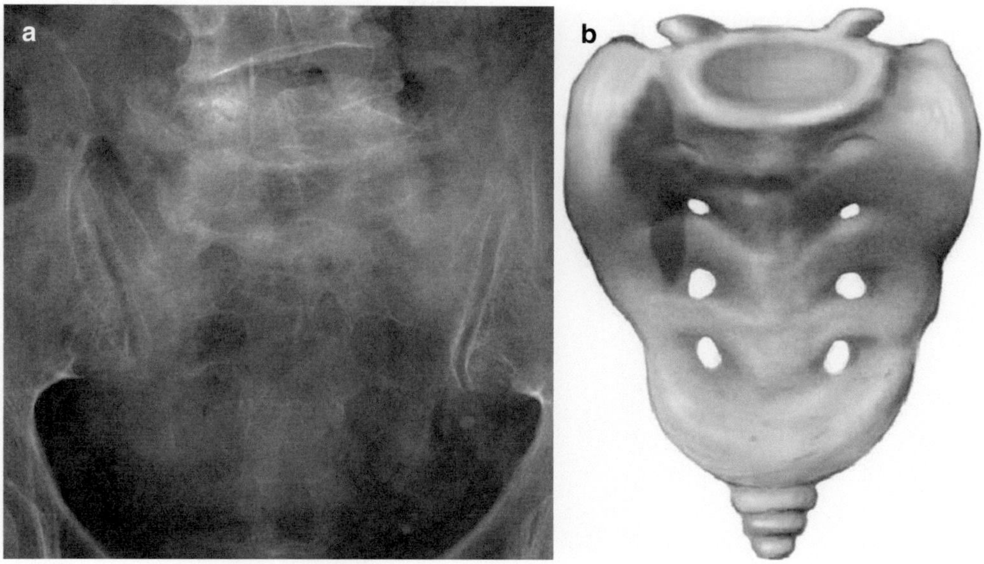

Fig. 18.30 (**a**) In the anteroposterior position, it shows the disordered structure and increased density of the right sacrum ala (**b**)

    11.2. CT (Fig. 18.30c–e)

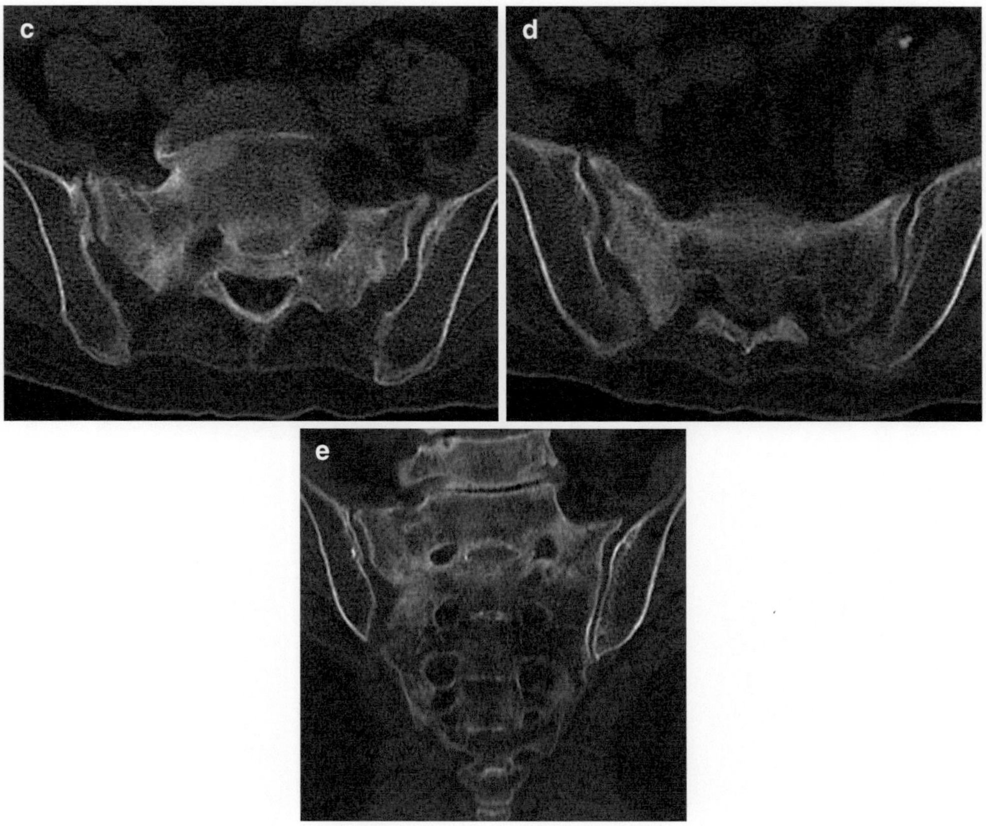

Fig. 18.30 (**c**, **d**) In horizontal axis, CT shows dense high-density lines in the I region of the right sacrum. (**e**) Reconstruction of coronal CT shows irregular high-density lines in bilateral sacrum I region walking along the bilateral sacroiliac joint. The upper margin of the bilateral sacrum was discontinuous, and it was more obvious the right side

12. Comparison of X-ray, CT, and MR of sacral failure fractures
    12.1. X-ray (Fig. 18.31a–d)

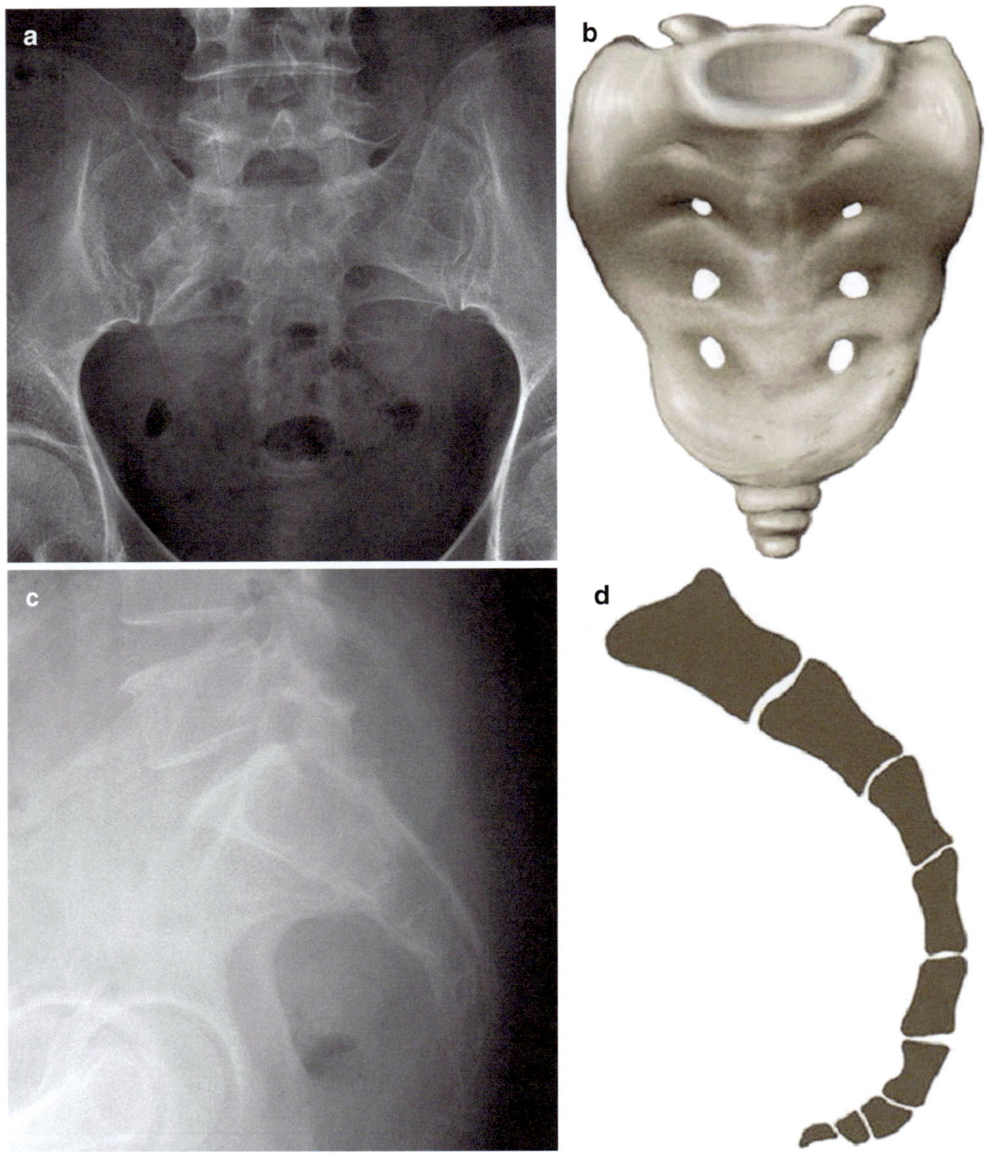

Fig. 18.31 (**a**, **c**) No positive signs were found on the X-ray. Schematic diagram (**b**, **d**)

12.2. CT (Fig. 18.31e, f)

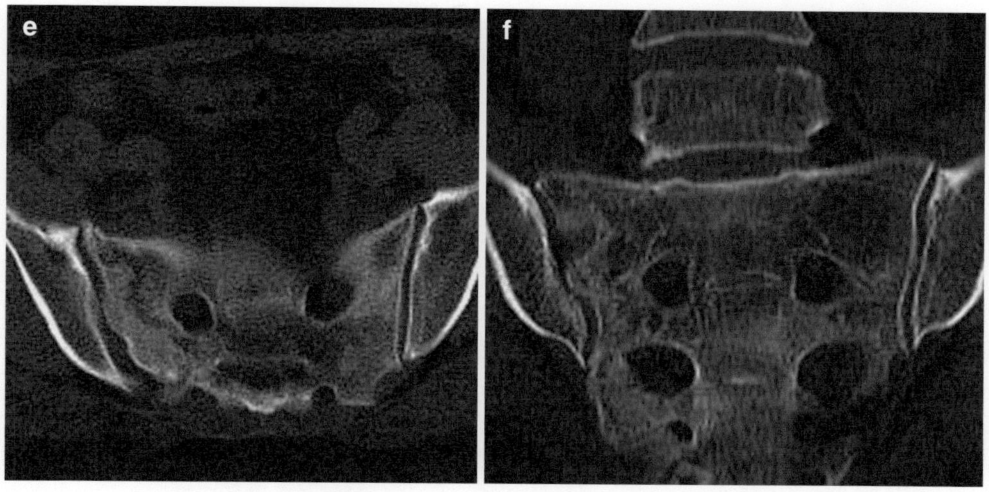

Fig. 18.31 (**e**, **f**) Coronal and cross-sectional view of CT shows the fracture line shadow of the right sacrum accessory, sclerosis on the edge of bone, and no shadow of paravertebral tumors

12.3. MR (Fig. 18.31g, h)

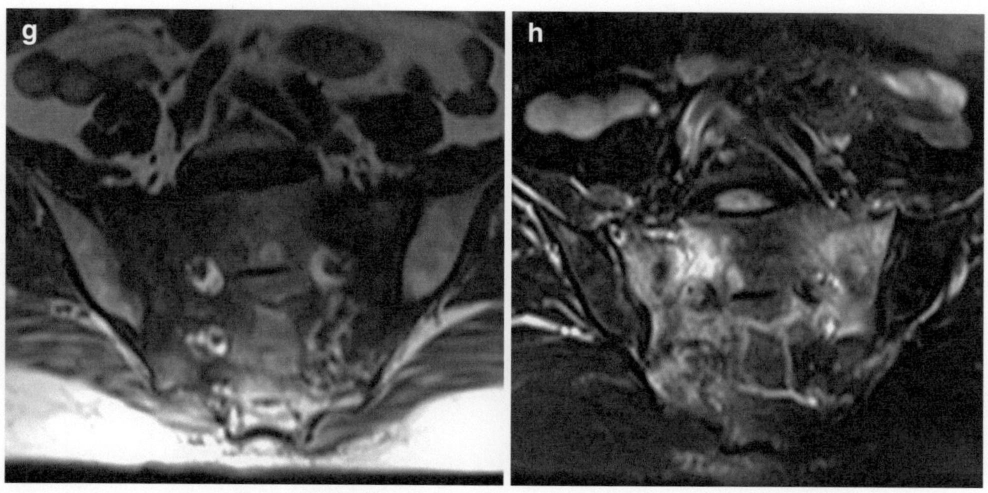

Fig. 18.31 (**g**) A 59-year-old female felt pain in bilateral hip more than 10 days. More than 20 days ago, she began to engage in a kind of physical labor (winding a windlass). Working about 5 hours a day, she felt pains in her bilateral hip. The coronal MR (T1WI) shows the bone marrow edema signal in the bilateral sacrum pterygium. (**h**) (Fat inhibition T2WI) It shows the patchy high signal in the attachment of bilateral sacrum. No heterocyst was found in the pathological biopsy

13. Comparison of X-ray and CT of sacral failure fracture
    13.1. X-ray (Fig. 18.32a, b)

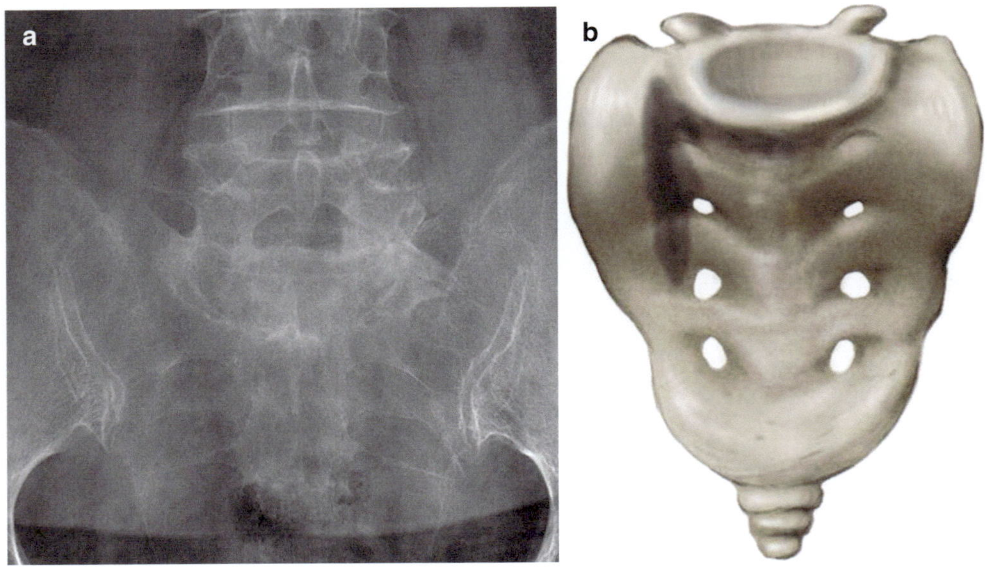

Fig. 18.32 (**a**) Slightly high density of bars in the right sacral vertebra and 1st sacral vertebra (**b**)

    13.2. CT (Fig. 18.32c, d)

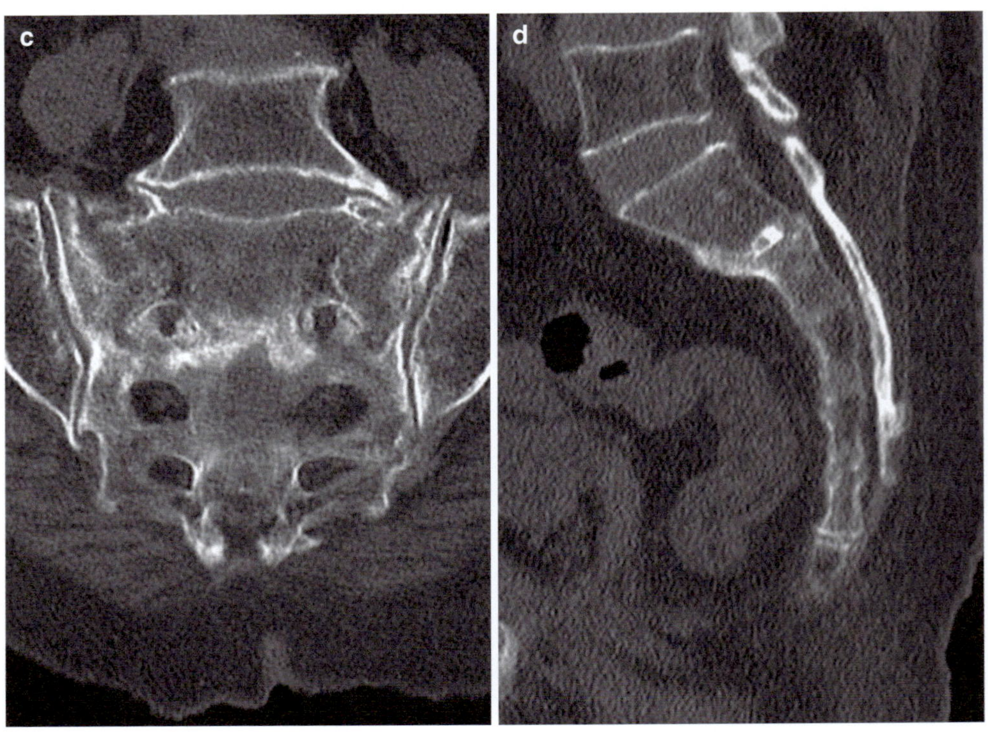

Fig. 18.32 (**c**, **d**) There were lumbosacral pains in 10 months after percutaneous vertebroplasty. Reconstruction of CT shows the discontinuity of sacral vertebral and left pubic branch, increased local bone density and shadow of the local fragment. MR images show local high signals in the sacrum and the left ramus of the pubis

14. Comparison of X-ray, CT, and MR of sacral failure fractures
    14.1. X-ray (Fig. 18.33a–d)

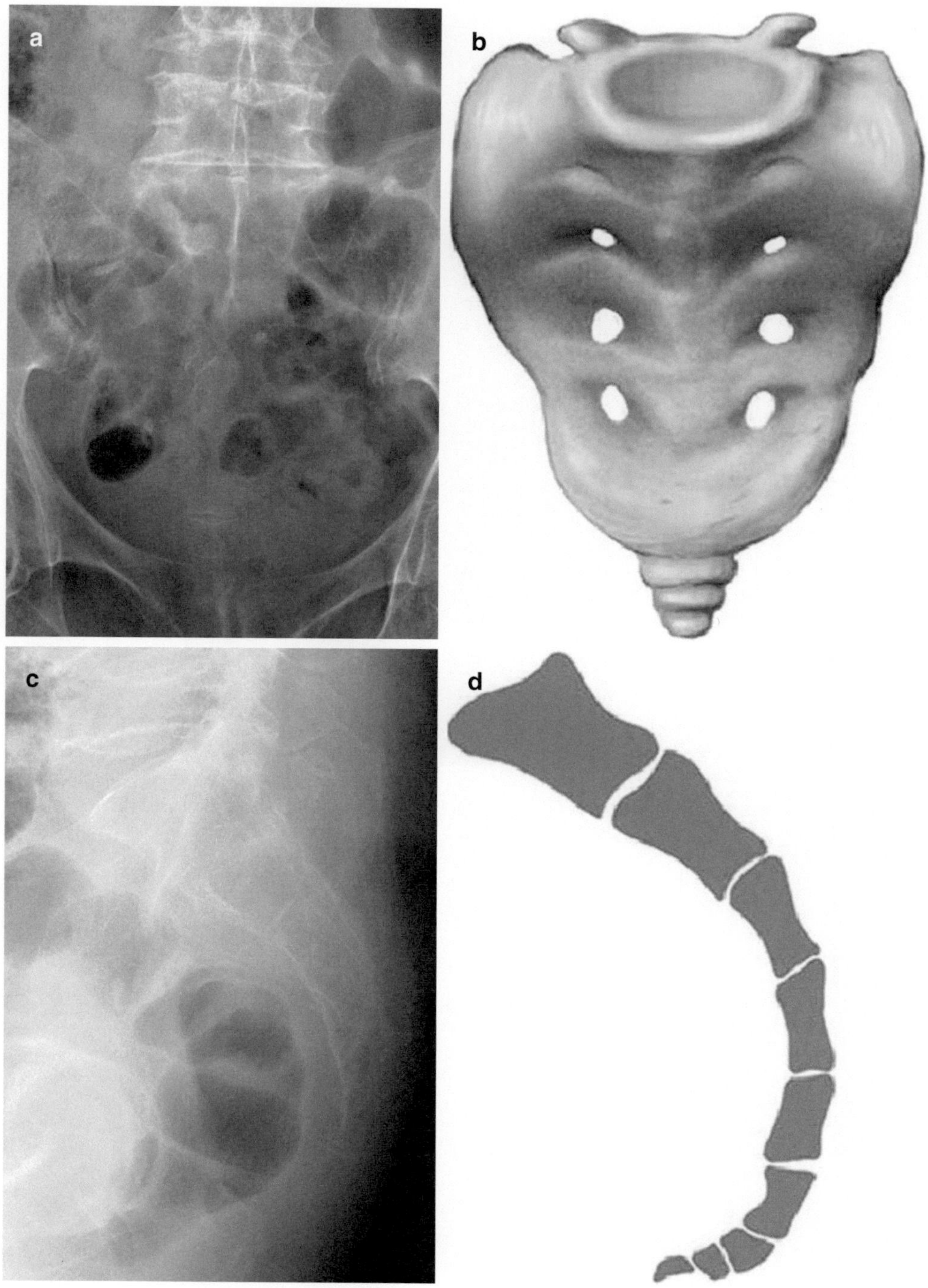

Fig. 18.33 (**a**, **c**) no obvious abnormality was observed (normal lateral position of sacrum). Schematic diagram (**b**, **d**)

14.2. CT (Fig. 18.33e)

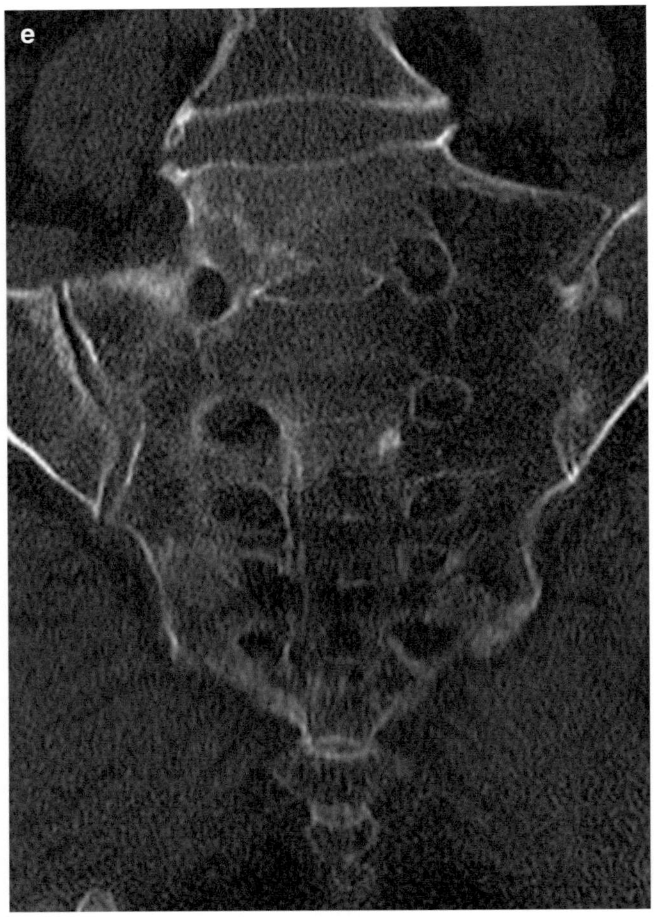

Fig. 18.33 (**e**) Reconstruction of coronal CT shows high-density images of sacral 1st vertebral body line

14.3. MR (Fig. 18.33f–h)

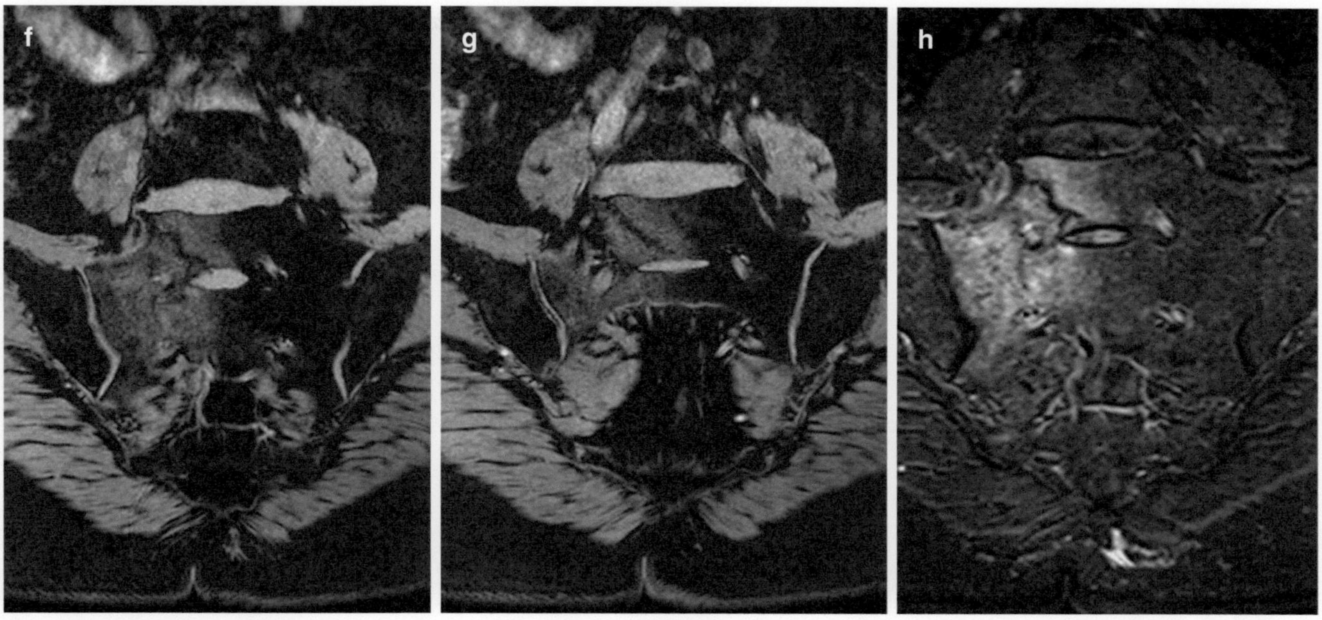

Fig. 18.33 (**f–h**) MR shows the low bar signal of sacral 1st vertebral body and the high signal shadow of T2 on the right of sacral 1st–3rd vertebral body

18.3 Summary

1. The spine and pelvis are the most common sites for pathological fractures. There are different kinds of pathologic fractures in different age groups. Acidophilic granuloma is more common in children, while giant cell tumor of bone is common in young adults. Metastatic tumors, multiple myeloma, osteoporosis, and hematologic disorders are all common in middle and old ages. Careful identification of each type is important and should be paid great attention.
2. Pathological fractures occur on the basis of bone damage caused by tumors, inflammation, and systemic diseases, and there is no definite history of trauma or minor trauma. For patients with lumbar and back pain, it is necessary to consider the possibility of the pathological fractures and apply appropriate X-ray, CT, and MRI scans to confirm the diagnosis.
3. Osteoporotic vertebral compression fracture shows a general reduction in bone density and typically manifested as double concave deformation of multiple vertebral body. MRI can identify old or fresh compression fractures in multiple deformed vertebral bodies.
4. Pathological compression fracture is caused by spinal tumors. The edge of the vertebral body is generally full and round, and damage of vertebral body or accessory can be seen. Tuberculosis is often seen with paravertebral abscess, compression, and destruction of adjacent vertebral body, and intervertebral disc was often involved. MRI plays an important role in the identification of pathological and common compression fractures.
5. Spinal fractures in patients with ankylosing spondylitis often have no obvious history of trauma and often form false joints.
6. Failure fractures often occur on both sides of the sacrum, and the fracture lines are usually parallel to the sacroiliac joint. The perisymphysis of the pubic ramus, pubic symphysis of the pelvis, and around the acetabulum are also the most common sites for failure fractures.
7. Pathological fractures should be highly suspected when there is no obvious history of trauma or minor trauma. CT or MRI can help determine whether a pathological fracture is present.

Part V

Cartilage and Epiphysis Injury

19 Cartilage and Osteochondral Injury

Jiashen Shao and Yingze Zhang

19.1 Normal Arthrosis Cartilage

The most common cartilage in the body is hyaline cartilage. It cannot be directly displayed on X-ray and CT, only on MRI. The normal shoulder, elbow, wrist, hip, and ankle joints have a uniform thickness of the cartilage and a smooth surface. The T1WI shows a medium signal intensity. The T2WI shows a high and uniform signal (Figs. 19.1, 19.2, 19.3, 19.4, and 19.5). The distribution of cartilage on the lateral tibia of normal knee joints is uneven. The thinnest and thickest partial in the outer side of the humerus is the front partial and the middle partial, respectively. Moreover, the back portion is also thick. The medial and lateral femoral condyle and the medial plateau of the tibia are uniform (Fig. 19.6). Normal knee cartilage is stratified in MRI (Fig. 19.7).

J. Shao · Y. Zhang (✉)
Department of Orthopaedics, The Third Hospital of Hebei Medical University, Shijiazhuang, Hebei, China

Y. Zhang (ed.), *Differential Diagnosis of Fracture*, https://doi.org/10.1007/978-981-13-8339-7_19

1. Normal shoulder articular cartilage and injured cartilage
   1.1. MRI (Fig. 19.1a–d)

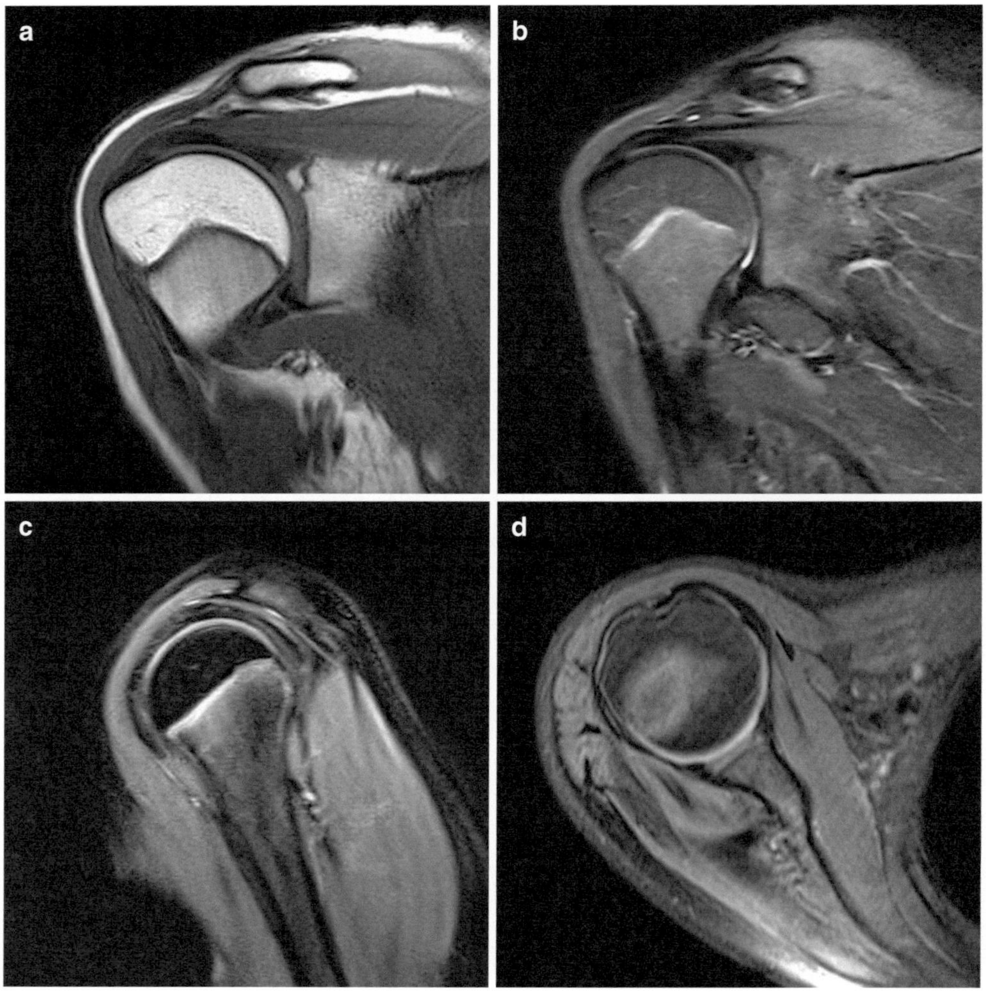

Fig. 19.1 (**a**) and (**b**) shows the oblique coronal plane T1WI and the fat suppression T2WI, respectively. (**c**, **d**) shows the oblique sagittal plane and transverse plane, respectively. Articular cartilage T1WI shows moderate signal intensity. Fat suppression T2WI shows high signal with smooth surface and uniform thickness

2. Normal elbow articular cartilage and injured cartilage
   2.1. MRI (Fig. 19.2a, b)

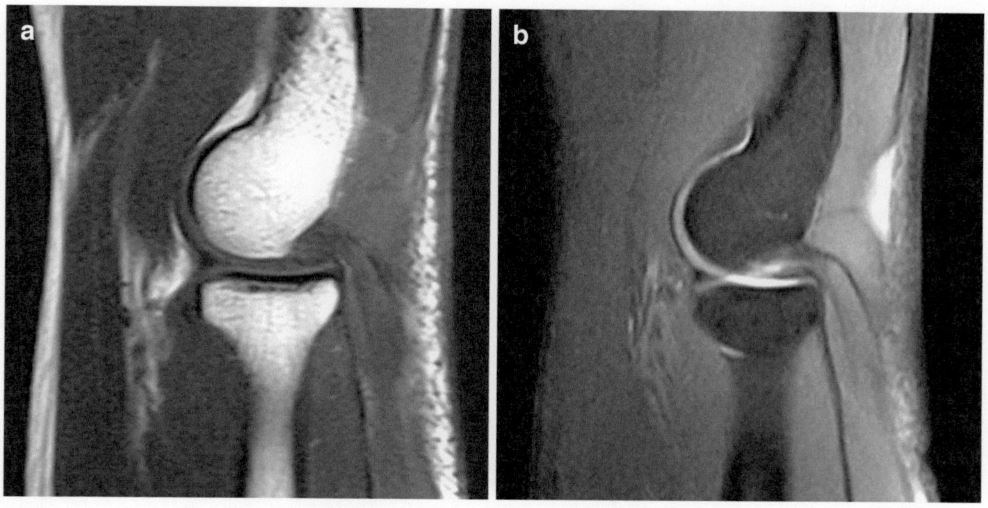

Fig. 19.2 (**a**, **b**) shows MRI sagittal T1WI and fat suppression T2WI, respectively. It shows that the distal humerus and the humeral head cartilage were thin and even with a smooth surface. T1WI shows moderate signal intensity. Fat suppression T2WI shows high signal

3. Normal elbow articular cartilage and injured cartilage
   3.1. MRI (Fig. 19.3a–d)

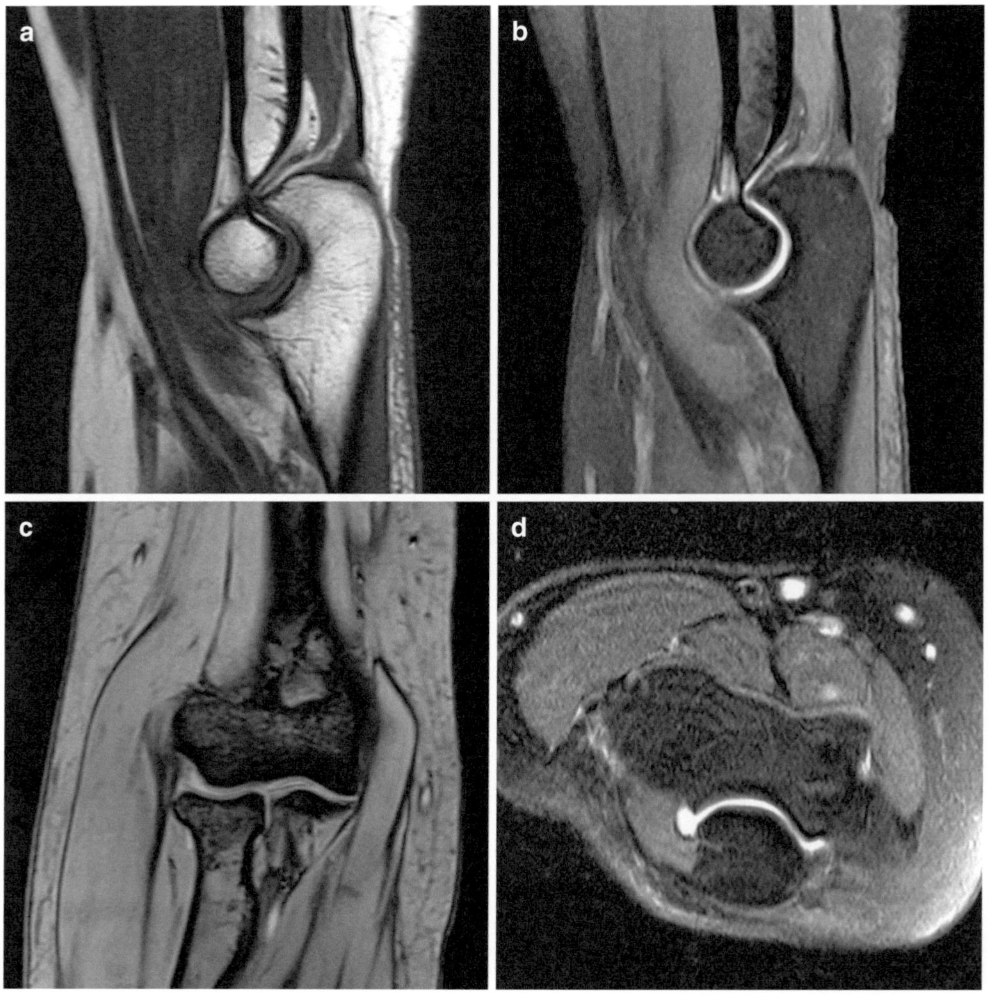

Fig. 19.3 (**a–d**) shows sagittal T1WI, fat-suppressed T2WI, coronal and transverse axis fat-suppressed T2WI, respectively. It shows that the distal end of the humerus, the olecranon, and the proximal humerus had a thin and uniform cartilage with a smooth surface. The T1WI shows moderate signal intensity and the fat suppression T2WI shows a high signal

4. Normal wrist joint cartilage and injured cartilage
   4.1. MRI (Fig. 19.4a, b)

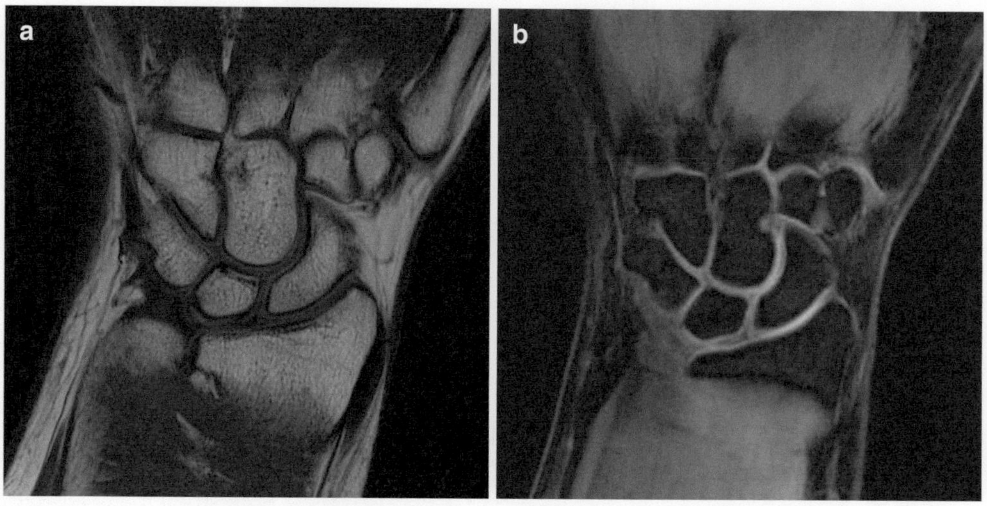

Fig. 19.4 (**a**, **b**) shows coronal T1WI and fat-suppressed T2WI, respectively. It shows the wrist joint, the intercarpal joint, and the ankle joint cartilage with uniform thickness and smooth surface. T1WI shows moderate signal intensity, and fat suppression T2WI shows high signal

5. Normal hip articular cartilage and injured cartilage
   5.1. MRI (Fig. 19.5a–d)

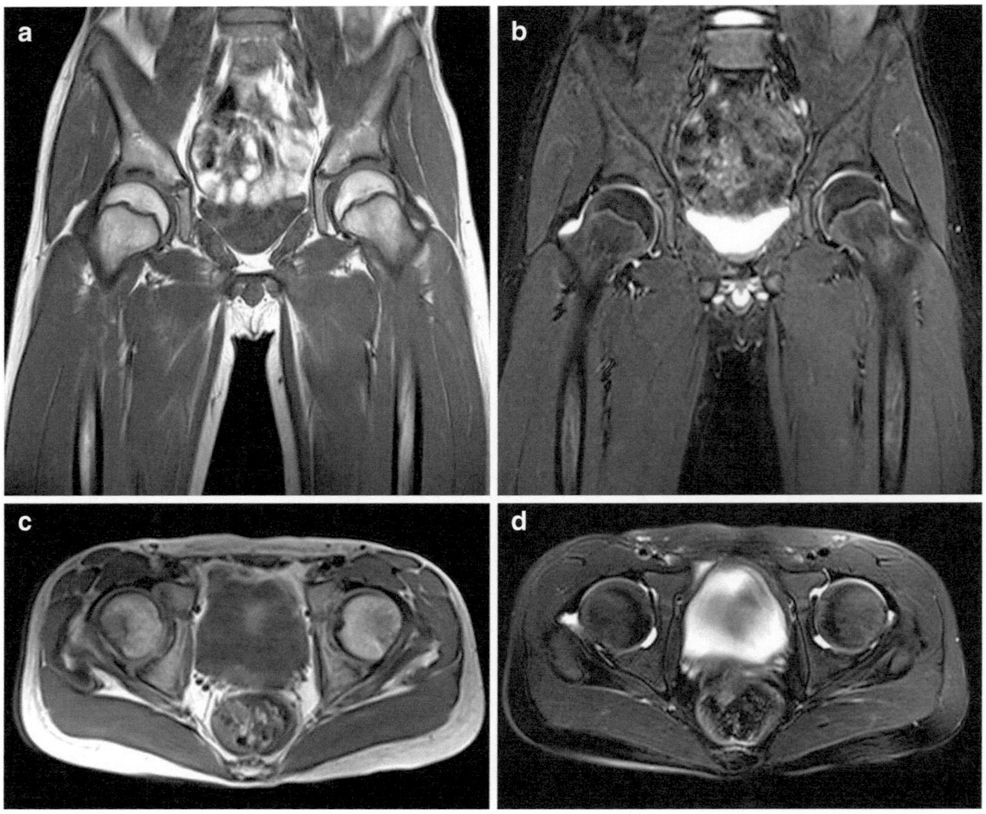

Fig. 19.5 (**a**, **b**) shows coronal T1WI and fat-suppressed T2WI, respectively. (**c**, **d**) are the transverse axis T1WI and the fat suppression T2WI, respectively. It shows that the hip articular cartilage was uniform in thickness and smooth in surface, with moderate signal intensity on T1WI and high signal on T2WI

6. Normal knee joint cartilage and injured cartilage
   6.1. MRI (Fig. 19.6a–f)

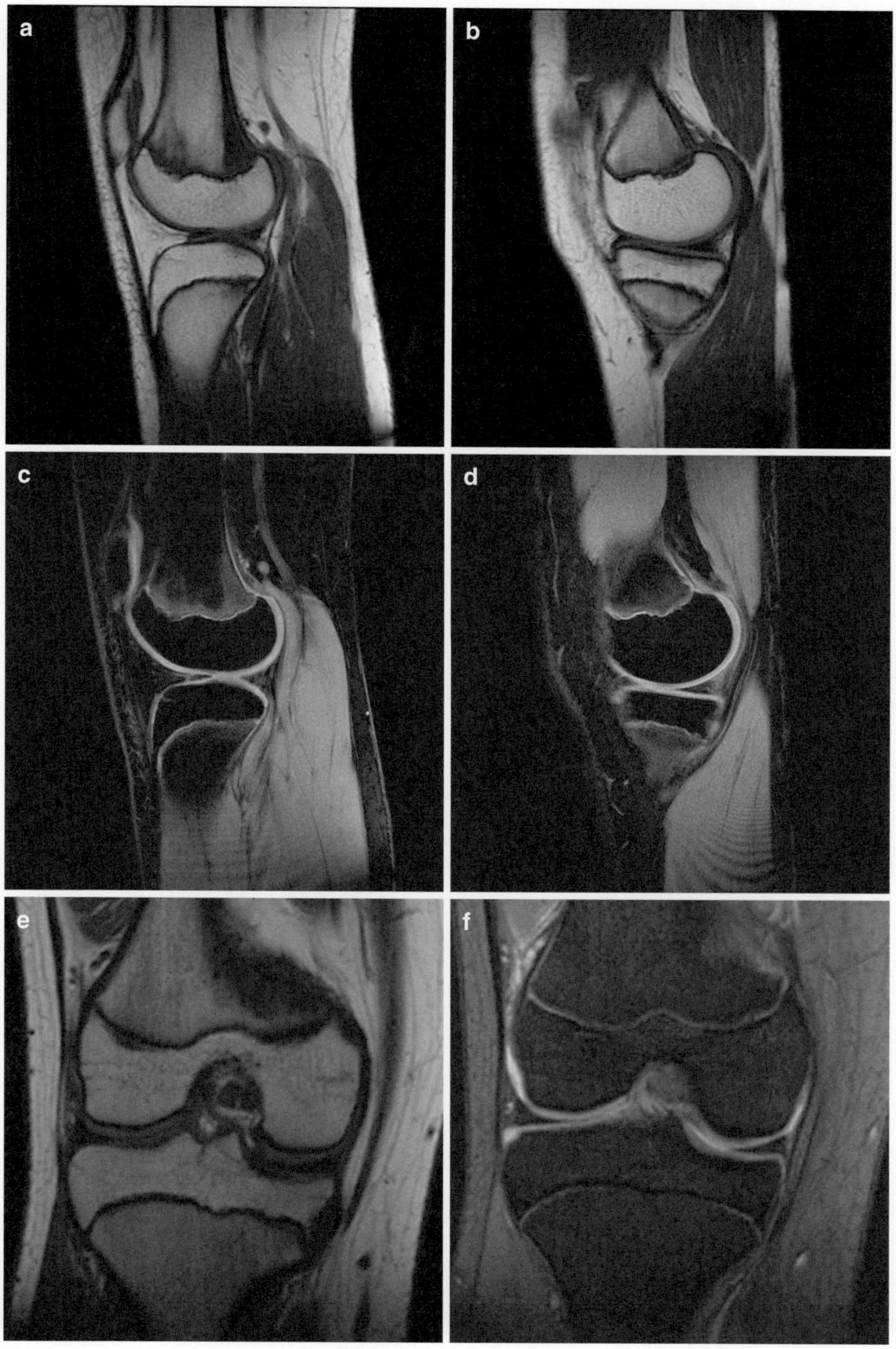

Fig. 19.6 (**a**, **b**) shows the sagittal plane T1WI. It shows the posterior border of the humerus, the internal and external femoral condyles, and the articular cartilage of the medial and lateral tibia. (**c**, **d**) shows sagittal fat inhibition T2WI. It shows that the articular cartilage is a high signal, the thickness of the lateral tibial plateau is inconsistent, and that of the internal and external condyle of the femur and the medial cartilage of the tibial plateau were uniform and the surface was smooth. (**e f**) shows the intermediate level coronal plane T1WI and fat suppression image of T2WI, respectively

7. Normal knee joint cartilage stratification and injured cartilage
   7.1. MRI (Fig. 19.7a, b)

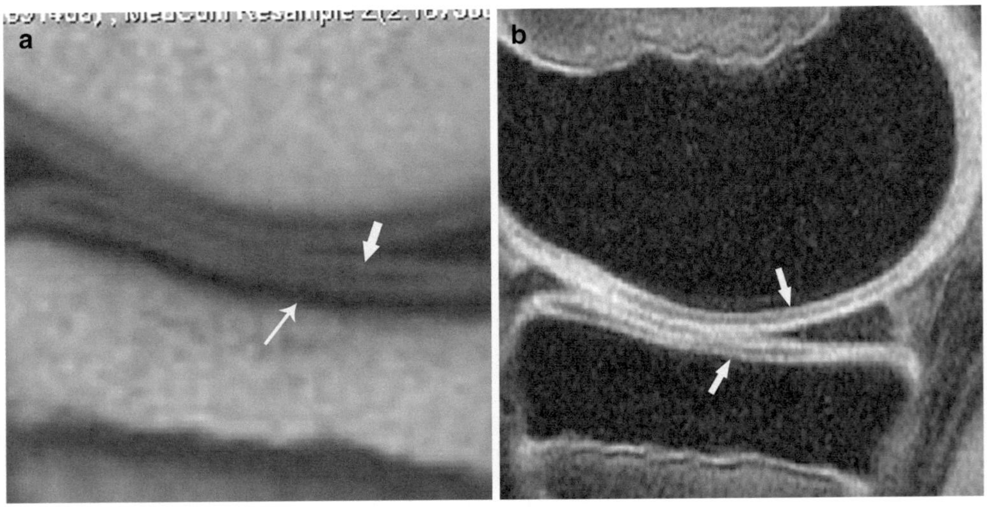

Fig. 19.7 (**a**) shows the MRI sagittal plane T1WI, showing the stratification of the medial plateau of the knee joint. It is divided into three layers. From the joint surface to the deep layer, it is medium signal, low signal and medium signal (rough white arrow), and deep cartilage low signal. The line is the surface of bony joint (white arrow). (**b**) Shows the sagittal fat-inhibiting image of T2WI, showing the stratification of the articular cartilage in the medial malleolus and medial tibial plateau, which is divided into three layers, with high signal, low signal, and high signal from the surface of the articular cartilage to the deep layer (rough white arrow)

8. Normal ankle articular cartilage and injured cartilage
   8.1. MRI (Fig. 19.8a–d)

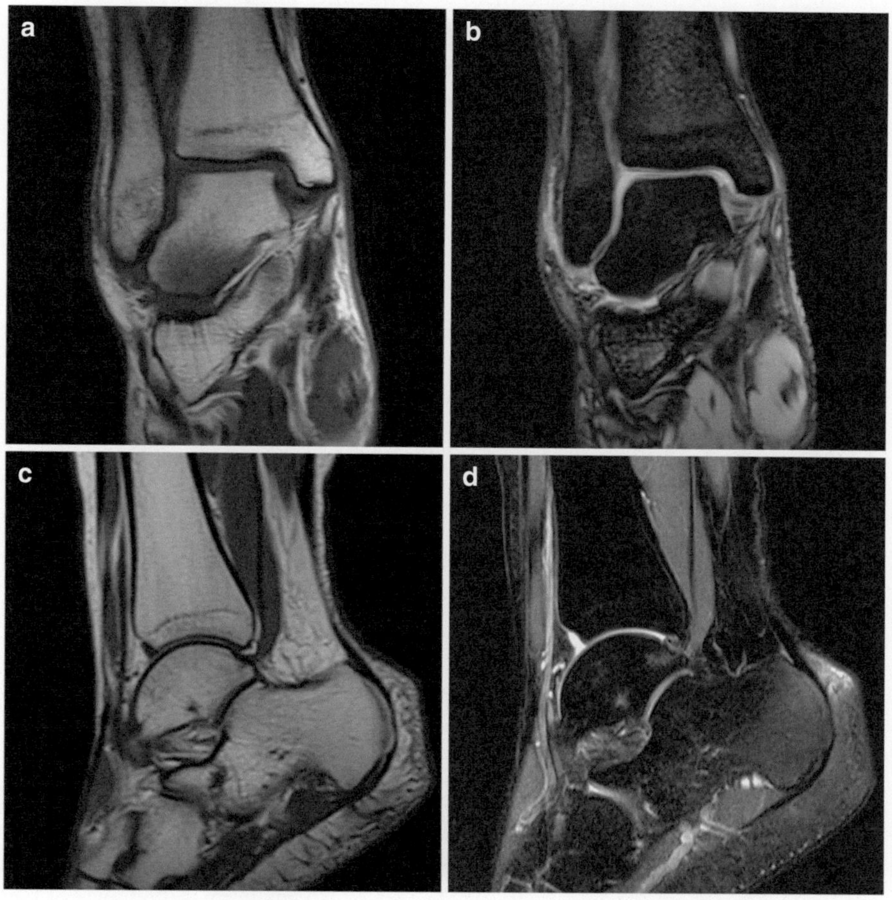

Fig. 19.8 (**a–d**) shows MRI coronal plane T1WI, fat suppression T2WI, sagittal T1WI, and fat suppression T2WI, respectively. It shows that the articular cartilage was thick and uniform with a smooth surface, T1WI shows moderate signal intensity, and fat suppression T2WI shows high signal

19.2 Acute Simple Articular Cartilage Fracture

Acute cartilage injury is defined as cartilage damage within 1 month of trauma, including simple cartilage fracture and osteochondral fracture. Simple cartilage fracture is defined as the articular cartilage continuity interrupted caused by trauma, while the subchondral bone is intact and there is no fracture. The morphology and low signal line of the subchondral on the MRI image were normal, whereas the "articular surface" seen on the X-ray was smooth. Osteochondral fracture is defined as the fracture of articular cartilage together with underneath subchondral bone fracture. Acute simple cartilage fractures are divided into three types:(1) A partial full-thickness defect of the cartilage, which the subchondral bone is visible via arthroscopy; (2) Part of the cartilage grinded and getting thinner; (3) The cartilage fracture is fissure-like, with the fracture being perpendicular or not perpendicular to the articular surface.

19.2.1 Injury Mechanism

Injury is caused by direct or indirect trauma to the cartilage articular surface. Sudden rotational force conducted on the joint surface.

19.2.2 Symptoms and Signs

The main symptom is pain, especially from the joint movement, either actively or passively. Localized swelling distension confined to the joint, occasionally joint lock can be detected. In the case of acute simple cartilage fractures, other structural injuries in the joints, such as the meniscus, cruciate ligament, patella support band, and collateral ligament injury, are often associated.

19.2.3 Differential Diagnosis of Imaging

MRI shows articular cartilage fracture or defect, bone marrow edema appeared in the adjacent site, and it was a map-like T1WI low signal and T2WI high signal area. X-ray and CT cannot show articular cartilage. Therefore, the distinction between simple cartilage fractures and osteochondral fractures is mainly based on MRI evaluation. Acute simple articular cartilage fractures are obscure, even the MRI scan also easily miss diagnosis of these fractures. Therefore, given some cases where the patient's severe clinical symptoms are inconsistent with the MRI findings, a great attention should be brought to the clinician to identify the definite diagnosis. Otherwise, it would delay the timely treatment, and even affect the prognosis, causing patients long-term pain and dysfunction of the knee joint.

1. Local full-thickness defects of knee articular cartilage and normal cartilage
    1.1. MRI (Fig. 19.9)

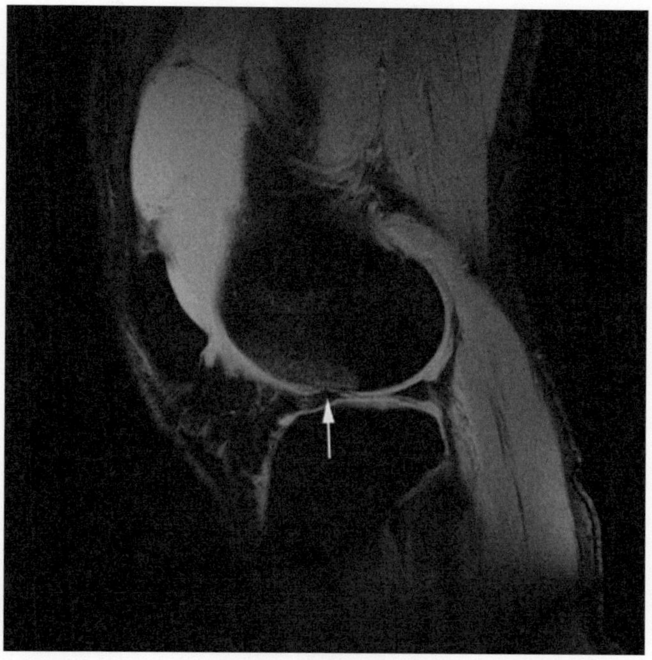

Fig. 19.9 MRI sagittal fat inhibited T2WI shows a 1.2 cm cartilage defect in the femoral condyle (white arrow). It can be seen that the subchondral bone marrow edema is flaky with high signal and the edges are blurred. Bones are visible under arthroscopy, and free cartilage pieces are visible in the joints

2. The localized full-thickness defect of the femoral condyle cartilage and normal cartilage
   2.1. MRI (Fig. 19.10)

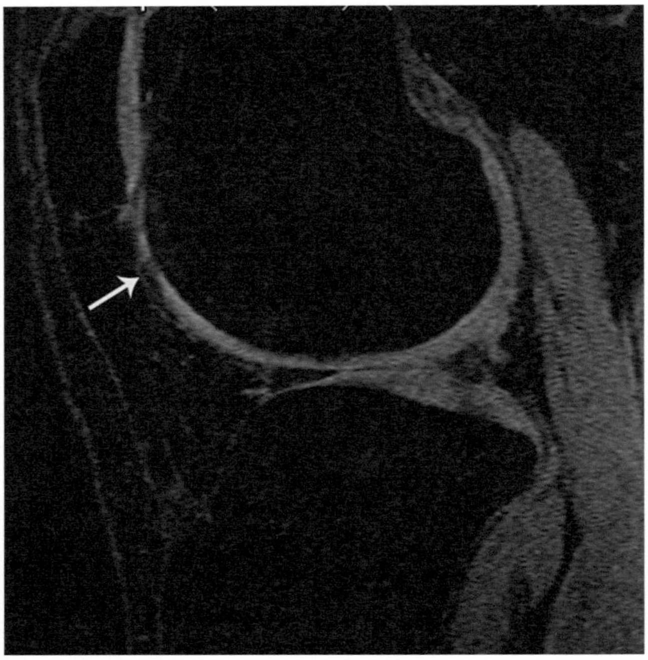

Fig. 19.10 MRI sagittal fat inhibits T2WI, which shows localized bone defects in the lateral femoral condyle (white arrows). Bones are visible under arthroscopy, and free cartilage pieces are visible in the joints

3. Full-thickness defects of knee articular cartilage and normal cartilage
   3.1. MRI (Fig. 19.11)

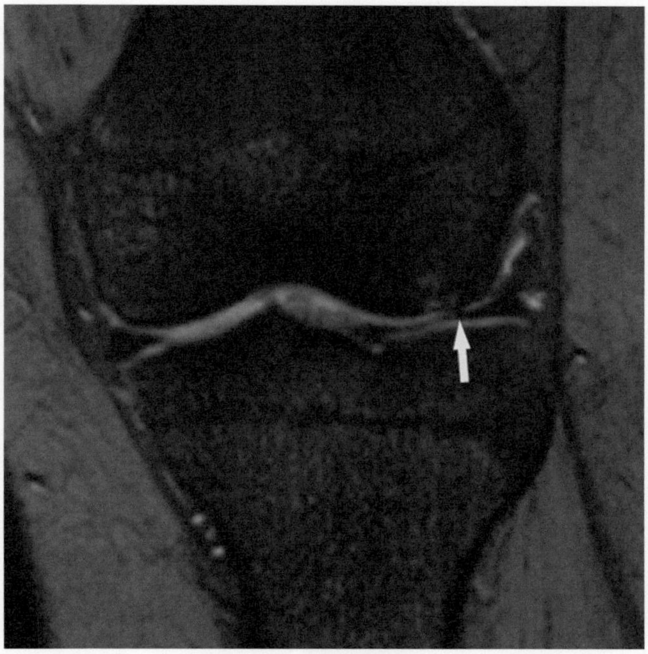

Fig. 19.11 MRI coronal plane T2WI shows localized cartilage defects of the left knee femoral condyle (white arrow). There is edema, which is flaky with high signal and blurred edges. The femoral condyle cartilage defect was found under arthroscopy examination. Approximately 8 mm of free cartilage flake can be seen in the joint

4. Partial cartilage defects of the knee joint and normal cartilage
   4.1. MRI (Fig. 19.12)

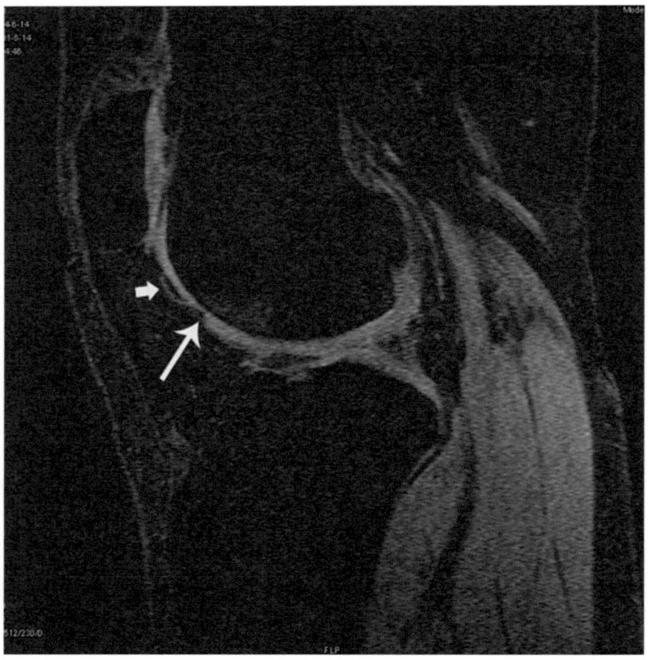

Fig. 19.12 MRI sagittal fat inhibited T2WI shows localized thinning and defect of the articular cartilage in front of the femoral condyle (white arrow). In front of the upper strip shadow (rough white arrow), equal to the cartilage signal, arthroscopy confirmed free bodys in the joint cavity

5. Partial defects of the tibial cartilage and normal cartilage
   5.1. MRI (Fig. 19.13a, b)

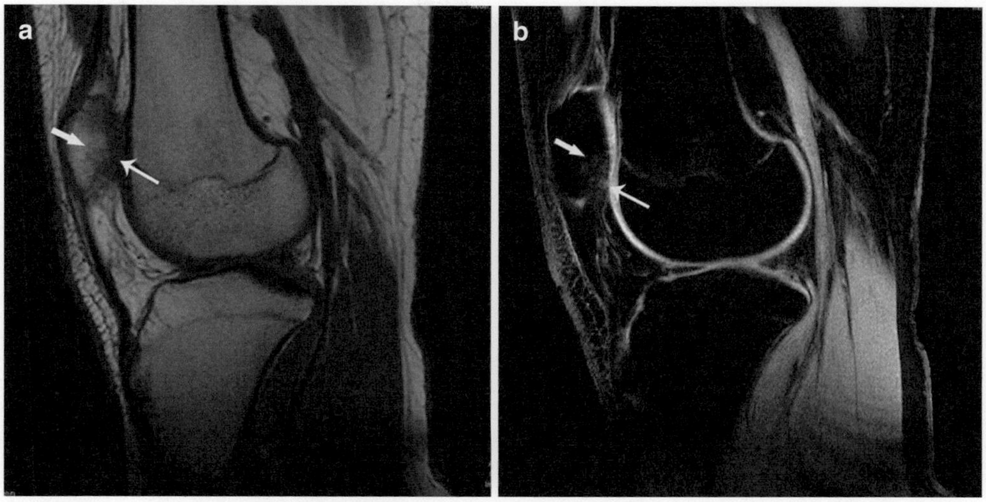

Fig. 19.13 (**a**, **b**) are sagittal T1WI and fat suppression T2WI, respectively. It shows a partial defect of the cartilage in the posterior border of the tibia (white arrow) and local intraosseous edema (thick arrow), which is a high signal of T1WI with low signal T2WI and blurred edges

6. Partial cartilage defects of the knee joint and normal cartilage
   6.1. MRI (Fig. 19.14)

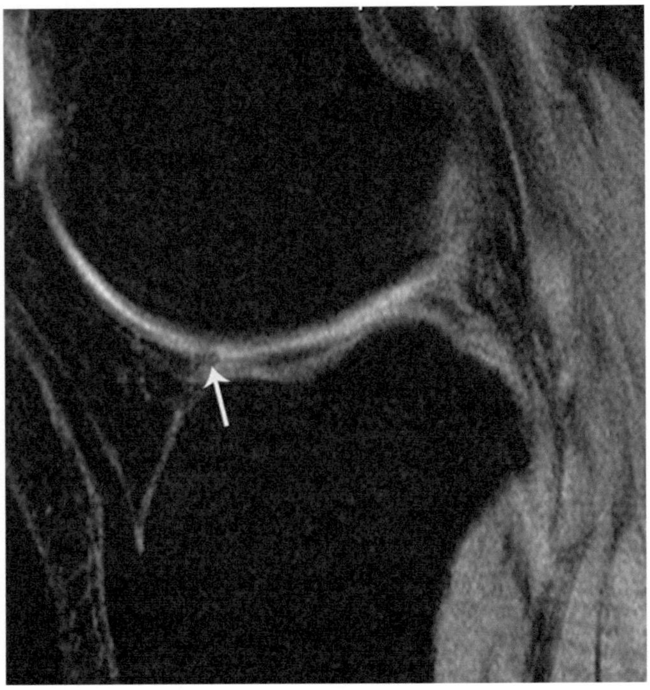

Fig. 19.14 MRI sagittal fat inhibits T2WI. It shows a partial defect in the cartilage of the femoral condyle (white arrow)

7. Posterior femoral condyle fracture of the knee joint and normal cartilage
   7.1. MRI (Fig. 19.15a–d)

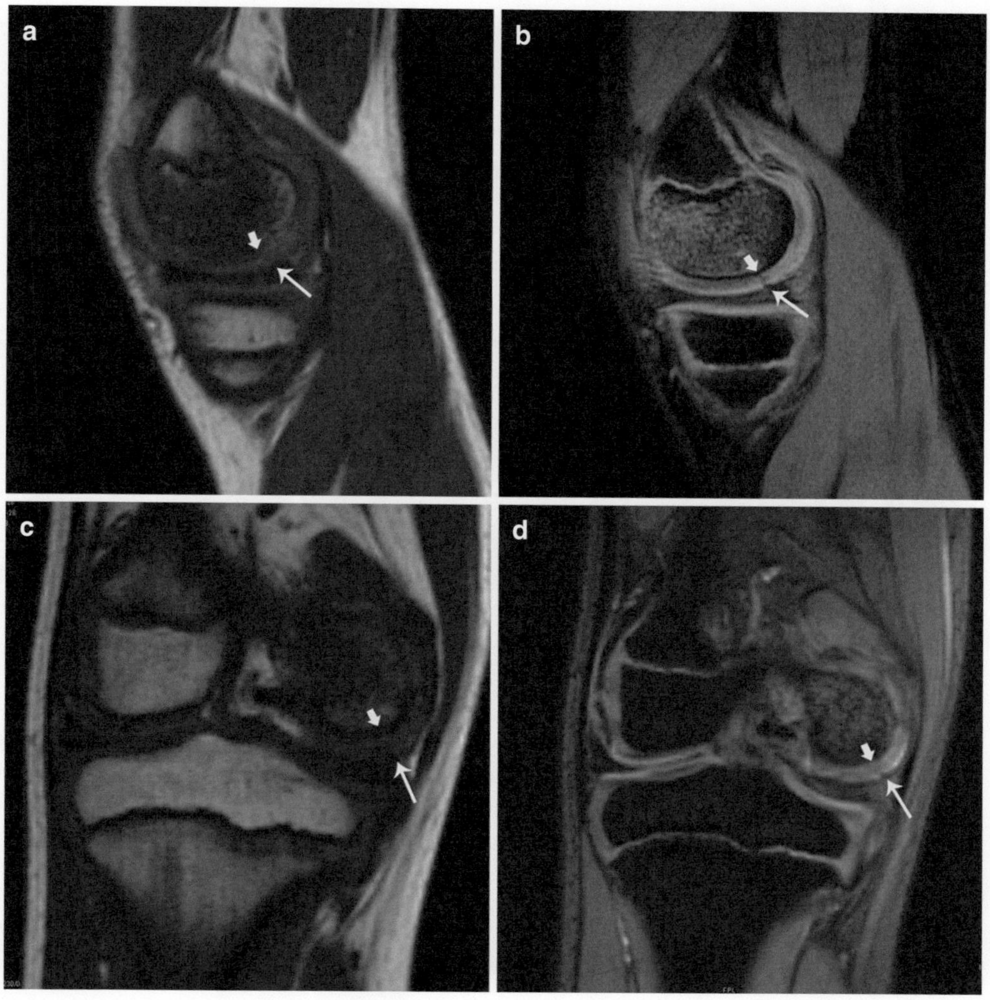

Fig. 19.15 (**a**, **b**) are sagittal T1WI and fat suppression T2WI, respectively. (**c**, **d**) are the coronal planes T1WI and T2WI, respectively. It shows that the cartilage fracture in the posterior femoral condyle is fissure-like (white arrow), and the fracture reaches the full layer of cartilage. Among them, cancellous bone edema is a long T1 and long T2 signal. The subchondral low signal band is smooth and intact with no breaks (white arrows)

19.3 Acute Joint Osteochondral Fracture

Acute joint osteochondral fracture is defined as the continuous interruption or defect of articular cartilage and subchondral bone caused by trauma. The fracture piece can be freed from the joint. It is divided into two types: osteochondral avulsion and osteochondral collapse.

19.3.1 Injury Mechanism

Direct or indirect trauma on the articular cartilage surface, causing the articular cartilage and the underlying bone to break.

19.3.2 Symptoms and Signs

The joint is painful with active or passive movement, the joint capsule is swelling, localized effusion, and joint lock can occur occasionally.

19.3.3 Diagnosis of Imaging

1. A continuous or localized defect in the articular cartilage and subchondral bone is shown on the MRI image; (2) There is bone marrow edema in the vicinity of the fractured area, which is irregularly long T1 and long T2 signal with blurred edges. X-ray plain film was mostly negative because the fracture flake was small and the articular cartilage cannot be seen on X-ray. We should perform CT and MRI scans with suspected acute osteochondral fractures. CT scan and multi-directional reconstruction images are sensitive to small fractures. MRI multi-directional, multi-sequence scans contribute to the display of articular cartilage defects. The femoral condyle and tibial plateau osteochondral fractures of the knee showed a clearer T2WI in the sagittal and coronal planes. T2WI of the transverse and sagittal planes of the tibial osteochondral fracture showed better. MRI is more likely to detect bone marrow contusion, and all cartilage lesions can be found. Therefore, pay attention to the identification of osteochondral injury and osteoarthritis.
2. MRI showed thin and uneven cartilage, patchy long T1 and long T2 signals in the subchondral bone, and the lesion was diffused, involving several articular surfaces (Fig. 19.20).

1. Acute osteochondral avulsion fracture and simple cartilage fracture of the femoral condyle of the knee
   1.1. CT (Fig. 19.16a–c)

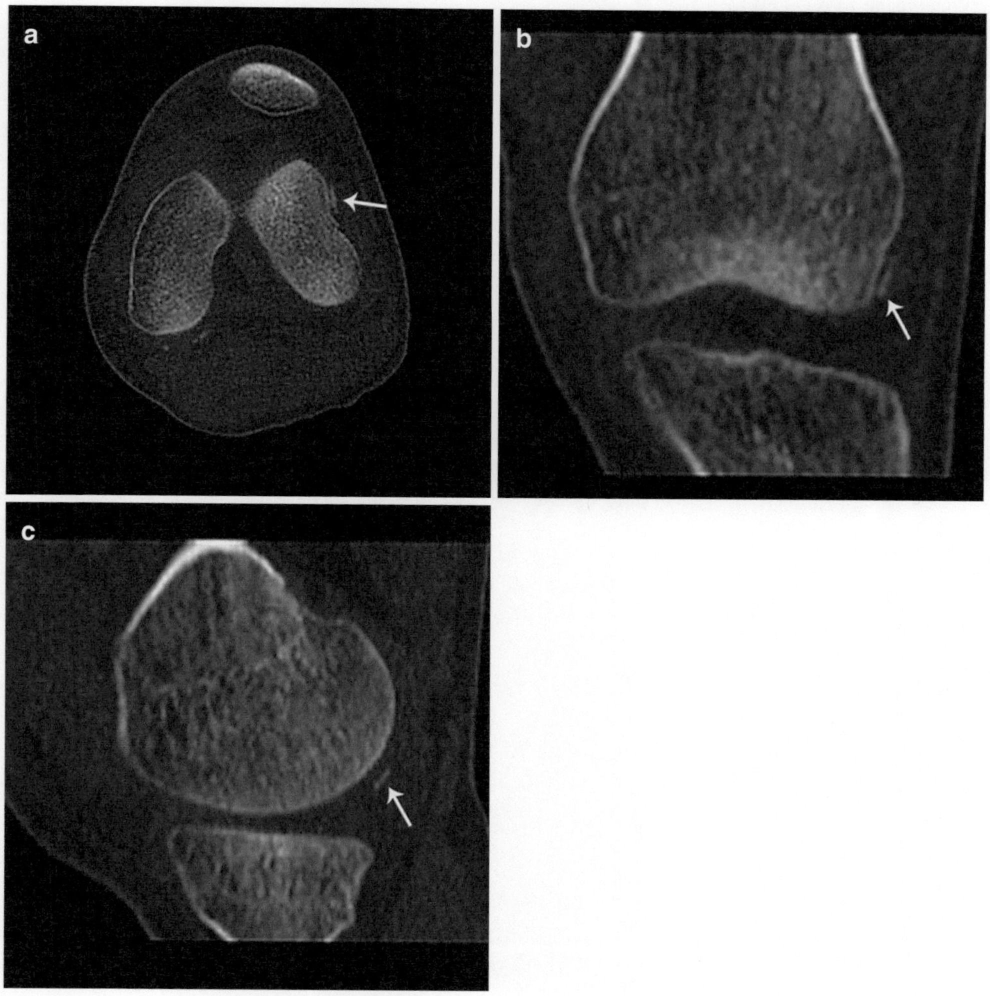

Fig. 19.16 (**a**–**c**) show images of CT plain transverse axis, coronal reconstruction, and sagittal reconstruction, respectively. It shows avulsed osteochondral slices (white arrows)

1.2. MRI (Fig. 19.16d–h)

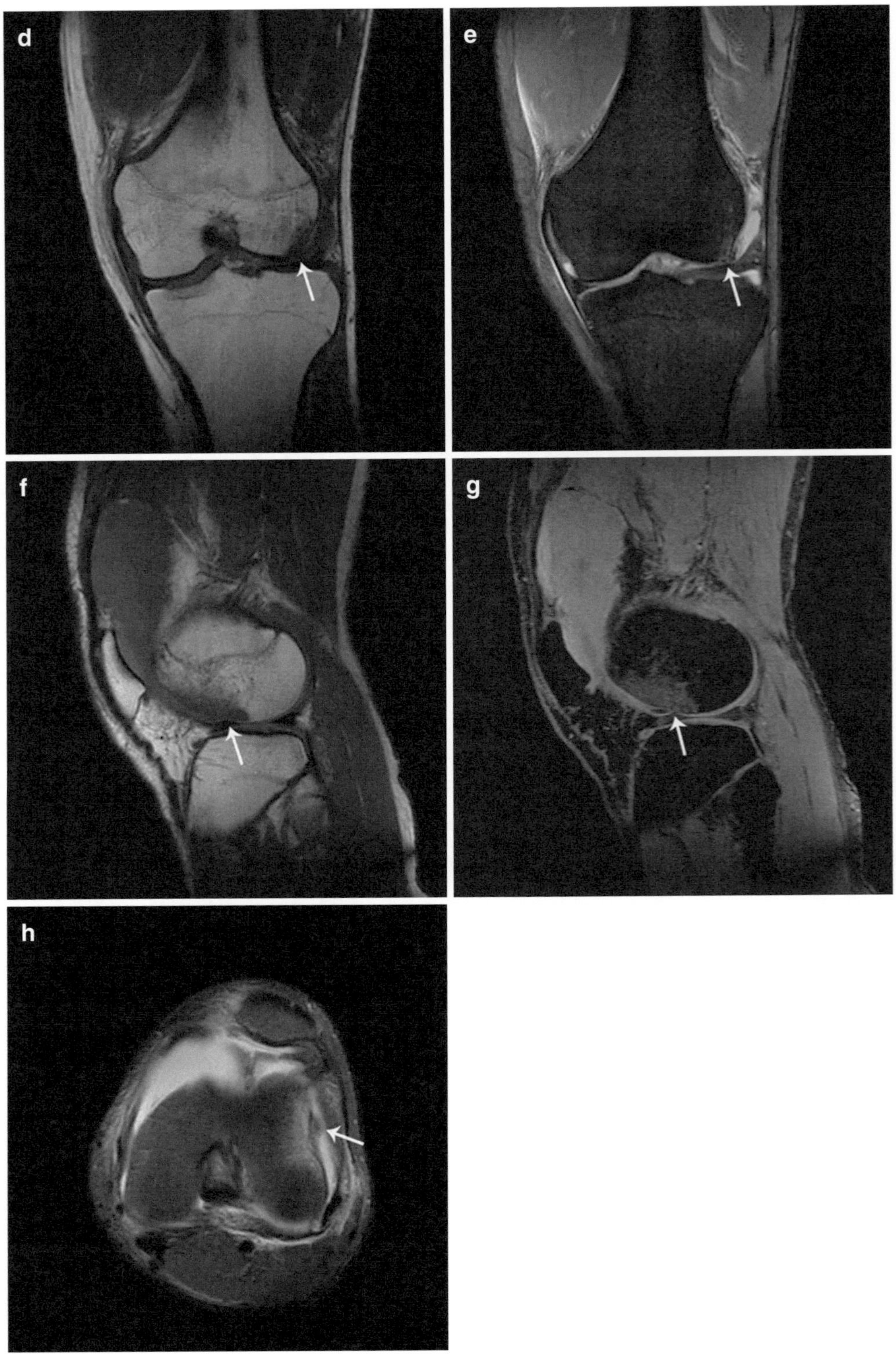

Fig. 19.16 (**d**–**h**) Show MRI coronal plane T1WI, T2WI, sagittal T1WI, fat suppression T2WI, and transverse axis fat suppression T2WI. It shows local cartilage and subchondral bone defects (white arrows), bone marrow edema, and massive blood accumulation in the joints

2. Femoral cartilage sag fracture and simple cartilage fracture
   2.1. MRI (Fig. 19.17a–d)

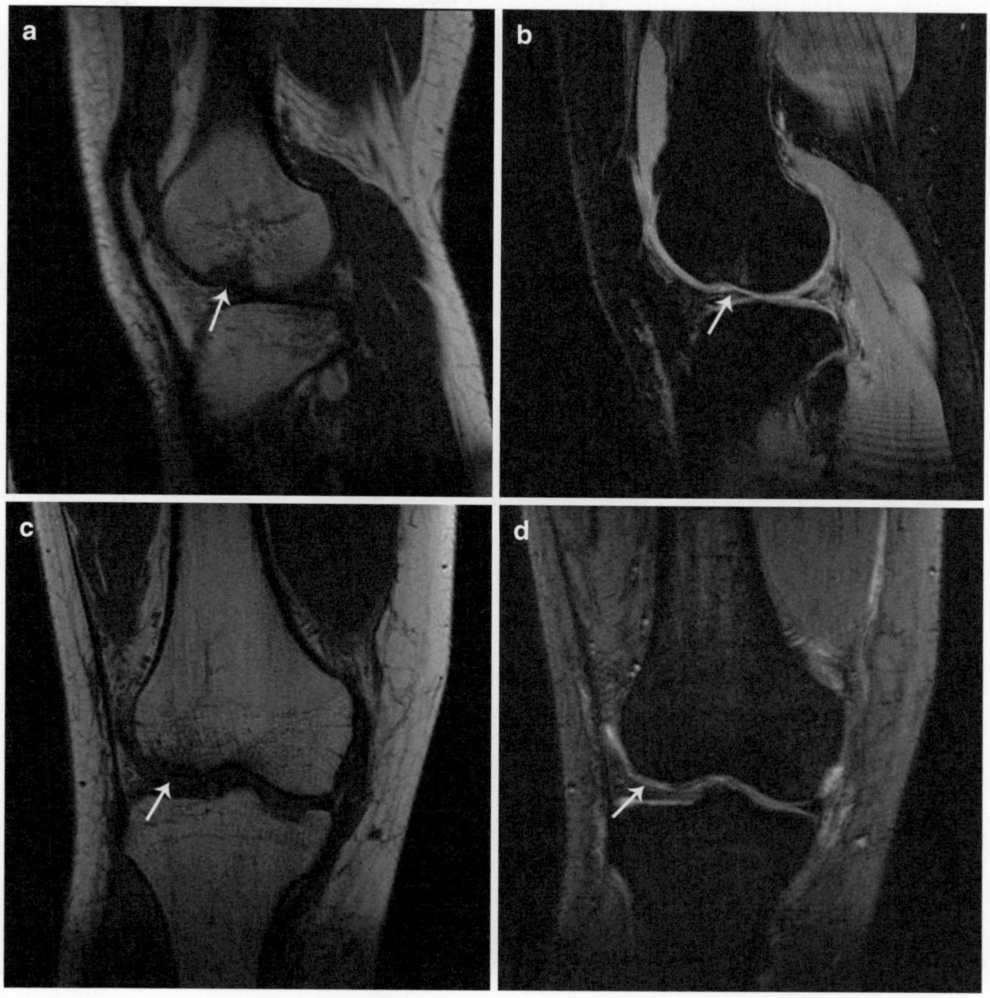

Fig. 19.17 (**a**, **b**) Show sagittal T1WI and fat suppression T2WI, respectively. (**c**, **d**) are coronal planes T1WI and T2WI, which show cartilage and subchondral bone fracture, invagination (white arrow), local bone marrow contusion, flaky long T1 and long T2 signal

3. Knee osteochondral depression and simple cartilage fracture
   3.1. X-Ray (Fig. 19.18a–d)

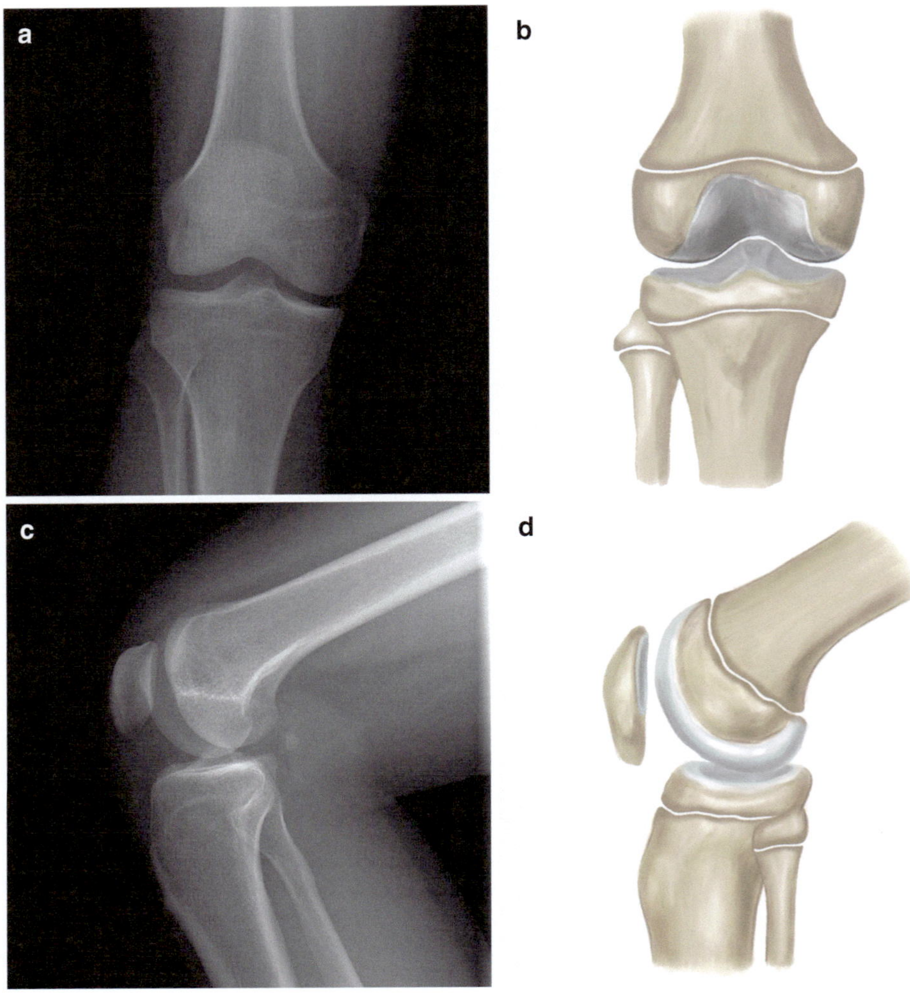

Fig. 19.18 (**a**, **c**) show the X-ray positive lateral slice, and there is no obvious abnormality in the bone (**b**, **d**)

   3.2. MRI (Fig. 19.18e, f)

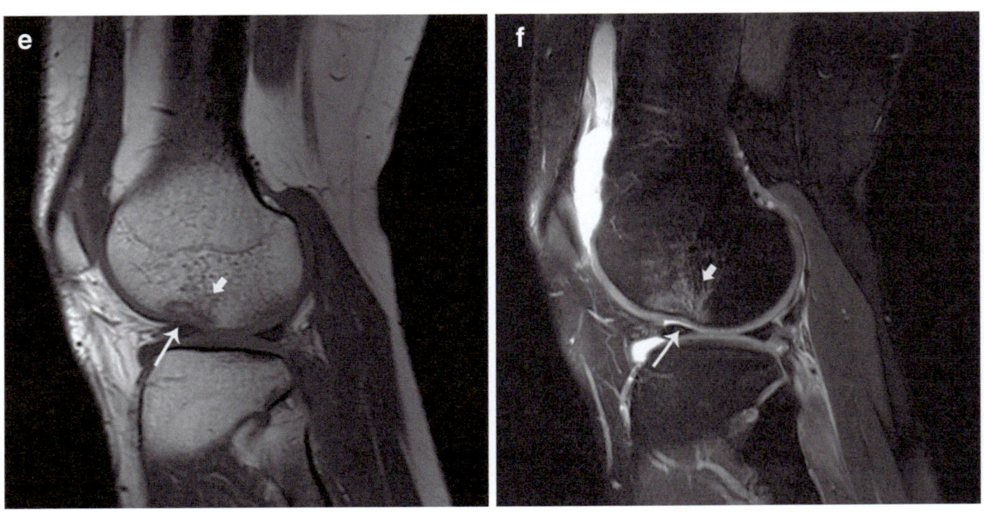

Fig. 19.18 (**e**, **f**) are sagittal T1WI and fat-suppressed T2WI, which show femoral cartilage and cortical fractures (white arrows), large bone marrow edema (rough white arrow) in the bone, showing a long T1 length T2 signal, blurred edges

4. Knee osteochondral avulsion fracture and simple cartilage fracture
   4.1. X-ray (Fig. 19.19a–d)

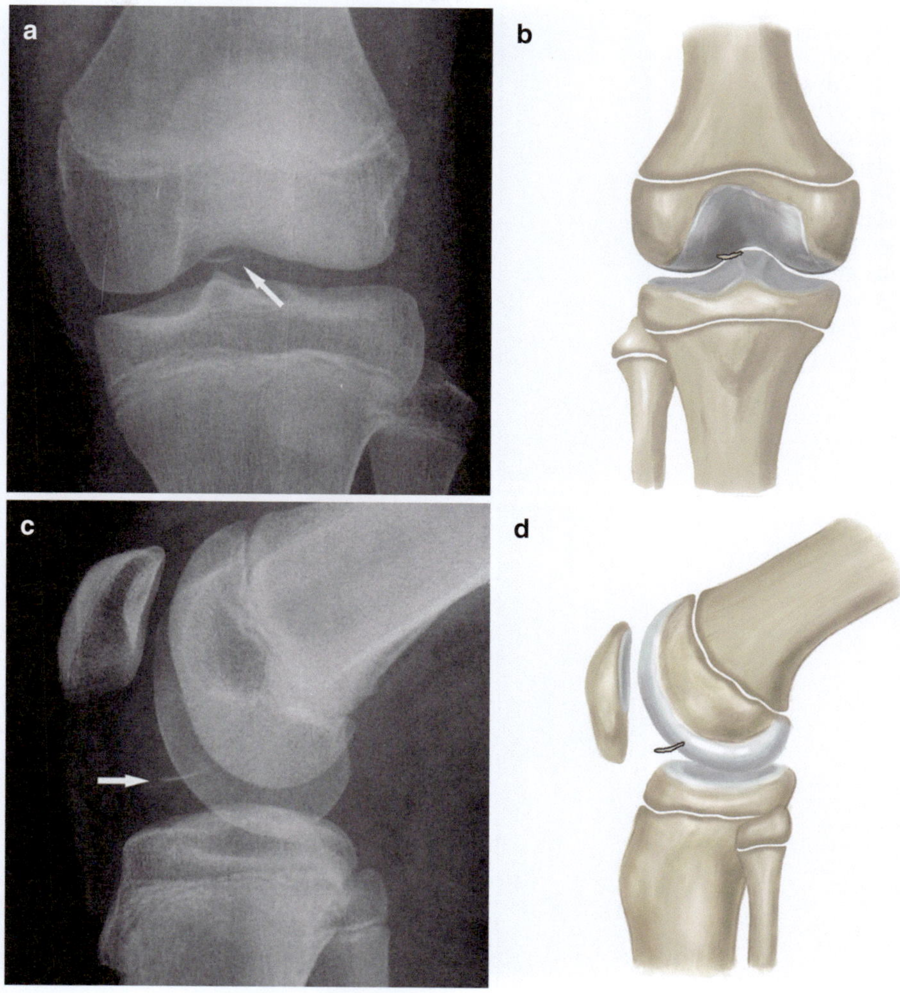

Fig. 19.19 (**a**, **c**) are the positive lateral radiographs of the left knee joint. It shows an image of the bone in the joint (white arrow). The schematic diagrams are shown in (**b**, **d**)

   4.2. MRI (Fig. 19.19e, f)

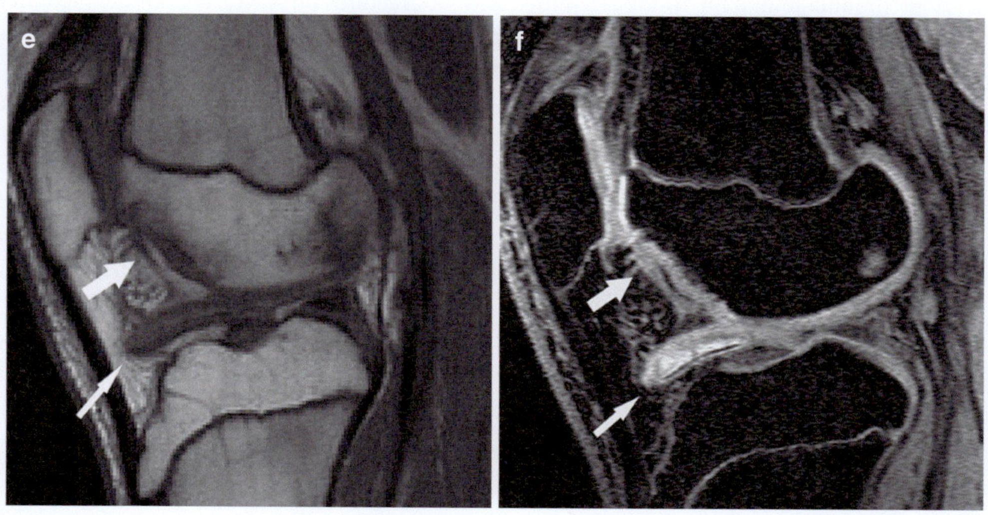

Fig. 19.19 (**e**, **f**) are MRI sagittal T1WI and fat suppression T2WI, respectively. It shows that the osteochondral fracture is separated but not yet free (white arrow), subchondral bone invagination (rough white arrow)

5. Knee osteoarthritis and cartilage damage
   5.1. MRI (Fig. 19.20a–d)

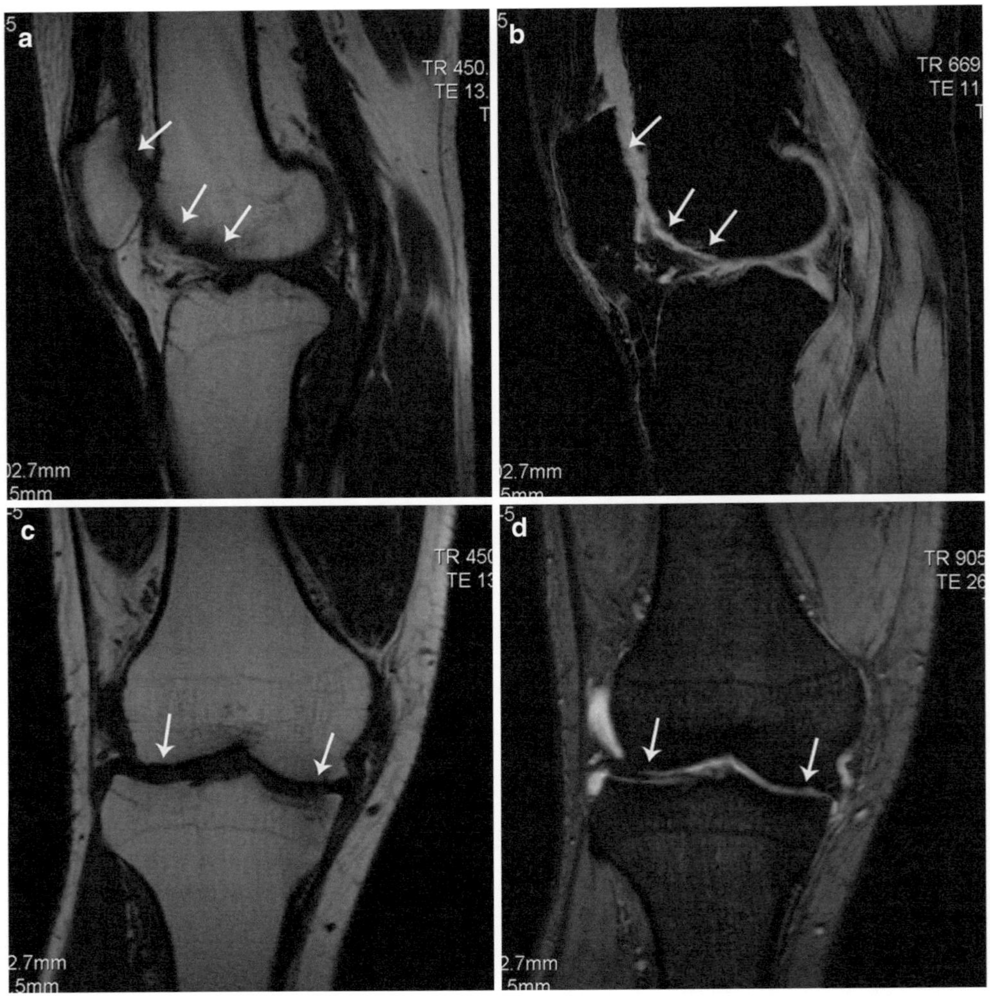

Fig. 19.20 (**a**, **b**) are MRI sagittal T1WI and fat suppression T2WI, respectively. (**c**, **d**) are the coronal planes T1WI and T2WI. It shows uneven thickness of the posterior border of the tibia and femoral condyle, and multiple patchy long T1 and long T2 signal (white arrow) in the subchondral bone without obvious bone marrow edema

19.4 Summary of the Points

1. Acute trauma joint pain, limited mobility, with no fractures on X-ray, are possible features of simple cartilage fracture or osteochondral fracture. CT and MRI should be performed to prevent missed diagnosis.
2. Cartilage damage includes both simple cartilage fractures and osteochondral fractures. A simple cartilage fracture refers to the continuous interruption of articular cartilage, while the subchondral bone morphology is intact. Osteochondral fracture refers to the continuous interruption or defect of articular cartilage and subchondral bone, which is characterized by avulsion of osteochondral piece free in the joint and collapse of osteochondral.
3. Articular cartilage is hyaline cartilage, X-ray film and CT scan cannot be displayed, and simple cartilage fracture is mainly diagnosed by MRI. Osteochondral fractures are mainly diagnosed according to CT and MRI. CT scan and multi-directional reconstruction images are sensitive to tiny fractures, and MRI contributes to the display of articular cartilage damage and bone marrow contusion.
4. In the case of articular cartilage or osteochondral fracture, often combined with other structural damage in the joint, such as the meniscus, tendons, ligaments and muscle tissue around the joints, comprehensive observation should be obtained.

Occult Fractures and Bone Contusion

20

Zekun Zhang and Yingze Zhang

20.1 Occult Fractures

Occult fracture refers to the discontinuity of trabecular bone and cortex, which is difficult to diagnose through routine X-ray film. CT and MRI may be required to make a definite diagnosis. These fractures often occur in covert areas with complex structures, whose treatment may be delayed if not diagnosed in time.

20.1.1 Identification of Injury Mechanism

Not available, but has clear trauma history.

20.1.2 Identification of Symptoms and Signs

It is difficult to get a definite diagnosis from posttraumatic pain in injured area because pain in these areas is not specific. For that reason, CT and MRI should be performed to avoid misdiagnosis when a fracture is suspected with a negative X-ray.

20.1.3 Imaging Differential Diagnosis

CT scans with reconstruction and MRI scans should be performed even if the non-fracture line appearance in the X-ray is not consistent with the symptoms, especially for the complex anatomical structures including joints and spine. CT scans and multiplanar reconstruction show low density of cancellous bone and cortical bone line. MRI scanning shows the low signal images of bone cortex and medullary cavity in linear, strip or network, with surrounding lamellar low signal in T1WI. T2WI shows high signal or linear low signal, surrounding chip high signal, edge can be clear or unclear. Bone marrow edema would disappear over 6–12 months.

Occult fracture should be differentiated from bone contusion. Fracture lines and displacement are always not accompanied by bone contusion, and self-healing could be accomplished within 2–3 months. However, fracture lines can be observed in cortex and trabeculae. Discontinuity of cortex could be clearly observed in MRI scan, especially in T1WI pattern. The direction and shape of fracture lines in T2WI are similar to those in T2WI because of the coverage of high signal edema. However, the scope of fracture lines in T2WI was smaller than that of T1WI.

Z. Zhang
CT/MRI Center, The Third Hospital of Hebei Medical University, Shijiazhuang, Hebei, China

Y. Zhang (✉)
Department of Orthopaedics, The Third Hospital of Hebei Medical University, Shijiazhuang, Hebei, China

Y. Zhang (ed.), *Differential Diagnosis of Fracture*, https://doi.org/10.1007/978-981-13-8339-7_20

1. Differential diagnosis of occult and no fractures in left tibial plateau
   1.1. X-ray (Fig. 20.1a–d)

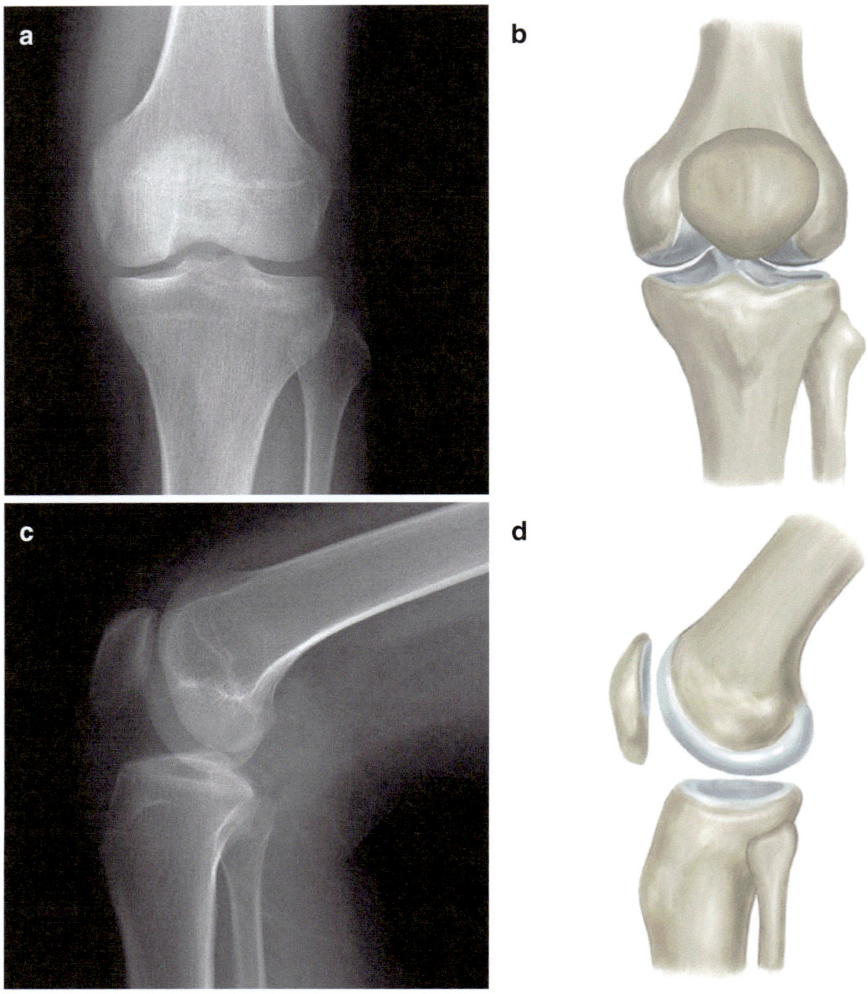

Fig. 20.1 There is no obvious fracture line in the anteroposterior and lateral projections/schematic diagram (**a**–**d**). However, pain symptom is obvious and MRI scan should be performed to make a definite diagnosis

1.2. MRI scan (Fig. 20.1e–h)

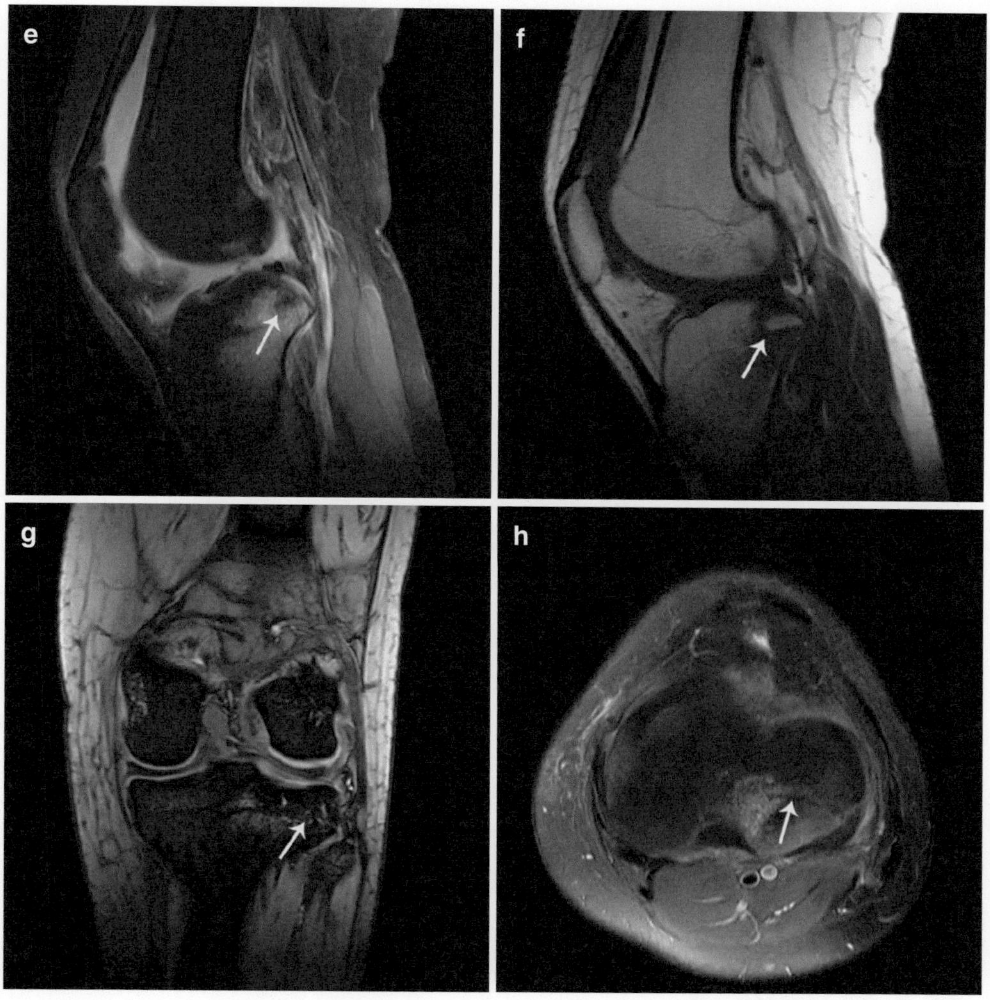

Fig. 20.1 MRI sagittal fat suppression T2WI, sagittal T1WI, coronal T2WI, and transverse axis fat suppression T2W are shown in (**e**–**h**), which show posterior fracture of the lateral tibia of the left knee. There is a short line length T1 long T2 signal (white arrow) surrounded by large flaky bone marrow edema with a long T1 long T2 signal and blurred edges

2. Differential diagnosis of occult and no fractures in tibial plateau
   2.1. X-ray (Fig. 20.2a–d)

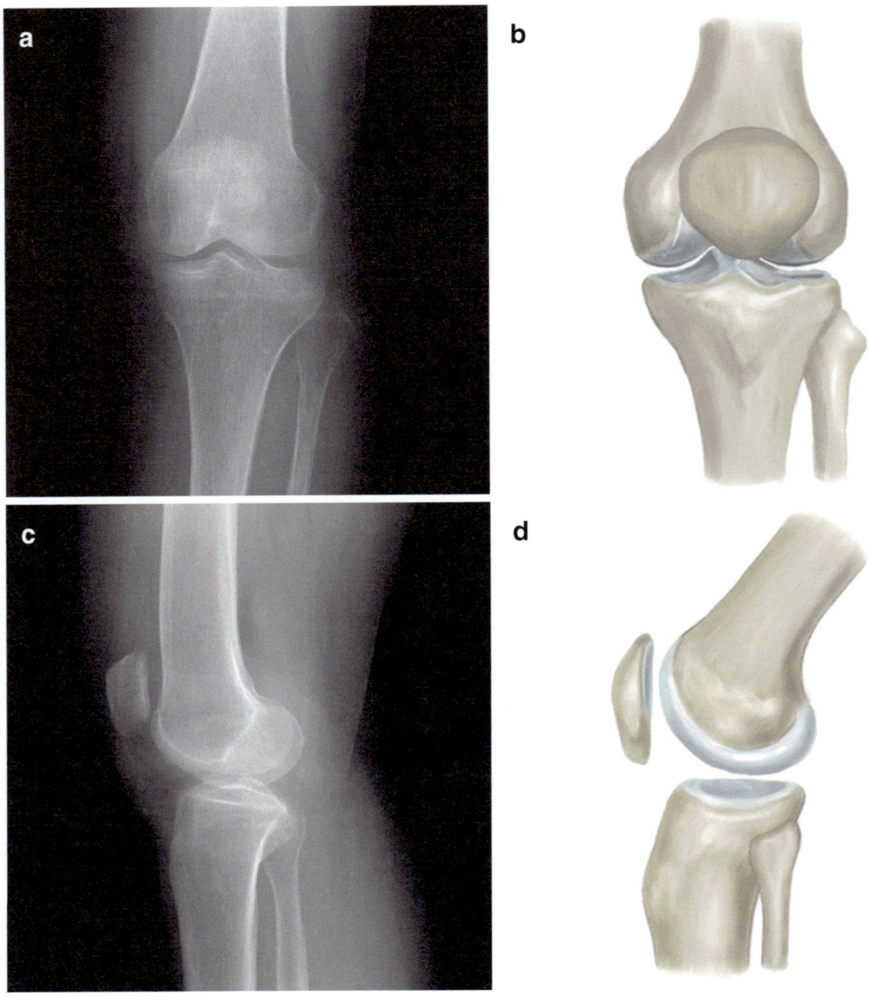

Fig. 20.2 Although there is no obvious fracture line in the anteroposterior and lateral projections/schematic diagram (**a**–**d**), pain symptom is obvious. Then, CT and MRI scan are performed

2.2. CT scan (Fig. 20.2e, f)

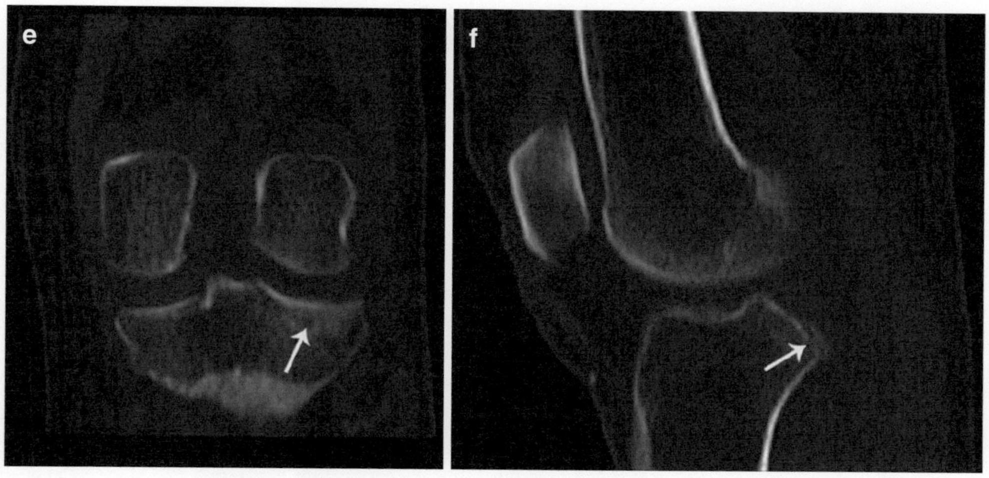

Fig. 20.2 Small fragment (white arrow) behind the left lateral tibial plateau could be observed in the coronal and sagittal CT scans (**e**, **f**)

2.3. MRI scan (Fig. 20.2g, h)

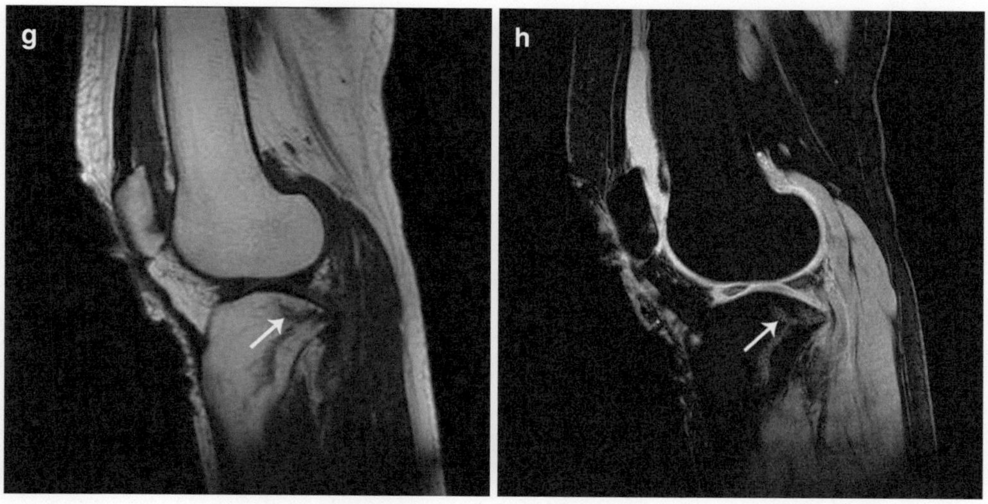

Fig. 20.2 T1WI and sagittal fat suppression T2WI MRI are presented in (**g**, **h**) showing the signal shadow of T1 and T2 of short line length (white arrow)

3. Differential diagnosis of occult and no fractures in patella
   3.1. CT scan (Fig. 20.3a, b)

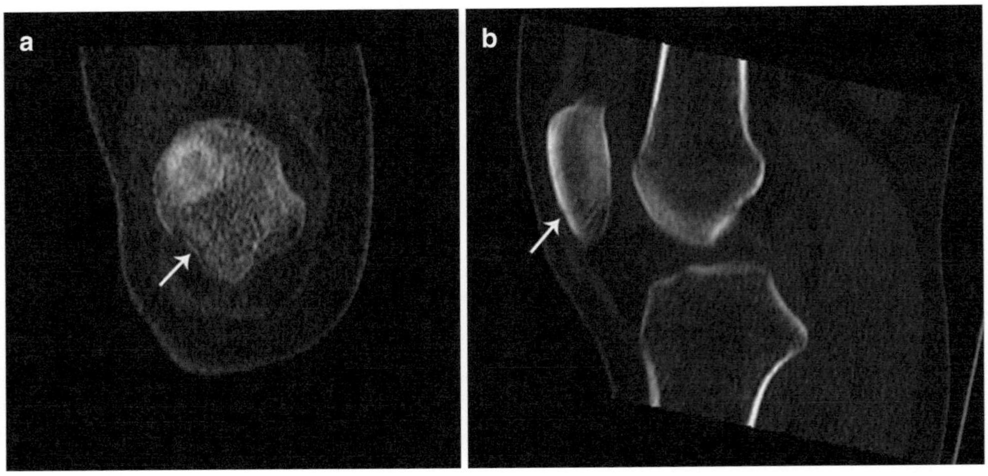

Fig. 20.3 A low-density image of the lower margin of patella (white arrow) could be observed in coronal CT scan (**a**). However, the fracture line in sagittal CT scan is not obvious (**b**)

   3.2. MRI scan (Fig. 20.3c, d)

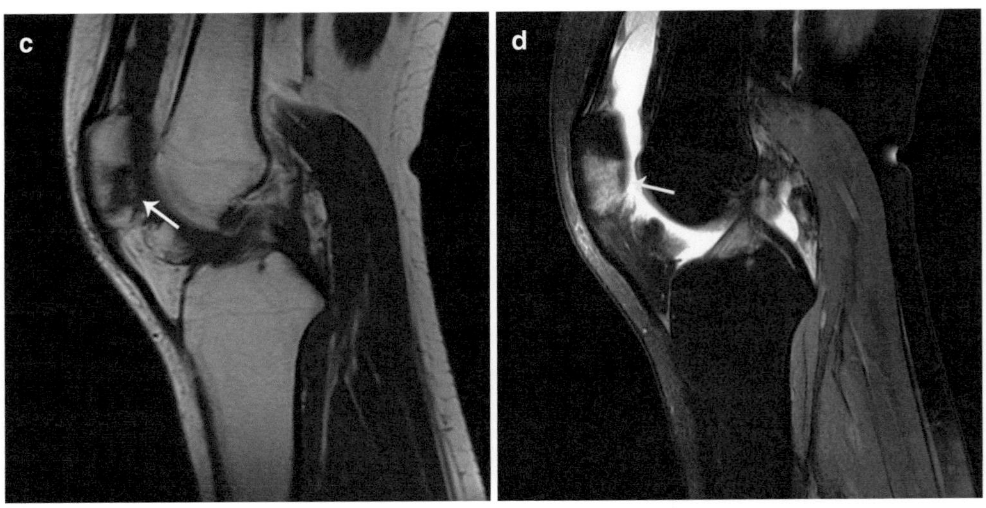

Fig. 20.3 T1WI and sagittal fat suppression T2WI MRI are presented in (**c**, **d**) showing short linear in length T1 and T2 signal shadow (white arrow) surrounded by large edema of bone marrow (**c**, **d**). There is massive intra-articular effusion (hematocele)

4. Differential diagnosis of right femoral intertrochanteric occult and no fractures
   4.1. X-ray (Fig. 20.4a, b)

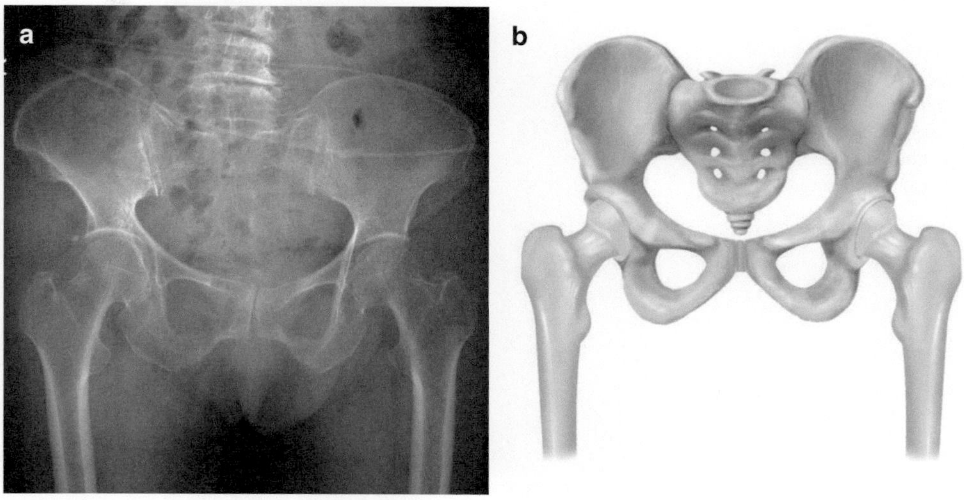

Fig. 20.4 Anteroposterior projection and schematic diagram (**a**, **b**) show there is no obvious fracture line in right hip

   4.2. CT scan (Fig. 20.4c)

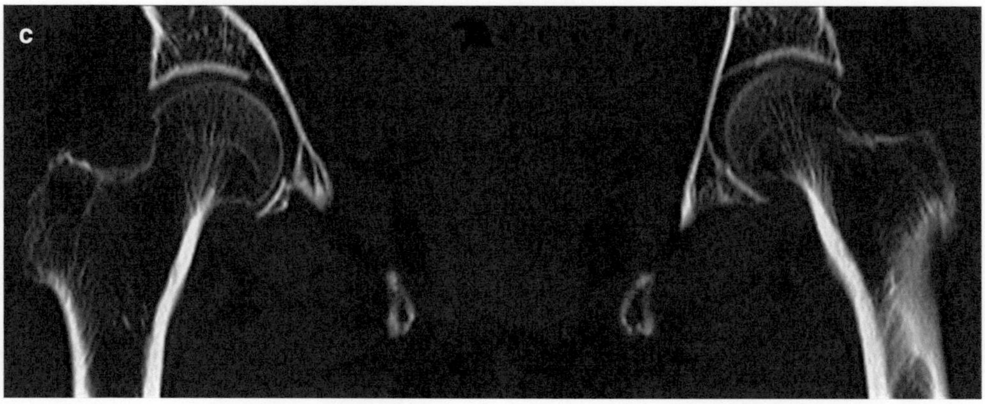

Fig. 20.4 CT coronal CT scans show that there is no obvious fracture line in the right hip joint (**c**). Thus, MRI scan is performed to make a definite diagnosis

   4.3. MRI scan (Fig. 20.4d, e)

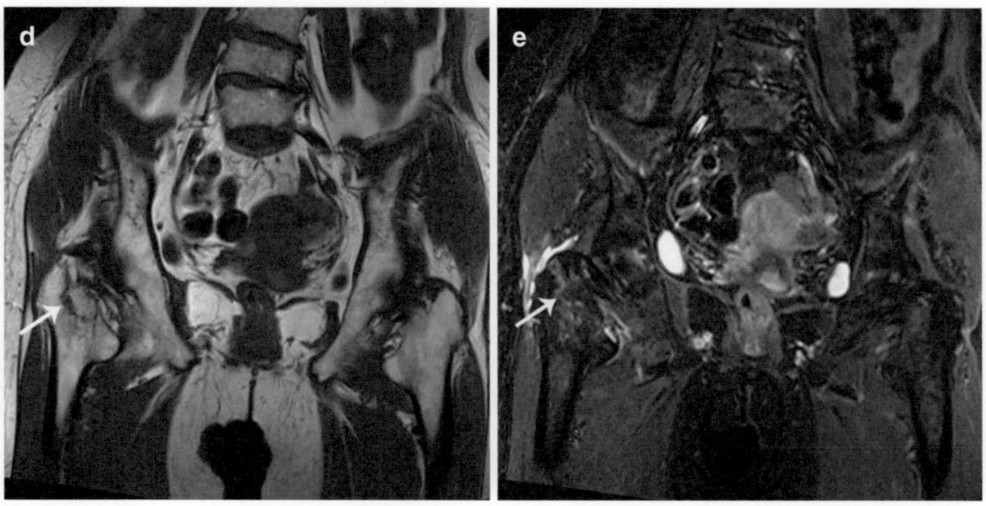

Fig. 20.4 T1WI and coronal fat inhibition T2WI MRI are presented in (**d**, **e**), showing right femoral intertrochanteric fracture. There is the signal shadow of T1 and T2 of short line length (white arrow) surrounded by swollen soft tissues

5. Differential diagnosis of occult and no fractures in distal fibula
   5.1. X-ray (Fig. 20.5a–d)

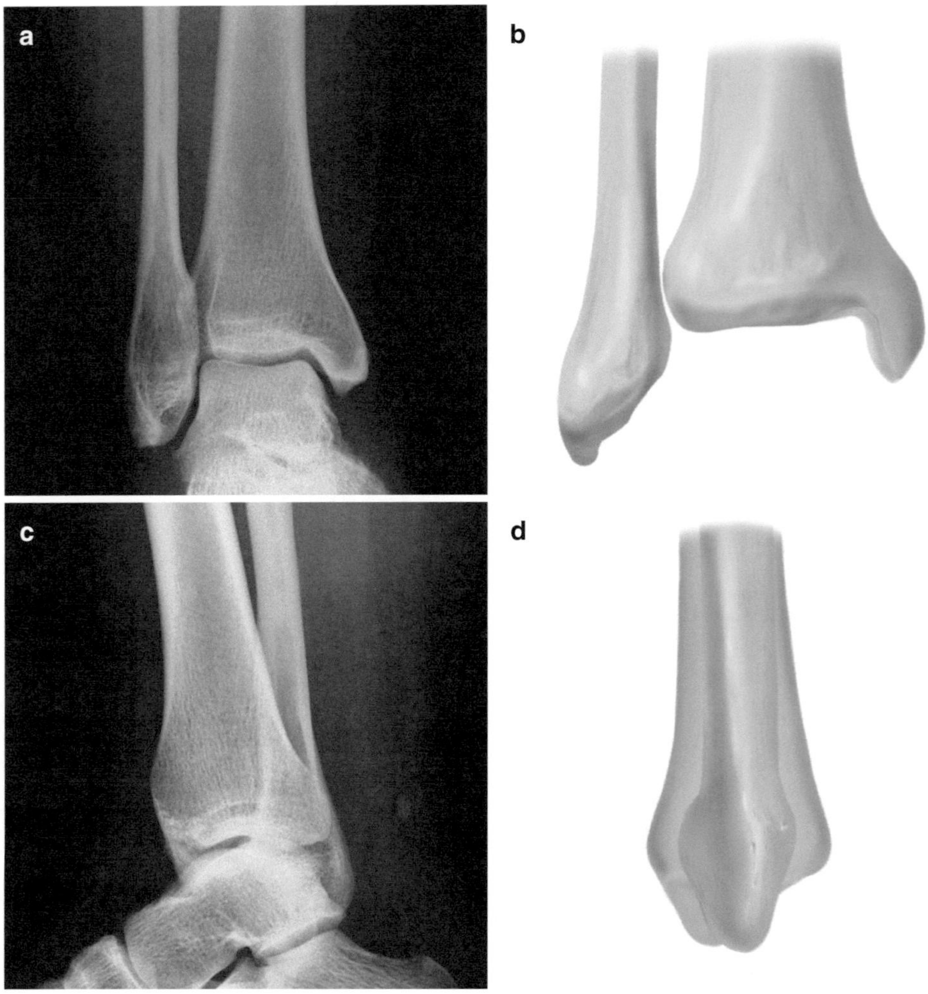

Fig. 20.5 There is no obvious fracture line in the anteroposterior and lateral projections/schematic diagram (**a**–**d**). However, pain symptom is obvious and MRI scan should be performed to make a definite diagnosis

   5.2. MRI scan (Fig. 20.5e, f)

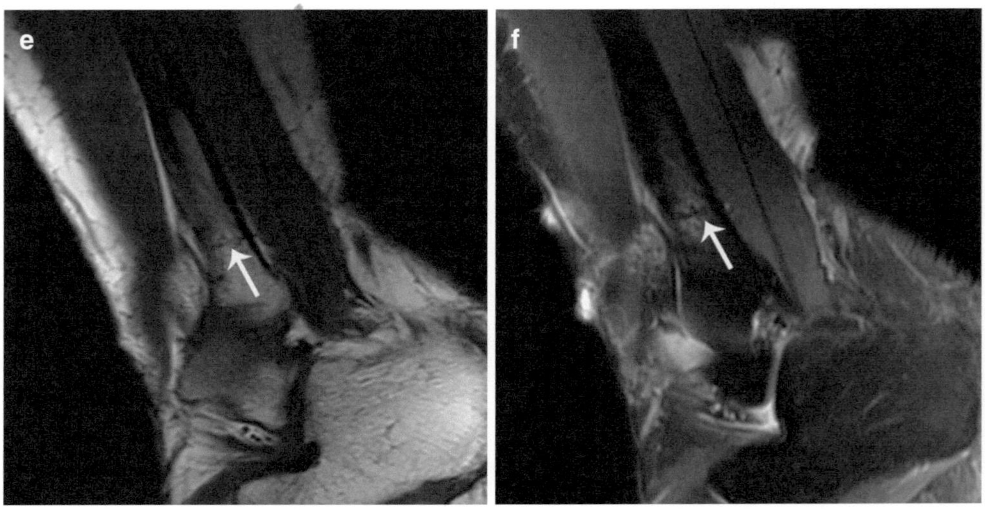

Fig. 20.5 T1WI and sagittal fat suppression T2WI MRI are presented in (**e**, **f**). There is a transverse low signal shadow (white arrow) with peripheral edema, T1WI low signal, T2WI high signal, fuzzy edge, meaning fracture of distal fibula

20.2 Bone Contusion

Bone contusion refers to bone marrow hemorrhage, edema, and microfracture of bone trabeculae caused by direct or indirect trauma, while the cortex is continuous. For occult bone contusion, positive appearance may not be observed in X-ray or CT scans; however, T1WI pattern of MRI shows speckle, map, or irregular shape low signal and T2WI pattern is high or equal signal, fuzzy boundary.

20.2.1 Identification of Injury Mechanism

Usually with a definitely trauma history.

20.2.2 Identification of Symptoms and Signs

Pain symptoms could be observed in trauma area; however, it is difficult to make a definite diagnosis because it lacks specificity.

20.2.3 Radiographic Differential Diagnosis

No positive sign could be observed in X-ray and CT scans; MRI showed low signal on T1WI and T2WI in cancellous bone lamellar or ground pattern, the edge is blurred, and no line signal is seen in it.

1. Differential diagnosis of bone contusion and normal bone in proximal radius
   1.1. X-ray (Fig. 20.6a–d)

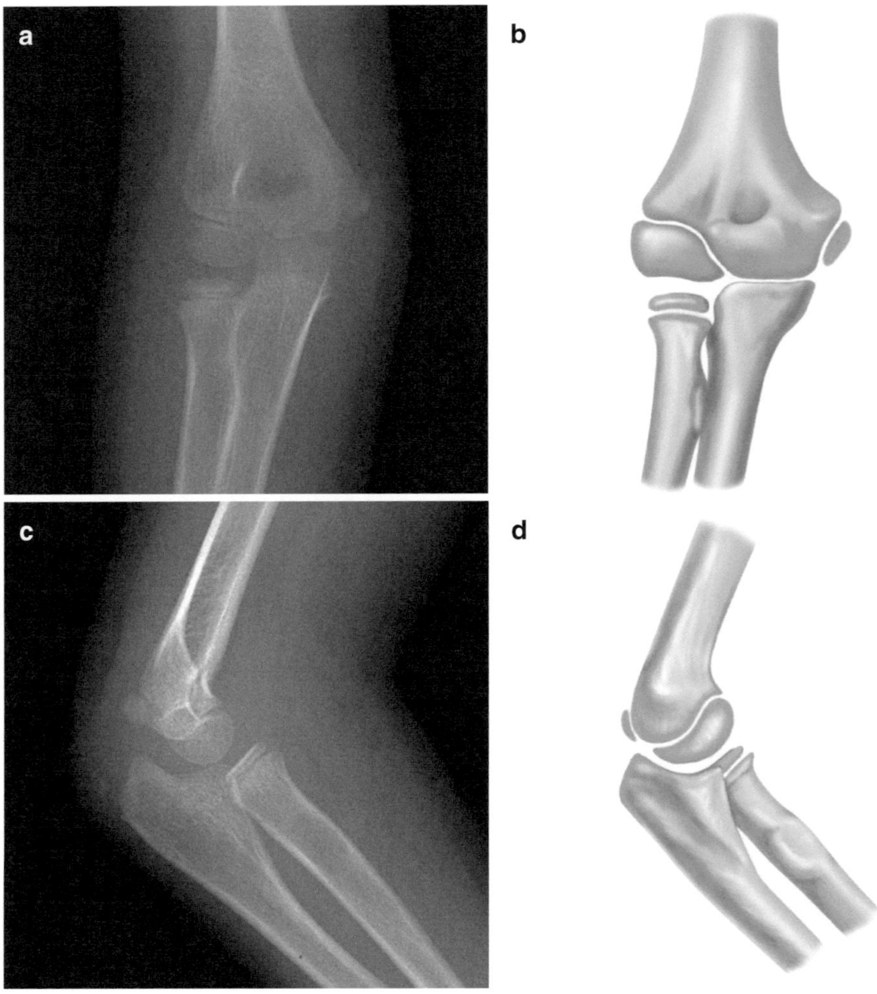

Fig. 20.6 There is no obvious fracture line in the anteroposterior and lateral projections/schematic diagram (**a**–**d**). However, pain symptom is obvious and MRI scan is conducted

   1.2. MRI scan (Fig. 20.6e, f)

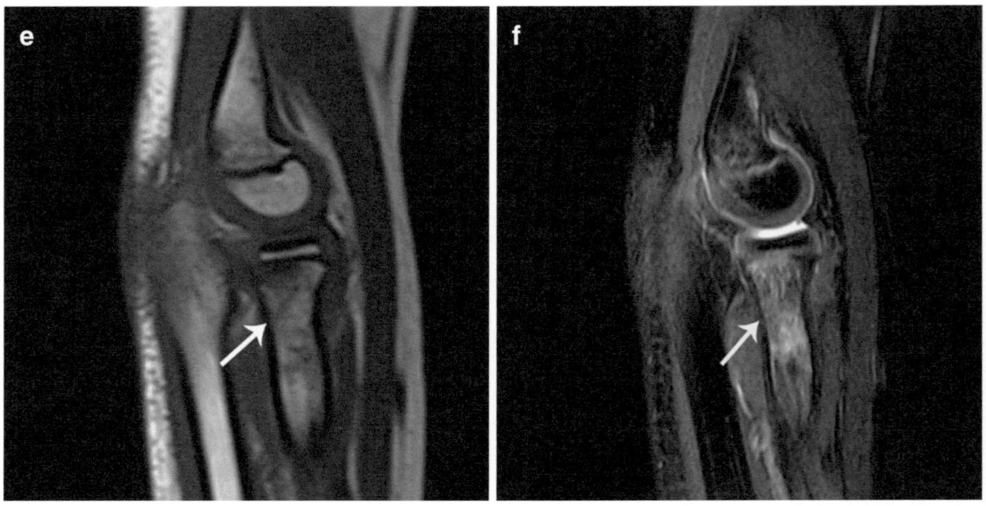

Fig. 20.6 T1WI and sagittal fat suppression T2WI MRI are presented in (**e**, **f**), showing diffuse long T1 long T2 signal shadow in the proximal radius bone, with blurred edges and intact cortex (white arrow)

2. Differential diagnosis of bone contusion and normal bone in the lateral condyle of right femur and lateral tibial plateau
   2.1. X-ray (Fig. 20.7a–d)

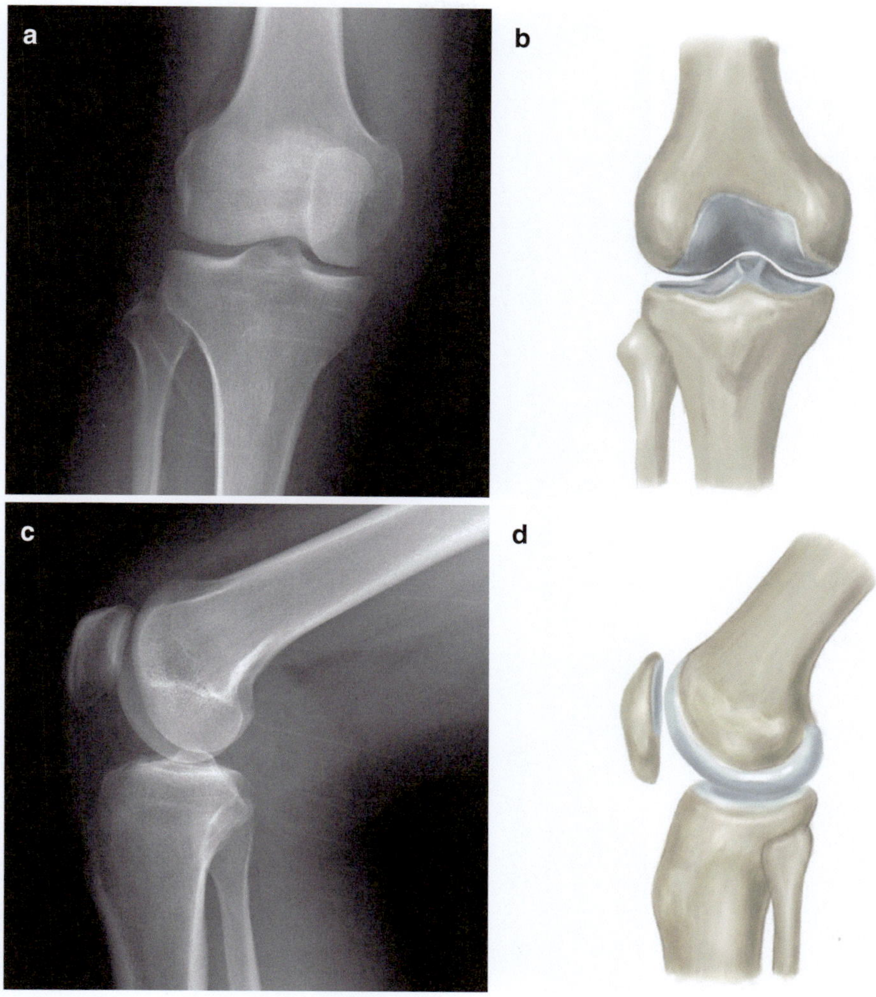

Fig. 20.7 There is no obvious fracture line in the anteroposterior and lateral projections/schematic diagram (**a–d**). MRI scan is performed to make a definite diagnosis because of pain symptom

   2.2. MRI scan (Fig. 20.7e, f)

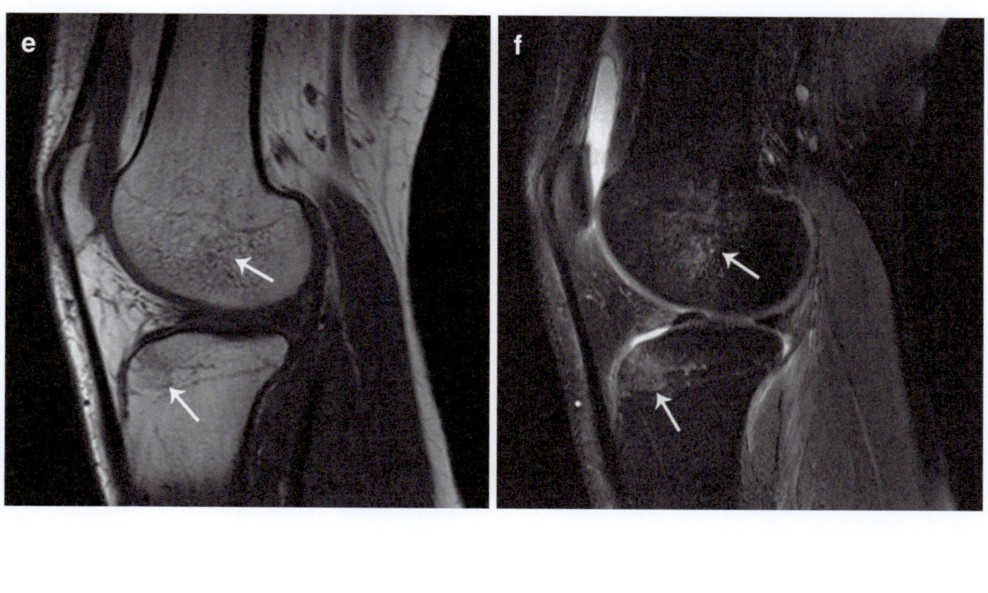

Fig. 20.7 T1WI and sagittal fat suppression T2WI MRI are presented in (**e, f**), showing the long patchy signal shadow with a fuzzy edge (white arrow) in lateral femoral condyle and tibia plateau

3. Differential diagnosis of bone contusion and normal bone in lateral femoral condyle
   3.1. X-ray (Fig. 20.8a–d)

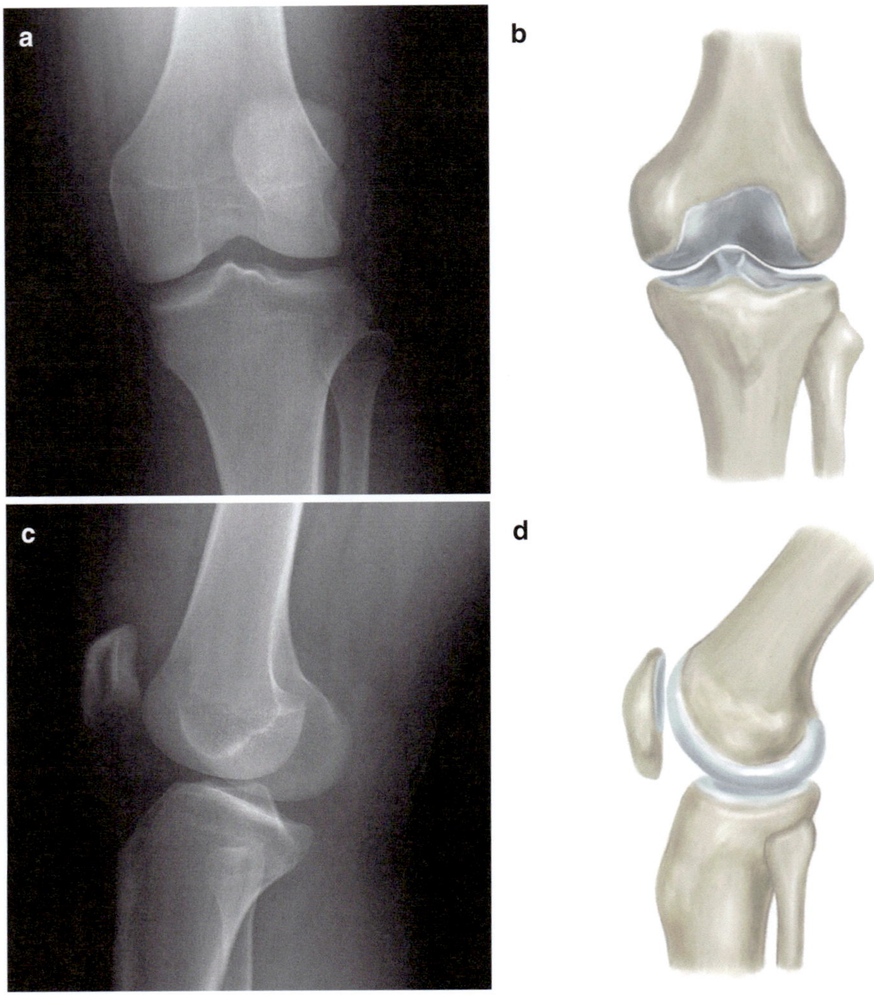

Fig. 20.8 There is no obvious fracture line in the anteroposterior and lateral projections/schematic diagram (**a**–**d**). CT and MRI scan are performed to make a definite diagnosis

3.2. CT scan (Fig. 20.8e, f)

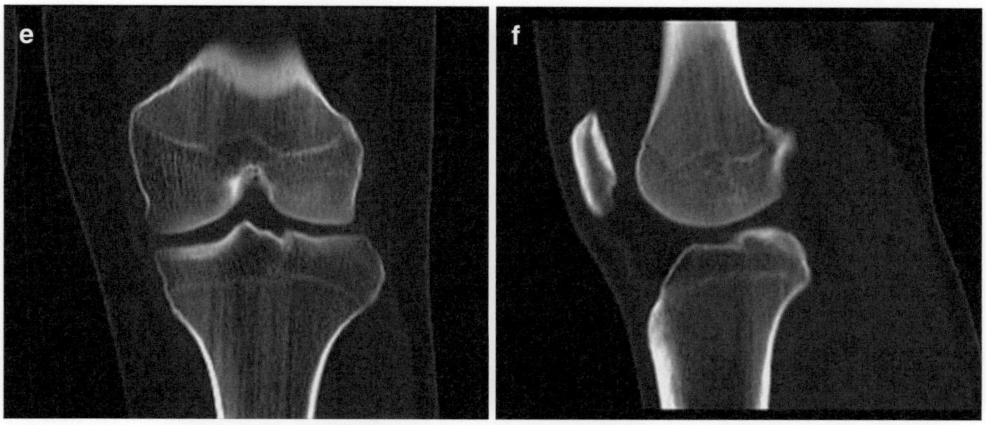

Fig. 20.8 There is no fracture line in coronal and sagittal knee CT scans (**e**, **f**)

3.3. MRI scan (Fig. 20.8g, h)

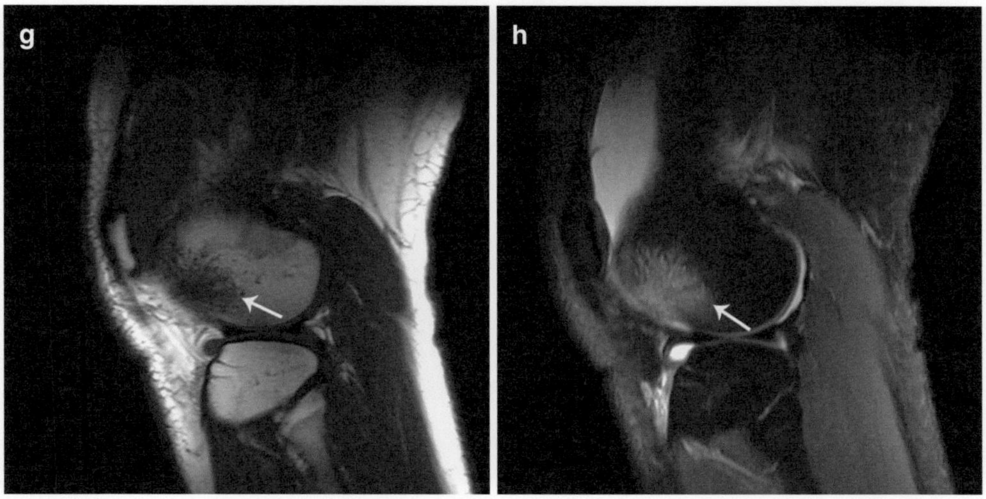

Fig. 20.8 T1WI and sagittal fat suppression T2WI MRI are presented in (**g**, **h**), showing the long patchy T1 and T2 signal shadow with a fuzzy edge (white arrow) in the lateral femoral condyle

4. Differential diagnosis of bone contusion and normal bone in tibial plateau
   4.1. X-ray (Fig. 20.9a–d)

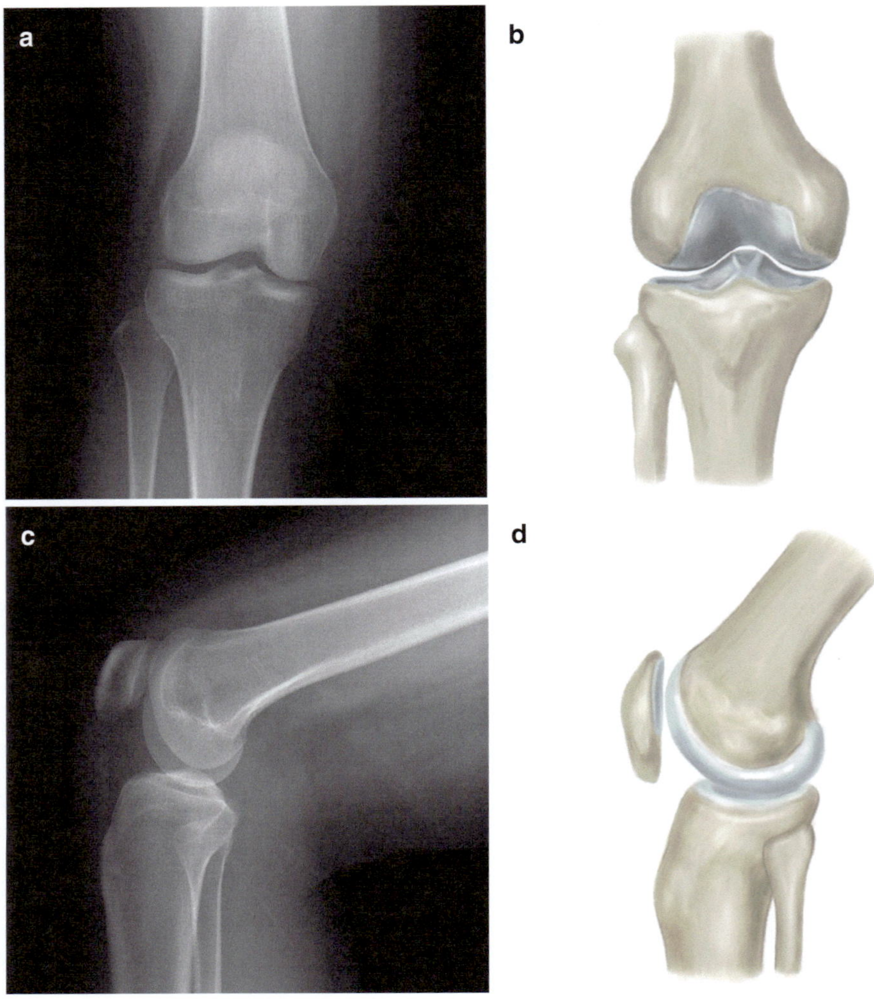

Fig. 20.9 There is no obvious fracture line in the anteroposterior and lateral projections/schematic diagram (**a**–**d**). CT and MRI scan are performed to make a definite diagnosis

4.2. CT scan (Fig. 20.9e, f)

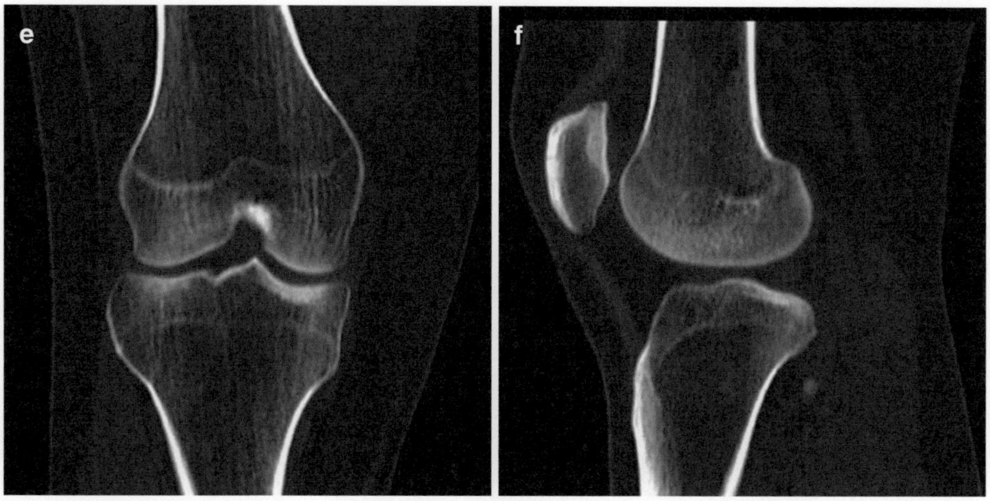

Fig. 20.9 There is no obvious fracture line in coronal and sagittal knee CT scans (**e**, **f**)

4.3. MRI scan (Fig. 20.9g, h)

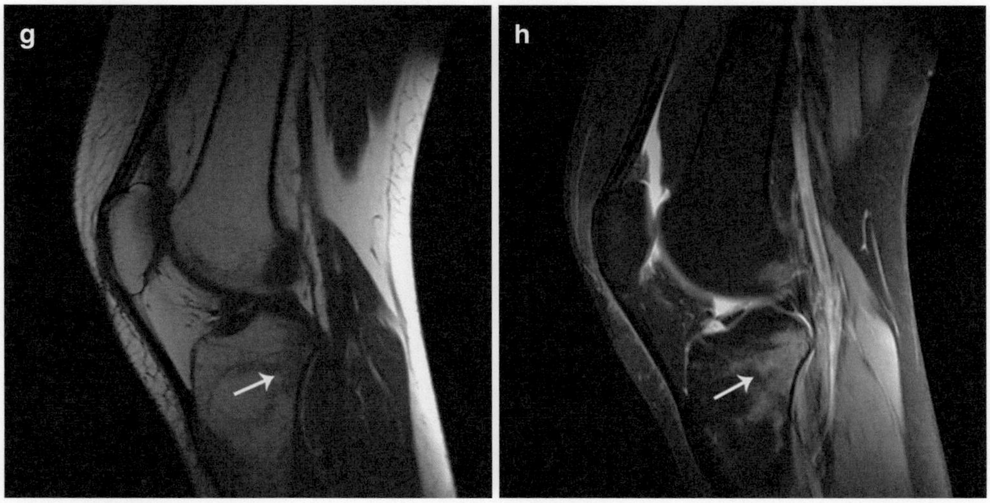

Fig. 20.9 T1WI and sagittal fat suppression T2WI MRI are presented in (**g**, **h**), showing long map T1 and T2 signal shadow with a fuzzy edge (white arrow) in proximal tibia. There is no short-line shadow in the knee MRI scan

5. Differential diagnosis of bone contusion and normal bone posterior distal tibia
   5.1. X-ray (Fig. 20.10a–d)

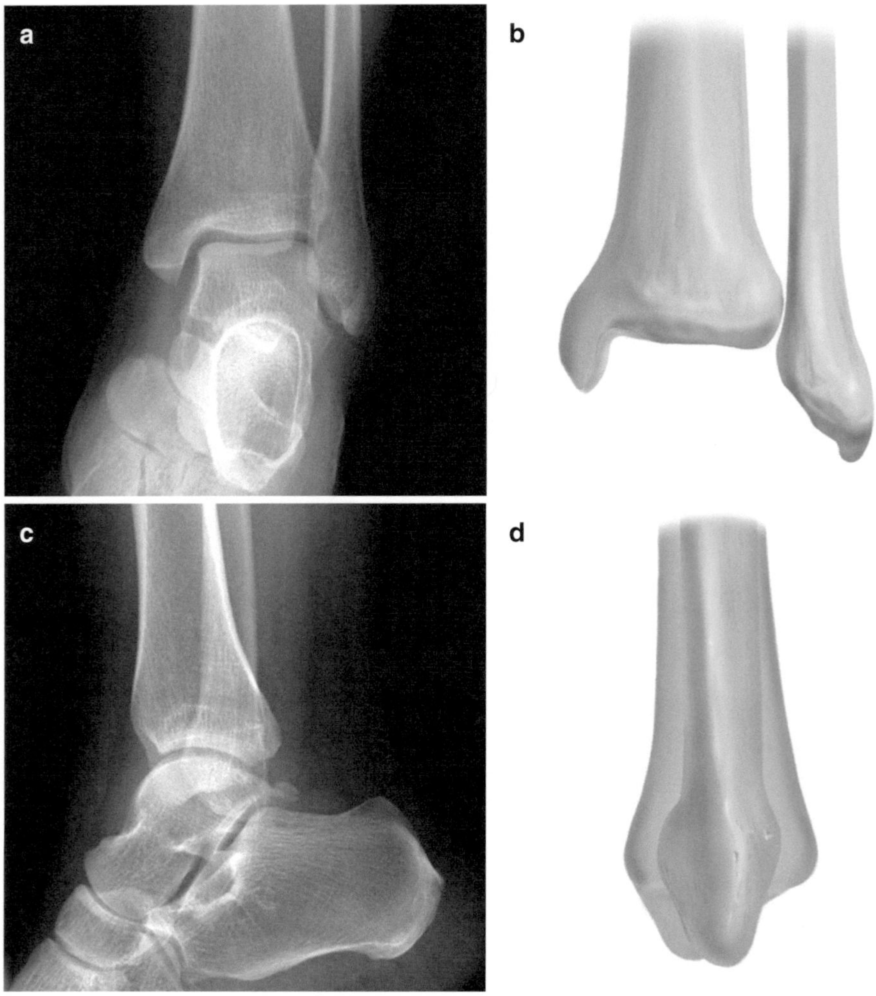

Fig. 20.10 There is no obvious fracture line in the anteroposterior and lateral projections/schematic diagram (**a**–**d**). MRI scan is performed to make a definite diagnosis

5.2. MRI scan (Fig. 20.10e–h)

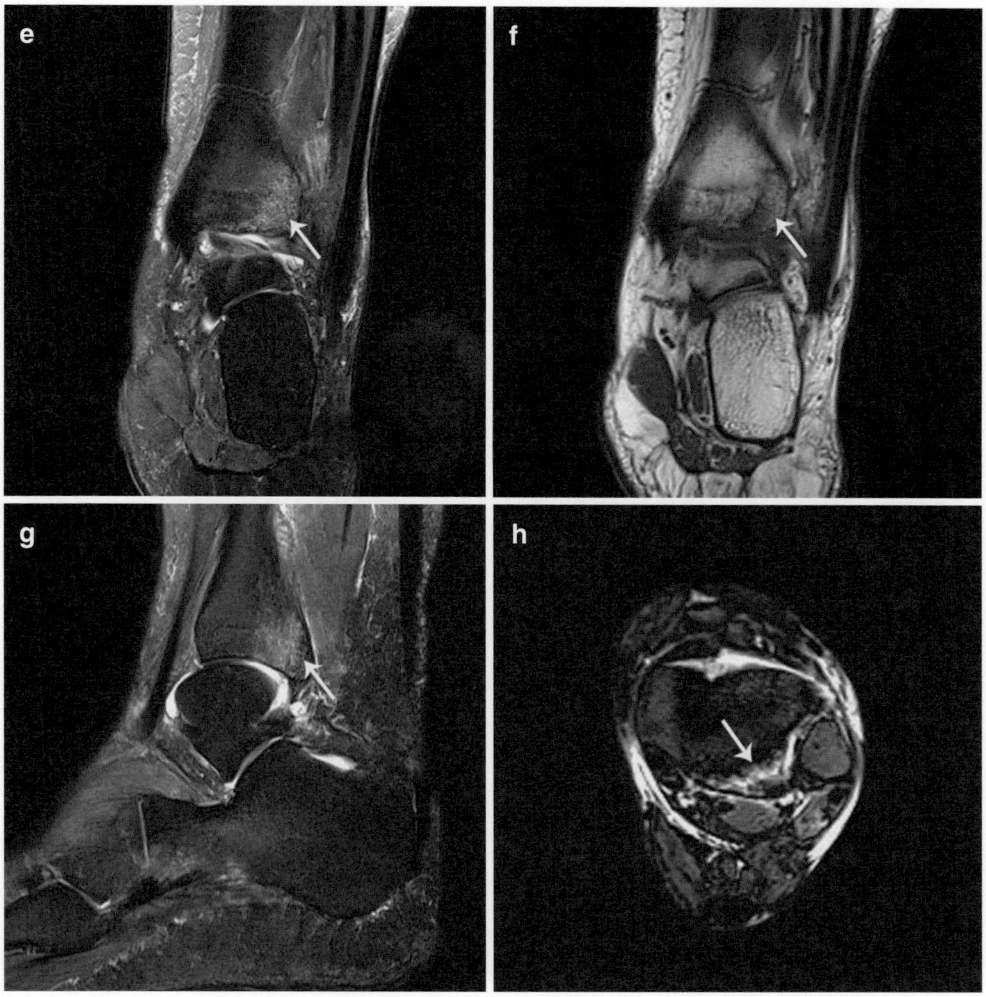

Fig. 20.10 (**e–h**) Show MRI CT scanning coronal fat inhibiting T2WI, T1WI, sagittal fat inhibiting T2WI, and horizontal axis fat inhibiting T2WI, respectively. It shows the patchy long T1 long T2 signal shadow with a fuzzy edge (white arrow) in the bone marrow of posterior distal tibia, surrounded by soft tissue swelling and small amount of fluid accumulation in the ankle joint

20.3 Summary

1. Occult fractures could be diagnosed by CT and MRI scan; however, it is not discoverable on X-ray. For the patients of significant trauma and pain with no fracture line in the X-ray, CT scans or MRI scan should be performed to make a definite diagnosis, especially in the areas with complex anatomical structures. Low density of cancellous bone and cortex could be showed in the CT scans and multiplanar MPR reconstruction. Linear, striate, or reticular low signal shadows of cortex and medullary space could be detected in T1WI MRI scan. However, high or low linear signal surrounded by lamellar hyper-signal bone marrow edema in T2WI scan.
2. Bone contusion, as a latent injury, showing the bone marrow hemorrhage, edema, and microfracture of bone trabeculae, but with the cortex being continuous. Fracture line could not be observed in the X-ray and CT scan. Lamellar, map, or irregular T1WI low signal could be seen in the cancellous bone. High signal shadow with a blurred edge and no obvious fracture line could be seen in the T2WI scan.
3. Occult fracture and bone contusion should be differentiated. Detachment of cortex is rarely involved for bone contusion, there is no need for special treatment and self-healing could be accomplished within 2–3 months. Fracture lines involve cortex and trabeculae for occult fractures. Fracture lines could be showed more clearly in the T1WI scan. However, fracture lines may be covered by high signal edema in T2WI scan. They are similar to the pathway and shape of low signal in the T1WI, which should be distinguished from each other.

21 Epiphyseal Injury and Early Closure of Epiphysis

Juan Wang and Yingze Zhang

21.1 Epiphyseal Injury

Epiphyseal cartilage plate injury, also known as epiphyseal injury, is a fracture across the epiphyseal cartilage plate. It is not only an isolated epiphyseal cartilage plate injury, but also syndesmotic injuries of epiphyseal cartilage plate, metaphysis, and epiphysis. It often causes partial epiphysis or total epiphysis or even partial metaphyseal displacement, which occurs diaphysis before the healing of the backbone and epiphysis. It is commonly seen in children 4–8 years old. Epiphyseal plate injury accounts for 15–30% of the long bone injury in children under 16 years of age, and about 1–2% of them have epiphyseal early closure. The classification of epiphyseal injury is of great significance in judging the prognosis and formulating treatment plans. Salter–Harris classification is divided epiphyseal injuries in children into five types. Type I: A separation through the physis (Fig. 21.1b); Type II: Fracture enters in the plane of the physis and exits through the metaphysis (Fig. 21.1c); Type III: Fracture enters in the plane of the physis and exits through the epiphysis (Fig. 21.1d); Type IV: Fracture across the physis, extending from the metaphysis to the epiphysis (Fig. 21.1e); Type V: Fracture is a crush injury resulting in injury to the physis (Fig. 21.1f).Type V injury under X-ray and CT imaging is not apparent and easily misdiagnosed, MRI is the only imaging method for early diagnosis of type V injury. Type III and IV injuries are prone to damage the growth layer, causing epiphyseal closure early, growth retardation, and progressive deformity. Type II and V can also cause epiphyseal closure early, but the incidence is low. The predilection sites of epiphyseal injury are: distal radius, medial epicondyle of the humerus, lateral humerus, proximal humerus, etc.

21.1.1 Identification of Injury Mechanism

The injury is caused by direct or indirect trauma. In addition, shear, avulsion, splitting, and squeezing force can cause epiphyseal injuries.

21.1.2 Identification of Symptoms and Signs

The most prominent symptoms are pain, swelling, and limited activity. Due to lack of specificity, they cannot be used for diagnosis. Therefore, if the child has pain in the metaphysis after injury, pay more attention when examining, and if necessary, X-ray, CT, or MRI is performed to prevent misdiagnosis.

J. Wang · Y. Zhang (✉)
Department of Orthopaedics, The Third Hospital of Hebei Medical University, Shijiazhuang, Hebei, China

Y. Zhang (ed.), *Differential Diagnosis of Fracture*, https://doi.org/10.1007/978-981-13-8339-7_21

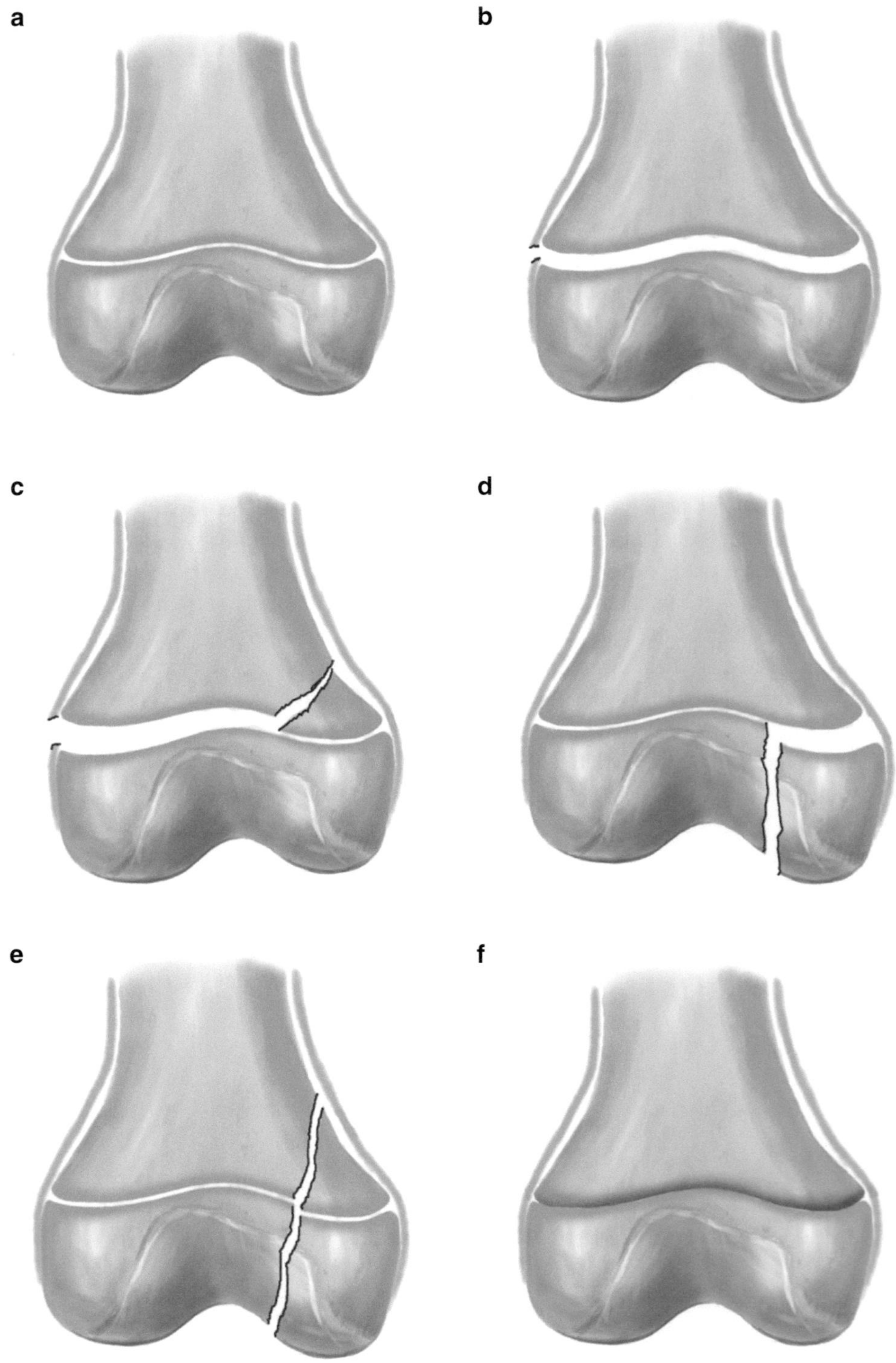

Fig. 21.1 Epiphysis of distal femur (**a**), Salter–Harris classification of epiphyseal injury (**b**–**f**)

21.1.3 Differential Diagnosis of Imaging

(1) The X-ray and CT of the epiphyseal cartilage plates show a low-density band between the epiphysis and the metaphysis. T1W1MRI image shows a moderate hypointensity and T2W1 MRI image shows a hyperintensity. When X-ray and CT scans are negative, but the symptoms and signs are apparent, MRI should be performed. MRI can clearly show the epiphysis and epiphyseal cartilage plate, which is more sensitive than X-ray and CT, and the classification is more accurate. (2) The non-ossified epiphysis is not visible on X-ray and CT, making it difficult to detect epiphyseal injuries. MRI

can directly show epiphyseal cartilage. (3) When fracture and epiphyseal injury exit at the same time, the fracture is obvious. While the epiphyseal injury is relatively light, be careful not to leave out the inconspicuous epiphyseal injury. (4) When there are multiple ossification centers in the epiphysis, it is important not to misdiagnose as a fracture of the epiphysis. (5) Familiarity with the time of occurrence and closure of the secondary ossification center of normal epiphysis is important, and attention should be paid to the contralateral alignment of the secondary ossification center and the metaphysis. It is also essential to identify the normal epiphysis and fracture in combination with children. If the epiphyseal injury is suspected, but the X-ray signs are not obvious, MRI should be performed. (6) When performing CT and MRI, the upper and lower levels are continuously observed from different scanning orientation.

21.1.4 Summary of Diagnosis Points

(1) History of trauma; (2) X-ray and CT showed a change in epiphyseal position with or without epiphyseal or metaphyseal fractures; (3) When there is no displacement of the epiphysis, there is no abnormal performance, sometimes showing that the epiphyseal line is enlarged or narrowed. (4) MRI showed that the epiphyseal position was abnormal and the epiphyseal cartilage plate is interrupted involving its injury. The normal uniform signal becomes uneven. Long T1 and long T2 signal can be visible at the epiphysis or metaphysis. When it comes to early closure of epiphysis, the high-signal epiphyseal cartilage plate on T2W1 MRI image is interrupted, during which low-signal trabecula is seen to pass-through.

21.1.4.1 Salter–Harris Type I:A Separation Through the Physis

1. Salter–Harris Type I:Identification of epiphyseal injury and non-injury
   1.1. X-ray (Fig. 21.2a–d)

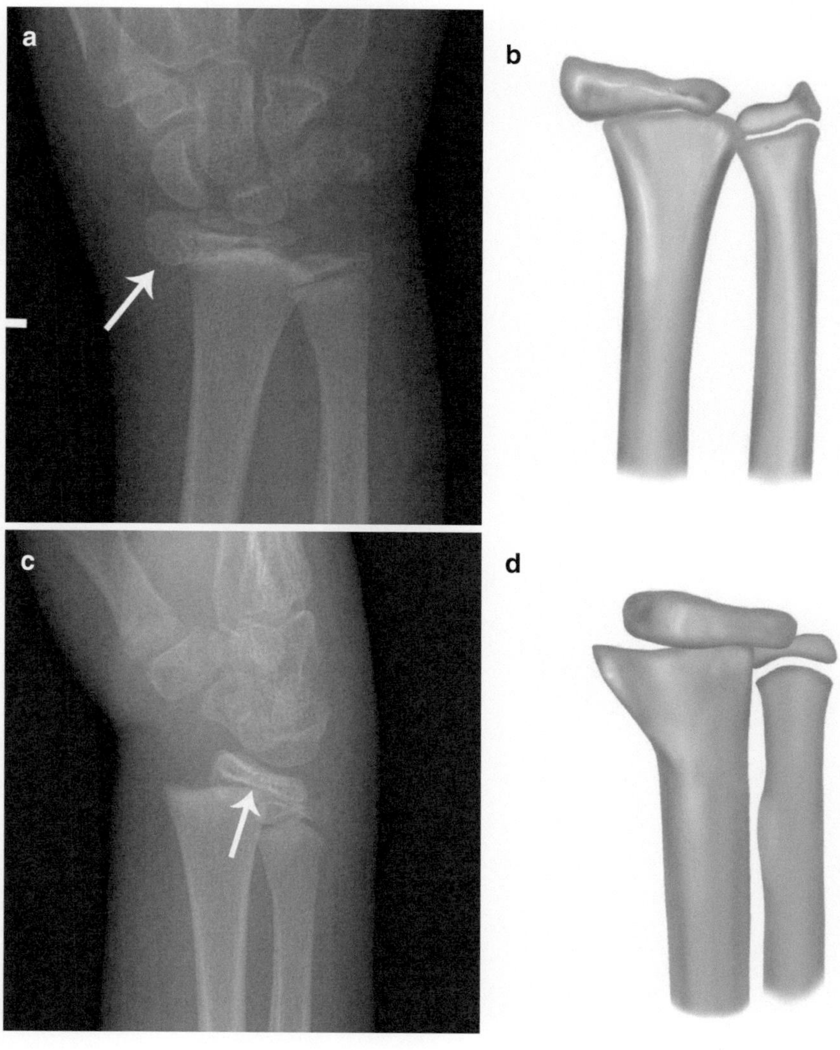

Fig. 21.2 (**a**, **c**) is the positive position and lateral position, respectively, and the epiphysis of the distal radius slips posteromedially (white arrow), schematic diagram (**b**, **d**)

1.2. CT (Fig. 21.2e)

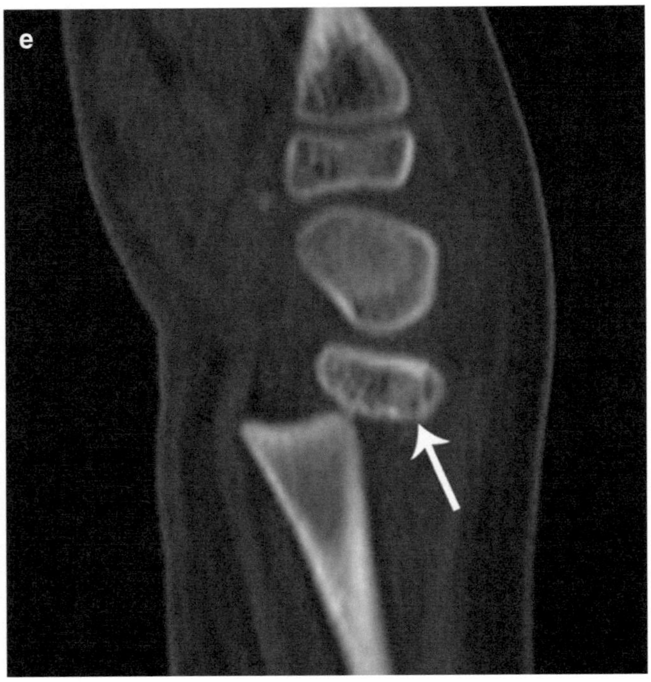

Fig. 21.2 (**e**) is the sagittal view, showing epiphyseal slips posteriorly (white arrow)

2. Right distal humerus of right elbow: Salter–Harris Type I:Identification of epiphyseal injury and non-injury
   2.1. MRI (Fig. 21.3a–c)

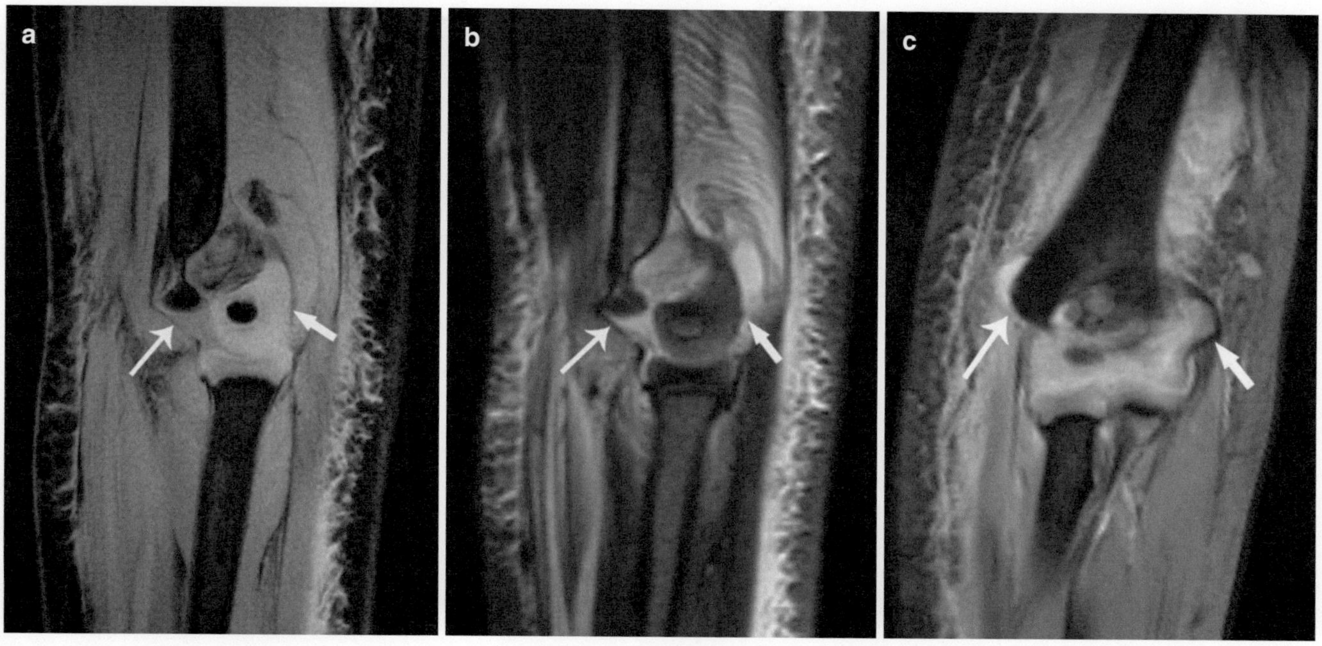

Fig. 21.3 (a–**c**), are respectively, MRI plain scan sagittal fat suppression T2WI, PDWI (proton density-weighted image), and coronal PDWI, showing the separation of the distal humerus epiphysis and posteromedial displacement of the epiphysis (rough white arrow), metaphysis (fine white arrow)

3. Medial epicondyle of the right humerus: Salter–Harris Type I:Identification of epiphyseal injury and non-injury
   3.1. X-ray (Fig. 21.4a–d)

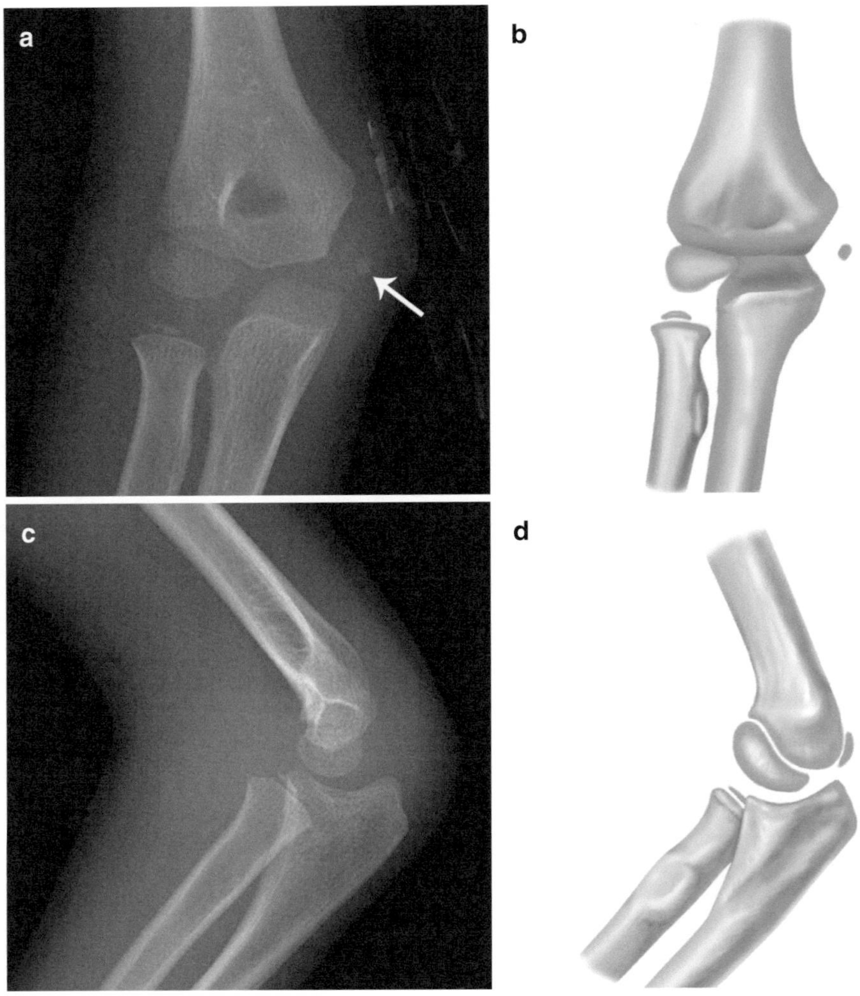

Fig. 21.4 (**a**) is the lateral position, showing the epiphysis of the medial epicondyle of the humerus slips. (**c**) shows unclear and schematic diagram (**b**, **d**). To further confirm the diagnosis, an MRI scan is performed

   3.2. MRI (Fig. 21.4e, f)

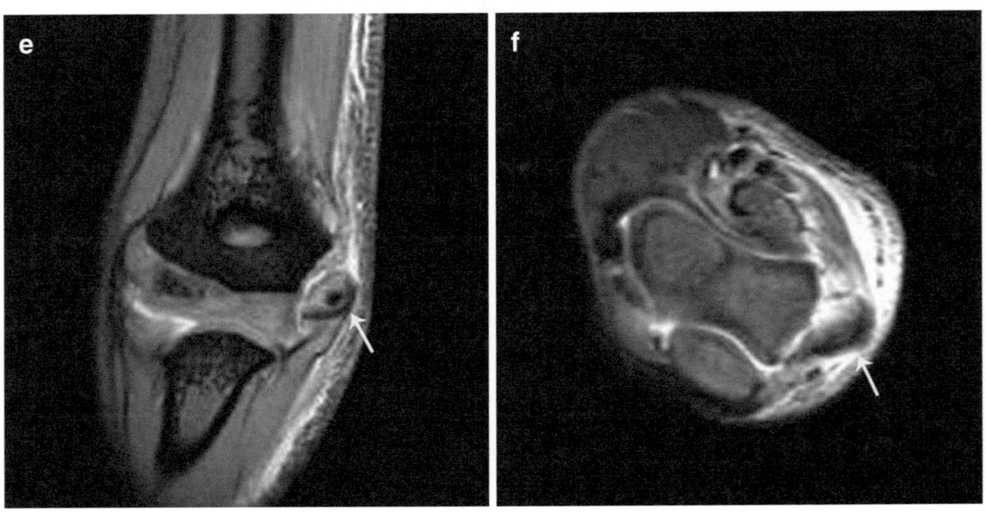

Fig. 21.4 (**e**, **f**) are, respectively, MRI coronal and transverse axis fat suppression T2WI, showing the epiphyseal separation of the medial epicondyle epiphysis (white arrow) and swelling of the surrounding soft tissue

4. Medial epicondyle of the left humerus: Salter-Harris Type I: Identification of epiphyseal injury and non-injury
   4.1. X-ray (Fig. 21.5a–d)

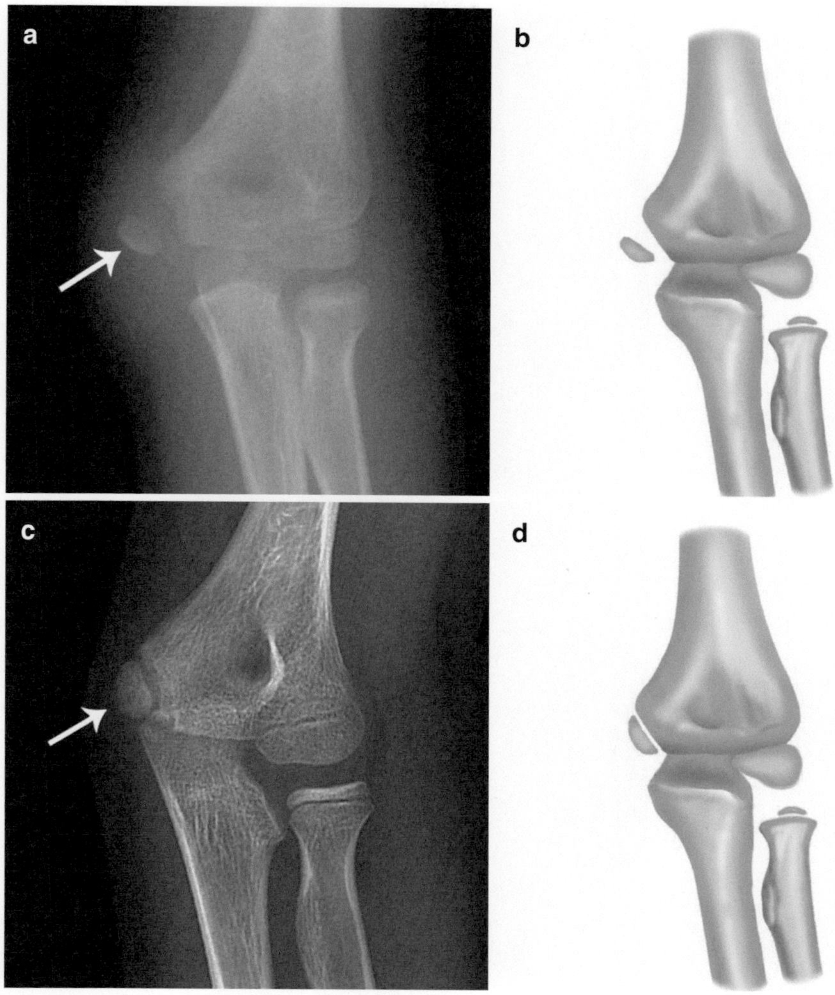

Fig. 21.5 (**a**) is a preoperative lateral position, showing epiphysis slippage of the medial epicondyle epiphysis and swelling of the surrounding soft tissue (white arrow) (**c**) is a schematic view of removal of the internal fixation after 3 months, showing that the epiphyseal position of the medial epicondyle of the humerus is normal (white arrow) and schematic diagram (**b**, **d**)

5. Distal tibia of the left ankle: Salter–Harris Type I epiphyseal injury
   5.1. X-ray (Fig. 21.6a–d)

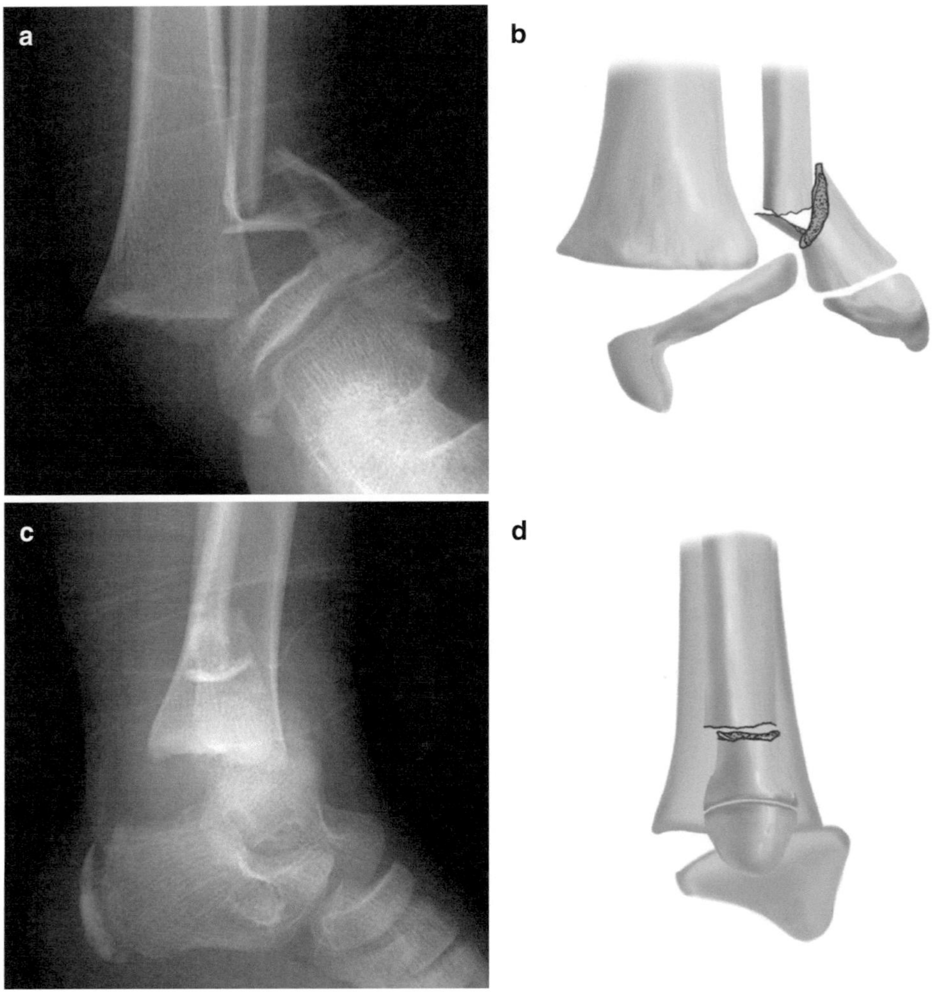

Fig. 21.6 (**a**, **c**) are, respectively, positive and lateral position, showing epiphysis slippage of the distal tibia with a fracture, and schematic diagram (**b**, **d**)

5.2. CT (Fig. 21.6e)

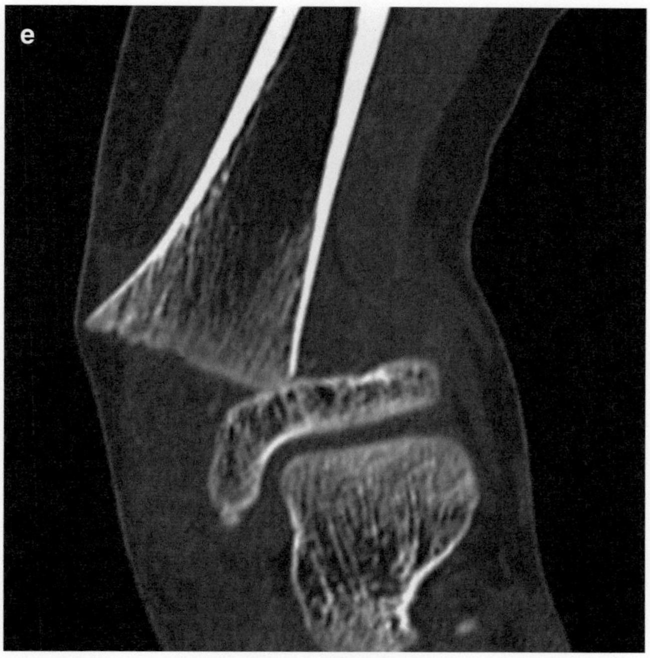

Fig. 21.6 (**e**) is the coronal plane, showing epiphysis slippage of distal tibia without epiphysis and metaphysis fracture

21.1.4.2 Type II: Fracture Enters in the Plane of the Physis and Exits Through the Metaphysis

6. Proximal first metacarpal: Identification of Salter–Harris Type II epiphyseal injury and Type I
   6.1. X-ray (Fig. 21.7a, b)

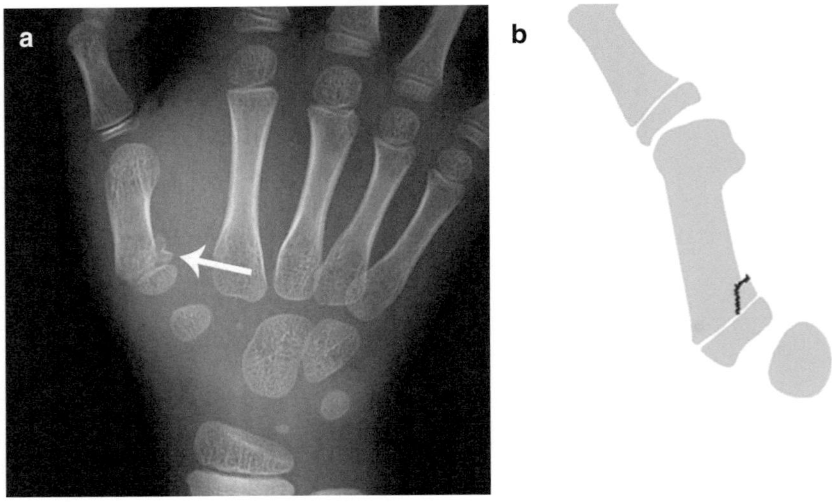

Fig. 21.7 (**a**) is the oblique position, showing epiphysis slippage anterolaterally of proximal first metacarpal, the metaphyseal fracture (white arrow), and the schematic diagram (**b**)

6.2. CT (Fig. 21.7c–e)

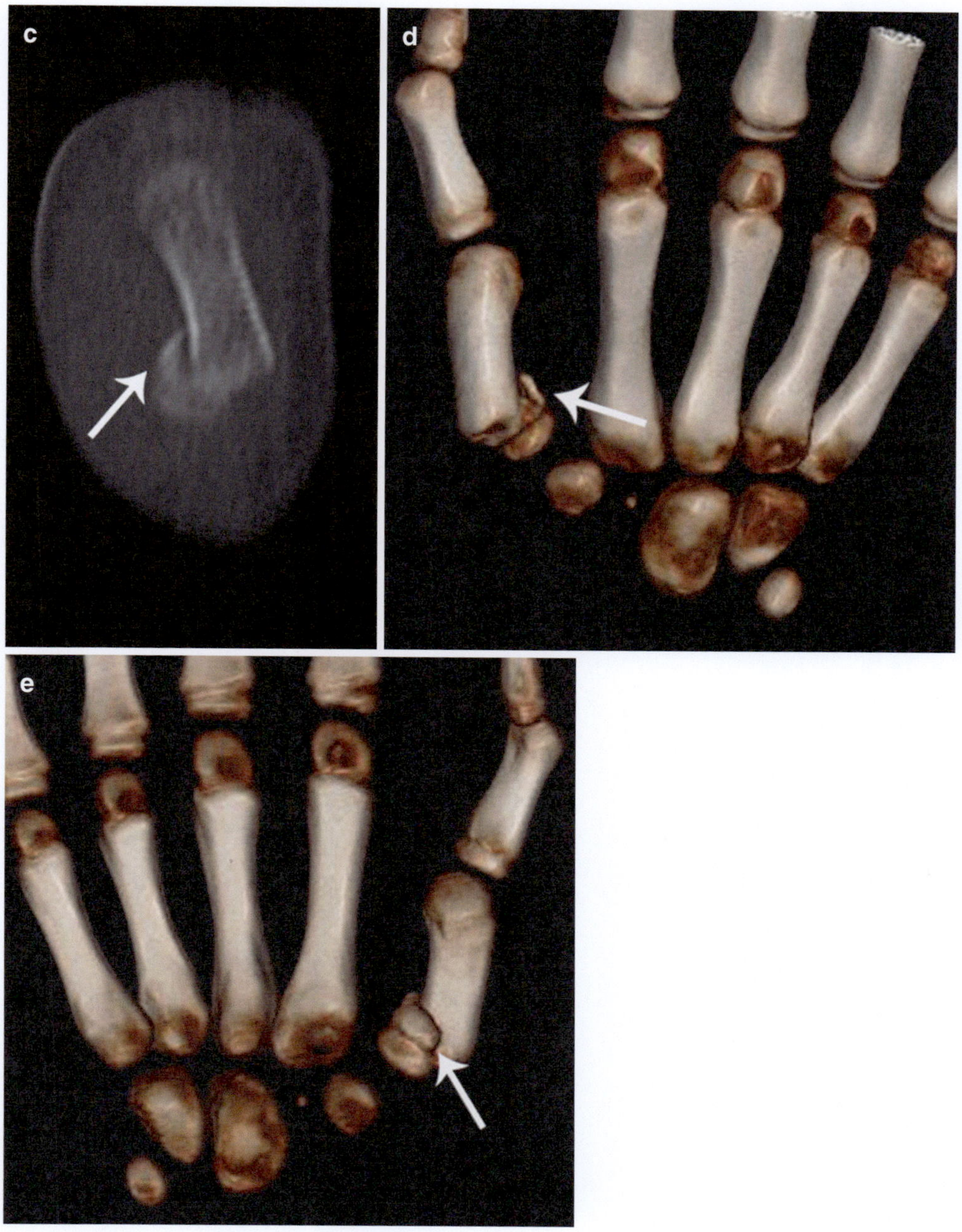

Fig. 21.7 (**c**) is the sagittal plane, (**d**, **e**) are, respectively, dorsal view and palmar view of three-dimensional reconstruction, showing epiphysis slippage anterolaterally of proximal first metacarpal and metaphyseal fracture (white arrow)

7. Bilateral distal radius: Identification of Salter–Harris Type II epiphyseal injury and Type I
   7.1. X-ray (Fig. 21.8a–h)

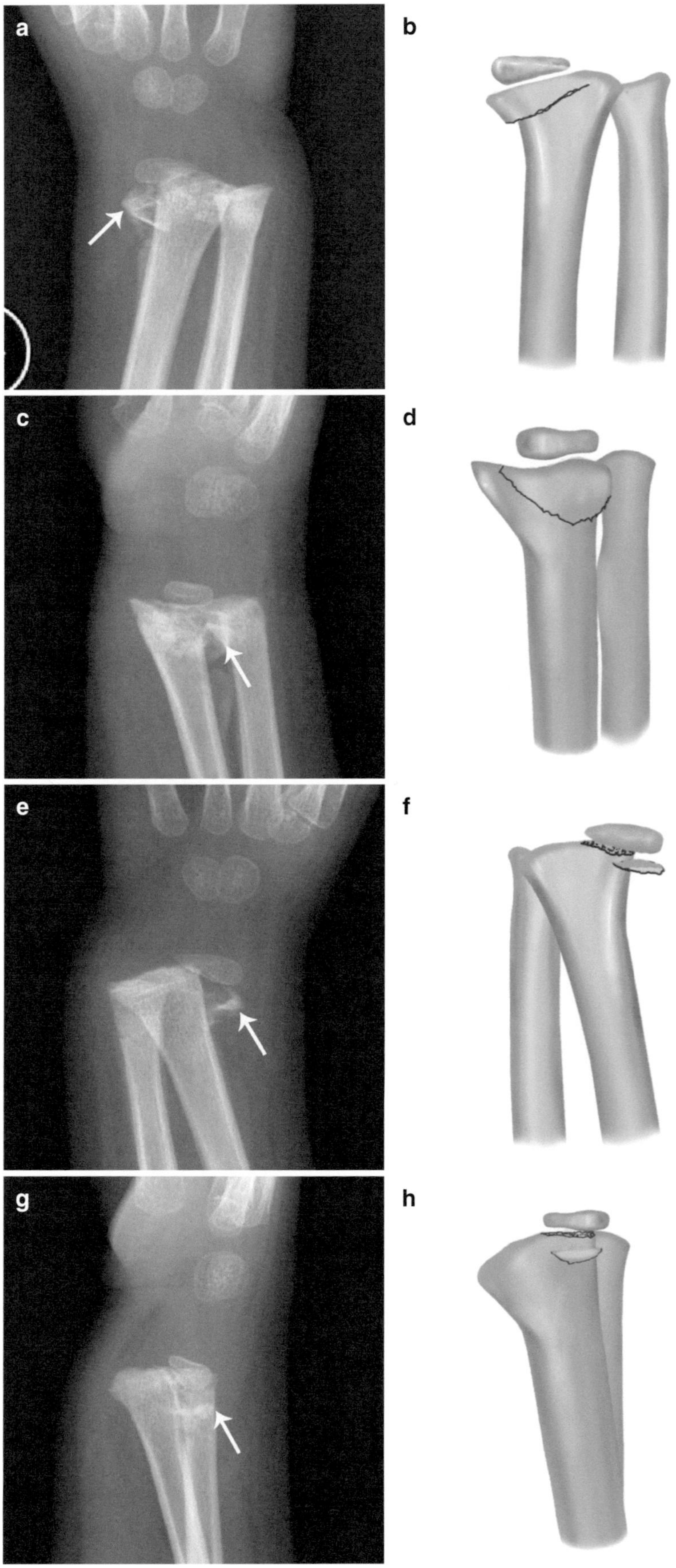

Fig. 21.8 (**a**, **c**) are, respectively, positive and lateral position of the left wrist, and the schematic diagram (**b**, **d**). (**e**, **g**) are, respectively, positive and lateral position of the right wrist, and the schematic diagram (**f**, **h**) showing epiphysis slippage of bilateral distal radius and metaphyseal fracture (white arrow). The epiphysis of bilateral distal ulna showed no secondary ossification center, so an MRI scan was conducted

7.2. MRI (Fig. 21.8i–l)

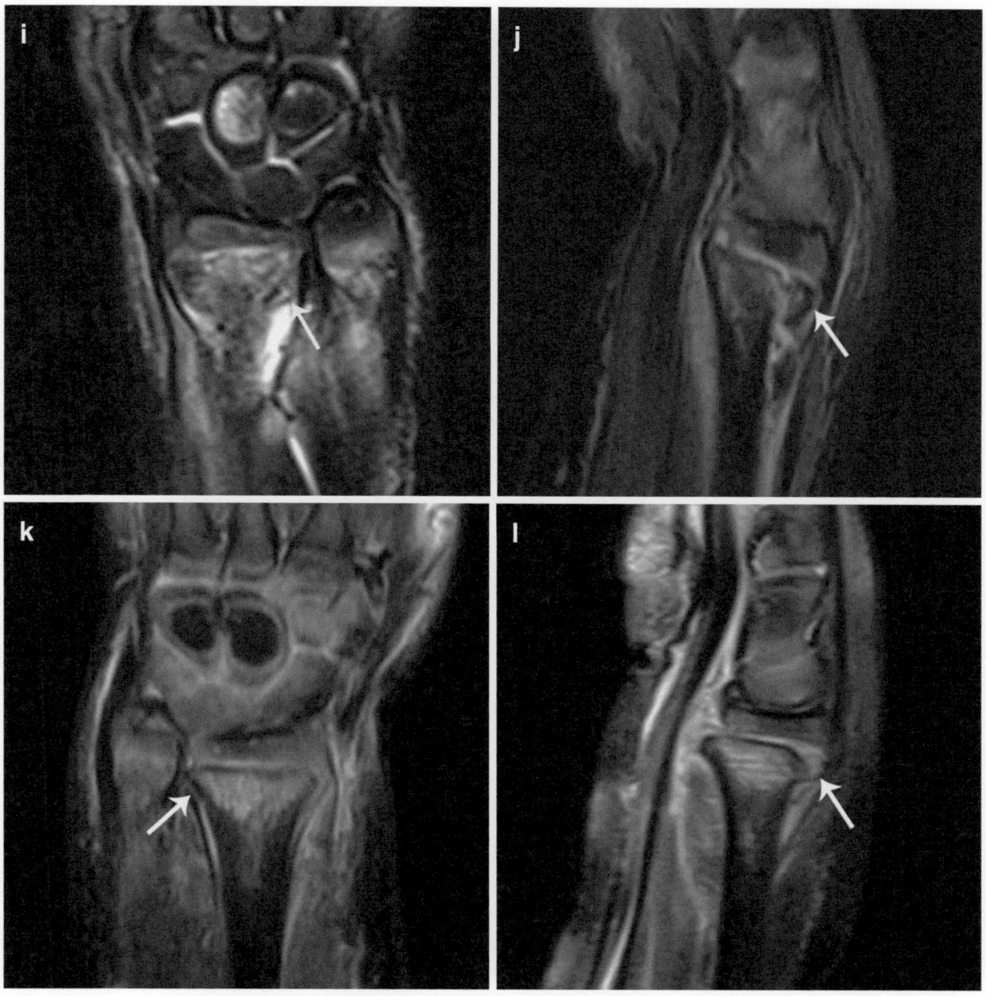

Fig. 21.8 (**i**, **j**) are, respectively, the left wrist MRI coronal and sagittal fat suppression T2WI, and (**k**, **l**) are, respectively, the right wrist coronal and sagittal fat suppression T2WI, showing epiphyseal slippage of bilateral distal radius, metaphyseal fracture (white arrow), bone marrow edema, and swelling around the soft tissue. The epiphysis position of bilateral distal ulna is normal

8. Left distal radius: Identification of Salter–Harris Type II epiphyseal injury and Type I
   8.1. X-ray (Fig. 21.9a–d)

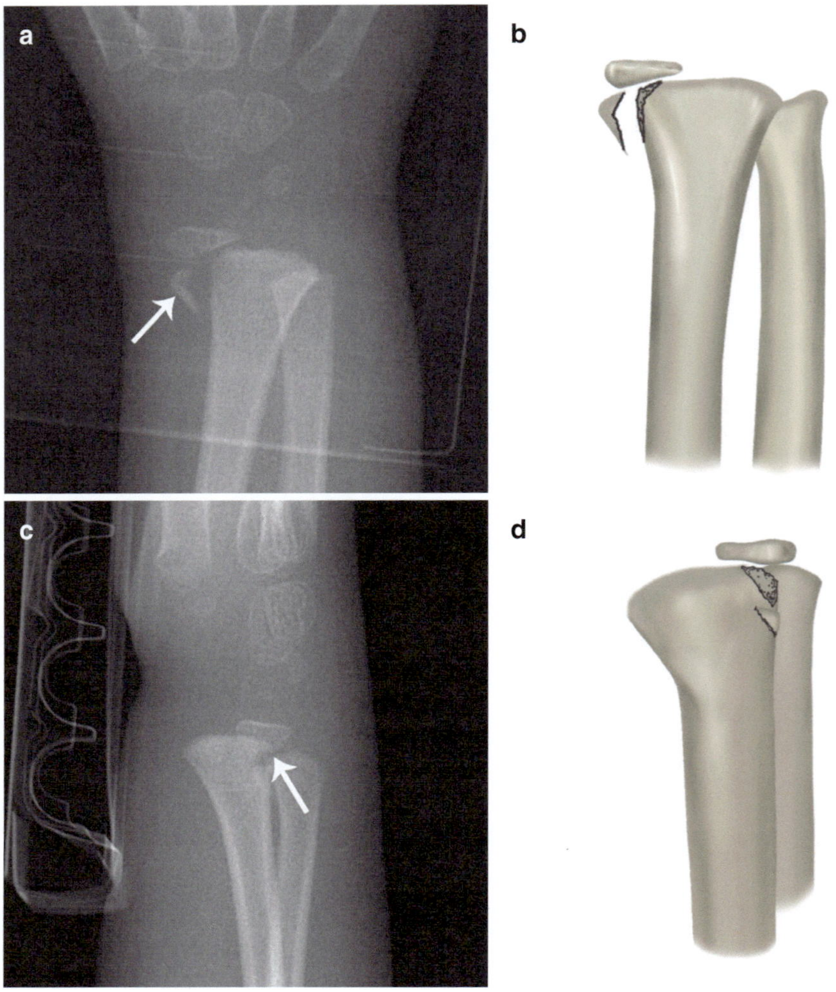

Fig. 21.9 (**a**, **c**) are, respectively, positive and lateral position, showing epiphysis separation of left distal radius, metaphyseal fracture (white arrow), and the schematic diagram (**b**, **d**)

   8.2. CT (Fig. 21.9e, f)

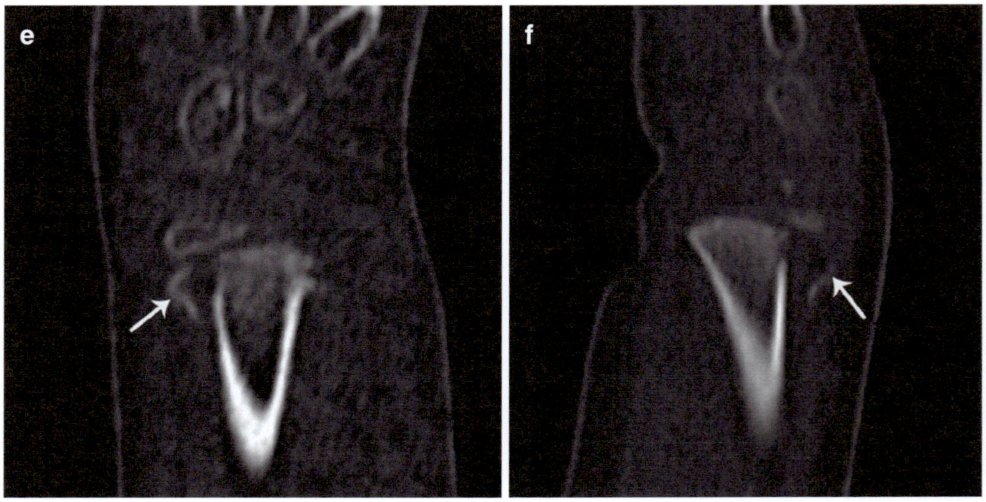

Fig. 21.9 (**e**, **f**) are, respectively, coronal plane and sagittal plane, showing epiphysis separation of the left distal radius and metaphyseal fracture (white arrow). Right radial head: Salter–Harris Type II: Identification of epiphyseal rotation and non-rotation (Fig. 21.10)

9. Right radial head: Salter–Harris Type II: Identification of epiphyseal rotation and non-rotation
   9.1. X-ray (Fig. 21.10a–d)

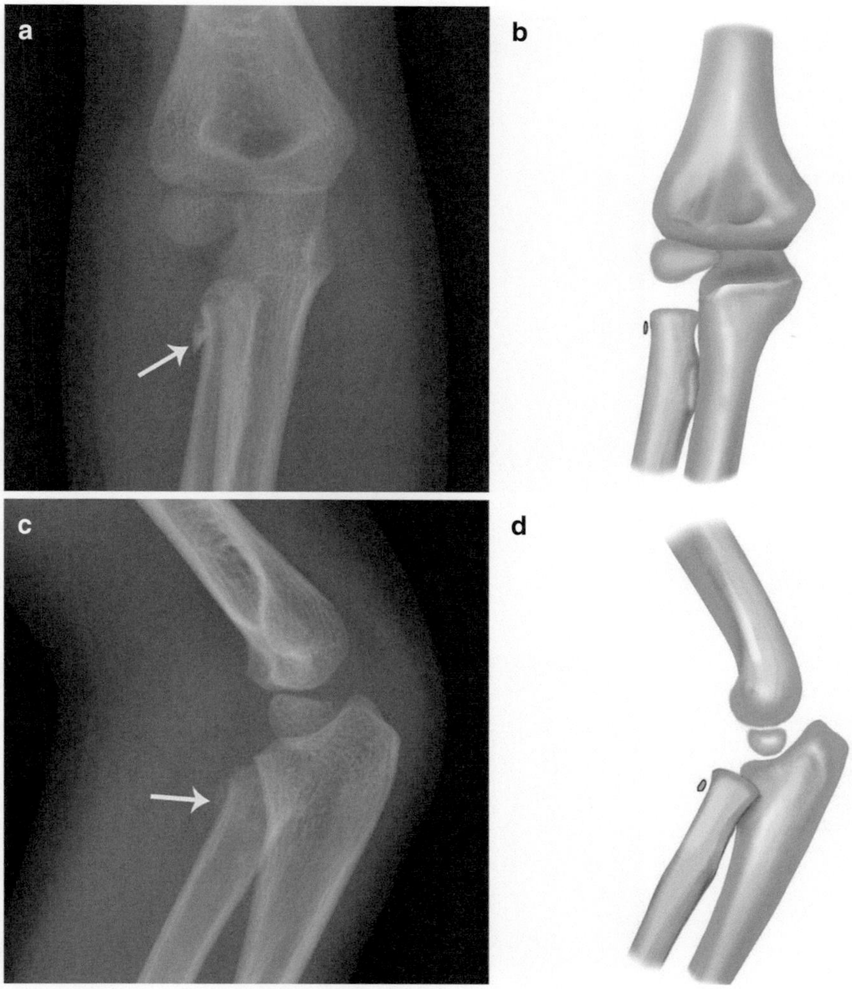

Fig. 21.10 (**a**, **c**) are, respectively, positive and lateral position, showing the metaphyseal fracture (rough white arrow) of the proximal radius, and the schematic diagram (**b**, **d**). The epiphyseal position was not clear, so MRI was conducted

   9.2. MRI (Fig. 21.10e, f)

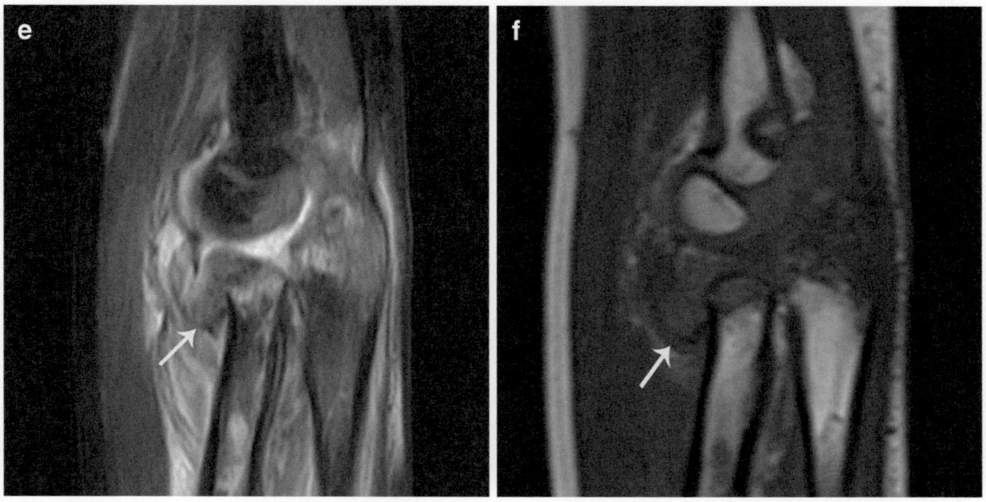

Fig. 21.10 (**e**, **f**) are sagittal fat suppression T2WI and T1WI, respectively, showing epiphysis separation of proximal radius. Turn laterally nearly 90° (white arrow), and visible medullary edema in the upper humerus and proximal ulna

10. Left radial head: Salter–Harris Type II: Identification of epiphyseal injury and non-injury
    10.1. CT (Fig. 21.11a, b)

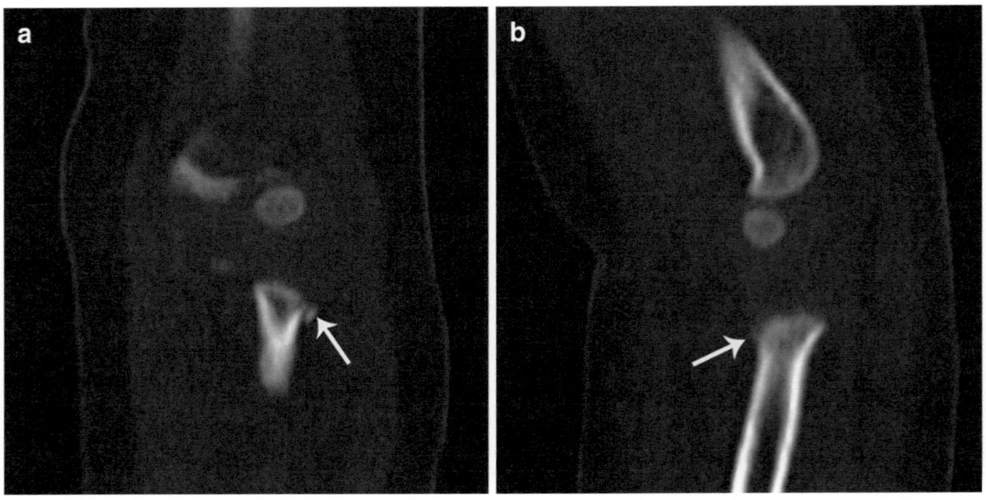

Fig. 21.11 (**a**, **b**) are, respectively, coronal plane and sagittal plane, showing metaphyseal fracture of radial head (white arrow). In order to display the epiphysis, an MRI scan is performed. In order to develop the epiphysis, MRI is performed

    10.2. MRI (Fig. 21.11c, d)

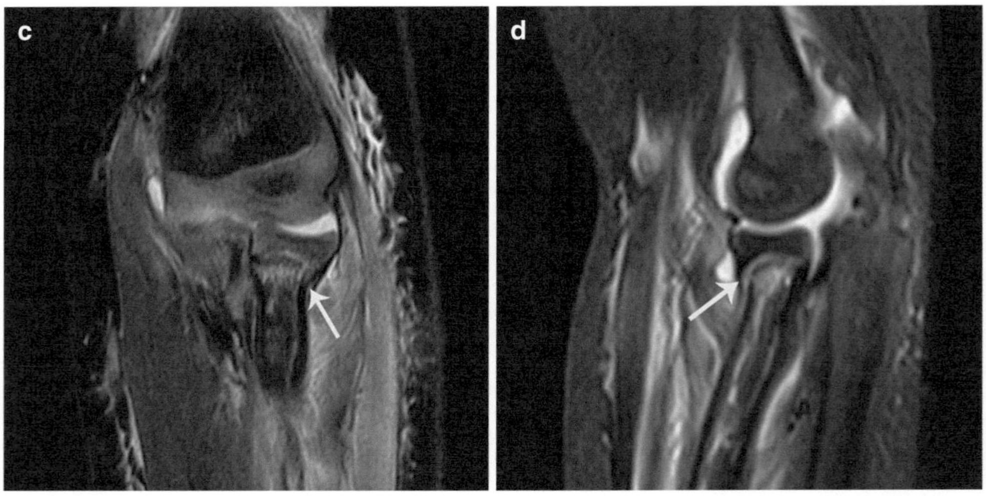

Fig. 21.11 (**c**, **d**) are, respectively, coronal plane and sagittal fat suppression T2W1, showing epiphysis of radial head with slight anterior displacement and metaphyseal fracture (white arrow)

11. Left proximal humerus: Salter–Harris Type II: identification of epiphyseal injury and non-injury
    11.1. X-ray (Fig. 21.12a–d)

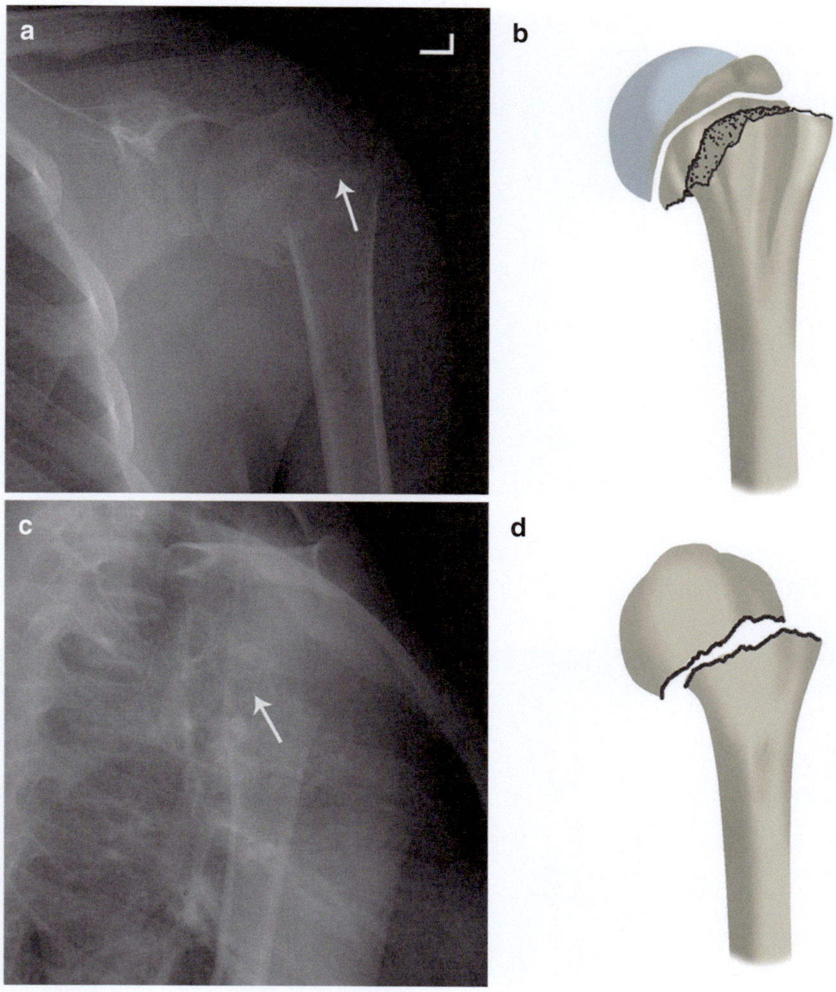

Fig. 21.12 (**a**, **c**) are, respectively, positive and lateral position, showing epiphysis slippage of proximal humerus with metaphyseal fracture (white arrow), and the schematic diagram (**b**, **d**).To further examine the epiphysis, CT was performed

    11.2. CT (Fig. 21.12e, f)

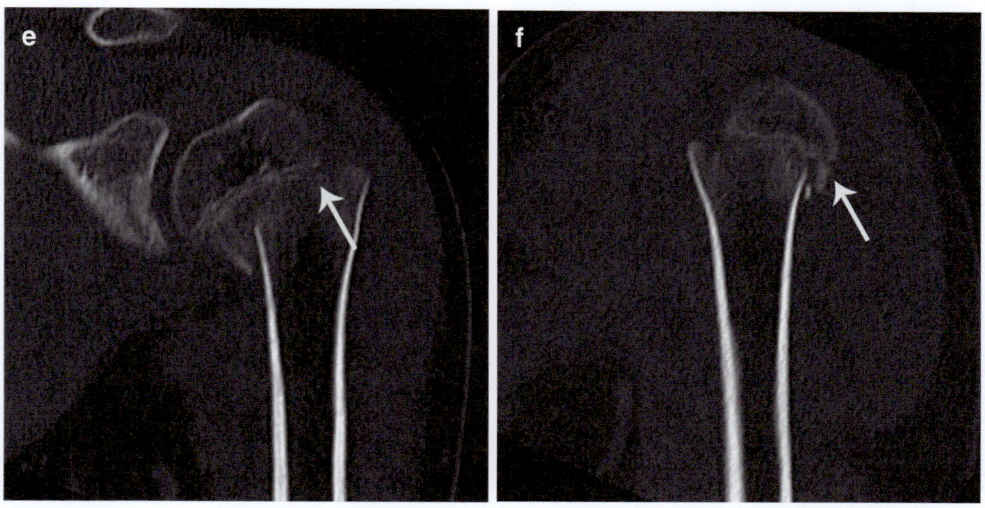

Fig. 21.12 (**e**, **f**) are, respectively, coronal plane and sagittal plane, showing epiphysis slippage of left proximal humerus with metaphyseal fracture (white arrow)

12. Left proximal humerus: Identification of Salter–Harris Type II epiphyseal injury and Type I
    12.1. X-ray (Fig. 21.13a, b)

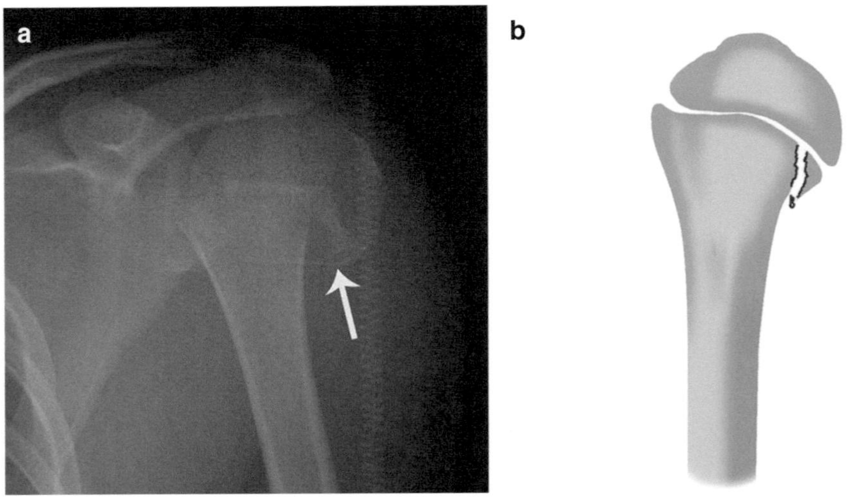

Fig. 21.13 (**a**) is positive position, showing epiphysis slippage of proximal humerus and metaphyseal fracture is not clear, and the schematic diagram (**b**)

12.2. CT (Fig. 21.13c, d)

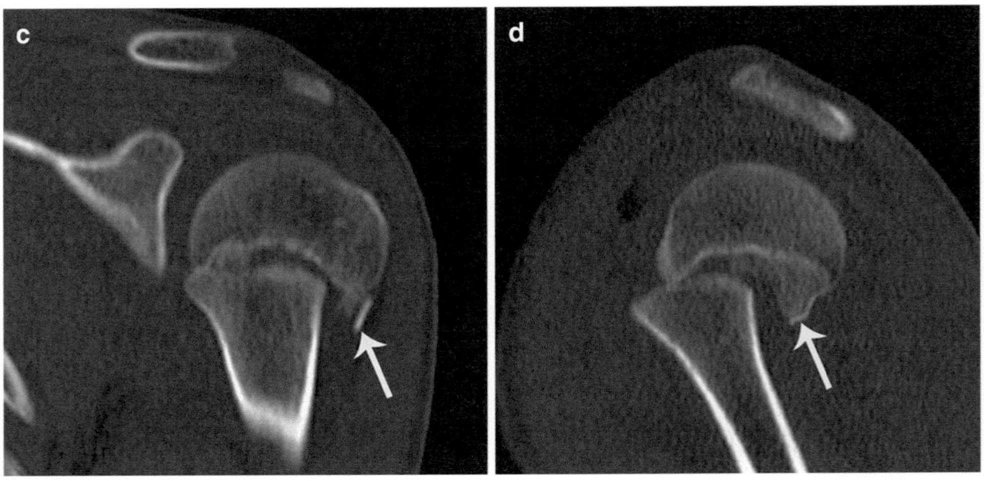

Fig. 21.13 (**c**, **d**) are, respectively, coronal and sagittal plane, showing epiphysis slippage of left proximal humerus with metaphyseal fracture (white arrow)

13. Right distal femur: Salter–Harris II epiphyseal injury
    13.1. X-ray (Fig. 21.14a–d)

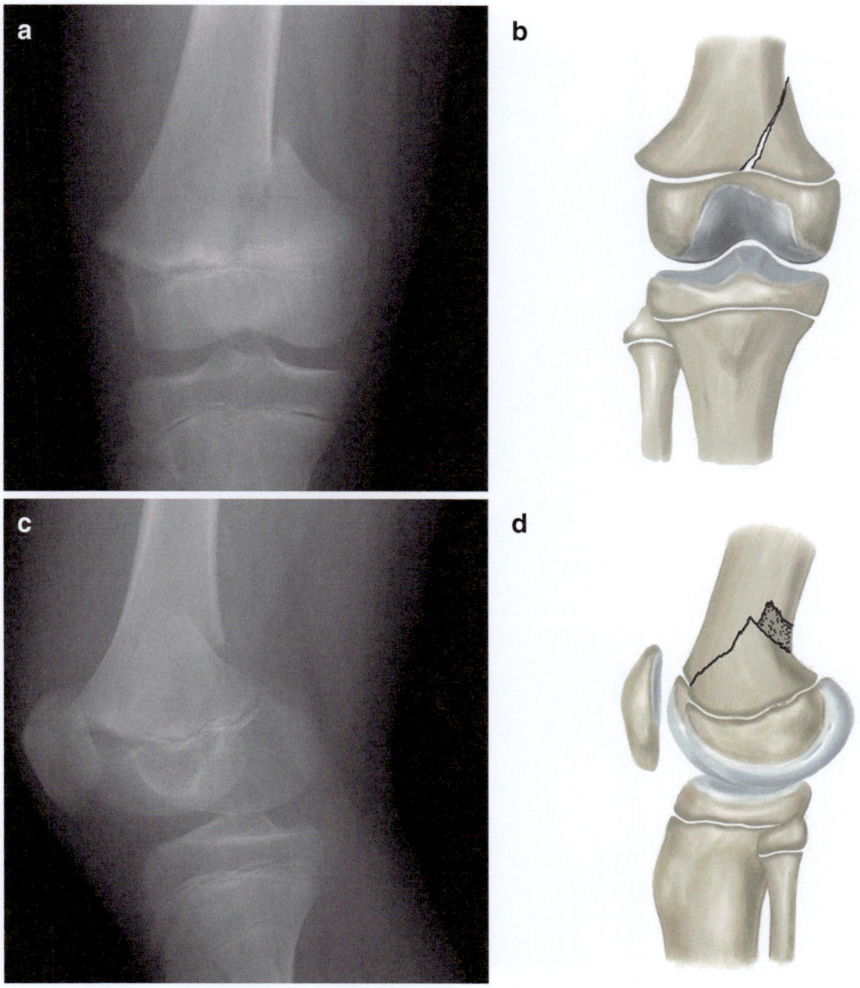

Fig. 21.14 (**a**, **c**) are, respectively, positive and lateral position, showing epiphysis separation of right distal femoral with slight interior displacement, metaphysis fracture and dislocation, and a schematic diagram (**b**, **d**).The anterior and posterior displacement of the epiphysis is unclear, so CT is performed

    13.2. CT (Fig. 21.14e, f)

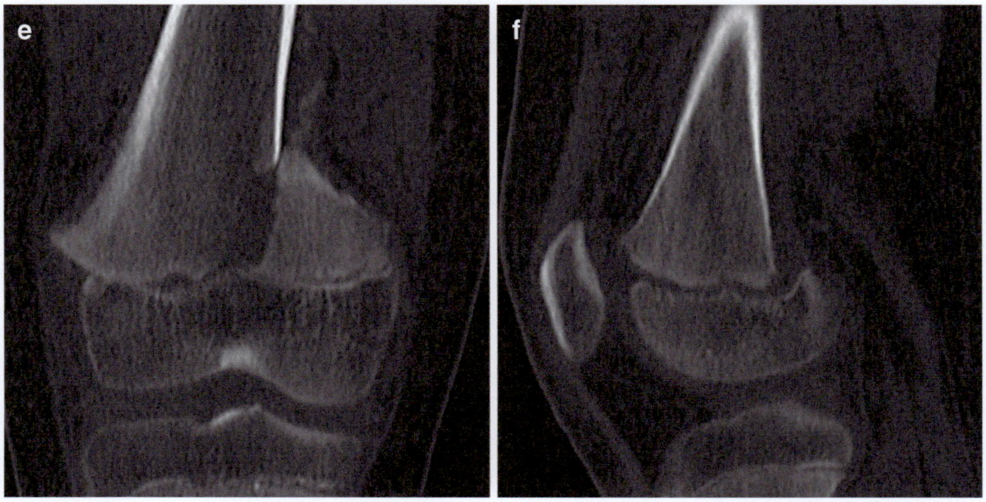

Fig. 21.14 (**e**, **f**) are, respectively, coronal and sagittal plane, showing epiphysis separation of right distal femoral with posterior displacement, and metaphyseal fracture and dislocation

14. Proximal right tibia: epiphysis and metaphyseal fracture of distal femur Identification of Salter–Harris Type II epiphyseal injury and Type I
    14.1. X-ray (Fig. 21.15a–d)

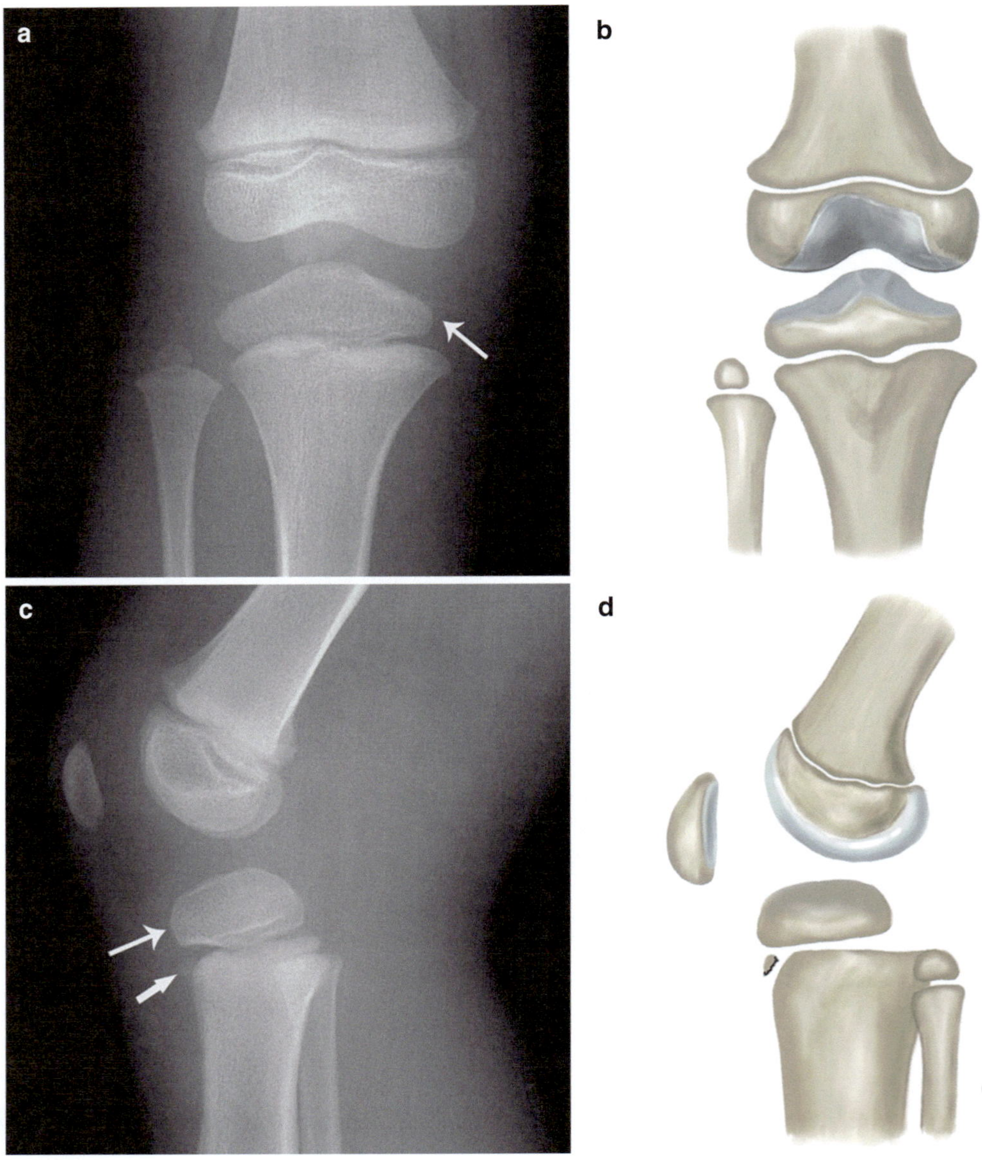

Fig. 21.15 (**a**) is the X-ray positive position, showing epiphysis exterior slippage of proximal tibia (fine white arrow) and the metaphyseal fracture is unclear. (**c**) is lateral position, showing epiphysis anterior displacement (fine white arrow), metaphyseal fracture (rough white arrow), and a schematic diagram (**d**)

15. Left distal tibia and fibula: Salter–Harris II epiphyseal injury
    15.1. CT (Fig. 21.16a–d)

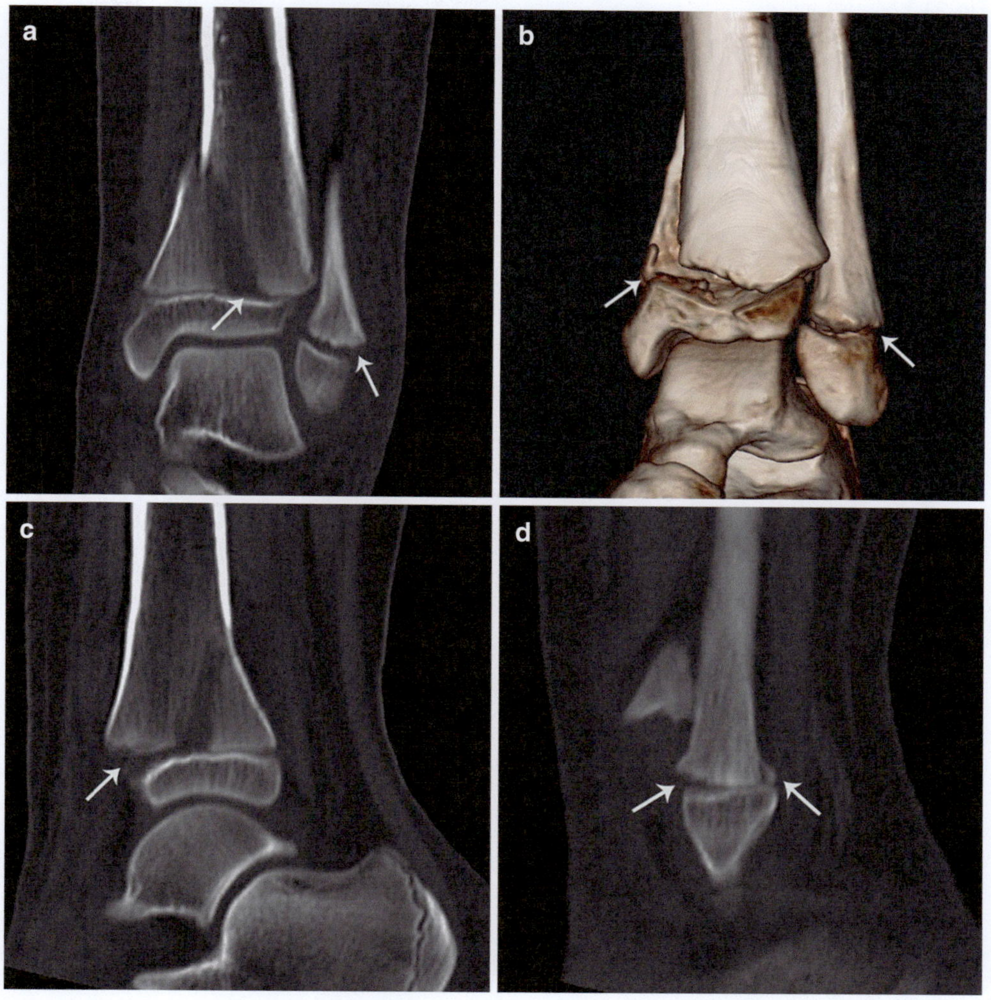

Fig. 21.16 (**a**) is the coronal reconstruction, (**b**) is the three-dimensional reconstruction, and (**b**, **d**) are sagittal reconstruction, showing epiphysis separation of distal tibia and fibula, and metaphyseal fracture (white arrow)

16. Left distal tibia: Identification of Salter–Harris Type II epiphyseal injury and Type I
    16.1. X-ray (Fig. 21.17a–d)

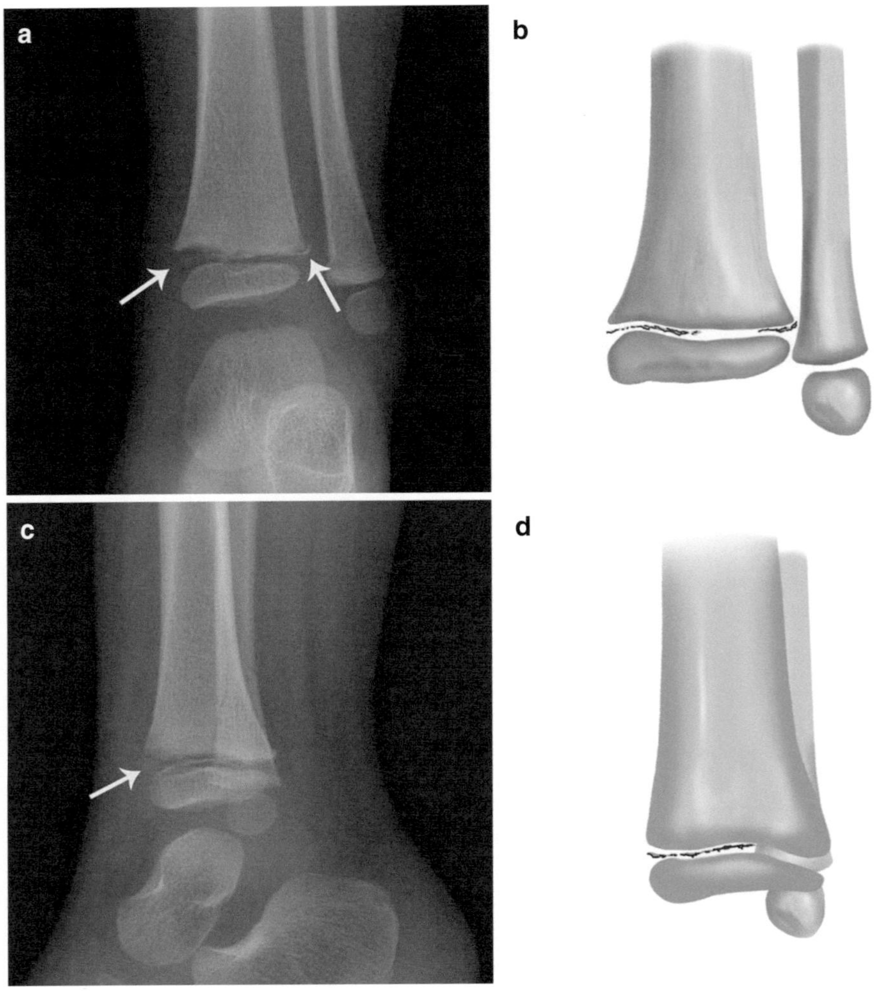

Fig. 21.17 (**a**, **c**) are, respectively, positive and lateral position, showing epiphysis separation of distal tibia, metaphyseal fracture (white arrow), and fracture line of the metaphysis is unclear, schematic diagram (**d**)

16.2. MRI (Fig. 21.17e, f)

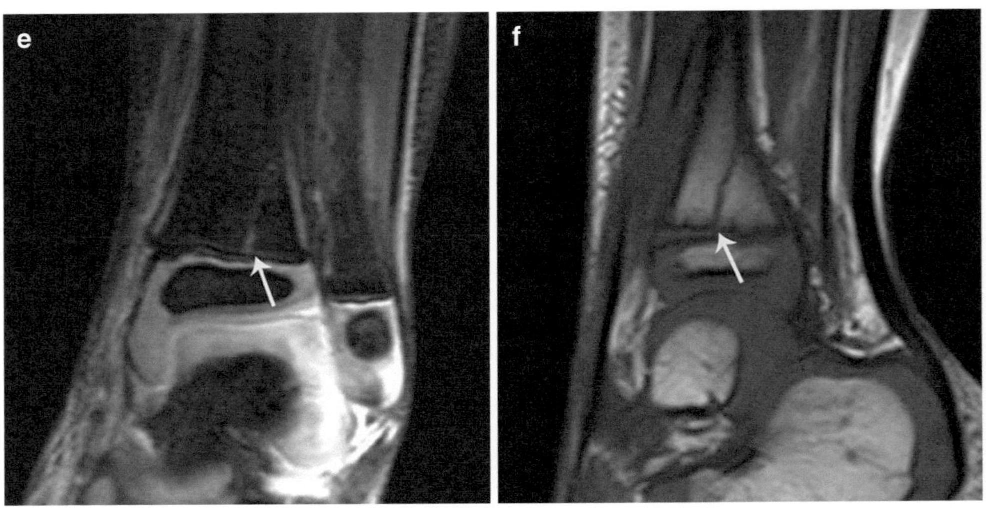

Fig. 21.17 (**e**, **f**) are coronal fat suppression T2WI and sagittal T1WI, respectively, showing slight separation of the distal tibia and metaphyseal fracture (white arrow)

21.1.4.3 Type III: Fracture Enters in the Plane of the Physis and Exits Through the Epiphysis

17. Left distal ulna: Identification of Salter–Harris Type III epiphyseal injury and Type II
    17.1. MRI (Fig. 21.18a–c)

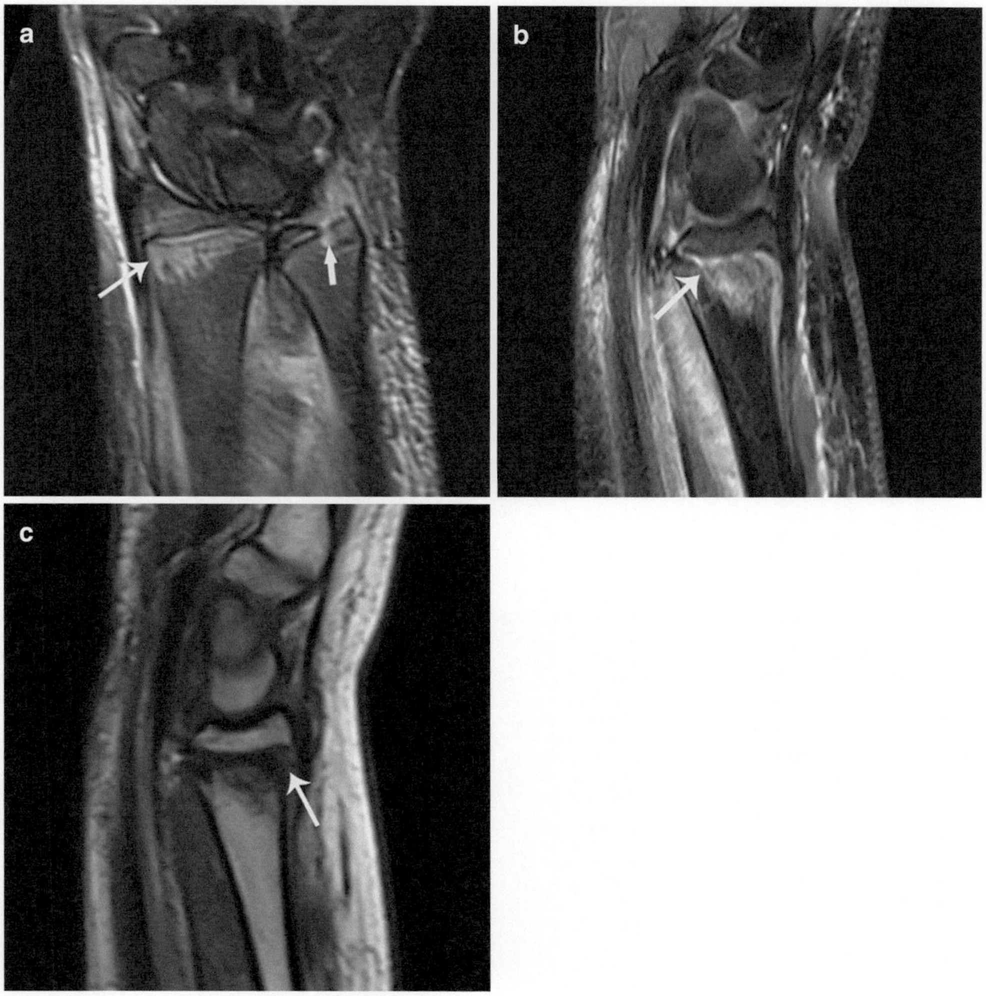

Fig. 21.18 (**a**) is coronal fat suppression T2W1, and (**b**, **c**) are sagittal fat suppression T2W1 and T1W1, showing epiphyseal fracture of the distal ulna involved the epiphyseal cartilage plate (rough white arrow), and slight separation of the distal radius with metaphyseal fracture (white arrow)

18. Right distal tibia: Identification of Salter–Harris Type III epiphyseal injury and Type II
    18.1. CT (Fig. 21.19a, b)

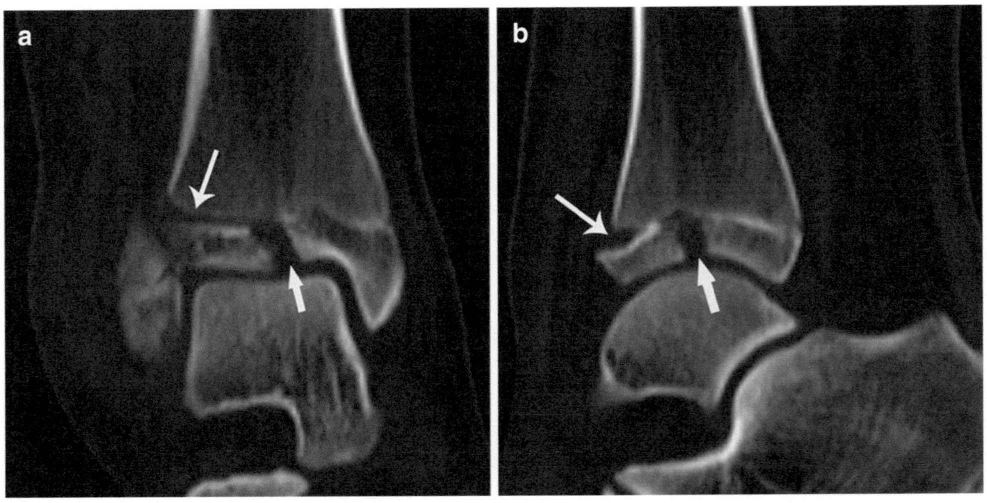

Fig. 21.19 (**a**, **b**) are coronal and sagittal plane reconstruction, showing epiphysis fracture of right distal tibia (rough white arrow) and the epiphyseal cartilage plate widening (fine white arrow)

18.2. MRI (Fig. 21.19c–f)

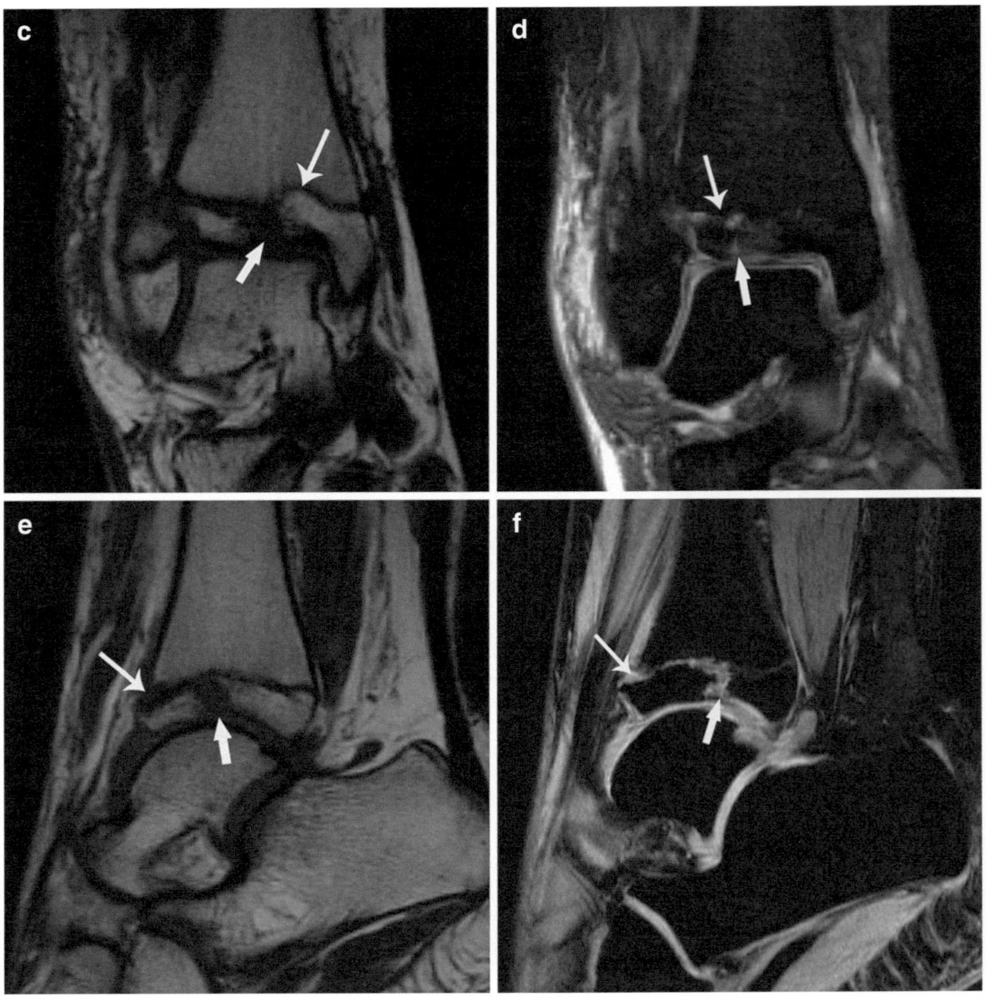

Fig. 21.19 (**c**–**f**) are MRI plain coronary T1W1, fat suppression T2W1, sagittal T1W1, and fat suppression T2W1, respectively, showing epiphysis fracture (rough white arrow) and uneven enlargement of epiphyseal cartilage plate (fine white arrow) and soft tissue of lateral malleolus swelling

19. Left distal tibia: Identification of Salter–Harris Type III epiphyseal injury and epiphyseal non-injury
    19.1. X-ray (Fig. 21.20a–d)

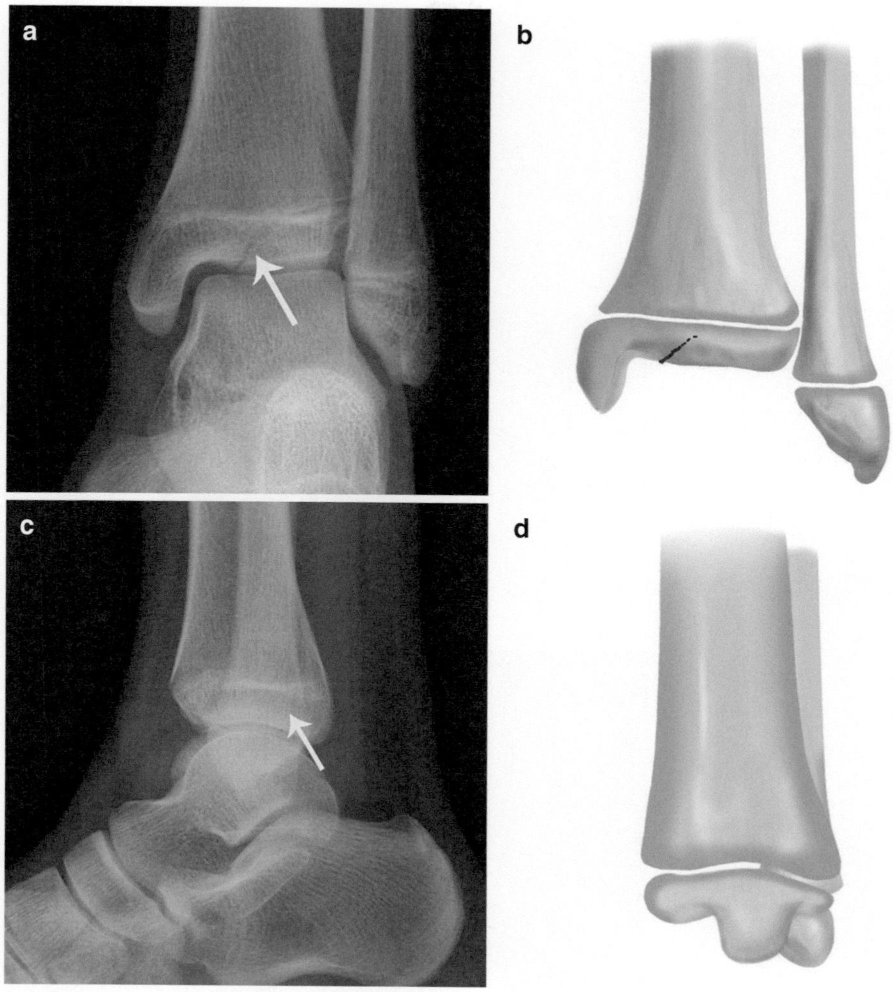

Fig. 21.20 (**a**, **c**) are positive and lateral position, respectively, showing epiphysis fracture of distal tibia (fine white arrow), epiphyseal cartilage plate injury is unclear, and the schematic diagram (**b**, **d**)

    19.2. CT (Fig. 21.20e, f)

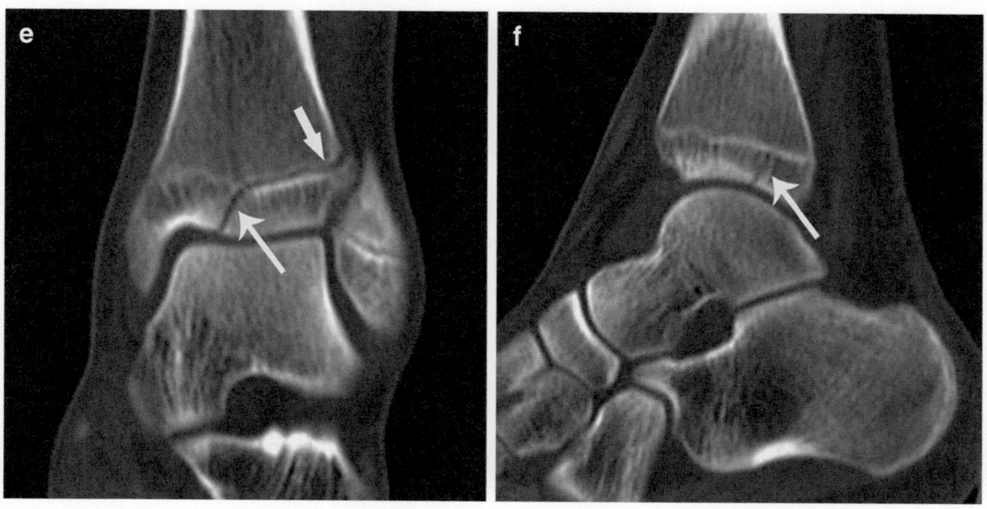

Fig. 21.20 (**e**, **f**) are coronal and sagittal plane reconstruction, respectively, showing epiphysis fracture of distal tibia (fine white arrow) and epiphyseal cartilage plate injury and widening (rough white arrow)

20. Identification of multiple ossification centers in the olecranon of elbow joint 19
    20.1. X-ray (Fig. 21.21a, b)

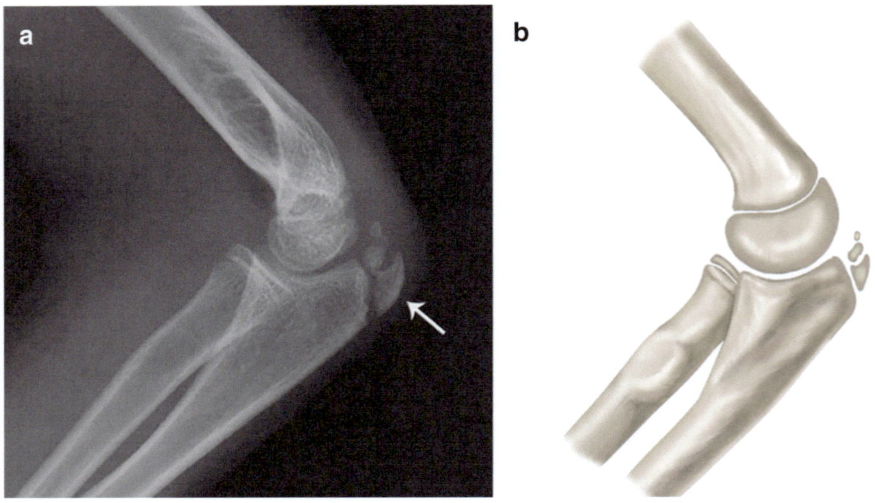

Fig. 21.21 (**a**) is the lateral position, showing multiple ossification centers in the olecranon (white arrow), and the schematic diagram (**b**)

    20.2. CT (Fig. 21.21c)

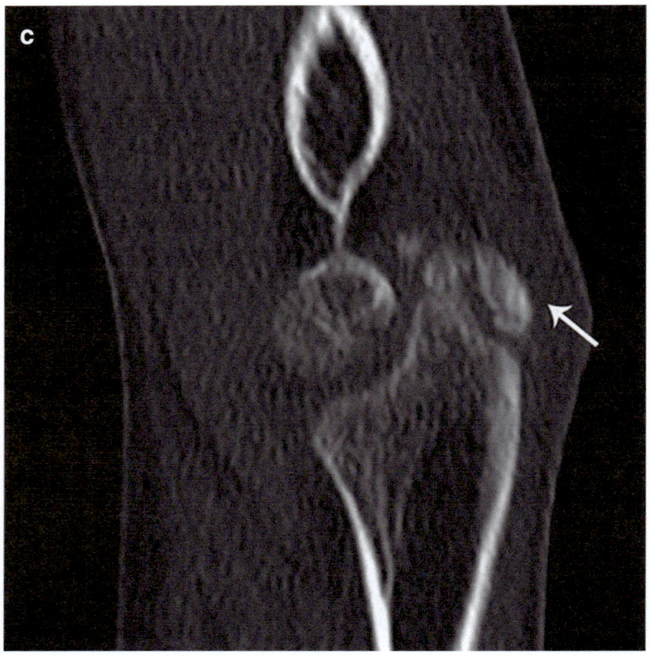

Fig. 21.21 (**c**) is the sagittal plane reconstruction, showing multiple ossification centers in the olecranon (white arrow)

21.1.4.4 Type IV: Fracture Across the Physis, Extending from the Metaphysis to the Epiphysis

21. Lateral condyle of right humerus: Identification of Salter–Harris Type IV epiphyseal injury and Type II
    21.1. X-ray (Fig. 21.22a–d)

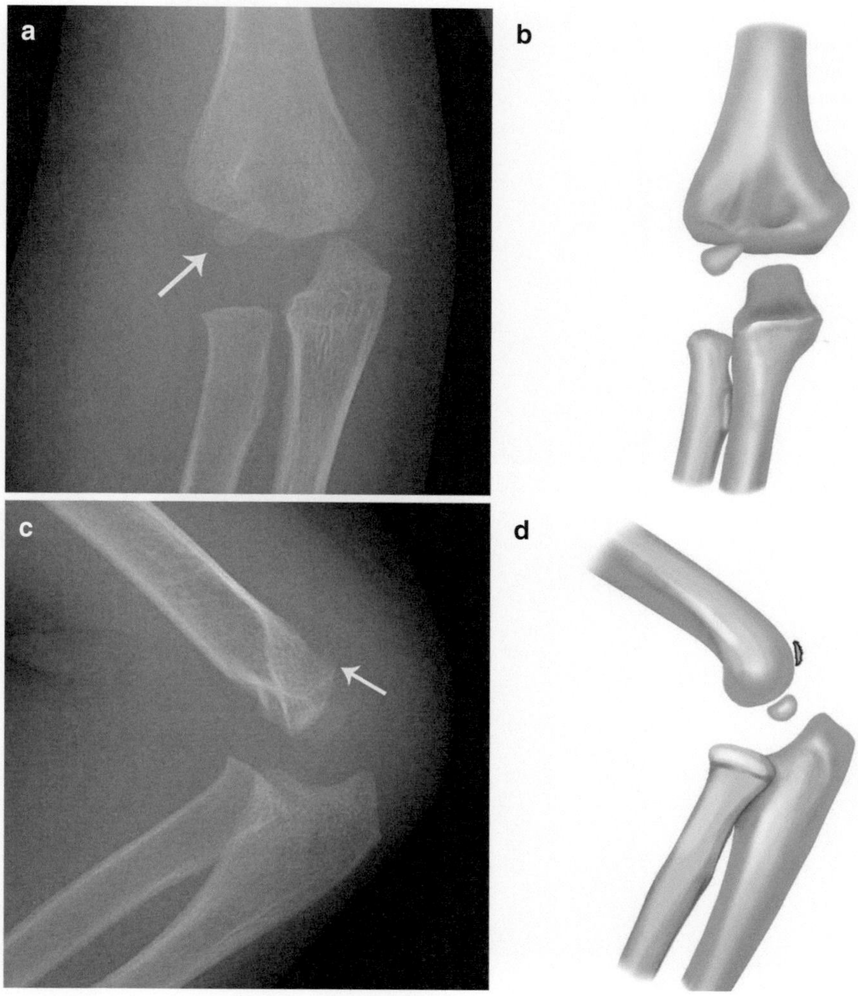

Fig. 21.22 (**a**, **c**) are positive and lateral position, respectively, showing the displacement of lateral condyle of humerus, metaphyseal fracture, and the schematic diagram (**b**, **d**)

    21.2. MRI (Fig. 21.22e, f)

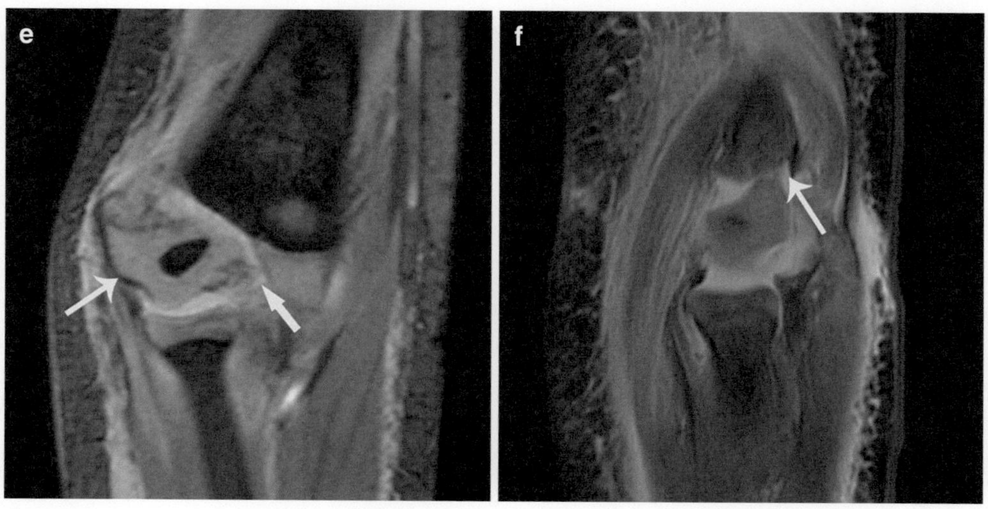

Fig. 21.22 (**e**, **f**) are MRI coronal T2W1 and sagittal fat suppression T2W1, respectively, showing dislocation of lateral condyle of humerus (fine white arrow), epiphyseal cartilage fracture of the trochlear, fracture line reaching the articular surface (rough white arrow), and surrounding soft tissue swelling

22. Lateral condyle of right humerus: Identification of Salter–Harris Type IV epiphyseal injury and Type II
    22.1. X-ray (Fig. 21.23a–d)

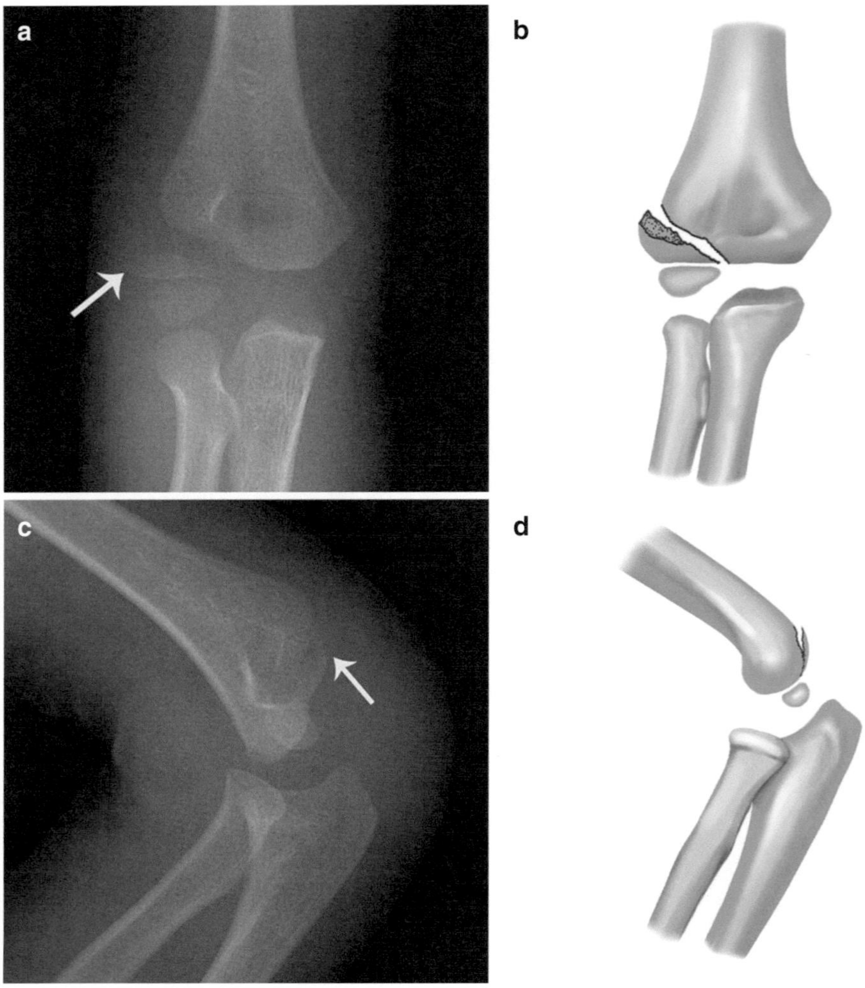

Fig. 21.23 (**a**, **c**) are positive and lateral position, respectively, showing epiphysis separation of lateral condyle of right humerus with metaphyseal fracture (fine white arrow), and the schematic diagram (**b**, **d**)

22.2. CT (Fig. 21.23e–h)

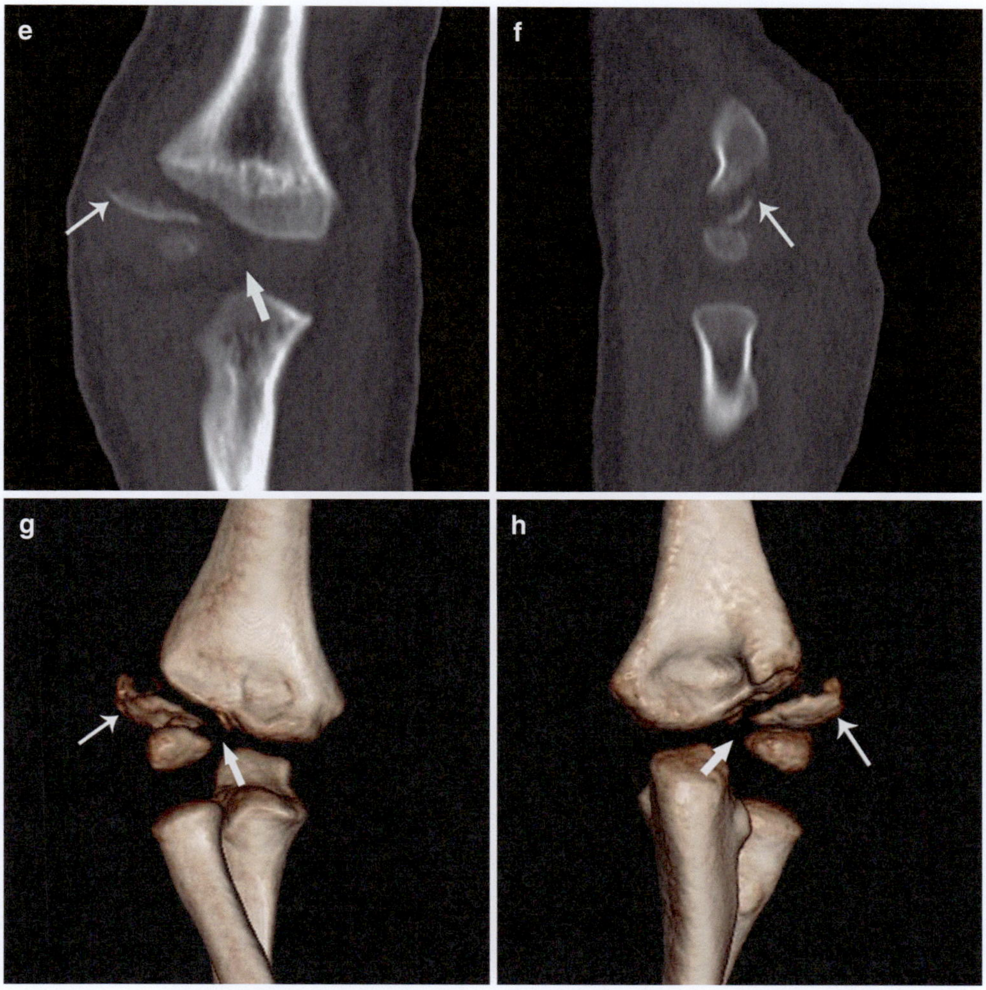

Fig. 21.23 (**e**, **f**) are coronal plane and sagittal plane reconstruction, respectively. (**g**, **h**) are anterior and posterior view of CT three-dimensional reconstruction, respectively, showing epiphysis separation of lateral condyle of right humerus with metaphyseal fracture (fine white arrow) and fracture line reaching the articular surface through trochlear (rough white arrow)

23. Left proximal tibia: Identification of Salter–Harris Type IV epiphyseal injury and epiphyseal non-injury
    23.1. X-ray (Fig. 21.24a–d)

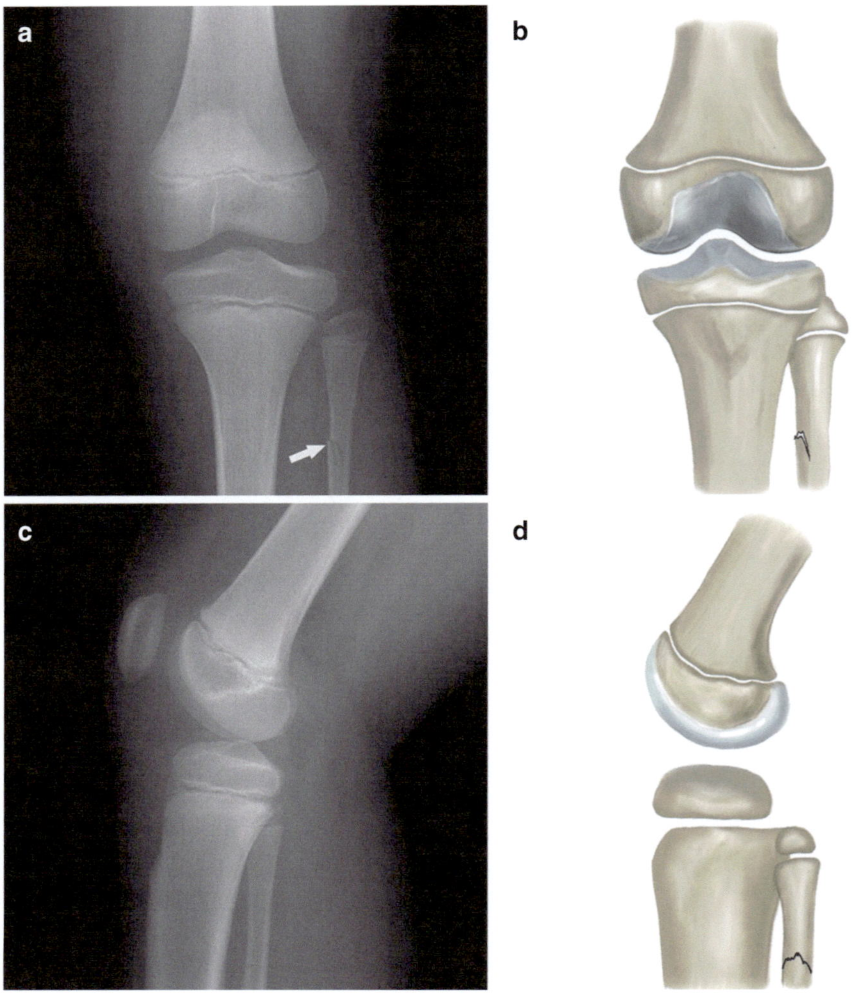

Fig. 21.24 (**a**, **c**) are positive and lateral position, respectively, showing the upper fibular fracture without dislocation (fine white arrow), and no obvious fracture of the proximal tibia, schematic diagram (**b**, **d**)

23.2. CT (Fig. 21.24e, f)

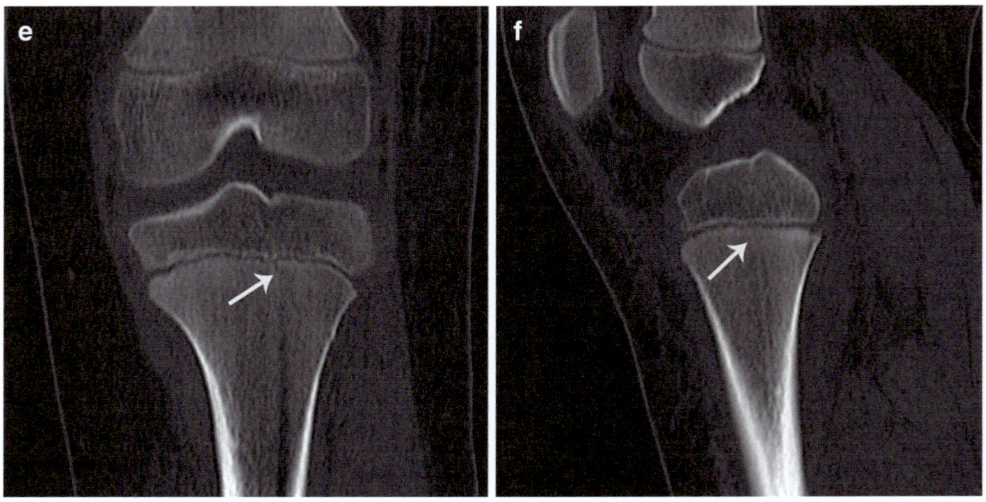

Fig. 21.24 (**e**, **f**) are coronal and sagittal plane reconstruction, respectively, showing metaphyseal fracture (fine white arrow)

23.3. MRI (Fig. 21.24g–j)

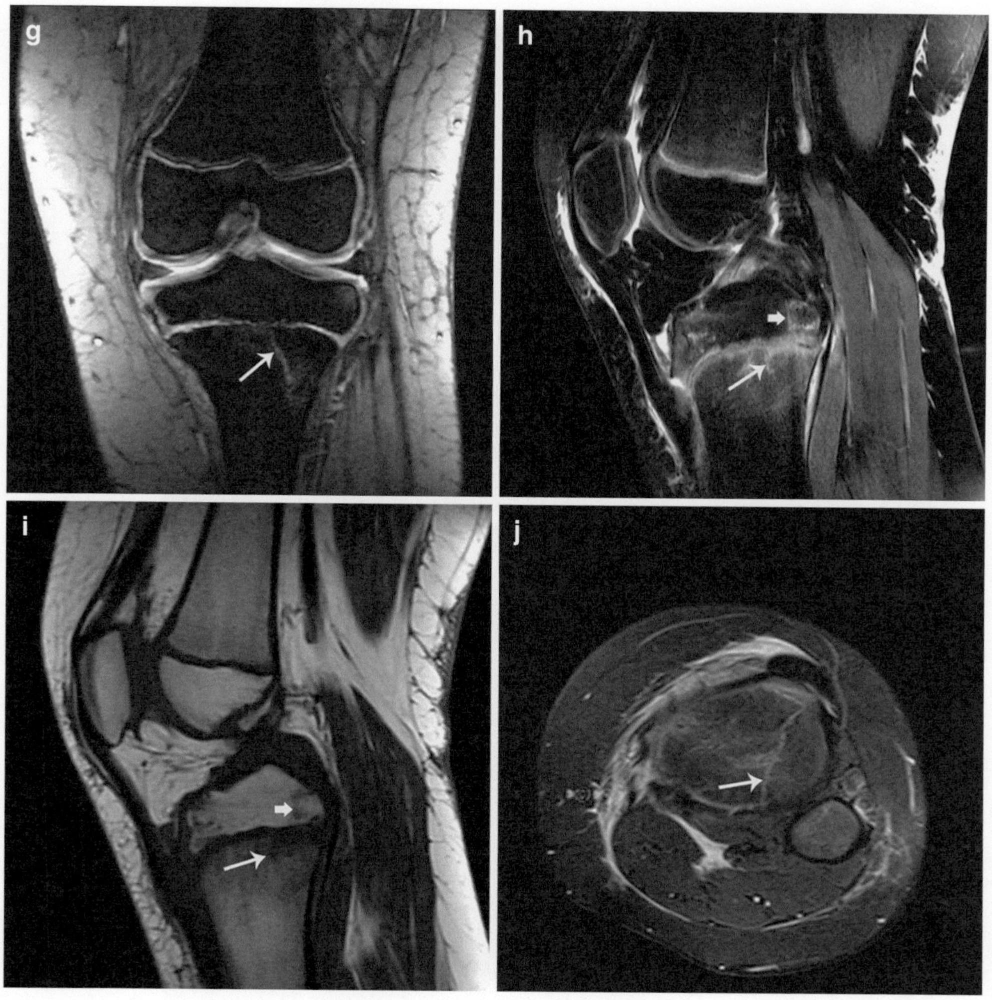

Fig. 21.24 (**g–j**) are MRI coronal T2W1, sagittal fat suppression T2W1, sagittal T1W1, and transverse axis fat suppression T2W1, showing metaphyseal fracture (fine white arrow) and epiphysis fracture, and the epiphyseal cartilage plate is uneven

24. Right distal femur: Identification of Salter–Harris Type IV epiphyseal injury and Type III
    24.1. X-ray (Fig. 21.25a–d)

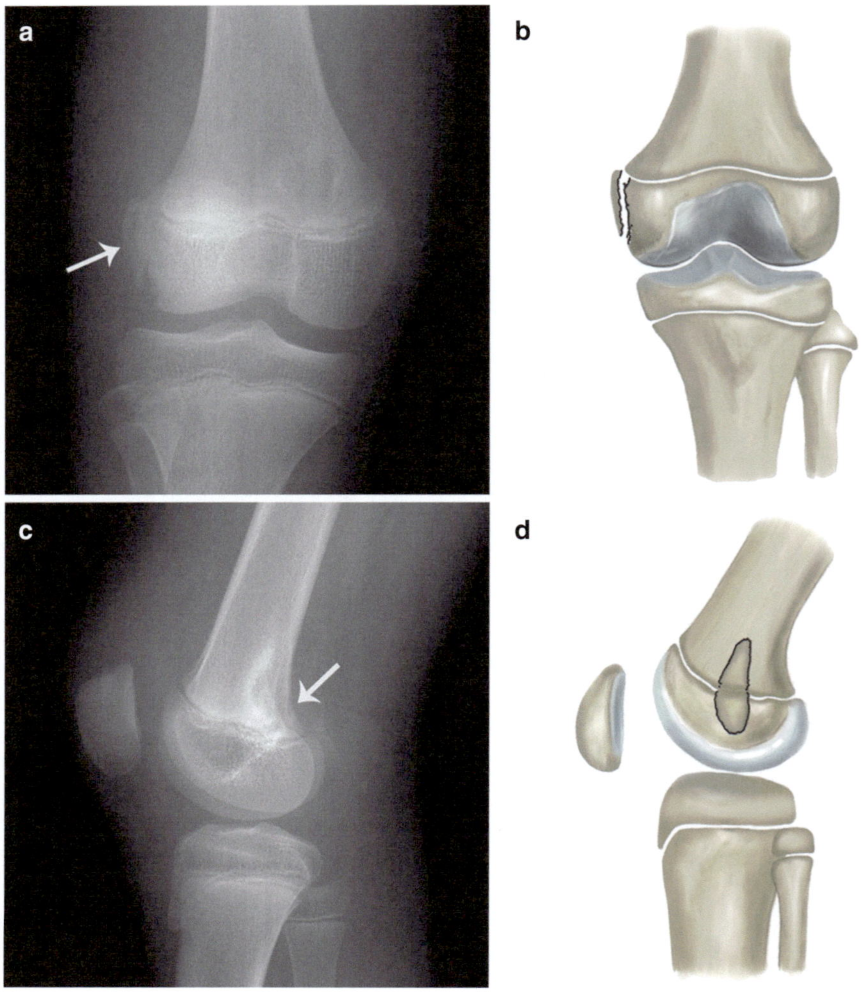

Fig. 21.25 (**a**, **c**) are positive and lateral position, respectively, showing the epiphyseal fracture of the lateral condyle of the right knee (white arrow) and the metaphyseal fracture is unclear, schematic diagram (**b**, **d**). The initially diagnosis was Type III on the basis of X-ray. For further diagnosis, CT and MRI were performed

24.2. CT (Fig. 21.25e)

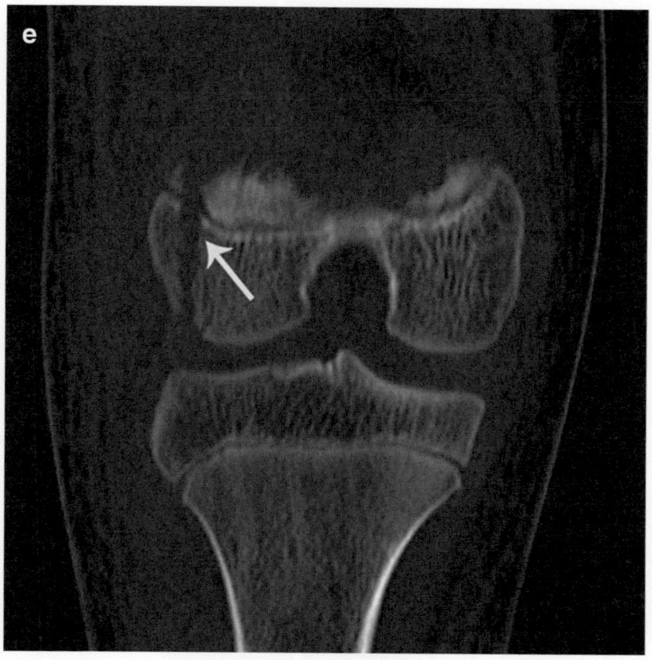

Fig. 21.25 (e) is the coronal plane reconstruction, showing lateral epiphysis and metaphyseal fracture of right distal femur, fracture line through epiphyseal cartilage plate (white arrow), and the diagnosis of Type IV epiphyseal injury

24.3. MRI (Fig. 21.25f)

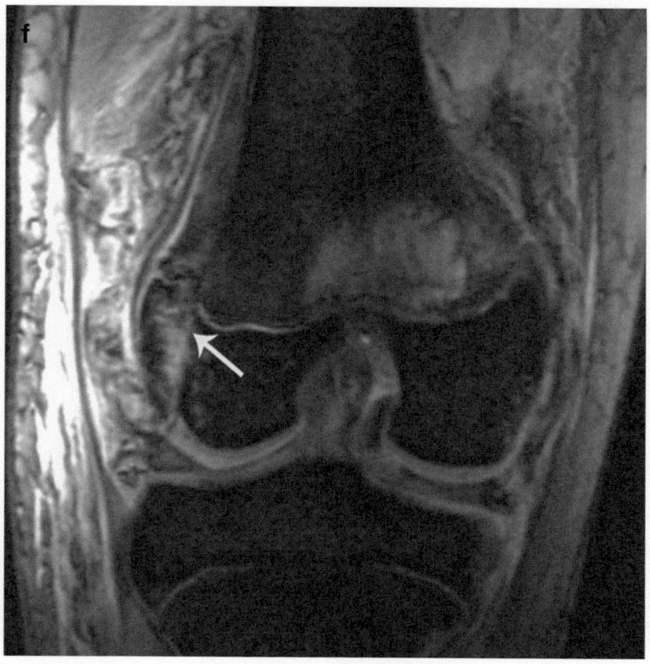

Fig. 21.25 (f) is MRI coronary T2W1, showing lateral epiphysis and metaphyseal fracture of right distal femur, fracture line through epiphyseal cartilage plate (white arrow) and the diagnosis of Type IV epiphyseal injury

25. Right distal femur: Identification of Salter–Harris Type IV epiphyseal injury and Type III
    25.1. X-ray (Fig. 21.26a–d)

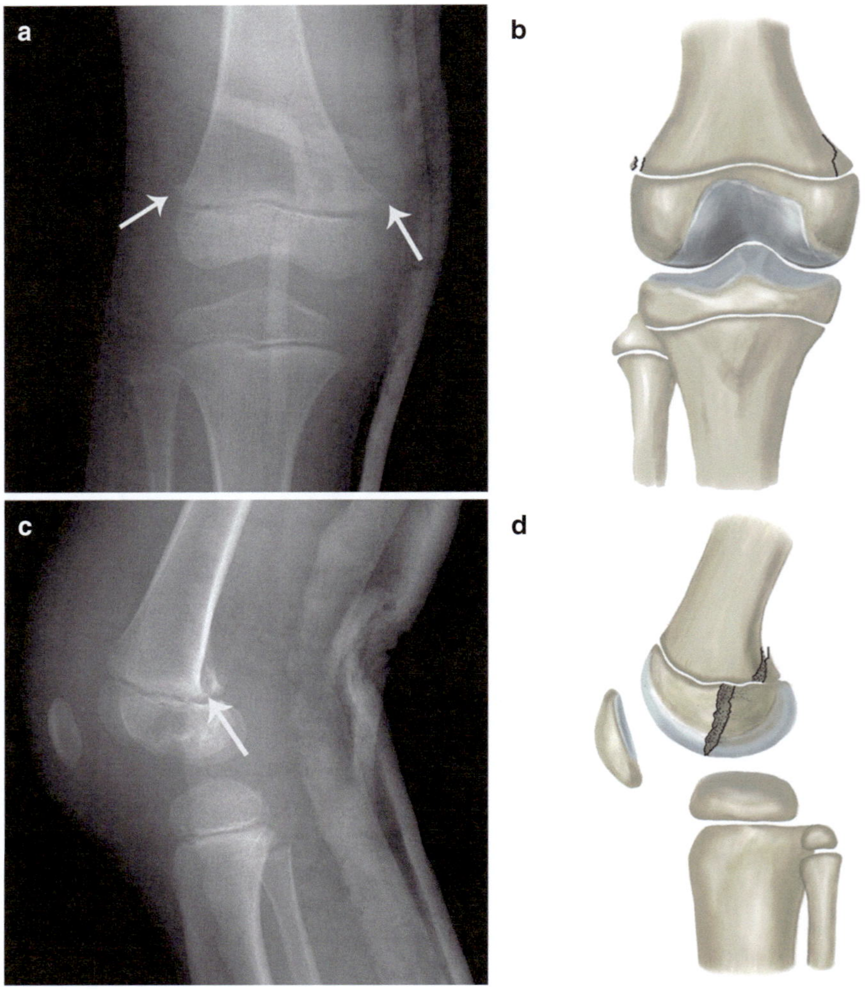

Fig. 21.26 (**a**, **c**) are positive and lateral through epiphyseal cartilage plate (white arposition, respectively, showing, fracture line through epiphyseal cartilage plate (white arrow), visible fixed shadow external plaster, schematic diagram (**b**, **d**)

25.2. CT (Fig. 21.26e–h)

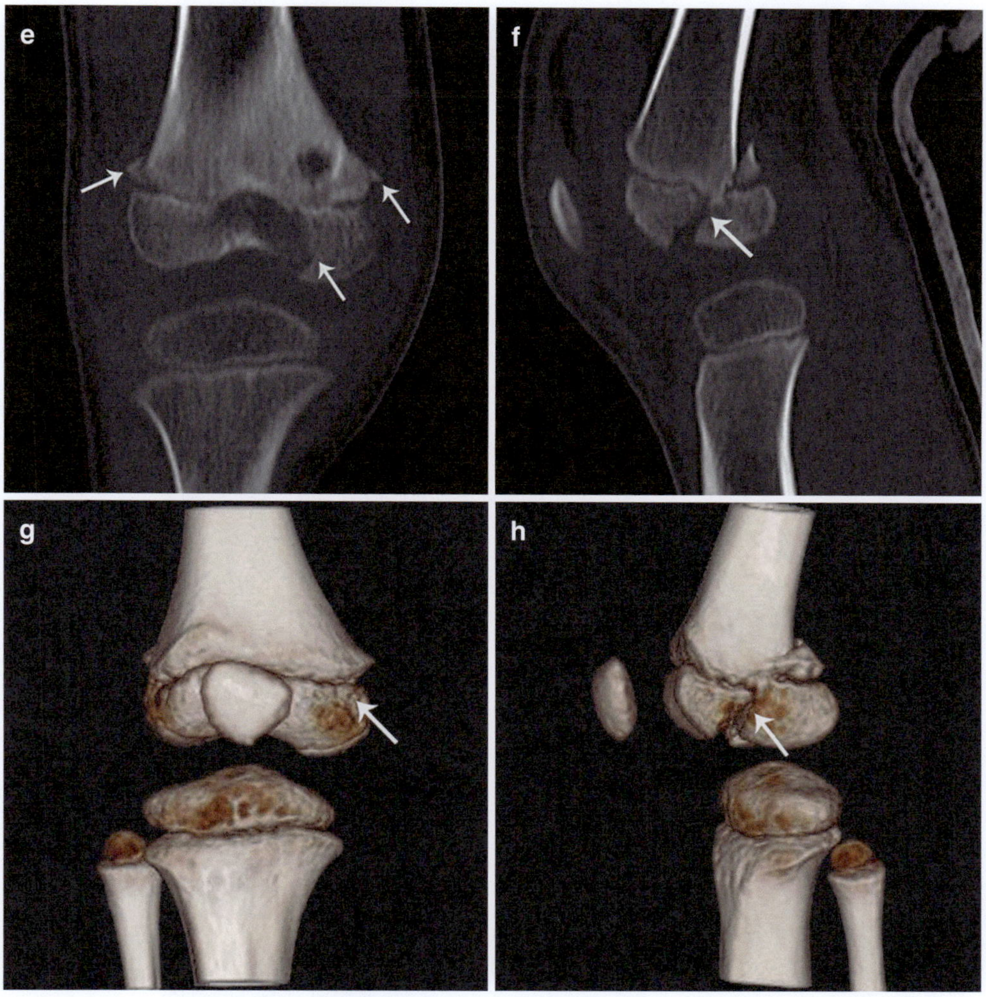

Fig. 21.26 (**e**, **f**) are, respectively, coronal plane and sagittal plane construction, showing epiphysis and metaphyseal fracture of right distal femur, fracture line through epiphyseal cartilage plate (white arrow). (**g**, **h**) are anterior and lateral view of the CT three-dimensional reconstruction, showing fracture line

25.3. MRI (Fig. 21.26i, j)

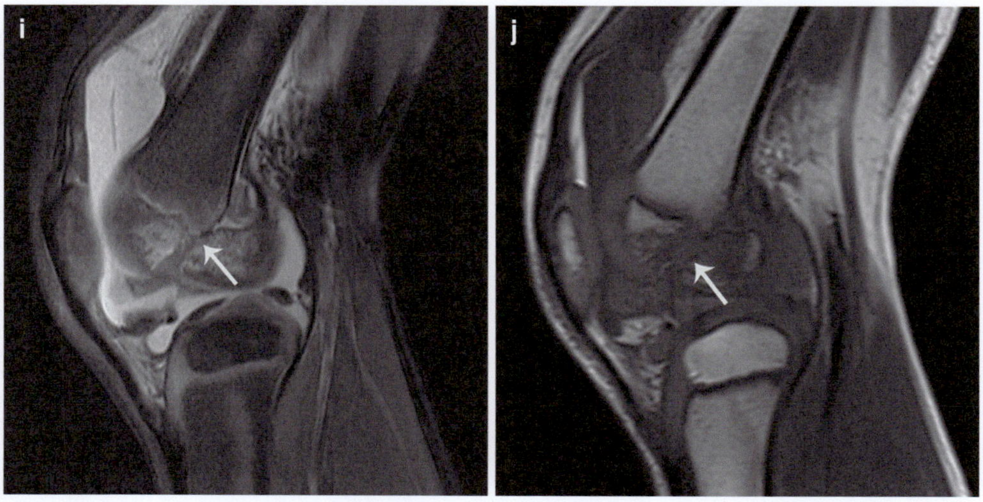

Fig. 21.26 (**i**, **j**) are MRI sagittal fat suppression T2W1 and T1W1, respectively, showing fracture line (white line), fracture and dislocation of epiphyseal cartilage plate, and massive fluid accumulation in the joints

26. Right distal fibula: Identification of Salter–Harris Type IV epiphyseal injury and Type III
    26.1. X-ray (Fig. 21.27a–d)

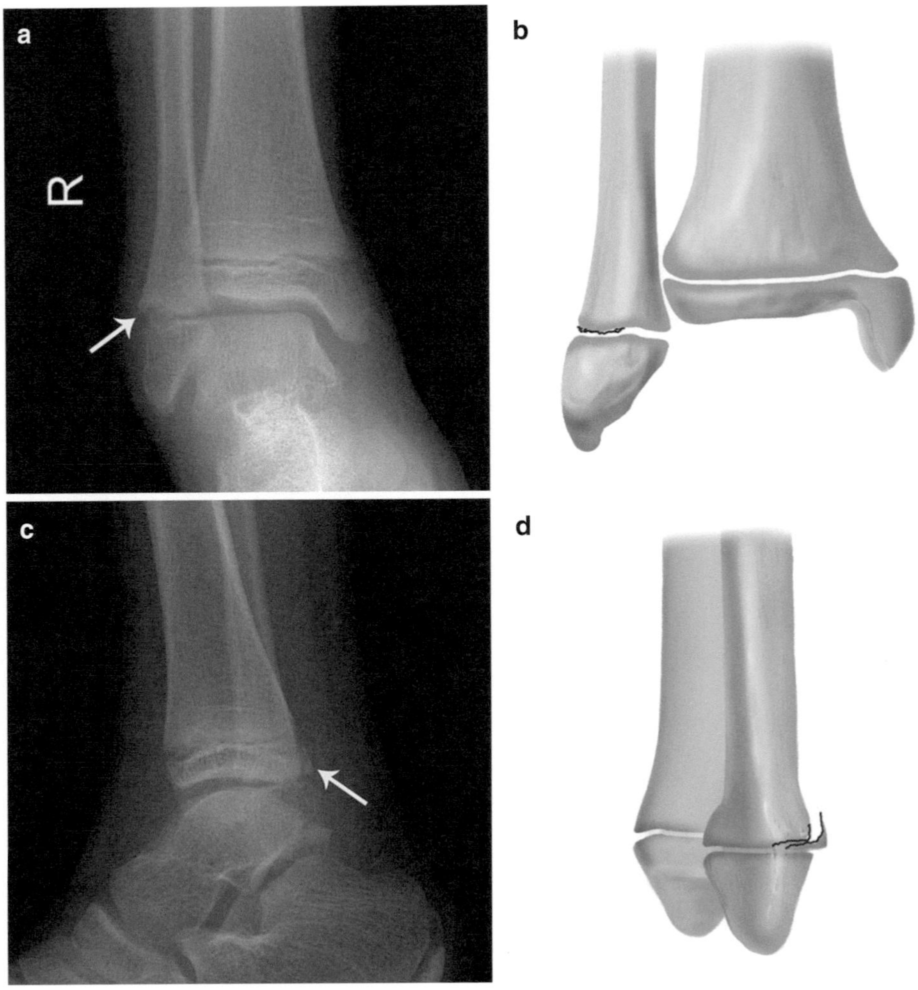

Fig. 21.27 (**a**) is the anteroposterior, showing the widening of the epiphyseal cartilage plate of distal fibula. (**c**) is the lateral position, showing metaphyseal fracture (white arrow), schematic diagram (**b**, **d**). The diagnosis is Type III on the basis of X-ray

    26.2. CT (Fig. 21.27e, f)

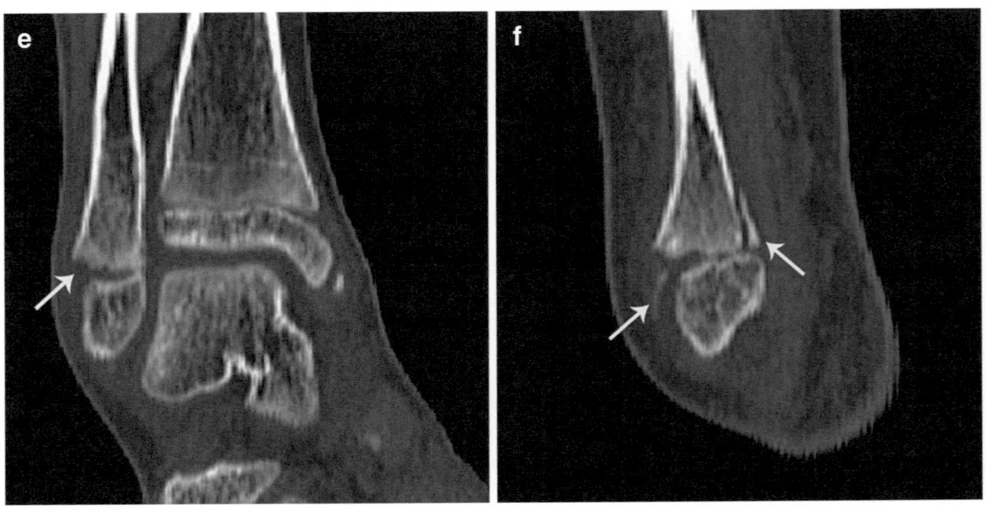

Fig. 21.27 (**e**, **f**) are CT coronal and sagittal plane reconstruction, showing the widening of the epiphyseal cartilage plate, the epiphysis, and metaphyseal fractures (white arrow), and the diagnosis is Type IV

27. Right distal tibia: Salter–Harris Type IV epiphyseal injury
    27.1. X-ray (Fig. 21.28a, b)

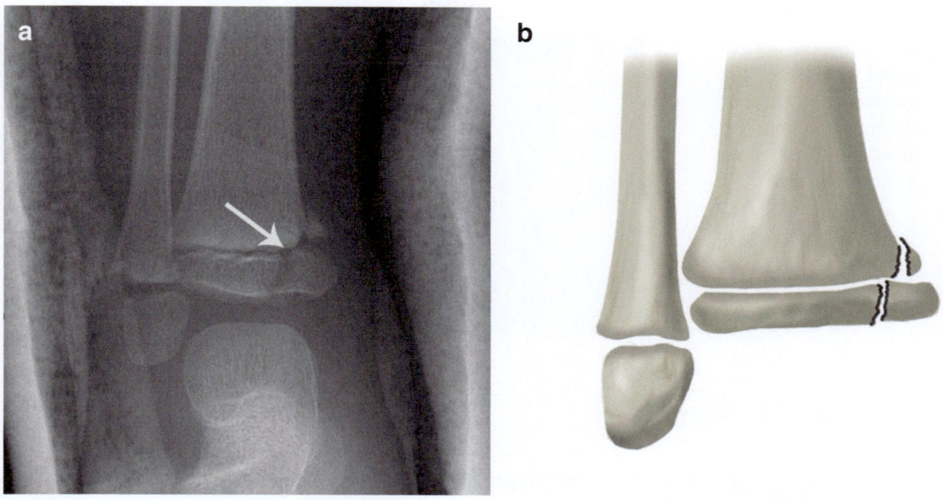

Fig. 21.28 (**a**) is the anteroposterior after plaster fixation, showing the distal tibia through the epiphyseal cartilage plate, involving the epiphysis and metaphyseal fracture (white arrow), and schematic diagram (**b**)

    27.2. CT (Fig. 21.28c–e)

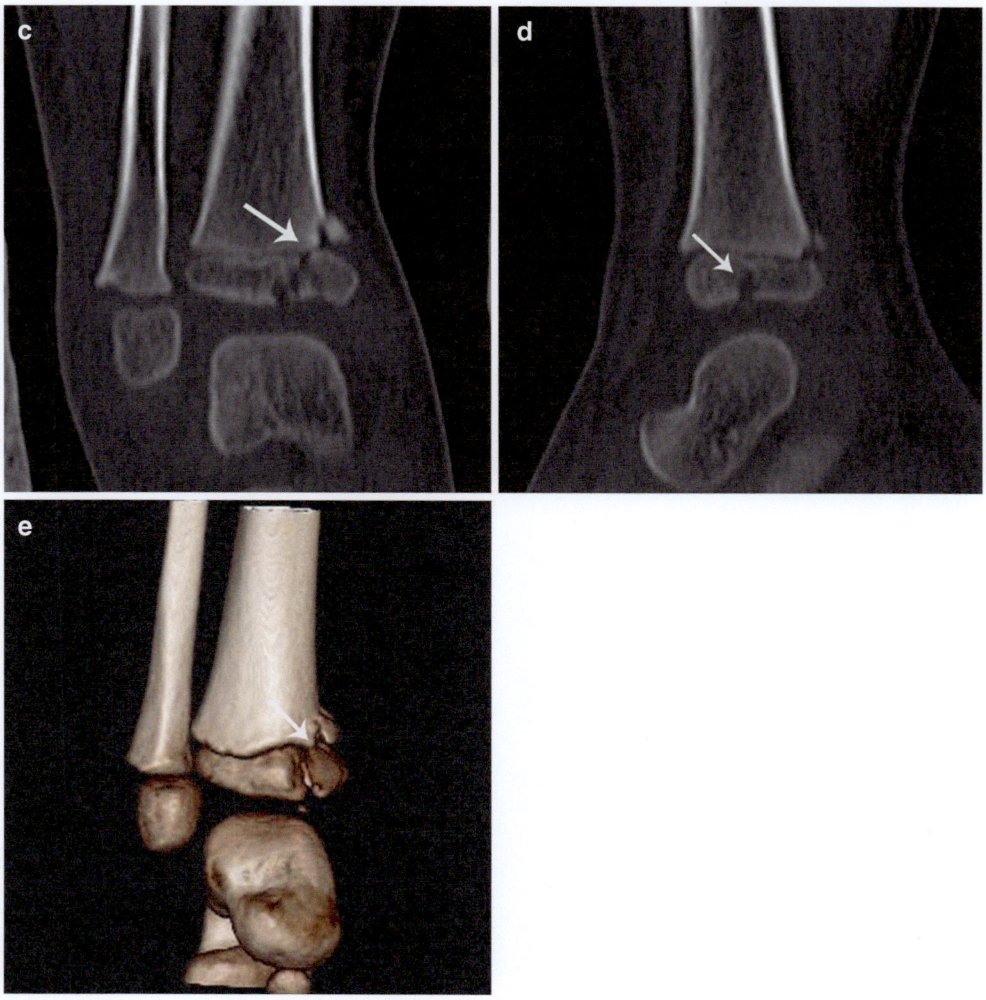

Fig. 21.28 (**c**–**e**) are CT coronal, sagittal, and three-dimensional reconstruction, respectively, showing the distal tibia through the epiphyseal cartilage plate, involving the epiphysis and metaphyseal fracture (white arrow)

21.1.4.5 Type V: Fracture is a Crush Injury Resulting in Injury to the Physis

28. Left proximal femur: Identification of Salter–Harris Type V epiphyseal injury and epiphyseal non-injury
    28.1. X-ray (Fig. 21.29a, b)

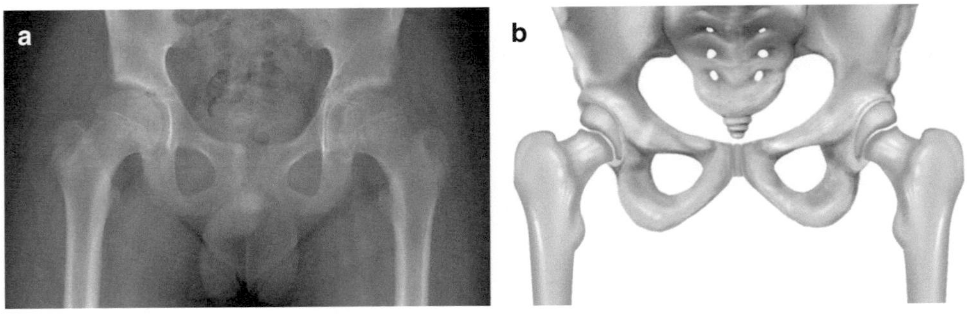

Fig. 21.29 (**a**) is the positive position, and there is no obvious abnormality in the bone, schematic diagram (**b**). For further definite diagnosis, CT scan was performed

    28.2. CT (Fig. 21.29c, d)

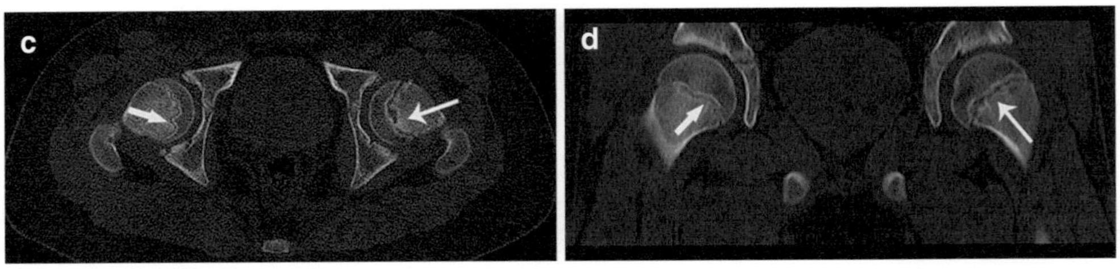

Fig. 21.29 (**c**, **d**) are the CT high-resolution scanning of the transverse and coronal plane, respectively. The epiphyseal cartilage plate of left proximal femur is widened and irregular (fine white arrow), and the epiphyseal cartilage plate of right proximal femur is normal (rough white arrow)

28.3. MRI (Fig. 21.29e–i)

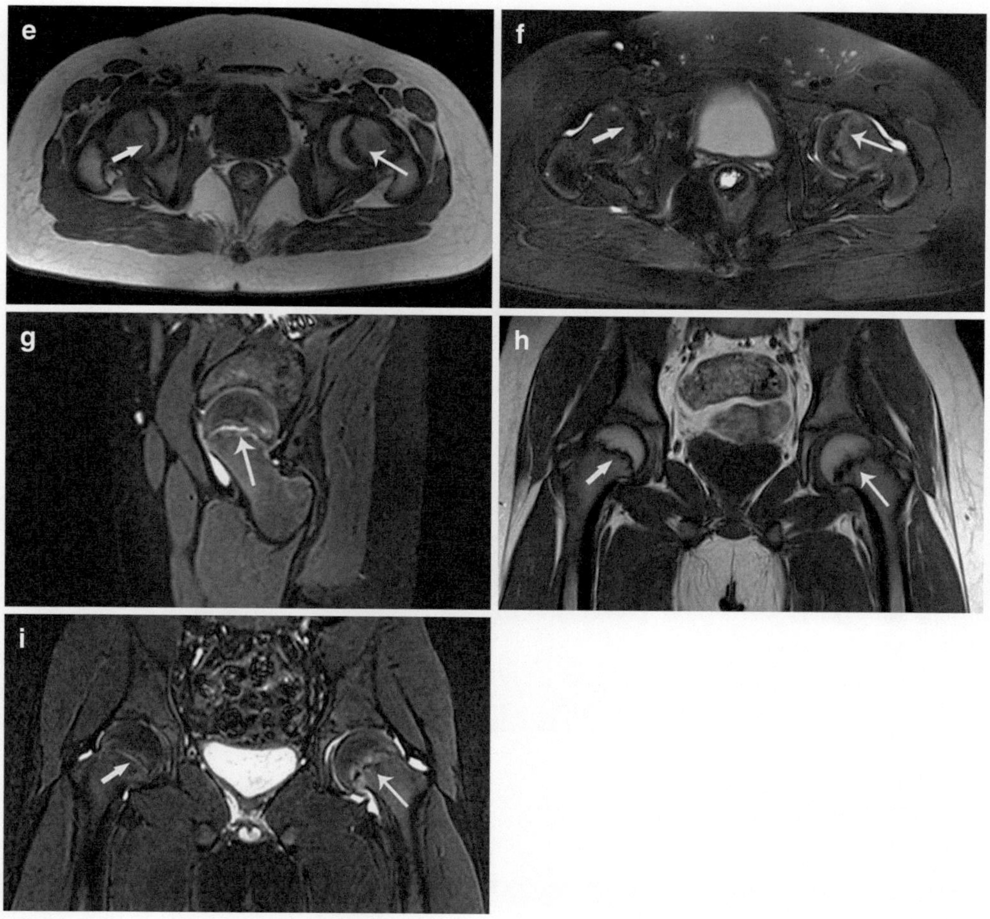

Fig. 21.29 (e–i) are MRI plain transverse axis T1W1, fat suppression T2W2, sagittal fat suppression T2W1, coronal T1W1, and fat suppression T2W1, respectively. It shows that the epiphyseal cartilage plate is widened and irregular of left proximal femur, the epiphyseal and metaphyseal signal is abnormal, and long T1 and T2 is seen but uneven (fine white arrow). The epiphyseal cartilage plate, epiphysis, and metaphysis are normal (rough white arrow)

29. Right proximal femur: Identification of Salter–Harris Type V epiphyseal injury and epiphyseal non-injury
    29.1. X-ray (Fig. 21.30a, b)

Fig. 21.30 (**a**) is the positive position, and there is no obvious abnormality in the epiphysis, schematic diagram (**b**). For further definite diagnosis, CT and MRI scan were performed

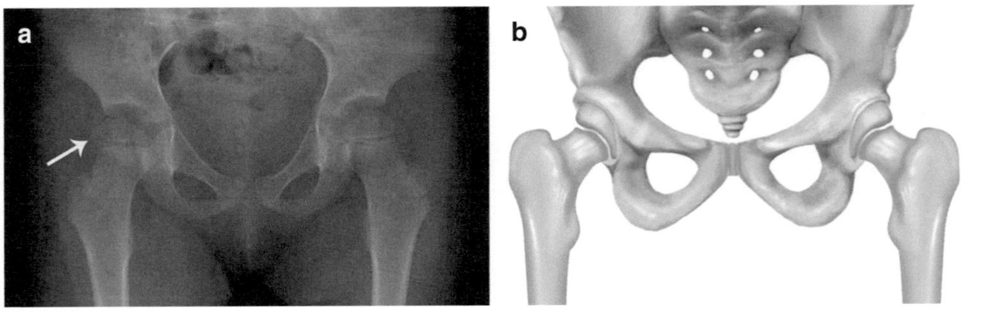

    29.2. CT (Fig. 21.30c, d)

Fig. 21.30 (**c**, **d**) are the transverse axial plane and coronal plane reconstruction, respectively, showing the epiphyseal cartilage plate is slightly wider and the metaphysis is irregular (white arrow)

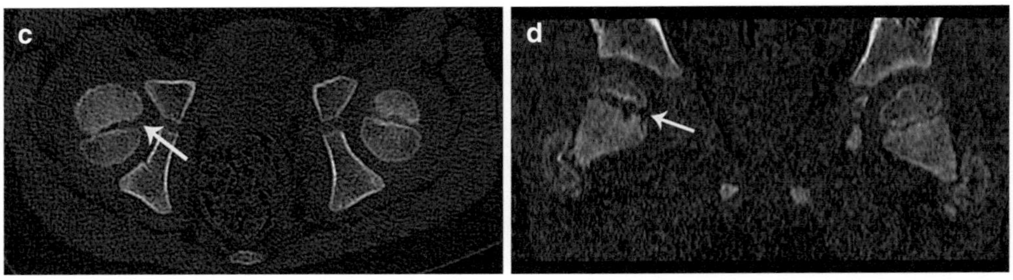

    29.3. MRI (Fig. 21.30e–g)

Fig. 21.30 (**e**, **g**) are MRI plain transverse axis fat suppression T2W1, coronal T1W1, and fat suppression T2W1, respectively, showing the epiphysis position of right femoral head is normal, the epiphyseal and metaphyseal signal is abnormal, and long T1, T2 (white arrow) and intraarticular effusion are seen

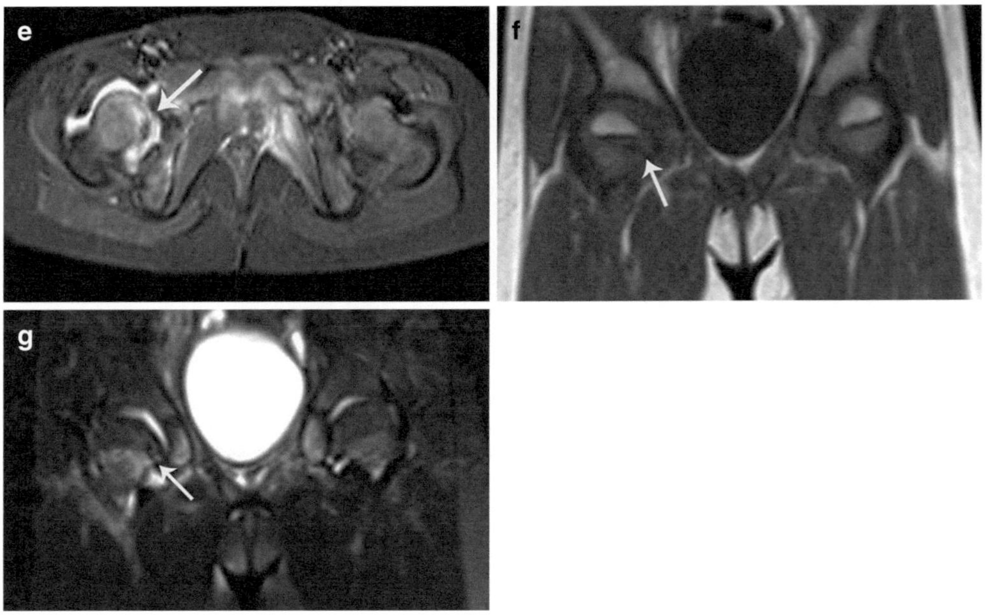

21.2 Early Closure of Epiphysis

21.2.1 Definition

Early closure of epiphysis, also known as early closure of epiphyseal plate, occurs when an epiphyseal cartilage plate injury of the immature bone in children leads to the formation of bone connection between the epiphysis and metaphysis, creating a bone bridge; which makes the whole or part of the epiphyseal plate closed early, resulting in limb shortening and/or deformity.

21.2.2 Classification

According to the extent of the epiphyseal cartilage plate closure, it can be divided into complete and partial early closure of epiphysis. Partial early closure of epiphysis can be divided into peripheral, central, and mixed type according to the position. The peripheral type is located on the edge of epiphyseal plate, the central type is located at the center or slightly eccentric of epiphyseal plate, and the mixed type is that two peripheral types of injuries are connected through the center, and the bone bridge is line-like on the horizontal axis.

21.2.3 Clinical Presentation

Complete early closure of epiphysis can lead to limb shortening. Generally, 1–2 years after injury, the limb is shortened by 1–2 cm. The partial peripheral type is located on the edge of epiphyseal plate, causing angular deformity of the limb in a short period of time. The central type is located at the center or slightly eccentric of epiphyseal plate, causing limb shortening and angular deformity.

21.2.4 Diagnosis Points

There are the history of trauma, limb shortening, and/or angular deformity. X-ray and CT showed complete or partial disappearance of the low-density area of the epiphyseal cartilage plate, forming a high-density bone bridge with or without limb deformity.

MRI showed that the thickness of the epiphyseal plate was thinner, and the immature bone bridge was the inner-line like, lumpy or irregular low signal. While the mature bone bridge was bone-like signal connecting the epiphysis and metaphysis.

21.2.5 Notes

(1) Epiphysis and cartilage plate injuries are common in children, accounting for about 6–30% of children's fractures, of which about 1–2% scan early closure of epiphysis, resulting in limb shortening and/or angular deformity. (2) The earlier closure of epiphysis, the more severe the deformity and the worse the prognosis will be. Therefore, early diagnosis and early treatment are very important. (3) CT and MRI scans can accurately show the location, extent, and scope of early closure of epiphysis, as well as the proportion of epiphyseal plate involved. (4) Classification of the traumatic early closure of epiphysis and other causes of early closure of epiphysis such as nutritional metabolic disorders (hypervitaminosis A, D), radiation injury, epiphyseal cartilage infection (suppurative, tuberculosis), epiphyseal cartilage burns and frost bite, Kashin–Beck disease, and fluorosis.

1. Left distal radius:part of the early closure of epiphysis
   1.1. X-ray (Fig. 21.31a–d)

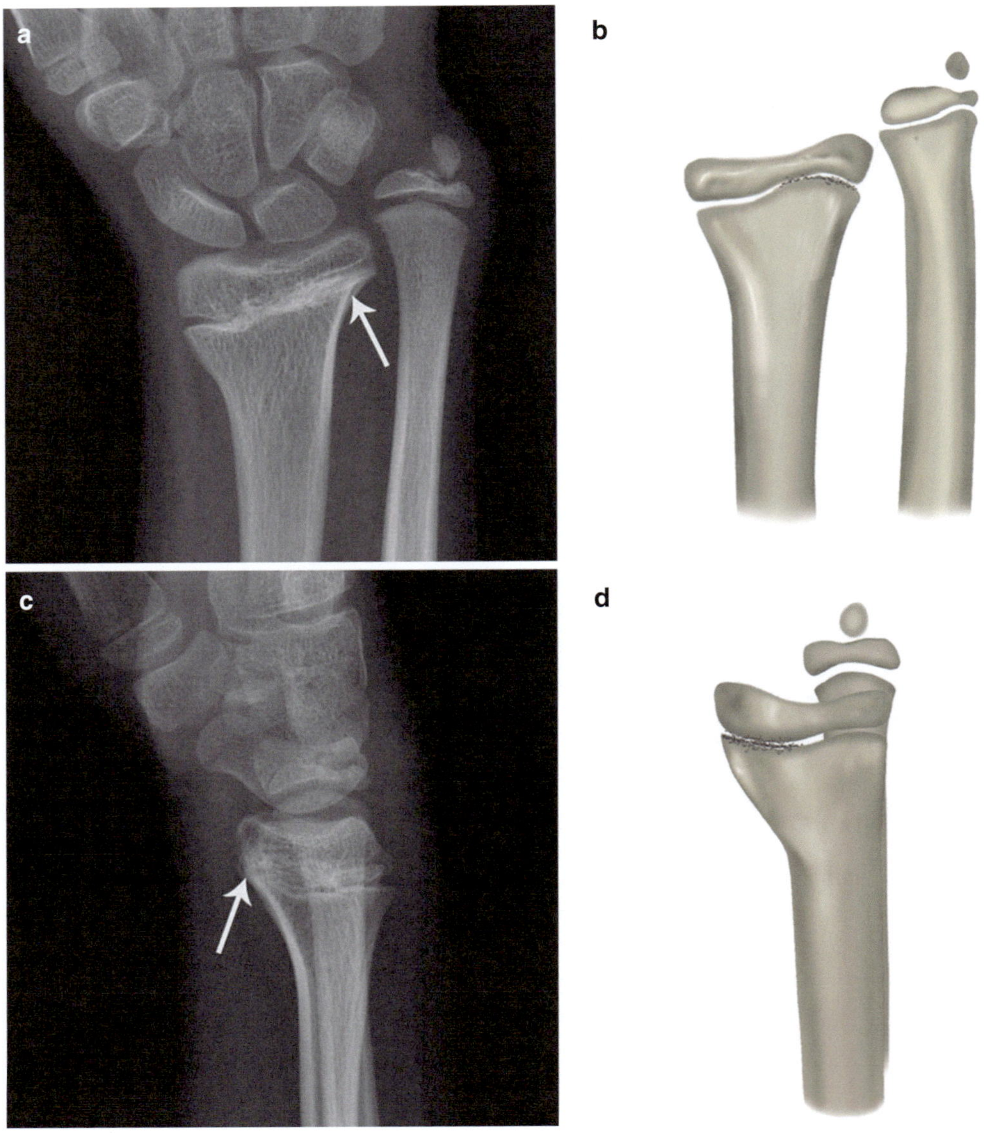

Fig. 21.31 (**a**, **c**) are positive and lateral position, respectively, showing part of the early closure of lateral epiphysis of distal radius (white arrow), resulting in deformity and shortening of the distal radius, and separation of the distal radioulnar joint, schematic diagram (**b**, **d**)

2. Left distal radius:part of the early closure of epiphysis
   2.1. X-ray (Fig. 21.32a–d)

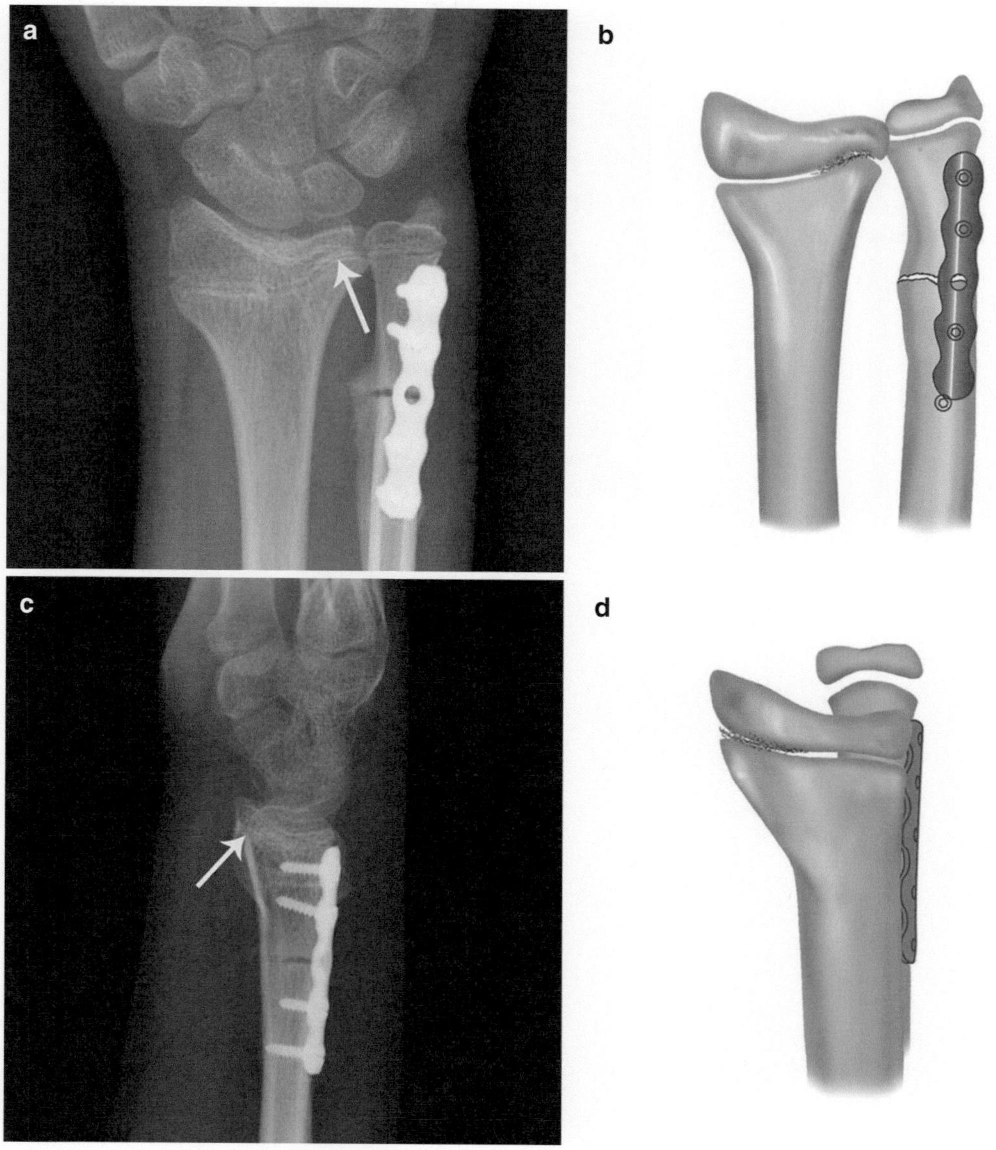

Fig. 21.32 (**a**, **c**) are positive and lateral position, respectively, showing the early closure of lateral epiphysis of distal radius (white arrow), after the internal fixation of posterior segment of ulna osteotomy, schematic diagram (**b**, **d**)

3. Early closure of epiphysis of right distal femur and formation of bone bridge
   3.1. MRI (Fig. 21.33a, b)

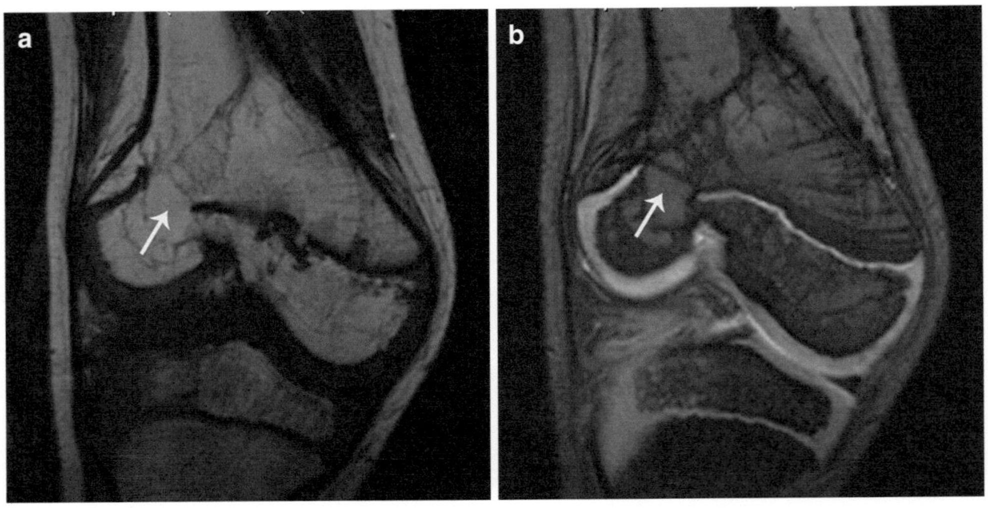

Fig. 21.33 (**a**, **b**) are coronal plane T1W1 and T2W1, respectively, showing partial disappearance of epiphyseal cartilage plate of distal femur and formation of bone bridge (white arrow), causing angular deformity of the distal femur, and schematic diagram

4. Early closure of epiphysis of left distal femur and formation of bone bridge
   4.1. MRI (Fig. 21.34a–d)

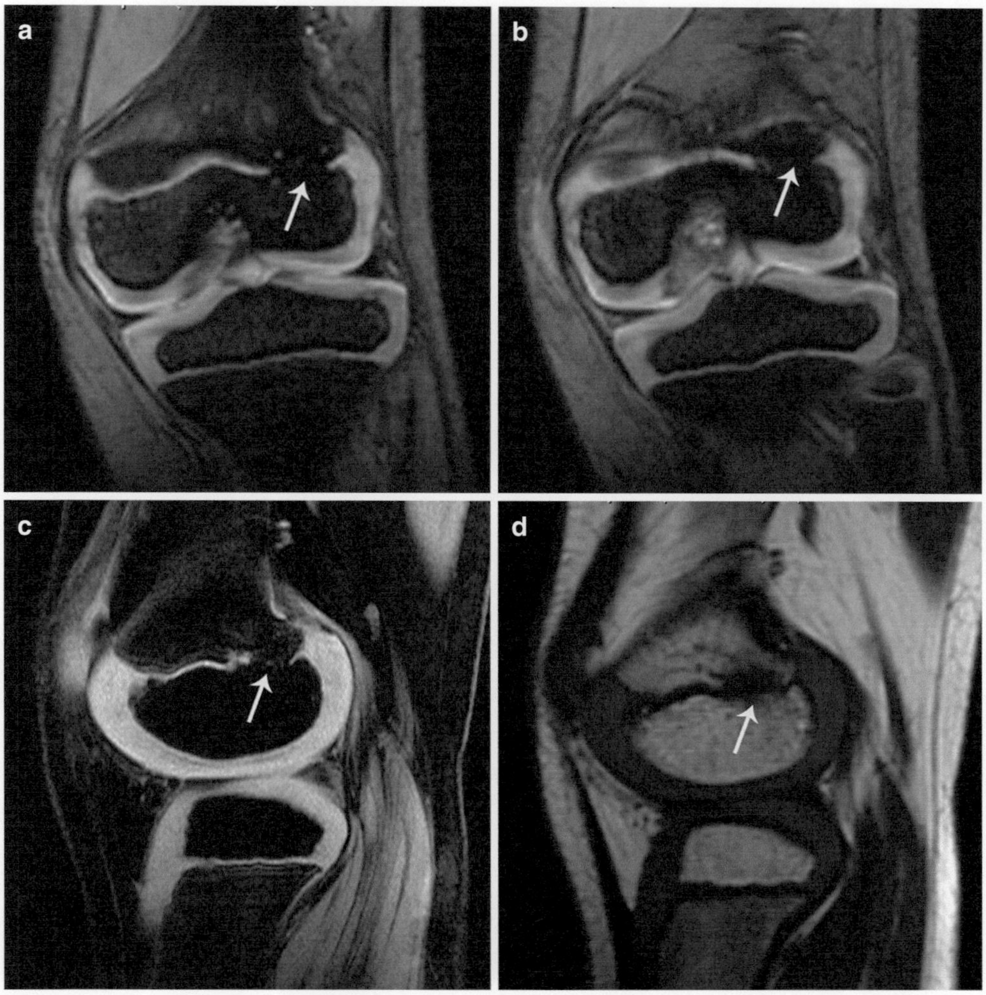

Fig. 21.34 (**a**, **b**) are coronal plane T2W1 at different levels, respectively. (**c**, **d**) are sagittal fat suppression T2W1 and T1W1, respectively, showing partial disappearance of epiphyseal cartilage plate of distal femur and formation of bone bridge (white arrow), resulting in skeletal deformity, and schematic diagram (**b**, **d**)

5. Early closure of the epiphysis of left femoral condyle
   5.1. X-ray (Fig. 21.35a, b)

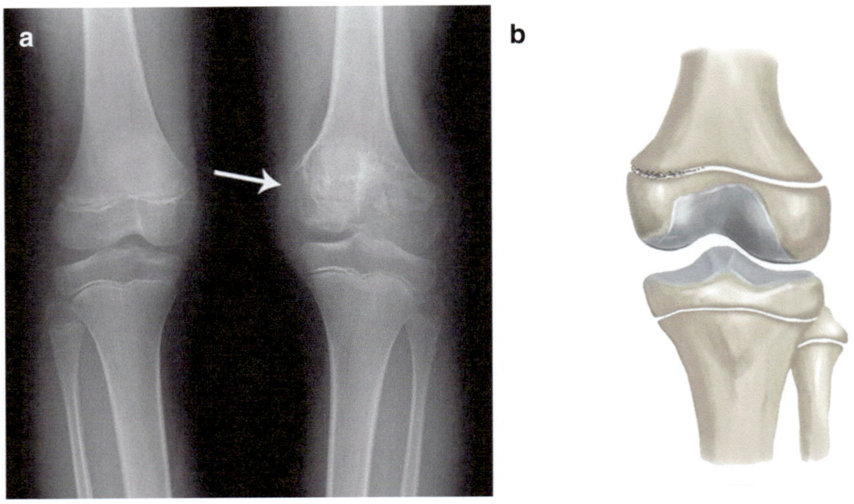

Fig. 21.35 (**a**) is positive position, showing anterior closure of epiphysis of left distal femur (white arrow), and schematic diagram (**b**)

   5.2. CT (Fig. 21.35c–e)

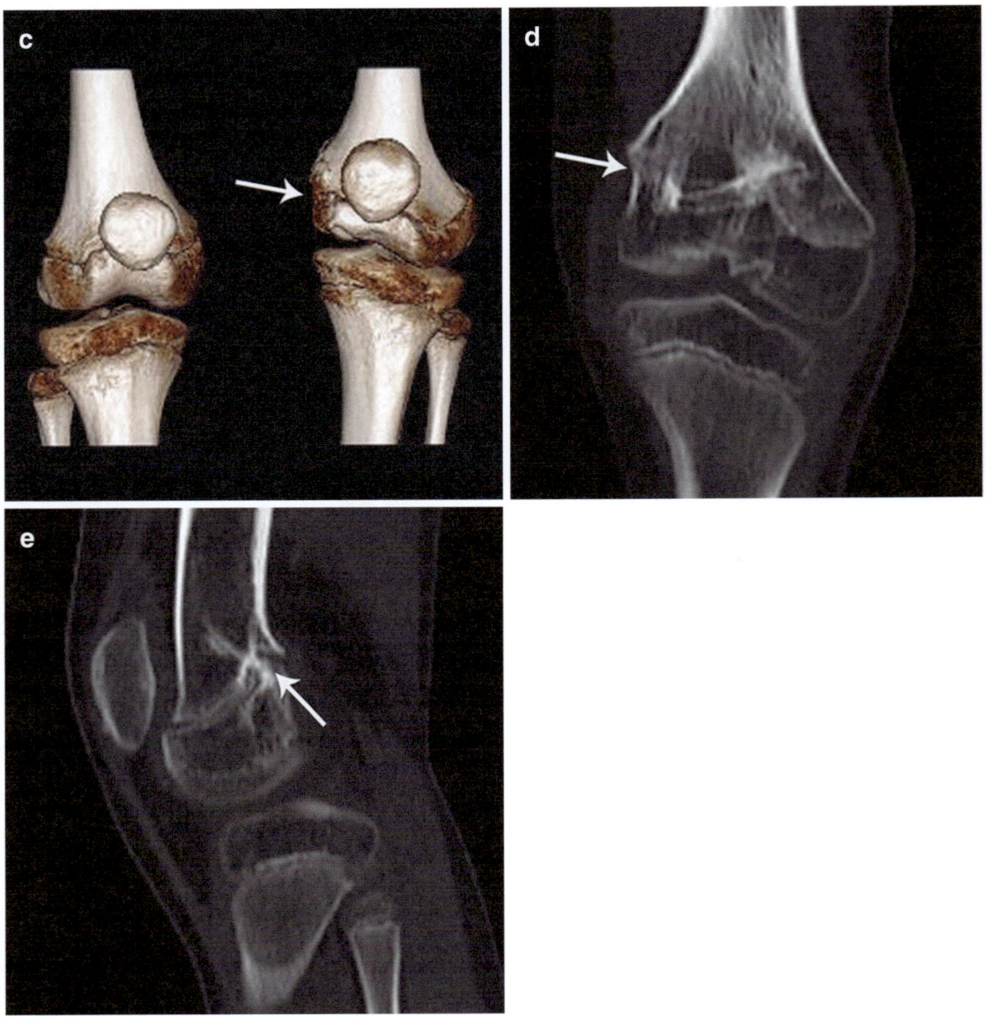

Fig. 21.35 (**c**) is the anterior view of the three-dimensional reconstruction. (**d**, **e**) are coronal and sagittal plane, respectively, showing posterior early closure of epiphysis of left distal femur (white arrow)

5.3. Postoperative X-ray plain film (Fig. 21.35f–i)

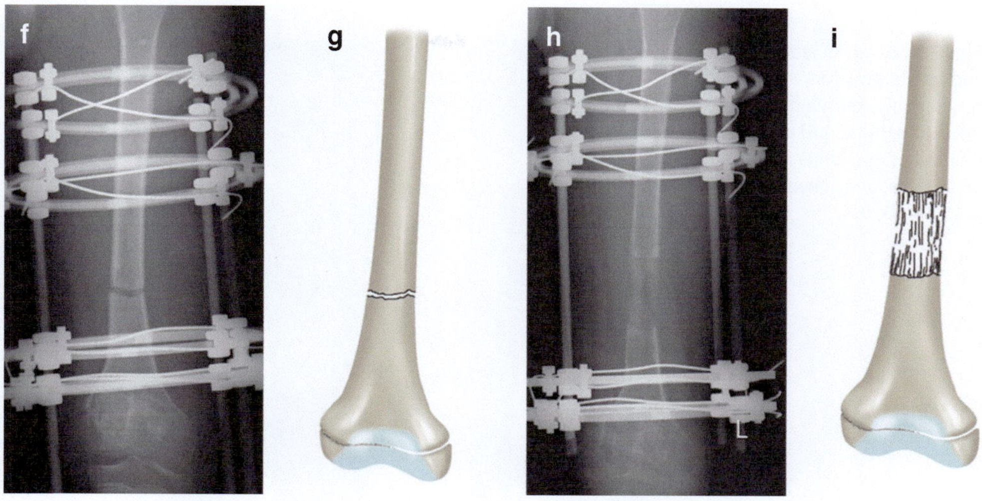

Fig. 21.35 (**f**) is 1 day after left lengthening femur, (**h**) is 3.5 months after lengthening, and schematic diagram (**g**–**i**)

6. Early closure of the epiphysis of right distal tibia
   6.1. X-ray (Fig. 21.36a–d)

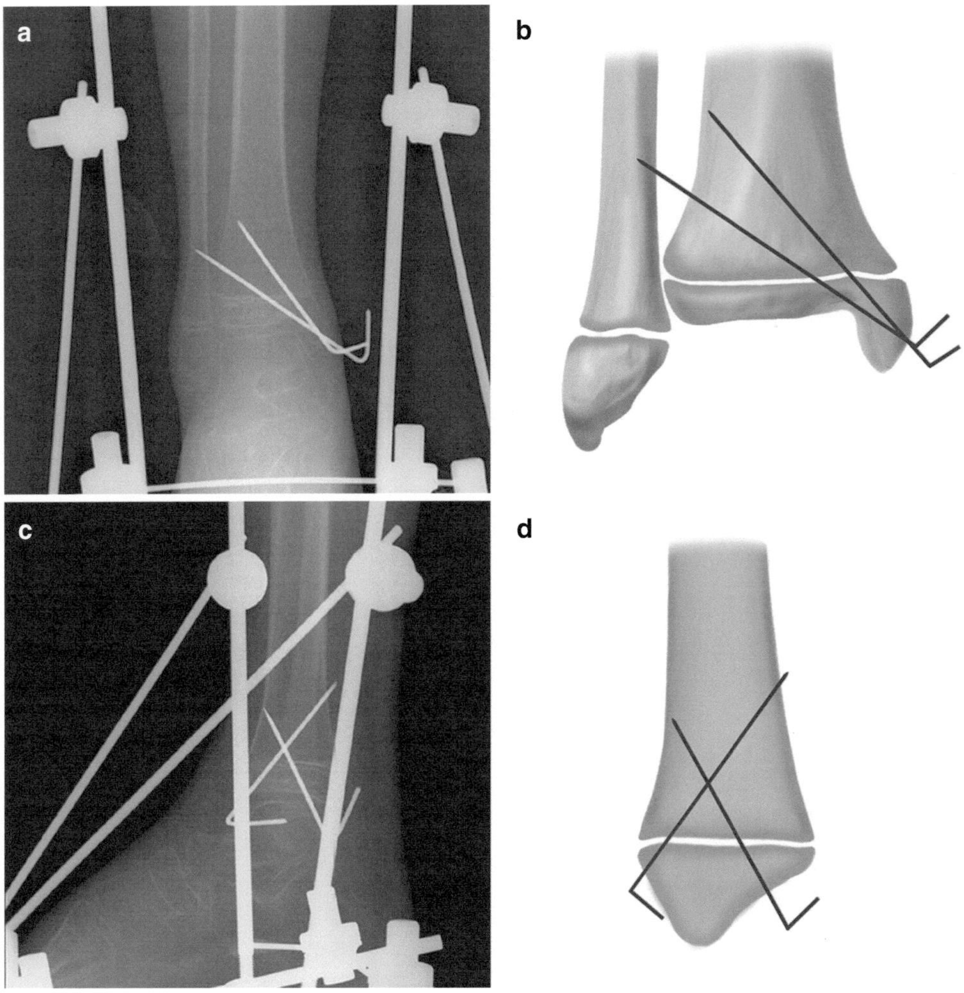

Fig. 21.36 (**a**, **c**) are positive and lateral position, respectively, showing after the internal fixation and external fixation of epiphysis injury of distal tibia, and schematic diagram (**b**, **d**)

6.2. Fig. 21.36e–h

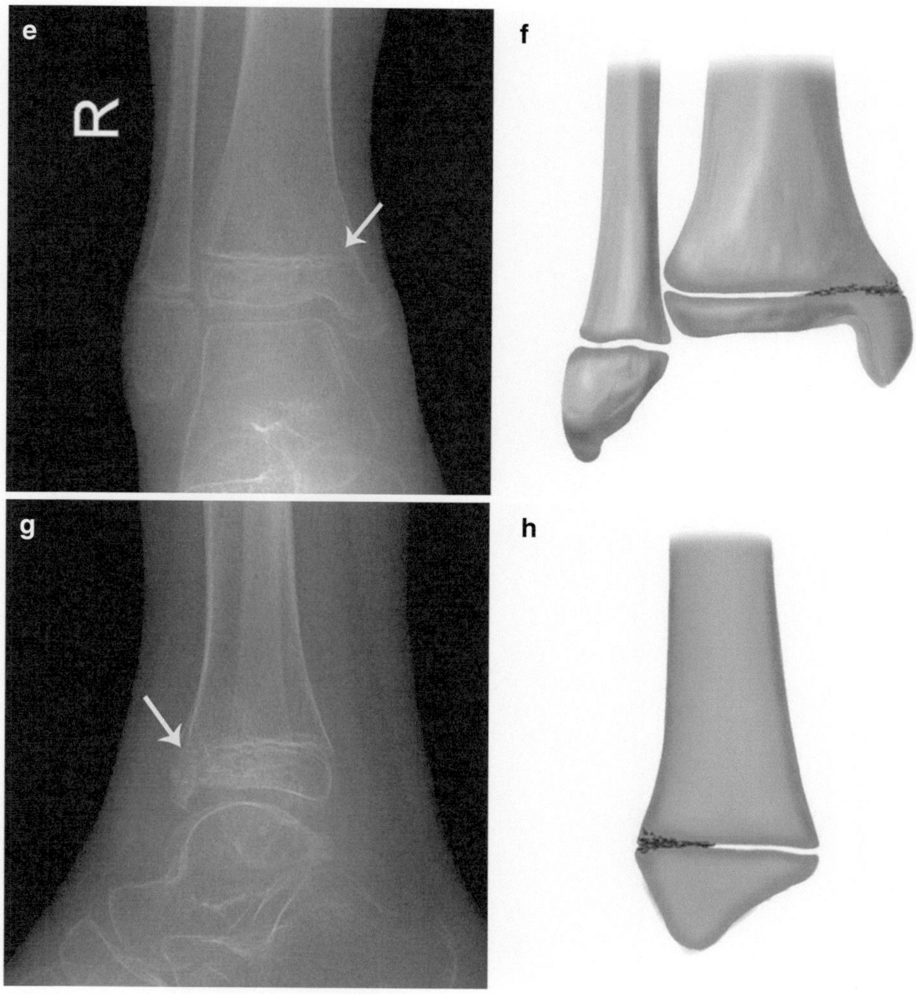

Fig. 21.36 (**e**, **g**) are the 5th week after internal fixation and removal of internal and external fixation, showing medial epiphyseal cartilage plate of distal radius is thinned, and schematic diagram (**f**–**h**)

6.3. Fig. 21.36i–l

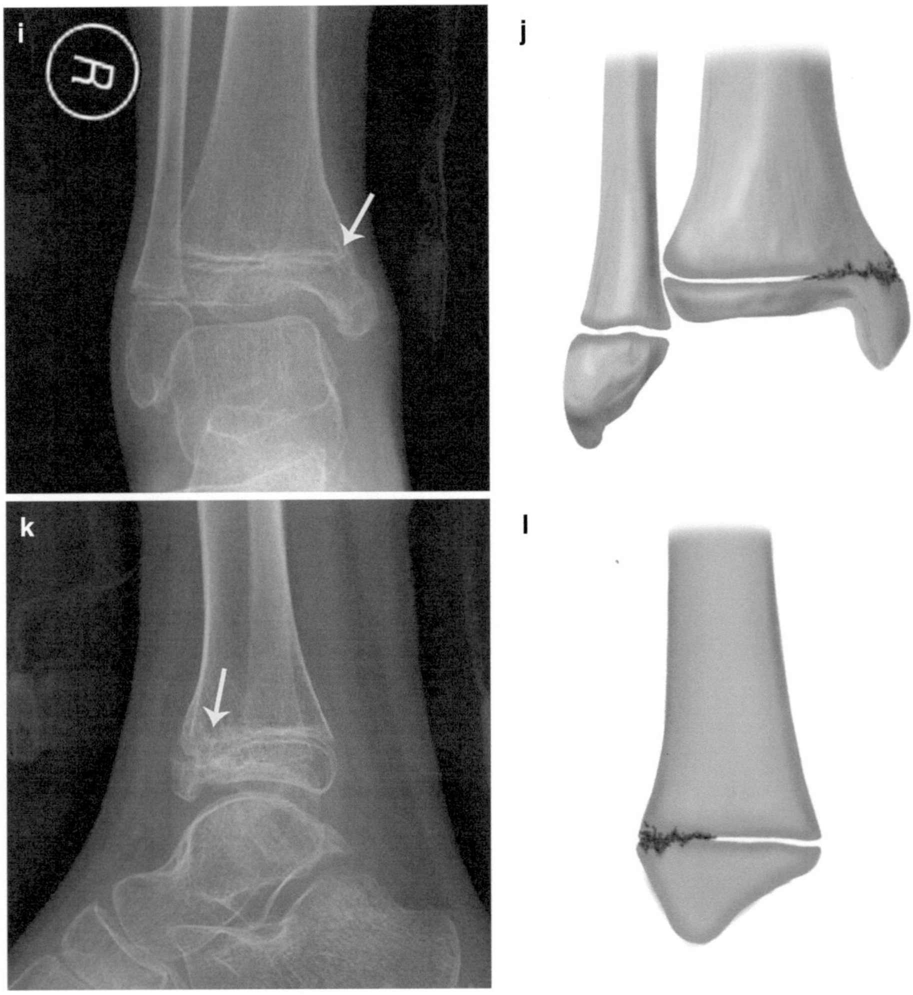

Fig. 21.36 (**i**, **k**) show the deformity of the distal radius at 3 months after internal fixation, and schematic diagram (**j**–**l**)

6.4. Fig. 21.36m–p

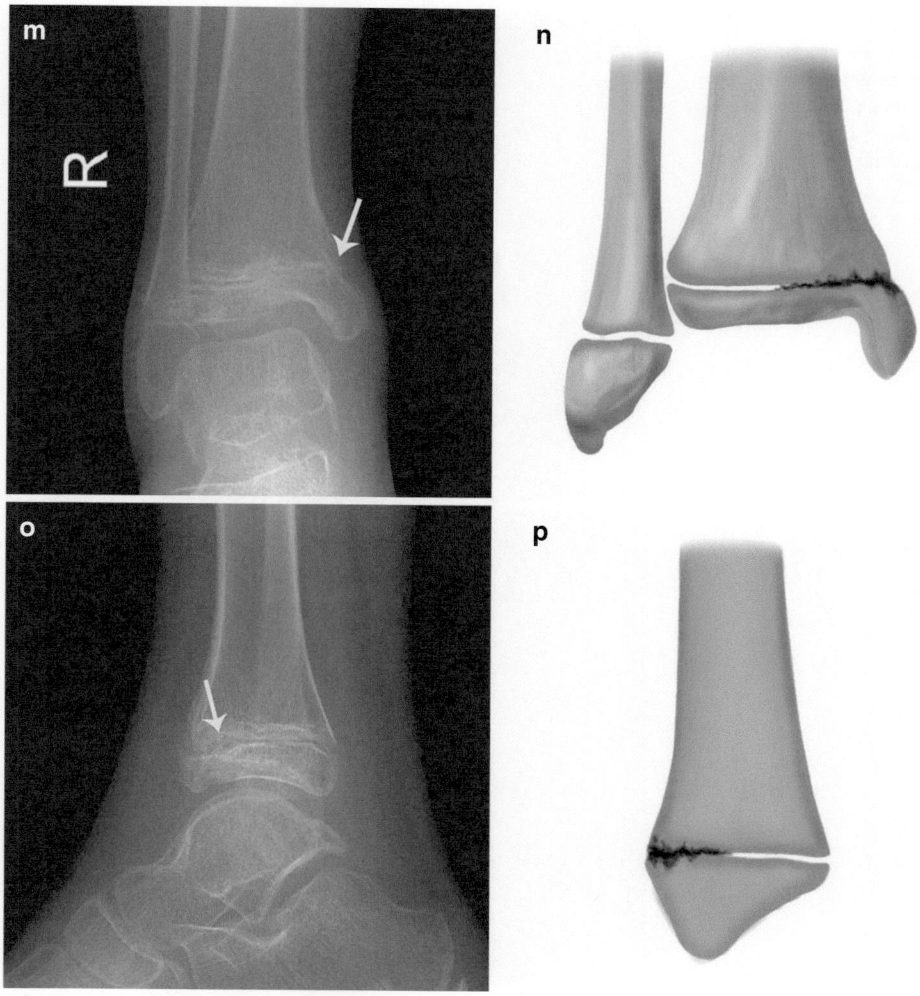

Fig. 21.36 (**m**, **o**) show the deformity of distal radius is aggravated at 3 months after internal fixation, and schematic diagram (**n**, **p**)

6.5. Fig. 21.36q–t

Fig. 21.36 (**q**, **s**) are epiphysis block procedure of distal fibula and 6 months after the medial epiphyseal release of the distal radius, and schematic diagram (**r**, **t**)

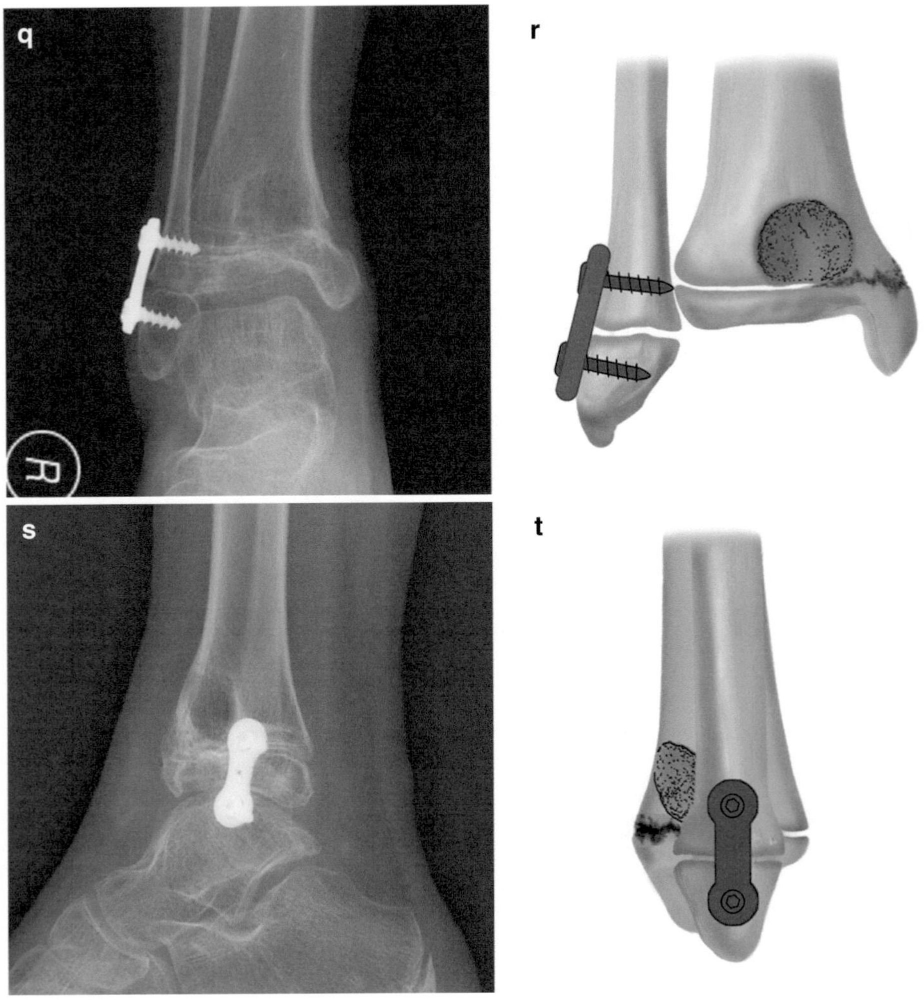

7. Early closure of the epiphysis of right distal tibia
   7.1. X-ray (Fig. 21.37a–d)

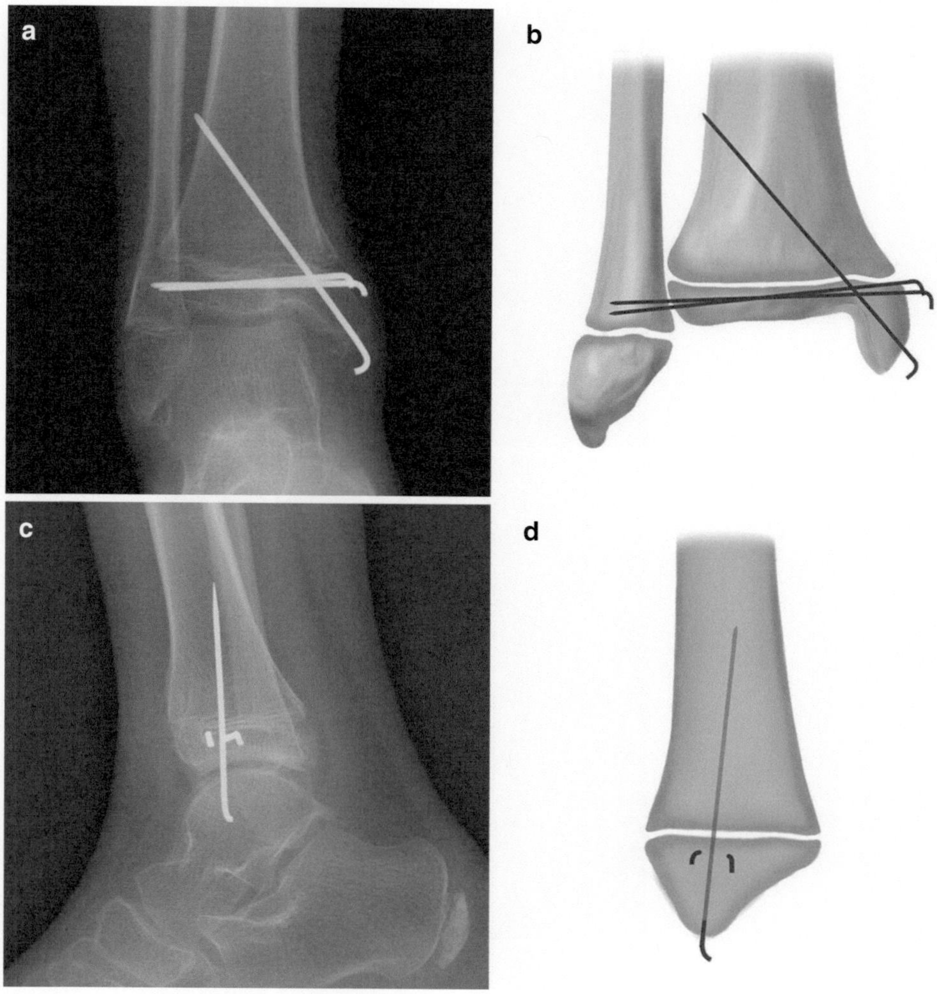

Fig. 21.37 (**a**, **c**) are the positive and lateral position, respectively, showing after the internal fixation of epiphyseal injury, and schematic diagram (**b**, **d**)

7.2. Fig. 21.37e–h

Fig. 21.37 (**e**, **g**) are 2 years after operation, showing the epiphyseal closure at the injury site, and schematic diagram (**f**, **h**)

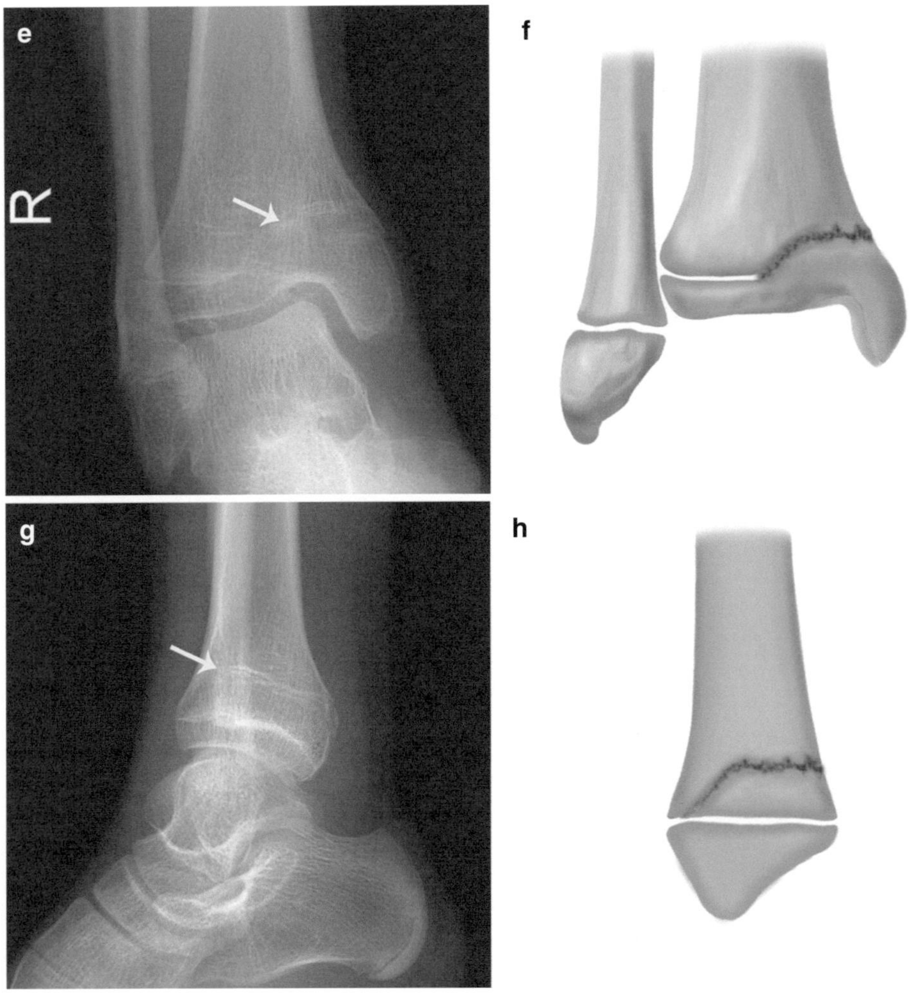

7.3. MRI (Fig. 21.37i, j)

Fig. 21.37 (**i**, **j**) are coronal plane T1WI and T2WI, respectively, showing epiphyseal closure and formation of bone bridge (arrow white)

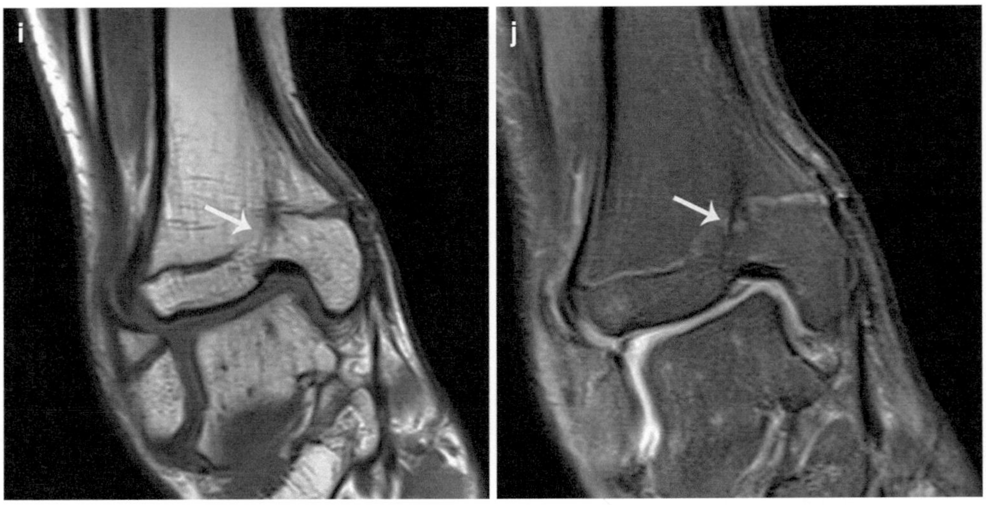

21.3 Summary of Key Points

1. Be familiar with the time of occurrence and closure of the secondary ossification center of normal epiphysis. Attention should be paid to the contralateral alignment of the secondary ossification center and the metaphysis, and identification of the normal epiphysis and fracture in combination with the age of the children. When there are multiple ossification centers in the epiphysis, it is important to not misdiagnose as a fracture of the epiphysis.
2. X-ray and CT show the normal epiphyseal cartilage plate was low-density band, and the non-ossified epiphysis was not developed. MRI can directly show the epiphysis and epiphyseal cartilage plates, which is similar to the articular cartilage signals. When X-ray and CT scans are negative, but the symptoms and signs are apparent for children with trauma, MRI should be performed.
3. When fracture and epiphyseal injury exit at the same time, the fracture is obvious. While the epiphyseal injury is relatively light, be careful not to leave out the inconspicuous epiphyseal injury.
4. Epiphyseal injury can cause early closure of the epiphyseal plate, which can be divided into complete and partial, causing limb shortening and / or angular deformity. Therefore, early diagnosis and early treatment are very important. CT and MRI scans can accurately show the location, extent, and scope of early closure of epiphysis. CT showed complete or partial disappearance of the low-density area of the epiphyseal cartilage plate, forming a high-density bone bridge with or without limb deformity. MRI showed that the thickness of the early closure of epiphyseal cartilage plate was thinner, and the high-signal epiphyseal cartilage plate on T2W1 is interrupted, during which low-signal trabecula is seen to pass-through. The immature bone bridge was the inner-line like, lumpy or irregular low signal, while the mature bone bridge was bone-like signal connecting the epiphysis and metaphysis.
5. When performing CT and MRI, the upper and lower levels are continuously observed from different scanning orientation.

Suggested Reading

1. Zhang Y, et al. Clinical Classification in Orthopaedics Trauma. Singapore: Springer Nature America Inc.; 2018.
2. 孙英彩, 崔建岭, 张英泽, 等.青少年急性单纯膝关节软骨骨折的MRI诊断. 中华放射学杂志, 2007, 41(12):1304-1308.
3. 孙英彩, 崔建岭, 彭志刚, 等.青少年急性膝关节软骨损伤的MRI表现. 实用放射学杂志, 2009, 25(12):72-75.
4. 张建军, 郑卓肇, 李选. 膝关节半月板后根部撕裂的MRI评价.中华放射学杂志, 2010年, 44(12):1300-1303.
5. England E, Wissman RD, Mehta K, et al. Cysts of the anterior horn lateral meniscus and the ACL: is there a relationship? Skeletal Radiol. 2014;44(3):369–73.
6. Walker B, Limbert A. Bilateral, simultaneous medial meniscus bucket handle tearsin a 23-year-old female. Case Rep Orthop. 2014, 11(9): Epub.

MIX
Papier aus verantwortungsvollen Quellen
Paper from responsible sources
FSC® C105338

If you have any concerns about our products,
you can contact us on
ProductSafety@springernature.com

In case Publisher is established outside the EU,
the EU authorized representative is:
Springer Nature Customer Service Center GmbH
Europaplatz 3, 69115 Heidelberg, Germany

Printed by Libri Plureos GmbH
in Hamburg, Germany